THE DISEASES OF OCCUPATIONS

THE DISEASES
OF OCCUPATIONS

DONALD HUNTER

C.B.E., D.Sc., M.D., F.R.C.P.

Consulting Physician
The London Hospital

THE ENGLISH UNIVERSITIES PRESS LTD
ST. PAUL'S HOUSE WARWICK LANE
LONDON E.C.4

First Printed 1955
Second Edition 1957
New Impression 1959
Third Edition 1962
New Impression (with corrections) 1964
Fourth Edition 1969

4ᵗʰ
~~Fifth~~ Edition
Copyright © 1969
Donald Hunter

SBN 340 04604 X

PRINTED AND BOUND IN ENGLAND
FOR THE ENGLISH UNIVERSITIES PRESS, LTD.,
BY HAZELL WATSON AND VINEY LTD., AYLESBURY

To the memory of
HUBERT M. TURNBULL, F.R.S.
with affection, gratitude and
deep respect

PREFACE

In this book it has been my purpose to review on a broad basis and with emphasis on its clinical aspects the problem of disease in relation to occupation. Every type of occupation is considered, whether it belongs to an industry or not. The work embodies the experience of twenty years' teaching and is designed to be of use to the student, the general practitioner and the consultant. The industrial medical officer and the works' chemist will need to consult books which are larger and more detailed than this.

The point of view is that of the general physician; unhappily I have never held a post as factory doctor. In using the clinical approach I have had always in mind the need to establish the subject on an academic footing, and I have merely put together something of what is known about occupational diseases, in order to lay down a basis upon which the practising doctor may build.

I have kept in mind the importance of describing the chemical composition of the materials handled in various occupations. Where I have described at length the use in industry of such harmless substances as chalk and limestone, the object has been to stress the fact that dirty and dusty conditions of working are not necessarily dangerous to health. In dealing with industrial poisons and dusts, I have given special emphasis to the mechanism by which poisoning occurs and the means of prevention used. Wherever possible, detailed descriptions of industrial processes and working conditions are given.

A large number of illustrations of factories and workshops is included with the object of giving at least an approximate idea of trade processes. The limitations of this method are, of course, realized. I have not been concerned solely with what happens in Great Britain: my review takes into account occupational disease in any part of the world. It follows that I have recorded certain descriptions of working conditions and diseases which I have not had the opportunity to study personally.

Some of the subject-matter refers to diseases which are rare or even obsolete. Thus I felt that it was worth while to describe phosphorus poisoning in detail, because history proves that very serious disease may sometimes exist in an industry without medical men knowing anything about it, and that every known hygienic measure may prove to be unavailing for the prevention of certain kinds of industrial poisoning.

Sometimes conditions unrelated to occupation have been described because of the light they throw upon what happens in industry. Injuries by lightning stroke and the disasters of Hiroshima and Nagasaki are examples of this. It has been necessary often to approach the subject historically, in order to show what has been achieved or what yet requires to be done.

The opening chapters depict in a disjointed way something of the historical, social and economic background of the occupations men follow. These chapters are amateur and merit the comment of Sir Robert Hutchison that to write about the history of medicine is itself a physical sign of cerebral arteriosclerosis in the writer.

In the preparation of this work I have had the valuable assistance of Dr. P. Lesley Bidstrup and Dr. Ian Lodge Patch. In addition I have had the help and advice of many other friends and colleagues, only a few of whom are mentioned in the text. I am particularly indebted to Dr. J. N. Agate, Dr. J. M. Barnes, Professor S. P. Bedson, Dr. J. A. Bonnell, Dr. E. Boyland, the late Dr. J. C. Bridge, Miss H. M. Buckell, the late Professor W. Bulloch, Mr. R. Drew, Dr. D. E. Freeland, Dr. J. R. Gilmour, Dr. H. C. Hamilton, Dr. D. G. Harvey, Dr. S. A. Henry, Mr. C. Hunter, Miss E. K. Hunter, the late Dr. H. Hunter, Mr. J. A. Hunter, Professor L. Hunter, Dr. M. E. F. Hunter, Dr. M. H. Jupe, Professor Sir Ernest Kennaway, Mr. E. King, Dr. C. A. Klein, Professor R. E. Lane, Mr. D. Lawford, Dr. W. H. Linnell, Dr. R. Lovell, Dr. E. R. A. Merewether, Dr. E. L. Middleton, the late Dr. G. Riddoch, Professor S. Russ, Professor Dorothy Russell, Dr. R. S. F. Schilling, Dr. W. A. M. Smart, Professor H. M. Turnbull, Dr. E. Williams and Dr. W. W. Woods.

I wish to express my appreciation of the generous treatment, both of myself and my staff, by the Medical Research Council. The equipment and maintenance of the Department for Research in Industrial Medicine at the London Hospital which I have the honour to direct has made possible a number of investigations described here in detail.

I am indebted to friends and colleagues in many parts of the world who have arranged for me to visit mines, shipyards and factories, as well as departments for research. It is a pleasure to acknowledge the kindness of executives in a great number of industrial firms who have supplied me with information and photographs, and given me free access to their works.

For many of the clinical photographs reproduced here, my thanks are due to the late Mr. H. J. Suggars, himself a victim of an occupational disease. Other excellent reproductions and all the charts are the work of Mr. H. S. Edwards. My grateful thanks are due to Mrs. Margaret Adams upon whom the arduous task of making accurate copies in type has mainly fallen. For help in reading the proofs I have to thank many friends and especially my clinical ward clerks.

Above all I am deeply grateful for the constant help, kindly interest, forbearance and devotion of my wife during the many years which were given to the task of writing this book.

DONALD HUNTER.

The London Hospital, E.1.
January, 1955.

PREFACE TO THE SECOND EDITION

I AM glad to have the opportunity of correcting and amplifying certain statements of fact. Some few additions have been made to the opening chapters on the history of the subject, eleven new illustrations have been added and the index has been enlarged and improved. The descriptions of poisoning by vanadium, manganese and cadmium have been brought up to date, the latter with the help of Dr. John Bonnell. New sections on thallium poisoning, on iron and steel foundries and on the hazards of work in sewers have been added. I am indebted to Dr. John Rogan for new information on the National Coal Board Medical Service and on the Coal Industry Social Welfare Organization. I wish to thank Dr. John Watkins-Pitchford for information bringing up to date the Industrial Injuries Scheme of the Ministry of Pensions and National Insurance. I am greatly indebted to the printers and publishers for the excellent work put into the production of the book.

DONALD HUNTER.

The London Hospital, E.1.
January, 1957.

PREFACE TO THE THIRD EDITION

AMENDMENTS and additions have been made to bring up to date the First Schedule, Part I of the Industrial Injuries (Prescribed Diseases) Regulations. Descriptions of the uses and toxic effects of acrylonitrile, hexachlorobenzene, hexachlorocyclohexane, metol, phenol, quinone and hydroquinone have been added. The so-called traumatic neurosis, Minamata disease and rheumatoid pneumoconiosis (Caplan's syndrome) have been described. Existing sections on poisoning by benzene and cadmium compounds, cysticercus epilepsy, injuries from animals, reptiles, insects and fish, louping ill, psittacosis and weavers' cough have been brought up to date. I am glad again to have had the opportunity of correcting and amplifying certain statements of fact. Nine new illustrations have been added and the index has been enlarged and improved. In the work of revision I have had the valuable assistance of four members of my staff, Dr. A. I. G. McLaughlin, Dr. G. Kazantzis, Mr. E. King and Mr. R. Drew. In addition, I have had the help and advice of many other friends and colleagues including help in reading the proofs from my clinical ward clerks. To all these people I am deeply grateful.

DONALD HUNTER.

The London Hospital, E.1.
November, 1961.

NOTE TO SECOND IMPRESSION

A new impression has given me the opportunity to make some corrections and additions to the text.

DONALD HUNTER.

The Middlesex Hospital, W.1.
December, 1963.

PREFACE TO THE FOURTH EDITION

EXTENSIVE revision has been made of the sections on man and his work, the effects of radiation, asbestosis, and injuries from animals, reptiles, insects and fish. Additions have been made to bring up to date the First Schedule, Part I of the Industrial Injuries (Prescribed Diseases) Regulations. New sections have been written on the uses and toxic effects of cobalt, toluylene di-*iso*cyanate, pentachlorphenol and dimethylnitrosamine together with paragraphs on brazing alloys and Q fever. Additions have been made to existing sections on poisoning by lead, mercury, arsenic, phosphorus, beryllium, cadmium, thallium and vanadium. I am glad again to have had the opportunity of correcting and amplifying certain statements of fact. The index has been enlarged and improved. In the work of revision I have had the valuable assistance of Dr. A. I. G. McLaughlin, Dr. John Bonnell, Dr. G. Kazantzis, Dr. André McLean, Dr. Elizabeth McLean and Mr. E. King. In addition I am deeply grateful for the help and advice of many other friends and colleagues including help in reading the proofs from my clinical ward clerks.

DONALD HUNTER.

Guy's Hospital, S.E.1.
October, 1968.

CONTENTS

VIII THE AROMATIC CARBON COMPOUNDS

IX THE ALIPHATIC CARBON COMPOUNDS

XV ACCIDENTS

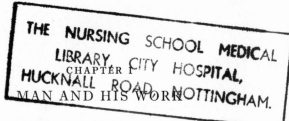

CHAPTER I

MAN AND HIS WORLD

OCCUPATIONS DETERMINED BY CLIMATE

THE occupations followed by different groups of mankind originally depended on geographical surroundings, for not all parts of the world are equally adapted to the needs of man. Broadly speaking, all land is either forest land, grassland or desert. Over the centuries each of these has led to the development of special occupations which have exercised the most profound influence on the lives of the races engaged in them.

Climate of the Tundra

The frozen desert surrounding the Arctic Ocean is known as the tundra in Russia and the Barren Lands in Canada. Buried in winter beneath a sheet of snow, it awakens with the tardy spring to a green life of great intensity. The sun melts the surface snow, but even in the height of summer it is powerless to penetrate more than a few inches into the permanently frozen soil. The surface soil is a thin layer affording nourishment only for those plants whose roots penetrate but a few inches. Stunted bushes such as cranberry and whortleberry grow abundantly half hidden among the moss which is the characteristic vegetation of the tundra. Huge tracts are covered by bog moss on the lower slopes and by reindeer moss on the higher ground, brightened in summer with flowers of all colours. For two-thirds of the year all vegetable life is hidden beneath the snow and the only traces of animal life are the footprints of fox or reindeer on its surface. The only important animal on the tundra is the reindeer (fig. 1). It is indifferent to cold and feeds on the reindeer moss, which it procures in winter by digging with its forefeet in the snow (Ratzel, 1898).

Fishing and the Hunting of Furred Animals

The tundra is inhabited by various races, which are of necessity very thinly scattered. The Eskimo are a coastal people deriving their sustenance entirely from the sea. In the tundra of the Old World we have Lapps and Finns in the west, and many similar tribes farther east, such as Yuraks, Samoyeds and Yakuts. Agriculture is, of course, impossible in a soil which scarcely thaws. In the three months of summer when the rivers melt, fish become abundant. Fishing and the hunting of small animals are the chief summer occupations, and the drying of fish for winter use is an important part of the women's work. The only occupation possible in winter is the hunting of furred animals on the edge of the forests which bound the tundra to the south.

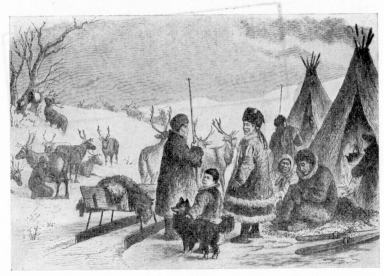

FIG. 1.—Samoyed Encampment in the Siberian Tundra
(*Drawn from life by G. Sundblad, 1898*)

Nomadic Mode of Life on the Tundra

The inhabitants lead a nomadic life, for reindeer cannot be kept in captivity and must be allowed to wander in quest of food. The owners are obliged to follow their herds from one feeding-ground to another, in order to obtain their milk for food and their services for draught. Hunting and fishing are likewise occupations which necessitate frequent moves, for game would soon be exhausted if they were always carried on over the same area. The division of labour between the sexes is that best suited to the mode of life. The men do most of the actual work of procuring food, by hunting and fishing. They also make and mend the necessary weapons. Women's work consists of making the most economical use of the supplies which the men procure. In summer, on the tundra, their task is to clean the fish caught and to dry any surplus for winter use. Their spare time is occupied in helping the children to collect berries and in watching that the reindeer do not stray too far to be milked.

Importance of the Reindeer to the Tundra Dweller

The importance of the reindeer both alive and dead can hardly be realized. In life it makes it possible to move freely from one part of the tundra to another. Dead, every portion of its carcase is valuable. The flesh supplies food, the bones and horns are used for implements, the tendons for thread and the skins when made into leather provide shelter and clothing. Prosperity is measured by the possession of reindeer. To have them is to be a rich man; to depend on fishing only is to be a poor one, and to live from hand to mouth (Herbertsen and Herbertsen, 1911).

Life in the Tropical Rain Forests

Primitive man was a forest dweller and there are tribes in tropical Africa, New Guinea and South America who still have forest homes. The impenetrable forests of the headwaters of the River Amazon limited the expansion of the Inca empire from the high plateaux of Peru and Bolivia eastwards into Brazil. This tropical rain forest, the *selvas*, is enormous covering 1,500,000 square miles of land; it has been well named the *green hell*. It is an evergreen forest containing an astonishing number of species of tree varying in height from 40 to 150 feet. It presents to the eye every conceivable shade of green, but the putrid odours which accompany its decay are horrible. The trees are usually hung with and interlaced by tree-perchers which include some of the most beautiful orchids in the world. Several hundred species of parasitic plants may live on a single large tree. But in the whole of Amazonia we must visualise this vast tract of selva punctuated by small localised patches of grassland and threaded by innumerable water-courses. Such a forest offers a poor home for man and the whole region is very sparsely peopled. The immigrant settlers now greatly outnumber the aboriginal peoples some of whom are still hostile to strangers. The native Indians include the Arawaks, the Caribs, the Tupis, the Tapuyus and the Boro. They subsist by collecting the fruits, nuts and roots of the forest as well as hides and skins. In addition they fish, snarl birds and small animals and carry out a little rudimentary cultivation. These aboriginal peoples live, for the most part, completely outside government control. Attempts are being made to civilise, protect and help them and to this end the Brazilian Government has instituted the Servico de Proteçao aos Indios. (Robinson, 1961.)

Occupations in the Temperate Forests and Great Plains

Life in the uncleared temperate forests of Canada and Siberia follows a definite type. Here the only occupations possible are those which utilize the raw materials of the forest, its animal life and its timber. The animals are clothed in thick fur, often of great beauty and therefore of commercial value. In Canada, fur hunting is actively carried on by trappers. Timber is required for poles, planking, joinery, furniture, plywood, veneers, and for the manufacture of paper and rayon, hence the value of the trade of lumbering. In the Siberian forest, fur hunting is more important than the trade in timber. The forests are uninhabited except on their fringes. Ostyak and Samoyed hunters penetrate a few miles into their gloomy depths, leaving their families on the edge. Their only exchangeable wealth consists of furs, which they barter to traders who periodically visit their settlements. Where the rainfall is insufficient to nourish forest trees, grass becomes the characteristic form of vegetation. These treeless lands are known by various names. In Asia, they are called steppes; in North America, prairies;

in South America, savannas, campos, llanos and pampas; in South Africa, veld; and in Australia, downs.

Inhabitants of the Steppes of the Old World

The steppes of the Old World are of peculiar interest not only on account of their vast extent but also because they have preserved almost unchanged for 5,000 years the mode of life described in the Hebrew scriptures. Their remoteness still retards the change from ancient to modern conditions. The horse herdsman of the great plains of Hungary is known as the csikós. The chief tribe of the Russian steppes is the so-called Kirghiz. This name is an uncomplimentary one, meaning freebooter. They call themselves Kazák or horsemen, which is the same word as Cossack. The domestication and breeding of animals is the only occupation for which the steppe is suitable, but the steppe-dwellers feel no envy for a life which cannot be theirs. They despise agriculture and the comforts and luxuries of a more advanced civilization. Their flocks and herds yield enough for all their needs. The wool of the sheep is made into felt for tent coverings, and camel's-hair cloth, such as John the Baptist wore, is also manufactured. Leather and hides are abundant, and provide shelter and raiment as well as bottles and other utensils. Rich rugs and carpets, whose beauty is proverbial, are also made from wool and hair, for the materials are abundant, and they are useful, easily portable and valuable as articles of exchange. Milk and flesh suffice for food, and the rich manage to procure flour and rice from trading caravans. The mode of life is essentially nomadic, the flocks are continually eating up the grass, though the skilful shepherd knows how to make it last as long as possible. First he sends the horses into the long grass, then these are driven a little farther and their place is taken by oxen and camels. When these can no longer manage to find food, the sheep are turned in, and for a while find abundant pasture on the short nibbled grass. But a day comes at length when even the sheep can no longer find food, and then all must move on (Herbertsen and Herbertsen, 1911).

Importance of the Horse to the Steppe-Shepherd

The flocks and herds of the steppe-shepherds are often of vast size. The wealthy possess hundreds of camels, thousands of horses and tens of thousands of sheep. Of these the horses are the most prized, and a man's wealth is measured by the number he owns. Without horses it would be impossible for the herdsman either to ride ahead and choose suitable halting-places, or to keep the vast flocks from straying beyond reach. Children are mounted at four years of age. They quickly become fearless riders, and soon learn to make themselves useful as mounted shepherds, keeping the droves from straying at will from the line of march. Obtaining everything from their herds and depending for nothing on outside supplies, the steppe-dwellers are proud and independent, and despise a settled life. No modern improvements are introduced into an occupation like shepherding, which is the same now as in the time of Abraham. These people are often reduced from wealth to poverty by unavoidable disasters, such as an unusually long and severe winter, prolonged drought, sudden storms or epizootics among the flocks. They are more highly developed than the tundra tribes. The more generous environment allows them to amass wealth, to supply the needs of the present and to provide for the future.

Occupations in the Grasslands of America and Australasia

The prairies of North America have been converted into extensive corn and wheat fields and large ranches where cattle breeding is a vast industry supplying the markets of the U.S.A. and Canada. Here the cowboy at one time lived the wild life of the mounted frontiersman and herdsman round-ing up the wild bison which he wrongly called buffalo, an error which persists to the present day. In returning to pastoral life the settlers of North European descent have not reverted to pastoral habits. This is largely because of the construction of railways which opened markets and removed the isolation of steppe life. Both the soil and the climate combined to make a success of this venture, and Chicago was predestined to become the leading meat packing and grain selling centre of the world. The richest grasslands of the continent of America are the pampas in the Argentine and Uruguay. As large as one-third of Europe, they produce quantities of meat, butter, hides and wool most of which is exported. The equestrian herdsmen, the gaucho of Argentine, the llanero of Venezuela, the sabanero of Costa Rica, and the vaquero of Mexico now no longer function as frontiersmen and, like the cowboy, have dwindled in numbers as cultivation has produced settled cattle ranches. The first settlers found no bison but there was wild cattle in plenty. Today of course famous breeds of livestock such as Angus, Hereford and Texas predominate. On the downs of Australia sheep and cattle stations have been formed by men and women of British origin, who retain the habits of settled life. The merino sheep has been bred with such success that Australian wool dominates the markets of the world. In 1788 there were 29 sheep in Australia; in 1965 there were 165 million! The downs of New Zealand produce beef, lamb, butter and cheese mainly for export.

EARLY WEAPONS AND TOOLS

Stone weapons were at first missiles thrown by hand and later hurled from slings. Then sharp edges and points of stones, shells, bones and horns were used for cutting and digging, thus making simple tools. These tools were first grasped in the hand, and later they were fitted into handles or shafts of bone or wood, generally by means of splicing (fig. 2). After this discovery, tools and weapons rapidly assumed different forms. Distinctive weapons appeared as spear- and arrow-heads; distinctive tools as axes,

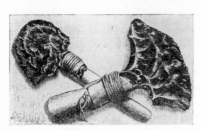

FIG. 2.—Obsidian Axes from Easter
Island

hammers, adzes, chisels, gimlets and
many others which are indispensable at every stage of civilization.

Bronze Weapons and Tools

The North American Indians
knew how to hammer copper but
not to smelt it. They were quite
ignorant of iron working. More than
15,000 years ago the Egyptians employed copper for utensils, weapons
and ornaments, and this knowledge
had spread throughout Europe by about 4000 B.C. The use of bronze dates
from remote antiquity. Bronze daggers of the later Minoan period, about
1500 B.C., have been found in graves in Mycenæ. The alloy contains 88
per cent copper and 12 per cent tin, and was probably discovered accidentally. It happens that in parts of Cornwall tin and copper minerals
occur together, and when in ancient times these minerals were smelted as
one charge, the rich golden-brown alloy produced was found to be harder
than either tin or copper and was thus more useful for making implements
(Jones, 1963). The lesser skill required for making bronze implements than
iron affords a reasonable explanation why the Bronze Age came before
the Iron Age.

Gold Mining in Ancient Egypt

The ancient Egyptians devoted great enterprise to the winning of gold,
both by conquest and by mining. According to Rosen (1943), Diodorus
Siculus, a Greek historian from Sicily, who visited Egypt in 50 B.C., gives
a detailed account of the Nubian gold mines under the Ptolemies.

> In the extremities of Egypt, on the frontiers of Arabia and Ethiopia,
> there is a country with many and large mines of gold, which is re-
> covered by much hard labour and expense. There the earth is of a
> black colour and is full of streaks and veins of a remarkable whiteness,
> the lustre of which surpasses the most brilliant natural products. From
> this earth those who have charge of the mining operations obtain the
> gold by means of a large number of workers, for the kings of Egypt
> collect condemned prisoners, prisoners of war and others who, beset
> by false accusations, have been in a fit of anger thrown into prison;
> these, sometimes alone, sometimes with their entire families, they
> send to the gold mines; partly to exact a just vengeance for crimes
> committed by the condemned, partly to secure for themselves a big
> revenue through their toil.
> Those who have been thus consigned are many, and all are fet-
> tered; they are held constantly at work by day and the whole night
> long without any rest, and are sedulously kept from any chance of

escape. For their guards are foreign soldiers, all speaking different languages, so the workers are unable either by speech or by friendly entreaty to corrupt those who watch them. The hardest of the earth that contains the gold is exposed to a fierce fire, so that it cracks, and then they apply hand labour to it; the rock that is soft and can be reduced by a moderate effort is worked by thousands of the luckless creatures with iron tools that are ordinarily used for cutting stone. The foreman, who distinguishes one sort of rock from another, instructs the workers in the whole business and assigns their tasks. Of those who are condemned to this disastrous life such as excel in strength of body pound the shining rock with iron hammers, applying not skill but sheer force to the work, and they drive galleries, though not in a straight line, but in the direction taken naturally by the glistening stone; these then, on account of the windings of these passages, live in darkness, and carry around lamps attached to their foreheads. In accordance with the peculiarities of the rock they have to get into all sorts of positions and throw on the floor the pieces they detach. And this they do without ceasing, to comply with the cruelty and blows of an overseer. The young children make their way through the galleries into the hollowed portions and throw up with great toil the fragments of broken stone, and bring it outdoors to the ground outside the entrance. . . . As these workers can take no care of their bodies and have not even a garment to hide their nakedness, there is no one, who seeing these luckless people would not pity them because of the excess of their misery, for there is no forgiveness or relaxation at all for the sick, or the maimed, or the old, or for women's weakness, but all with blows are compelled to stick to their labour until worn out they die in servitude. Thus the poor wretches ever account the future more dreadful than the present because of the excess of their punishment and look to death as more desirable than life.

This description, notable for the horrors which it depicts, presents a picture of ancient mining, which in its essential details remained unchanged throughout the whole period of antiquity.

Slavery and Forced Labour in the Mines

The miner of antiquity was almost always a slave. The slaves were recruited from condemned criminals, prisoners-of-war and, when the supply of workers ran short, forced labour was employed. Innocent individuals, sometimes entire families or tribes, were exiled to the mines. The miners worked in chains, practically naked and, as Diodorus mentions, guarded by foreign mercenaries with whom they were unable to talk. The lash of the overseer drove them to their arduous labour. The workers were divided into three groups; the strongest adult men did the actual work of breaking the rock, and handled pick and pitching-tool; children carried the broken ore out of the mine, and the women and old men were employed to grind it by hand. When the rock was too hard to be attacked with quarrying tools, the method of fire-setting was employed. This procedure, which is also mentioned by Pliny and other writers of antiquity, consisted in placing a fire against the ore face and then pouring water on the heated rock. On cooling rapidly, the rock cracked and was easily broken loose with the usual tools. The implements employed were of bronze and stone.

The Metal Worker in Mythology

In Greek mythology Hephaistos was the god of fire and became the divine smith and patron of craftsmen. His cult reached Athens about 600 B.C. In epic poetry he is a pathetic figure, lame and unkempt in appearance. In Homer his skill in metallurgy is often mentioned, his forge being on Olympus, where he is served by images of golden handmaids whom he has animated. He was the most industrious of all the gods, renowned in particular for the famous *Arms of Achilles* which he forged at the request of the hero's mother, the sea nymph Thetis. Vulcan, the Roman god of iron, brass and devouring flame also was ugly, misshapen and lame. The legendary genealogy of Tubal-Cain is recorded in the Old Testament. Lamech, a descendant of Cain, had three sons Jabal, Jubal and Tubal, to whom are attributed the development of pastoral civilization, music and metal work respectively.

Why were the Smith-gods lame?

Myths similar to those of ancient Greece and Rome are found in relation to the Teutonic Wieland who also was lame, to the Scandinavian Völundr, lord of the elves, and to the Finnish Smith-god Ilmarinen. English legend makes Wayland the Smith the mythical hero of the skilled metal worker, and local tradition has placed his forge in a cave close to the White Horse in Berkshire. Enough is known of the metallurgy of antiquity to make it clear that some of the copper and brass vessels made in ancient times were harder because they contained arsenic. But attempts in modern times (Rosner, 1955) to show that the smith-gods were lame because of arsenical poisoning are too far-fetched to be taken seriously, violating as they do the cardinal principles of clinical method. Besides, many versions of the old legends show that the child was crippled from birth and was cast out by an angry father to live upon his own resources. Surely it is likely that at an early stage of society the trade of a smith came to be regarded by common consent as suitable for the lame.

Early Use of Iron

Man learned the use of iron nearly 6,000 years ago. It was already being made in China, Mesopotamia and Egypt about 4000 B.C., some 2,000 years before it reached Greece and the countries along the Danube. Between 1000 B.C. and A.D. 100 its use spread into Western Europe, Scandinavia and Ireland. We learn from Cæsar that iron was used in Britain in pre-Roman days.

> The Britons use either bronze or iron rings, determined at a certain weight, as their money. In the maritime regions iron is produced but the quantity of it is small.

Hæmatite mining in the Lake District has revealed stone hammer-heads and a bronze implement in a working at Stainton-in-Furness, a deer-horn pick at Grange-over-Sands as well as pre-Roman coins (Fell, 1908).

Iron Weapons and Tools

Iron weapons and tools gradually replaced bronze, stone and horn implements (fig. 3). The discovery of iron occurred in early times, and at first by chance, when iron ore was heated in a charcoal fire. As the fire died down, a spongy lump of iron remained which could be hammered into shape and used for tools and weapons. Our metallurgical forefathers found that when a high wind was blowing their fires burnt faster and hotter and the iron was produced more rapidly, so eventually bellows were

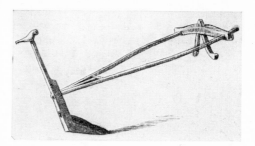

FIG. 3.—Iron Plough used by the Triamans of Bencoolen
(*After Ratzel*)

used to increase the supply of air (Alexander and Street, 1951). Such primitive forced-draught furnaces are still in use in parts of India and Africa. The use of iron is known to most African tribes except the Bushmen, and most Negroes are excellent metal workers (fig. 4). Since ancient times tribes such as the Tibbu of the Sahara have used throwing irons as hunting implements (fig. 5). Some tribes, otherwise advanced, like the Pacific islanders, have no knowledge of metal working mainly because metals are not found on coral islands. The use of iron was, however, known in New Guinea, whither it was probably introduced by Malays. The Malays are excellent smiths, and make many beautiful metal weapons, like the terrible curved kris or dagger. In India, metal weapons in strange and horrible forms are everywhere made by Hindu smiths.

GREEK PREJUDICE AGAINST MANUAL LABOUR

Studies in social history have revealed certain points of interest as to the attitude of ancient Greece to those citizens who plied a mechanical

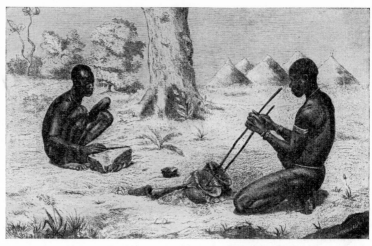

FIG. 4.—Bari Coppersmiths using Primitive Bellows
(*Drawn from life by Richard Buchta*)

trade. In 1941, in a delightful oration delivered before the Royal Institution of Great Britain, Professor Benjamin Farrington of University College,

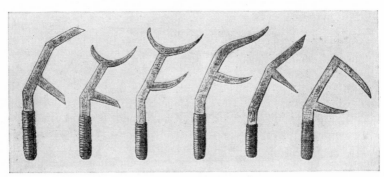

FIG. 5.—Throwing Irons used since Ancient Times as Hunting Implements by Tribes such as the Tibbu of the Sahara
(*After Nachtigal*)

Swansea, spoke of the prejudice of the ancient Greeks against manual labour and of the decline in social status of the manual labourer which accompanied the growth of civilization.

Social Stigma of the Mechanical Arts

He pointed out how Xenophon in his treatise called *Œconomicus* represented Socrates as delivering the following judgement on manual work and
the manual worker.

> What are called the mechanical arts, carry a social stigma and are
> rightly dishonoured in our cities. For these arts damage the bodies of
> those who work at them or who have charge of them, by compelling
> the workers to a sedentary life and to an indoor life, by compelling
> them, indeed, in some cases to spend the whole day by the fire. This
> physical degeneration results also in deterioration of the soul. Further-
> more, the workers at these trades simply have not got the time to
> perform the offices of friendship or of citizenship. Consequently, they
> are looked upon as bad friends and bad patriots. And in some cities,
> especially the warlike ones, it is not legal for a citizen to ply a mechan-
> ical trade.

The Diseases of Occupations Ignored

Obviously a social division so deep as this, a cleavage which when complete made it impossible for the same man to be both worker and citizen,
could not be without effect on the science and practice of medicine, which
touch the life of every man. But the nature of this effect remained inadequately explored until Professor Farrington undertook the task. He
discussed fully the limitations of ancient medical science and practice in
respect of the type of person and the type of disease it habitually dealt with
and habitually neglected. Roughly speaking, the working man was neglected in ancient medical practice and the occupational diseases ignored in
medical science.

Class Limitations of Hippocratic Medicine

Undoubtedly Hippocratic medicine was limited in its application to a
section of the people. A treatise like *Airs, Waters, Places* was written for
citizen doctors with citizen patients in view, and those, too, of the leisured
class. The Hippocratic medicine, we are informed by all competent in-
quirers, rested on the concept of a balance between the living organism and
its environment. It regarded sickness as an effort to restore a disturbed
equilibrium, and the duty of the physician was to co-operate with nature
in her efforts to secure a readjustment. Therefore the Hippocratic doctor,
who was frequently, perhaps even normally, itinerant, was taught to study,
as he came to each new locality, the major features of the environment of
his future patients.

The Environment of the Aristocrat

This is the subject of *Airs, Waters, Places*. As the title indicates, it was
the natural features of the place he was taught specially to observe—the

climate, the situation, the quality of the water. He was also given hints as to the kind of constitution he might expect to find in the inhabitants of a town living under conditions of oriental despotism as contrasted with those enjoying the privileges of Greek liberty. That is to say, even the political environment of a patient was to be taken into consideration by the Hippocratic doctor. Historians have been very properly impressed with the comprehensive outlook of the ancient medical manual. But, if we look at it carefully, we can see that it is deficient, professing to be a treatise on environment and yet omitting what may be described as the most important element in the environment from the point of view of health and disease, the regular occupation of the man.

The Food of the Wealthy

If we turn to the four books of the Hippocratic treatise called *Regimen*, we find that the author of this much admired and very important treatise developed a theory that health depends upon a balance of food and exercise. But the foods which he discusses hardly suggest the diet of a potter or a peasant, and the exercise which he recommends has nothing to do with work. Thus it would be a mistake to suppose that beef, goat, kid, pork, mutton, lamb, ass, horse, dog, puppy, wild boar, deer, hare, fox and hedgehog all formed a normal part of the diet of the working man, slave or free, any more than doves, partridges, pigeons, cocks, turtles, geese, ducks and other marsh or river fowl.

Counsels as to Exercise

And it would equally be a mistake to suppose that the following counsels as to exercise were addressed to the working man:

> Exercises should be many and of all kinds; running on the double track increased gradually; wrestling after being oiled, begun with light exercises and gradually made long; sharp walks after exercises, short walks in the sun after dinner; many walks in the early morning, quiet to begin with, increasing till they are violent and then gently finishing.

The following advice also seems not to be addressed to the worker:

> These patients ought to take their baths warm, to sleep on a soft bed, to get drunk once or twice but not to excess, to have sexual intercourse after a moderate indulgence in wine, and to slack off their exercises, except walking.

Progress awaits the Revival of Learning

But Hippocrates was not alone in his neglect of the working man; the possibility that occupational factors could be of importance in explaining a given illness was ignored all through the Dark Ages. More than 2,000 years were to elapse before the Revival of Learning brought this idea to the notice of men. It occurred as a revolutionary innovation (p. 35) made by Ramazzini, the Father of Occupational Medicine. In his

De Morbis Artificum Diatriba (1713) he made a striking addition to the art of diagnosis, giving to doctors the simple practical advice that to the questions recommended by Hippocrates they should add one more, to ask the patient to describe his occupation.

TRADITIONAL TRADES AND CRAFTS

The craftsmanship of the men who worked in metals had its counterpart in other fields of effort such as agriculture (fig. 6) and textiles (fig. 7). Many traditional crafts involved the empirical use of chemical substances. It is not unfair to claim that at the dawn of the Christian era and, indeed, for some centuries afterwards, chemistry did not greatly differ from its state of two thousand

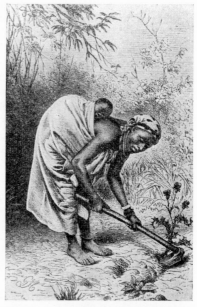

FIG. 6.—Loango Negress at Field Work
(*After Falkenstein*)

years earlier. Yet at the very earliest times of which we have a record a considerable number of chemical processes had been discovered and many substances with which we are familiar today were even then in daily use. Among the metals available were copper, silver, gold, iron, tin, lead and mercury. Among the salts in general use were common salt, alum, soda, nitre, sal ammoniac and potash. Sulphur, limestone, lime, malachite, quartz and fuller's earth were familiar minerals. Among organic substances in use were various vegetable dyes, sugar, products of alcoholic and acetic fermentation, oils, fats and waxes.

Methods of Fire Making

The discovery of fire making is one of the great landmarks in the history of man.

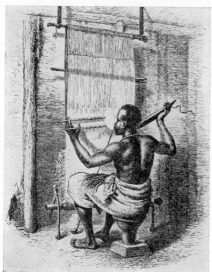

FIG. 7.—A Weaver of Ishogo
(*After du Chaillu*)

D.O.—2

Without fire life would be impossible except in the most favoured climates, and then only under the rudest conditions. The simplest method of obtaining fire is by friction—for example, some Malay tribes rub split bamboo together. The Polynesians make one stick drive a groove along another placed beneath it. This sort of fire drill is used by Bushmen and other tribes. The Eskimo improve on this method by fastening a cord round the drilling stick to make it rotate more rapidly. All these methods quickly produce fire in experienced hands. Success depends partly on the choice of wood and still more on practice. The next method is by striking a spark into dry tinder. The Fuegians strike sparks with flint flakes from lumps of iron pyrites into the down of birds and blow them into a flame.

The Art of the Potter

The discovery of fire satisfied a new set of wants, including those of the cook. For cooking utensils a great variety of materials are suitable. Naturally, metal vessels became important among those tribes which under-

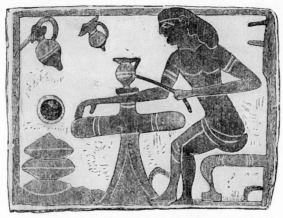

FIG. 8.—A Potter's Wheel of Ancient Egypt

stood metal working. Not only are they fireproof, but also they are far more durable than any others. The possession of pottery is often taken to imply a high state of progress, but we must not assume that its absence means a low stage of civilization, for it is unknown to many advanced races of Pacific islanders. They use vessels of wood and of coconut shell, and their method of boiling water is by dropping into it stones made red-hot in the fire. The Hottentots made clay vessels which were sun-dried and fired. The Negroes are expert potters, and the art is universal among the Malays, though their pottery is not well fired and is therefore too soft. The art of the potter was known to the Indians of both North and South America, who, in many cases, produced excellent specimens, glazed by various processes. The potter's wheel was known to the ancient Egyptians (fig. 8), but it is still unknown to a great number of the pottery-making races of the present day. In the first Egyptian Dynasty blue glazes were made for pottery with the help of copper salts. By roasting malachite, $CuCO_3.Cu(OH)_2$, with sand, a coloured frit known as Egyptian blue, $CaO.CuO.4SiO_2$, was made. This was used with soda for making a blue glaze on faience.

The Use of Glass

Glass was an accidental discovery of the Phœnicians. At one time a merchant ship laden with saltpetre, KNO_3, was wrecked on the Phœnician coast and some of the cargo washed ashore. Later the sailors found transparent stones where their fire had been. Some of the nitre had mingled and fused with the sand on the beach and formed crude glass. The Egyptians

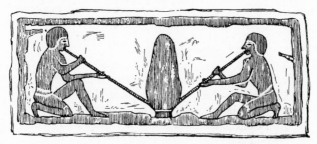

FIG. 9.—Glass Blowers of Thebes

used soda, Na_2CO_3, obtained under the name of natron from various natural deposits, and with this they made glass ornaments before the Hebrew exodus (fig. 9). The art was probably brought to Britain by the Roman invaders. Because of its great cost, glass making for many years was confined to the production of ornaments. In the thirteenth century flat glass probably made by casting began to be used for cathedral windows, and rich nobles eventually employed it in the windows of their castles instead of oiled paper. For a long time it was very precious, and owners upon taking a journey often took the window-panes out of the frames and locked them up to prevent them from being damaged or stolen while they were away.

The Empirical Use of Alum

In the preparation of leather it has been known since the earliest times that unless the hide is carefully treated after being stripped from the beast it rapidly becomes hard and useless. The value of alum for this purpose was discovered very early in man's history. By a natural accident this chemical substance is available in a state of high purity from many sources. Chemical analysis of ancient leather goods shows the presence of aluminium in quantities sufficiently high to make it very probable that this substance was used in their preparation. The *Iliad*, for example, describes the preparation of leather, and leather of the period of Homer has been proved to contain a good deal of aluminium. The first written reference to alum is in the Ebers Papyrus, and this suggests that it has been in continuous use for roughly 4,000 years. It was valued as a mordant in dyeing, but when used for this purpose it must be of high purity. Since much of the natural mineral contains traces of iron which would stain any fabric dipped in it, we may suppose that the Egyptians were familiar with the process of re-crystallizing alum from water in order to purify it.

Rock Alum and Roman Alum

In the fifteenth century there was a large Turkish Mediterranean trade in dyed fabrics and wool in which alum was employed as a mordant. At that time alum was obtained from Roc in Syria, which was in the possession of the Turks, hence the name rock alum, which is still in use for the finest kinds. In a descriptions of imports brought from Italy to England by the Genoese in *The Libelle of Englyshe Polycye* (1436) rock alum is mentioned.

> silk, and pepir blake
> They bringe wyth hem, and of wood great plente,
> Wolle, oyle, woad-aschen, by vessels in the sea,
> Coton, roch-alum, and gode golde of Jene.
> And they be charged wyth wolle ageyne, I wene,
> And wollene clothe of owres of colours alle.

At the fall of Constantinople in 1462, Giovanni di Castro, who had made a fortune by dyeing Italian cloth using Turkish alum as a mordant, fled to Italy. He discovered alum on Papal territory at Tolfa where there is a local deposit of alunite or alum stone, $K_2SO_4.Al_2(SO_4)_3.4Al(OH)_3$, which has remained in use to within the present century. It is insoluble in water, but on calcination it gives a residuum of alumina, mixed with ferric oxide as impurity, and potash alum, $K_2SO_4.Al_2(SO_4)_3.24H_2O$, passes into solution when the mass is digested with water. Alum prepared in this way is called Roman alum and it is handled in commerce crystallized in cubes. Pope Pius II monopolized the trade in alum and made any interference with it a sin punishable by excommunication. His works employed 8,000 men, and they produced for him an annual revenue of 100,000 gold florins.

Alum on a Yorkshire Estate

In Great Britain the manufacture of alum was established in Dorset, the Isle of Wight and Yorkshire. The manor of Longhull, in Yorkshire, belonged for generations to the Chaloner family. It was granted to Sir Thomas Chaloner in the reign of Queen Mary. His son, also Sir Thomas, is reputed to be the man who first established the manufacture of alum in England. The ruins of many of the works he built are still to be seen in the neighbourhood of Whitby and Guisborough. When Sir Thomas Chaloner was travelling in Italy it is said that he was struck by the re-semblance of the soil about the Papal alum works at Tolfa to the soil of

Guisborough, and also by the fact that in both places the leaves of the trees were of a special pale green colour. On his return to England about the year 1600 he began works here, but in order to learn the secrets of the industry he had to bribe some of the Pope's workmen to enter his service, and he smuggled them out of Italy hidden in barrels on board his ship.

A Papal Curse

For this it is said that Sir Thomas Chaloner was solemnly cursed by the Pope (Bett, 1950). The curse was made in the name of God the Father, the Son, and the Holy Spirit, in the name of the Virgin Mary, in the name of angels and archangels, of cherubim and seraphim, of patriarchs, prophets, apostles, evangelists and saints. He was cursed in the house, in the church, in the field, in the highway, in the path, in the wood, in the water; in living, in dying; in eating, in drinking, in hunger, in thirst, in fasting, in sleep, in walking, in standing, in sitting, in lying, in working, in resting; in the hair of his head, in his brains, in his temples, in his ears, in his eyebrows, in his eyes, in his cheeks, in his jaws, in his teeth, in his lips, in his throat, in his breast, in his heart, in his fingers, in his hips, in his knees, in his legs, in his feet and in his toe-nails. But despite papal denunciation the manufacture extended considerably and the method continued largely unchanged until the middle of the nineteenth century.

Alum from Coal-shale

In 1845, when sulphuric acid became available on a large scale (see p. 84), a completely new and much more economical method of manufacturing alum was discovered by a fortunate accident. A Scottish chemist, Peter Spence, had been seeking for a means of making alum from coal-shale, but discouraged by lack of success he was on the point of turning his energy in other directions. By a mischance a beaker of liquor was left in his laboratory overnight and he noticed crystals of alum which had settled out by next morning. By his method the weight of aluminous raw material required per ton of alum was reduced from about 100 tons to less than one ton. The time required for the process was greatly shortened and the old method of manufacture gradually died out.

Pigments and Dyes in Early Use

Early painters worked mainly with mineral pigments. Vermilion, identical in composition with mineral cinnabar, HgS, was prepared by the Chinese many centuries ago and used as a durable bright red pigment. The Greeks and Romans decorated some of their buildings and statues with red lead or minium, Pb_3O_4. For yellow tints they used orpiment or King's yellow, which is arsenic sulphide, As_2S_3. Egyptian blue was known to the Romans as cœruleum (see p. 14). Chalk and gypsum, terra alba, were used for white pigments, and carbon for black. The oxides of iron known as earth pigments have been used all over the world from remote times. They vary in colour from pale yellow through red to crimson, brown and black. Yellow ochre is the hydrated oxide, $Fe_2O_3.H_2O$, which becomes red on dehydration, forming burnt ochre, Fe_2O_3. Red ochre is a mixture of hæmatite with clay. From Sienna in Italy came raw sienna, a brownish-yellow pigment readily converted to burnt sienna, which is a rich orange-brown. Red oxide of iron called Spanish oxide was obtained from Malaga, from the Persian Gulf a similar pigment called Gulf red was exported and Devonshire produced Brixham red. The dyes used in ancient times came from sea molluscs, plants and insects. The preparation of the dyes with which alum was used as a mordant entailed a certain skill in chemical manipulation. Much dyeing was no doubt done by means of extracts of local herbs and lichens just as it is today in the Outer Hebrides for the making of Harris tweed. Such vegetable dyes were few in number and of unexciting hues. Of more brilliant and powerful dyes we have better knowledge.

Sepia and Tyrian Purple

In the ancient world two dyes, sepia and Tyrian purple, were obtained from sea molluscs. The ink of the common European cuttlefish, *Sepia officinalis*, is the source of the brown pigment used by water-colour artists

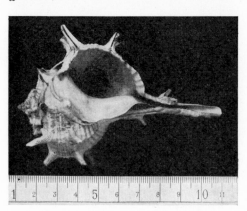

FIG. 10.—Shell of *Murex brandaris*
(*Scale in centimetres*)

and known as sepia. The ink is secreted into a sac communicating with the anal canal, and when in danger the cuttlefish discharges it forcibly, in order that the dark cloud formed in the water may act as a screen against its enemies. But sepia was of little importance in comparison with the brilliant Tyrian purple, or murex purple, which came from the rock whelk, *Murex brandaris*, a shellfish of the Eastern Mediterranean (fig. 10). The source of the dye was the hypobranchial gland, whose function it is to clear out particles from the mantle cavity of the mollusc. The secretion is colourless and stinks because it contains bromine. It rapidly goes blue on exposure to air and light. Even 3,000 years ago this dye was of much importance and was named Tyrian purple after the city of Tyre, where, according to legend, it was discovered. In the Roman Empire it became known as Royal or Imperial purple and only the wealthiest people could be "clothed in purple and fine linen" or "born to the purple." At one time it cost £60 an ounce, and because it was so valuable its manufacture in the Roman Empire was made an imperial monopoly and great purple factories were established all over the Mediterranean. It was not until 1909 that it was shown to be 6:6[1] dibrom indigo (fig. 61). There is now no demand for it, as other blues are preferred.

Indigo, Archil and Woad

Three other blue dyes were obtained from plants. The use of the indigo plant as the source of a dye seems to have been familiar to the people of India, China, Persia and Egypt since ancient times. The dye is the leaf juice of the indigo plant, which has been left to develop a blue colour on keeping. The plant is called *Indigofera anil*, the second word being derived from the Sanskrit, *nila*, dark-blue. Dyeing with indigo was improved in the eighteenth century by adding ferrous sulphate and lime to the vat. Until about 1850 the fields of India grew indigo plants which sold yearly to the value of £5,000,000, but the Badische Anilin und Soda Fabrik spent 20 years and a vast fortune to synthesize indigo from naphthalene, and by 1913 India was producing practically none and was free to raise food over the area released. Very ancient too is the use of a violet dye resulting from the action of ammonia as stale urine on certain lichens found in Asia Minor. These are known as archil, orchil or orchilla weed and one of them, *Roccella tinctoria*, is still used to make blue litmus paper. Litmus was referred to by Pliny as of service in reinforcing the shade of Tyrian purple. In Europe, up to the middle of the seventeenth century, the woad plant, *Isatis tinctoria*, was in great demand as a blue dye.

Safflower, Madder and Kermes

Of the three red dyes used in ancient times, two came from plants and one from an insect. The safflower or bastard saffron, *Carthamus tinctorius*, was for centuries cultivated for the red dye in its leaves. It was used in ancient Egypt to dye mummy cloths and in England to colour government red tape. It is still used mixed with powdered talc in the preparation of toilet rouge. Madder is the red root of *Rubia tinctorum*. Fabrics dyed with it were found in Tutankhamen's tomb and in other Egyptian tombs as far back as 3000 B.C. Large quantities were exported from Smyrna all over the world as Turkey red. Up to a late date in the nineteenth century, large areas of France were devoted to its cultivation. It was not until 1868 that its structure was determined; it was called alizarin and synthesized from anthracene (fig. 61). Biblical scarlet or kermes was a discovery of Phœnicians in Palestine and was known before Moses. It was made from a female wingless insect, *Coccus ilicis*, formerly supposed to be a berry and found on the leaves of the kermes oak, *Quercus coccifera*. In the fifteenth century kermes was replaced by cochineal (see p. 86).

Weld, Young Fustic, Turmeric and Cutch

From a remote period at least four plants have been used as sources of yellow dyes. Weld is extracted from a plant called *Reseda luteola*. It is the oldest European dyestuff known and was used by the Gauls in the time of Julius Cæsar. But it was not until about 1912 that Arthur George Perkin identified the yellow dye as a tetrahydroxyflavone (see p. 152). Young fustic comes from the wood of the Venetian sumach, *Rhus cotinus*; Pliny refers to the use of cotinus as a yellow dye. Turmeric is obtained from the tuberous rhizomes of *Circuma longa*, a native of Southern Asia. It owes its colour to a yellow crystalline substance, *curcumin*. Cutch or catechu is obtained from the wood of *Acacai catechu*, a native of India. For dyeing and tanning, this substance has been in use in India from the most remote period, but it was introduced into Europe only in the nineteenth century.

Roger Bacon and Berthold Schwarz

The earliest of the great scientists of England, Roger Bacon (1214–92), was born in Ilchester. He became a Franciscan monk, and in 1242 in a Latin text he made known the composition of gunpowder, the oldest explosive. It is, of course, a mixture of charcoal, sulphur and saltpetre (KNO_3). According to a mediæval legend, another monk, the mysterious Berthold Schwarz of the Black Forest, first used it as a propellent. The date of his invention of the first firearms is unknown, but it was probably 1330, and sixteen years later cannon shot was used at the battle of Crécy. The change in the art of warfare from the use of spears and bows and arrows to small arms and cannon opened up many new trades. Not only were forging and foundry methods improved, but also greater skill was required in the building of fortifications. The influence of powder and shot on the art of war changed mediæval feudalism. It provided better methods for the protection of life and property, and enabled industry and the arts to advance at an accelerated pace.

Gunpowder as a Blasting Explosive

In 1627 at Schemnitz, Caspar Weindl, a Tirolean, introduced the use of gunpowder for underground blasting. In England it was first used in the Cornish tin mines in 1689. Today, except in coal mines, blasting is still largely done with black powder which differs very little from the original gunpowder of the thirteenth century. In Great Britain, 3,500 tons of black powder are made annually and most of this is used for blasting. It was not until 1865 that the agelong position held by gunpowder as a blasting explosive was undermined by the researches of Nobel on nitroglycerine which led to his invention of dynamite (see p. 585).

THE MEDIÆVAL GILDS

The thirteenth century which gave to the world Thomas Aquinas and Dante made great contributions to civilization. It was the pre-Renaissance period and it took a great part in the rise of education, the origin of universities, and the awakening of science, engineering, architecture, painting and music. The work of its artisans was astonishing. As a result of their crafts-manship beautiful cathedrals were built and perfection was attained in the art of glass making, so that in colour and design the stained-glass windows of the period were of unsurpassed beauty. This era produced skilled men whose work has never been excelled. There were sculptors in stone, wood carvers, silversmiths, goldsmiths and decorative ironsmiths, who were artists of unusual creative ability.

Origin of the Mediæval Gilds

The form of industrial organization which controlled the activities of these workers in the towns was the localized gild. The origin of the medi-æval gilds has been traced to the eighth century in England and to the eleventh century in France, Norway and the Netherlands. They were voluntary associations formed for the mutual aid and protection of their members. The merchant and craft fraternities were closely connected with municipal government. The gild merchant came into existence soon after the Norman Conquest. Its chief function was to regulate the trade monopoly conveyed to a borough by the royal grant of *gilda mercatoria*. When the King be-stowed upon the tanners or weavers or any other body of artisans the right to have a gild, they secured the monopoly of working and trading in their branch of industry.

Creation of Craft Gilds

With every creation of a craft fraternity the gild merchant was weakened and its sphere of activity was diminished, though the new bodies were sub-sidiary to the older and larger fraternity. In the earlier stages of the craft gild, masters, apprentices and journeymen were more or less of one class. They shared their meals in the same shop and, though poor by modern standards, they were a proud fraternity, the skilled men of the trade. Their gild represented their common interest and, subject to the general control of the municipality, it managed the affairs of the craft within the town, fixing prices, wages and conditions of work to the general satisfaction of masters and men (Trevelyan, 1942).

Formation of Yeoman Gilds

In the early part of the fourteenth century things changed because the expansion of trade led to further division of labour and the masters became more and more engaged in organizing the business and selling the goods. The distinction between employer and employed was becoming more marked. There were occasional strikes for higher wages inside the gild, and in some cases the formation of yeomen gilds to champion the interest of the employees and perform the fighting functions of a modern trade union. There was at no time a general struggle in England between the gild mer-chant and the craft gilds, though in a few towns there seems to have been some friction between merchants and artisans. In London the craft gilds are historically represented by the Livery Companies.

D.O.—2*

The Gilds of Continental Europe

There is no exact parallel in England to the great Continental revolution of the thirteenth and fourteenth centuries, by which the crafts threw off the yoke of patrician government and secured more independence in the management of their own affairs and more participation in the civic administration. The main causes of these conflicts on the Continent were the monopoly of power by the patricians, acts of violence committed by them, their bad management of the finances and their partisan administration of justice. In some Continental towns the victory of the artisans in the fourteenth century was so complete that the whole civic constitution was remodelled, with the craft fraternities as a basis.

The Statutes of Labourers

In England when Edward III's Statutes of Labourers had attempted in vain to fix a maximum wage for the whole country, national control began to impinge upon municipal control. In the reign of Elizabeth I the emphasis on national control was even greater and the town economy ultimately gave place to a national economy. In the process of change the Justices of the Peace carried out national control of wages and prices without attempting to impose everywhere a fixed maximum wage. Under Edward VI there had been confiscating legislation against gild property, and this caused a decline of the craft gilds. And then in the first Elizabethan Age there came a wave of joyous nationalism in which men no longer felt their first loyalty owing to town or gild but to Queen and country.

The Statute of Artificers (1563)

The Statute of Artificers (1563) laid down that every craftsman in England had for seven years to learn his craft under a responsible master. It was based on the supposition that the average man was without sufficient judgement or experience to govern himself until after the age of twenty-four. Having then served his apprenticeship, he was at liberty to marry and either to set up a business of his own or to become a journeyman for hire. On the whole the apprentice system served society well. Apprenticeship was the very practical answer made by our ancestors to the problem of technical education after the school years. But the system was destroyed in the nineteenth century by the industrial revolution and nothing worth having was provided to replace it.

Assistance to Sick and Poor Members

At an early date workmen organized themselves into societies for mutual aid and assistance. The oldest known mutual-aid society is that of the miners of Goslar in the Harz Mountains which received a charter from Friedrich I in 1188. These organizations multiplied in the thirteenth century under such names as *Bruderschaften* or *Knappschaften*. Whenever a member of the brotherhood fell ill he received a certain sum of money, and when a member died, four solidi were contributed to the funeral expenses.

The weekly contribution of each member was one denar (Rosen, 1943). In England the craft gilds performed the functions of friendly societies, benefit societies and sick societies. Thus the charter granted by Richard II to the furriers of Norwich created the Gild of the Peltyers in Norwich. In this document

> it is ordeyned . . . yat quat broyer or syster, be goddis sonde, falle in mischefe or mys-ese, and have nout to helpen hemselfe, he schal han almesse of eueri broyer and syster euery woke, lastende his myschefe . . . But if it be his foly, he schal nout han of ye elme.

Respect was shown for the dead by a procession of the members of the gild at the funeral, burial service and by offerings at mass (Legge, 1920).

Insistence on Honest Workmanship

In addition to assistance to sick and poor members of a gild, great stress was laid on the use of good materials and on proper and honest workmanship. Inspectors known as searchers were appointed to enforce the ordinances as to workmanship and to stamp the articles made as being of the quality and nature which they claimed to be. This system survives in the hall-marks stamped upon articles of gold and silver. Rooms still exist in the Guild Halls of Norwich and Witney in which every piece of cloth produced was inspected and stamped by the aulnagers of the gild. Each gild had its own seal, sometimes in the form of a coat of arms, which was attached to the article made to assure the buyer of the soundness of his purchase.

A System founded on Family Life

One aim of the gild was to limit competition, and this was done by forbidding any master to have more than one apprentice in order that work should be equally distributed. The whole gild was bound by certain customs and ordinances. The system was largely founded on family life. The master was allowed to bring up his children in his trade. His apprentice had to be formally inscribed and had to sign on for seven years, during all of which time he had to live as one of the family in the house of his master, sharing his food and the family life. Hours of work were very long, from 5 o'clock in the morning in winter and 6 in summer to 7 at night, with perhaps three hours off for meal-times. Work by artificial light was often prohibited. The desire to shorten the working day showed itself early, and in some ordinances we find work forbidden on one half-day a week. Holidays were fixed by the Church festivals, of which there were plenty. In all there were 275 working days in the year. Work was forbidden on Sundays, on holy days and on the evenings before them. The apprentice had usually to be indoors by 9 o'clock at night.

Beauty of the Gild Halls

In looking through the charters of gilds of various crafts, no matter from what town or country, one is impressed by the emphasis placed upon pride in the gild and pride in workmanship. Generous contributions were made to chapels and chantries, and on the gild hall was expended all the talent of all the crafts combined. The beauty of the buildings, and the details of the internal fittings, are still to be seen in the Guild Halls of London, Westminster, York, Lavenham and Exeter. Pride in the workman's tools and in the merchant's mark is expressed and emphasized,

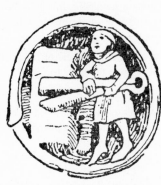

FIG. 11.—Mark of Mediæval Tailors' Gild carved in Stone

or they are emblazoned on shields, carved in stone or wood or set in stained glass (fig. 11). The merchant and craftsman chose to have beautiful things and to make them of the best.

The Festival of the Patron Saint

In many cases men combining in a gild for a benevolent, a useful or even a convivial purpose gave a religious tinge to their proceedings by invoking the blessing of a saint on their association (Mantoux, 1928). The day of days to the members of a gild was the festival of their patron saint, when the warden of the year was elected. Then all the members, attired in their livery suits, would assemble at the gild hall and go in procession to attend mass, celebrated by their chaplain at the gild chapel in the parish church.

Banquets, Morris Dances and Miracle Plays

Later, with their wives and families, they dined in state, showing their wealth in plate upon their sideboards. Finally, as epilogue to the banquet and business, the day would end either with a Miracle Play or with Morris dancing. The subject of a Miracle Play was often related to the trade followed by a gild. Thus the shipwrights, fishermen and fishmongers would enact the story of God foretelling Noah in the ark with his wife and divers animals; and the goldsmiths and moneymakers, the three kings from the East offering gifts (Legge, 1920). In our day in London, survivals of these customs are seen in the Lord Mayor's Show, the Queen's opening of Parliament and banquets at the Mansion House and Guildhall. In provincial towns the pageantry survives in the figures of dignitaries such as the Master Cutler of Sheffield.

EARLY OCCUPATIONAL MEDICINE

Throughout the mediæval period there were no contributions to the subject of occupational diseases and it is not until the sixteenth century that we find definite information relating to diseases of miners and of workmen in dangerous trades. It was in the middle of the sixteenth century that two remarkable men, Agricola and Paracelsus wrote on the subject of miners' diseases, and at the close of the seventeenth century came the classical work of Ramazzini, the Father of Occupational Medicine.

Metalliferous Mining in Bohemia and Silesia

In 965 silver was discovered near Goslar and mining began in the Harz mountains. Between 1100 and 1300 important discoveries of precious metals were made in the Erzgebirge. During the thirteenth century silver began to be mined in Bohemia and gold in Silesia, and for 300 years mining became an important industry in Central Europe. This meant that the Germans supplied Europe with the precious metals needed for currency and as a result they became the leaders of the commercial world. The mines of Schneeberg were opened in 1410, and in 1516 rich veins of silver were discovered at Joachimstal on the southern slopes of the Erzgebirge. In Bohemia in 1519 a silver coin worth 3 marks, about 2s. 11d., was minted at Joachimsthal. It became known as the *Joachimsthaler* and later as the *Thaler*. The word was corrupted in English to *daller* and about 1553 to *dollar*.

Georgius Agricola, 1494-1555

The classic description of metalliferous mining in Central Europe in the sixteenth century is to be found in *De Re Metallica* by Georg Bauer, who

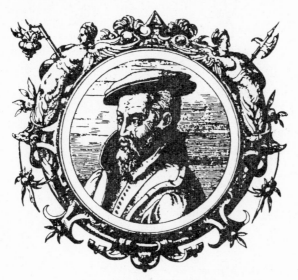

FIG. 12.—Georgius Agricola (Georg Bauer), 1494–1555

was more commonly known as Georgius Agricola (fig. 12). He was born at Glauchau in Saxony at the very beginning of the Revival of Learning. The printing press had been first used forty years before, Luther was a babe of one year, Erasmus was still a student, Columbus had just discovered

America and three years were to elapse before Vasco da Gama rounded the Cape of Good Hope. At the age of twenty Agricola went to Leipzig to study Latin and Greek for three years, and he then taught these subjects in a municipal school in Germany. Between the ages of thirty and thirty-three he studied philosophy, medicine and the natural sciences in Italy, attending the universities of Bologna, Venice and perhaps Padua. In 1526 he was appointed official physician to the mining town of Joachimsthal.

GEORGII AGRICOLAE

DE RE METALLICA LIBRI XII▸ QVI▸
bus Officia, Inſtrumenta, Machinæ, ac omnia deniĉ ad Metalli-
cam ſpectantia, non modo luculentiſſimè deſcribuntur, ſed & per
effigies, ſuis locis inſertas, adiunctis Latinis, Germaniciſĉ appel-
lationibus ita ob oculos ponuntur, ut clarius tradi non poſſint.

EIVSDEM

DE ANIMANTIBVS SVBTERRANEIS Liber, ab Autore re-
cognitus:cum Indicibus diuerſis, quicquid in opere tractatum eſt,
pulchrè demonſtrantibus.

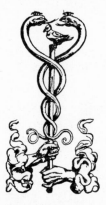

BASILEAE   M▸ D▸ LVI▸

Cum Priuilegio Imperatoris in annos v.
& Galliarum Regis ad Sexennium.

FIG. 13.—Title Page of *De Re Metallica*, 1556

De Re Metallica, 1556

De Re Metallica was published in 1556, a year after the death of Agricola (fig. 13). It is a scholarly work consisting of twelve books which deal with every aspect of mining and with the associated smelting and refining of gold and silver. The fifth book deals with the actual mining underground. The art of surveying in the mine, the different kinds of ores to be found, the types of shafts and how to sink them are all fully described. The sixth book describes the various tools and implements fully. It gives a complete account of the machinery employed for ventilation, pumping and winding. Drainage was effected by means of a continuous chain of buckets operated by a foot tread-wheel. The book ends with an account of the diseases and accidents prevalent among the miners and the means available to guard against them.

Ventilation of the Mines

The ill effects of poor ventilation were known from practical experience. Agricola says:

Miners pay the greatest attention to these matters just as much as to digging or they should do so. Air indeed becomes stagnant both in tunnels and in shafts. I will now speak of ventilating machines. If a shaft is very deep and no tunnel reaches to it, or no drift from another shaft connects with it, or when a tunnel is of great length and no shaft reaches to it, then the air does not replenish itself. In such a case it weights heavily on the miners, causing them to breathe with difficulty, and sometimes they are even suffocated and burning lamps are also extinguished. There is therefore a necessity for machines which enable the miners to breathe easily and carry on their work.

Several types of ventilating machines were employed to force air into the mine workings. Agricola speaks of powerful blowing machines and he mentions the use of bellows. He also describes another ventilating machine consisting of a cylindrical barrel, within which four wings rotated.

Accidents in the Mines

Accidents were by no means rare. Miners slipped from the ladders into the shafts and broke their limbs or their necks, or they fell into the sump at the bottom of the shafts where they were drowned. Falls of ground imperilled their lives, and major tragedies sometimes occurred, as on the occasion when Remmelsburg near Goslar subsided, killing 400 men. The actual methods of mining ore had changed very little from the days of ancient Egypt (see p. 5), except that the hammers, picks, blocks and wedges were of iron instead of stone or bronze. Where these tools were of no avail, the method of fire-setting was used. Agricola was well aware that fire-setting had its perils.

While the heated veins and rock are giving forth a fetid vapour and the shafts or tunnels are emitting fumes, the miners and other workmen do not go down in the mines lest the stench affect their health or actually kill them. The Bergmeister in order to prevent workmen from being suffocated gives no one permission to break veins or rock by fire in shafts or tunnels where it is possible for the poisonous vapours and smoke to permeate the veins and pass through into neighbouring mines.

Diseases of the Lungs in the Miners

In the last part of his sixth book Agricola discusses those ailments which attack the joints, the lungs and the eyes of miners. The accounts he gives are rambling and lack precision; it is clear that the idea of diseases specifically caused by particular occupations had not, in his day, entered men's minds. His description of the harmful effects of the dust inhaled is of a suppurating disease of the lungs with a visible and progressive emaciation. It is probable that silicosis, tuberculosis and carcinoma of the lung were involved in the conditions he describes.

On the other hand some mines are so dry that they are entirely devoid of water and this dryness causes the workmen even greater harm, for the dust, which is stirred and beaten up by digging, penetrates into the windpipe and lungs, and produces difficulty in breathing and the disease which the Greeks called asthma. If the dust has corrosive qualities, it eats away the lungs, and implants consumption in the body. In the mines of the Carpathian Mountains women are found who have married seven husbands, all of whom this terrible consumption has carried off to a premature death.

To protect the miners against dust Agricola advises purification of the air in the mine by ventilating machines and the use of loose veils over the faces of the miners.

Demons of the Mines in German Mythology

In Agricola's day it was not considered unnatural for the miners to come across demons in the mine workings. These were usually considered to be jolly and of kindly intent rather than cruel or evil. They were either little boys or dwarfed men, and they did little harm beyond chattering and extinguishing the miners' lamps (see p. 649). Agricola wrote of them in his *De Animantibus Subterraneis* and told how demons of ferocious aspect were expelled and put to flight by prayer and fasting. In his great work *Deutsche Mythologie* (1835), Jacob Grimm (1785–1863), the philologist, perpetuated the folk-lore which surrounded these demons of the mines. In the enchanting *Kinder und Hausmärchen* (1812), which he wrote with

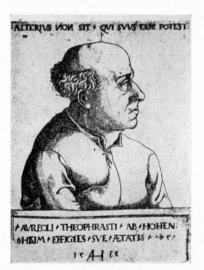

FIG. 14.—Paracelsus, 1493–1541

his brother Wilhelm, he relates the story of the persecuted child princess befriended by dwarfs who lived in the woods and worked in the mines nearby. In our time this story has been delightfully rendered into animated cartoons by Walt Disney in his *Snow White and the Seven Dwarfs*.

Paracelsus, 1493–1541

In 1567, eleven years after the publication of Agricola's treatise, there appeared the first monograph devoted to the occupational diseases of mine and smelter workers. The author of this work was Aureolus Theophrastus Bombastus von Hohenheim, usually known as Paracelsus (fig. 14). The book, published posthumously, was entitled *Von der Bergsucht und anderen Bergkrankheiten*. Paracelsus was born in Switzerland at Einsiedeln near Schwyz. His father was a doctor, an able, well-educated man who had considerable experience of chemistry and metallurgy. In 1502 he was called to be town physician to

Villach where the Tyrolese alchemist Sigismund Függer owned mines and maintained a mining school. From him the young Paracelsus received his first instruction in the extraction of drugs from plants and in the methods of identifying metals and producing chemical compounds.

His Popularity during his Wanderings

Paracelsus studied medicine under Leoniceno in Ferrara. Like all other medical students of his day he read the Greek and Arab authors, the chief authority being Galen. Having obtained his medical degree in 1515, he wandered for many years all over Europe, enlisting in various armies and visiting numerous countries as far apart as England and Turkey. During his wanderings he came into contact with people in every walk of life, and wherever he went he sought knowledge not only from the learned abbots and bishops but also from barbers, gipsies, midwives, executioners and fortune-tellers. He learned a great deal about medical practice, and incidentally acquired an unusual knowledge of folk-medicine and a permanent taste for low company. He thought and spoke in the language of the people and was popular as no other physician before him. Finally returning to Strassburg in 1526 he began to practise medicine, but in 1527 he became town physician in Basel and lecturer at the university.

His Contempt for Medical Scholasticism

In the substance and manner of his teaching Paracelsus soon revealed his intention of reforming and rejuvenating medical theory and practice. Contrary to custom he held his lectures in German and not in Latin; he also wrote many of his books in his mother tongue. His lectures were very popular and soon became overcrowded. Imbued with a lifelong reverence for Hippocrates, implanted by his teachers in Italy, he began his campaign of reform by publicly burning the works of Galen and Ibn Sina. Instead of commenting upon the ancients, the customary manner of instruction at the time, he preferred to base his lectures on his own experiences. His popularity soon aroused the envy of his colleagues, and his attitude of derision and contempt for medical scholasticism added to his unpopularity with established authority. He had a truculent independent spirit and was one of the few writers who ever advanced medicine by quarrelling about it. Far in advance of his time, Paracelsus taught physicians to substitute chemical therapeutics for alchemy. He made opium, mercury, lead, sulphur, iron, arsenic, copper sulphate and potassium sulphate part of the pharmacopœia.

His Death in a Tavern Brawl

In 1528 he was forced to leave Basel and the next year found him in Nuremberg where he published the work in which he established the use of mercury in the treatment of syphilis. But the university authorities prohibited any further printing of his books and he set off again on his wanderings, visiting Scandinavia and Saxony. In 1536 he reached Augsburg and

then Innsbruck, where there was an epidemic of bubonic plague. He practised all over Germany and Austria with varying success and in 1538 he
lived at Klagenfurt in Carinthia. Two years later he was invited to work
in Salzburg by Prince Ernst of Bavaria. His hope of finding a haven of
contentment was fulfilled but briefly, for in 1541 he met his end from a
wound in a tavern brawl in Salzburg.

His Experience of Mining and Metallurgy

We have seen how Paracelsus while only a boy learned chemistry,
metallurgy, pharmacy and botany from his father in the mining centre of
Villach. Soon after he qualified in medicine he was employed for five years
in the smelting plant at Schwaz, in Tyrol. Later on, during his journeys
through Hungary, Denmark and Sweden, he learned about the mines of
those countries. About 1533 he passed through the industrialized Inn
valley which contained many mines, and it is likely that conditions in the
mines and the diseases of miners awakened his interest then (Sudhoff,
1936). But in 1537 the management of the Függer mines called him back
to Villach to take charge of the metallurgical work there. It is evident that
Paracelsus had ample opportunity to study the mining industry, to observe
the diseases of miners and to study the effects of various minerals and
metals on the human organism.

Tartarus, Mercury, Sulphur and Salt

In order to understand his views upon the toxicology of metals one
must look to the theories held by alchemists long before this time. For
example, the theory of the tartarus diseases was introduced into Europe
from the Orient in the thirteenth century. Tartarus was a general term comprising all forms of precipitation or sedimentation. According to Paracelsus
the tartarus itself was not a simple substance but a mixture of mercury,
sulphur and salt. We are not to think of these three substances as identical
with those we know today but rather as the three basic categories of matter.
The names allude to the reactions of substances when exposed to heat;
sulphur is that which burns, quicksilver that which evaporates and salt
that which resists heat. There are as many kinds of mercury, sulphur and
salt as there are substances.

His Concept of the Pathology of Miners' Lung

He knew that work in certain mines gave rise to dyspnœa, cough and
even cachexia, and he thought that these symptoms were due to the climate
or vapour of the mines. It is striking, however, that he refers to no protective
apparatus such as the veils to be worn by miners mentioned by Agricola.
Nor does Paracelsus pay any special attention to dust as a causative factor
in the diseases of miners (Rosen, 1943). Although he makes correct clinical
observations, he then turns to weird alchemical theories to explain them.
For example, he strives hard to make the respiratory diseases of miners fit
the theory of the tartarus.

The lung sickness comes through the power of the stars, in that their peculiar characters are boiled out, which settle on the lungs in three different ways: in a mercurial manner like a sublimated smoke that coagulates, like a salt spirit, which passes from resolution to co-agulation, and thirdly, like a sulphur, which is precipitated on the walls by roasting.

He goes on to identify this process with the slow deposition in a barrel of clear wine of a layer of wine-stone or tartarus.

Diseases of Smelter Workers and Metallurgists

In the second and third books of *Von der Bergsucht*, Paracelsus describes the diseases of smelter workers and metallurgists. The numerous correct observations that he made are evidence of his own experiences in the mines and metal refineries. He was well acquainted with the Tyrol, Carinthia and Carniola regions where mercury was mined and refined. He recognized the poisonous effects of various metals and differentiated acute and chronic poisoning. In his detailed description of mercurialism, he mentions most of the important symptoms. Although his monograph was only a beginning, there can be no doubt it was an important one. His work is unique in the literature of the sixteenth century and it exerted a definite influence for at least 150 years after it was written (Sudhoff, 1936).

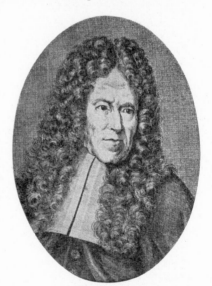

FIG. 15.—Bernardino Ramazzini, 1633–1714

The Father of Occupational Medicine

Exactly a hundred years after Paracelsus began his study of the toxicology of metals in the valley of the Inn there was born in Italy in 1633 a babe who was to become a great pioneer of the seventeenth century and the Father of Occupational Medicine. Ramazzini lived to the age of eighty-one (fig. 15). The first edition of the work to which he owes his immortality *De Morbis Artificum Diatriba* was published in 1700 when he was sixty-seven years of age (fig. 16). Sigerist (1936) says that this book is to the history of occupational diseases what the *De Fabrica Humani Corporis* (1543) of Vesalius is to anatomy, Harvey's *De Motu Cordis* (1628) to physiology and Morgagni's *De Sedibus et Causis Morborum* (1761) to pathology.

Bernardino Ramazzini, 1633–1714

Ramazzini was born at Carpi near Modena. He studied philosophy and medicine at the University of Parma, where he took his medical degree in 1659. After practising for twelve years in Rome and in Carpi, he was appointed in 1671 professor of medicine in the newly restored University of Modena. He worked there for thirty years, eighteen of which were spent at the University. He made accurate studies in epidemiology, describing the outbreak of lathyrism at Modena in 1690 as well as several outbreaks of malaria. No doubt he would be astonished could he know that his fame today is based not upon his *Constitutiones Epidemicæ* but upon his work on occupational diseases. Equally he might be somewhat surprised to learn that, since 1907, his countrymen in Florence have published in his honour a journal of social hygiene known as *Il Ramazzini*.

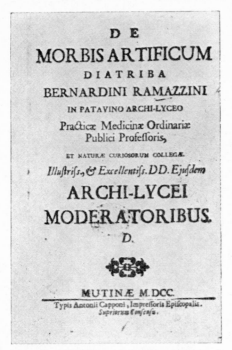

FIG. 16.—Title Page of the First Edition of Ramazzini's *De Morbis Artificum Diatriba*, 1700

The Chair of Medicine in Padua

In 1700 he accepted the call of the Venetian Senate to the chair of medicine in Padua (fig. 17), and his fame spread rapidly throughout Italy and all over Europe. About 1703 he began to lose the sight of both eyes, presumably as a result of retinal arteriosclerosis. His grandsons helped him, especially with his reading and writing, but in 1707, at the age of seventy-four, he asked leave of Venice to retire. Instead he was promoted to the great distinction of being President of the Venetian College and told that he need not lecture if he felt indisposed (fig. 18). On his eighty-first birthday, as he was preparing in the afternoon to go to lecture to his students, he was seized with apoplexy and died within twelve hours. He was buried in the church of the Nuns of St. Helena in Padua but in an unknown grave.

His Personal Appearance and Habits

From the writings of his nephew we know that he was lean and dark-complexioned, with black curly hair and attractive dark eyes. He was a hard worker and keen observer, paid little attention to the affairs of his household and avoided games as one would a mad dog or a snake. He was active and walked so fast that his regular escort of students could hardly keep up with him. His hair became prematurely white, but was hidden by an elegant and becoming wig. He liked to dress well and suitably, but scorned doctors who were soft or self-seeking. When he had anything to do in public he was timid and nervous, especially at first. He eagerly cultivated friendships with the learned, and with so much affection and homage that they paid him honour at all times. At work his chief asset was a capacity for exact observation which enabled him, in spite of the lack of knowledge of anatomy, physiology, chemistry and bacteriology of his time, to arrive at surprisingly accurate conclusions. Unlike Paracelsus he was a singularly untravelled man, and there is no evidence that he ever left Italy or, indeed, ever went farther than Rome.

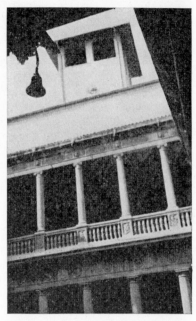

Fig. 17.—Courtyard of the University of Padua, built in 1552 by Andrea Della Valle

The Man who cleaned the Cesspits in Modena

In the town of Modena where Ramazzini lived, the inhabitants of the tall, crowded houses, acting up to the best sanitary standards of the time, saw to it that the cesspits, which were connected with the drains that ran in different directions through the streets, should be cleaned out in each house once in every three years. And so Ramazzini wrote:

> On one occasion when that work was going forward in our house, I observed one of the labourers making extraordinary exertions to get through with his task. I pitied him on account of the cruel nature of the work and asked him why he toiled so feverishly and did not try to avoid exhaustion by working at a slower pace. Whereupon the poor fellow lifted his eyes up out of the pit, fixed them upon me and said: "No one who has not tried it can imagine what it costs to spend more than four hours in this place. It is as bad as going blind."

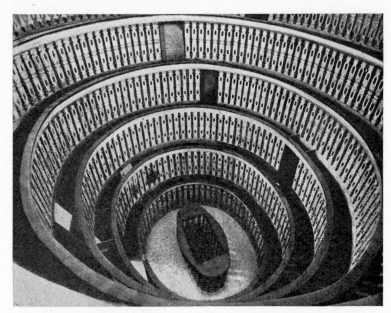

FIG. 18.—Anatomical Theatre of Fabricius of Acquapendente in the
University of Padua (1594)

Visits to the Lowliest Workshops

The inquiry thus auspiciously begun bore a rich fruit. Ramazzini did
not forget that cleaner of privies. He was profoundly convinced of the importance of the mechanical arts for the progress of civilization, but he was
equally impressed by the wretched conditions of those engaged in these
arts. He said he had to confess that many arts are the cause of grave injury
to those who practise them, and that many an artisan has looked to his
craft as a means to support life and raise a family, but all he has got from it
is some deadly disease, with the result that he has departed this life cursing
the craft to which he has applied himself.

> Medicine, like jurisprudence, should make a contribution to the
> well-being of workers and see to it that, so far as possible, they should
> exercise their callings without harm. So I for my part have done what
> I could and have not thought it unbecoming to make my way into the
> lowliest workshops and study the mysteries of the mechanic arts.

Dirty and Dangerous Trades

In the course of carrying out his resolve Ramazzini inquired into the
conditions of work and the occupational diseases of the following types of
workers: miners of metals, healers by inunction, chemists, potters, tinsmiths, glass workers and mirror makers, painters, sulphur workers, blacksmiths, workers with gypsum and lime, apothecaries, cleaners of privies

and cesspits, fullers, oil pressers, tanners, cheese makers and other workers at dirty trades, tobacco workers, corpse carriers, midwives, wet-nurses, vintners and brewers, bakers and millers, starch makers, sifters and measurers of grain, stone cutters, laundresses, workers who handle flax, hemp and silk, bathmen, salt makers, workers who stand, sedentary workers, runners, grooms, porters, athletes, those who strain their eyes over fine work, voice trainers, singers, farmers, fishermen, soldiers, learned men, nuns, printers, scribes and notaries, confectioners, weavers, coppersmiths, carpenters, grinders of razors and lancets, brick makers, well diggers, sailors and rowers, hunters and soap makers.

Faulty Posture and Want of Ventilation

Perhaps Ramazzini erred in attributing disease to trades which were merely offensive to the sense of smell; certainly he was wrong in imputing fever to limewashed walls, but he fully realized many things which would today come under the heading of welfare recommendations. For example, he counsels rest intervals in work of prolonged duration and dwells much on the need for exercise and change of posture, being convinced of the importance of faulty posture in producing ill health in many trades. He condemns want of ventilation and unsuitable temperatures and urges that workers in dusty trades should, in default of any known exhaust system, work in spacious rooms with their backs to the draught and should wash their faces, rinse out their mouths with water and quit work in such trades immediately symptoms of respiratory disease show that the lungs are threatened. His advocacy of personal cleanliness and protective clothing is described on p. 767.

A Striking Addition to the Hippocratic Art

As one result of his inquiries we find Ramazzini, among other wise counsels, making a striking addition to the Hippocratic art:

> When a doctor visits a working-class home he should be content to sit on a three-legged stool, if there isn't a gilded chair, and he should take time for his examination; and to the questions recommended by Hippocrates, he should add one more—What is your occupation?

Did ever a man announce with more point or with less fuss a revolutionary innovation? In one innocent-sounding sentence we find that Ramazzini characterizes and supersedes the medical science and the medical practice of two thousand years (Farrington, 1942). This simple piece of practical advice throws a strong light on our industrial civilization. In the main it is only when dealing with the common people that the doctor must think of the dangerous trades. Ramazzini made this his motto—*Medici munus plebeios curantis est interrogare quas artes exerceant.*

This Monstrous Social Paradox

Thus there are whole groups of diseases which do not affect the privileged classes of society but only those who labour in workshop, factory or

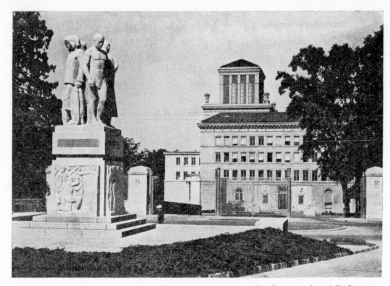

Fig. 19.—Memorial to Albert Thomas in front of the International Labour Office, Geneva

mine. For a long time the work of these men, which is indispensable to the prosperity of the community, brought them nothing but physical, intellectual and moral poverty. But men like Albert Thomas (fig. 19) have awakened the conscience of the modern world to this monstrous social paradox. Too much misery lies behind many humble daily tasks; they lead to much unnecessary physical, and hence also moral, suffering. It was Pierre Hamp who wrote:

> We live on the sufferings of others. Everyone makes life a torment for some of his fellow men. How many people earn their living pleasantly? Many do so in unpleasant and often intolerable conditions. To love one's occupation is to be happy, but where are the occupations which one can love?

The Domestic Woollen Industry

From time immemorial England, a country of pasture, has bred sheep and sold their wool. A large part of it was sold abroad especially to merchants in Flemish towns. The woollen industry developed and prospered from the reign of Edward III onwards, spread to the towns and villages and became the main source of wealth to whole populations. Until nearly the end of the eighteenth century it was surrounded with great prestige and was referred to as the great staple trade of the kingdom.

Broadcloths, Calimancoes and Worsteds

In *A Tour Through the Whole Island of Great Britain* (1724) Daniel Defoe found the yeomen in the villages of Kent, while still owning and cultivating land, weaving the fine cloth known as Kentish broadcloth. In Essex he found Colchester famous for its druggets, stuffs worn by nuns and friars. In Suffolk coarse woollen goods called says and calimancoes were made, and in Norfolk long staple wool was used to make worsteds. In the counties of Lincoln, Nottingham and Leicester the making of woollen stockings, either by hand or on frames, created a fairly extensive trade.

Blankets, Flannels and Serges

In Gloucestershire, Stroud was famous for its fine scarlet woollens, and Witney in Oxfordshire sent blankets as far as America. Salisbury Plain was the land of flannels and fine cloths which were made in Malmesbury, Chippenham, Calne, Trowbridge, Devizes and Salisbury. In Devonshire the serge industry was vigorous and thriving. Barnstaple imported Irish wool, which was made into cloth in Crediton, Honiton, Tiverton, Cullompton and Ottery Saint Mary and marketed in Exeter.

Shalloons, Druggets and Ratteens

The West Riding of Yorkshire was peopled all along the Pennines by spinners and weavers grouped round Wakefield and Halifax, where coarse materials called kerseys and shalloons, serges of Châlons, were made. These towns, as well as Huddersfield and Bradford, marketed their goods in Leeds. In Westmorland, Kendal made druggets and ratteens, and in Lancashire wool had been spun and woven long before cotton ever made its appearance in England. From this it will be seen that the woollen industry was essentially rural and was far from being localized (Mantoux, 1928).

The Weaver's Cottage

It was impossible to go far without meeting it, spreading as it did through small towns interspersed by innumerable villages, hamlets and scattered houses. The weaver's cottage, often in unhealthy surroundings, had few and narrow windows, very little furniture and even fewer ornaments. The main, and sometimes the only, room did duty both for kitchen and for workshop. There stood the loom of the weaver, who lived and worked there. That loom, which can still be found in country districts, had changed very little since the days of antiquity.

The Warp and the Woof

The threads forming the warp of the fabric were fastened parallel on a double frame, of which the two ends rose and fell alternately and were worked by two pedals; to make the woof, the weaver threw the shuttle between them, from one hand to the other. As early as 1733, an ingenious device had enabled the shuttle to be thrown and brought back with one hand. The use of this improvement, however, spread rather slowly. The rest of the apparatus was still simpler.

Carding and Spinning

Carding was done by hand, but in addition to the hand-carding brushes there was one card, immovable, fixed to a wooden support. For spinning, the hand or foot spinning wheel which had been in use since the sixteenth century was employed; even the distaff and spindle, as old as the textile industry itself, often were in use. The small man could easily provide himself with these cheap implements.

Fulling and Teazling

At his door was water for removing the grease from the wool and for washing the cloth. If he wanted to dye the fabric he had woven, a tub or two was enough. As for the things which could not be done without special and costly plant, these were the object of separate undertakings. For instance, for fulling and teazling wool there were water mills, to which all the neighbouring manufacturers brought their cloth. They were called public mills, as they could be used by everyone for a fixed payment.

Division of Labour within the Family

To match these simple tools there was an equally simple organization of labour. If the weaver's family was large enough, it did everything, its members dividing all the minor operations amongst themselves, the wife and daughters at the spinning wheel, the boys carding the wool, while the man worked the shuttle. This is the classic picture of that patriarchal state of industry. As a matter of fact, these extremely simple conditions were but rarely found. They were altered by the frequent necessity of getting part of the wool spun outside. One loom, working regularly, was reckoned to provide work for five or six spinners. In order to find them, the weaver had sometimes to go far afield. He went from house to house, until he had distributed all his wool.

The First Specialization

It was in this way that specialization first came about. There were houses where only spinning was done. In others, several weaving looms were gathered together; and the weaver, while still remaining an artisan working with his hands, had under him a small number of hired hands. Thus the weaver, in the cottage which was both his dwelling-place and his workshop, controlled production, and did not depend on a capitalist, since he owned not only the tools but the raw material. The woven fabric he sold himself in the market of the nearest town. The aspect of that market alone would be enough to show how the means of production were scattered amongst this multitude of small independent producers.

Emergence of Capitalism

The weaver was also, last but not least, a landed proprietor. His house stood in an enclosure of a few acres. In 1724 Defoe wrote that a manufacturer must have one or two horses, to fetch wool and foodstuffs in town, to bring the wool to the spinner and the cloth, once woven, to the fulling mill, and finally to take the pieces to the market; he noticed, moreover, that most clothiers kept a cow or two, to supply their family with milk, and fed them on the plots of land surrounding their houses. The witnesses who gave evidence before the Parliamentary Committee of 1806 expressed themselves in similar terms.

The Domestic System

This small property increased the means of the working manufacturer. He could hardly cultivate; when he tried ploughing he ran the risk of losing all he made on the sale of his cloth. But he could raise poultry, a few head of cattle, the horse which took his goods to the market or on which he rode to neighbouring villages in search of spinners. Although agriculture was not his main occupation, part of his living was derived from the land, this being a further element of his independence. To this method of production the term *domestic system* has been applied (Mantoux, 1928).

ENGLAND IN TRANSITION

The period round about 1750 and 1760 which looms so large in accounts of the industrial revolution marks a turning-point in social history. Developments in religion, literature, science, industry and politics were all acting and reacting on one another and preparing the way for the modern world.

Fall in the Death-rate

In the course of the eighteenth century the population of England and Wales rose from five and a half to nine millions. This increase represented a rather larger birth-rate and a reduced death-rate. It was due to more abundant food, more regular employment, a decline in gin drinking and improvements in public hygiene such as abolition of the window tax (1851). The founding of lying-in hospitals, foundling hospitals, orphanages, general hospitals and dispensaries also were factors. Improved midwifery and advances in preventive and curative medicine played their part.

More Food and Regular Employment

The great advance in agriculture during the eighteenth century gave more abundant food to many, though not to all. The advance in locomotion and the changes in industrial method gave more employment and higher wages, and brought more numerous and more varied articles of purchase within the cottager's reach. It is true that the industrial and agricultural revolution had some most unhappy effects on society and on the amenities of life in village and town. It did not always make for content, possibly not on the average for happiness. But it certainly provided more food and clothing and other articles per head of the population, though their distribution was scandalously unequal. And this greater abundance, by lengthening human life, was one cause why the population continued to rise (Trevelyan, 1942).

Decline in Gin Drinking

At the height of the gin-drinking era, between 1740 and 1742, the burials in the London region had been twice as many as the baptisms! The capital had been supplied with inhabitants by the unfailing stream of immigrants from the healthier and more sober countryside.

> Distilling had been encouraged by the Government as a remedy for the over-production of corn, which was then thought to be a danger to the whole agricultural interest. "The distillers are the farmers' great friends," said a pamphleteer in 1736, "what would become of our corn *injured by bad harvests* were it not for the Distillers?" But the over-production of gin (which was very cheap, fiery and poisonous) was found to be threatening the very existence of the race, and there was a succession of Acts to check the consumption of spirits. It is interesting to note that one (in 1736) which amounted practically to prohibition was a complete failure—it led to riot and murder, and could not be enforced. So the attempt was given up and the method adopted which has been followed more or less ever since: to make spirits dearer and to make the conditions of sale decent. A beginning was made on these lines in 1751, and after this spirit drinking declined, crimes of violence diminished and health improved (George, 1953).

The campaign against gin is important not only because it was effective, but because it was one of the first attempts to get a measure of social reform by putting pressure on Parliament. Petitions from doctors, magistrates and industrial towns were backed up by Press propaganda. Fielding wrote a famous pamphlet on the connexion between drink, crime and poverty. Hogarth published his *Gin Lane* engraving, which depicts a scene in the parish of St. Giles. In all this there was nothing whatever of the spirit of temperance reform, a movement as yet unborn. There is no doubt that the change for the better was very great; the decline of spirit drinking had a direct affect on the death-rate and especially on infant mortality.

Evolution of the Police Court

The new humanitarianism also produced the novel, a literary development which, like Methodism, was connected with the increasing influence of the middle class. In her *England in Transition* (1953), Dorothy George describes how:

> By a strange coincidence, this development of the novel was brought into direct as well as indirect relation with social history through Henry Fielding.
> His appointment as a salaried justice of the peace for Westminster in 1749 was in its way as epoch-making as the appearance of *Tom*

Jones in the same year. He was succeeded at Bow Street in 1754 by his half-brother the blind Sir John, who ruled there till his death in 1780. Out of Bow Street developed the police-court, on the lines laid down by the Fieldings. Indeed, the traditions of the modern police-court, as the poor man's court of justice, derive directly from Bow Street and the Fieldings. In their day the court was what it is now, a court of conciliation, a place where the poor could get free advice on points of law. It is worth noting that the practice of collecting funds for hard cases coming to the notice of the magistrates was begun by Henry Fielding. He was the first of a succession of London magistrates who were active social reformers with an expert knowledge of the difficulties of the poor. The old sort of London magistrate had preyed on the poor, the new sort protected the poor.

The Religious Revival under Wesley

The religious revival under Wesley was a spiritual revolution compar-able with the revolution in industry. In its early stages Methodism was highly emotional, intolerant and puritanical in its gospel of unremitting work and in distrust of all amusement. It was a democratic movement, its chief appeal being in the industrial towns, mining villages and seaports, where it was a great civilizing and educating influence. Its influence spread far outside its own congregations and gave rise to the evangelical movement in the Church of England. By 1760 Methodism was easily the most highly co-ordinated body of opinion in the country, the most fervent, the most dynamic. Had it been bent on revolution in Church or State, nothing could have stopped it (Plumb, 1950). By 1784 in a span of twenty-five years, 356 Methodist chapels had been built in places where there were practically no churches. Methodism was an important current in the rising tide of humanitarianism and it played a great part in helping the bewildered masses to bear the hardships of the industrial revolution.

Foundation of Hospitals

The hospitals of the Middle Ages had been intended as places of refuge for the sick poor. The idea behind the hospital movement of the eighteenth century was that hospitals would be centres for acquiring and spreading medical knowledge (fig. 20).

The great improvement in professional skill was supported by the foundation of Hospitals, in which the age of Philanthropy gave sober expression to its feelings, just as the age of Faith had sung its soul in the stones of cloisters and Cathedral aisles. Lying-in hospitals were founded in the principal towns. County hospitals for all sorts of patients were set up. In the capital, between 1720 and 1745, Guy's, Westminster, St. George's, London and Middlesex Hospitals were all founded: the mediæval St. Thomas's had been rebuilt in the reign of Anne, and at Bart's teaching and practice were improving apace. In the course of 125 years after 1700, no less than 154 new hospitals and

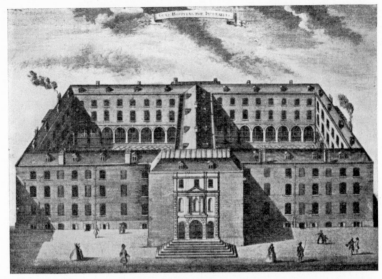

Fig. 20.—Guy's Hospital, London, 1725
(*Engraving by John Bowles*)

dispensaries were established in Britain. These were not municipal undertakings—municipal life was then at its lowest ebb; they were the outcome of individual initiative and of co-ordinated voluntary effort and subscription (Trevelyan, 1942).

But since hygiene and sanitation were in their infancy, hospitals in these early days must not be credited with too direct a share in the saving of life.

Filthy State of Hospitals

Pictures of eighteenth-century hospitals show the patients two in a bed and the workhouses were far worse. Shoreditch parish complained that their workhouse was so crowded that thirty-nine children had to sleep in three beds. Sir William Blizard of the London Hospital wrote his *Suggestions for the Improvement of Hospitals and Other Charitable Institutions* in 1796. In Paris the old Hôtel Dieu was a veritable hotbed of disease. There were some 1,220 beds, most of which contained from four to six patients, and also about 486 beds for single patients. The larger halls contained over 800 patients crowded on pallets or often lying about miserably on heaps of straw, which was in vile condition. Vermin and filth abounded and the ventilation was abominable. The same was true of the Allgemeines Krankenhaus in Vienna (fig. 21) and the Moscow Hospital.

Mortality in Hospitals

In such conditions communicable diseases spread from bed to bed and from patient to patient, and surgical wounds became infected. Gas

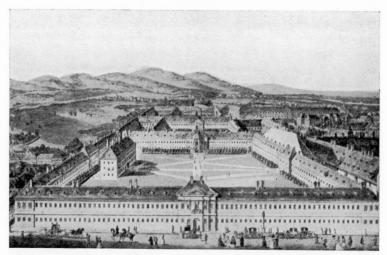

FIG. 21.—Allgemeines Krankenhaus, Vienna, 1793

gangrene (hospital gangrene), typhus (hospital fever) and puerperal fever (child-bed fever) were responsible for many deaths. The average mortality was 20 per cent, and recovery from surgical operations was, in the nature of things, a rarity. But hospitals remained notorious for uncleanliness and general danger to life well into the nineteenth century; indeed, there are persons alive today who recall the horror in which they were held. The real angel of purity and cleanliness was Florence Nightingale, and there was no such thing as surgical cleanliness before the time of Lister.

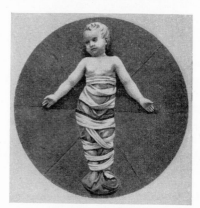

FIG. 22.—Terracotta Medallion of a Swaddled Infant
(*By A. Della Robbia, from the Loggia of the Foundling Hospital, Florence*)

Foundling Hospitals

At the same time the growing benevolence of the age was moved to cope with the appalling infant mortality among the poor and especially among deserted bastard children (fig. 22). At the beginning of the century there was a terrible mortality among infants and young children. A baby born in one of the big towns had about one chance in three of reaching the age of a year, and the odds that it would die before it was five were about the same. Under the insanitary conditions prevailing in the poorer parts of the towns or wherever large numbers of people were herded together, as in the workhouses, the mortality was even more dreadful. The picture of the fate of infants handed over to the tender mercies of parish nurses was grim. In one parish, out of a total of 3,000 no less than 2,960 died before reaching the age when they could be placed as apprentices. Jonas Hanway and Thomas Coram did much to reduce these evils. Coram was a sea captain who, with the warm understanding of a sailor, agitated the project of a Foundling Hospital and at length obtained a charter from George II. In 1745 the hospital was completed

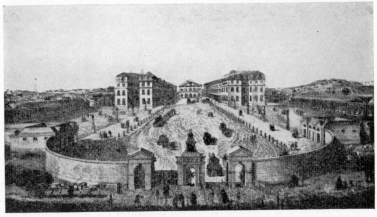

FIG. 23.—The Foundling Hospital, London
(*From an Eighteenth-century Engraving*)

and opened (fig. 23). Many infant lives were saved and many deserted children were brought up and apprenticed to trades.

The Diet and Clothing of Children

Many things were wrong with the feeding and clothing of children. George Armstrong, who founded the first Dispensary for Sick Children in London (1769), speaks of a feeding-bottle in which the teat was made from the finger of a glove of linen or thin leather. Occasionally a small piece of sponge was used as a teat or placed inside the glove finger. Considerable use was made of paps prepared from flour or bread with water or milk. Sometimes rice flour or arrowroot was used. When sweetened or slightly spiced, they were called panadas. Such methods were responsible for many deaths since the linen teat or sponges attached to the primitive feeding-bottles were breeding-grounds for bacteria. In 1762 the London physician, William Cadogan, at a time when babies were heavily swaddled to keep them from chills and to straighten their limbs, insisted that they were not hot-bed plants and that the lighter and looser their clothing the better they would be. He even dared to suggest that deformities were more likely to be caused than cured by binding and swaddling. Turning to the feeding of children and heaping heresy on heresy, he completely rejected the old belief that fruit and vegetables are dangerous for children. As soon as they were able to live on bread and butter and a little meat, he wanted them to have raw, baked or stewed fruit and all the produce of the kitchen garden. Cadogan was a remarkable man and nearly two centuries ahead of his time.

Inoculation against Smallpox

At the beginning of the century smallpox had been the scourge most dreaded as destructive of life or beauty in that its survivors showed permanent disfigurement, the pock-marking of the face with scars. Human inoculation of variolous material or *variolation* dates back to ancient times, certainly to the school of Salerno, and most Oriental peoples knew about it. It was taken up in England by Sir Hans Sloane in 1717. The woman traveller, Lady Mary Wortley Montagu, had her children inoculated, her three-year-old son in Turkey in 1718 and her five-year-old daughter in England in 1721. The remedy was suspected as unnatural and impious; it excited great opposition and even threats of hanging. Nevertheless, an inoculation hospital was set up in London and the method made some headway in reducing the ravages of the disease. But smallpox still carried off a thirteenth of each generation until, at the close of the century, Jenner discovered vaccination.

John Hunter and Edward Jenner

Edward Jenner (1749–1823), a practising doctor with fair hair, blue eyes and a handsome figure, lived the life of a typical English country gentleman (fig. 24). His active mind concerned itself with many things. He was interested in geology and botany and wrote about the hibernation of hedgehogs and distemper in dogs. Above all he was a master of accurate observation, for he recorded in detail the curious nesting habits of the cuckoo and wrote *On the Migration of Birds*, 1823. Born in Berkeley,

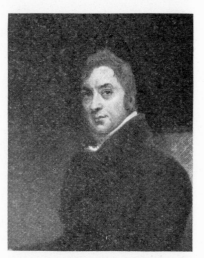

FIG. 24.—Edward Jenner, 1749–1823

Gloucestershire, he became apprenticed to a Bristol surgeon and in 1770 went to London as a pupil of John Hunter. It had long been a popular belief in Gloucestershire that dairymaids who had had cowpox from milking an infected cow could never get smallpox. On learning of this fact from a milkmaid Jenner conceived the idea of applying it on a grand scale in the prevention of the disease. He wrote about it to his friend and benefactor, John Hunter, whose advice was: "Don't think, try; be patient, be accurate."

Vaccination against Smallpox

In 1778, on returning to his home in Berkeley, Jenner began to collect his observations, and on 14th May 1796 performed his first vaccination upon an eight-year-old country boy, James Phipps, using matter from the cowpox vesicles on the hand of the milkmaid Sarah Nelmes. The experiment was put to the test by inoculating Phipps with material from smallpox vesicles on 1st July. No eruption appeared: he was immune. And so immunotherapy became a reality and serotherapy was born. By 1798 Jenner had twenty-three cases which he described in his work, *An Inquiry into the Causes and Effects of the Variolæ Vaccinæ* (fig. 25). The merit of Jenner's work rests on the fact that he set out with the hope of making his thesis a permanent working principle in science and he succeeded. Like Newton, Harvey, Sydenham, Darwin and Lister, he is one of the great men of purely Saxon genius, a happy combination of rare common sense with extreme simplicity of mind and character (Garrison, 1929). His method rapidly came into general use and was highly successful. Thus in Holland and Prussia, where vaccination was made compulsory, the mortality curve of smallpox was shown to approach zero as its limit.

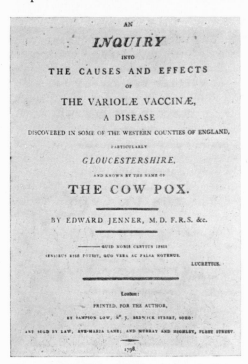

Fig. 25.—Title Page of *An Inquiry into the Causes and Effects of the Variolæ Vaccinæ*, 1798

First Light on Puerperal Fever

The publication of Jenner's work on vaccination coincided with the first major advance in knowledge about the ætiology of puerperal fever. Both occurred in the last decade of the eighteenth century—those fertile years that produced the French Revolution and so many other notable events. It was Alexander Gordon who first threw real light on the ætiology of the disease. As a young man in Aberdeen he was doing most of the obstetric work of that city in the latter years of the eighteenth century. He made two observations which were important—the first, that the disease

was in some way related to erysipelas; the other, that it was being transmitted to women in labour by doctors and midwives. Gordon (1795), in
his report on 28 cases, declared that he himself had been the unwitting
agent in several instances, and he gave the names of several midwives, and
the circumstances in which he believed they had transmitted the disease.
This very forthright document did not make him popular in Aberdeen,
and he found it expedient to leave that city and take service in the Navy,
where there was no obstetric practice. He died of tuberculosis at the early
age of 48. There is little evidence that Gordon's thesis became widely
known or was accepted among obstetricians of his day (Colebrook, 1956).
The further work on the cause of the disease was published by Oliver
Wendell Holmes in 1843 and by Ignaz Semmelweis in 1861. The turning
point in the history of puerperal infection came in 1935 when the discovery
by Gerhard Domagk of the action of red prontosil on streptococci enabled
Leonard Colebrook to show that the use of sulphanilamide can reduce the
case mortality of the disease almost to nothing (Colebrook and Purdie,
1937).

Rapid Expansion of the Lower Middle Classes

The steady growth of the population after 1740 had a tonic effect on
the economy of Great Britain. In his *England in the Eighteenth Century*
(1950), J. H. Plumb says:

> It increased the home market, provided more labour and swelled
> the growing, man-eating towns. Yet perhaps the most important
> effect was the survival of more children of the middle and lower
> middle class parents than ever before. This was the greatest stimulant
> of all. With some education, a little capital, occasionally an influential
> relative, the expanding world offered them endless opportunities of
> advancement. The early industrial capitalists—Watt, Wedgwood,
> Arkwright, Fielden, Peel, Wilkinson, and a score of others—all
> emerged from the lower middle classes. And, of course, there were
> hundreds who failed. But without a rapidly expanding lower middle
> class with sufficient education and technical background the Indus-
> trial Revolution would have been impossible. This and a growing
> labour force, adequate capital, and expanding markets were the pre-
> requisites; they provided the opportunities to which human ingenuity
> and skill readily responded.

Geographical Distribution of the People

In the first half of the eighteenth century the geographical distribution
of the people of England was rapidly altering and was already tending towards the form which it has since maintained. Nevertheless, by the middle
of the century Lancashire was showing but little sign of her particular
industrial future, for

at the coronation of George III, in 1761, representatives of the principal trades of Manchester walked in procession through the streets; tailors marched in the pageant, worsted weavers, woolcombers, shoemakers, dyers, joiners, silk weavers and hatters; but there were no cotton weavers or manufacturers (Hammond and Hammond, 1919).

On the other hand, the West Riding of Yorkshire was already a seat of coarse woollen manufacture, the Midland pottery and hardware industries were becoming important, and the serious development of the North-eastern coalfields had already begun.

THE AGRICULTURAL REVOLUTION

It is important to notice that the potteries and the cotton industry were established on a large scale while England was still depending on canals and roads for transport. In consequence of the agrarian revolution there was a great development of road making and canal making in the eighteenth century. The revolution, which increased rapidly the system of large tenant farming, with landlords applying their capital to improvement, made farming much more productive. It was effected partly by Enclosure Acts, which set up commissioners to enclose the common fields and the common wastes.

A Peculiar Theory of Cultivation

Agricultural progress in the form of discoveries to improve crops and stock came at the very beginning of the eighteenth century. Among the most celebrated of the agricultural reformers was Jethro Tull (1674–1741), a law student who, at the age of twenty-five, took to farming with considerable success. In place of a changeless tradition he substituted methods based on observation and deduction. Unhappily he held to a peculiar theory of cultivation. Believing that plants could obtain nutriment only in the form of tiny particles, which he called atoms, he advocated and practised on his farm near Hungerford a constant pulverization of the soil by deep working; and to facilitate this he invented, or developed, in 1714, a horse-drawn hoe. His *Horse-hoeing Husbandry* was published in 1731.

Retrograde Teachings of Jethro Tull

In many respects his teaching was retrograde. He was an opponent of the use of manures. About 1701 he invented and perfected a machine drill, but his practice of sowing in drills wide apart, though economical of seed, was wasteful of land. And his hostility to rotation, supported as it was by a claim to have grown wheat for thirteen successive years on the same land, set back the movement to progressive farming in many parts of England. Ashton (1948) holds that Tull was a crank, and that his importance in the history of agriculture has been vastly exaggerated. It was not from his farms in Berkshire, but from those of the large-scale proprietors of Norfolk, that the real innovations came.

The Norfolk System of Agriculture

What is known as the Norfolk system was a series of inter-related technical, economic and legal processes, combined on an enclosed farm. Like every other innovation of such magnitude, it was the work of many minds and hands. It included the introduction to sandy soils of marl and clay, the rotation of crops, the growing of turnips, clover and new grasses, the production of grain and cattle rather than of sheep, and cultivation by tenants, under long leases, on large-scale holdings. Some of its features were derived from the example of continental Europe, for Norfolk, with its textile and fishing trades, had close connexions with the Netherlands. But most of them were the product of an indigenous race of energetic landlords and cultivators. Thomas Coke, Lord Lovell (1697–1755), predecessor of the famous Coke of Norfolk, was active in the use of marls, the draining of marshes and the practice of rotation of crops now familiar to everybody as turnips, barley, clover and wheat. Viscount Townshend (1674–1738), by popularizing the turnip as a field crop, became known as Turnip Towns-hend.

Four-course Rotation of Crops

The Norfolk system introduced the four-course rotation of crops, namely turnips, barley, clover and wheat, in place of the three-course rotation, namely winter crop, spring crop, and fallow of the old Midlands system. The cultivation of grasses and turnips meant that areas of what had been permanent pasture could be brought under the plough; and, since cattle could not be maintained through the winter, the supply of natural fertilizer for the cereal and root crops was increased. But the transition to *convertible husbandry* was very slow; the open-field system, with its concentration on grain, rather than livestock, died hard. In no part of Britain, not even in Norfolk itself, were the innovations adopted on a large scale.

The Famous Coke of Norfolk

But the man who turned West Norfolk into the most profitable wheat-growing district of England was Thomas William Coke, first Earl of Leicester of the second creation (1754–1842), who lived at Holkham Hall. Eight years before Coke succeeded to the inheritance, Arthur Young visited the district. In *A Six Weeks' Tour through the Southern Counties of England* (1768) he remarked that:

> All the country from Holkham to Houghton was a wild sheep-walk, before the spirit of improvement seized the inhabitants, and this spirit has wrought amazing effects: for instead of boundless wilds and uncultivated wastes, inhabited by scarcely anything but sheep, the country is all cut into enclosures, cultivated in a most husband-like manner, richly manured, well peopled and yielding a hundred times the produce it did in its former state.

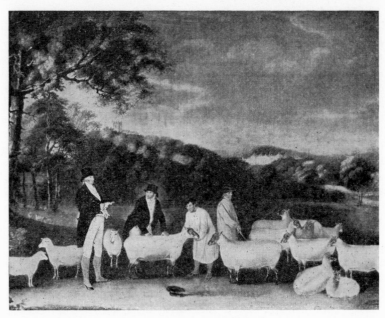

FIG. 26.—Coke of Holkham inspecting his Southdown sheep, with Holkham
Hall in the background

The Holkham Sheep-shearings

However, much still remained to be done, and Coke's attention was
drawn to the matter by the refusal of one of his tenants to renew the lease
of his land at five shillings an acre because he could not make it pay. The
landlord resolved to farm the land himself and he invited farmers from
neighbouring districts to meet on his property once a year to suggest improvements. These annual meetings became known as the Holkham Sheepshearings, and finally attracted agriculturists from all over the country and
even from countries abroad (fig. 26).

A New System of Leases

By expending vast sums of money on the improvement of his estate,
Coke found it possible by 1787 to grow wheat where only rye had been
grown before. His farmers, with the conservatism of their kind, showed
some reluctance to follow his example, and he systematically granted them
long leases by which alone they could feel secure and be encouraged in
careful, persevering efforts. He looked upon himself as an educator and
included clauses in the leases by which the tenant was no longer free to
cultivate the land as he chose, but had to adopt some, at least, of his landlord's ideas.

The Best Kind of Landlord

No detail of farming escaped the personal attention of Coke, and he stands out in English agricultural history as the best kind of landlord, who lives on his land and spares no effort to improve it. His popularity with his tenants, to whom he had brought a new prosperity, was enormous, and the name *Coke of Norfolk* or *Coke of Holkham* was famous all over England. In his own neighbourhood he was known as *King Tom*.

Improvements in Stock-breeding

Coke's contemporary, Robert Bakewell (1725–95), carried out breeding experiments which became the pattern for modern times. He began a systematic improvement of the domestic species, and succeeded, thanks to ingenious crossings. In fact, he initiated the methods of artificial selection, a close study of which was to reveal to Darwin some of the general laws of biology. In 1710 the average weight of oxen sold on Smithfield market was 370 lb., that of calves 50 lb., of sheep 38 lb. By 1795, through the efforts of Bakewell and his followers, the figures had risen respectively to 800 lb., 150 lb. and 80 lb.

Famous Breeds of Livestock

Certain famous breeds of cattle, such as the Dishley and the Durham oxen, date from that period and, better than any document, their build shows what aim the eighteenth-century stock-breeders had in view; the slender bones, short limbs, small head and horns are evidence of the care they took to suppress whatsoever did not conduce to the enormous quantity and superior quality of the flesh which was needed for beef (Mantoux, 1928). Coke experimented widely with livestock. His cattle were first Bakewell's Leicester breed of Longhorns, but these were abandoned for Devons as more satisfactory. He tried the new Leicester breed of sheep, then the Merinos and eventually adopted the Southdowns. He crossed the Suffolk breed of pigs with the Neapolitan, thereby greatly improving the quality of the meat.

SILK-THROWING BY WATER POWER

The introduction of machinery into the textile industries of England began not with cotton but with silk. In the last years of the seventeenth century a colony of Huguenot workmen driven from France by the repeal of the Edict of Nantes settled in Spitalfields and started to weave silk. Since the English climate put the cultivation of the mulberry leaf and the rearing of silkworms out of the question, raw silk had to be imported from Italy and France.

Italian Machines for throwing Silk

It arrived in the form of thrown silk—that is, silk already made into thread by twisting together the filaments from the cocoons. Rumour said

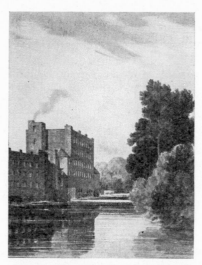

FIG. 27.—Lombe's Silk Mill at Derby, 1809
(From a water-colour by Matilda Lowry, afterwards Mrs. Heming)

that in Italy there were machines for throwing silk, and certainly one Vittorio Zonca had described such machines in a thesis entitled *Nuovo Teatro di Macchine ed Edifici,* and published in Padua in 1621. From drawings smuggled into England from Italy, silk-throwing machines worked by a water-wheel were set up by Thomas Lombe in a mill in Derby in 1718. This was a fully fledged textile factory of particular interest because it was the prototype of the Lancashire cotton mill of the nineteenth century, the large water-wheel being replaced, of course, by tall chimneys (George, 1953).

The Famous Silk Mill in Derby

It was the first factory building in England; its size surprised everyone and it became one of the sights of the country (fig. 27). It was a huge, six-storied, stone-built block 500 feet long and with 468 windows. By the early nineteenth century it had something of the character of an ancient monument. The machines were cylindrical and they rotated on vertical axes. Several rows of bobbins set on the circumference received the threads and by a rapid rotary movement gave them the necessary twist. At the top, the thrown silk was automatically wound on a winder, all ready to be made up into hanks for sale.

Accuracy and Rapidity of Work

Successive generations of visitors described with admiration the complicated machinery, which yet made the process of twisting and winding the silk so simple that it was chiefly done by women and children. The 22,586 wheels which made up the machines, the accuarcy and rapidity of the work and the delicacy of the processes could not but make a vivid impression on people who had never seen anything of the kind before. Centres of production grew up in London, Derby, Stockport, Congleton, Macclesfield and Coventry.

Further Technical Progress Stops

By 1750 the factory system was actually in being, and since no one had yet dreamed that the employment of women and children was other than beneficial to society, no one had complained that few of the factory hands were men. But nowhere was there any industrial change comparable to that produced later on in Lancashire by the invention of cotton-spinning machines. The real reason for the secondary position held by the early silk industry was that technical progress stopped with the setting up of silk-throwing machines.

Failure of the Silk Industry to Survive

In the weaving and in the finishing of the material, the old processes were maintained, together with the system of small-scale production. In spite of protective measures the silk industry could not survive the compe-

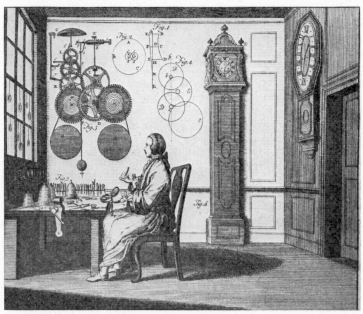

FIG. 28.—A Print entitled *The Art of Makeing Clocks and Watches*
(*Universal Magazine, London 1748*)

tition of France and Italy, whose production was aided by better natural conditions and experience of the trade. The Spitalfields weavers, with their coalitions, strikes and riots, worked at home. Their employers were merchants and contractors rather than manufacturers. The industrial revolution had not yet begun, but by building his silk factory in Derby Sir Thomas Lombe had already pointed the way (Mantoux, 1928).

NAVIGATION AND THE CHRONOMETER

The forerunners of the steam engine and of machine tools as we know them today are to be found in the optical instruments of the seventeenth and eighteenth centuries. The millwrights who made water-wheels and the craftsmen who made clocks and ultimately chronometers formed the advance guard of the industrial revolution (fig. 28). The intellectual ferment of the eighteenth century found the scientific technique of Newton already well developed, but with applications which had yet scarcely gone beyond astronomy. It had, however, become manifest to intelligent scientists that the new mathematics was going to have a profound effect on the other sciences. The first field in which this came to pass was that of navigation and of clock making.

The Problem of Longitude

Navigation is an art which dates from ancient times, but it had one conspicuous weakness until the 1730s. The problem of determining latitude was always an easy one, even in the days of the Greeks. It is simply the problem of determining the angular height of the celestial pole. This may be done roughly by taking the pole star as the actual pole of the heavens, and it may be done with precision by further refinements which locate the centre of the apparent circular path of the pole star. On the other hand, the problem of longitudes is always more difficult and can be solved only by a comparison of local time with some standard time such as that of Greenwich. In order to do this, we must either carry Greenwich time with us on a chronometer or we must find some heavenly body other than the sun to take the place of a chronometer.

Every Voyage an Adventure

Before either of these two methods had become available for the practical navigator, he was considerably hampered in his techniques of navigation. He was accustomed to sail along the coast until he reached the latitude he wanted. Then he would strike out on an east or west course, along a parallel of latitude, until he saw land. Except by an approximate dead-reckoning, he could not tell how far he was along the course. It was therefore a matter of great importance to him that he should not come unawares on a dangerous coast. Having made his landfall, he again sailed along the coast until he came to his destination. It will be seen that in these circumstances every voyage was very much of an adventure. Nevertheless, this was the pattern of voyages for many centuries. It can be recognized in the course taken by Columbus.

Design of an Accurate Ship's Chronometer

This slow and risky procedure was not satisfactory for the admiralties of the eighteenth century. There was great competition between England and France for the supremacy of the seas, and the advantage of better navigation was a serious one. It is not surprising that both governments offered large rewards for an accurate technique of finding longitudes. In the end, these prizes were awarded in both countries for two very different achievements. One was the design of an accurate ship's chronometer—that is, of a clock sufficiently well constructed and compensated to be able to keep time within a few seconds during a voyage in which it was subject to the continual violent motion of the ship. The other was the construction of good mathematical tables of the motion of the moon, which enabled the navigator to use the moon as the clock with which to check the apparent motion of the sun. These two methods have dominated all navigation until the recent development of radio and radar techniques.

The Clock Makers and Optical-instrument Makers

Accordingly, the craftsmen whose work paved the way for the machines of the industrial revolution consisted on the one hand of clock makers, who used the new mathematics of Newton in the design of their pendulums and their balance wheels; and, on the other hand, of optical-instrument makers, with their sextants and their telescopes. The two trades had much in common. They both demanded the construction of accurate circles and accurate straight lines, and the graduation of these in degrees or in inches. Their tools were the lathe and the dividing engine. These machine tools for delicate work were the forerunners of the machine-tool industry of the present day just as the men who used them were the ancestors of our modern fitters, turners and pattern makers.

The Genealogy of the Turret Lathe

It is an interesting reflection that every tool has a genealogy, and that it is descended from the tools by which it has itself been constructed. The clock-makers' lathes of the eighteenth century have led through a clear historical chain of intermediate tools to the turret lathes of the present day. In order to construct a great turret lathe, it is clearly impossible to depend on the unaided human hand for the pouring of the metal, for the placing of the castings on the instruments to machine them and, above all, for the power needed in the task of machining them. These must be done through machines that have themselves been manufactured by other machines, and it is only through many stages of this that one reaches back to the original hand or foot lathes of the eighteenth century. It is natural that those who were to develop new inventions were either clockmakers or scientific-instrument makers themselves, or called on such craftsmen to help them. Watt, for instance, was a scientific-instrument maker (Wiener, 1950).

THE REVOLUTION IN IRON

The manufacture of iron originally depended on charcoal. From the fourteenth to the seventeenth century, Sussex was the important iron-smelting district of England; the great forests which then covered the Wealds of Kent and Sussex and the Forest of Dean were felled to provide charcoal for the furnaces.

Importance of Sussex Charcoal

The guns that battered the Spanish Armada and the railings that still stand round parts of St. Paul's Cathedral were cast from Sussex iron (Jones, 1943). Although various Acts were passed by Elizabeth I limiting the felling of trees, the rapidly diminishing English forests became unable to supply wood in adequate quantities, more especially because of the increased demand for timber for naval use. Coal could not be used in smelting because its chemical action rendered the metal brittle. Coke smelting was first practised by Abraham Darby in 1709 at Colebrookdale near Wolverhampton, and his son improved the process. Eventually the use of charcoal ceased, though it was not until 1920 that the last British charcoal iron furnace at Backbarrow near Windermere was modernized and adapted to the use of coke as fuel.

Abundance of Coal and Iron

The iron-working trades prospered under iron masters such as John Roebuck, Matthew Boulton, the Wilkinsons, Richard Crawshay and Samuel Walker. When coal took the place of charcoal, the iron manufacturer could set up his plant in the neighbourhood of a coal field. So the industrial revolution created the Black Country and enabled England to turn to account the good fortune which had given her an abundance of coal and iron conveniently placed near her ports. Before the middle of the eighteenth century iron was handled in small pieces and hammered and wrought into shape. It was material for a craftsman. Quality and treatment were enormously dependent upon the experience and sagacity of the individual iron worker. In the sixteenth century the largest masses of iron that could be dealt with in these conditions amounted at the most to two or three tons.

Coke Smelting and the Blast Furnace

Because of its metallurgical inferiority the ancient world could never have used steam. Even the most primitive steam engine could not develop before sheet iron was available. The early engines seen through the modern eye are very pitiful and clumsy bits of ironmongery, but they were the utmost that metallurgical science could do (Wells, 1920). The blast furnace arose in the eighteenth century (fig. 29) and developed with the use of coke (fig. 30). Rolled-sheet iron was first made in 1728 and rolled rods and bars in 1763. Benjamin Huntsman discovered a method of making steel in crucibles in 1750 and started using it on a large scale near Sheffield in 1772.

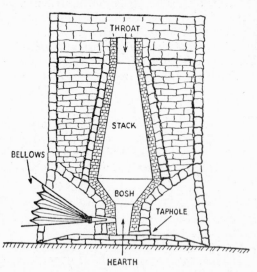

FIG. 29.—Early Eighteenth-century Blast Furnace
(*By courtesy of Mr. D. J. O. Brandt*)

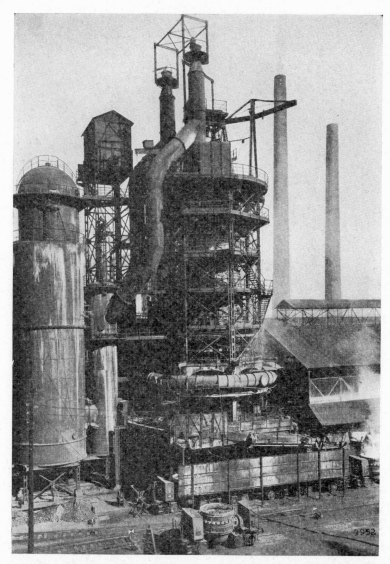

FIG. 30.—Part of Modern Blast Furnace at Ostrava, Czechoslovakia
(By courtesy of Vitkovice Steel Industries)

Wrought Iron and Steel

Henry Cort's invention of a puddling and rolling process was exploited from 1784 onwards. The Bessemer process (1856) and the open-hearth furnace (1864), in which steel and every sort of iron could be melted, purified and cast, led to production upon a scale hitherto unheard of (fig. 31). Nothing in the previous practical advances of mankind is comparable in

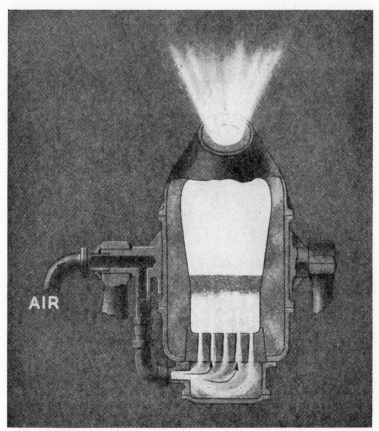

FIG. 31.—Arrangement of Modern Bessemer Converter
(*By courtesy of Mr. D. J. O. Brandt*)

its consequences to the complete mastery over the enormous masses of
steel and iron and over their texture and quality which man has now
achieved. The railways and early engines of all sorts were the mere
first triumphs of the new metallurgical methods. Presently came ships
of iron and steel, vast bridges and a new way of building with steel upon
a gigantic scale. Before the nineteenth century there were no ships in the
world much over 2,000 tons burthen, while in 1938 a 50,000-ton passenger
liner scarcely caused surprise. Today the seas are dotted with oil tankers
the average tonnage of which has doubled between 1957 and 1967. The
world had 237 tankers in construction in 1967; of these 89 exceeded
100,000 tons and 6 supertankers were of 276,000 tons.

BIBLIOGRAPHY

AGRICOLA, G. (1556), *De Re Metallica*, Basel, transl. by H. C. Hoover and
L. H. Hoover, 1912, *The Mining Magazine*, London.

ALEXANDER, W., and STREET, A. (1951), *Metals in the Service of Man*, Penguin Books, London.

ASHTON, T. S. (1948), *The Industrial Revolution, 1760–1830*, Oxford University Press, London.

BETT, H. (1950), *English Legends*, Batsford, London.

BLIZARD, W. (1796), *Suggestions for the Improvement of Hospitals and Other Charitable Institutions*, Dilly, London.

COLEBROOK, L. (1956), *Brit. med. J.*, **1**, 247.

COLEBROOK, L., and PURDIE, A. W. (1937), *Lancet*, **2**, 1237, 1291.

DOMAGK, G. (1935), *Dtsch. med. Wschr.*, **61**, 250.

FELL, A. (1908), *The Early Iron Industry of Furness*, Hume Kitchin, Ulverston.

GARRISON, F. H. (1929), *An Introduction to the History of Medicine*, 4th ed., Saunders, Philadelphia.

GEORGE, D. (1953), *England in Transition*, Penguin Books, London.

GORDON, A. (1795), Reference not traced. Printed later as an appendix to *A Treatise on the Epidemic Puerperal Fever*, Campbell, W. (1822) Edinburgh.

HAMMOND, J. L., and HAMMOND, B. (1919), *The Skilled Labourer*, Longmans, Green; London.

HERBERTSEN, A. J., and HERBERTSEN, F. D. (1911), *Man and His Work*, Adam and Charles Black, London.

HOLMES, O. W. (1843), *New Engl. Quart. J. Med.*, **1**, 503.

JENNER, E. (1798), *An Enquiry into the Causes and Effects of the Variolæ Vaccinæ*, London.

JONES, W. R. (1963), *Minerals in Industry*, 4th ed., Penguin Books, London.

LEGGE, T. M. (1920), *J. Industr. Hyg.*, **1**, 475, 550.

MANTOUX, P. (1928), *The Industrial Revolution in the Eighteenth Century*, Jonathan Cape, London.

PARACELSUS, T. (1567), *Von der Bergsucht*, Dilingen.

PLUMB, J. H. (1950), *England in the Eighteenth Century*, Penguin Books, London.

RAMAZZINI, B. (1713), *De Morbis Artificum Diatriba*, Geneva, translated by W. C. Wright, 1940, Univ. of Chicago Press, Chicago.

RATZEL, F. (1898), *The History of Mankind*, translated from the second German Edition, Macmillan, London.

ROBINSON, H. (1961), *Latin America*, Macdonald & Evans, London.

ROSEN, G. (1943), *The History of Miners' Diseases*, Schuman's, New York.

ROSNER, E. (1955), *Forschungen und Fortschritte*, **29**, 362.

SEMMELWEIS, I. P. (1861), *Die Aetiologie, der Begriff und die Prophylaxis des Kindbettfiebers*, Budapest and Vienna.

SIGERIST, H. E. (1936), *Bull. New York Acad. Med.*, **12**, 603.

SUDHOFF, K. (1936), *Paracelsus*, Bibliogr. Institut, Leipzig.

TREVELYAN, G. M. (1942), *English Social History*, Longmans, Green; New York.

WELLS, H. G. (1920), *The Outline of History*, Cassell, London.

WIENER, N. (1950), *The Human Use of Human Beings*, Eyre and Spottiswoode, London.

ZONCA, V. (1621), *Nuovo Teatro di Macchine ed Edifici*, Padua.

CHAPTER II

THE INDUSTRIAL REVOLUTION, 1760–1830

THE complex series of events which changed the face of England between the years 1760 and 1830 has been aptly compared to a revolution. The term *die industrielle Revolution* was used as early as 1845 by Friedrich Engels in his *Die Lage der arbeitenden Klasse in England*, but the credit for originating the comparison is generally ascribed to Arnold Toynbee, whose book, unfinished when he died, was published in 1884 under the title *Lectures on the Industrial Revolution in England*.

The Term accepted in Common Speech

Whether the name is appropriate has been much debated. Clearly the changes which took place were not merely industrial but also social and intellectual, and equally they did not occur with the suddenness of a revolution. But the great inventions which distinguished these years played so decisive a part in creating the new kind of society that the term industrial revolution is not too violent a description of the changes they produced. It is now an established phrase like the Renaissance, or the Middle Ages, with a well-understood meaning (Hammond, 1929).

Ownership of the Means of Production

Although the characteristic external indication of industrial change in the eighteenth century was the introduction of machinery into the process of production, the industrial revolution in fact had deeper roots in two factors, namely, the development of the exchange of commodities or commerce, and the resulting division of labour. These involved the application of capital to production in increasing quantities. The merchant whose function had previously been purely that of middleman found that in an expanding market he could make bigger and quicker profits if he owned the means of production.

Division of Labour

In the woollen and iron goods trades this development took place at any time during the century without outwardly in any way affecting the traditional domestic system of production. The individual spinner or weaver became a contractor using his master's tools and producing yarn or cloth at a piece-work rate. This system had existed, though exceptionally, in the sixteenth century, under one Jack of Newbury, whose organizing genius made its success possible. The increased demand of the eighteenth century made the new form of organization necessary, though it by no means excluded the traditional independent domestic worker from the market.

Large-scale Application of Capital

The important point is that the divorce of the worker from the ownership of the means of production, which is synonymous with the large-scale application of capital, existed before the technical revolution, and the introduction of machinery completed the process of industrial change. However, in the cotton industry, although the simplest forms of machinery such as Kay's flying shuttle and Hargreaves' spinning jenny could be, and were, employed by the individual worker, the more complicated machines and processes invented later could only be exploited in factories by the capital of the new merchant-manufacturer class. It is to be emphasized that these three phases of production—the domestic system, manufacture and the factory system—existed concurrently even in the rapidly developing cotton trade up to and beyond the end of the eighteenth century.

Expansion of the Domestic Woollen Industry

Machinery, however, though it consummated the industrial revolution and accelerated the divorce of workers and means of production, was not its starting-point. In 1750 in the West Riding a man owning four or five looms was an exception and the large majority of weavers combined their trade with agriculture on a small scale. In that year the town of Halifax had 5,000 inhabitants, though the parish numbered 50,000. Yet the market of Leeds, where the weavers overflowed from the Cloth Halls into the streets, provides proof of widespread activity in the woollen trade. The continually increasing demand combined with commercial expansion and diminishing prices assured the development of machine industry on a large scale.

Advance in the New Cotton Industry

This development, however, was retarded in the established industries because of prejudice in the trade and in government and the traditional regulations governing both labour and exports. Hence the initial advance came in cotton, a new and unfettered product. Cotton had become fashionable with the growth of Indian trade which followed the amalgamation of the two rival East India Companies in 1708. So much so that the woollen trade asked Parliament to limit the import of Indian cottons, and prohibitions were enacted between 1715 and 1720. This gave the necessary stimulus to the production of cotton cloth in England.

Kay's Flying Shuttle

The first successful invention was the flying shuttle patented by John Kay in 1733, while working in his father's wool business in Colchester. By pulling a cord, the weaver could send the shuttle carrying the weft to and fro through the gap known as the *shed* in the warp. Besides speeding up the work, this enabled a weaver, working alone, to weave broad cloth that had previously required two men at the loom. As with all inventions during the period, it aroused the powerful opposition of the workers involved and the inventor derived no profit from it. Nevertheless, by 1760 its use had become general and the different processes of the industry became unbalanced, since weaving became proportionately faster and easier than spinning and there was a constant shortage of thread. The spinning machine patented in 1738 by Wyatt and Paul was a failure, chiefly because of lack of capital, and the problem became increasingly acute until the invention by Hargreaves in 1770 of a simple manual-powered spinning machine which worked several spindles at once.

Hargreaves' Spinning Jenny

James Hargreaves was a Blackburn weaver and his device was probably called *jenny* after his wife. His first machine was a small one, but even this could twist eight threads at once. For a time he kept his invention a secret, but other spinners noticed that his family produced great quantities of yarn, and they broke into the house and smashed the machines. Hargreaves then moved to Nottingham, where there was a cotton-stocking industry. There he set up a small spinning factory, and made machines which would spin sixteen, twenty, and then thirty threads, and in due course a hundred and twenty threads; but the jenny was a small and compact machine, which, like the spinning-wheel which it replaced, was normally used in cottages.

The Heyday of the Domestic Cotton Industry

The spinning jenny was simple and inexpensive, and its introduction did not substantially affect either the domestic or the manufacturing systems. Its extensive use brought about a rapid rise in the production of thread with a corresponding fall in price. The import figures for raw cotton show how great was this expansion before the introduction of machinery on a factory scale—in 1751, 3,000,000 lb.; in 1771, 4,760,000 lb.; and in 1781, 5,300,000 lb. This was the heyday of domestic industry; the demand for weaving became so great that loomshops were established wherever a roof was available (Hunter, 1948). However, in 1770, the year of Hargreaves' patent, a Lancashire barber, Richard Arkwright, also secured a patent for a spinning machine.

Arkwright's Spinning Machine

Arkwright's spinning frame was bigger and heavier than the jenny and was too big to be worked by hand in a cottage room. It was able to produce thread strong enough for use as warp, which Hargreaves' machine had been unable to do. Because the new machine was worked by water power it became known as the *water-frame*. Arkwright was an organizer of genius, and it was his exploitation of the greatly increased division and concentration of labour made possible by machinery which brought about the vast and rapid growth of the factory system. His first factory employed 300 hands; the grant of further patents for carding, combing, water-frame and roving-frame machines enabled him to expand rapidly, so that by 1785 he had more than half a dozen establishments in Nottinghamshire, Derbyshire and Lancashire. In that year he lost his patent rights in a legal action, and the greatest factory expansion followed as other capitalists copied his method. But on the whole Arkwright was the most successful of the early inventors. He became a millionaire and a baronet, and ranks in history as the founder of the modern factory system.

Crompton's Spinning Mule

Although it was now possible to make textiles entirely of cotton without a warp of linen or of wool, English cotton goods remained coarser than those imported from the East until another invention was made. This was a machine designed in 1775 after years of hard work and poverty by Samuel Crompton, a cotton spinner of Bolton. It was a superior device driven by water power which spun finer and stronger thread than either Hargreaves' spinning jenny or Arkwright's water-frame. As it was a cross between these two machines it was called a *mule*. The machine enabled even fine muslins to be made in England, so that there was no longer any need to import them from the East. But Crompton was most unfortunate. Jealous spinners broke into his house and tried to wreck his machine, and manufacturers stole his invention so that he died penniless. But with his mule, spinning moved from cottage to factory and from village to town. Although this change was completed early in the nineteenth century an improved version of Crompton's invention, the self-acting mule, is still the basis of the premier industry of Lancashire today (Derry and Jarman, 1956).

Cartwright's Power Loom

In 1784 imports of raw cotton amounted to 11,480,000 lb. (well over double the 1781 figure), but by 1789 this was nearly trebled at 32,580,000 lb. A further improvement was effected on the introduction of Crompton's mule, but this machine again upset the balance of processes, which was not restored until the power loom invented by Edmund Cartwright, a clergyman, came into use after 1800. The inventor had set up a factory in 1787, which failed largely because of the hostility of the weavers who feared a reduction of their high wages. Even after 1800 its use in the industry was only gradually extended; in 1839 the handloom weavers were still numerous enough to attract a Parliamentary investigation. Nevertheless, the factory system was well established, though still dependent on water power and therefore concentrated at the base of the Pennines in East Lancashire and Derbyshire. Mechanically the cotton trade had reached its full development apart from the expansion made possible by steam power. Watt's inventions in turn were made practicable only because of the complete transformation of the iron and steel industry brought about in 1709 by the use of coke in place of charcoal for smelting.

Advent of Steam Power

Thus by the time of Watt's partnership with Boulton in 1778 the iron and steel trade was in a position to carry out his specifications with the necessary accuracy. Watt's engines rapidly replaced the inefficient Newcomen pumps, and in 1781 he patented his rotary-motion engine. This development, together with the initial introduction of machinery on a large scale, are the decisive events in the Industrial Revolution. Steam power was initially used in metal-working mills, but spread to spinning mills and other factories in 1785. The mill owners, who had previously depended entirely on water power, were now able to set up factories wherever coal was easily obtainable. This achievement solved their chief remaining problem—the scarcity of labour. The position of a factory was now governed no longer by the availability of water power. The coal supply was guaranteed, throughout the Midlands at any rate, by the tremendous improvement in communications and especially of canals which had occurred since 1750 (Hunter, 1948).

THE CANALS

Although geographically well adapted to a complete system of navigable waterways, England remained far behind other countries in building canals. This neglect is explained by the existence of so many seaports on navigable estuaries and by the fact that no inland town is really far from the sea. Until 1759 England had no single canal—150 years after the construction of the first canal in France and eighty years after the building of the canal which connects the Mediterranean with the Atlantic (Mantoux, 1928).

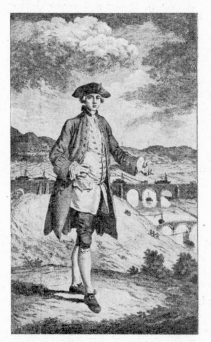

FIG. 32.—Francis Egerton, Third Duke of Bridgewater, and his Canal
(*From a print of 1767*)

The Bridgewater Canal

A small stretch of canal between Worsley and Manchester has been called the cradle of England's modern industrial strength. At the time it was built, many large landed proprietors were striving to develop the trade of the areas from which they derived their personal incomes. Foremost among these was Francis Egerton, third Duke of Bridgewater, who laid out a fortune on the development of his coal pits and canals (fig. 32). According to Malet (1961) it was in

1759 that the Duke, tired of London society and disappointed in love, took up a project that his father had formed to construct a canal from his coal pits at Worsley to the growing town of Manchester, a few miles away. What made the *Canal Duke* mortgage his estates for more than £300,000 and then live and swear like a navvy nobody knows; maybe it was his rejection by the beautiful Elizabeth Gunning; maybe it was a moment of truth when he saw the splendid aqueducts of the Montesana Canal near Milan; maybe he was hypomanic and stumbled on his project by accident: whatever was the motive, the result for his country as well as his family was profoundly enriching.

The Work of James Brindley

The engineer who constructed this canal was James Brindley (1716–72), a most remarkable man who later designed and nearly completed the Grand Trunk. He was an unlettered millwright who retained to the last a rough demeanour and worked all his life without written calculations or drawings. He overcame many difficult obstacles and by the summer of 1761, his task being complete, it was possible to deliver coal in Manchester at half the cost at which it had previously been brought by road. The canal was later extended to Liverpool, a town to which in 1760 there was no carriage road. The Bridgewater Canal is still in use, and now incorporates one of the most remarkable examples of canal engineering in Great Britain—the great swing aqueduct at Barton by which it is carried over the Manchester Ship Canal.

Josiah Wedgwood and the Grand Trunk

The success of the Bridgewater Canal stimulated manufacturers and speculators throughout the country, and the next thirty years saw a tremendous boom in canal construction. First of the great canals of this era was the Trent and Mersey, then known as the Grand Trunk, which was built by Brindley at the instigation of Josiah Wedgwood to supply the potteries (fig. 33). The clay and flint for this industry had formerly to be brought

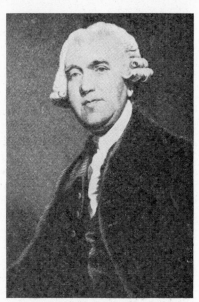

FIG. 33.—Josiah Wedgwood, 1730–1795

from the south by sea, either to Chester or up the Severn, and carried thence by packhorse to the factories, the finished products being similarly distributed. The Grand Trunk connected the Trent at Wilden Ferry with the

Mersey near Runcorn Gap, following a course between those two points best suited to the factories it was to serve, and it completely revolutionized the industry, not only on account of its convenience but also because the smoothness of water transport was ideally suited for the carriage of frangible goods and brought about a substantial reduction in breakages (fig. 34).

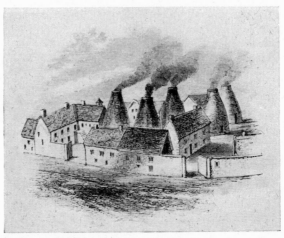

FIG. 34.—The Brick House or Bell Works, Burslem, where Josiah Wedgwood made Useful as distinct from Ornamental Ware from 1766 to 1773

A Complete Web of Rivers and Canals

The subsequent efforts of canal builders can be traced without difficulty on the map, since their natural desire, trade having for so long followed the course of rivers, was to link rivers together by building canals over the intervening watersheds and so provide a through route from one side of the country to the other. From the Grand Trunk was built the Staffordshire and Worcestershire Canal, which linked both the Trent and Mersey with the Severn at Stourport; and the Oxford and Coventry canals, which joined the same rivers with the Thames at Oxford. So the web grew. The next threads were woven across the Pennines by the Leeds and Liverpool Canal, which linked the Mersey with the Aire and Calder Navigations of Yorkshire, and the Huddersfield Canal, linking Manchester with the Calder on a more southerly line. Lastly, after the turn of the century, the southern links were added by two canals built to connect the Bristol Avon with the Thames—the Kennet and Avon at Reading and the Wilts and Berks at Abingdon; and a third, the Thames and Severn, to provide a direct link between these two great rivers.

The Grand Junction Canal

The final link in this great chain of inland waterways was joined in 1805, when the Grand Junction Canal was built to link the Thames near

London with the Grand Trunk, thus providing a through route up the heart of England. North, south, east and west, the great waterways were now complete, and in between them smaller canals were added by degrees until there was hardly an industry in England which could not send its products to any part of the country by waterway. Curiously enough, the heart of this great network of waterways is not, as in the case of road and rail transport, London, but Birmingham, a fact principally responsible for the initial prosperity of that town.

The Navvies invade the Countryside

The cutting of all these canals was carried out by a mobile army of unskilled labour known as *inland navigators* or *navvies*. They worked in gangs that moved from place to place alternately making roads and digging canals. In the next generation their work was to construct embankments and tunnels for railways.

> In the North, the Irish were found in their ranks in great numbers; but in the South they consisted almost entirely of the surplus labour of English villages, which in those parts had fewer outlets to factories and mines. Some highly paid engineers were officers in the army of navvies, and were specially numerous and highly rewarded when it came to railway construction and the piercing of tunnels. But as a whole the "navvies" were among the least skilled, the most ignorant and the least well paid of the new industrial classes. They were the nomads of the new world, and their muscular strength laid its foundations (Trevelyan, 1942).

The navvies invaded the countryside in such numbers that English village life, which had remained undisturbed for centuries, was completely disrupted. The wages offered also attracted so many agricultural labourers to the camps that a Bill had to be introduced in 1793 to prohibit work on the construction of canals during harvest time, lest there should be insufficient men available to gather the crops.

John Smeaton and the Civil Engineers

The problems encountered in constructing the canals also brought into being a new professional class—the civil engineers. Before the canals were built, the modern science of road making was almost unknown, the railways were still undreamt of and there was in consequence no necessity for such a class. Outstanding names in canal engineering were those of Telford, Brindley, Smeaton, the Rennies, Jessop, Mylne, Whitworth and Cubitt, men who, working in the days before the Ordnance Survey, when the land was almost unknown, worked carefully over the ground, took correct levels, and knew enough geology to avoid the worst disasters. John Smeaton (1724–92), who attended Leeds Grammar School as a boy and became F.R.S. before he was thirty, had studied the canals and bridges of the Netherlands. He founded the first society for the profession, and from this the Institution of Civil Engineers was developed in 1818, with Telford as president.

The Lack of Accurate Surveys

More than one projected canal had to be abandoned and the share-holders' money lost for want of an accurate survey of the proposed route. Many difficulties faced these men in making navigable waterways, seventy or a hundred miles in length, up hill and down dale, across almost unknown country. Tunnels had to be built, bridges to carry roads over the canals, and aqueducts to carry the canals themselves over rivers and valleys. To name only one example the aqueduct which was built by Telford to carry the Ellesmere Canal, now the Shropshire Union, over the valley of the Dee is over a thousand feet long. To overcome sudden rises in level ingenious alternatives to locks were invented, such as the inclined plane and the canal lift.

The Decline of the Canals

Although the early history of the canals was fortunate enough, their subsequent record is a gloomy one of gradual decline and fall. The trade was there, the transport facilities were adequate, if not exceptional, and the possibilities of economical transport must have appeared immense, but with rare exceptions their proprietors made insufficient effort to overcome the competition of the railways. Those canals constructed between 1760 and 1790 were almost uniformly successful. They were built cheaply and through areas which were ready for industrial development, and they there-fore immediately attracted a large trade. The Duke of Bridgewater's canal, for example, cost £220,000 to construct, but by 1792 was bringing in a revenue of £80,000 per annum from freight.

The Great Slump of 1825

By 1820, most of the present canal system, and many navigations now derelict, had been built. But the great slump of 1825 was really the end of the canal era. Railway competition soon became serious. A few canal com-panies started to improve their services, and nearly all made drastic cuts in their charges, thus further reducing their revenues, but modernization, which would have been the only answer, was made impossible by the fact that the capital necessary was now flowing to their competitors. Many canal companies sold themselves to the railways almost immediately, seventeen companies being thus swallowed up in the year 1846 alone, and some founded railways on their own account (Eyre and Hadfield, 1945).

The Canal Boat Worker of 1960

In view of this decline of the canals it is not surprising that in 1960 the worker in other forms of transport outnumbers the canal boat worker by more than 1,000 to 1. Thus the 1951 census for England and Wales showed 1,331,334 persons employed in transport including 680,862 on road trans-port, 262,676 on railway transport, 177,831 on water transport, and 5,915 on air transport. Of the water transport workers 67,940 were dock labourers, 9,387 were wharfingers and stevedores and 12,332 were classed as barge-men, boatmen and tugmen. In this last group probably only 1,120 work on the canals and other inland waterways. The flat-bottomed freight-boats on our canals and lesser rivers are smaller and much narrower than the lighters of the Thames and Mersey (p. 1117). The men and women who form their crews work either for British Transport Waterways or for independent carrier companies. They refer to their craft as canal boats or narrow boats but not as barges. They are insular in their outlook and resent change and interference just as they resent being called bargees. In many of the areas where they can tie up their narrow boats in a lay-by the local authority provides the service of a full-time nurse and also of baths, toilets and laundries. The families can consult the local general practitioners and hospitals and the mothers can avail themselves of the maternity and child welfare services. Owing to the nomadic life they lead the attendance of their children at school is liable to be intermittent and therefore unsatisfactory.

THE ROADS

An important effect of the agricultural revolution was that roads came to be greatly improved. They were in a very bad state, especially in clay country, and it was necessary to construct new ones and reconstruct old ones in order to enable corn and other agricultural products to be taken to the towns. In 1745 military necessity compelled the Government to assist in this process, for it proved impossible to concentrate an army to oppose the advance of Charles Edward Stuart, the Young Pretender, from Scotland (Hunter, 1948).

Making the Traffic conform to the Road

In the first half of the eighteenth century, Acts had been passed to regulate such things as the weight of the loads to be carried, the number of horses to a wagon and the breadth of the rim of the wheel. It was really a policy of making the traffic conform to the road. After 1750, however, attempts were made to adapt the roads to the traffic. The number of turnpikes increased rapidly and in the north several engineers did much to increase the carrying capacity of the highway. Among the pioneers was John Metcalf (1717–1810) who constructed many new roads in England, laying bunches of heather as a foundation where the subsoil was soft. He made his roads with convex surfaces and dug ditches to carry off the water, which was the chief enemy of the road maker, as of the miner (Ashton, 1948). He was known as *Blind Jack of Knaresborough*, having been blinded by smallpox at the age of six, but this did not prevent him from doing thirty years of productive work in Yorkshire, Lancashire and Derbyshire.

Thomas Telford and John L. McAdam

The most noted of the civil engineers to give us roads, bridges, canals and docks was Thomas Telford (1757–1834) who began his work as road surveyor in Shropshire. He advocated solid foundations to roads and gave them a moderately cambered surface. He built the Caledonian Canal (1804), the Conway Bridge (1822), the beautiful Menai Bridge (1825) and St. Katherine's Dock, London (1828). In Scotland alone he constructed

920 miles of road and more than 1,200 bridges. As a result of his work traders and travellers were enabled to move freely between England and Scotland. But Telford's best known work was the London to Holyhead road, along the line of the old Roman Watling Street which he extended from Shrewsbury through the Welsh mountains and across Anglesey (Derry and Jarman, 1956). His contemporary in Scotland, John Loudon McAdam (1756–1836), gave his name to the system of road making which utilizes broken stone pressed so as to form a kind of arch. At a later date tar was added to the stone, and the tar-macadam road is still with us. McAdam was Surveyor-General to the London Turnpikes and his work as the first great transport administrator revolutionized travel.

The Statutory Turnpike Trusts

Wagons superseded pack horses over much of the country; the number of public and private vehicles increased beyond measure and about 1830 England passed into the era of flying coaches and busy wayside inns. From 1763 onwards the governing class threw itself into road development and statutory turnpike trusts were set up all over the country for that purpose (Hammond, 1929). If the changes in the roads were of less moment to industry than those in the waterways, their effects on internal trade were significant: the commercial traveller appeared; the Royal Mail became a more efficient channel of correspondence; and the processes of placing orders and remitting money were made more simple and speedy.

THE STEAM ENGINE

In mediæval mining the water draining into the pit bottom was raised to the surface by an endless chain of pots worked either by a human treadmill, a water-wheel or a windmill. In 1698 to help this problem in the Cornish tin mines Thomas Savery devised a pumping engine which involved the use of steam. Erected in a recess in the pit shaft, this consisted simply of a boiler and a condenser fitted with pipes, one of which ran down the shaft to the sump and the other to the surface. The vacuum created by condensation of the steam sucked the water from the sump; and injection of fresh steam from the boiler forced it up the eduction pipe to ground level. But the waste of energy involved in bringing steam into direct contact with cold water was enormous.

The Newcomen Engine

It was to avoid this that an ironmonger of Dartmouth, Thomas Newcomen (1663–1729), invented, in 1708, an entirely different form of self-acting atmospheric engine. A great beam of timber, pivoted high above the ground on a solid piece of masonry, was given freedom to swing vertically through the arc of a circle. At one end the beam was connected to a piston which moved up and down, as steam was first injected, and then condensed, in the cylinder. These movements were transmitted to the beam, and so to the pump rods attached to the opposite end of it, by movement of which the water was drawn up a pipe in the mine shaft. Many modifications and additions were made by Newcomen and his successors. First employed at collieries in the Midlands, the contrivance was soon adopted elsewhere, and by 1765 there were about a hundred engines at work in the northern coalfield.

The Defect of the Atmospheric Engine

Until the sixties of the eighteenth century, Newcomen's engine remained a contrivance for the useful but limited purpose of pumping water. It is true that the water, raised to a height, could be used to drive a wheel and so to work machines of various kinds; but the expenditure of energy involved in the process was great. At the University of Glasgow, in his class on Natural Philosophy, John Anderson was making use of a model of the engine. Working nearby at his shop within the precincts of the University, James Watt (1736-1819), a mathematical-instrument maker, was called upon to repair the model. He saw that the chief defect of the atmospheric engine arose from the alternate injection and condensation of steam; in order to prevent the steam from condensing before the piston had completed its upward stroke, it was necessary to keep the cylinder warm; but, equally, in order to condense the steam for the return stroke, it was necessary for it to be cold. The sudden changes in the temperature of the cylinder wall meant that a great amount of potential energy ran to waste.

Use of a Separate Condenser

Fortunately at this time the sciences were not so specialized as to be out of contact with the language, thought and practice of ordinary men, and there was much coming and going between the laboratory and the workshop. Watt had had many conversations with the Professor of Chemistry, the famous Joseph Black (1728-99), and with John Anderson, John Robison and other members of the University about these things and had pondered deeply on them for many months. Then in 1765 he hit on the solution of introducing a separate condenser which could be kept permanently cool while the cylinder could be kept permanently hot. Within a few weeks a model was made, but many years were to pass before the technical difficulties of translating this into a full-scale engine were overcome.

Experiments financed by John Roebuck

Watt's experiments were financed by John Roebuck, who held a share in the patent which was taken out in 1769. But the Carron ironworks could not supply the skilled artisans whose help was essential, and most of Watt's own energies had to be given to earning a living by work as a surveyor and civil engineer. In 1774, however, Roebuck, whose affairs had become embarrassed, transferred his share in the patent to Matthew Boulton (1728-1809), and James Watt left Scotland for Birmingham. Here he had the support of a man, already well established in business, endowed with a sanguine temperament and driven by an ambition which extended far beyond that of merely making money.

Partnership with Matthew Boulton

At Boulton's Soho works there were the craftsmen Watt needed to make the valves and other delicate parts of the engine. Not far away was the Coalbrookdale ironworks, with its long experience of producing castings for the atmospheric engine, and near at hand, at Bradley, was the great ironmaster, John Wilkinson (1728–1808), whose patent, of 1774, for boring cannon could be adapted to boring cylinders with an accuracy that had not hitherto been attained. Watt was fortunate in his associates. The researches of Black, who laid down the first principles, the capital and enterprise of Boulton, the ingenuity of Wilkinson, the technical skill of Murdoch, Southern and a host of obscure artificers were all necessary to the making of the steam engine.

The Single-acting Reciprocating Engine

In 1775 Parliament extended Watt's patent for a further quarter of a century to 1800. During the first six years of this period the engine remained a single-acting device for producing a reciprocating stroke. It had an efficiency four times that of the atmospheric engine, and was used extensively for pumping water at reservoirs, brine works, breweries and distilleries, and in the metal mines of Cornwall. In the iron industry the contrivance was used to raise water to turn the great wheels which operated the bellows, forge hammers and rolling mills; and, even at this first stage of development, it had important effects on output.

The Double-acting Rotative Engine

Had Watt done no more than this he would have established a claim to a place in the front rank of British inventors. But he could not rest satisfied with having made improvements, however great, in what was little more than a steam pump. His mind had long been busy with the idea of converting the to-and-fro action into a rotary movement, capable of turning machinery, and this was made possible by a number of devices, including the sun-and-planet, a patent for which was taken out in 1781. In the following year came the double-acting rotative engine, in which the expansive force of steam was applied to both sides of the piston, in 1784 the parallel motion, and in 1788 the beautiful device of the governor, which gave the greater regularity and smoothness of working essential in a prime mover for the more delicate and intricate of industrial processes.

A Technological Revolution Afoot

The introduction of the rotative engine was a momentous event. Coinciding in time as it did with that of Cort's puddling and rolling of iron, and following closely on the inventions of Arkwright and Crompton, it completely transformed the conditions of life for hundreds of thousands of men and women. After 1783, when the first of the new engines was erected to work a hammer for John Wilkinson at Bradley, it became clear that a technological revolution was afoot in Britain. Before their patents expired in 1800, Boulton and Watt had built and put into operation about 500 engines of both types. The new form of power and, no less, the new transmitting mechanisms by which this was made to do work previously done by hand and muscle were the pivot on which industry swung into the modern age (Ashton, 1948).

Richard Trevithick (1771–1833)

After Watt's patent expired, the Cornish engineer Richard Trevithick developed a high-pressure engine, and in 1803 he tested a steam carriage on several journeys through the streets of London. Public highways, however, proved to be unsuited to locomotive traffic, and Trevithick's experiment bore no immediate fruit. The possibility of running wheeled vehicles on *plateways* was put into practice with the opening of the Surrey Iron Railway in 1805. The plateways had many disadvantages and further progress was obstructed by the curious belief that a smooth wheel would not bite on a smooth rail. Nevertheless, wrought-iron rails were introduced in 1810, and by 1812 flanged wheels were in use in conjunction with them.

THE RAILWAYS

Before the beginning of the nineteenth century the quantity of goods that could be carried overland was limited by the strength of a team of bullocks or horses. Only when loads were heavy and there was much to be moved was it necessary to have anything more than a horse, a cart and a rough track. In the sixteenth century, when the mines o. Saxony and Bohemia were the industrial centre of the world, baulks of wood were laid down to facilitate the movement of the wagons carrying the ore.

Wagons with Wooden Wheels

At first such wagons had wooden wheels. Sometimes use was made of self-acting inclines on which loaded wagons running downhill pulled empty wagons up to the top. Otherwise on all the early railroads traction was by horses. In England wagon-ways were used to carry coal to the rivers or ports, and as the mines near the coast or rivers became exhausted these were extended inland. The lengthening of the tracks brought engineering problems which have faced railway builders ever since, for the wagon-ways no less than the main lines today had to have gentle gradients. Early in the eighteenth century, plates of cast iron were fixed to the wooden rails at curves or other points of exceptional friction, and later the rails were made more durable by facing them with strips of iron.

The Surrey Iron Railway

In 1767 Richard Reynolds constructed from Coalbrookdale to the Severn the first plateway in which the rails were of cast iron and were furnished with flanges to hold the wheels to the lines. So far the rails had been used almost exclusively about coal mines, ironstone quarries and iron works. But in 1805 the first railway in London was opened. It was a plateway with wagons drawn by horses, and was called the Surrey Iron Railway. It was built along the river Wandle and carried goods from Croydon to a spacious and busy wharf on the Thames at Wandsworth. Subsequently, plateways were built over large areas because the wagons employed could also run on an ordinary road. But their great disadvantage was that stones and dirt accumulated in the metal angle of the plates and they were gradually abandoned. In 1789 the famous engineer John Smeaton transferred the flange from the rail to the wheel. Wrought-iron rails were introduced about 1810, and rails supported by chairs were designed as early as 1797. By the year 1812 horse-drawn carriages with flanged wheels were running on iron rails supported by chairs.

George Stephenson (1781–1848)

We have seen how Trevithick in 1803 drove through the streets of London a steam carriage powered by a high-pressure engine (p. 72). Shortly after this the colliery engine-wright George Stephenson raised the efficiency of the locomotive by increasing the draught to the fire-box; and when in 1821 a railway was constructed from Stockton to Darlington, Stephenson was engaged as engineer and his locomotive was used for traction. In 1826 he was appointed engineer to the Liverpool and Manchester Railway, being put in charge not only of the building of the railway but of the locomotive power as well. This gave him his chance to bring steam transport to a practical success. At first the directors of the railway did not know whether to use stationary engines, which would pull the trains along by ropes, or locomotive engines.

The Triumph of the *Rocket*

In order to decide, they offered a prize of £500 for a locomotive engine which should be a great improvement upon those in use at the time. The competition was held in 1829 on a level stretch of railway at Rainhill, about nine miles from Liverpool. There was a grandstand, a crowd of at least 10,000 people, and 200 men acted as special constables. The locomotive *Rocket*, built by George and Robert Stephenson, won the prize, reaching a speed of thirty miles an hour amidst great excitement. This was the culminating triumph of the technical revolution; the effects of the locomotive railway on the economic life of Britain were profound. Within five years the first railways of continental Europe began to be opened in Bohemia and Bavaria, always with Stephenson locomotives.

Rapid Growth of the Railways

The period between 1830 and 1850 saw the rapid growth of railways and steamships. Although the first passenger railways used horses, the steam locomotive was to be seen all over the country by 1835. In his *England in the Nineteenth Century*, D. Thomson writes:

> The background noises to all the seething movements of reform were not only the whirring and clatter of the cotton mills, but the clanging of permanent ways and the hissing of the new locomotives. When the Duke of Wellington attended the opening of the new Man-

chester and Liverpool Railway in September 1830, he witnessed an event as important in its own way as the Battle of Waterloo which he had won fifteen years before. It symbolized the conquest of space and of parochialism. "Parliamentary Reform must follow soon after the opening of this road," wrote a Manchester man of the time. "A million of persons will pass over it in the course of this year, and see that hitherto unseen village of Newton; and they must be convinced of the absurdity of its sending two members to Parliament, whilst Manchester sends none." Between 1825 and 1835 fifty-four Railway Acts of all kinds went through Parliament. During the two years 1836–7 thirty-nine more bills for new lines in Great Britain were passed, and these were the boom years of railway construction, which added over 1,000 miles to the railroads of the country. A second big boom came in the years 1844–7, and by 1848 some 5,000 miles of railways were working in the United Kingdom, of which less than 400 were in Ireland. Fierce resistance came from the canal companies and from the turnpike trusts and coaching interests that ran the roads. Here again was a big conflict of interests, but everywhere the railroads won. The demand for coal and iron which this vast construction caused stimulated the development of the heavy industries, encouraged the rise of big contractors, and offered employment to thousands ranging from the gangs of navvies who laid the tracks to the drivers, firemen and other staffs which ran the lines. A great new industry was born in little more than twenty years.

With the capital which flowed into the new companies the railways could afford the best of everything. The standards of comfort and luxury were high for those days. The passengers had first consideration, and the health and welfare of the railway servants were left to the discretion of local officials. The obvious result was that extremes of good and bad management occurred.

Building the Great Main Lines

The engineering methods used to build the railways were relatively simple. Although locomotives were employed to some extent for haulage, the main work was done by men with pick and shovel. Rock was attacked with gunpowder, and stationary pumping engines were often installed for draining tunnels and cuttings. In *Dombey and Son* (1846–8) Charles Dickens described the building of the great cutting from Camden Town to Euston.

Houses were knocked down; streets broken through and stopped; deep pits and trenches dug in the ground; enormous heaps of earth and clay thrown up; buildings that were undermined and shaking, propped by great beams of wood. Here, a chaos of carts, overthrown and jumbled together, lay topsy-turvy at the bottom of a steep unnatural hill; there, confused treasures of iron soaked and rusted in something that had accidentally become a pond. Everywhere were bridges that led nowhere; thoroughfares that were wholly impassible; Babel towers of chimneys, wanting half their height; temporary wooden houses and enclosures, in the most unlikely situations; carcasses of ragged tenements, and fragments of unfinished walls and arches, and piles of scaffolding, and wilderness of bricks, and giant forms of cranes, and tripods straddling above nothing. There were a hundred thousand shapes and substances of incompleteness, wildly mingled out of their places, upside down, burrowing in the earth, aspiring in the air, mouldering in the water, and unintelligible as any dream. Hot springs and fiery eruptions . . . lent their contributions of confusion to the scene. Boiling water hissed and heaved within dilapidated walls; whence also, the glare and roar of flames came issuing forth; and mounds of ashes blocked up rights of way, and wholly changed the law and custom of the neighbourhood.

In short, the yet unfinished and unopened railroad was in progress; and from the very core of all this dire disorder, trailed smoothly away, upon its mighty course of civilisation and improvement.

The great main lines could never have been built at this time save for the mass of labour that was available. The population of the towns had grown faster than the factories which had created them. There was poverty and unemployment all over the country. Employers regarded combinations of workers to secure higher wages as an interference with the laws of God, and all such actions were ruthlessly repressed. So it was that railways were able to make tens of thousands of men work for low wages under conditions unequalled since the Pharaohs built the pyramids of Egypt.

The Great Western Railway

Of the early main lines, the Great Western was the most remarkable. It was built by Isambard Kingdom Brunel (1806–59), one of the greatest engineers of the nineteenth century and designer of the first transatlantic steamer. He was bold, direct, imaginative, a rugged individualist and a genius. Within a fortnight of the passing of its Act in 1835, Brunel persuaded the directors to allow him to make the distance between the rails seven feet instead of the usual four feet eight and a half inches. He considered that the West Country would be the exclusive preserve of the Great Western, and that almost all traffic would be to and from London. North and south traffic would be negligible, so the break of gauge would be unimportant. Alternatively, he argued that all other railways would sooner or later have to be altered to meet his new standard, for he thought the broad gauge would mean faster, more comfortable and safer travel. Brunel laid out the best main line in Britain, with few curves, and almost level except for two gradients at Wootton Bassett and through the Box Tunnel.

Failure of the Broad Gauge

The Great Western was opened throughout its length in 1841. Within three years the difficulties of a break of gauge had become acute. The line from Bristol to Gloucester was broad gauge, from Gloucester on to Birmingham narrow gauge. Passengers and goods had to be transferred at Gloucester, which was in a state of permanent confusion, encouraged as much as possible by the narrow-gauge party, who wished to prove that the broad gauge was a failure. Finally the narrow-gauge party bought up the broad-gauge line from Gloucester to Bristol and thus decisively defeated the broad gauge, which lingered on till 1892.

The Atmospheric Railway

Brunel did not stop at the broad gauge. He adopted a system of power different from anything which had been used before when he laid out the South Devon Railway. This was the atmospheric system, by which trains were hauled by a piston running in a pipe laid between the lines. The air in front of the piston was exhausted by pumping installations built at intervals along the line, and the piston with its train was sucked forward. The atmospheric railway had some of the advantages of an electric railway, with a central source of power, the possibility of a dense service of trains, and no smoke or dust. But it also had fatal disadvantages. The piston inside the pipe had to be attached to the train outside the pipe. To do this, the pipe had a slit from end to end, through which an arm projected from the piston. The slit was sealed in front and behind by a leather flap which opened to allow the arm to pass. This was a failure. The flap could not be kept airtight because the leather perished. Rats attacked it. Water collected in the pipe. The atmospheric railway had to be abandoned, with a loss of hundreds of thousands of pounds. Brunel died in 1859, just after completing one of his greatest railway works, still one of the great monuments of Britain, the Royal Albert Bridge over the Tamar estuary at Saltash, west of Plymouth (Elton, 1947).

Advent of the Driver's Cab

Engines of the first fifty years were built for utility only, with no thought for the health of the driver and fireman. The first ones merely had a platform upon which the crew stood to drive and fire the engine. Speeds were slow and distances short, and there was little demand for protection. A primitive windscreen was added, then tarpaulins were used as a roof in wet weather. It was not until 1859 that the cab appeared. In that year George Stephenson built his first engine with a cab for the Oxford, Worcester and Wolverhampton Railway, and in 1860 his firm built two further locomotives with spacious cabs for the Stockton and Darlington's long extension over the Pennines. The drivers objected to this innovation, which was designed to protect them from the stormy weather of the fells, on the grounds that visibility was obstructed, that they were too comfortable and that this might cause them to fall asleep. This last objection was not so ridiculous as might at first appear, for a spell of twenty hours on duty was not uncommon and, if held up by snow, the crew might be on duty for two or three days, for they were obliged to remain on the engine from the time it left the depot until its return. Following these protests, engines built for the same line in 1862 had no cabs. During the 'sixties, however, cabs came into use on other lines and were appreciated, so that in the 'seventies the use of cabs became general, except on underground and suburban lines (Hughes, 1952).

Signalling Systems

The earliest light signal was a candle burning in the window of a point watchman's house, it having been agreed with the driver that the presence of a light meant that he had to stop. With the advent of the semaphore signal, coloured lights were adopted for night signalling, on most lines a red light for stop and a white light for proceed. Owing to the danger for a white light alongside the railway being mistaken for a signal to proceed, the use of a white light was discontinued and a green light was introduced. In 1855 attention was drawn to the fact that disasters on the railroad might be due to colour-blind drivers being unable to distinguish between the coloured light signals. There was at this time considerable public alarm regarding the frequency of accidents that Queen Victoria herself in appointing a Royal Commission went so far as to suggest that a director of the railway company should travel on every train.

Tests for Defects in Colour Vision

As a result of a railway accident at Lagerlunda, Holmgren in 1876 devised his wool test for the railway employees of Sweden, and thereafter tests for colour blindness became obligatory in the railway services of most countries. Since in the transport industries safety is the first consideration, there exists what is possibly the only point on which all authorities on colour vision agree, namely that men with defective colour vision should not be employed on the traffic staff. Already this means that nearly 10 per cent of male applicants for employment are unacceptable, and with improved methods of testing this proportion may increase. Tests for colour vision should invariably be carried out after an accident when the subsequent inquiry reveals that a member of the staff may have been responsible (Norman, 1949).

CHEMISTRY

In early times chemistry remained an empirical art followed for such practical ends as the carrying out of metallurgical processes (fig. 35). Many facts were understood, but scarcely any chemical theory existed. By the seventeenth century, however, the time was ripe for a great change. After centuries of unquestioning acceptance of so-called facts which had never been confirmed, the western world was in an inquiring frame of mind. In 1610 Francis Bacon, in his *Novum Organum*, stressed the importance of first collecting all available facts, either by observation or by experiment, and then trying to formulate theories to account for them. Bacon had little use for facts as such except when they could be fitted into a common framework; he believed, too, that knowledge should be applied to allow man to master nature.

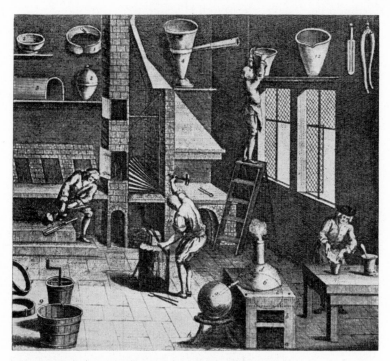

FIG. 35.—Refiners of Gold and Silver at Work
(*Universal Magazine, London, 1747*)

Robert Boyle and the Royal Society

Bacon's teaching did not lose its momentum with his death in 1626, for in the following year was born Robert Boyle, a man well fitted to succeed him. Boyle may truly be called the father of modern chemistry. He disputed the four-element theory which had survived since the time of Aristotle and defined an element in essentially the same way as we do to-day—namely, as a substance which cannot by any means be broken down into simpler ones. He challenged the mysticism and obscure writing of the alchemists, so often a cloak for ignorance, and expressed himself freely and lucidly. He stated bluntly that "he that hath seen it hath more reason to believe it, than he that hath not." His views were clearly set out in *The Sceptical Chymist*. While Boyle was at the height of his powers, there occurred, in 1660, an event of most far-reaching scientific importance. This was the foundation in London of the Royal Society, formed specifically for the study of natural phenomena. This event has a double significance in relation to the advancement of chemistry; on the one hand it denotes the existence of a considerable body of men pledged to advance scientific knowledge, on the other it gave these men a very valuable means of exchanging views (Williams, 1953).

Hermann Boerhaave, the Dutch Hippocrates

This growth of interest in science was not peculiar to Britain; on the continent of Europe, too, the study of chemistry was advancing rapidly (fig. 36). Of course, the teaching of chemistry began in the medical schools.

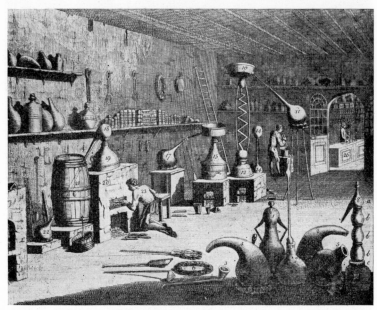

Fig. 36.—A Print entitled *A First View of Practical Chymiftry*, showing the Orderly Arrangement of an Eighteenth-century Laboratory and Apothecary's Shop. The Books bear the Names of Paracelsus, Lemery and Boerhaave. The Zigzag Fractionating Column made of Tin was used to obtain Spirit of Wine from Brandy

(*Universal Magazine, London, 1747*)

Early in the eighteenth century the Leyden School rose to the premier position in Europe under Hermann Boerhaave (1668–1738). Known as the Dutch Hippocrates, he was probably the most erudite and versatile figure of his day. In 1701 he became lector in medicine in the University of Leyden, and by 1709 his reputation was such that he was appointed to the chairs of Medicine and Botany. In 1718 he strengthened his position when he was elected also to the chair of Chemistry. In medicine, Boerhaave became the first great exponent of clinical teaching.

The Chemistry of the Pre-oxygen Era

His text book of chemistry, the *Elementa Chemiæ*, is restrained in tone, clearly written and at the same time the most complete and least biased exposition of chemistry known to the pre-oxygen era. With the immense industry and application which characterized him, Boerhaave collected his data from every conceivable source, and gave for the first time in the history of chemistry an orderly exposition of its theory and a detailed account of its practice. As a man of wide culture he depicted it liberally as a science as well as an art and showed its bearing upon the activities of everyday life.

The modern student of historical chemistry may thus use the *Elementa Chemiæ* as a window enabling him to take a backward look into eighteenth-century chemistry, using the eyes of an informed and reflective observer of that day. In the wider world of 1732, seen only in one aspect through this magic casement, Bentley, Swift, and Congreve, like Boerhaave himself, were approaching old age; Bach, Handel, Pope, Voltaire and Hogarth were in their prime; Benjamin Franklin, Fielding, Linnæus, Chatham, Johnson and Rousseau were young men; David Garrick, Joshua Reynolds and Adam Smith were boys; Goldsmith, James Cook, Black, Cavendish, Haydn and George Washington were infants. It was a world of good literature, good architecture and good music. For chemistry, it was an age of suspense, an age which might well be called the induction period of the chemical revolution (Read, 1947).

Joseph Priestley and the Lunar Society

It is not surprising that the process of combustion, which from time immemorial had provided man with such vital necessities as heat and light and the means of cooking food and smelting metals, excited a lively curiosity. Not until the Industrial Revolution had already begun to change the face of England was any plausible hypothesis put forward to explain this fundamentally important process. Joseph Priestley (1733–1804) was born in a Yorkshire farmhouse and educated for the ministry (fig. 37). He drifted through several changes of faith, and finally ended as a Unitarian minister to a meeting-house in Cheshire. While there, he came in contact with such famous men as James Watt, the inventor of the steam engine, Erasmus Darwin, the grandfather of Charles, and William Withering, the botanist and physician who discovered the value of digitalis. All these people belonged to the Lunar Society, which met in Leamington. He wrote essays on education, a long monograph on electricity and a treatise on government, as well as numerous theological tracts.

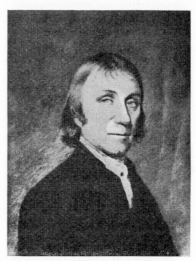

FIG. 37.—Joseph Priestley, 1733–1804

The Isolation of Oxygen, 1774

At one time he lived next to a brewery and became interested in the nature of the gas given off in fermentation. This he found to be carbon dioxide. While experimenting on this he isolated oxygen or *dephlogisticated air*, as he called it. This was on 1st August 1774, when he extracted a gas from calcined mercury. What surprised him more than he could express was that a candle burned in this air with a remarkably vigorous flame. In 1794 he wrote:

> It is this ingredient in the atmospheric air that enables it to support combustion and animal life. By means of it most intense heat may be produced and in the purest of it animals will live nearly five times as long as in an equal quantity of atmospheric air. In respiration part of this air passing the membranes of the lungs unites with the blood and imparts to it its florid colour, while the remainder, uniting with phlogiston exhaled from venous blood, forms mixed air. It is dephlogisticated air combined with water that enables fishes to live in it.

During the French Revolution his radical opinions so enraged his fellow townsmen that they burned his house, destroying his library, scientific apparatus and notes of experiments. Following a series of such persecutions, he sailed to America where, after ten years, he died in a town in Pennsylvania.

Lavoisier and the Reign of Terror

It was a great Frenchman who first realized that combustion is a process of combination with oxygen. Antoine-Laurent Lavoisier (1743–94) was a martyr of the French Revolution. In the Reign of Terror he was condemned to the guillotine. It is true that he held the hated office of Government Collector of Taxes, but when his merits as a scientist were pointed out, the President of the Revolutionary Tribunal sent him to his death with the cynical phrase: "The Republic no longer has any use for men of science." The great chemist met his death calmly and with dignity, and his body was placed in an unmarked grave. "It took but a moment to cut off that head," said Lagrange, "though a hundred years, perhaps, will be required to produce another like it." Two years later the people of France realized what a crime had been committed against the intellectual world, and the nation took part in a solemn funeral ceremony.

Chemical Union, a New Conception

Helped by his wife (figs. 38 and 39), Lavoisier was able through the use of quantitative methods to overthrow the doctrines of phlogiston and to establish the elemental character of oxygen which previously had been isolated by Mayow, Priestley and Scheele. For Priestley and the others oxygen was still only air which had lost phlogiston, and hydrogen, which they called *inflammable air*, was possibly even phlogiston itself. The plausibility of the phlogiston theory had clouded the vision of chemists for a whole century and it was Lavoisier's tremendous achievement to show that air was a mixture containing oxygen which was capable of uniting with hydrogen to form water or with a metal to form a calx. Therewith he introduced the essentially new conception of chemical union between elements to form compounds, new substances, as distinguished from mere mixtures, and thus he laid a firm foundation on which all modern chemistry has been built. The earlier observations of Joseph Black and Stephen Hales, as well as those of Priestley and Cavendish, fitted naturally into Lavoisier's clear and coherent picture, and a new era began.

The Great Facts of Respiration

Much of modern physiology has been built on his work. With a few poignant phrases he outlined the great facts of respiration: absorption of oxygen through the lungs with liberation of carbon dioxide which he called *fixed air*. He also gave conviction to the then unproved suspicion that respiration of living

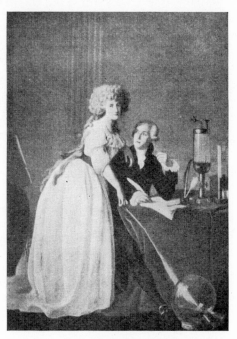

FIG. 38.—Lavoisier and his Wife
(*After David*)
Portrait in the library of the Rockefeller Institute for Medical Research, New York

bodies was analogous to combustion, and that both resulted from union with oxygen in the air. This great Frenchman showed how fully he understood the significance of these facts by commenting on the irony of the circumstance that those who work hardest are usually the least able to afford the food to support their labour. Lavoisier had opened an entirely new era in the study of nutrition, the era of quantitative experiments and therefore the scientific era. He had lived for his fellow men without thought of personal profit. He died when he was only fifty-one because he opposed the revolutionaries in their desire to suppress the French Academy of Sciences and the other learned societies of France (fig. 40).

John Dalton and the Atomic Theory

These excursions into chemical theory were of great practical importance, for they were accompanied by a great increase in the number of sub-

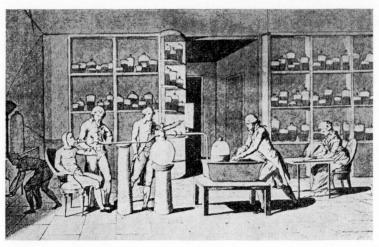

Fig. 39.—Lavoisier works in his Laboratory, assisted by his Wife

stances known to chemists. In Sweden, for example, Scheele investigated hydrofluoric acid, chlorine, manganese, barium, oxalic and citric acids, and many other new substances. Priestley developed special techniques for handling gases; among those he studied were hydrochloric acid, sulphur dioxide, nitric oxide and ammonia. At Glasgow, Joseph Black carried out important research, establishing the relationship between a number of important basic or alkaline substances, including limestone, lime, magnesium carbonate, magnesia and soda. All these great advances in practical and theoretical chemistry paved the way for John Dalton's atomic theory, which for more than a century has profoundly influenced every kind of chemical thought.

The Lead-chamber Process for Sulphuric Acid

In the course of the Industrial Revolution the rapid increase in the number of textile mills brought about a proportionate increase in the quantity of chemicals, such as soaps, mordants, alkalis and acids, needed for processing textiles. In the first half of the eighteenth century the manufacture of sulphuric acid had been firmly established on a considerable scale. There was a sulphuric-acid works in Richmond as early as 1736. The acid was made by dry-distilling iron sulphate; later by heating nitre and sulphur. The lead-chamber process was invented in 1746 by John Roebuck (1718–94). He was born in Sheffield and studied medicine in Edinburgh. As a medical student he was imbued with a taste for chemistry by William Cullen and Joseph Black, and finally graduated M.D. at Leyden in 1742, four years after the death of Boerhaave. Although he started to practise medicine in Birmingham, he soon gave this up because of his greater interest in chemistry and especially its practical applications. The lead-chamber process had no serious competitor until 1875, when rival plants

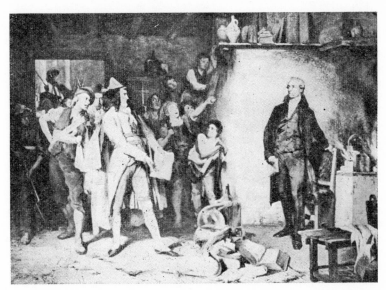

FIG. 40.—Arrest of Lavoisier by Order of the French Revolutionary Tribunal

using the contact process appeared. This process greatly helped forward the new organic chemical industry which followed upon the discovery of the first synthetic dyestuff in Britain in 1856.

The Leblanc Soda Process

As the Industrial Revolution gained in impetus, the supply of natural alkali made from burning certain plants became inadequate to meet the need. It was in France, prevented by war from importing soda freely, that the situation first became acute and that active steps were taken to relieve it. In 1775 the French Government, through the Academy of Sciences, offered a prize of 100,000 francs for the first person to put forward a satisfactory industrial process for converting sodium chloride into the much-needed sodium carbonate. The prize was finally awarded in 1790 to Nicholas Leblanc. His process consisted in treating salt with sulphuric acid, thus obtaining sodium sulphate and, at the same time, clouds of hydrochloric-acid gas. By roasting the sodium sulphate with limestone and coal, a mixture known as *black ash* was obtained; this consisted primarily of soda and calcium sulphide. The soda was extracted from the black ash with water, from which it was subsequently crystallized.

Soap and Bleaching Powder

Soap making had to be expanded rapidly to meet the almost insatiable demands of the new textile factories. It is not known exactly when commercial soap making was first established in Britain, but at least one factory existed as early as 1703. The raw materials used were natural fats and oils, and alkalis of vegetable origin. Even as late as 1834, when the Leblanc process for making sodium carbonate from salt was firmly established, Britain imported no less than 12,000 tons of plant ash from Spain. As to bleaching, although Roebuck had shown that linen could be bleached with sulphurous acid, the method of exposure to the sun in bleach fields was still mainly used. In 1785 Berthollet discovered the powerful bleaching action of chlorine first made by Scheele in 1774. Glasgow took this up and in 1799 Charles Tennant showed that chlorine could be absorbed by lime, yielding bleaching powder (Williams, 1953).

The Dyeing of Fabrics

As a result of the discovery of Mexico and South America by the Spaniards at the end of the fifteenth century, many important dyes indigenous to those countries, especially old fustic, logwood and cochineal, became available in Europe. Old fustic is the wood of *Cladrastis tinctoria*, used as a yellow dye. Logwood comes from the *Hæmatoxylon campechianum*, which has been cultivated extensively in Jamaica since 1715. At first it was used with a chromium mordant to dye silk black, but *logwood black* was largely superseded by a chemical process making use of red iron oxide, gallic acid and tannin. But logwood has again come into use in our time for dyeing nylon. The chemical composition of hæmatoxylin was not established until 1810; not until after the middle of the nineteenth century were the first synthetic dyes produced from coal tar. Kermes was replaced by the richer cochineal, and the employment of weld, young fustic, catechu and turmeric greatly decreased (p. 19). From the seventeenth century onwards, new mordants were discovered and the dye-houses of Europe became important customers of the chemical industry. Considerable use was made of alum (p. 15), tannin, gallic acid, ferrous sulphate and other salts of iron, tin and chromium.

Cochineal replaces Kermes

The dyeing properties of cochineal are ten times stronger than those of kermes (p. 19). The Incas were skilled in the art of dyeing, and the scarlet dye cochineal was known in Mexico long before the Spaniards got there, and was introduced into Spain by Fernandez in 1519. It is the natural colouring matter of the female insect, *Dactylopius coccus*, which feeds on prickly pear, *Opuntia monocantha*, in Mexico and Peru. The insects, one female to 200 males, are brushed from the plants into bags and then immersed in hot water. The dried female insect contains eggs, larvæ and the red pigment carminic acid, or cochinealin. Carmine alum lake is obtained from cochineal by precipitation with alum. In 1630 the Dutch chemist Drebbel discovered how to dye wool a brilliant scarlet colour, using cochineal with a tin salt and tartaric acid. This process was adopted for dyeing at the Gobelin works in Paris and for British army tunics, the first works for this purpose being erected in Bow, London, in 1643. It was not until 1920 that the composition of carminic acid was determined; it is a complicated hydroxy-anthraquinone derivative.

Cochineal for Australia

The demand for cochineal as a dye was the indirect cause of the disastrous spread of prickly pear in Australia. In May 1787 Commodore Arthur Phillip sailed from the Solent with a fleet of eleven small ships crammed with 1,400 people, more than half of them convicts, with warders and marines to keep them in order. It was one of the great voyages of history, made possible by the splendid seamanship of Phillip, who, as Captain-General and Governor, was to become the founder of New South Wales. Putting in at Rio de Janeiro in August 1787 he took on board some prickly-pear plants, together with the cochineal insects, *Dactylopius coccus*, which they harboured. He hoped in this way to establish in his new colony a cochineal industry that would provide the red dye necessary for the military uniforms of those days; but there is no record of the plants or their insect parasites after their arrival at Port Jackson in January 1788.

The Tragedy of the Prickly Pear

The plant introduced on this occasion, *Opuntia monocantha*, was probably harmless; the dangerous species were brought in later from time to time as plant curiosities. By about 1917 prickly pear had formed an almost impenetrable barrier over some twenty million acres in Queensland, and in some areas the weight of pear rose to 800 tons per acre. Settlement retreated before the oncoming wall of prickly vegetation, and holdings and homesteads lying in the line of advance had to be abandoned. In 1925 *Cactoblastis cactorum* was deliberately introduced from Argentina in an attempt at biological control, and by 1928 it had become evident that this insect was able to bring about the complete destruction of *O. inermis* and *O. stricta*. Some three thousand million eggs were released in the infested areas and the effect was phenomenal. By 1933 the prickly-pear territory had been transformed as though by magic from a wilderness to a scene of prosperous endeavour (Read, 1947).

Inorganic Pigments

By the end of the eighteenth century several newly discovered chemical substances such as Scheele's green, copper aceto-arsenite and chrome yellow, lead chromate, had been added to traditional pigments such as white lead, red lead, verdigris and Naples yellow, lead antimonate. Following the example of the Princess Charlotte, about 1800 it became fashionable to use lead chromate as a yellow paint for all kinds of carriages. Another valuable pigment dating from about this time is Prussian blue, ferric ferrocyanide. By mixing this with lead chromate, the brilliant Brunswick green was made. About 1845 zinc oxide came into use as a white pigment and, of course, it has the advantage of not blackening in air containing traces of hydrogen sulphide. This increase in the range and quality of the pigments available was accompanied by an increasing skill in making durable paints.

Humphry Davy inhales Nitrous Oxide

Humphry Davy (1778–1829) was a Cornishman born at Penzance. At the age of twenty he obtained an appointment in Dr. Thomas Beddoes' Pneumatic Institution in Bristol, which had been founded by this former student of Joseph Black for studying the medicinal effects of gases. The year was 1798, and, on his way to Bristol on 4th October, Davy met at Okehampton the public coach decorated with laurels and ribbons which was bearing westwards the news of Nelson's victory in the Battle of the Nile. Having carried out his dramatic experiments on the inhalation of nitrous oxide at the age of twenty, at twenty-two he took London by storm through his brilliant lectures at the Royal Institution; at twenty-four he was elected to the Royal Society; and at twenty-eight he discovered potassium. Davy was a contemporary of the French chemist Gay-Lussac, and of the Swede, Berzelius, who were destined to open a new era—that of organic chemistry.

Opening of the Era of Organic Chemistry

In Gay-Lussac's private laboratory, the young Liebig collaborated with his chief in researches on the salts of fulminic acid and in 1824 the composition of this acid was established. Meanwhile Wöhler was working in Stockholm with Berzelius and almost at the same time determined the composition of cyanic acid. The astonishing conclusion was reached that these two distinct substances have the same ultimate chemical composition: they possess the same elements combined together in the same proportions, and yet they exhibit widely different properties. This revolutionary idea was unpalatable to the somewhat rigid Berzelius, until four years later, in 1828, Wöhler showed that a similar relationship exists between ammonium cyanate and urea, and that the first of these substances can actually be transformed into the second. Convinced at last, Berzelius in 1830 coined the word *isomerism* to denote the new phenomenon. Wöhler's work on urea had an even greater significance, for he had now prepared artificially for the first time one of the most typical products of animal metabolism, thus striking the first blow at the prevailing theory of the operation of an imagined vital force in the production of organic substances. And so the Industrial Revolution saw the birth of organic chemistry.

BIBLIOGRAPHY

Ashton, T. S. (1948), *The Industrial Revolution, 1760–1830*, Oxford University Press, London.

Derry, T. K., and Jarman, T. L. (1956), *The Making of Modern Britain*, John Murray, London.

Elton, A. (1947), *British Railways*, Collins, London.

Eyre, F., and Hadfield, C. (1945), *English Rivers and Canals*, Collins, London.

HAMMOND, J. L. (1929), *Encyl. Brit.*, **12**, 303, 14th ed., London.
HOLMGREN, A. F. (1876), *Upsala Lakaref.* Förh., **12**, 171.
HUGHES, G. O. (1952), *Trans. assoc. indust. med. off.*, **1**, 196.
HUNTER, J. A. (1948), *The Industrial Revolution in the Eighteenth Century*, unpublished essay.
MALET, H. (1961), *The Canal Duke*, Phœnix House, London.
MANTOUX, P. (1928), *The Industrial Revolution in the Eighteenth Century*, Jonathan Cape, London.
NORMAN, L. (1949), *Proc. Ninth Internat. Congr. Industr. Med.*, London, Wright, Bristol, p. 1060.
READ, J. (1947), *Humour and Humanism in Chemistry*, G. Bell and Sons, London.
TREVELYAN, G. M. (1942), *English Social History*, Longmans, Green, New York.
WILLIAMS, T. I. (1953), *The Chemical Industry*, Penguin Books, London.

CHAPTER III

SOCIAL REFORMS IN THE NINETEENTH CENTURY

Evil State of the Towns

The Industrial Revolution found Great Britain without any effective system of local government. The country districts were in the hands of country gentlemen acting as magistrates, and the towns were unorganized for any of the more important purposes of administration. But the sloth and ignorance which had led to overcrowding, filth, cholera and typhus were to give way under a campaign for public health and hygiene. In the twenty-year period prior to 1855 the towns of Great Britain were transformed as a result of schemes for town planning, slum clearance, the scavenging and paving of streets, the building of waterworks and water mains, of sewers and sewage disposal plants, of burial grounds and even of public parks.

Life in the New Towns Hideous and Squalid

Just as coal was the foundation of Britain's industrial wealth so also was it the cause of the smoky pall which lay over most of the large industrial towns, descending as a relentless deposit of dirt on the face of Britain. Remorselessly, in the course of the nineteenth century, the old London of Canaletto, with its clear skies and glistening white stonework, was blotted out. The ships, towers, domes, theatres and temples which Wordsworth had beheld in wonder upon Westminster Bridge were no longer all bright and glittering in the smokeless air half a century later (Wilson, 1954). The plight of towns in the Midlands and the North was even worse. As the textile and metal industries expanded, their uncontrolled growth made the new town life hideous and squalid.

In *Hard Times* (1854) Charles Dickens describes such a town.

> Coketown, to which Messrs. Bounderby and Gradgrind now walked, was a triumph of fact; it had no greater taint of fancy in it than Mrs. Gradgrind herself. Let us strike the key-note, Coketown, before pursuing our tune.
>
> It was a town of red brick, or of brick that would have been red if the smoke and ashes had allowed it; but as matters stood it was a town of unnatural red and black like the painted face of a savage. It was a town of machinery and tall chimneys, out of which interminable serpents of smoke trailed themselves for ever and ever, and never got uncoiled. It had a black canal in it, and a river that ran purple with ill-smelling dye, and vast piles of building full of windows where there

was a rattling and a trembling all day long, and where the piston of the steam engine worked monotonously up and down, like the head of an elephant in a state of melancholy madness. It contained several large streets all very like one another, and many small streets still more like one another, inhabited by people equally like one another, who all went in and out at the same hours, with the same sound upon the same pavements, to do the same work, and to whom every day was the same as yesterday and tomorrow, and every year the counterpart of the last and the next.

Typhus in the Industrial Towns

In the first two decades of the nineteenth century the population of Manchester increased from 94,000 to 160,000, of Bolton from 29,000 to 50,000 and of Lancashire from 672,000 to 1,052,000. But these Lancashire towns were at first just a collection of villages administratively quite unable to handle their new problems. In *The Age of Elegance* (1950), Arthur Bryant writes:

> The houses were put up by jerry-builders as cheaply as possible, with bricks so thin that neighbours could hear one another speaking, with roofs and floors supported by planks, without water pipes or drains. As late as 1842 four out of five houses in Birmingham were without water. In the sinister, sunless city beside the filthy Sheaf, whose forges, set against the black Derbyshire hills, made the world's finest cutlery, Bamford and his wife Mina were driven from their inn by the bugs which swarmed off the dirty walls and bedding. Fever caused more deaths in the industrial towns every year than Wellington's armies suffered in the Peninsular War. Thousands, particularly where the Irish bog-trotters congregated in search of subsistence, lived in fœtid cellars and airless courts. Within a few months of their migration from a moorland village to Manchester, Bamford's entire family was stricken down by typhus.

Overcrowding in the Old Towns

The cholera epidemic of 1832 called public attention to the subject of the towns and led to a series of inquiries which threw a vivid light on the conditions of town life. Though the new districts and the new houses were squalid and unsightly, it is a nice question whether they were any worse than the older districts round which they grew. Certainly the worst overcrowding was to be found in the old quarters of existing towns, especially Manchester, Liverpool, Newcastle and London. The *window tax*, first imposed as a temporary measure in 1696, still served to discourage proper lighting and ventilation. Architects and builders of any houses bigger than small cottages were naturally encouraged to devise structures with as few openings as possible. In most new houses, privies, closets, passages, cellars and roofs were left without ventilation. The tax was finally repealed in 1851.

Disposal of Solid Human Refuse

The disposal of refuse created an increasingly desperate problem. In the country, human excrement was hoarded and prized and farmers were glad to pay for it. In *The Bleak Age* (1934), J. L. and Barbara Hammond describe in some detail the state of affairs in the early nineteenth century.

Contentment, no doubt, sat spinning at her cottage door, with a rich dung-heap beside her, which would either serve to make her potato patch more productive or would bring a few shillings from a neighbouring farmer. So long as there were not too many other cottages with similar heaps close by, and provided that the heap did not drain into the well, no one was much the worse; but when similar heaps were scattered about in the crowded quarters of Birmingham, or Leeds, or Liverpool, the consequences were dangerous as well as disgusting.

As the towns grew, the demand for this manure fell off. The cost of cartage to more distant fields swallowed up all profit, and it became necessary to pay to have middens or cesspools cleared out.

Regular Dumping Grounds in London

London had regular dumping grounds on sites where now stand Belgrave Square, Hyde Park Gardens and University College, Gower Street. The problem of what to do with London refuse became acute as building spread to cover these regular dumping grounds. Meanwhile the spread of water sanitation was changing the nature of the problem. The use of water to flush away refuse led to an increase in the number of cesspools. Filth and corruption were at any rate out of sight, dug in the earth, and though the solid matter had to be cleared out at intervals, the liquid took care of itself by soaking away. London became a honeycomb of cesspools and its spring water acquired a peculiar colour and taste for which coal gas was considered responsible! About 1834 the increasing use of baths made the problem more difficult, for cesspools filled up too rapidly. A disastrous solution presented itself, namely, to connect house drainage with the existing sewers and let everything be washed away together!

The Serpentine becomes a Cesspool

Sewers were first established in 1532 by Henry VIII. They were constructed to carry off water from marshes and low-lying places, and for three centuries they were managed by some hundred different authorities, many of them grossly inefficient. And then, in 1840, as a result of the new system, the Thames was made a great cesspool instead of each person having one of his own (fig. 41). The Serpentine itself, intended by the original designer of Kensington Gardens and Hyde Park as an ornamental water, became an open sewer draining Kilburn, Paddington and Bayswater. Thus it became a scandal upon the greatest metropolis in the world, that the only place in which the public could bathe was an open

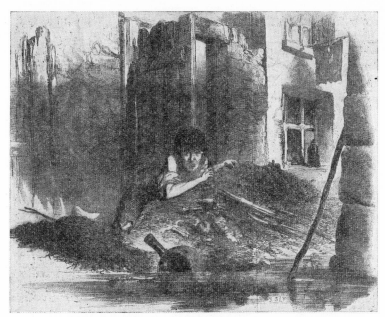

Fig. 41.—Open sewer on Thames-side near Lambeth in 1846

drain to a populous district, the filthy bed of which when disturbed caused the most unwholesome and disgusting effluvia imaginable.

Contamination of Rivers and Canals

Where a river ran through a manufacturing town and was used for water power, the results were particularly disastrous. As the flow was stopped by dams or weirs, a series of huge open cesspools was created. Leeds, Bradford, Halifax, Sheffield, Coventry, Derby, Birmingham, Manchester—all suffered alike. For those who lived near its banks the famous Bridgewater Canal was associated not with the triumph of engineering skill, but with disgusting odours of which the victims complained to the trustees. Even where no dams obstructed the flow, a slow stream produced much the same effect. Thus the sewers of Bolton emptied themselves into the small rivers, which wound sluggishly through the town and yielded to the air in their passage the most offensive smells.

Offensive Sewer Gases invade Houses

Apart from the contamination of rivers and streams, the new use of sewers for house drainage produced volumes of sewer gas which escaped through the gratings of the street drains. Proposals to provide shafts for ventilation in place of the street gullies were disregarded. The escape of sewer gas into the streets was offensive to rich and poor alike, but in other respects the poor were less exposed to the nuisance than the well-to-do, whose houses were connected with the sewers under the new system. When he had big fires lighted and the doors and windows shut to warm his house for a party, the rich man whose drains were imperfectly trapped was treated to a greater concentration of the offensive odour in proportion to the greater draught created.

Campaign for Public Hygiene, 1838

The campaign for public health and hygiene began in 1838, and the man who took the first step was the great lawyer-sanitarian Sir Edwin Chadwick (1800–90). By showing how the census and bills of mortality could be used to diagnose public ailments, he initiated the sanitary era of public hygiene. His inquiries included building, town planning, sewers, water supplies, burial grounds, open spaces, lodging-houses and slums. As secretary of the Poor Law Commission set up by Lord Grey's Government in 1834 he became better known to history than any of the men to whom he gave his disobedient service. Edwin Chadwick had expected to be a Commissioner, and his natural intolerance of the opinions of others was encouraged by his conviction that a subordinate office hardly gave his talents room to turn round.

Investigation of Complicated Abuses

The most successful work he did in the next ten years was not in administration, where his want of sympathy and his quarrelsome temperament made him a dangerous guide, but in the investigation and analysis of complicated abuses in which he excelled. Looking at the power and courage with which he brought abuses to light, Chadwick may be regarded as the chief benefactor of his age, but on the other hand, if one dwells on the fate of any plan of reform that fell into his hands one can regard him as the evil genius of his time. This ruthless and unpopular man used for his purpose an unpopular institution. In 1838 the Poor Law Commission published a report calling attention to the vast burden thrown on the rates by sickness and epidemics, the result of the absence of good sanitation. The report contained striking evidence of the evil state of housing in the East End of London, and Chadwick had a question asked in the House of Lords requesting permission to make a similar return for the whole of England. The request was granted.

Edwin Chadwick's Celebrated Report

Chadwick set to work and within four years the Poor Law Commission published his justly celebrated *Report on the Sanitary Conditions of the Labouring Population of Great Britain* (1842):

> Such is the absence of civic economy in some of our towns that their condition in respect to cleanliness is almost as bad as that of an encamped horde, or an undisciplined soldiery. Whilst the houses, streets, courts, lanes and streams are polluted and rendered pestilential, the civic officers have generally contented themselves with the most barbarous expedients, or sit still amidst the pollution, with the resigna-

tion of Turkish fatalists, under the supposed destiny of the prevalent ignorance, sloth and filth.

The whole family of the labouring man in the manufacturing towns rise early, before daylight in winter-time, to go to their work; they toil hard, and they return to their houses late at night. It is a serious inconvenience, as well as discomfort to them to have to fetch water at a distance out of doors from the pump or the river on every occasion that it may be wanted, whether it may be in cold, in rain, or in snow. The minor comforts of cleanliness are, of course, foregone, to avoid the immediate and greater discomforts of having to fetch the water. It is only when the infant enters upon breathing existence, and when the man has ceased to breathe—at the moment of birth and at the hour of death—that he is really well washed.

Vital Statistics and Epidemiology

The earliest of the modern work on statistics was the famous *Essay on the Principle of Population* (1798) by the English clergyman Thomas Robert Malthus (1766–1834), in which he claimed that food supply and birth-rate increase in arithmetical and geometrical ratios respectively so that poverty is the natural result of increased population. In England vital statistics began with William Farr (1807–83) who in 1839, at the instance of Chadwick, was appointed compiler of abstracts in the new General Register Office in Somerset House, London. In 1866 he first stated that the curve of an epidemic at first ascends rapidly then slopes slowly to a maximum, to fall more rapidly than it mounted (Farr's law). He had already plotted this curve for the smallpox epidemic of 1840, and from it he had predicted correctly the early subsidence of the devastating outbreak of cattle plague in 1865–6. In 1851 the work of Farr led to the publication for the first time of the Registrar General's Occupational Mortality Supplement. Such tabulations of occupational mortality have been issued subsequently at ten-year intervals. For the last hundred years in England and Wales it has therefore been possible to tabulate the deaths of men according to the occupations which are recorded on the death certificates. Bringing these numbers of deaths, by age and certified cause, into relation with the numbers of men following different occupations, as recorded in the decennial census, gives, in terms of mortality, some indication and measure of special occupation hazards. In the Supplement to the Thirty-fifth Annual Report Farr pointed out that the mortality of needle manufacturers at 35 to 45 was excessively high and that earthenware manufacture was one of the unhealthiest trades in England.

Medical Statistics

But Pierre Charles Alexandre Louis (1787–1872), a clinician and a contemporary of Armand Trousseau in Paris, was the first to apply the numerical method in clinical medicine. Thus he was the founder of medical as opposed to vital statistics. He made statistical studies of diphtheria, phthisis, typhoid and yellow fever. He applied his methods to the study of prognosis and treatment. Thus by statistical proof that blood-letting is of little value in pneumonia he did away with its abuse in that disease. Societies grew up to discuss his work but the *méthode numérique* hardly survived him in his own country, although its spiritual children lived on in other lands. Happily, in Great Britain the universities and schools of hygiene and public health made posts for medical statisticians and epidemiologists. Nineteenth-century Britain produced Charles Creighton, Sir Francis Galton and Karl Pearson. But the employment of statisticians in the planning and carrying out of researches in occupational health was delayed until well into the twentieth century. And even today the systematic use of statistical methods has not become part of routine hospital work. Had Louis succeeded in persuading the great French clinical teachers of the early nineteenth century to attempt a systematic statistical evaluation of their hospital records we might have had statisticians on the staffs of our teaching hospitals today.

Outbreaks of Cholera

Regulation of public hygiene was forced upon the attention of legislators by outbreaks of epidemic disease, especially cholera. Endemic in India for centuries it became pandemic in Asia during 1816–30 and reached England in 1831. An Act of Parliament designed to check the grossest abuses of filth was passed in the year 1848, but this statute and its immediate successors were so circumscribed as to interfere as little as possible with the trade and profit of those who produced filth. Neither was there any interference with the vested interests of the private water companies or the sewer companies. The epidemics of 1849 and 1854 were particularly severe in Newcastle and in London; in both towns overcrowding and the inadequacy of sewers and water supplies were responsible for disgusting conditions of life among the labouring people. Cecil Woodham-Smith in her *Florence Nightingale*, gives this description:

> In the summer of 1854 cholera broke out in London, particularly in the miserable, undrained slums round St. Giles, to the west of Drury Lane. The hospitals were overcrowded, many nurses died, many, afraid of infection, ran away. In August Miss Nightingale went as a volunteer to the Middlesex Hospital to superintend the nursing of cholera patients. The authorities at the Middlesex Hospital were obliged to send out their usual patients in order to take in the patients brought in every half hour from the Soho district, Broad Street, etc., chiefly fallen women of the district. . . . The prostitutes came in perpetually—poor creatures staggering off their beat ! It took worse hold of them than of any. Miss Nightingale was up day and night, undressing them. . . . putting on turpentine stupes, etc., herself, to as many as she could manage. The women were filthy and drunken, crazed with terror and pain, and the rate of mortality was very high. All through the night wretched shrieking creatures were being carried in.

The Broad Street Pump

The crucial test of the means of spread of cholera took place in London, and it was John Snow (1813–58) who made the experiment (fig. 42). The issue was made relatively simple by the fact that, shortly before the 1854–5 epidemic the Lambeth Water Company had removed their waterworks to Thames Ditton well above the tidal reaches of the Thames, thus obtaining a supply of water quite free from the sewage of London. On the other hand, the Southwark and Vauxhall Water Company continued to supply unfiltered water from the Thames at London Bridge. In a fantastic personal inquiry into every death taking place in the districts served by both companies, Snow found that the fatalities from cholera during the epidemic were 14 times greater in people drinking the Southwark supply than in those

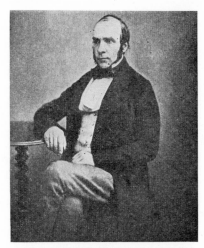

FIG. 42.—John Snow, 1813–1858
(*By courtesy of the Wellcome Historical Medical Museum*)

drinking the Thames Ditton supply. Snow's short treatise *On the Mode of Communication of Cholera, 1855*, includes the figures of his most famous field study, that of the Broad Street pump. The evidence which he built up to incriminate the pump lay principally in the geographical distribution of the deaths around it and in the fact that almost all the dead had used the pump water. Snow's claim to fame does not rest on the removal of the pump handle, for his figures show that the end of the epidemic was not dramatically determined by its removal. The deaths had already been declining from a very marked peak for at least five days. The freedom from epidemic cholera which Great Britain has enjoyed for nearly a century we owe to the untiring zeal, logical thinking and acute observations of John Snow in his statistical approach to the problem he undertook to solve.

Town Life made Healthy

Chadwick inaugurated a new and ambitious effort in which he and his contemporaries succeeded in making town life healthy and tolerable, not merely for the rich but for all classes. However unhappy his plans, he deserves the utmost credit for that bold initiative. He worked with many doctors, one of whom, Thomas Southwood Smith (1788–1861), had, like himself, been private secretary to Jeremy Bentham. Dr. Southwood Smith (fig. 43) took steps to interest the Home Secretary, Lord Normanby, in the cause of sanitary reform. A visit to the slums of Whitechapel and Bethnal Green in the East End of London made Normanby as ardent for reform as Southwood Smith himself. Dr. J. P. Kay, afterwards Sir James P. Kay-Shuttleworth (1804–77), wrote on overcrowding of the cotton workers in Manchester, on the training of pauper children and on public education.

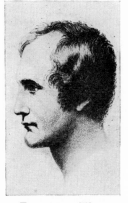

FIG. 43. — Thomas Southwood Smith, 1788–1861
(*After Margaret Gillies*)

Sir John Simon (1816–1904)

The *Towns Improvement Clauses Act* of 1847 not only dealt with improvements in paving, drainage, cleansing, and lighting, but gave power to large towns to appoint whole-time medical officers independent of private practice. *The City Sewers Act* of 1848 gave power to the City of London to appoint a medical officer of health and John Simon took up this office. Born in 1816, he was the sixth of fourteen children, and was more than half French. Qualifying in 1838, Simon decided on a surgical career, and during the next ten years he held posts as a surgeon and as a pathologist. For his pathological work he was elected to the Royal Society at the age of twenty-nine. Supported by a brilliant team of colleagues, he built up a system of public health which was the envy of the world. He was in effect preaching the importance of public health as an administrative entity, and the creation of a Ministry of Health. He came to an arrangement with the Registrar-General whereby he was provided each Monday with the death returns for the City for the previous week. He instituted a system of weekly inspections, with a follow-up of all nuisances. In the few years of his tenure of the office enormous improvements were effected in drainage, water supply, the abatement of nuisances, in scavenging, and in general cleanliness. He says himself that "at a time when cesspools were still almost universal in the Metropolis, and while, in the mansions of the west end, they were regarded as equally sacred with the wine-cellars, they had been abolished, for rich and poor, throughout all the square mile of the City."

Simon's Classic Annual Reports

In dealing with water supply he laid down the postulates that every house, and every floor of a tenement, should be separately supplied; that every privy should have a sufficient supply; that every court should have a standcock; and that the supply should always be uninterrupted. He stated that there were 138 slaughterhouses in the City, and in 58 of these slaughtering occurred in vaults and cellars. He was convinced that both slaughterhouses and other offensive trades should be excluded from the Metropolis. The five annual reports which Simon wrote while he was at the City are classics of public health administration. As examples of vigorous, fearless prose in official reports they can seldom have been equalled. Besides, they show an unusual quality in that they make medical arithmetic readable. On 7th May 1948 the Corporation of London commemorated the centenary of the first Public Health Act and of the appointment of Sir John Simon as first Medical Officer of Health for the City. Thanks were rendered to the enlightened members of the City Corporation in 1848–54, for these were the men who first really accepted Chadwick's principles and who gave Simon the opportunities which he so quickly grasped (Underwood, 1948).

Powers given to Local Authorities

Other reformers were Joseph Hume, who advocated the preservation of open spaces for recreation, R. A. Slaney, who worked to improve the plight of the housewife in the slums of towns, and Joseph Toynbee, who was tireless in his educational and propagandist work for the health of towns. Lord Shaftesbury worked ceaselessly for the Health of Towns Association, and he brought before the House of Lords the hardships and overcrowding caused by the railway schemes. Lord Morpeth gave local authorities powers to construct waterworks and gasworks, and appointed local surveyors and inspectors of nuisances. Charles Dickens was a ringleader upholding the cause of social reform in the world of literature. In 1841 J. T. Delane became editor of *The Times* and from then onwards this newspaper was a powerful and steadfast friend to the cause of public health.

Modern Equipment and Amenities

Struggling gallantly against great difficulties, these few men taught the nation, however slowly, the lesson of the Chartist agitation. The Acts they put on the Statute Book between 1845 and 1854 showed that Parliament had become aware of a problem to which the statesmen of the 'thirties had been blind. In the 'thirties the English town was a raw settlement where men and women lived as men and women lived in the gold-rush. Twenty years later some of these towns were busy constructing waterworks and sewage-disposal plants and paving and scavenging their neglected streets. A few of them were making public parks, and in 1852 Manchester opened the first public library.

The Metropolitan Board of Works

Chadwick continued to advocate a main drainage system for London and he and others put forward various schemes. In 1847 the first Metropolitan Commission of Sewers was appointed, and between 1848 and 1855 a further five commissions followed, but without deciding on a definite scheme. Then in the latter year the Government, spurred by intolerable conditions, appointed the Metropolitan Board of Works charged with the primary duties of maintaining the main sewers and of preventing sewage from entering the Thames within the London area. The Board's engineer, Sir Joseph Bazalgette, was able in due course to carry out his scheme of intercepting sewers to carry the flow to discharge points down-river at Barking on the north bank and at Crossness on the south, involving the construction of 100 miles of large diameter sewers and of four pumping stations. The Northern Outfall works were completed in 1864, the Southern in 1865 and the whole scheme was completed in 1875. The Metropolitan Board of Works continued in existence until the responsibilities were taken over by the newly-formed London County Council in 1889.

THE CHARTIST MOVEMENT

The spread of social distress and economic upheaval, combined with the various conflicts of economic interest, created what was called the condition of England question. To this question various men and various movements gave very varied answers. Besides the philanthropists, such as Robert Owen and Lord Shaftesbury, there were the artisan reformers, Francis Place (1771–1854) and William Lovett (1800–77), and a large number of lesser figures. The social history of this period can be understood largely through the lives and achievements of these men. But behind the reflections of the new social thinkers, the experiments of the philanthropists and the successes of the popular leaders, there was fermenting a new spirit of discontent. Life in the new industrial towns, the discipline of the factories and the strenuous, incessant activity of the mines and mills, in which men were harnessed to machines, all meant great problems of human adjustment.

Machine Breaking in the Hosiery Trade

The setting-up of new machines often led to riots by bands of machine-breakers. In 1811 in the hosiery trade of the Midlands such an organized movement occurred as a protest against the new inhuman competition of human labour. It became known as the Luddite Movement because it was carried out in the name of Ned Ludd, a mythical leader of Sherwood Forest linked up with the name of Robin Hood as the friend of the poor. The movement was skilfully directed by leaders who, working in secret, established an extraordinary hold over the framework-knitters of Nottingham whose standard of life was being beaten down by new methods of production. The trouble centred on the making of a new cheap kind of hose at less than the recognized rates of pay, and the use of a new wide frame which reduced the number of workers employed. The Luddite remedy was to intimidate the offending employers by breaking the obnoxious frames (Cole, 1925).

The Luddite Movement

The Luddites remained active from 1811 to 1816, when in various districts they vented their rage on the particular kind of machinery which seemed to threaten their employment. Their activities were not confined to the stocking frames of Nottingham. In Lancashire the Luddites were hand-loom weavers; they succeeded at the third attempt in burning a steam-loom factory at Westhoughton in 1812. In Yorkshire it was the *croppers* who were Luddites. These were skilled workmen who cropped the nap on the cloth to give it a smooth surface; they objected to the use of the shearing frame which replaced their work. A number of machine-breakers were hanged and others transported to Botany Bay in Australia, but the leaders were never brought to trial and the employers were compelled to raise wages.

Agitation for Reform of Parliament

During the Napoleonic Wars there had been a great deal of distress both among agricultural workers and in the factory districts. To counter the strikes and machine-breaking disturbances there had been persecution and repression, which had really continued from the days of panic which followed the French Revolution. The repression which accompanied the textile strikes of 1818 strengthened the following of the political reformers. Weavers and spinners, convinced that they could do nothing by strikes in face of police prosecution and military force, turned to the agitation for the reform of Parliament. Great reform meetings were held throughout the industrial districts.

The Massacre of Peterloo

One of these meetings, held in St. Peter's Fields, Manchester, in 1819, has become known as the Massacre of Peterloo. The demonstrators, estimated at 60,000 strong, were unarmed and marched in an orderly way to St. Peter's Fields, chiefly to hear the famous radical orator Hunt. No warning was given in advance that the meeting would be regarded as illegal, but after the vast multitude had assembled, the Yeomanry were ordered to force their way through the crowd to arrest Hunt. He made no resistance, but the Yeomanry struck out at the crowd and the order was given to charge. Frightful confusion followed. Eleven persons were killed and some 400, including 100 women, were injured by sabre cuts and by trampling. The demonstrators fled, leaving their dead and wounded behind them. These casualties, which deeply impressed the public mind, were at least inflicted in hot blood. But in the winter of 1830–31 the farm labourers of the Southern counties of England demonstrated against threshing machines which seemed to them to be connected with starvation wages. His Majesty's judges sent three to the gallows and 420 to penal settlements in Australia. The Peterloo massacre raised a fury of protest in the country, and many people who were not Radicals supported the protest. But the Government passed further repressive measures in which even constitutional agitation was forbidden.

The Chartist Movement

The Chartist Movement (1834–48) was a working-class movement seeking higher wages and better conditions, the repeal of the obnoxious Poor Law Act, the passing of a better Factory Act and many other reforms. It was a programme that Cartwright and Cobbett had preached, but formulated with more exactness and elaboration. Its roots were partly political and partly economic, and to some extent it was a consequence of the failure of Owen's experiments in trade unionism. Disillusioned elements of Owen's union joined hands with radical movements among the well-to-do London artisans and with the movements of mass-discontent in Lancashire and Yorkshire. All fused together to produce one of the most dynamic movements of working-class agitation so far known in England. In 1836 William Lovett founded the London Working Men's Association of respectable and self-educated artisans. Two years later he and Francis Place drew up the *People's Charter* as the political programme of their society.

The People's Charter

The six points of the Charter were (i) manhood suffrage, (ii) vote by ballot, (iii) annual Parliaments annually elected, (iv) the abolition of the property qualification for members of Parliament, (v) payment of members and (vi) equal electoral districts, rearranged after each decennial census. These points were the common stock of all radical reformers. Differences within the Chartist Movement arose not over the programme but over the measures to be adopted in order to secure its acceptance.

In his novel, *Sybil, or The Two Nations* (1845), Disraeli gives an excellent description of Chartism.

> "Well, society may be in its infancy," said Egremont, slightly smiling; "but say what you like, our Queen reigns over the greatest nation that ever existed."
>
> "Which nation?" asked the younger stranger, "for she reigns over two."
>
> The stranger paused; Egremont was silent, but looked inquiringly.
>
> "Yes," resumed the younger stranger after a moment's interval. "Two nations; between whom there is no intercourse and no sympathy; who are as ignorant of each other's habits, thoughts, and feelings, as if they were dwellers in different zones, or inhabitants of different planets; who are formed by a different breeding, are fed by a different food, are ordered by different manners, and are not governed by the same laws."
>
> "You speak of——" said Egremont, hesitatingly.
>
> "The Rich and the Poor."

The two delegates of the National Convention stared at each other, as if to express their surprise that a dweller in such an abode should ever have permitted them to enter it; but ere either of them could venture to speak, Lord Valentine made his appearance.

He was a young man, above the middle height, slender, broad-shouldered, small-waisted, of a graceful presence; he was very fair, with dark blue eyes, bright and intelligent, and features of classic precision; a small Greek cap crowned his long light-brown hair, and he was enveloped in a morning robe of Indian shawls.

"Well, gentlemen," said his lordship, as he invited them to be seated, in a clear and cheerful voice, and with an unaffected tone of frankness which put his guests at their ease; "I promised to see you; well, what have you got to say?"

The delegates made their accustomed statement; they wished to pledge no one; all that the people desired was a respectful discussion of their claims; the national petition, signed by nearly a million and a half of the flower of the working classes, was shortly to be presented to the House of Commons, praying the House to take into consideration the five points in which the working classes deemed their best interests involved; to wit, universal suffrage, vote by ballot, annual Parliaments, salaried members, and the abolition of the property qualification.

"And supposing these five points conceded," said Lord Valentine, "what do you mean to do?"

"The people then being at length really represented," replied one of the delegates, "they would decide upon the measures which the interests of the great majority require. The Aristocracy of England have had for three centuries the exercise of power; for the last century and a half that exercise has been uncontrolled; they form at this moment the most prosperous class that the history of the world can furnish; as rich as the Roman senators, with sources of convenience and enjoyment which modern science could alone supply. All this is not denied. Your order stands before Europe the most gorgeous of existing spectacles; though you have of late years dexterously thrown some of the odium of your policy upon that middle class which you despise, and who are despicable only because they imitate you, your tenure of power is not in reality impaired. You govern us still with absolute authority,—and you govern the most miserable people on the face of the globe."

"And is this a fair description of the people of England?" said Lord Valentine. "A flash of rhetoric, I presume, that would place them lower than the Portuguese or the Poles, the serfs of Russia or the Lazzaroni of Naples."

"Infinitely lower," said the delegate, "for they are not only degraded, but conscious of their degradation. They no longer believe in any innate difference between the governing and the governed classes of this country. They are sufficiently enlightened to feel they are victims. Compared with the privileged classes of their own land, they are in a lower state than any other population compared with its privileged classes. All is relative, my lord, and believe me, the relations of the working classes of England to its privileged orders are relations of enmity, and therefore of peril."

"The people must have leaders," said Lord Valentine.

"And they have found them," said the delegate.

Thomas Attwood and Feargus O'Connor

If the moderate demands of Lovett seemed more radical then than now, his movement was soon joined by forces which do not even appear moderate to us. There was, first, the Birmingham Political Union, dating from 1816, which was revived by Thomas Attwood (1783–1856). Attwood was something of a novelty, a very radical banker; though his views on currency made him very unorthodox even as a banker. The Birmingham Union sponsored the People's Charter and called for a National Petition on its behalf. This meant intensive drives of big public meetings, propagandist societies and general popular agitation, and as such was distrusted by many of the Londoners who supported Lovett. The Chartist Movement was joined, too, by a third and still more demagogic movement, led by the hot-headed Irish landowner Feargus O'Connor (1794–1855), whose Leeds paper the *Northern Star* became the official Chartist organ. On this tripod basis—London, Birmingham and Leeds—the Chartists organized big meetings all through the year 1838, some of them involving exciting torchlight processions at night, and most of them enabling the hungry, indignant and often ignorant populace of the distressed northern countries to hear the fiery speeches of J. R. Stephens, James B. O'Brien and Richard Oastler. *The Charter* became the battle-cry of a nation-wide movement, and something of a religion which was expected to bring universal salvation.

The National Petition presented to Parliament

The climax of the Chartist agitation was the National Convention, which was gathered together in Westminster Palace Yard, very near the Houses of Parliament, in the spring of 1839. Its accompaniment was the organization of a monster petition, for which hundreds of thousands of signatures were collected. The Convention was deeply split over what to do if Parliament should reject the petition. Lovett and his southern followers urged a further campaign of peaceful agitation and popular education; O'Connor and his northern supporters urged violent reprisals. A Polish exile published articles on revolutionary tactics, and pamphlets were sold on how best to build barricades. There was a tang of civil war in the air. In May the Convention moved to Birmingham, and in July the petition, with nearly a million and a quarter signatures, was rejected by the Commons. Despite the riots, local strikes and even insurrection which accompanied these events, the firm wisdom of Lord John Russell as Home Secretary and the solid sense of the working-class artisans prevented anything worse.

The Ultimate Fall of Chartism

During the 1840s the National Charter Association kept alive the principles of the movement, and in 1842 a second petition was presented and again rejected. In 1848, the year of revolutions in Europe, a third petition was prepared and the movement fell increasingly into the hands of O'Connor and the extremists. So many of the alleged signatures were forged and the threatened monster procession to Parliament was such a fiasco that the whole movement faded into nothing. Chartism in this second phase after 1839, although more violent in tone, was never so serious and solid a movement as in its earlier phase. The middle classes were diverted from interest in Chartism to support for the Anti-Corn-Law League; the artisans reverted to peaceful agitation; and large sections of the working classes began to turn to trade unionism. Latterly only the cranks, the rabble and portions of the industrial wage earners remained faithful to Chartism, and it came to an end in general apathy and ridicule, killed partly by reviving trade and greater prosperity.

Radicalism moving towards Socialism

The failure of Chartism as a political movement was more apparent than real. Five of the six points were fully incorporated in due course into the working constitution of England by 1918. It drew the attention of all classes to the condition of England question, and that attention was never subsequently lost. John Stuart Mill's *Political Economy*, which appeared in 1848, showed how far radicalism was moving towards socialism. Chartism stirred the social conscience of the Victorian people, and its whole commotion severely shook their hardening complacency. Routed in 1848, it left a deep and permanent mark on English history. It was the first widespread and sustained effort of working-class self-help; it was directed to the cause of parliamentary democracy and constitutional reform; and the impetus it gave to eventual political reform on the one hand and to trade union organization on the other was never wasted. All these three facts about it give it lasting importance (Thomson, 1950).

CHILD LABOUR AND APPRENTICESHIP

We have seen (p. 22) how the gild system of apprenticeship was based on family life. Under the Statute of Artificers which had become law in 1563 in the reign of Elizabeth I, the apprentice lived in his master's house and, in theory at least, was his pupil, his unpaid servant and a member of his family. The apprentice was to obey all his master's lawful commands, all his time and labour were to be at his master's disposal. In return for his work he was to be taught a trade, fed and lodged, and sometimes clothed. The lot of the poor boy was, of course, very different from this. He was apprenticed for labour and not for education and admission to an exclusive trade. In some trades apprentices were taken in great numbers as a source of cheap labour, with the inevitable result that the poorer the boy the more undesirable was the trade which offered as well as the master.

The Fate of the Parish Apprentice

The surprising thing about the apprentice system is not that it often worked badly but that it sometimes worked well. The worst part of the system was that it weighted the scales so heavily against the poor and friendless child. Apprenticeship was the common lot of the poor-law child. Neither was the untaught child from a poor home or the streets a desirable inmate of a respectable household, and only the least eligible masters were available. The lot of the parish apprentice was particularly hard. He was generally bound very young and had to serve for a very long term. The usual object of the parish officers was to find a master, any master, no matter of what trade but to take especial care that he lived in another parish.

Spinning Schools and Workhouses

Although the apprenticeship clauses of the Statute of Artificers of 1563 were repealed in 1814, parish apprenticeship was not affected and lasted until 1844. We have seen (p. 52) how generations of visitors admired the Derby silk mill, where the work was done chiefly by women and children. The idea that the children of the poor should live with their parents had been as remote from the conceptions of the early eighteenth-century philanthropists as from the notions of Elizabethan statesmen. Spinning schools, workhouses and apprenticeship had all been regarded as the alternative to vice, vagrancy, crime or at the best running wild and getting into mischief (George, 1953).

Grave Social Consequences of the New System

As the Industrial Revolution developed, the apprenticeship system went into decay. It was no longer suited to industrial conditions, the seven years' term was too long and it was being modified spontaneously by indentures for shorter terms. Although the Lancashire district had a source close to hand in Ireland the employers had great difficulty in getting labour. The new factory discipline and the prospect of work lasting up to eighteen hours a day repelled both those who had previously been engaged in domestic industry and small workshops and those who had left the land. The social consequences to the subjects of the new system were grave indeed and fell with particular severity on the women and children, who were driven by two circumstances into the new factories. The women were enticed by inflated wages and the children were conscripted by the existing poor-law apprenticeship (fig. 44).

Helpless Children sold into Slavery

Both women and children were helpless to protect themselves against the demands and cupidity of the employers of cheap labour. From the workhouses of London, Manchester and Liverpool contractors collected the orphans and unwanted children of improvident and irresponsible parents and packed them off in wagons and barges to the industrial towns of the north. Often they were sold for £5 apiece to the mill owners, who were so anxious to obtain an unlimited supply of cheap labour that they were not averse to accepting one idiot child with every twelve sane. They went not only to the cotton mills but to any employer, however brutal, and to any employment, however dangerous and degrading (fig. 45).

Graphic Picture in Prose of Gross Cruelty to Children

The picture of what happened was clearly described by Frances Trollope in *The Life and Adventures of Michael Armstrong, the Factory Boy* (1840).

Exactly at the bottom of the hill began a long, closely-packed double row of miserable dwellings, crowded to excess by the population drawn together by the neighbouring factories. There was a squalid, untrimmed look about them all, that spoke fully as much of want of care as of want of cash in the unthrifty tribe who dwelt there. The very vilest rags were hanging before most of the doors, as demonstration that washing of garments was occasionally resorted to within. Crawling infants, half-starved cats, mangy curs, and fowls that looked as if each particular feather had been used as a scavanger's broom, shared the dust and the sunshine between them, while an odour, which seemed compounded of a multitude of villainous smells, all reeking together into one, floated over them.

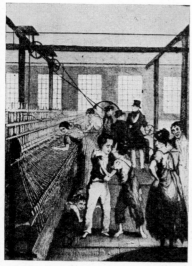

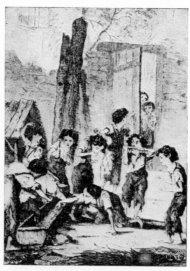

Fig. 44.—Child Labour in the Textile Factories. The Well-dressed Visitors contrast with Ragged Apprentices and Slatternly Workers. Note the Small Child crawling under the Self-acting Spinning Mule.

Fig. 45.—Half-starved Factory Children fed on Water Porridge and Oaten Cake scrambling for Tit-bits at the Pig Trough in the Farmyard adjoining the Factory.

(*Life and Adventures of Michael Armstrong, the Factory Boy, by Frances Trollope, 1840*)

"You are not big enough take care of her, my poor child. Why don't you go to the factory, and let one of the bigger ones stay at home?"

"They won't have me now, 'cause of this."—And as she spake, the child held up a little shrivelled right hand, three fingers of which had a joint deficient. "I can't piece now, and so they won't let me come."

"And Sophy won't let me go, 'cause of this," said the little one, slipping her arm out of a bedgown (which was the only garment she had), and displaying the limb swollen and discoloured, from some violent contusion.

"My poor little creature! how did you do this?" said Mary, tenderly, taking the little hand in hers, and examining the frightful bruise.

"'Twas the billy-roller," said the little girl, in an accent that seemed to insinuate that the young lady was more than commonly dull of apprehension.

"But how did it happen, my child? Did some part of the machinery go over you?"

"No!—That was me," cried the elder, with a loud voice, and again holding up her demolished fingers. "'Twas the stretcher's billy-roller as smashed Becky."

"'Twas 'cause I was sleepy," said the little one, beginning to cry.

"But these bruises could not be the effect of beating," said Mary, again examining the arm, "it is quite impossible."

"Why, ma'am, the billy-roller as they beats 'em with, is a stick big enough to kill with; and many and many is the baby that has been crippled by it."

Picture to yourself a bleak winter's morning, Miss Brotherton, when the mother of factory children must be up hours and hours before the sun to rouse her half-rested little ones; and nervously watching her rude clock till the dreaded moment comes, must shake the little creatures, whose slumber the very beast of the field might teach her to watch over and guard, till they awake, and starting in terror from their short sleep, ask if the hour be come? The wretched mother and the wretched child then vie with each other in their trembling haste to seize the tattered mill-clothes, and to put them on. The mother dreads the fine of one-quarter of the infant's daily wages, which would be levied, should it arrive but a minute too late, and the poor child dreads the strap, which, in addition, is as surely the punishment for delay. Miss Brotherton, I have seen with my own eyes the assembling of some hundreds of factory children before the still un-

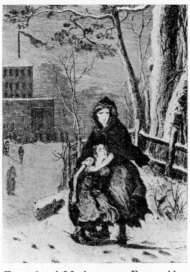

FIG. 46.—A Mother urges Forward her Benumbed and Exhausted Child in order to avoid the Fine for Being Late at the Mill
Life and Adventures of Michael Armstrong, the Factory Boy, by Frances Trollope, 1840)

opened doors of their prison-house, while the lingering darkness of a winter's night had yet to last three hours. The ground was covered deep with snow, and a cutting wind blew whistling through the long line of old Scotch firs which bordered an enclosure beside the road. As I scudded on beneath them, my eye caught the little figures of a multitude of children, made distinctly visible, even by that dim light, by the strong relief in which their dark garments showed themselves against the snow. A few steps farther brought me in full view of the factory gates, and then I perceived considerably above two hundred of these miserable little victims to avarice all huddled together on the ground, and seemingly half buried in the drift that was blown against them. I stood still and gazed upon them—I knew full well what, and how great was the terror which had brought them there too soon, and in my heart of hearts I cursed the boasted manufacturing wealth of England, which running in this direction at least, in a most darkened narrow channel, gives power, *lawless and irresistible*, to overwhelm and crush the land it pretends to fructify. While still spell-bound by this appalling picture, I was startled by the sound of a low moaning from the other side of the road, at a short distance from me, and turning towards it perceived a woman bending over a little girl who appeared sinking to the ground. A few rapid steps brought me close to them, and I found on examination that the child was so benumbed and exhausted as to be totally incapable of pursuing her way—it was her *mother* who was urging her forward, and who even then seemed more intent upon saving a fine, than on the obvious sufferings of her sinking child. I know, poor wretch, that little choice was left her, and that the inevitable consequence of saving her from the factory, and leading her gently home to such shelter as her father's roof could give, would be to watch her perish there for want of food (fig. 46).

No Legal Provision for their Welfare

These children were virtually sold into slavery, for though theoretically a record had to be kept by the parish overseers of their prospective masters and their indentures

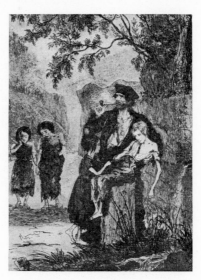

FIG. 47.—A Father faces the Loss of Earnings about to ensue from the Death of his Starving Son

(*Life and Adventures of Michael Armstrong, the Factory Boy, by Frances Trollope, 1840*)

had to be signed by a magistrate, these were no real safeguards, and in reality there was no legal provision made for their welfare. The responsibilities for their housing, feeding and clothing, to say nothing of their schooling, lay but lightly on the shoulders of the mill owners, who were concerned only with extracting the last ounce of labour, and knew that if one child fell out there was always another waiting to take his place (fig. 47).

Public Concern expressed in Poetry

Public concern in this problem was stimulated by Elizabeth Barrett Browning in a charming poem, *The Cry of the Children* (1843):

> "For oh," say the children, "we are weary,
> And we cannot run or leap—
> If we cared for any meadows, it were merely
> To drop down in them and sleep.
> Our knees tremble sorely in the stooping—
> We fall upon our faces, trying to go;
> And, underneath our heavy eyelids drooping,
> The reddest flower would look as pale as snow.
> For, all day, we drag our burden tiring,
> Through the coal-dark, underground—
> Or, all day, we drive the wheels of iron
> In the factories, round and round.
>
> "For, all day, the wheels are droning, turning,—
> Their wind comes in our faces,—
> Till our hearts turn,—our head, with pulses burning,
> And the walls turn in their places—
> Turns the sky in the high window blank and reeling—
> Turns the long light that droppeth down the wall—
> Turn the black flies that crawl along the ceiling—
> All are turning, all the day, and we with all—
> And all day, the iron wheels are droning;
> And sometimes we could pray,
> 'O ye wheels,' (breaking out in a mad moaning)
> 'Stop! be silent for today!' "

Kindness to Children in some Apprentice Houses

Here and there exceptional public-spirited employers effectively considered the interests of the children and conducted their factories with kindness. The achievements of Robert Owen at New Lanark are well known. At the apprentice houses run by Samuel Oldknow, a cotton spinner at Mellor, and by the Gregs at Styal, children were well fed, well housed and taught, and kindly treated. In these early factories, men like these sowed the seeds of the future state education of children and of the regulation of child labour.

Exploitation of Child Labour regarded as an Outrage

What was new and revolutionary was that for the first time the excessive toil of children was regarded as an outrage and not as something to be admired. By 1792 the country was richer and the toil of children no longer seemed the best safeguard against poverty and vagrancy. Public opinion had begun to reflect not only the attitude of the employing classes but also of the workers. And it was the sense of something monstrous in the factory system which directed attention to the yet more monstrous exploitation of the labour of young children (George, 1953).

Typhus Epidemics in Factories

The gaunt barracks where these young workers lived, sometimes in very overcrowded conditions, were frequently visited by epidemics of typhus, known as *factory fever*, and it was one such visitation in 1784 in the mills of Radcliffe near Manchester which paved the way towards public inquiry and eventual legislation. These mills belonged to Sir Robert Peel the elder, then Home Secretary who, declaring himself aghast at the conditions in his own factories, by his subsequent championship of the cause of the factory children has earned the title of *the father of industrial legislation*. This particular epidemic was accorded much publicity by the medical inquiry instituted by the Lancashire justices, who wisely chose Dr. Thomas Percival, a Manchester practitioner, to lead the group of doctors charged with this duty. As educationalist, mathematician and pioneer, he was the friend of Voltaire and Condorcet and the leader of that long line of doctors who fought for the health of the factory worker.

A Report to the Magistrates of Manchester

In their report to the magistrates Percival and his colleagues gave it as their opinion that the infection was "supported, diffused and aggravated by the ready communication of contagion to numbers crowded together; ... and by the injury done to young persons through confinement and too-long-continued labour: to which several evils the cotton mills have given occasion." They advocated shorter hours, prohibition of night-work and opportunities for education and "the active recreations of childhood." These revolutionary suggestions so impressed the justices that they resolved in future not to sign indentures to masters who would work their apprentices more than ten hours a day, or at night. In 1795 Dr. Percival and his associates formed themselves into the Manchester Board of Health to undertake voluntarily the supervision of the mills in the Manchester area, and they drew up a further report recommending that legislation should be passed to regulate the hours and conditions of work in factories.

HEALTH AND MORALS OF APPRENTICES ACT, 1802

It was this report and the gradually awakening interest in the sad plight of the apprentices that finally induced Sir Robert Peel to introduce into Parliament the Bill which eventually, with very little opposition, became law as the *Health and Morals of Apprentices Act, 1802.*

A Local System of Voluntary Factory Inspection

This Act contained regulations for the work of apprentices in cotton and woollen factories, but established no restriction as to their age. It fixed the maximum hours of work at twelve a day, forbade night work and ordered the walls of the factories to be washed twice a year and the rooms to be ventilated. It also established a local system of voluntary factory inspection by which *visitors* had the right to "direct the adoption of such sanitary regulations as they might on advice think proper." But visitors

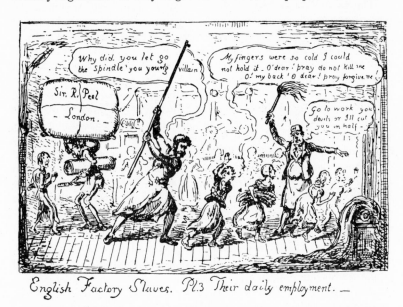

FIG. 48.—Engraving from a Book entitled *The Condition of the West Indian Slave Contrasted with that of the Infant Slave in our English Factories*, by Robert Cruikshank. Published about 1833 by W. Kidd, London

were rarely appointed and still more rarely were they active. Although it soon became a dead letter, it is interesting that this Act not only marks the beginning of a flood of industrial legislation which is still in motion, but its provisions cover nearly all the aspects of factory life which future statutes were to regulate.

Decline in the Demand for Pauper Children

As steam superseded water as a driving-power for machinery, so the demand for pauper children declined. When factories were no longer confined to the hills and valleys, but could be built in any convenient spot and preferably near centres of population, it was found that the supply of free children was equal to that culled from the workhouses. Although in 1802 there were still some 20,000 apprentices employed in mills, the case for the free children was already being taken up with enthusiasm, and by 1816 Parliament was able to pass an Act prohibiting the export of apprentices farther than forty miles from the parish to which they belonged. In the same year the first Parliamentary Committee to investigate child labour was set up, with Sir Robert Peel as Chairman (fig. 48).

Memorandum to the Peel Committee

In a memorandum to the Committee Peel said that the advent of steam had made the 1802 Act a dead letter owing to the substitution of the local poor for parish paupers, and continued:

> I most anxiously press upon the Committee that unless some Parliamentary interference takes place, the benefits of the Apprentice Bill will be entirely lost, the practice of employing parish apprentices will cease, their place will be wholly supplied by other children, between whom and their masters no permanent contract is likely to exist, and for whose good treatment there will not be the slightest security. . . . Gentlemen, if parish apprentices were formerly deemed worthy of the care of Parliament, I trust you will not withhold from the unprotected children of the present day an equal measure of mercy, as they have no masters who are obliged to support them in sickness or during unfavourable periods of trade.

The Peel Committee took evidence from forty-seven witnesses, of whom eight were doctors and twenty-eight were textile manufacturers. But the people who really mattered, the operatives, and more especially the children, were not represented.

The Factory Act, 1819

It is therefore not surprising that in the subsequent *Factory Act, 1819*, few concessions were made. It stipulated nine years as the minimum age for the employment of children and it limited their working hours, but it did not apply to all textile factories. But one important principle it did establish. Parliament, in the teeth of violent opposition, had won the right to extend the law to workers other than bound apprentices, and as the opponents of the Bill so rightly judged, this was indeed the thin end of the wedge. Though the Bill was badly mutilated, the weak and feeble Act which emerged was to become the Magna Carta of childhood; thereafter the protection of the children of the poor, first from toil and then from bodily starvation and ignorance, began.

THE TEN HOURS MOVEMENT

The *Factory Act, 1819*, served to bring the question of the mills before the public eye, and there was an increasing demand for investigation and control of the many abuses which were becoming evident. The first moves came not from the workers themselves, which is not surprising in view of the almost universal illiteracy of the labouring classes, but from public-spirited men who, wishing to establish good conditions in their own factories, found themselves placed at a disadvantage by the cut-throat practices of their competitors. The demand for legislation to restrict the exploitation of child labour was made first by them, and the popular clamour and widespread agitation which characterized subsequent Bills was not really canalized into an effective weapon until the birth of the *Ten Hours Movement*, which sought to reduce the hours of all workers—men, women and children alike. The struggle for the Ten Hours Bill was long and cruel, and lasted from 1830 to 1847. In its later years groups of ragged children went about the towns chanting—

> We will have the Ten Hours Bill;
> Yes we will, yes we will.

Jeremy Bentham and Robert Owen

Robert Owen, himself a cotton manufacturer, was one of the early heroes of this conflict, the first of a long line of humanitarians who fought for the education and health of factory workers (fig. 49). Both Owen and Pitt were converted to free trade by the work of Adam Smith, the professor-economist of Glasgow, who moved the industrial world in 1776 by his great book *Enquiry into the Nature and Causes of the Wealth of Nations*, in which he holds that labour, being the source of national wealth, must have freedom to pursue its own course of interest. Owen was taught his factory principles by his business partner, Jeremy Bentham, the father of English law reform,

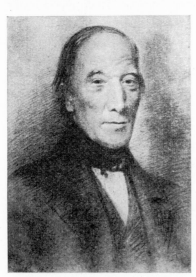

who in 1789 wrote his *Introduction to Principles of Morals and Legislation*. In this book he inspired the whole world with his doctrine of utility, the aim of which was to prevent mischief, pain, evil or unhappiness. He claimed that the object of all legislation must be the greatest happiness of the greatest number.

Model Mills at New Lanark

Owen made experiments in the formation of a human society of a new kind. His work was based on his conviction that environment makes character and that environment is under human control. Being a thoroughly competent business man he made a number of inno-

FIG. 49.—Robert Owen, 1771–1858

vations in the cotton-spinning industry and acquired a fair fortune at an early age. He was distressed by the waste of human possibilities among his workers, and he set himself to improve their condition and the relations of employer and employed. This he sought to do first at his Manchester factory and afterwards at New Lanark. According to the unanimous testimony of all who visited his model mills, the results achieved by Owen were singularly good. But in spite of this universal admiration the world refused to imitate the New Lanark mills (Trevelyan, 1942).

A System of Educational Philanthropy

Connected with his mills were about 2,000 people, 500 of whom were children, most of them brought at the age of five or six from the poor-houses of Edinburgh and Glasgow. Having found when he arrived in New Lanark that crime and vice were common, education and sanitation neglected and housing conditions intolerable, he set himself to ameliorate these evils. He greatly improved the workers' houses, and mainly by his personal influence trained them to habits of order, cleanliness and thrift. In 1813 he published *A New View of Society, or Essays on the Principle of the Formation of the Human Character*, in which he expounded the principles on which his system of educational philanthropy was based.

The Path to a Better Industrialism

Between 1800 and 1828 he achieved very considerable things: he reduced the hours of labour, made his factory sanitary and agreeable, abolished the employment of very young children, improved the training of his workers, provided unemployment pay during a period of trade depression, established a system of schools and made New Lanark a model of a better industrialism, while at the same time sustaining its commercial prosperity. He wrote vigorously to defend the mass of mankind against the charges of intemperance and improvidence which were held to justify the economic iniquities of the time. And he set himself to a propaganda of the views that New Lanark had justified. But, unfortunately, in the earlier years of the nineteenth century State control in the interest of the working classes was not an idea congenial to the rulers of Britain and they turned a deaf ear to Robert Owen.

The Founder of Infant Schools in Britain

He achieved his greatest success in the education of the young, to which he devoted special attention. He was the founder of infant schools in Britain. Children entering his model mills at New Lanark were sent to school in one of the buildings and were fed in a public kitchen in another. Owen pointed out that parents did not hesitate to sacrifice the well-being of their children, by putting them to occupations by which the constitution of their minds and bodies was rendered greatly inferior to what it might and ought to be under a system of common foresight and humanity. The children brought up on his system—which included instruction through the eye as well as the ear, country walks, nature study, singing and dancing—were graceful, genial and unconstrained.

The Owenite Community Experiments

For a time he seemed to have captured the imagination of the world. *The Times* and *Morning Post* supported his proposals for the cure of pauperism. He recommended that communities of about 1,200 people each should be settled on plots of land up to 1,500 acres, all living in one large building in the form of a square, with public kitchen and mess rooms. Each family should have its own private apartments and the entire care of the children until the age of three, after which they should be brought up by the community. New Lanark itself became a much frequented place of pilgrimage for social reformers, statesmen and royal personages, including the Grand Duke Nicholas of Russia who succeeded Alexander I as Tsar, and Owen's steadfast friend the Duke of Kent, son of George III and father of Queen Victoria.

A Counter-attack upon Robert Owen

But all the haters of change, all who were jealous of the poor and all the employers who were likely to be troubled by his projects were waiting for an excuse to counter-attack him, and they found it in the expression of his religious opinions which were hostile to official Christianity, and through those he was successfully discredited. Of four Owenite communities in England, Scotland, Ireland and America, that in Indiana, U.S.A., begun in 1825, was wound up after three years and Owen lost £40,000, which was four-fifths of his fortune.

The First Benevolent Business Organization

His work at New Lanark had been, he felt, only a trial upon a small working model. What could be done for one industrial community could be done, he held, for every industrial community in the country; he advocated a resettlement of the industrial population in townships on the New Lanark plan. Owen's experiments and suggestions ranged very widely, and do not fall under any single formula. There was nothing doctrinaire about him. His New Lanark experiment was the first of a number of benevolent businesses in the world; Lord Leverhulme's Port Sunlight, the Cadburys' Bourneville and the Ford businesses in America are contemporary instances.

Fight for Reform by the Seventh Earl of Shaftesbury

Another champion of the *Ten Hours Movement* was Anthony Ashley Cooper, at first Viscount Ashley and afterwards the seventh Earl of Shaftesbury, a life-long apostle and exponent of practical altruism who never ceased to fight for reform. His contemporaries in the House of Lords, some of whom owned the mills, the mines and the land, remained for a long time apathetic and deaf to his appeals. The ruling doctrine of the time was that progress was measured by trade and profits, that popular misery could be cured only by encouraging capital; that the needs of the new industrial system must govern and limit the development of social life. No mill owner thought he could afford fair wages, especially as new machinery was paid for out of profits. The wages of industrial workers were forced down lower and lower and longer hours were worked. Hunger and hatred made Chartism a mass movement of the working classes. Religion and money making had contrived to get on the same side, and it was possible at one and the same time to be very rich, very greedy, very cruel and very orthodox. So long as the factory owners professed to fear God, continued to hold morning prayers with their families and attended church or chapel on Sunday they considered their duty to their fellow men well done.

A Spirit of Humanitarianism

In combating this situation, men like Percival and Shaftesbury introduced many reforms, but their chief contribution was a spirit of humanitarianism and an understanding of the health and social requirements of the worker. Nor were all the employers flint-hearted. David Dale and Robert Owen set the classical example of beneficent autocracy in industry, and men like Josiah Wedgwood, Matthew Boulton and John Wilkinson retained a high standard in their treatment of workers and in their business methods.

Opposition by Powerful Employers

Nevertheless, many powerful employers resisted legal action, declaring that the new laws would destroy industry. They were supported by the economists of the time, who rejected any interference by the State with economics and advocated a general policy to let things alone. To this policy French economists had given the name *laissez faire, laissez aller*—that is free enterprise in no way influenced or hindered by the State. It was a long struggle in which Robert Owen, Lord Shaftesbury, Sadler, Oastler and Cobbett tried to persuade those of their own social class that the health and welfare of the people must be placed before money making. For every new bill the struggle had to be renewed, and even if the principle of the legislative measures was recognized as justifiable, the ensuing law was generally adopted only with serious restrictions which could not be eliminated until many years later. In consequence of this opposition the laws following the Act of 1802 were limited to the work of children (1819, 1825, 1829 and 1831). Some of the laws for the protection of children contained regulations which later became helpful for adult workers also. More important in this respect was the Act of 1833, which enforced the appointment of factory inspectors (Teleky, 1948).

Early Medical Supervision

In 1830 an employer in worsted spinning who was perturbed by the public concern about children being crippled by the long hours and conditions of factory life consulted Robert Baker, a surgeon in Leeds, who advised that a medical officer should be appointed to visit the factory daily and watch the effects of work on the children's health. It is interesting that this first recorded instance of recommending medical supervision for a general purpose came from a medical man who was destined to become a junior inspector or superintendent of factories in 1834, serving under Robert Rickards, one of the four original inspectors under the Factory Act of 1833. In 1858 he was promoted to be inspector. Another example of medical supervision for a general purpose occurred in 1842 in Scotland, when the report of the Poor Law Commissioners, of which Edwin Chadwick was secretary, on sanitary conditions of the labouring population of Great Britain recorded that Mr. James Smith, Managing Director of the cotton mills at Deanston in Perthshire, retained the services of a medical man to inspect the workpeople from time to time, to give them advice and, as far as possible, to prevent disease (Henry, 1944).

Report of the Sadler Committee

In 1831 a Select Committee was set up by the House of Commons under the chairmanship of Michael Sadler, a Yorkshire business man and mill owner, a Member of Parliament and one of the early protagonists of factory reform, to inquire into the condition of children in factories. It was Robert Owen and Percival who brought Sadler into the reform movement; he in his turn inspired Lord Shaftesbury. Before the Sadler Committee nearly twenty medical witnesses alone were examined, besides very many manufacturers, magistrates, clergymen and others who might be expected to be able to contribute information. Nor were the operatives themselves forgotten:

> Before this Committee there files a long procession of workers—
> men and women, girls and boys. Stunted, diseased, deformed, degraded, they pass across the stage, each with the tale of his wronged life, a living picture of man's cruelty to man, a pitiless indictment of those rulers who, in their days of unabated power, had abandoned the weak to the rapacity of the strong.

Criticisms of the Sadler Report

Though this dreary picture of cruelty, misery, disease and deformity among the factory children is generally accepted as authentic many authors have pointed out that it was biased and really referred to abuses which had largely disappeared in the first thirty years of the century. They regard it as particularly unfair because these years "had been accompanied by considerable material improvements and advances, both within and outside the factories, and these changes had been followed by adjustments in social standards. Sadler was making desperate efforts to get his Ten Hours Bill through Parliament. He exercised the greatest energy to get his case complete by the end of the session and then, ignoring the demands of justice, he immediately published the evidence" (Hutt, 1926) "and gave to the world such a mass of *ex-parte* statements, and gross falsehoods and columnies . . . as probably never before found their way into any public document" (Greg, 1837). Even Engels (1892) wrote of the Report that it "was emphatically partisan, composed by strong enemies of the factory system for party ends . . . Sadler permitted himself to be betrayed by his noble enthusiasm into the most distorted and erroneous statements."

Nature and Incidence of Deformities in Children

The most impressive of the condemnations of the early factory system is the charge that it produced deformities and stunted growth in children. Since, however, at that time the means to recognise or to differentiate between rickets, congenital talipes, spastic diplegia, the infantile hemiplegias and the palsies of poliomyelitis did not exist it must have been a great temptation to blame the factories for producing them. The Committee made no systematic inquiry into the incidence of deformities in both factory and non-factory populations. To test the charge that factory children were stunted, Cowell, one of the commissioners, took the trouble *to ascertain their ages* and then measure and weigh them. Their average height was found to be identical with that of non-factory children. Their average weight was slightly less. Cowell attributed this to the relative lightness of their work. Nor, supposing there *had been* a larger proportion of deformity or malnutrition among the factory children, was any inquiry made as to whether children who were insufficiently strong for other employments were sent to the cotton factories because of the lightness of the work there (Hutt, 1926).

THE BIRTH OF INDUSTRIAL MEDICINE IN ENGLAND

Whereas, through Ramazzini, the idea of asking a patient what is his occupation had birth in Italy, industrial medicine itself was born in England. Because the Industrial Revolution began in England it naturally came about that English doctors were the first to assume responsibility for the health of the worker in industry. The special task of investigating the health hazards in various occupations began early in the nineteenth century in the West Riding of Yorkshire and in Lancashire, when Charles Turner Thackrah, a clinician who practised in Leeds, decided to devote his life to preventive medicine of a new kind.

Charles Turner Thackrah, 1795–1833

The manufacturing activities of Leeds at that time, as today, were very varied, and at least 128 trades and occupations existed there. The reason for such a diversity of manufactures was, as the Hammonds have pointed out, that Leeds, like certain other northern cities, was not the creation of the Industrial Revolution: it was a town of antiquity already renowned as the centre of special industries and trades. Such a town was not thrown up by the Industrial Revolution, but rather overwhelmed by it; its population increased from 60,000 to 130,000 between 1801 and 1831. Thackrah expounded his work in a short book of 220 pages published in 1831 with the title *The Effects of the Principal Arts, Trades and Professions, and of Civic States and Habits of Living, on Health and Longevity, with Suggestions*

*for the Removal of many of the Agents which produce Disease and shorten the
Duration of Life.* It was the first treatise of any kind to be written in England on this subject. For comprehensiveness, first-hand clinical experience
and constructive proposals for improvements, Thackrah's monograph is
superior to that of Ramazzini. It attracted attention from both medical
men and laymen at the time that it appeared, and there is no doubt that it
played an important part in stimulating the factory and health legislation
which mitigated some of the worst features of the Industrial Revolution.

A Pupil of Sir Astley Cooper

Thackrah was born in Yorkshire in 1795 and became apprenticed to a
prominent local practitioner (fig. 50). Like the more ambitious of his contemporaries he came to London, then the only serious centre for medical
education in England, to complete
his training in one of the larger
hospitals. At that time the clinical
staff at Guy's Hospital was the
most active centre of research in
London, and through their publications they were gaining both a
national and international reputation for their hospital. Sir Astley
Cooper, his immediate teacher
and the inspirer of much of his
work, was at the height of his
powers and Thackrah remained in
this stimulating atmosphere for
several years as one of his assistants. During these years Bright,
Addison and Hodgkin, who had
all been attracted to Guy's shortly
after their graduation at Edinburgh, were his contemporaries.
After leaving Guy's, Thackrah
returned to Yorkshire and settled
in practice at Leeds. In 1826 he
opened the Leeds School of
Anatomy, which soon became so successful that it grew into the complete
medical school from which the present Leeds University School of
Medicine has developed. Thackrah may thus be regarded as one of the
founders of provincial medical education in England, and as one of the
vigorous and successful opponents of the claims to monopoly which had
long been maintained by the two Royal Colleges in London (Wright, 1945).

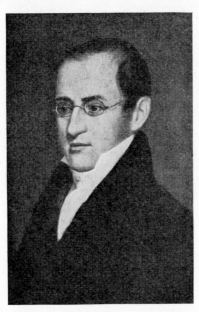

Fig. 50.—Charles Turner Thackrah,
1795–1833

The State of the Artisans in Manufacture

What directed Thackrah's interest to industrial diseases is not clearly
known. It is possible that it resulted from some personal contact with

Robert Owen, who visited Leeds during Thackrah's apprenticeship to study the methods of working of the local factories and the condition of their employees, and the two men exchanged views at the time. Most probably Thackrah's interest in the medical aspects of the problem were the combined result both of his own professional activities amongst the poorer classes in Leeds and of Owen's forceful representation of the urgency of reform. Whatever might have been the impetus, the results of his activities materialized in a small volume which appeared in 1830, and which was soon followed by a much larger and definitive second edition in 1831, a year before his death. His own intentions in publishing the book may be learned from the two following paragraphs:

> The object of this paper is to excite the public attention to the subject. Myself and my pupils have personally and carefully inspected the state of the artisans in most kinds of manufacture, examined the agencies believed to be injurious, conversed on the subjects with masters, overlookers, and the more intelligent workmen, and obtained many tables illustrating the characters of the disorders prevalent in the several kinds of employ. It will be remembered that the subject is new. I have had therefore to enter a new track without guide or assistance.

> Most persons, who reflect on the subject, will be inclined to admit that our employments are in a considerable degree injurious to health: but they believe, or profess to believe, that the evils cannot be counteracted, and urge that an investigation of such evils can produce only pain and discontent. From a reference to fact and observations I reply, that in many of our occupations, the injurious agents might be immediately removed or diminished. Evils are suffered to exist, even when the means of correction are known and easily applied. Thoughtlessness or apathy is the only obstacle to success.

Postural Deformities in Young Children

The book is divided into four sections, which deal successively with operatives, dealers or shop-keepers, merchants and master manufacturers, and professional men. Much the longest and most interesting section deals with the operatives. Before proceeding to diseases associated with particular trades, two of the more general of Thackrah's comments deserve attention: the employment of children, and the frequent references to bad occupational postures as sources of disability. The severity of the conditions of child labour, especially in cotton mills, had been lessened at the time Thackrah wrote, but that they had been far from eliminated can be seen from his comments upon work in the flax mills.

> Children from seven to fifteen years of age go to work at half-past five in the morning, and leave at seven in the evening, or at half-past six and leave at eight, and thus spend twelve hours a day, for five or six years, in an atmosphere of flax dust. Serious injury from such

employment we should expect at any age, but especially during the period of growth. The employment of young children in any labour is wrong. The term of physical growth ought not to be a term of physical exertion. Light and varied motions should be the only effort, motions excited by the will, not by the taskmaster, the run and the leap of an unshackled spirit. How different is the scene in a manu-facturing district! No man of humanity can reflect without distress on the state of thousands of children, many from six to seven years of age, roused from their beds at an early hour, hurried to the mills and kept there, with an interval of only forty minutes, till a late hour at night: kept, moreover, in an atmosphere impure, not only as the air of a town, not only defective in ventilation, but as loaded also with noxious dust. Health! Cleanliness! Mental improvement! How are they regarded? Recreation is out of the question. There is scarcely time for meals. The very period of sleep, so necessary for the young, is too often abridged. Nay, children are sometimes worked even in the night!

Pulmonary Tuberculosis in Tailors

Bad posture at work, though by no means confined to the textile trade and its various branches, was particularly prevalent amongst persons fol-lowing such occupations. It was probably the large numbers of such tradesmen in Leeds in his time that drew Thackrah's attention the more forcibly to the disabilities and deformities that resulted from it. Weavers, burlers, cloth-drawers and especially tailors are remarked upon unfavour-ably.

We see no plump and rosy tailors: none of fine form and strong muscle. The spine is generally curved. Pulmonary consumption is also frequent. Let a hole be made in a board of the circumference of the tailor's body, and let his seat be placed below it. The eyes and the hands will then be sufficiently near his work: his spine will not be un-naturally bent, and his chest and abdomen will be free.

Lung Disease in Miners and Grinders of Metals

Thackrah wrote of the dust diseases of the lungs affecting miners and grinders of metals.

In the mines in the North of England, the workmen, I am in-formed, suffer considerably when employed in ore in the sandstone, but are sensible of no inconvenience where the ore is in limestone. I am indebted to an intelligent friend for the following information: The reason they assign is, that the latter is full of vertical and other fissures, which allow the superincumbent beds of water to percolate through the roof of the mine: whilst the sandstone strata, which are impervious to water, preserve the mine quite dry: consequently, the minute particles of rock formed by blasting or the pickaxe are kept in a dry state within the sandstone mine, forming, as it were, an atmosphere of dust, which the miner is constantly inhaling. Miners rarely work for more than six hours a day, yet they seldom attain the age of forty. A parallel case to that of the miners occurs in the grinders of Sheffield. Dr. Knight, in the *North of England Medical Journal*, states that the fork-grinders, who use a dry grindstone, die at the age of 28 or 32, while the table-knife grinders, who work on wet stones, survive to between 40 and 50.

In both trades, mining and grinding, Thackrah comments on the common association of dust inhalation and tuberculosis. Amongst the men filing iron castings to remove burnt-on sand, pulmonary diseases were prevalent. To protect such workmen he recommends, in addition to proper ventilation, the introduction of suitable magnetic mouthpieces.

Lead Poisoning in Glaze Dippers

Amongst other specific industrial diseases discussed by Thackrah, perhaps the most important were those associated with chronic lead poisoning amongst house-painters and the potters making glazed ware. Such men were frequently attacked with colic, suffered from constipation and ultimately developed lead palsy. Thackrah made specific recommendations for the elimination of lead poisoning as a trade disease amongst pottery workers.

Could not the process be effected without the immersion of the hands in the metallic solution? Or could it not be effected by a machine? Or could not some article less noxious be substituted for the lead? I am told, indeed, by an intelligent manufacturer of earthenware in Leeds, that the comparative cheapness of the leaden glaze is the chief recommendation. Surely humanity forbids that the health of workmen, and that of the poor at large, should be sacrificed to the saving of halfpence in the price of pots. The total disuse of lead in glaze is highly desirable.

A Great Contribution to Preventive Medicine

Thackrah's work in the field of occupational hygiene has never failed of recognition. He was undoubtedly an able and energetic man with a strong social sense, vigorous, pertinacious and courageous, and was determined that his findings should be made widely known at a time when the advocacy of reforms was even less popular than usual. The publication of such a volume from a member of the medical profession, with the prestige that special technical knowledge gave him, considerably aided the parliamentary advocates for the limitation of factory abuses.

Sir John Simon, the first Chief Medical Officer to the Local Government Board (now the Ministry of Health), referred to Thackrah's work as being comparable as a contribution to preventive medicine with the work of Jenner on smallpox. He wrote:

This special service of investigating health in various branches of industry, Thackrah set himself to render: not under any official obligation or inducement, nor with any subvention from Government, but as his own free gift to a public cause. Not less meritorious than the assiduity and the care for truth with which he collected his facts were the unprejudiced good sense and moderation with which he weighed them; and the service thus rendered by Thackrah deserves grateful recognition. By his eminently trustworthy book, he, more than fifty years ago, made it a matter of common knowledge, and of State responsibility, that, with certain of our chief industries, special influences, often of an evidently removable kind, are apt to be associated, which, if permitted to remain, give painful disease and premature disablement or death of the employed persons.

Untimely Death of Thackrah

Thackrah's crowded life was brought to an untimely end by his death from tuberculosis in 1833 at the age of thirty-seven. Sir Thomas Legge (1920) wrote:

I believe that Thackrah's early death retarded the progress of industrial medicine and surgery and the amelioration of conditions of employment for half a century. Had he lived his clinical knowledge and experience would have given prominence in legislation to the need for medical supervision in the factory and workshop by practitioners having the necessary knowledge of the home conditions of the workers and the maladies attributable to industrial life in its widest sense.

THE FACTORY ACT, 1833

In spite of the Report of the Sadler Committee, which ran to six hundred pages and half a million words, Parliament declared itself unsatisfied that a case had been made out for further legislative interference, and two years later a Royal Commission on the Employment of Children in Factories was established. The Commissioners, both lay and medical, travelled all over the country collecting evidence, and in their final report came down heavily on the side of reform. The *Factory Act, 1833*, which followed swiftly on the Commissioners' Report was the first really effective legislative measure in the industrial field. It was entitled *An Act to Regulate the Labour of Children in the Mills and Factories of the United Kingdom*. It applied to all textile factories where steam or water power was used, including flax, hemp and silk. It forbade night work for those under eighteen and restricted their hours to twelve a day and sixty-nine a week; factory schools were established and all children under the age of thirteen were required to attend for at least two hours a day. The minimum age was set at nine. Prior to the passing of this Act the age of a child was established by a certificate, often very dubious, from the parent; but by the Act of 1833 a certificate of age was required from a medical man to the effect that a child was of the ordinary strength and appearance of a child exceeding nine years or other specified age.

A Factory Inspectorate established

But the most important provision of all was the establishment of a Factory Inspectorate to administer the Act. The *Factory Acts of 1819 and 1825* had left the voluntary local system of factory inspection by visitors unchanged, but now the principle of enforcement of the law by means of statutory inspection was introduced and the first four inspectors were appointed. They were Leonard Horner, Thomas J. Howell, Robert Rickards and Robert J. Saunders. These men were given the power of entry into all factories covered by the Act, power of prosecution of recalcitrant owners and, in particular, responsibility for setting up and inspecting factory schools. The country was fortunate in that the early holders of office were men of great moral courage and a wide experience of affairs, and the importance of their contributions to later reform cannot be over-emphasized. Indeed, it would be difficult to point to a single legislative measure of importance relating to the health of factory workers from that day to this which has not been initiated in whole or in part by the Factory Department.

Accidents to Mill-hands

The Commissioners' Report of 1833 had drawn attention to the prevalence of serious accidents to mill-hands, particularly to children, and, on account of their long and voluminous skirts, to women also, and this question was also being taken up by the inspectors in their bi-annual reports. There could be no doubt about the serious accidents occurring, but on the matter of curtailment of hours their champions among the factory workers were accused of hiding behind the skirts of the women and of carrying on a thinly veiled campaign to control the hours of all men workers. There was some truth in this, for the work of men, women and children was so intimately connected that it was difficult to see how one group could be made subject to legislation without interfering with the rest. Be that as it may, the controversy dragged on through many reverses for upwards of twenty years until in 1847 an *Act to Limit the Hours of Young Persons and Females in Factories* was passed, which prohibited the employment of a young person or female for more than ten hours a day or fifty-eight a week. By a curious oversight, children—that is, those under thirteen—were left out of the provisions of the Act (Swanston, 1949).

The Certifying Factory Surgeon

Although the factory inspectors tried to arrange as far as possible for one medical man in each district to perform the duty of certifying surgeon, they had no statutory powers to back them. Eleven years later, by the Act of 1844, power was given to them to appoint a sufficient number of practising medical men to be certifying surgeons for the purpose of examining young persons brought before them for certification, though it was still possible for certificates to be given by persons other than the certifying surgeon provided there was a counter-signature by a Justice of the Peace.

The Act also established the half-time system for children under thirteen to enable them to attend school, the obligation to fence dangerous machinery, the inclusion of women in the limitation of hours imposed on young persons and children and the prohibition of cleaning machinery while in motion.

A Twelve-hour Day in Textile Mills

The one retrograde step in this Act was the reduction of the minimum age from nine years to eight, reluctantly conceded by Lord Shaftesbury, the promoter of the Bill, in order to gain his other points. In the years following the passage of this Act, the inspectors found that evasion of the relay system, which had been introduced to overcome the disparity between men's and women's hours, was difficult to prevent, and so in 1850 a normal working day of twelve hours was fixed, to include at least one hour and a half for meals. These results represent a very notable achievement in the education of public opinion, for legislation to be successful must perforce follow in the wake of general experience and reflect the accepted views of the majority rather than the revolutionary ideas of a few enthusiasts, for a bad law is worse than no law at all. By now the principle of interference by the Legislature between employer and employed for the good of the latter had been established; very young children were excluded from the textile mills; it was no longer legal to work women and children at night or for more than a prescribed period during the day; a weekly holiday was compulsory; safety measures were in force in an attempt to reduce the serious accidents due to machinery and, finally, the principle of the need for education had been recognized.

DREADFUL CONDITIONS IN MANY TRADES

During the second half of the nineteenth century the Factory Acts were extended to embrace the whole manufacturing field, and, in addition, legislation was directed not only against unhealthy conditions of work in general but also against the specific disease-producing factors in the different trades. The widespread interest aroused by the legislation in the textile industry was by this time spreading to other trades. By the *Print Works Act, 1845*, the ancillary process of textile printing had been regulated, but so far none of the other staple industries of the country had been touched. In Parliament from time to time the attention of the Government had been drawn, both by supporters and detractors of the various factory Bills, to the dreadful conditions still existing in the potteries, the paper and printing trades, the steel industries of Sheffield and many other trades.

The Children's Employment Commission of 1861

Many employers were demanding legislation to remedy unsatisfactory conditions, notably the great pottery manufacturers, of whom some twenty-six sent a petition to the Home Secretary in 1862. The effect of the textile legislation had been to reduce very considerably the number of children working in the regulated factories, but in many other industries enormous numbers were still employed, many at a very early age. In 1861 a Children's Employment Commission began an investigation of a variety of un-regulated industries and a series of reports was issued between 1863 and 1867, notably on the lucifer-match industry, paper staining and the manu-facture of percussion caps, cutlery grinding and the potteries. In all these there were specific and well-known hazards.

Deaths from Phthisis in Cutlers and Potters

The cause for the greatest alarm was the mortality from pulmonary diseases in the potteries and among the cutlery workers. "In Sheffield," wrote Dr. Arnold Knight of that city in 1844, "there are some 2,500 grinders at work. About 150 are fork grinders; these die between the 28th and 32nd year. The razor grinders, who grind wet, die between the 45th and 50th year." Dr. E. H. Greenhow, in the third Public Health Re-port of 1860, noted the increased deaths from pulmonary affection in the potteries, and potters were described by Dr. J. T. Arlidge of the North Staffordshire Infirmary as a "degenerated population both physically and morally . . . prone to chest disease. One form would appear peculiar to them and is known as potters' asthma and potters' consumption."

The Dread of Poisoning from Phosphorus and Arsenic

The lucifer-match trade, in which women and girls were almost ex-clusively employed, had by this time achieved much notoriety on account of the dreaded phosphorus necrosis or phossy jaw. This affliction, with its all-too-obvious disfigurement, its long-drawn-out agony and the fact that it so frequently attacked young girls, demanded control by its very appear-ance, and it is the only industrial disease which has been virtually abolished by international prohibition (see p. 381). The staining of paper and textiles, harmless occupations today, at that time involved the use of the green arsenites of copper (see p. 334). These pigments were incorporated so loosely into paper and textiles that a considerable hazard was present, not only to the operatives themselves, but to those who used the finished article. In the manufacture of percussion caps, a trade employing practically no men, there was a constant danger of injury from explosion.

Special Regulations for Dangerous Trades

The Commissioners made individual recommendations for each in-dustry they investigated, but the gist of all their reports was the need for the extension of legislation. As a result, in the *Factories and Workshops Act, 1867*, a large number of previously unregulated industries were brought under control. This Act also authorized employers to make special regu-lations for dangerous trades, subject to the approval of the Secretary of State, and for the first time certain classes of workers were definitely ex-cluded from particular processes. Thus no boy under twelve and no woman was to be employed in melting or annealing glass, no child under eleven was to grind metal, and no protected person was to take meals in any part of a glass factory. But the first Act of Parliament to be directed against a specific occupational disease was the *Factories (Prevention of Lead Poisoning) Act, 1883* (see p. 236). As the forerunner of our present-day scheme of prescribed diseases (see p. 200), this Act marks the opening of the modern era in legislation aimed to protect the workers in all dangerous trades.

THE MINES ACT, 1842

Although the squalid abominations of the Industrial Revolution had been at last seriously attacked in the *Factory Act, 1833,* this Act had not affected the mines, where abuses similar to those in the factories had existed long before the Industrial Revolution had begun. But an eddy of the main tide penetrated even into the coalfields. Inspectors had been sent out to inquire into the working of the Factory Act, and one of these undertook an inquiry into the colliery population of the district assigned to him. Further publicity was given to the condition of the miners' children by the report on schools in South Wales made in 1840 by Seymour Tremenheere.

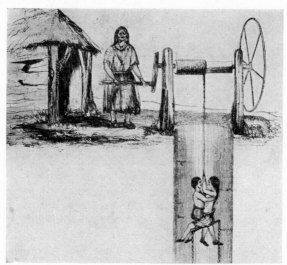

Fig. 51.—One of the Pictures which shocked Victorian
England
(*Children's Employment Commission, First Report, 1842*)

Royal Commission on the Employment of Children in the Mines

These and similar reports attracted the attention of Lord Shaftesbury, and at his instance was appointed in 1840 a Royal Commission on the employment of children in mines and manufactures. The *Children's Employment Commission, First Report, 1842,* dealt with mines. It was written in a clear, sober and convincing style, and the effect of the moving tale it told was set off by pictures, more vivid than the language of the Commissioners, drawn on the spot from women and children at work. This innovation was due to Dr. Southwood Smith, who argued that Members of Parliament who might think themselves too busy to read the text of the report would turn over its pages to glance at the illustrations. The Report threw a glaring light upon the darker side of the social history of the time and shocked both the humanity and the delicacy of Victorian England (fig. 51).

Solitary Confinement in the Darkness of the Coal Pits

In every district except North Staffordshire, where the younger children were needed in the Potteries, the employment of children of seven was common; in many pits children were employed at six, in some at five, and in one case a baby of three was found working underground. Such babies were sometimes taken down into the pits to keep the rats from their father's food. The youngest children, both boys and girls, were employed as trappers; that is, they were in charge of the ventilating doors in the galleries, on the opening and closing of which the safety of the mine depended. Such a boy would sit in a small cell with a cord in his hand in darkness and solitude for twelve hours or longer at a time. The solitude was periodically interrupted while the trucks and the rats went by.

Rats, Mice and Beetles in the Pits

In parts of the pits besides rats the miner had to contend with mice and beetles.

When I worked in the pits as a driver-lad, I used to leave my jacket hanging on a nail outside my pony's stall. At the end of my shift, I took care to shake the coat vigorously. A beetle or two always fell out. My father who was a horse-keeper had worked underground in the stables where beetles moved in masses up the walls and they hung from the ceiling like prunes. They were at their worst when they tried to walk across the arched roof of the stall. Then they would dangle above a man's head, or worse still, above the bent back of a horse-keeper who was glistening with sweat as he brushed and curry-combed a pony. The stables were infested with mice. Cats were the only way of keeping the numbers down. There were so many mice that after the first few days the cat usually gave up eating them and got its food from the horse-keepers. But the cat never gave up hunting. It killed for pleasure and we found dead mice everywhere. Yet few of us ever saw the cats, and even the men who fed them only saw them at bait time. Then they'd come sidling into the horse- keeper's cabin, their tails erect and their eyes glowing in the lamplight like green bubbles. The rest of the time they mooched around the corn bins or prowled around the loose-boxes. Their relationship with the pit pony which caught them in its manger was often lethal (Hitchin, 1967).

Haulage of Trucks by Children on All Fours

Being cheaper than horses, children were harnessed with chains to heavy trucks of coal which they hauled like dogs on all fours. As the passages were often low and narrow, it was necessary to use very small children for this purpose. On this point the Report states:

In many mines which are at present worked, the main gates are only from 24 to 30 inches high, and in some parts of these mines the passages do not exceed 18 inches in height. In this case not only is the employment of very young children absolutely indispensable to the working of the mine, but even the youngest children must necessarily work in a bent position of the body.

Another task carried out by children was that of pumping water in the under-bottom of coal pits, a job that kept them standing ankle-deep in water for twelve hours.

A Child Engineman of Nine

In certain districts children were used for the particularly responsible duty of winding-engineman.

In Derbyshire and parts of Lancashire and Cheshire it was the custom to employ them as enginemen to let down and draw up the cages in which the population of the pit descended to its depths and returned to the upper air. A "man of discretion" required 30s. a week wages; these substitutes only cost 5s. or 7s. a week. Accidents were, of course, frequent —on one occasion three lives were lost because a child engineman of nine turned away to look at a mouse at a critical moment—and the Chief Constable of Oldham said that the coroners declined to bring in verdicts of gross neglect from pity for the children (Hammond and Hammond, 1923).

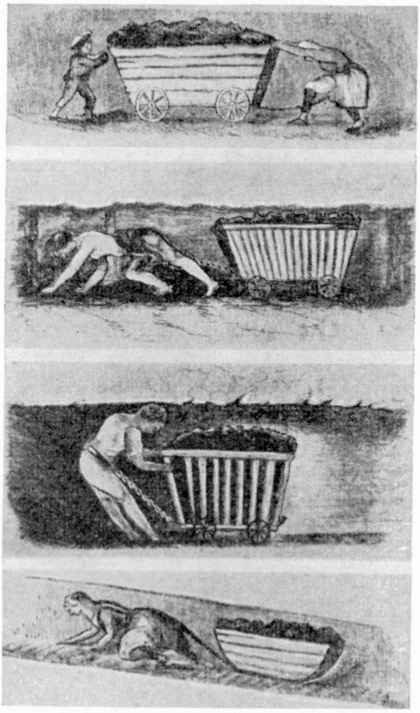

FIG. 52.—Children hauled Trucks of Coal and Women almost naked were harnessed like Horses to Coal Trucks
(*Children's Employment Commission, First Report, 1842*)

Women carry Coal in Baskets on their Backs

The employment of girls and women was confined to certain mining districts. In Yorkshire the women were hired by the men and were content with smaller wages than men wanted. Harnessed like a horse to a coal truck and almost naked, a woman would show all a horse's determination to keep ahead of her rivals (fig. 52). In Scotland women were also used to

carry coal in baskets on their backs up steep ladders and along the passages
from the workings to the
pit bottom (fig. 53); in
some cases girls of six were
found carrying half a hundredweight of coal (fig. 54).

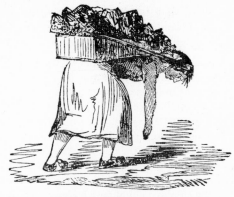

The employment of
women offended an
instinct that was still
more powerful. The
picture of men and
women working to-
gether in the mines,
almost naked, under re-
pulsive and degrading
conditions, outraged
the sense of decency of

FIG. 53.—In Scotland Women were used to carry
Coal in Baskets on their Backs
(*Children's Employment Commission, First Report,
1842*)

the House of Commons even more than the story of human misery
had outraged its sense of pity. This was almost the only feature of
the arrangements brought to light by the Commission for which no
one was ready with an apology (Hammond and Hammond, 1923).

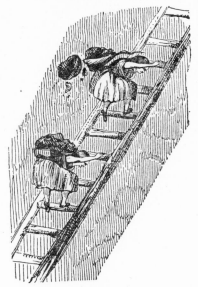

FIG. 54.—In some Cases Girls of six were
found carrying Half a Hundredweight
of Coal up a Ladder
(*Children's Employment Commission, First
Report, 1842*)

Cruelty to Workhouse Appren-
tices

The hours worked by the children varied from one district to
another. They were seldom less
than twelve and often they were
sixteen. In some cases children
had been known to remain in the
pit for thirty-six hours while
working double shifts.

Of the cruelty to which
children were exposed, employed by men, brought up in
this rough school, screened
from notice, and hard pressed
to earn their living, ample
proof was forthcoming. The
worst victims were workhouse
apprentices, bound from the
age of eight or nine for twelve
years, employed in large
numbers in South Staffordshire, Lancashire and in the

West Riding. These unhappy boys could be forced into places where miners would not allow their children to be used, and in case of refusal were taken before magistrates and sent to prison (Hammond and Hammond, 1923).

Passing of the Mines Act, 1842

Such was the indignation of the country over the Report, that Lord Shaftesbury was able to strike his blow at once (fig. 55). His speech in the House of Commons, arranging and presenting the facts set out in the Report with admirable skill, occupied two hours. Its effect was overwhelming and many members were reduced to tears. In the House of Lords, in spite of bitter opposition from the great coal owners, the Bill was passed but in an amended form. In the end the Act was a very moderate measure. The employment of women and girls underground was indeed absolutely prohibited, but boys were still to be allowed to enter the mines at the age of ten, the employment of parish apprentices was still to go on, and boys were to be allowed to act as winding-enginemen at fifteen. Although provision was made for the appointment of inspectors, they were not to be allowed to examine the underground workings but only the state and condition of the persons working in the mines. Thus, to his great shame and disappointment, was Lord Shaftesbury's Bill mutilated.

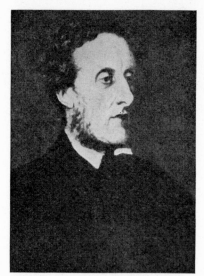

FIG. 55.—Anthony Ashley-Cooper, Seventh Earl of Shaftesbury, 1801–85

Principle of Government Inspection

The Act of 1842 marked the beginning of a new era in mining by establishing the principles of Government inspection and State interference in the conduct of the industry. These principles were gradually extended by the passage of successive *Mines Regulation Acts* in 1850, 1855, 1860, 1862, 1872, 1887 and 1911, and other Mines Acts dealing with specific problems. In this way there has been evolved a comprehensive code of mining law touching every aspect of mining practice, and designed to ensure, as far as practicable, the safety, health and well-being of all mine workers. The history of mining legislation in Britain reveals the gradual recognition of the importance and rights of the mine worker and of the increasing interest and concern of the State in his protection and well-being, culminating in the passage of the *Coal Industry Nationalization Act* in 1946.

THE TRUCK ACTS

During 500 years many laws have been enacted to protect workers from being under any pressure to spend their wages to their disadvantage. They were called Truck Acts, the word *truck* being derived from the French *troc* meaning *barter*. The first Act of the kind was made in 1464 in the reign of Edward IV. It was applied to woollen clothworkers only. The Act of 1701, passed in the reign of Queen Anne, extended the truck regulations to woollen, linen, fustian, cotton and iron manufacture.

Mining Communities Remote from Shops

During the eighteenth century the truck system developed rapidly in response to a real need. Many mining communities were remote from towns with adequate shopping facilities and the mine owners often established their own shops, usually in conjunction with a public-house near the pithead. It was then a simple matter for the miner to get into the debt of his employer. The Truck Acts were adopted owing to the abuses which arose, in the first place from the truck-shops, owned by employers, out of which wages were paid in the form of goods or where the workers were constrained to spend their nominally cash wages; and, in the second place, from the habit of making oppressive and arbitrary deductions from wages. The workers referred to the trashy goods obtained at the truck shops as *tommy* and to the shops as *tommy shops*. Tommy is an old name used by soldiers, sailors and workmen for food or bread. The rubbishy nature of the goods supplied added to our language the expression *tommy-rot* which now means *nonsense, bosh,* or *twaddle*.

The Truck Act, 1831

During the early part of the nineteenth century the Potteries and the Black Country were strongholds of the truck system, but it never obtained a firm footing in Northumberland and Durham. At this time strenuous efforts were made in Great Britain to eradicate the system, and after three years of agitation Lord Hatherton obtained the *Truck Act, 1831*. This law proved ineffectual, and in 1843 the Midland Mining Commission found truck still prevalent in the coalfields.

Report of the Midland Mining Commission, 1843

It is upon the report of this Commission that Benjamin Disraeli in his novel *Sybil, or The Two Nations* (1845) makes coal miners while drinking beer in a public-house describe the effects of the truck-shops.

"The question is," said Nixon, looking round with a magisterial air, "what is wages? I say, 'tain't sugar, 'tain't tea, 'tain't bacon. I don't think it's candles; but of this I be sure, 'tain't waistcoats."

Here there was a general groan.

"Comrades," continued Nixon, "you know what has happened; you know as how Juggins applied for his balance after his tommy-book was paid up, and that incarnate nigger Diggs has made him take two waistcoats. Now the question rises, what is a collier to do with waistcoats? Pawn 'em I s'pose to Diggs's son-in-law, next to his father's shop, and sell the ticket for sixpence. Now there's the question; keep to the question; the question is waistcoats and tommy; first waistcoats and then tommy."

"I have been making a pound a week these two months past," said another, "but as I'm a sinner saved, I have never seen the young queen's picture yet."

"And I have been obliged to pay the doctor for my poor wife in tommy," said another. " 'Doctor,' I said, says I, 'I blush to do it, but all I have got is tommy, and what shall it be, bacon or cheese?' 'Cheese at tenpence a pound,' says he, for he is a thorough Christian, 'I'll take the tommy as I find it.' "

"Juggins has got his rent to pay and is afeard of the bums," said Nixon; "and he has got two waistcoats!"

"Besides," said another, "Diggs's tommy is only open once a week and if you're not there in time, you go over for another seven days. And it's such a distance, and he keeps a body there such a time—it's always a day's work for my poor woman; she can't do nothing after it, what with the waiting and the standing and the cussing of Master Joseph Diggs,—for he do swear at the women, when they rush in for the first turn, most fearful."

"They do say he's a shocking little dog."

Evils of the Tommy-shops

Disraeli makes it clear that his descriptions of the tommy-shop are written from his own observations.

The door of Mr. Diggs's tommy-shop opened. The rush was like the advance into the pit of a theatre when the drama existed; pushing, squeezing, fighting, tearing, shrieking. On a high seat, guarded by rails from all contact, sat Mr. Diggs, senior, with a bland smile on his sanctified countenance, a pen behind his ear, and recommending his constrained customers in honeyed tones to be patient and orderly. Behind the substantial counter, which was an impregnable fortification, was his popular son, Master Joseph; a short, ill favoured cur, with a spirit of vulgar oppression and malicious mischief stamped on his visage. His black, greasy, lank hair, his pug nose, his coarse red face, and his projecting tusks, contrasted with the mild and lengthened countenance of his father, who looked very much like a wolf in sheep's clothing.

For the first five minutes Master Joseph did nothing but blaspheme and swear at his customers, occasionally leaning over the counter and cuffing the women in the van or lugging some girl by the hair. . . .

"Don't make a brawling here," said Master Joseph, "or I'll jump over this here counter and knock you down, like nothink. What did you say, woman? are you deaf? what did you say? how much best tea do you want?"

"I don't want any, sir."

"You never want best tea; you must take three ounces of best tea, or you shan't have nothing. If you say another word, I'll put you down four. You tall gal, what's your name, you keep back there, or I'll fetch you such a cut as'll keep you at home till next reckoning. . . ."

"Cuss them; I'll keep them quiet": and so he took up a yard measure, and, leaning over the counter, hit right and left.

"Oh! you little monster!" exclaimed a woman, "you have put out my baby's eye."

There was a murmur; almost a groan. "Whose baby's hurt?" asked Master Joseph, in a softened tone.

"Mine, sir," said an indignant voice; "Mary Church."

"Oh! Mary Church, is it!" said the malicious imp; "then I'll put Mary Church down for half a pound of best arrowroot; that's the finest thing in the world for babbies, and will cure you of bringing your cussed monkeys here, as if you all thought our shop was a hinfant school."

The story ends in a glorious riot in which the outraged mob advances in anger upon Diggs's tommy-shop and burns it to the ground.

Unfair Deductions from Wages

Between 1840 and 1870 stricter enforcement of the law gradually displaced the truck system. In 1871 it was prevalent only in the West of Scotland and South Wales. By 1887 truck payments were declared illegal except in the case of agricultural and domestic workers. In that year factory inspectors took over the administration of the Truck Acts in factories and found that payment of goods for labour was a passing practice. One of the curses of the wage system in factories lay in unfair deductions from workers' wages so that they were sometimes reduced almost to nothing, as in the case of a girl earning 22s. 6d. a week having 20s. deducted for spoilt work.

Rules Governing Deductions from Wages

In the first place the Truck Acts make all payment of wages otherwise than in current coin of the realm illegal. If any wages are paid in a manner contravening this rule the transaction is entirely void. In the second place the Acts render illegal any contract requiring the workman to spend any part of his wages in any particular manner or at any particular shop. A workman may not be dismissed for spending or failing to spend his wages at any particular place. In the third place the Truck Act, 1896, regulates deductions from wages. It requires the terms of any contract authorizing the employer to impose disciplinary fines and deduct the amount from wages to be posted up where they can be easily seen. The amount deducted, whether as a disciplinary fine or in respect of bad work, must, moreover, be fair and reasonable, having regard to all the circumstances of the case. The most recent Truck Act (1940) permits an employer to contract to pay a weekly wage and deduct for meals provided, but forbids a contract for a sum in wages plus meals to a stated value.

THE SWEATING SYSTEM

Sweating is a term applied to underpaid and overworked labour. It originated early in the nineteenth century when it was known as *the contract system*. Many trades were involved but the limelight was first turned upon those impoverished immigrants from Russia, Poland and the Baltic States who were employed in the east end of London in tailoring, mantle-making, shirt making, furriery, cabinet-making and the manufacture of matches (see p. 380). When contracts were given to suppliers of clothing for the army and navy, the contractors handed the work over to sub-contractors. The oppressive conditions which arose in the trade spread to the manufacture of ready-made and made-to-measure clothing. Whereas previously the practice had been for garments to be made up by workers directly employed by the master tailor, the new scheme brought people possessing little skill into competition with the regular craftsmen. As a result of this a fall in wages occurred and affected the whole body of workmen in the trade. From 1843 there was a general outcry against the sweating system and this mounted in intensity during forty-five years until the *Consolidating Factories and Workshops Act*, 1878, drew into the field of control all factories and many workshops. Even then there was still a large number of small work-places, notably domestic and men's workshops, which the arm of the law did not reach and over which the inspectors had no jurisdiction. Many of these were in the sweated industries, those trades which were unorganized, often restricted to certain localities, combining bad working conditions, long hours and low wages.

Vigorous Agitation against the Sweating System

Thomas Hood (1799–1845), British humorist and poet, dedicated some of his best efforts to the cause and sufferings of the workers of the world. *The Bridge of Sighs* and the *Song of the Labourer* pictured the appalling conditions of the industrial worker of his day. *The Song of the Shirt*, which appeared anonymously in the Christmas number of *Punch*, 1843, told in moving verse the horrors of sweated labour in domestic industry, where a woman might have to stitch shirts at the rate of sevenpence a dozen, finding her own sewing cotton!

The Song of the Shirt

Work—work—work!
Till the brain begins to swim;
Work—work—work

Till the eyes are heavy and dim!
Seam, and gusset, and band,
  Band, and gusset, and seam,
Till over the buttons I fall asleep
  And sew them on in a dream!

Work—work—work!
  My labour never flags;
And what are its wages? A bed of straw,
  A crust of bread—and rags.
That shattered roof, and this naked floor,
  A table, a broken chair,
And a wall so blank my shadow I thank
  For sometimes falling there!

Oh! but for one short hour!
  A respite however brief!
No blessed leisure for Love or Hope,
  But only time for Grief!
A little weeping would ease my heart,
  But in their briny bed
My tears must stop, for every drop
  Hinders needle and thread!

With fingers weary and worn,
  With eyelids heavy and red,
A Woman sat in unwomanly rags
  Plying her needle and thread—

Stitch—stitch—stitch!
  In poverty, hunger, and dirt,
And still with a voice of dolorous pitch—
Would that its tone could reach the rich—
  She sang this "Song of the Shirt"!

In 1850 the *Morning Chronicle* started a series of articles which vigorously attacked the system of sweated labour. These were followed by Charles Kingsley's pamphlet *Cheap Clothes and Nasty* and by his novel *Alton Locke*, 1849. In 1889 the sufferings of women nail-and-chain makers in Cradley Heath were disclosed, and in the same year an Anti-Sweating League was formed.

Salient Points of the Sweating System

The salient points of the sweating system were:

(1) In these trades there existed a middleman, known as a *sweater* or *fogger*, whose business was to obtain unfinished work from a factory, farm it out to individual workers, who finished the job, pay them, and in his turn receive payment from the manufacturer to whom he returned the finished

work. The sweater made his profit out of the worker, not the manufacturer.

(2) The work so farmed out was done in private houses, or in hired
rooms of workshops attached to houses, and often presided over by the
sweater himself. Often whole families worked together, a single room doing
duty as workroom, living-room and bedroom.

(3) Workshops could be inspected only by Factory Inspectors if they
contained hired labour, therefore where stalls or hearths were hired by the
workers themselves, as in the cutlery and nail-and-chain trades, they were
outside the jurisdiction of the law.

(4) Competition for work was severe and wages were further debased
by the influx of foreign workers, especially by Jewish refugees from Eastern
Europe. These people, accustomed to a very much lower standard of living
than the British worker, so reduced wages that starvation levels soon pre-
vailed in a dozen different trades.

(5) The indifference of employers to the welfare of the work-people
resulted in the continuance of deplorable conditions of work and rates of
pay.

(6) The employment of married women who were content to accept
minimum wages below the subsistence level further reduced the rates for
the different jobs, and in many of these industries women were extensively
employed.

(7) The evils of the sweating system can be summarized as a rate of
wages inadequate to the necessities of the workers, or inappropriate to the
work carried out, excessive hours of labour, and the insanitary state of the
houses in which much of the work was done.

Private Inquiry by *The Lancet*

Attention was drawn to this state of affairs by *The Lancet* which
in 1884, started a private inquiry into certain industries. It sent its own
Sanitary Commissioner, Mr. Adolphe Smith, to visit the sweated workshops in different parts of the country and published his reports in the
form of leading articles during the next few years. In 1889 a Select Committee was set up by the House of Lords under the chairmanship of Lord
Dunraven to investigate conditions in a number of different industries.
This Committee inquired into the trades of bespoke tailoring, cutlery,
shirt making, chain and nail making, boots and shoes, harness and
accoutrements, guns, locks, nuts and bolts, and cabinet making and upholstery. One extract from the evidence will suffice to show the sort of
conditions their Lordships unearthed.

House of Lords Committee, 1889

Dr. Edward Squire, with reference to the tailoring trade in Soho,
London, stated:

> There is a room about twelve or fourteen feet by ten, and eight
> feet high, as near as I could judge it with my eye; in this room there is

a large bed, the only bed in the room; on which the mother of the family was dying of consumption; although it was summer there was a large fire in the room before which the husband was at work as a tailor, pressing cloth and so of course filling the air with steam; beside him there was his son, also at work; and playing on the floor there were two or three children; all crowded into a room which would properly contain two or three people at the most, with due consideration for health.

The space in that room averages about one hundred and sixty cubic feet per person.

Domestic Industry notoriously difficult to Regulate

Dr. Squire also said that the mortality rate for phthisis among tailors was one in four, against one in ten for the general population. He suggested 500 cubic feet as the minimum space required for each individual. In the nail-and-chain trade the employment of women on the *oliver* or heavy sledge hammer was condemned as being much too arduous. It was pointed out that in some of the subsidiary clothing industries, such as glove making, very young children were being employed for long hours. Domestic industry, notoriously difficult to regulate, was here revealed in all its horrors; men were earning ten shillings a week as cutlers, and women sevenpence a dozen for sewing shirts.

Remedies proposed by the Lords Committee

The remedies proposed by the Lords Committee included the exclusion of women from unsuitable work, extension of the sanitary provisions of the Factories Act to all workshops and the appointment of additional inspectors with an extension of their powers of entry. Lists of outworkers were to be kept by all occupiers for inspection when necessary, and there was to be a stricter enforcement of the Truck Acts. Furthermore, the Committee specifically recommended a minimum wage for Government contract work, and an extension of co-operative societies and combination among workers. Many of these recommendations were implemented in subsequent statutes beginning with the *Trade Boards Act, 1909*. By establishing machinery for fixing minimum rates in unorganized industries, these laws ultimately helped to remove the evils of sweating. Nevertheless, home work is bound to remain very largely beyond the reach of legislation and therefore a potential field for exploitation, particularly of women (Swanston, 1949).

THE CLIMBING BOYS

During the reign of Elizabeth I shortage of wood led to an expansion of coal mining. New industries, such as the manufacture of glass, came into being and all required coal. Cast-iron firebacks for coal fires were manufactured at the Sussex forges. In 1577 Harrison, Canon of Windsor and

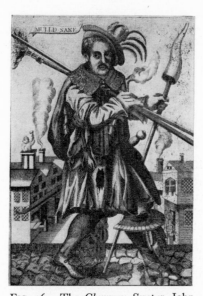

FIG. 56.—The *Chymney Sweper*, John Cottington, nicknamed *Mull'd Sake*, 1604–59

rector of Radwinter, in his *Description of England*, recorded that chimneys had become general even in cottages, while bricks were being used for building houses in place of wood and in competition with stone. By 1578 brewers, dyers, hatmakers and others had for some time past altered their furnaces and firing places to suit sea coal—that is, coal transported to districts approachable by sea, mainly London, the Thames Valley, the Trent, the Severn, the Humber, the Tyne and sea-coast towns.

A Fashion for Long and Tortuous Chimneys, 1666

At the end of the sixteenth century the *Chymney Sweper* became important. Henry (1946) reminds us that John Cottington, nicknamed *Mull'd Sake* (fig. 56), was born in Cheapside in 1604 and was put out by the parish overseers as apprentice to a sweep at the age of eight, but ran away after five years to work on his own and became a notorious thief and murderer until he was hanged in 1659 at the age of fifty-five at Smithfield Rounds. After the Great Fire of London in 1666, the unfortunate and short-sighted practice of building long, narrow, tortuous chimneys came into fashion, requiring the increased use of child assistants or *climbing boys*. The employment of these children was cruelly exploited more and more throughout the eighteenth century.

Jonas Hanway suggests Licences for Apprentices, 1773

In 1773 Jonas Hanway, traveller and philanthropist, drew attention to the miserable condition of the climbing boys, and suggested that no chimney sweep should be allowed to take an apprentice without an annual licence. The child apprentices, who had to be small to negotiate flues only 7 inches in diameter, were stolen for the purpose or were sold by their parents for a few pounds. They were driven up the chimneys and sometimes forced to climb by means of a fire of straw lighted beneath them. Submerged in soot in narrow or horizontal flues, many were suffocated. They usually slept in cellars with a bag of soot for a bed and another for a coverlet (Hammond and Hammond, 1917). It is not surprising that some of the boys never washed at all but just dusted themselves in the morning, nor is it remarkable that they were covered with lice. It was part of the duty of the child apprentice to advertise his master by crying the streets. This street cry, and also the bed of soot, is recorded in a poem by Blake in the first verse.

William Blake records their Plight in Verse, 1789

In his *Songs of Innocence* (1789), William Blake wrote:

The Chimney-Sweeper

When my mother died I was very young,
And my father sold me while yet my tongue
Could scarcely cry "'weep! 'weep! 'weep! 'weep!"
So your chimneys I sweep, and in soot I sleep.

There's little Tom Dacre, who cried when his head,
That curled like a lamb's back, was shaved; so I said,
"Hush, Tom! never mind it, for, when your head's bare,
You know that the soot cannot spoil your white hair."

And so he was quiet, and that very night,
As Tom was a-sleeping, he had such a sight!—
That thousands of sweepers, Dick, Joe, Ned and Jack,
Were all of them locked up in coffins of black.

And by came an Angel, who had a bright key,
And he opened the coffins, and set them all free;
Then down a green plain, leaping, laughing, they run,
And wash in a river, and shine in the sun.

Then naked and white, all their bags left behind,
They rise upon clouds, and sport in the wind;
And the Angel told Tom, if he'd be a good boy,
He'd have God for his father, and never want joy.

And so Tom awoke, and we rose in the dark,
And got with our bags and our brushes to work.
Though the morning was cold, Tom was happy and warm:
So, if all do their duty, they need not fear harm.

And in his *Songs of Experience* (1794), he wrote:

The Chimney-Sweeper

A little black thing among the snow,
Crying "'weep! 'weep!" in notes of woe!
"Where are thy father and mother? Say!"
"They are both gone up to the church to pray.

"Because I was happy upon the heath,
And smiled among the winter's snow,
They clothed me in the clothes of death,
And taught me to sing the notes of woe.

"And because I am happy and dance and sing,
They think they have done me no injury,
And are gone to praise God and his priest and king,
Who make up a heaven of our misery."

Charles Lamb praises the Boys, 1823

In one of his *Essays of Elia* (1823), Charles Lamb wrote *The Praise of Chimney-Sweepers*:

I like to meet a sweep—understand me—not a grown sweeper—old chimney-sweepers are by no means attractive—but one of those tender novices, blooming through their first nigritude, the maternal washings not quite effaced from the cheek—such as come forth with the dawn, or somewhat earlier, with their little professional notes sounding like the peep-peep of a young sparrow; or liker to the matin lark should I pronounce them, in their aerial ascents not seldom anticipating the sunrise?

I have a kindly yearning towards these dim specks—poor blots—innocent blacknesses——

I reverence these young Africans of our own growth—these almost clergy imps, who sport their cloth without assumption; and from their little pulpits (the tops of chimneys), in the nipping air of a December morning, preach a lesson of patience to mankind (fig. 57).

My pleasant friend Jem White instituted an annual feast of chimney-sweepers, at which it was his pleasure to officiate as host and waiter. It was a solemn supper held in Smithfield, upon the yearly return of the fair of St. Bartholomew. Cards were issued a week before to the master-sweeps in and about the metropolis, confining the invitation to their younger fry.

The guests assembled about seven. In those little temporary parlours three tables were spread with napery, not so fine as substantial, and at every board a comely hostess presided with her pan of hissing sausages. The nostrils of the young rogues dilated at the savour.

How genteelly he would deal about the small ale, as if it were wine, naming the brewer, and protesting if it were not good, he

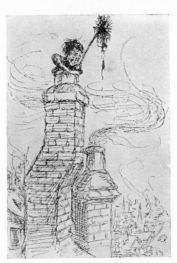

FIG. 57.—Illustration to an Essay by Charles Lamb

should lose their custom; with a special recommendation to wipe the lip before drinking. Then we had our toasts—"the King,"—"the Cloth,"—which, whether they understood or not, was equally diverting and flattering; and for a crowning sentiment, which never failed, "May the Brush supersede the Laurel!"

Futile Act of 1814

By 1819 it had been amply proved that all but a few difficult chimneys could be swept, and better swept, by suitable mechanical brushes and that the difficult chimneys were the very chimneys most dangerous for boys. It had also been proved that special brushes if properly worked brought certainly no more, and probably less, dirt into rooms than the boys brought but that master-sweeps when using machines would often purposely smother the furniture with soot in order to prejudice housewives and servants against them. In 1814 an Act had been placed on the Statute Book forbidding the climbing of chimneys by children, and yet in the 'sixties the employment of boys for the purpose was actually increasing. Year after year children were bought and sold to a life of dirt and suffering, ending for many of them by the dreadful chimney-sweep's cancer. Year after year a child or two from the miserable number reaped local notoriety by being asphyxiated in a flue. Year after year persons otherwise kindly and humane continued to have their chimneys swept by children. The child's tender skin had to be hardened for the work. This was done close by a hot fire by rubbing the elbows and knees with the strongest brine. The master sweep stood over the children with a cane or coaxed them by the promise of a halfpenny if they would stand a few more rubs. At first they came back from their work with their arms and legs covered with raw areas and with their knees bleeding from wounds where the skin had been torn away. Then they were rubbed with brine again and set off up another chimney!

Charles Dickens takes up the Fight, 1837

In 1834 the reformed Parliament passed a mild Act, forbidding the binding as apprentice of any boy under ten, and ordering that before apprenticeship a boy was to be examined by two magistrates, and was not to be bound unless *willing and desirous to follow the Business of a Chimney Sweeper*. Charles Dickens immortalized this Act in the scene in *Oliver Twist* (1837), where Oliver, before being bound to the villainous master-sweep, Gamfield, appears before two old magistrates.

"Well," said the old gentlemen, "I suppose he's fond of chimney-sweeping?" "He doats on it, your worship," replied Bumble; giving Oliver a sly pinch, to intimate that he had better not say he didn't.

Oliver is only saved from his fate by the accident that the short-sighted magistrate, in searching for the ink-bottle, catches sight of his terrified face.

Dead Letter Act of 1834

The Act of 1834 also ordered that in future new flues, unless they were circular, measuring 12 inches in diameter, were to measure 14 inches by

9 inches, so that the danger of suffocation or jamming should be diminished. Directions were also given about angles, and a penalty of £100 laid down for failure to conform to these building regulations; but as no machinery was indicated by which these provisions could be carried out, they were a dead letter.

Charles Kingsley's Climbing Boy, 1863

In 1863 Charles Kingsley wrote *Water Babies*, making the small, ill-treated and ill-behaved Tom, the climbing boy, its central figure (fig. 58).

Once upon a time there was a little chimney-sweep, and his name was Tom. That is a short name, and you have heard it before, so you will not have much trouble in remembering it. He lived in a great town in the North country, where there were plenty of chimneys to sweep and plenty of money for Tom to earn and his master to spend. He could not read or write, and did not care to do either; and he never washed himself, for there was no water up the court where he lived. He had never been taught to say his prayers. He never had heard of God, or of Christ, except in words which you never have heard, and which it would have been well if he had never heard. He cried half his life, and laughed the other half. He cried when he had to climb the dark flues, rubbing his poor knees and elbows raw; and when the soot got into his eyes, which it did every day in the week; and when his master beat him, which he did every day in the week; and when he had not enough to eat, which happened every day in the week likewise. And he laughed the other half of the day, when he was tossing halfpennies with the other boys, or playing leap-frog over the posts, or bowling stones at the horses' legs as they trotted by, which last was excellent fun, when there was a wall at hand behind which to hide. As for chimney-sweeping, and being hungry, and being beaten, he took all that for the way of the world, like the rain and snow and thunder, and stood manfully with his back to it till it was over, as his old donkey did to a hailstorm; and then shook

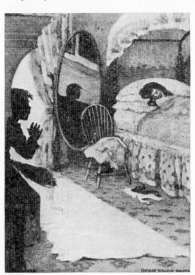

Fig. 58.—Tom, the Climbing Boy, in Charles Kingsley's *Water Babies*, 1863
(*After Jessie Willcox Smith*)

his ears and was as jolly as ever; and thought of the fine times coming, when he would be a man, and a master sweep, and sit in the public-house with a quart of beer and a long pipe, and play cards for silver money, and wear velveteens and ankle-jacks, and keep a white bulldog with one grey ear, and carry her puppies in his pocket, just like a man. And he would have apprentices, one, two, three, if he could. How he would bully them, and knock them about, just as his master did to him; and make them carry home the soot sacks, while he rode before them on his donkey, with a pipe in his mouth and a flower in his button-hole, like a king at the head of his army. Yes, there were good times coming; and, when his master let him have a pull at the leavings of his beer, Tom was the jolliest boy in the whole town.

Lord Shaftesbury victorious in 1875

In 1875 victory over this evil was at last secured, although 102 years had passed since Hanway had first brought it before the public. The struggle is vividly described by J. L. and Barbara Hammond in *Lord Shaftesbury* (1923):

A Bill introduced by Shaftesbury in 1875 brought these scandals to an end. The Bill proposed that no chimney-sweep should be allowed to carry on his trade without a licence from the police, to be renewed annually. For offences against the Acts of 1840 and 1864, sweeps could be deprived of the licence, and, most important of all, it was declared to be the business of the police to enforce those Acts.

Thus Shaftesbury removed at last from our social life a disgrace that was peculiar to the British Isles. That he succeeded, after all his exertions, by adopting a method which had been considered in 1788, when men and women were still hung for petty theft, reflects at once on the conscience of the Victorian age and on his own sense for practical remedies. But his perseverance and his humanity stand out in sharp contrast to the apathy of the politicians and the cynicism of the magistrates, and had he done nothing else in the course of his long life, he would have lived in history by this record alone.

BIBLIOGRAPHY

ARLIDGE, J. T. (1892), *The Hygiene, Diseases and Mortality of Occupations*, Percival, London.

BLAKE, W. (1789), *Songs of Innocence*, London ; (1794), *Songs of Experience*, London.

BROWNING, E. B. (1843), *The Cry of the Children*, Palgrave's Golden Treasury, Macmillan, London.

BRYANT, A. (1950), *The Age of Elegance*, Collins, London.

COLE, G. D. H. (1925), *A Short History of the British Working Class Movement, 1789–1927*, Vol. I, London.

DICKENS, C. (1854), *Hard Times*, London.

DISRAELI, B. (1845), *Sybil, or the Two Nations*, London.

ENGELS, F. (1892), *Condition of the Working Classes in 1844*, London, p. 170.

GREG, R. H. (1837), *The Factory Question*, Cobbett, London.

HAMMOND, J. L., and HAMMOND, B. (1917), *The Town Labourer*, Longmans, Green, London; (1923), *Lord Shaftesbury*, Penguin Books, London; (1934), *The Bleak Age*, Penguin Books, London.

HENRY, S. A. (1944), *Public Health*, **57**, 121 ; (1946), *Cancer of the Scrotum in Relation to Occupation*, Oxford University Press, London.

HITCHIN, G. (1967), *The Listener*, **78**, 242, London.

HOOD, T. (1843), *Punch*, **5**, 260, London.

HUTT, W. H. (1926), *Economica*, **6**, 78.

KINGSLEY, C. (1849), *Alton Locke*, London; (1863), *Water Babies*, London.

LAMB, C. (1823), *Essays of Elia*, London.

LEGGE, T. M. (1920), *J. industr. Hyg.*, **1**, 578.

STATHAM, I. C. F. (1951), *Coalmining*, English Universities Press, London.

SWANSTON, C. (1949), *Proc. Ninth Internat. Congr. Industr. Med.*, *London*, Wright, Bristol, p. 966.

TELEKY, L. (1948), *History of Factory and Mine Hygiene*, Columbia University Press, New York.

THOMSON, D. (1950), *England in the Nineteenth Century*, Penguin Books, London.

TREVELYAN, G. M. (1942), *English Social History*, Longmans, Green; New York.

TROLLOPE, F. (1840), *The Life and Adventures of Michael Armstrong, the Factory Boy*, Colburn, London.

UNDERWOOD, E. A. (1948), *Brit. med. J.*, **1**, 890.

WELLS, H. G. (1920), *The Outline of History*, Cassell, London.

WILSON, C. (1954), *The History of Unilever*, Cassell, London.

WOODHAM-SMITH, CECIL (1950), *Florence Nightingale*, Constable, London.

WRIGHT, G. P. (1945), *Guy's Hospital Gazette*, **59**, 301.

CHAPTER IV

HEALTH OF THE WORKER IN THE TWENTIETH CENTURY

SOCIALLY and historically the conditions and life of the industrial worker lie near the foundation of the well-being of an industrial people. In England that vital issue was raised at the beginning of the Industrial Revolution in the middle of the eighteenth century, and it has remained with us, increasing in magnitude and complexity as the population and the various industries have expanded. Its development is one of the most impressive in our social annals. Its lessons of triumph and failure have been carried to the ends of the earth. For England was the first of the civilized nations to embark, all unwittingly, upon a rapid and unforeseen evolution of industrial enterprise. In some ways she has been surpassed by her foreign competitors, but she remains the originator of mechanical invention by a whole people. For it was England which first learned the great principles of restricting the hours of labour, of safeguarding the health of the factory worker, of exploring the effect of occupation upon health, and of the prevention of its ills and accidents. It was England also which contrived methods of State control in the form of the Factory Acts.

THE PROGRESS OF SCIENCE AFTER 1830

In order to understand the occupational diseases of the twentieth century it is necessary to know something of the progress of science in the modern period—that is, from the end of the Industrial Revolution about 1830 to the present time. Certain points in this progress will be touched upon under the headings (a) chemistry, (b) engineering and (c) metallurgy.

(a) Chemistry

We have seen (p. 88) how the close of the Industrial Revolution coincided with the birth of organic chemistry in the synthesis of urea (1828). From that date new branches of chemical industry gradually emerged along with studies of the aromatic, aliphatic, naphthene and olefine hydrocarbons in that order. The chemistry of the coal-tar derivatives (p. 506) and electro-chemistry (p. 303) were developments of the first half of the nineteenth century. Nitroglycerine (p. 584) and the nitrocelluloses (p. 590) came in the second half of the nineteenth century. The halogenated hydrocarbons (p. 594) and the petroleum chemical industry (p. 154) were developments of the twentieth century.

Hydrochloric-acid Gas a Public Nuisance

In 1830 noxious fumes from chemical works became a public nuisance. Legislation was introduced to control them, until today the provisions of the *Alkali Act* apply to innumerable chemical processes. We have seen (p. 85) how the Leblanc process came into being in France in 1790. In England it was set up on a large scale both in Liverpool and at St. Helens. The escape of large quantities of hydrochloric-acid gas caused much annoyance and destruction of vegetation in the neighbourhood, and the local landowners sought redress in the courts. The problem was solved in 1830 by William Gossage, who knocked the floor out of a derelict stone windmill near his factory, filled the interior with brushwood and passed the waste gas upward against a descending stream of water which effectively washed out the acid. Gossage patented his invention in 1836. The Leblanc process was worked with great success for more than a century. The ammonia-soda process appeared only in 1873, when John Brunner and Ludwig Mond began to operate their plant in Winnington, Cheshire (Williams, 1935).

The Alkali Works Regulations Act, 1906

This Act is a consolidation and extension of earlier Acts with similar titles. The Act of 1863 dealt with alkali works only; manufacturers were required to absorb at least 95 per cent of the hydrochloric acid in their waste gases. Subsequent extensions of the Act up to 1906 brought within its scope a wide range of chemical processes. Finally, power was included in the *Public Health Act, 1926*, to extend the provisions of the Alkali Act to any other chemical processes which are considered to cause serious pollution. A public inquiry is held before each extension, and the authority of an order laid before Parliament is required for any extension. As now extended, the provisions of the Act apply to about 2,000 chemical processes in 1,000 works.

The Registration of Chemical Works

The Alkali Act calls for registration of all works which are subject to its provisions, and the registration is renewed annually. Before a works can be registered, the Chief Alkali Works Inspector has to be satisfied that the works are provided with the best means which are practicable to prevent the escape of noxious and offensive gases and to render such gases harmless and inoffensive. In some cases the Act lays down standards for the amount of fume which may be emitted, namely 4 grains of sulphur trioxide per cubic foot from sulphuric-acid works, 1·5 grains of sulphur trioxide per cubic foot from works concentrating sulphuric acid and 0·2 grains of hydrochloric acid per cubic foot from hydrochloric-acid works. The Act leaves it to the Chief Inspector to decide what are the best practicable means of dealing with a case of emission of fume. In the last resort, where there is no completely satisfactory method of treating the fumes to render them harmless, the knowledge of the effect of the height of a chimney on dispersion of fume is applied in dealing with the residue after such treatment as may be possible.

Staff of the Inspectorate

The staff of the Inspectorate under the Alkali Act is attached in England to the Ministry of Housing and Local Government and in Scotland to the Department of Health for Scotland. In England and Wales the staff consists of one Chief Inspector, one Deputy Chief and seven District Inspectors. They are recruited from men who have had about ten years' experience in responsible positions in chemical industry. There is close co-operation between the chemical industry and the inspectors, so that prosecutions have rarely been necessary. Factories in the possession of the Crown, such as certain explosives factories, are not subject in law to the provisions of the Alkali Act, but in practice there is a working arrangement that they comply with them. On the other hand, factories in the possession of public boards, such as the nationalized industries, are subject in law to its provisions. Any air pollution from the chemical industry which falls outside the scope of the Alkali Act comes, together with general industrial air pollution, under the provisions of the Public Health Act. Local Authorities are responsible for administering these provisions, but in cases of any technical complexity they generally seek the advice of the Alkali Works Inspectorate (Damon, 1953).

The Beaver Committee and the Clean Air Act, 1956

In 1954 the Beaver Committee recommended that, "in the case of certain industrial processes in which the prevention of dark smoke, grit, or harmful gases present special technical difficulties, responsibility for ensuring that the best practicable means of prevention are used at all times should be vested in the Alkali Inspectorate and the Provisions of the *Alkali Acts* should be extended accordingly." The Government accepted this recommendation, and, as a result of the *Clean Air Act of 1956*, the responsibilities of the inspectorates were greatly increased on 1st June 1958. Then the *Alkali Act* was extended to cover eleven more classes of works which include many metallurgical processes, power stations, gas and coke works, coal-fired producer gas plants, certain types of ceramic kilns, and coal-burning lime kilns. Although such an increased load could well have crippled the inspectorate, in 1958 the Chief Alkali Inspectors in the *95th Annual Report* claimed that they had shouldered the burden with no signs of administrative collapse. They report an increase of registered works from 872 at the end of 1957 to 2,160 at the end of 1958, and state that the number of separate processes at the works has increased from 1,733 to 3,412. In its advisory capacity the inspectorate has inherited vast technological problems in the prevention of serious air pollution. The iron and steel and the ceramics industries, for example, are beset with problems which are admitted at present to be almost insoluble and demand the continuance of intensive research, which the inspectorate must actively encourage. The Chief Inspectors gallantly acknowledge their formidable responsibilities and report the establishment of good liaison with the new industries. In 1956 Sir Hugh Beaver paid tribute to the inspectorate, which, he says, "owes much of its undoubted and beneficial influence to the fairness and friendliness of its approach", but he states emphatically that "all industrial pollution should be subject to a continuous and sharp challenge".

Chemistry of the Aromatic Compounds: The First Aniline Dye

We have already discussed (p. 88) the emergence of organic chemistry towards the end of the Industrial Revolution. The second half of the nineteenth century was marked by spectacular advances in coal-tar chemistry. Organic chemistry rests upon the theory of molecular structure pro-

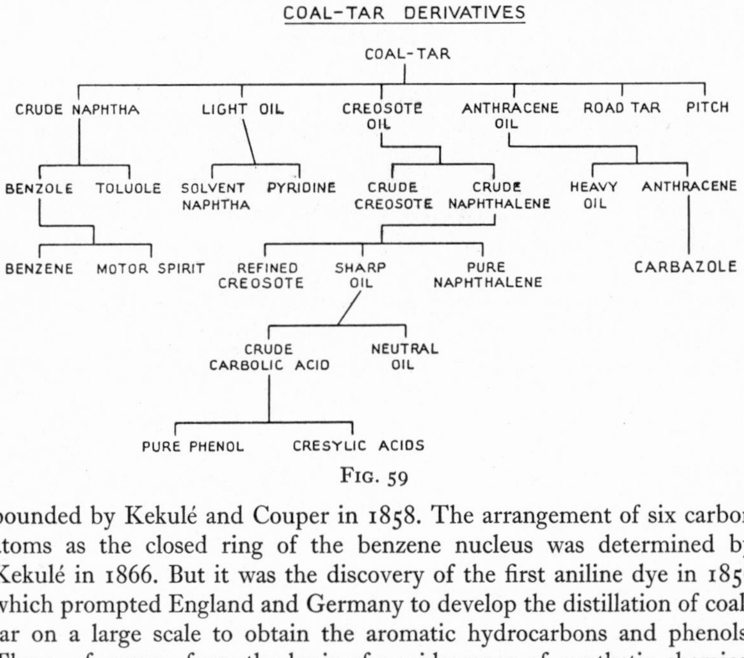

FIG. 59

pounded by Kekulé and Couper in 1858. The arrangement of six carbon atoms as the closed ring of the benzene nucleus was determined by Kekulé in 1866. But it was the discovery of the first aniline dye in 1856 which prompted England and Germany to develop the distillation of coal-tar on a large scale to obtain the aromatic hydrocarbons and phenols. These, of course, form the basis of a wide range of synthetic chemical substances, which make up a large branch of the chemical industry today (fig. 59).

Sir William Henry Perkin, 1838–1907

Although picric acid had been used previously to dye fabrics yellow, the dramatic colouring produced by aniline purple is always referred to as the first aniline dye. In 1845 August Wilhelm von Hofmann (1818–92), German chemist and pupil of Liebig, accepted the invitation of the Prince Consort to become the first director of the new Royal College of Chemistry in Oxford Street, London. This was later absorbed into the Imperial College of Science, South Kensington. His first research was upon coal-tar and it established the chemical composition of aniline. In the Easter vacation of 1856 a pupil of von Hofmann, William Henry Perkin (1838–1907), decided to synthesize quinine! Having left the City of London School at the age of 15 he was only 18 at the time. The work was independently contrived and was carried out in the attic of his father's house in Shadwell, London. He oxidized aniline with chromic acid and washed the resulting tarry mass with alcohol. A purple solution resulted. This he called aniline purple or mauveine. It was the first synthetic dye (fig. 60). In 1857 he devised a process for its commercial manufacture and the Perkin family founded at Greenford Green a company to exploit it.

The young Perkin was inspired with a sense of mission and he never faltered when this took him into the unfamiliar realms of chemical technology and commerce. Mauve proved to be a fast dye for silks and cottons and was a great success. It was used to colour the lilac penny postage stamp of Queen Victoria's reign. In 1869 Perkin and Sons made one ton of alizarin paste, and in 1873, 435 tons (fig. 61). But in 1874 the family sold the Greenford works, and after his retirement from business at thirty-six Perkin devoted himself to pure research.

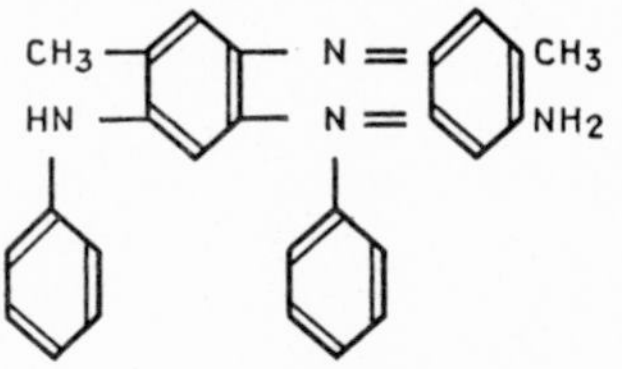

ANILINE PURPLE

MAUVEINE

FIG. 60

The Perkin Family of Organic Chemists

This historic discovery marked the birth of the synthetic dyestuffs industry and the greater part of the organic chemical industry of the world. From these small beginnings have sprung dyes, explosives, insecticides, perfumes, flavouring essences and pharmaceutical substances, textile and rubber chemicals, as well as plastics and synthetic fibres, for Perkin's discovery turned organic chemistry from an academic study into a matter of world-wide industrial importance. Three sons of Sir William Perkin inherited various aspects of the genius of their father and like him became chemists. William Henry Perkin, jun. (1860–1929) after working some time in his father's laboratory in London joined the brilliant group that clustered round Adolf von Baeyer in Munich. He studied brazilin, hæmatoxylin and complex alkaloids such as berberine, strychnine and brucine. As a lecturer and teacher generally he was extremely successful, especially because of a clear lucidity of exposition. As Waynflete professor of chemistry he produced in Oxford a change of attitude to chemistry, establishing there a strong school of original research. Like his father he was admitted into the Fellowship of the Royal Society. Arthur George Perkin (1861–1937) worked in the Dyeing Department of the Yorkshire College, later the University of Leeds. For a long period of years he studied the constituents of dyewoods and other sources of natural colouring matters. Thus he improved the method of isolation of luteolin from the natural yellow dye weld (see pp. 19, 86) and showed that it is a tetrahydroxyflavone. Perkin's third son, Frederick Mollwo Perkin (1870–1928), collaborated with his brother Arthur in many researches and became a successful technical consultant. It should be noted that all the Perkins were musicians and there was a family orchestra of almost professional calibre (Robinson, 1956).

Fire and Explosion in the Early Coal-tar Industry

Another of Hofmann's pupils, Charles Blachford Mansfield, undertook a systematic study of coal-tar. He devised a still for fractionating tar oils by the reflux principle, and in this way he isolated benzene and characterized it with great precision. His paper, *Researches on Coal Tar, Part 1* (1849), is therefore of considerable historic interest. He also isolated toluene and two higher homologues. Unhappily, he never lived to complete his work, for in 1855 when he was only thirty-five years of age he met with an accident in London due to the ignition of hydrocarbons he was distilling; he was burnt so severely that he died. About 1868 Edward Chambers Nicholson, another of Hofmann's pupils, improved the large-scale production of nitrobenzene and aniline by replacing glass flasks with cast-iron stills. In the pioneer years serious damage was done in one chemical works by the explosion of aniline machines, and in another works the nitration shed was usually referred to among the workmen as the shooting gallery, owing to accidents which occasionally befell the plant and operators.

Dye Intermediates

Synthetic dyes, which have almost entirely replaced natural dyes in the textile industry, are largely manufactured from the products of the distillation of coal-tar, the principal raw materials being benzene, naphthalene, toluene and anthracene (fig. 59). From these relatively simple organic compounds, a wide range of complex *intermediates* is manufactured. These are made in a number of stages; the first and simpler compounds, such as aniline, nitrobenzene and nitrotoluene, are known as *primaries* and are made in very large quantities.

NATURAL DYESTUFFS

I   MADDER, root of *RUBIA TINCTORUM*

TURKEY RED, 3000 B.C.

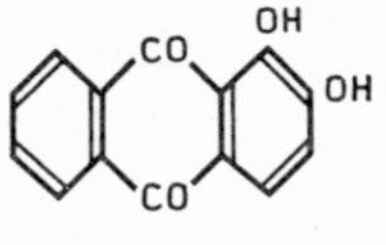

ALIZARIN, 1868 A.D.

II *MUREX BRANDARIS* :   A ROCK-WHELK

TYRIAN PURPLE, 3000 B.C.

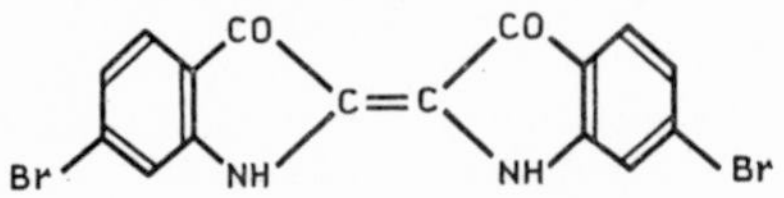

DI-BROM INDIGO, 1890 A.D.

FIG. 61

Predominance of the German Colour Industry

In 1906, on the jubilee of his discovery of mauveine, Perkin was knighted. On this occasion Carl Duisberg, afterwards Director-in-Chief of the Interessen Gemeinschaft, made a speech in which he said that the predominance of the German colour industry was due to fundamental differences between the two countries as regards national temperament and

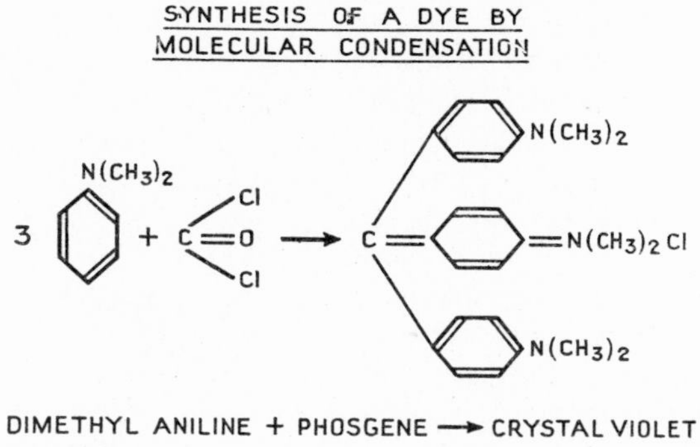

SYNTHESIS OF A DYE BY
MOLECULAR CONDENSATION

DIMETHYL ANILINE + PHOSGENE ⟶ CRYSTAL VIOLET

FIG. 62

outlook. In 1914 Great Britain was the greatest textile-producing country in the world. In that year the dye-making trade, worth £2,000,000, subserved the needs of a textile trade worth £200,000,000; 80 per cent of the dyes were imported and even the 20 per cent of home-made dyes were largely produced from foreign intermediates. In 1914 the misuse of the German chemical industry to make war taught England and the United States of America to develop adequate chemical industries of their own.

Perfumes and Flavouring Essences

A particularly interesting branch of the organic chemical industry is that concerned with the preparation of perfumes and flavouring essences. Many of these are derived from natural sources such as flowers and plants. For example, citral, citronellal and cinnamaldehyde are aromatic substances extracted from oils of lemon grass, citronella and cassia respectively. From oil of caraway is derived a substance known as carvone, which is used in making kümmel and other liqueurs. Many of these natural products are now made synthetically; in addition, the organic chemist can now offer a wide range of pleasantly aromatic substances which are unknown in nature. This branch of the industry may be said to have had its beginnings in Britain, for as long ago as 1868 Perkin synthesized coumarin, a valuable natural aromatic substance largely responsible for the odour of newly mown hay. Natural coumarin is obtained from the tonka bean; it is used for scenting tobacco, soap and cosmetics. A number of artificial musks are made by treating a coal-tar hydrocarbon with nitric acid. A substance known as terpineol, a lilac-like perfume much used in the soap industry, is

made from pinene, contained in oil of turpentine, by a series of complicated chemical transformations. Vanillin, which gives natural vanilla its
characteristic flavour, is made in considerable quantities from eugenol,
which comprises almost the whole of oil of cloves, and from waste products of the manufacture of wood pulp. From oil of anise is obtained a
substance called anethole; this can be transformed into anisaldehyde,
which has an odour of hawthorn (Williams, 1953).

Chemistry of Aliphatic Compounds

One of the earliest developments in modern chemical industry was
based on the development of nitroglycerine, dynamite and cordite (see
p. 585). For civil engineering, especially building tunnels, and for blasting
rock and soil to provide raw materials such as coal and limestone for industry, high explosives are in constant demand. In 1938 Great Britain
used 21,000 tons of high explosives for blasting, a great part of it in coal
mines where 63 million shots were fired in the course of one year. Today
the production of nitrocellulose and cellulose acetate is even more important for the manufacture of lacquers and plastics than for explosives
(p. 590).

The Petroleum Chemical Industry

The use of petroleum as a raw material resembles that of coal. As might
be expected from the existence of immense deposits of petroleum within
its own frontiers, the United States of America has taken a leading part in
this new industry and already uses two million tons annually for this purpose. In Great Britain, although the petroleum chemical industry is of
comparatively recent growth, it is already producing many chemical substances originally derived from other sources such as coal and agricultural
products. In spite of the stable chemical nature of paraffin hydrocarbons,
processes have been developed for their oxidation, chlorination and nitration, thus producing a wide variety of substances. Whereas the destructive
distillation of wood is still carried out to produce methyl alcohol and acetone, and the fermentation of carbohydrates is still used in the production
of ethyl, propyl and butyl alcohols, the petroleum industry now makes all
these substances from natural gas and the gases derived from the cracking
of petroleum.

Chemistry of the Olefines

Crude petroleum is a mixture of aliphatic, aromatic and naphthene
hydrocarbons, and certain of these are extracted and used directly for
chemical production, but the main source of chemical substances is a
further type of hydrocarbon—the olefine or unsaturated type, which is
produced by processes such as cracking. This process consists of heating a
petroleum product to a high temperature and pressure, causing large molecules, such as decane, $C_{10}H_{22}$, to break up into smaller ones such as octane,
C_8H_{18}, liberating ethylene, C_2H_4. Besides ethylene, other gases containing

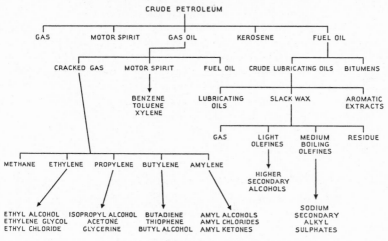

FIG. 63

high proportions of olefines such as propylene, butylene and amylene are liberated by cracking (fig. 63). Lately, five cracking plants have been erected in Great Britain, aimed primarily at ethylene production. As a result the consumption of ethylene has increased tenfold since 1950. It now stands at 70,000 tons annually and is still increasing. In the plastics industry, ethylene is polymerized under 1,500 atmospheres pressure to make *polythene* (p. 161). Xylene, necessary for the manufacture of *terylene*, is being made from petroleum (Williams, 1953).

Synthetic Detergents

Soap making is one of the oldest of chemical industries, but today soap has many rivals in the shape of synthetic detergents. These are the more significant in a world which is short of fats and alkalis. The very long-chain paraffin hydrocarbons which form paraffin wax can be separated from petroleum by chilling or by solvent precipitation, and then cracked to give olefines. A special variety of the latter process is the production of higher olefines for conversion to synthetic detergents by sulphonation and neutralization. These are termed sodium secondary alkyl sulphates and form the basis of *teepol*. They are surface active agents or wetting agents with properties like soap, but because they form soluble calcium salts they have the advantage of lathering even in hard water. Since they do not form a scum comparable to the calcium soaps, they are ideal for removing dirt and grease, especially from wool and hair, and as ingredients of shampoos. In the United States of America synthetic detergents are now made to the extent of 350,000 tons a year, a figure roughly equivalent to one-quarter of the normal soap production.

(b) Engineering

An important step in the building up of a specialized engineering industry was taken in 1795 when Boulton and Watt ceased merely to supervise the construction of engines and established the Soho Foundry in Birmingham. Similar engineering workshops grew up in London. Between them they devised more precise methods for the planing, drilling, cutting and turning of metals. As a result of these advances in technique, there arose in the second half of the nineteenth century a big engineering and machine-tool industry. This was the process which turned the average Englishman from a countryman into an urban industrial worker, thereby creating a new era in English history.

James Nasmyth and Henry Bessemer

In some respects the more important of the results of Watt's discoveries was the use of machines for making machines. For how could he make good steam engines, if he had no means of boring a true cylinder or of turning a true piston-rod or of planing a valve face? After 1820, with the rapidly growing demand for machinery from all parts of the world, the importance of mechanical engineering grew at a rapid rate. The scope and power of the industry were increased by a series of inventions such as James Nasmyth's steam hammer in 1838, and by discoveries associated with the names of Henry Bessemer (1856), the brothers Siemens (1866) and Snelus (1879), which created the modern steel manufacture (see p. 57). All the metal industries were helped further by the chemical discoveries of which Michael Faraday had made a beginning in 1826, discoveries that created in their turn the successful chemical industries of Lancashire and Cheshire.

England as the Workshop of the World

The effect of all this energy in scientific pursuits and industrial enterprises was to make England the leading representative of the new civilization: the workshop of the world. The heavy industries were growing fast. By 1871 more than three-quarters of a million were employed in metal, engineering and shipbuilding trades. The development of machinery meant that 106,000 were engaged in making machines. The years of Gladstone's first Ministry were marked by a big boom in trade. There was an almost universal inflation of credit and business, as well as of prices. This was the period when Britain enjoyed to the full the economic benefits of having become the workshop of the world. Her total exports in 1850 were worth £71,000,000; in 1870 they were worth nearly £200,000,000. Modern Britain—industrialized, mechanized and urbanized—was coming into being. Already suburbanism, at least around London, had begun: more than 3,254,000 people lived in the capital, constituting a city of unprecedented size (Thomson, 1950).

Stimulus from the Railways

As we have already seen, in England, where the sea was nowhere very far distant, an Industrial Revolution had occurred before the railways, because canals and roads could give access to the ports. In the two countries where industrial expansion was most rapid in the latter half of the nineteenth century—Germany and the United States—the industrial revolution began with the introduction of the railway. The demand for railways abroad underlay the boom in iron, steel and coal in England. It was mechanical engineering that received the greatest stimulus from railway expansion, and when the world wanted railways, docks and ships, England was ready with the plant, the experience, the capital and the skill. Hence it was to English capital and English labour that the world turned for the task. But there was this difference between the early days of the revolution, when England sold piece-goods all over the world, and the later, when she sold railways; for the railways she sold were turning peasant into industrial societies, and it was certain that when this change had taken place, England's preponderant share in the trade of the world would decline. When the twentieth century opened, England had powerful industrial rivals both in and out of Europe (Hammond, 1929).

Use of Steel on a Massive Scale

During the twentieth century, building with steel has been carried out on a gigantic scale. The Forth Bridge and Sydney Harbour Bridge each contains over 50,000 tons of steel. In Great Britain alone, over ten million tons of iron and steel are used in our railway line system and two million tons in locomotives. A liner such as the *Queen Mary* is made with about 80,000 tons of steel, compared with only a few hundred tons of all other metals. As an illustration of the scale of manufacture of iron and steel, four large blast furnaces today can produce in one year a million tons of pig iron from which steel is made. In the year 1954 steel production in Great Britain reached the record figure of nearly nineteen million tons.

Open-cast Mining of Iron Ore

The open-cast mining of iron ore is being carried out by what has been called the robber economy of the twentieth century. It is to be seen in its worst form in the open country of the East Midlands. Here, along the foot of an escarpment which runs from the Humber down into Northamptonshire and on into Oxfordshire, are immense deposits of iron ore, the most extensive and valuable in Britain. The ore is *siderite* or *spathic iron ore*, ferrous carbonate, $FeCO_3$, containing only 48 per cent of iron, but although it is low-grade, it is comparitively accessible and is worked cheaply by open-cast methods. The biggest workings are around Scunthorpe in Lincolnshire, and around Kettering and Corby in Northamptonshire. Already more than 3,000 acres in Northamptonshire are completely derelict, a monstrous waste-land which may be seen near Corby (fig. 64).

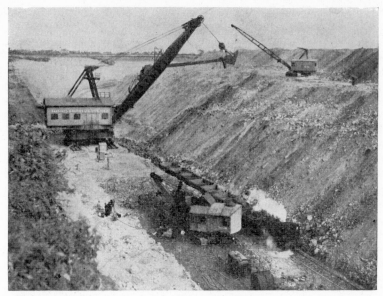

FIG. 64.—Open-cast Iron-ore Mining. The Large Shovel is removing Overburden, the Lower Shovel is digging out the actual Ironstone
(*B.I.S.F., by courtesy of Mr. D. J. O. Brandt*)

Vast Farmlands Derelict

Because the reserves of iron ore are so enormous, the possibility remains of another 90,000 acres being devastated in the county of Northamptonshire alone, most of it valuable farmland. In such a small country as England, closely packed with 50,000,000 people, every acre of land has a number of competing uses—for example, housing, farming and recreation. And yet, owing to the rapidity with which the ore is uncovered and the increasing depth at which it lies, it is said to be technically impossible to replace the soil cover in many places. The enormous rifts created by mechanical excavators may be seen in many parts of Lincolnshire, Rutland, Leicestershire and Northamptonshire.

The Robber Economy of the Twentieth Century

Although the quarrying of ironstone has gone on spasmodically since Domesday at least, nearly all this development is the work of the last hundred years, and most of it of the last two generations. In 1921 Corby was a village of about 1,600 people, whereas in 1951 it had 12,000 people. As one of the new towns to be created under the *New Towns Act of 1946*, it aims to have a population of 40,000 all dependent on one industry. In 1951, Scunthorpe, at the northern end of the iron-ore belt, was a borough with more than 50,000 people. In 1842 it was described as a village and township, pleasantly seated on an eastern declivity of the Wolds, with a population of 249 and a little under a thousand acres of fertile land, complete with its farmers, its village blacksmith, wheelwright, corn miller, mason, tailor, shoemaker, bricklayer, carrier and victualler. It was a typical Midland village living entirely off its fertile land. Now, with its great ironworks, it has multiplied itself two hundred times over in a hundred years.

The Amalgamated Society of Engineers

In 1851 was formed the famous Amalgamated Society of Engineers, with some 11,000 members, including nearly all the engineering unions. Thus the new unions, based on particular kinds of skilled industrial labour, grew up on a firmer basis than the old. They were stronger financially and more open in their discussions and activity. They were still, like their predecessors, hampered by legal restrictions and prohibitions, but they were not driven into behaving like secret societies. Insurance and social benefits were a large part of their work, as well as collective bargaining with employers. An embryonic trades union congress met in Manchester in 1868, and represented some 118,000 trade unionists. About 1873 the unions were given greater legal protection, both for their own internal funds and organization and for their favourite methods of collective bargaining and peaceful picketing. When Gladstone formed his first Ministry, trade unionism was an accepted and well-established feature of English industrial life. That its growth was relatively so smooth and peaceful was largely due to the victories won by the defunct unions of the days of Owen and to the repeal of the Combination Laws in 1824-5. They could now grow in step with the development of industrialization, as part of it and of English life.

Electrical Power applied to Industry

A second phase in engineering began with the application of electrical power to practical problems of transmission and traction. When the electric motor was first employed in industry, it was used merely as an alternative device for carrying out existing techniques. In the twentieth century the typical picture of a factory is no longer a line of shafting supplemented by pulleys and belts. The electric motor is a mode of distributing power which is very convenient to construct in small sizes so that the individual machine may have its motor. The change from the old system to the new is still going on. For example, in 1951 a jute mill was opened in Dundee in which every machine had an individual drive from a separate motor. In the whole factory there were 204 electric motors totalling 1,447 horse-powei. The transmission losses in the wiring of such a factory are low, and the efficiency of the motor itself high. The connexion of the motor with its wiring is not necessarily rigid, nor does it consist of many parts. Moreover, should it be so desired a single piece of machinery may contain several motors each introducing power at the proper place. Since power can be readily made available in country districts, factories need no longer be crowded together in towns, and where necessary industry can return to the old domestic type within the worker's own house (Wiener, 1950).

The Internal-combustion Engine

In 1889 Hiram Maxim built an aeroplane driven by steam engines. It weighed three tons and its crash occurred just as a further revolution ushered in a new type of engine. This was the internal-combustion engine, in which the expansive force of an explosive mixture replaced that of steam. The light, highly efficient engines that were thus made possible were applied to the motor car and developed at last to reach such a pitch of lightness and efficiency as to render flight through the air a practical achievement. The first aeroplane flight was made by the Wright brothers in 1903, and in 1906 a new discovery occurred in metallurgy which made possible the performance first of Zeppelins and other rigid airships and then of aeroplanes as we know them. The discovery was that of aluminium alloys (p. 163), which are so light that structures made with them are stronger than steel but only half the weight. But both the Wright brothers and Count Zeppelin would have been helpless without the internal-combustion engine as a source of motive power.

The Jet-turbine Aeroplane Engine

In the Second World War the invention of the jet-turbine aeroplane engine was brought to practical success by systematic research upon non-ferrous alloys (p. 165). Improvements were made until nickel, chromium, aluminium alloys and others were produced capable of withstanding great stresses at very high temperatures and at the same time of resisting corrosion by the products of combustion. Without these alloys the civilian and military jet aircraft of today could not have attained their present performances.

The Emergence of Chemical Engineering

The first half of the twentieth century saw the emergence of chemical engineering as a profession; this occurred concurrently with the expansion of chemical industry. In the years before 1914 German chemical industry was built up by chemists collaborating with mechanical and civil engineers. Consequently, German chemical plant of that time, and even of a later period, tended to take a similar form to the chemical laboratory apparatus used in research, except for an increase in size. The corresponding modern plant is entirely different because the task of carrying out chemical operations efficiently on a large scale is approached as a problem in its own right. The work is done by chemical engineers whose interests embrace chemistry, physics, mechanical and civil engineering, architecture and economics. The foundations of this new profession were laid in the Massachusetts Institute of Technology in Boston about 1920, and Britain followed this lead in 1922 by founding an Institution of Chemical Engineers (Pearson, 1954).

Polymerizing Gases to make Plastics

We have seen (p. 154) how the petroleum industry produces unsaturated hydrocarbons as by-products of the cracking process. New uses were soon found for these substances, and in 1933 Gibson and Fawcett polymerized ethylene under extreme pressure to produce the plastic *polyethylene*, which is usually called *polythene*. The large-scale production of this substance was a difficult task because ethylene had to be heated to 200° C. at pressures varying between 1,000 and 1,500 atmospheres, conditions similar to those produced in a 15-inch naval gun. In 1939, after many explosions and pipe-bursts, the engineers of Imperial Chemical Industries, Limited, solved this problem and handed the world's first polythene plant over to the works in time to meet the wartime needs of radar. Without polythene the Allied land, sea and airborne radar systems could not have developed as they did in a fashion far superior to anything Germany could produce. The Germans used polystyrene in their radar-location apparatus. It is not flexible and proved inferior as an insulator (Hunter, 1954). Polythene has found a unique place as a high-frequency insulator in the equipment of wireless, television, radar and electronic control apparatus. It is ideal for piping in chemical works, cold-water tubing, surgical drainage tubing, domestic refrigerator trays, kitchen bowls and packaging film. In 1953 K. Ziegler of Mülheim made polythene at low pressures using titanium chloride as a catalyst. In 1954 G. Natta of Milan, following up the work of Ziegler, was able to polymerize propylene to make *polypropylene* and butylene to make *polybutylene*. It is expected that these two new hydrocarbon polymers will find wide application in textiles (Gibbs, 1961).

(c) Metallurgy

Great advances have been made in the art and science of producing metals, their heat treatment, alloying, casting, forging, cutting, welding and fabricating, together with their study by the aid of the microscope.

Native Alloys

Osmiridium is a native alloy mined in Tasmania and South Africa. It contains iridium, osmium, platinum, ruthenium and rhodium. Native alloys are also found in metallic meteorites; they sometimes contain electrum, an alloy of gold and silver. Alloys of iron and nickel, with small quantities of cobalt and chromium, are common constituents of meteorites. At the end of the eighteenth century such a meteorite landed near Cape York in Greenland, and for a hundred years Eskimo hunters used to break off pieces and fashion the alloy into weapons and tools. There was still a mass of nearly forty tons remaining when this meteorite was taken to a museum.

Metallurgy of the Romans in Britain

We have seen (p. 6) how the occurrence in the same mother rock of the ores of tin and copper led to the fortuitous manufacture of bronze, consisting of copper with about one part in ten of tin. It seems clear that metal workers of antiquity understood that if higher contents of tin were used the alloy was harder, while less tin gave a softer alloy, so that for different purposes bronzes with varying tin contents were deliberately produced. By the time the Romans came to Britain they were using iron and bronze for weapons, tools and farming implements; copper for vessels and ornaments; lead for water pipes, baths and coffins; tin, gold and silver for ornaments; and silver, brass and bronze for coinage.

Fourteenth-century Swords of Alloy Steels

The use of steel in China has been traced as far back as 2550 B.C., and certainly the production by empirical methods of steel for sword blades dates back many centuries. The scarcity of copper and the abundance of iron in India makes it probable that with the Hindus the Iron Age was not preceded by a Bronze Age. The process of smelting iron was early practised in the East, and the Hindus acquired considerable skill in the manufacture of wrought iron and steel. This knowledge and skill was carried by emigrants to Damascus, and soon after the downfall of the Roman Empire the manufacture of iron developed in Spain. The famous sword blades of Toledo and Bilbao were the products of Spanish artisans using their peculiar Catalan forge. Mohammedan swords were famous in antiquity for their magnificent blades of Damascene and Toledo steel; some of the extant pieces date back to the fourteenth century. In a similar way in ancient times, Japanese swords acquired a strong individuality, and one of these, dating back to about 1330, has been found to contain molybdenum. It is conceivable that the steel for this sword was fashioned out of the iron in a meteorite.

Nature of Alloys

Two or more metals when fused together usually form a homogeneous liquid; when this solidifies the resulting metallic substance is an alloy. It may be either a solid solution or a pure chemical compound. Of the elements blended, all need not be metals; thus steel is an alloy of iron and carbon. Alloys composed of two major ingredients are called binary alloys and those composed of three ingredients are called ternary alloys.

Reasons for Alloying

In the pure state, certain metals are possessed of only a low tensile strength and are soft and malleable. A particular metal may have properties of great value while being deficient in some other special respect, and the purpose of alloying is to remedy this deficiency. Thus aluminium is light in weight and has good corrosion resistance but is not strong; its alloys combine strength with lightness. Various alloy steels are stronger, harder and tougher than iron; others have special magnetic properties or show increased strength at high temperatures or resist oxidation to the extent of being stainless. Certain beryllium-copper alloys have six times the tensile strength of copper (see p. 429). Antimony is added to lead to harden it, and lead-antimony alloys are used for type-metal, accumulator plates, cable coverings, toy soldiers, ornamental castings and bullets (see p. 234). Lead-tin alloys are used as soft solders and lead-bronze alloys to make bearing-metals for motor-car and aeroplane engines (see p. 234). Stainless chromium-nickel steel is extensively used in the chemical industry because it is resistant to corrosion. Alloying may improve the casting properties or machining properties of a metal; thus tellurium-copper is much easier to work on a lathe than copper itself.

Alloys of every Type

In engineering, nickel-base alloys of great strength and able to resist severe stresses at 900° C. have been devised for use in jet-turbine aircraft engines (see p. 467). Columbium (Cb), formerly known as niobium (Nb), has become important in certain alloy steels, and because of its great corrosion resistance and high melting-point it is used in gas turbines and turbo-superchargers. Beryllium alloys are now in wide use. When 2 per cent of beryllium is added to copper, the alloy produced is hard, corrosion-resistant, non-rusting, non-sparking, non-magnetic and of great tensile strength (see p. 429). When copper is alloyed with 1 per cent of cadmium, the strength and wear resistance are greatly improved without serious impairment of electrical conductivity (see p. 446). In chemistry, cobalt-thorium catalysts are employed in the synthetic production of petrol from coal. In dental surgery, pasty amalgams of mercury, silver and tin are used for fillings in teeth. For jewellery, gold alloyed with palladium or nickel is known as *white gold* (see p. 481).

Silver Alloy Brazing

Low temperature brazing is brazing in the temperature range 600° C. to 850° C. using filler metals based mainly on silver and copper. Of 17 silver brazing alloys in regular use 7 contain cadmium as well as silver and copper (see p. 446). This process is also called silver brazing, silver soldering or hard soldering. It is straightforward for 27 alloys and metals namely cobalt, copper, copper-beryllium, copper-cadmium, copper-, chromium, copper-palladium, copper-silver, copper-tin (bronze), copper-zinc (brass), copper-zinc-nickel, gold, gold alloys, iridium, wrought iron, carbon steel, low alloy steels, mild steel, nickel-beryllium, nickel-silver (German silver, properly nickel-brass), palladium, palladium alloys, platinum, platinum alloys, rhodium, ruthenium, silver and silver alloys. As to the trades concerned in its use it is employed extensively in the manufacture of jewellery, in the joining together of copper pipes and in the manufacture of metal rings (of copper, iron, molybdenum, silver, nickel, tantalum, titanium and tungsten). It is used in the manufacture of refrigerators, motor car petrol tanks, suspension assemblies and wind-screen wiper motors. The electrical industry employs the method for joining electrical assemblies, for the construction of the rotors of induction electric motors and for the assembly of motor armatures. It is used to solder the joints of domestic copper hot water cylinders and to secure cemented tungsten carbide bits to steel drills.

Commercial Production of Steel Alloys

Experiments in the production of steel alloys began with nickel in 1853, and nickel steels came into full commercial use about 1888. They are of high tensile strength and show superior resistance to shock, so that the engineer can design various parts of considerably smaller size than would otherwise be possible. Production of chromium steel began in 1865 and the Eads Bridge built over the Mississippi in 1874 was the first bridge in the world to be built in alloy steel. Chromium is now an essential component of high-speed steel, many of the engineering steels, stainless steels and a large proportion of other corrosion-resistant alloys. The era of alloy steel tools was opened in 1868 when Robert Musket deliberately added tungsten to steel, and since that date chromium, molybdenum and vanadium also have been used. In 1888 Sir Robert Hadfield demonstrated that addition of manganese to steel made it tough and strong. Two main types of alloy containing 1 per cent and 12 per cent of manganese respectively are widely used (see p. 459). In 1889 Hadfield invented silicon steel and showed that it had magnetic properties superior to those of iron. It came into use for electromagnet and transformer stampings. The use of *stalloy* containing 4 per cent of silicon for the cores of electrical transformers has saved millions of tons of coal every year. Vanadium and then titanium were first used about 1907 to make steel alloys with superior resistance to oxidation. For making stainless-steel alloys, molybdenum was first used in 1900 and chromium-nickel in 1912. Cobalt steels were introduced about 1920 and boron steels about 1948.

The Discovery of Age-hardening

In 1880 aluminium was an expensive curiosity worth £7 an ounce and modern metallurgy was scarcely born. Yet by 1943 the annual world output of aluminium had reached two million tons and the price had dropped to 1s. 2d. a pound, making possible the modern aeroplane. Over three-quarters of the weight of the frame of a modern aircraft consists of aluminium alloys, and so does 43·6 per cent of the weight of the Rolls-Royce Merlin aero-engine. In the early days of the twentieth century Dr. Alfred Wilm, a German research metallurgist, was investigating the effect of additions of small quantities of copper and other metals to aluminium in the hope of improving the strength of wrought light-alloy bars and sheets. He tried various combinations and different forms of heat-treatment until, in the autumn of 1906, a revolutionary discovery was made, more or less by accident. An aluminium alloy containing 3·5 per cent copper and 0·5 per cent magnesium was heated and then quenched, and finally tested on a Friday. The results were not particularly impressive. Early in the next week, some doubt was expressed about the accuracy of the tests, so the same pieces of the alloy were tried again. To Wilm's surprise the hardness and strength were much higher than the values already obtained and this led him to perform a series of experiments on the effect of storing the alloy for different periods after heating and quenching. The gradual rise in strength which he discovered, reaching completion in this type of alloy in four or five days, has now become known as *age-hardening*. We now know that a similar phenomenon occurs in numerous alloys both ferrous and non-ferrous. In 1909 Wilm gave to the Durener Metal Works at Duren sole rights to work his patents; hence the name *duralumin* (Alexander and Street, 1951).

The Discovery of Stainless Steel

The discovery of stainless steel is a well-known story. In 1913 Harry Brearley of Sheffield was experimenting with alloy steels for gun barrels and among the samples which he threw aside as being unsuitable was one containing about 14 per cent chromium. Some months later he saw the pile of scrap test pieces and noticed that most of the steels had rusted, but the chromium steel was still bright. This led to the development of stainless steels, as typified by our present-day cutlery which contains chromium 18, nickel 8, tungsten 1 and titanium 1. It was later found that a still more corrosion- and heat-resisting steel with up to about 20 per cent chromium and 10 per cent nickel had many uses in the kitchen, in chemical industry and in bone and joint surgery. With still higher chromium and nickel contents such alloys are used for furnace parts, chemical plant equipment and pump parts.

Alloys of Iron and Nickel

Ferro-nickel alloys have a wide range of magnetic, electrical and thermal properties, depending on the percentage of nickel used. In 1896 Dr. Charles E. Guillaume, of the International Bureau of Weights and Measures of Paris, discovered *invar*, an alloy of iron and nickel which has the property of expanding only to a minute extent with changes of temperature (see p. 466). Nickel features in two alloys used as permanent magnets which are far more powerful than any type of steel magnet. In 1925 nickel cast-irons began to be used giving increased hardness, resistance to wear and strength, together with good machining properties. Brake drums, cylinder liners for internal-combustion engines and cold pressing dies are examples of articles that have been improved by the use of nickel cast-iron.

Non-ferrous Alloys

Happily in Great Britain the light-metals industry was founded upon modern metallurgical research, and it continues to be developed on a scientific foundation. Useful non-ferrous alloys of every description are constantly tested and put into use; by 1950 metallurgists had described 4,600 such alloys. In 1905 Ambrose Monell, President of the International Nickel Company, suggested that the mixed ore from Sudbury, Ontario, should be smelted direct, thus giving a natural alloy of nickel with copper and small quantities of iron, manganese, silicon and carbon. This useful alloy is known as *Monel metal* (see p. 467). Nickel-chromium alloys are or great importance. The alloy nickel 80, chromium 20 possesses a high resistance to the passage of electricity, coupled with resistance to corrosion and to scaling at red heat. It is used for making resistance wires for electric fires, ovens and furnaces.

The Nimonic Series

From the highest grades of nickel-chrome resistance wire an improved series of alloys was developed in the Second World War for use in jet-turbine aeroplane engines (see p. 467). These alloys, known as *Nimonic 75*, *Nimonic 80* and *Nimonic 90*, are capable of withstanding great stresses at temperatures between 750° and 900° C. and at the same time of resisting corrosion by the products of combustion. Cobalt-base alloys also have useful strength at high temperatures. One of these, containing approximately cobalt 67, chromium 28 and molybdenum 5, has been prepared for use in gas-turbine engines. A variation of this alloy known as *vitallium* is used in orthopædic surgery in view of its resistance to corrosion by body fluids.

Metallurgy of the Future

Cæsium, columbium, tantalum, titanium and zirconium are metals, each of which already occupies a special place for specific uses. In the future new alloys will certainly be developed, not so much binary alloys as complex alloys of carefully controlled composition which will be heat-treated to attain optimum properties. In the past, new alloys have been discovered in two ways; some, like stainless steel and duralumin, were found largely by accident, while others, such as the magnesium-zirconium alloys and the zinc-base die-casting alloys, were the result of planned research. Both these methods are bound to continue, but obviously as more is learnt about the fundamental principles of metallurgy, planned research with a definite goal will predominate. At present it is still not possible to foretell with certainty the properties of an alloy made by blending two or more metals of known properties. Metallurgists have been working empirically on the problem for years, but it is only recently that physicists and mathematicians have become interested in theoretical metallurgy, and as a result of their work it may eventually be possible to specify from theoretical considerations the composition and heat-treatment of an alloy needed to provide certain desired properties.

THE RISE OF SOCIALISM

The Founder of Modern Socialism in Britain

It is in connexion with the work of Robert Owen that the word *socialism* first arose about 1827. He is generally regarded as the founder of modern socialism. A point to note about this early socialism is that it was not at first at all democratic. The democratic idea came later. Its early form was patriarchal; it was something up to which the workers were to be educated by liberally disposed employers and leaders. The first socialism was not a workers' movement; it was a masters' movement. Throughout its history the ideology of socialism has been the work mainly of men who were not themselves working men. Tolstoy was a Russian count and Kropotkin was a Russian prince; Saint Simon was a French count and Robert Owen was a cotton manufacturer; Charles Booth was a Liverpool shipowner; Karl Marx married into a family of Prussian aristocrats, and his collaborator Friedrich Engels was the son of a Lancashire cotton spinner; Lenin was an exiled member of a land-owning family and Beatrice Webb the daughter of a capitalist.

Socialism in France

The work of Claude Henri de Rouvroy, Comte de Saint-Simon, attracted little attention while he lived, and it was only after his death that his influence became considerable and that he became known as the founder of French socialism. In his greatest work, the *Nouveau Christianisme* (1825), he endeavours to resolve Christianity into its essential elements and finally propounds the precept:

> The whole of society ought to strive towards the amelioration of the moral and physical existence of the poorest class; society ought to organize itself in the way best adapted for attaining this end.

Pierre Joseph Proudhon of Besançon held a bursary in his native town and within two years he greatly displeased the academy which had granted it by publishing in 1840 *Qu'est-ce la propriété?* which contained the famous words "La propriété, c'est le vol." In the middle of the nineteenth century more and more people became stirred by the dream of universal social justice and saw the supreme evil in private property and the accumulation of wealth by the few.

Economic Doctrines of Karl Marx

But the advocate of world revolution was Karl Marx, an irascible German Jew of great scholarly attainments. He banished God from socialism and emphasized materialism to the point of making it a new religion. In 1847, with his friend Friedrich Engels, he wrote a pamphlet entitled *Manifest der Kommunisten*, which stated:

> The proletarians have nothing to lose but their chains. They have a world to win. Working men of all countries, unite!

He pointed out that property so far as it was power was being gathered together into relatively few hands—those of the capitalist owners. Against these men the workers were bound to develop a common *class consciousness* of the conflict of their interests with those of the rich men.

Marxist Doctrine of Surplus Value

In the massive volumes of *Das Kapital* (1867) his doctrine of *surplus value* is elaborately expounded. In the class struggle the capitalist class is the exploiter and the labouring class the exploited, which will in time over-throw its rulers. The extraction of surplus value from the workers is the means by which the capitalist exploitation is accomplished. By a day's work the labourer produces more than enough for the subsistence of him-self and his family. The capitalist after paying him a subsistence wage is able to keep for himself the rest of the labourer's product. This residue, the fund from which rent, interest and profits are drawn, Marx calls surplus value.

Marx carries the Day against Owen

According to Marx there would be a social revolution in which labour would seize everything organized and owned by capitalism. In the new system State capitalism would replace private-owner capitalism. This marks a great stride away from the socialism of Owen, who looked to the common sense of men of all classes to reorganize the casual and faulty political, economic and social structure. The subsequent history of social-ism was chequered between the British tradition of Owen and the German class-feeling of Marx. But, on the whole, it was Marx who carried the day against Owen, and the general disposition of socialists throughout the world was to look to the organization of labour, and labour only, to supply the fighting forces against the private owner (Wells, 1920).

Leninist-Marxism attempts World Revolution

Karl Marx quarelled with fellow-socialists who rejected his teaching: all who were not wholly for him were against him. After his death in 1883 and until the triumph of Lenin there was incessant disagreement among the Social Democrats of Europe as to the true meaning and proper application of the Marxian teaching. The Russian Marxists quarrelled with the German Marxists and no less bitterly among themselves. In 1903 they split into Bolsheviks and Mensheviks. The Bolsheviks won and in 1917 Lenin adapted Marxism to foster revolution thus altering the face of Russia and the world. Leninist-Marxism remained unchallenged until the Chinese revolution of 1948. Now China, also claiming Lenin as its prophet, offers the Mao Tse-tung version of Marxism as the only true faith (Crankshaw, 1967).

The Fabians reject the Marxian Doctrine

Meanwhile in Great Britain what was called Fabian Socialism, the exposition of socialism by the London Fabian Society, within less than a year of the death of Karl Marx began to make its appeal to reasonable men of all classes. The Society was founded on 4th January 1884 and its first tract, published a few weeks later, was *Why are the Many Poor?* The founders were nine young people who named themselves after Quintus

Fabius Maximus, surnamed Cunctator, from his cautious tactics in the war against Hannibal. They realized that "long taking of counsel" would be necessary before they could achieve their ambitious object of "reconstructing society in accordance with the highest moral possibilities." The revolutionary socialism of the period was Marxian, but the Fabians rejected the Marxian doctrine both in economics and in politics, holding that socialism was not a scheme to be adopted on the morrow of the revolution, but a principle already partially embodied in municipal government. One of their number, William Clarke, was right in saying that the economic evolution they were seeking to encourage was "proceeding silently every day, practically independent of our individual desires and prejudices."

New Type of Social Legislation

But it went deeper than that. In a lecture on *Liberal Legislation and Freedom of Contract* (1880), T. H. Green had restated liberal theory so that it could comprehend the new type of social legislation. He and the Fabians represented the changed climate of opinion in which people looked to the use of the legislative power of the State to improve the social order. It was this idea which the Fabians worked out in detail in their tracts and pamphlets on everything from pawnshops to laundries and tramways to gas works.

Fabian Essays in Socialism

In the first three years of its life the society was joined by George Bernard Shaw, Sidney Webb, Sydney Oliver, Graham Wallas and by Mrs. Annie Besant. In 1889 the society published a volume of essays by these five, with two others, entitled *Fabian Essays in Socialism*. These essays were widely read and led to the foundation of Fabian Societies throughout England which, however, a few years later were mostly turned into branches of the new Independent Labour Party. The Fabian Society rarely had more than 2,000 members at one time, but, partly through affiliated societies at the universities, many people who entered politics passed through its ranks, and the plays and writings of its leading members brought its docrines before a wide public.

Fabian Socialism permeates the Middle Classes

"We are all socialists nowadays," said the Prince of Wales in 1895. It was the Fabians who made quite sure that he was right. They worked incessantly, especially in the middle-class drawing-rooms of London, trying to change society by influencing their equals. Beatrice Webb wrote in her diary: "Our hope lies in permeating the young middle-class man." Their success was extraordinary, and nobody who studies the years from 1884 to 1914 can fail to notice the influence of the Webbs in even the most unexpected quarters. Sidney Webb and the Fabians found in the doctrine of "the inevitability of gradualness," a device which, they hoped and believed, would reconcile with existing institutions the demands of the new labouring classes. Socialists of diverse brands looked forward to a commonwealth wherein co-operatives, trade unions or industrial guilds would achieve harmony through a socialist reorganization of society (Thomson, 1950).

The Pattern set by Sidney Webb and G. D. H. Cole

The history of the Fabian Society could almost be written in terms of two men: Sidney Webb in the first generation, G. D. H. Cole in the second. Of course many others contributed decisively. Bernard Shaw put the tracts into good English, drew a crowd for the Fabian lectures, and provided the money for the office premises. Beatrice Webb was, in some ways, even more essentially Fabian than her husband. All the same, Webb and Cole set the pattern (Cole, 1961). Though a few working-men got into the Society by mistake, the Fabians were really the snob section of the Labour movement. The typical Fabian had an independent income, great intellectual energy, enlightened views on almost every topic, the capacity to quarrel without intolerance and usually too much leisure.

EMPLOYMENT OF SCHOOL CHILDREN AND YOUNG PERSONS

The education of factory children had made no great strides since schooling was first required under the Act of 1833, but there was a growing volume of opinion that education should be made available to all, and this feeling was being publicly voiced as a result of the *Reform Act, 1867*, which gave the vote to the urban working classes. The ensuing *Elementary Education Act, 1870*, abolished factory schools and set up in all districts School Boards under a central body, the Board of Education, to provide education for all children. These local Boards were empowered, but not compelled, to pass by-laws requiring the attendance at school of all children between the ages of five and thirteen.

Children kept out of Factories and Mines

In progressive districts, therefore, children were kept out of the factories and mines until the latter age. This Act was the first of the great Education Acts and marked the beginning of a change in public opinion. The primary importance of work for the child was superseded by a growing belief in the necessity of education; yet it was fifty years before the incompatibility of the two demands was finally recognized. A few years later, in 1874, a further Act was passed which, incredible as it may seem after all the experience which had gone before, applied only to textile factories. The minimum age was raised to ten years, and children had to attend recognized schools. The certificate of entry was changed from one of age to one of fitness, and continuous employment for protected persons was limited to four and a half hours.

Wage-earning Children

At the end of the nineteenth century attention became focused on those children of school age who were also gainfully employed. In 1899 the

Committee on Wage-earning Children had estimated that at least 144,000 children were employed out of school hours for wages, of which 40,000 were working more than twenty hours a week, 3,000 were working for more than forty hours and some were working from fifty to sixty hours a week. The minimum age of entry into factories had been raised to eleven in 1891 and to twelve in 1901, and from twelve to thirteen half-time school attendance was still required, and it was during this transition from all school to all work that children were being forced beyond their strength. Younger children as well were working at each end of the day and attending school in between.

Poverty and Excessive Child Labour

The 1897 Committee discovered children who were getting up at three o'clock in the morning, and others working until ten o'clock at night, chiefly in unorganized trades on which there was no check, and, provided they made the necessary eight or ten appearances weekly in school, their other work could not be controlled. The reason for this excessive child labour was in nearly every case family poverty. From a survey of 1,500 families both in London and the provinces in 1901, it was evident that a proportion of the population was subsisting on negligible incomes, augmented in many cases by poor relief.

Studies of Child Labour

The Inter-Departmental Committee on the Employment of School Children, which was set up in 1901, studied child labour in factory and home, industrial work, in mines and quarries, in shops, in agricultural and domestic work, in street employment and in odd trades such as places of entertainment and ships and canal boats. It was estimated that a total of 300,000 children were in gainful employment. One of the main evils of child employment was non-attendance at school or an inability to absorb instruction owing to sleepiness when the child did attend, and there are frequent references in the minutes of evidence to backwardness in children as a result of this interrupted education.

Value of Work in Moderation

It seems to have been generally accepted by the Committee that work in moderation was beneficial, and the members were unanimous in agreeing that from twenty to twenty-five hours' labour a week on top of school would do a child no harm. Domestic work, running errands, milking cows and milk rounds were all approved as being suitable jobs for young children. The Committee was no doubt swayed by the undoubted fact that many working children were better fed by their employers than they would be at home, and that only too often the only alternative to work was gambling for buttons on the kerbstone.

Lack of Facilities for Physical Recreation in Towns

The report draws attention to the lack of facilities for physical recreation in towns, and also the lack of practical training in manual work. Nevertheless, in reading the evidence and report today, one cannot help being struck by the lack of appreciation of the needs of childhood and adolescence and the ignorance of the physiological demands of the growing individual. There is nowhere in the report any mention of the long hours of sleep required by children, and the recommendation that a child with incipient phthisis might benefit from the fresh air of an early milk round would shock the modern clinician.

Keeping Children usefully Employed

The final recommendations of this Committee, which were to form the basis of much of the legislation relating to children and young persons of this century, reflect the prevailing opinion that work was permissible provided it was properly controlled, and that it was better to keep a child usefully employed for a few hours a day than to have him loafing about the streets; that it was better to break in children gradually to the industrial milieu than to plunge them headlong into it at fourteen; and that unhealthy occupations, including night work, should be prohibited. Poverty should not be used as an excuse for absence from school or work, and Local Authorities should be authorized to make by-laws controlling employment.

Regulation of Employment

The first Act of Parliament specifically relating to the employment of children was placed on the Statute Book in 1903. Street trading was prohibited under the age of eleven, night work was forbidden and any occupation which was likely to be injurious to health or to interfere with education was also banned. As recommended by the Committee, Local Authorities were given powers under this Act to regulate employment in their areas, and they have retained these powers under all subsequent Acts. Further legislation in 1933 and 1938 has attempted to control employment in many miscellaneous and unregulated trades by prescribing daily and weekly hours of work, overtime and night work, periods of continuous employment, holidays, and particularly by legislating against double employment of an excessive nature.

Employment under Twelve Illegal

It is now illegal to employ a child in any paid capacity under twelve years of age, and the hours during which he may work outside school-time are severely limited. The employment of young persons in shops is subject to the provisions of the 1938 Act, which brings working conditions into line with those prescribed under factory legislation. By raising the compulsory school age to fourteen in 1918 and finally to sixteen in 1945, the Education Acts have abolished the half-time system and have introduced a scheme for further education at County Colleges up to the age of eighteen. So the gradual introduction to industry envisaged in 1901 is become a reality but, and this is the difference between the old and the new conception, at the expense of work and not at the expense of school (Swanston, 1949).

Young Persons in Industry

Since 1918 there have been no children in industry, only young persons. Their employment is regulated chiefly by the *Factories Act, 1937*, and by the Regulations made under this Statute. Generally speaking, the following are the chief controls demanded:

(1) Hours of work are restricted to nine a day and forty-eight a week (forty-four for those under sixteen).

(2) Night work is forbidden (with certain exceptions in the case of boys of sixteen and over), and overtime is strictly controlled. Holidays are prescribed, and so are working periods and periods of continuous employment.

(3) Certificates of fitness are required for all those under sixteen years of age on their first entry into an industry.

(4) There are certain regulations relating to the cleaning of moving machinery, working of dangerous machines and lifting of weights.

(5) There are twenty-one distinct processes from which all or certain youngsters are excluded, of which twelve relate to work with lead, or lead compounds.

Women in Industry

Recent legislation relating to women in industry has closely followed that prescribed for young persons in relation to hours of work, overtime and night work, and the cleaning of moving machinery. They must not be employed in certain lead processes nor in the casting of brass. They cannot work below ground in mines. They must not be knowingly employed within four weeks of childbirth (1891), though there are no restrictions whatever on the employment of pregnant women. Apart from these legal restrictions, women can be, and in times of national emergency are, employed in almost every occupation normally followed by men.

EXPANSION OF THE FACTORY INSPECTORATE

The various Factory Acts and Regulations would have been useless unless their execution in the factories had been provided for by an efficient system of factory inspection. Factory inspectors were charged with the enforcement of factory laws and had in addition the duty of persuading the management and the workers in factories to reduce nuisances. A very important task of the inspectors was to bring about a further development of new laws by studying the actual working conditions and their effects on health.

Qualifications and Duties of a Factory Inspector

A factory inspector must be a person of integrity who is by character well able to stand up to the employer. To become an inspector a man or woman must be either a graduate of a university or must hold the qualification of a recognized school of engineering. In 1929, among twenty-nine accepted candidates, twenty-six had university degrees. A candidate must pass oral and written examinations, attend lectures and work for some weeks with an older inspector. After two years on probation, the candidate is required to pass an examination on factory law and the sanitary sciences before being appointed. Inspectors must treat as confidential all information concerning installations in factories and may discuss them outside the factory only in official reports and at legal prosecutions. Relations between inspectors, management and workers have improved during the course of the years. At first factory inspectors reported much resistance from managements, many attempts at deception and also disagreeable incidents. In 1966 only 160 people were prosecuted for failing to comply with cleanliness standards, or to take adequate precautions against dust or toxic materials. This represents a big improvement over the opening years of the twentieth century, when there were from 3,000 to 4,000 offences every year. The factory inspector of today has been aptly described as a friendly adviser, whose advice is backed by the knowledge that he has the power to enforce his recommendations. But the TUC criticizes the inspectorate for its permissive attitude and insists that they should use their powers for prosecution with more vigour.

The Chief Inspector of Factories

The *Factories and Workshop Act, 1878*, created a centralized system of factory inspection with a Chief Inspector in London. The first man to hold this office was Alexander Redgrave. In 1884, there were, in addition to this Chief Inspector in London, five superintending inspectors, thirty inspectors and ten juniors distributed throughout the country. In 1893 the first woman inspector was appointed. It was not until 1896 that the services of a medical man, Arthur Whitelegge, Medical Officer of Health for the West Riding of Yorkshire, who became Sir Arthur Whitelegge, were enlisted for the post of Chief Inspector, and, although he did not so act in a medical capacity, it was no doubt as a result of his advice that the post of Medical Inspector was created in 1898, and Thomas Morison Legge, who later became Sir Thomas Legge, was appointed. In 1902 the first electrical inspector was appointed, and in 1903 the first inspector for dangerous trades. Each of these individual appointments has since been expanded into a body of several inspectors. In 1910 the authorized staff of inspectors and assistants consisted of 200 persons, in 1939 of 320, in 1944 of 440 persons. In that year 317,040 inspection visits and 63,852 other official visits were made to factories. In 1966 there were 482 inspectors. The establishment is 533 and there are something like 250,000 places of work to visit. Most factories reckon to see an inspector once in every four years! There is little if any follow-up work. Surely a far larger body of factory inspectors is urgently required.

Thomas Morison Legge, 1863–1932

Born in Hong Kong, Legge came as a boy to England, where his father, Dr. James Legge, was appointed Professor of Chinese in Oxford. The boy attended Magdalen College School, went to Bonn to learn German and then joined Trinity College, Oxford, as a commoner. He completed his medical education at St. Bartholomew's Hospital, graduated B.M., B.Ch. in 1890 and obtained the D.M. in 1894. Wishing to study preventive medicine, he paid a series of visits to the capitals of France, Germany, Belgium, Sweden, Norway and Denmark, and wrote his first book, *Public Health in European Capitals*, in 1896. After working under Arthur Newsholme, Medical Officer of Health for Brighton, he was appointed in 1898 the first Medical Inspector of Factories and began what may be described as his life's work.

Lead Poisoning and Lead Absorption

In the early part of his career in the Factory Department of the Home Office he was chiefly engaged in studying and dealing with the prevention of lead poisoning, the disease with which, more than any other, his name will always be associated. In 1912, with Dr. K. W. Goadby, he wrote a book entitled *Lead Poisoning and Lead Absorption*. In subsequent years he investigated anthrax, glass-blowers' cataract, industrial cancer of the skin, toxic jaundice and poisoning by phosphorus, arsenic and

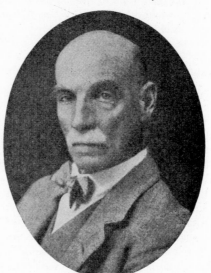

FIG. 65.—Thomas Morison Legge, 1863–1932

mercury. His vast knowledge of his subject was recognized both at home and abroad; indeed, it is difficult to think of an industrial disease on which he could not speak with authority and experience. He was appointed C.B.E. in 1924 and was knighted in 1925. He laid stress on the need for better education in occupational medicine as part of the curriculum in medical schools and was untiring in giving lectures to medical students in many hospitals. As a lecturer he showed a good sense of proportion as well as a sense of humour. He often punctuated his subject with historical anecdotes of great interest (fig. 65).

Artistic Influence of Oxford and of William Morris

His love of foreign languages facilitated his studies of the history of his subject, and his knowledge of German gave us his excellent translation of Rambousek's *Industrial Poisoning from Fumes, Gases, and Poisons of Manufacturing Processes*. There was a strong artistic side to his nature, strengthened by his upbringing in Oxford in the atmosphere of William Morris (1834–96), Dante Gabriel Rossetti and Edward Burne-Jones. He admired the work of these men, who protested against the ugliness of Victorian commercialism, asserting the necessity for natural decoration and pure colour in chintzes, carpets, metalwork and stained glass. The *Kelmscott Chaucer*, decidedly the crowning glory of Morris's printing-press, was finished in June 1896 after five years' planning. Legge also admired the work of the Belgian sculptor of labour, Constantin Meunier, and his artistic eye sought and found much beauty in industry. He was never happier than when in his spare time after a day's work he was making a water-colour drawing of slag-heaps, cranes on the Clyde or kilns at Hanley. But his chief hobby was the study and collection of mediæval stained glass, and he was an accepted authority on Trade Guild windows.

The Geneva White Lead Convention, 1921

In 1921 Legge went to Geneva as representative of the British Government at the International Labour Conference organized by M. Albert Thomas. He there helped to draft the original White-lead Paint Convention which prohibited its use for the internal painting of buildings. In 1926, taking the view that Regulations for the inside painting of buildings should be given a fair trial before adopting the drastic remedy of prohibition, the British Government refused to ratify the Geneva White Lead Convention. Believing the drastic method to be indispensable, Legge felt that he could not bring himself to administer a method of prevention from which he could not foresee satisfactory results. He therefore resigned his appointment as H.M. Senior Medical Inspector of Factories. The fact that he was a Civil Servant and could in no sense be responsible for any policy which a higher authority deemed advisable did not appeal to him on this occasion. In retirement he felt keenly the loss of contact with both employer and worker in the factory.

Medical Adviser to the Trades Union Congress

It was therefore with real pleasure that he accepted in 1929 the post of Medical Adviser to the Trades Union Congress. In the three years which followed he wrote his book on *Industrial Maladies*, and when he realized that his death might befall before the book was ready for the press, left directions that his colleague, Dr. S. A. Henry, should edit the work. And so passed a great Englishman, one of the finest of our civil servants, a man who by his energy, intellectual integrity and common sense achieved more for the protection of the worker against injury and disease than anybody else in all history. His life work lives on, to the greatest benefit of the worker in industry throughout the world.

MEDICAL SUPERVISION IN INDUSTRY

Medical service in industry may be statutory or voluntary, continual or periodic, permanent or temporary, and it may be for a purely specific or for a general purpose. We have seen (p. 117) that medical supervision was first recommended in 1830 and that the *Factory Act, 1844*, created the post of Certifying Factory Surgeon (see p. 125).

Certificate of Fitness

Under the Act of 1844, in addition to age the Certifying Factory Surgeon had to certify that the child or young person was not incapacitated by disease or bodily infirmity from working daily in the factory concerned for the time allowed by the Act. The Act of 1901 gave the certifying surgeon the same power as an inspector to inspect the process at which it was proposed to employ the worker in question, and to qualify his certificate of fitness, if he thought advisable, by conditions as to the work to be performed, and now also as to re-examination even up to the age of eighteen. For a number of years a few surgeons have voluntarily co-operated with a local Juvenile Employment Committee by forwarding a summary of the conditions on a card provided by the committee, so that the young person could be advised of a factory where such conditions were available when not so at the factory first concerned. Today the initial examination must take place within fourteen days of beginning work, and when performed at the factory must be in suitably furnished premises provided for the examination. Power is also given to grant a provisional certificate for a period of twenty-one days pending results of advice or receipt of any further information the surgeon may desire, as, for example, the school medical record, which he is entitled to obtain from the requisite educational authority. Further, he must record his findings on an official form or card provided by the Department. Thus at last we have a true certificate of fitness.

Rejection of Young Persons Examined

An analysis of 1,387,342 examinations of young persons for the four years 1939 to 1942 shows rejection in nearly 3 per cent; passing with conditions in over 4 per cent, or provisionally in well under 1 per cent, mainly pending the result of advice rather than of the school certificate. While the percentage of refusals at re-examination of those under sixteen is nearly seven, for those over sixteen it is only just above one. The main causes of refusal are pediculosis in 43 per cent, eye defects 20 per cent and skin diseases 11 per cent. The statutory duty for certifying surgeons to investigate and report on all accidents in any factory for which they had been appointed to grant certificates of age was introduced also by the Act of 1844. The *Consolidating Act, 1878*, introduced a disciplinary measure, as the Secretary of State was authorized to make rules to govern the office of certifying surgeon. The Act of 1891 placed a new obligation on the surgeon of making an annual report.

Periodic Examination

After the passing of the *Factory Act, 1891*, Special Rules were applied to industries where dangerous materials were handled and injurious effects known to be produced. Under the Special Rules for the Enamelling of Iron Plates, the employer was required to send to a doctor, at his own expense, any worker complaining of any illness apparently due to his employment. In the amended Rules of 1900 for Lucifer Match Factories the *Appointed Dentist* came upon the scene with his initial examination within twenty-eight days, quarterly examination and reference of cases of suspected necrosis of the jaw to the certifying surgeon. The Act of 1898 introduced the great principle of notification of industrial diseases. The investigation of such cases added to the duties of the certifying surgeon, and entailed not only a clinical examination of the injured person but also a thorough examination of the process at which he was engaged, thus giving the certifying surgeon the unique opportunity of continually increasing his knowledge of industrial medicine while providing the Factory Department with valuable information. The *Factory Act, 1901*, introduced the principle of periodic examination of young persons to ensure that certain work of an unusual nature was not causing injury to health. Under the Act, male young persons of fourteen years of age and upwards were permitted under certain conditions to perform shift work which necessitated work at night, because the process was necessarily continuous, as in paper, glass and metal works, provided that they were examined periodically every six months by the certifying surgeon. By the *Factories Act, 1937*, the principle of an initial medical examination at the factory, within fourteen days of employment, was added, and the periodic examination now takes place within the first three months and thereafter six-monthly, with the power of suspension by the surgeon if the work appears to be injuring the health of the young person. It is calculated that slightly over 2 per cent are refused at the initial or subsequent examinations.

Certificate under the Workmen's Compensation Act

But this was not the only addition to the surgeon's labours, for in 1906 his services were enlisted by the Home Office for a new duty outside the province of the Factory Acts for the purpose of giving a certificate of disablement under the Workmen's Compensation Act to any workmen suffering from one of the diseases, of which there were ultimately forty-three, scheduled under that Act. Many of these diseases occur elsewhere than in factories—for example, ankylostomiasis, nystagmus, inflammation of the synovia of the wrist joint and tendon sheaths, and the conditions of acute bursitis known as beat hand, beat elbow and beat knee in coal miners. Other examples are chimney-sweep's scrotal cancer, the glanders of those caring for horses and the cramp of telegraphists and writers. Such pulmonary diseases as silicosis and asbestosis are in a separate category and are dealt with by special schemes, which include examination by members of the Silicosis Board. Certain diseases subject to benefit, such as dermatitis produced by dust or liquids, cataract in glass workers or in those exposed to rays from molten and red-hot metal, poisoning by diethylene dioxide, and poisoning by methyl bromide or tricresyl or triphenyl phosphate, are not notifiable.

Examining Surgeon and Appointed Surgeon

When the new Factories Act reached the Statute Book in 1937, not only did it raise the status of a workshop to that of a factory, but it added greatly to the power and prestige of the certifying surgeon, whose title was altered to that of *Examining Surgeon*, though the original title of *Certifying Surgeon* still remained. With the introduction, after the 1891 Act, of *Special Rules* for dangerous trades, which were gradually replaced by *Regulations* applicable to all such factories after 1901, a new statutory medical figure came upon the scene in 1899, the *Appointed Surgeon*.

Regulations for Dangerous Trades

The Appointed Surgeon was employed for the *weekly* examination under the amended White Lead Rules and the *monthly* examination under the Regulations for the Manufacture of Electric Accumulators in 1903, of Paints and Colours in 1907, for Lead Smelting in 1911, of Indiarubber and for Chemical Works in 1922, and the *quarterly* examination under Regulations for the Heading of Yarn, dyed by means of a lead compound, in 1907, for Vitreous Enamelling in 1908 and for Tinning of Metal Hollow Ware in 1909. When the Electric Accumulator Regulations were amended in 1925, the principle of examination *before* beginning work was instituted, as the first examination must take place within seven days before or after beginning work. Under Regulations for painting of vehicles in 1926, and the Lead Paint Regulations, 1927, made under the *Lead Paint (Protection against Poisoning) Act, 1926*, there are normally no periodic medical examinations, but the Chief Inspector has power to require them under certain conditions if he thinks fit. The Chromium Plating Regulations, 1931, require a *fortnightly* examination and, finally, the *Factories (Luminizing Health and Safety Provision) Order, 1942*, provides for an *initial* and *quarterly* medical examination of those persons of sixteen years of age and over who are allowed to be employed in the process of luminizing with radio-active material (Henry, 1944).

The Pottery Regulations, 1913

Under the Pottery Regulations, 1913, in addition to the monthly periodic medical examination of certain workers in contact with lead, further duties of a special nature were imposed on the certifying surgeon. These related to certain processes of a strenuous nature, such as the carrying of clay or other systematic carrying or lifting work. Male or female young persons aged fourteen to eighteen are allowed to perform these duties, only provided that the certifying surgeon gives within seven days of beginning the work a *certificate of permission to work*, specifying the maximum weight to be carried. Further, the young person must be re-examined twice in the first period of six months and once in each period of six months thereafter till the age of eighteen is reached. A similar certificate of permission to work has to be obtained by a female employed in a pottery as a wheel turner to a thrower or in wedging of clay, and she must be re-examined at a later date if the surgeon considers it necessary. In 1921 another statutory examination for a specific purpose was created. This is the quarterly examination of women and young persons who are permitted under certain conditions to work in certain processes involving the use of lead compounds, and was prescribed by an Order under the *Women and Young Persons Lead Processes Act, 1920*, which, although later repealed, was incorporated in the *Factories Act, 1937*.

Voluntary Medical Services

The service of a medical man who may be required by the employer to be on call for accidents or for giving advice on questions of pension or compensation, especially if the firm carries its own insurance, cannot be described as supervision, but reference must be made to schemes of treatment either provided free or to which the employers and employed contribute. An important example of free treatment in Great Britain is provided by the Post Office Medical Service of Her Majesty's Mails. The scheme, which is described in No. 31 of the Post Office Green Papers, is a combination of free medical treatment at the surgery or at the home and examination for suitability for entry into employment and for pension. This service was introduced as early as 1855, when Dr. Waller Augustus Lewis was appointed as whole-time medical officer at Headquarters in London, and has so expanded that there are now eight medical officers, including five women, under the Chief Medical Officer, and 2,600 part-time medical officers in other parts of the country.

Hospitals maintained by Industry

Again, there are examples of a hospital being maintained by a colliery or a railway, while one large glassworks had, in the past, a small hospital with an orthopædic surgeon and a staff of nurses for the main purpose of suturing severed nerves and tendons. The earliest example of a scheme to which employer and employed contributed jointly is that of the Crowley Iron Undertakings in Sussex in the eighteenth century, where a doctor, a schoolmaster and a clergyman were retained jointly by employer and employed. Another example of interest is that of a Railway Medical Fund Society founded in 1847, which is a self-supporting and autonomous institution, including hospital treatment, receiving important aid from the railway company. Finally, some colliery companies have a hospital used by employees and members of their families or of other firms, supported by a levy from the workers and the grant from the Miners' Welfare Fund, which was endowed by a tax on coal in 1920 and is best known for its pit-head baths.

Supervision for Special Risks

A medical examination is advisable to exclude unsuitable persons from taking up work in compressed air, or on railways with special reference to eyesight, including night and colour vision. Consequently the railways have some fourteen whole-time and six part-time medical officers mainly for this specific purpose, in addition to others used on an area basis as required. Many firms have been persuaded to institute a periodic examination as a preventive measure where some toxic product is involved. In the case of workers in cancer-producing substances such as pitch, tar, mineral oil or even arsenic, the object of examination cannot be so much to prevent the disease as to discover it at the earliest stage when it can be treated with the best chance of recovery. Such periodic medical examinations have been instituted for pitch-briquette workers, tar distillers, paraffin or shale-oil refiners, and arsenical sheep-dip workers, while in certain large gas works and chemical works whole-time medical officers are employed. Such examinations must, of course, have the consent of employer and employed. Sometimes, although the employer willingly offers to provide and finance such supervision, there are workers who are suspicious that the examination, although intended only for a specific purpose, may result in some other defect being found which will be prejudicial to their employment and lead to their discharge; it is therefore most important if the scheme is to be successful that the management and doctor should reassure them on this point.

Poisoning by T.N.T. and Lead

During the First World War it was realized by the Ministry of Munitions that certain processes, such as filling shells with T.N.T., could not be met completely by regulating the process, and that it was essential to have not periodic but continual medical supervision. The Ministry of Supply in the Second World War enlisted for this purpose the services of more than twenty-five part-time, and sixty whole-time, doctors, including twenty-four women, under a Chief Medical Officer at Headquarters. About 1924, when there was a general increase of lead poisoning throughout Great Britain, one large firm manufacturing accumulators came to the conclusion in their wisdom that, although statutory periodic medical examination was in force under Regulations, it would be advisable o go further and institute continual supervision, by appointing a whole-time works medical officer. This was done in 1927, and it ultimately resulted in a reduction in the number of notified cases of lead poisoning throughout the whole accumulator trade. It therefore forms an outstanding example of true supervision. Lastly, we must not forget the special periodic medical examinations of the Silicosis Board (Henry, 1944).

The Works Doctor

The adoption, from about 1900, of whole-time medical supervision for a general purpose was comparatively slow, being mainly confined to a few larger firms manufacturing foodstuffs or engaged in engineering. Since the Order of 1940 came into force and the advantages were increasingly realized, adoption without direction rapidly increased, the larger firms engaging the services of one or more whole-time medical officers and the smaller firms a part-time medical officer, whether he be the examining surgeon or other medical man of the firm's choice. In some cases, where his time permits, one doctor may be employed part-time by more than one firm. Hence, in spite of the shortage of medical men, there were, at the end of 1943, 926 works medical officers, including 63 women, of whom 176 were whole-time in 209 factories, and 750 part-time in 1,155 factories. By the end of 1953 these figures had risen to 186 whole-time and 1,101 part-time works doctors (Table I).

TABLE I

Health Services in Factories

Appointed factory doctors { Full-time	. .	227
Part-time	. .	1,732
Industrial medical officers { Full-time	. .	186
Part-time	. .	1,101
Industrial State-registered nurses .	. .	2,250
Inspectors of factories:		
On ordinary duties	. . . .	346
Medical inspectors	. . . .	13
Electrical inspectors	. . . .	14
Engineering and chemical inspectors	.	18
Canteen advisers .	. . . .	20
Personnel management advisers	. .	19

Duties in the Workroom as well as in the Ambulance Room

The duties of a works' medical officer for a general purpose will differ according to the prevailing conditions and the type of industry. A memorandum issued by the Factory Department has, however, suggested certain broad principles for guidance. But there is one essential rule. His home should be mainly in the workroom among the workers, rather than in the ambulance room. Thus only can he investigate the causes of accidents and learn to offer the best medical advice to management and workmen. He must co-operate with the worker's family doctor, the local hospital, the examining surgeon, the Medical Officer of Health, the school medical officer, the tuberculosis officer, the Silicosis Board and the Factory Department. The advantage of a whole-time works' medical officer being on the honorary staff of a hospital cannot be over-estimated. He or she is concerned with innumerable auxiliary or special services connected with the health of the factory worker. These include dentistry, ophthalmology, pathology, gynæcology, radiology, radiotherapy, chiropody and manicure.

Health Education of the Worker

Health education of the worker by means of classes, posters, films and exhibitions are the concern of the medical officer and his colleague the State-registered nurse, but in any effort to use the factory population for the purpose of enlightenment or prevention of a particular disease which is common to the general population, it should be made quite clear to the worker that it is not an industrial disease. The works' medical officer will promote schemes of physical training for purposes of health, rest-break schemes for the fatigued worker, and rehabilitation and retraining of the injured worker with proper allocation to suitable work (see p. 186). Finally, both doctor and nurse are necessary members, together with employers and employed, of any advisory health committee which may exist in the factory (Henry, 1944).

Appointed Factory Doctor

The appointed surgeon is now known by the name of appointed factory doctor and as everybody knows he is the very backbone of the health services in factories. He examines young persons entering industry and advises both the employer and the employee in cases where a disease or disability is likely to be affected by working conditions. His other duties have been outlined in the four previous pages. Naturally his duties are added to from time to time as in the case of the obligation for workers exposed to lead to have a periodic hæmoglobin estimation (*The Lead Processes, Medical Examinations Regulations*, 1964). His numerical strength approaches 2,000. In 1966 the Ministry of Labour proposed a complete alteration in the appointed factory doctor system whereby the 2,000 or so general practitioners forming the appointed factory doctor service would be replaced by 100 full- or part-time A doctors specializing in industrial health. The Royal College of Physicians hopes that these A doctors of the future will hold its Membership diploma. But will such new-style specialists be forthcoming in adequate numbers? There are many who think not. The T.U.C., standing out for a nation-wide occupational health service, takes comfort in the proposed new constitution of the appointed factory doctor system. But this raises many questions long left unsettled. Should general practitioners come into the factories or should an occupational health service be linked to the hospitals? The envisaged 100 A doctors will serve only that part of the working population covered by the Factories Act, whereas those covered by the Shops, Offices and Railway Premises Act will be left out, as will many other groups of workers, such as fishermen. It is wrong to fragment the care of the national health in this way. Many doctors feel that the public health officers of the Ministry of Health should take over the responsibility. How otherwise can a health service claim to be national and comprehensive if it ignores the factories and workshops where so many men and women spend so much of their time (Shearer, 1967).

The Pioneer Industrial Nurse

To the imagination of the family of Colman of Norwich can be attributed the creation of industrial nursing, for in 1878 Mrs. Jeremiah Colman appointed Philippa Flowerday to work in the mustard mill of J. and J. Colman at Carrow. She was engaged to act as district nurse for 26s. a week. All morning she helped the doctor at the Dispensary of the Carrow Works Self-help Medical Club, formed by Mrs. Colman in 1872. Later in the day she visited the sick workers in their homes, where she looked after their nursing and social needs. Little is known of the actual duties of this pioneer industrial nurse except that through her work she linked the factory and the home, a principle which is often forgotten today in the more highly specialized nursing services which have subsequently developed (Charley, 1949).

Industrial Nursing Certificate

The principle is now accepted that industrial nursing is a special branch of public health nursing and that the influence of the nurse, if given full expression, can raise the standard of factory life wherever she comes into contact with it. In 1932 a course of training for an Industrial Nursing Certificate was established jointly by the Royal College of Nursing and Bedford College for Women in the University of London. In 1940, when Mr. Ernest Bevin became Minister of Labour and National Service, he prompted the Government to make available training grants for nurses taking the course at the College. The Universities of Cardiff, Liverpool, Leeds, Glasgow and Bristol have since given facilities for training. In 1943, during the peak effort in the Second World War, there were 8,385 nurses in industry, some two-thirds of whom were State-registered. In addition to work in factories, the nurse finds herself in mining, at docks and fishing ports, on the canals, in air transport, in sea-going liners and in the hop-fields and agriculture.

Her Influence on Factory Life

In a factory the nurse holds a responsible position. She fosters goodwill and confidence and takes an intelligent interest and pride in the fortunes of the firm for which she works. In certain cases she acts as welfare supervisor, and often she gives advice to the canteen manageress on the question of special diets. She will expect free access to the factory through the works manager. If there is no medical officer she will expect to co-operate with the personnel officer in pre-employment interviews and examinations by the examining surgeon. She has a valuable contribution to make to the Safety Committee and should always be consulted by the Safety Officer on accident investigations. Among juvenile employees her work is especially full of promise, for where general education is part of a factory scheme she may be called upon to teach the subjects of general and personal hygiene (Mann, 1946).

THE FACTORIES ACT OF 1961

In addition to consolidating the Factories Acts, 1937 to 1959, the *Factories Act*, 1961, strengthened the provisions for safety and health of employed persons and the requirements for first-aid installations. Important safety measures include regulations for the construction of machinery. These specify that every set-screw and bolt on a revolving shaft shall be sunk and that gearing shall be encased. Any person selling or renting a machine that does not comply with the requirements of the law shall be fined. If illnesses occurring in a factory are traceable to the nature of a particular job or if by reason of changes in any process the risk of injury arises, the Secretary of State is authorized to require arrangements for the medical supervision of the endangered persons. He also is authorized to prescribe the maximum weights to be lifted, carried or moved by any class of person, and to require the attending physician to report all industrial diseases, not just those enumerated in earlier laws.

Factory Orders, 1944

Factory Orders, 1944, published by the Ministry of Labour and National Service, is a book of 388 pages. Under general provisions it includes five on health (cleanliness, lighting); eight on safety (hoists, chains and cranes); and three on welfare (first aid). There are also twenty-two welfare regulations for particular trades (cement works, bakeries, laundries, sugar factories and so on), and forty-eight for safety and health in particular trades. Other regulations concern lead paint, the employment of women and young persons in lead processes, notification and investigation of accidents and industrial diseases, and homework. These rules and regulations show not only the tendency to make provisions against all the important causes of accidents and industrial diseases but, even more, the tendency to adapt all regulations to the special peculiarities of the work and to make the provisions as clear and definite as possible.

Notification of Industrial Diseases

From 1878 until 1940 provisions for the control of dangerous trades were made by the Home Office, and subsequently by the Ministry of Labour and National Service. Early knowledge of certain industrial diseases was obtained by placing an obligation on the medical practitioner to notify the Chief Inspector of Factories, and on the employer to notify both the district inspector of factories and certifying surgeon, now the appointed factory doctor. Since 1896 an increasing number of diseases has been made notifiable. Under the Factories Act, 1961, the Chief Inspector of Factories must be informed of poisoning arising under sixteen headings:

Lead poisoning	Compressed-air illness
Phosphorus poisoning	Anthrax
Manganese poisoning	Toxic jaundice
Arsenical poisoning	Toxic anæmia
Mercurial poisoning	Epitheliomatous ulceration or
Carbon disulphide poisoning	Chrome ulceration
Aniline poisoning	Beryllium poisoning
Chronic benzene poisoning	Cadmium poisoning

By the *Lead Paint (Protection against Poisoning) Act, 1926*, the practitioner must notify any case of lead poisoning contracted in painting any building. The aims of the Factories Act, 1961, and of the National Insurance (Industrial Injuries) Act, 1965, are, of course, quite different. The former is concerned with the prevention and control of occupational accidents and diseases, and the latter with those workers affected by occupational accidents or prescribed diseases. Notification is an important ancillary in the prevention and control of occupational accidents and of certain occupational diseases. Thus we find that the list of diseases prescribed under the Industrial Injuries Act is longer than that of the diseases required to be notified under the Factories Act, and in some cases they are described differently.

Personnel Services and Canteens

The Second World War saw the compulsory establishment of personnel services in certain prescribed factories (*Factories (Medical and Welfare Services) Order, 1940*, and the *Factories (Canteens) Orders, 1942 and 1943*). It is probable that the future will see industrial legislation focused on the individual rather than on a particular section of industry. There will also be a shift of emphasis from toxic and accident hazards to the personal needs of workers, both as individuals and as members of a group. But it is well to remember that only by the strictest measures of control, sometimes enforced by law, have industrial diseases and injuries due to accidents been reduced in the past, and regulations will still be needed, not so much to protect the worker from his employer, as to help the latter, who cannot be expected to know all the details of the numerous hazardous processes to be found in modern industry.

THE DISABLED PERSONS (EMPLOYMENT) ACT, 1944

The shortage of labour during the Second World War became so acute that in 1941 a committee known as the *Inter-departmental Committee on the Rehabilitation and Resettlement of Disabled Persons* was appointed under the chairmanship of Mr. George Tomlinson, M.P. The recommendations of the *Tomlinson Report (1942)* were set before Parliament and were accepted almost unaltered in a new Act known as the *Disabled Persons (Employment) Act, 1944*, in which the nation accepted the principle that any disability, medical or surgical, constitutes a claim upon the State for assistance, both financial and by way of treatment and rehabilitation, so that the disabled person can be reinstated, when possible, into useful work. The Act defines a disabled person as one who—

> on account of injury, disease or congenital deformity is substantially handicapped in obtaining or keeping employment, or in undertaking work of a kind which apart from that injury, disease or deformity would be suited to his age, experience and qualifications.

Such persons are entitled to apply for registration; and if accepted as disabled, they are assisted in various ways by the Ministry of Labour and National Service to obtain suitable work.

Register of Disabled Persons

Since September 1945 a register of disabled persons has been maintained at all local offices of the Ministry of Labour. Registration is voluntary and application is made by disabled persons. To be accepted the following obligations have to be fulfilled:— (a) The worker's disability must come within the definition laid down, (b) the disablement is likely to last for at least six months, and (c) the applicant must be ordinarily resident in Great Britain. Medical evidence may be necessary before an application is accepted, but rejection can only be made by the Disablement Advisory Committee which has the assistance of medical advice. Registration may be for one to five years and may be renewed. A person may be removed from the register if he fails to satisfy the definition, or if there is persistent and unreasonable refusal to take up suitable work, or if there is refusal without reasonable cause to complete a course of vocational training. Employers are required to engage a proportion of registered disabled persons, this usually amounts to 3 per cent when twenty or more men are employed. Certain industries, for example fishing fleets, are required to employ 0·1 per cent only of disabled persons.

Disablement Resettlement Officers

There are some 800,000 names on the register, about half of these disabled persons being surgical cases. The medical group numbers just under one-third, and a group of patients with psychiatric symptoms makes up about 5 per cent of the total. The work of lift attendants and car park attendants is known as *designated employment* and these jobs can be filled only by men who are on the register of disabled persons. The work of the Ministry is carried out by local officers known as *Disablement Resettlement Officers (D.R.O.)* who maintain a close co-operation with hospitals, training institutions and local industries. When necessary, patients are visited in hospital or at home and advised as to the proper steps to be taken to secure treatment, training and placement.

Industrial Rehabilitation Centres

The Ministry of Labour has set up training centres at which disabled persons are tested for vocational aptitude and instructed in suitable trades.

All the facilities provided at such industrial rehabilitation centres are free of cost to the trainee, who is paid his travelling expenses and maintenance allowances for his dependants. The training of disabled persons in Government Training Centres is carried out, where possible, side by side with that of the able-bodied, so that the former may learn to work together with the latter. Those so seriously handicapped as to require a period of training of six months or more may be sent to one of the residential centres specially equipped for dealing with such cases, such as Queen Elizabeth's Training College for the Disabled, Leatherhead; St. Loyes College, Exeter; or the Sir John Priestman Hospital, Finchale Abbey, near Durham, all of which are run by private voluntary organizations.

Sheltered Employment in Remploy Factories

It was to meet the needs of cases of severe disablement that the Disabled Persons Employment Corporation (Remploy) was set up by Act of Parliament in 1945 as a non-profit-making company. It now runs ninety factories and employs over 6,000 severely disabled workers. The main disability groups into which these workers fall are tuberculosis (11·4 per cent), injuries and diseases of the lower limbs (8·9 per cent), diseases of the heart or circulation (8·3 per cent), diseases of the lungs other than tuberculosis (8·2 per cent) and epilepsy (7·7 per cent). The principal trade groups included in the 90 factories are 20 for domestic furniture, 17 for general woodworking, 12 for cardboard box making, printing and bookbinding, 12 for protective clothing and textile sewing, 9 for engineering, 7 for knitwear and 6 for leatherwork. There is also a separate home-work group. The conditions of employment are a 44-hour week at a standard rate of wage for all trades which is settled by negotiations with the trade unions. Annual sales have increased from £12,000 in 1947 to £3,204,000 in 1957 and Government assistance from £7,000 in 1945–46 to £2,737,000 in 1956–57. Remploy has already provided employment for nearly 13,000 men and women, most of whom would otherwise have had little prospect of obtaining it (Edwards, 1958).

Hospitals and Industry

Rehabilitation should be based as far as possible on economic considerations, so that the individual obtains at the earliest possible opportunity both work and reward (Stewart, 1946). Hospital services deal in the main with anatomical and functional recovery. With good hospital treatment the need for special measures of rehabilitation decreases, so that on economic grounds industry is fundamentally interested in future hospital policy. Many hospitals have ventured into the social field by changing the outlook and work of the almoner, but closer contacts with industry are still required.

Social Service Departments in Hospitals

The policy of setting up social service departments in hospitals is gradually providing an important link with industry; the function of the almoner is changing, and her increasing contact with managements, on behalf of the sick and injured worker, will be a real advance in hospital service. Industry itself frequently needs contact with hospitals; it must have knowledge, for instance, of the progress of key men under treatment, or it may wish to offer special facilities to an injured man to assist his recovery; this can best be done through the social service department of the hospital. Hospitals should consider the possibility of appointing their own industrial liaison officers, persons with practical experience of factory work, who would not only provide a link with the patient's employer but would advise the physician or surgeon concerning the physical and mental requirements of different occupations.

The Contribution of Management

In addition to efficient hospital treatment and close contact between the almoner's department and industry, the co-operation of the employer is necessary for full resettlement (Stewart, 1949). The promise of continued employment can remove the fear of insecurity, which is a potent means of retarding recovery. Many disabled workers already in employment are unwilling to put their names on the register of disabled persons for fear of losing their jobs, and because of a natural dislike of being classified as disabled.

Alternative Work under Medical Supervision

A promise of alternative work can be made if the employee is unfit for his previous job, but, to be effective, this must be true alternative work under medical supervision and not light work specially created as a charity. The possibility of retraining for alternative work should be considered. This can only be done in the larger firms where such jobs are available. Government Training Centres and certain extra-industrial centres can, theoretically, cover the remainder of industry. It is important that employers should appreciate the fact that a man cannot be unfit one day and on the next, in a different environment, be really fit for full work. The goodwill of managers and foremen, who are the real executives of industry, must therefore be obtained for the worker during what is often an awkward phase in recovery—that period of time between being signed off by the insurance practitioner or the hospital and his return to his original occupation.

Responsibility of Personnel Management

It is a primary responsibility of personnel management to play a part in the supervision of the return of the sick or injured worker to work. In the larger firms, personnel management and medical services work in close collaboration. In the small industrial unit—for example, the factory with less than 300–400 employees—there is usually no special official appointed as personnel or welfare officer, and supervision therefore becomes the direct responsibility of the works' manager. Because the majority of firms come within the small category, and because over 50 per cent of the factory workers are employed in units of 250 or less, the education of works' managers and foremen in the meaning of rehabilitation and the part they must play in it becomes increasingly important.

Objections to Light Work

Whereas firms may appreciate the need for *light or alternative work*, the provision of such work is difficult in industry as a whole, and in the small organization it is frequently impossible. In larger firms a number of jobs may be especially allocated for convalescent sick and injured patients as part of general welfare schemes. The main criticism of this is that patients are often under inadequate medical supervision, and that this allocation may become no more than a method of dumping or losing unwanted workers for so-called philanthropic motives. Objections to alternative or light work can be summed up as follows. It is frequently hit-or-miss therapy; it is difficult to find in the majority of industries; it is difficult to keep under medical control, and may retard functional recovery; it is frequently disliked by managers, foremen and by workers themselves, for the productive effort of the industrial unit—the gang or team—may be hampered by the presence of a semi-fit man; managers and foremen may resent the increase in overhead expenses; and the patient is apt to be permanently lost sight of in the works.

The Contribution of the Industrial Medical Officer

In firms in which an industrial medical officer is employed, supervision of the return of the injured or sick worker to his job is one of his primary duties and is a main reason for further extension of occupational health services (Stewart, 1946). Among other things he can obtain accurate information of the incidence of sickness and accidents and of the progress of sick and injured workers; he can review progress with hospital staffs and with medical practitioners. He should regard the local hospital as his base and make close contacts with it, for health departments in industry should regard themselves in certain respects as outposts of hospitals and should not work in isolation. He can develop an adequate follow-up service and here the help of a good nurse is of much importance; and he can build up a library of job references with a view to more effective placement.

Special Rehabilitation Workshops

The whole-time industrial medical officer should investigate the possibility of setting up, in his own organization, a special workshop for the rehabilitation of selected sick and injured workers. Selection could be made in collaboration with hospital physicians and surgeons, who might act in a consultative capacity in this respect and so themselves learn something of industrial conditions. The potential medical contribution to industrial rehabilitation is thus great, particularly in larger firms. This type of workshop, within industry itself, provides one good answer to the problem of rehabilitation, but it should essentially develop as a part of an occupational health service. The Austin and Vauxhall experiments are examples of this.

The Worker relieved from Anxiety

Employees other than those disabled by accident are admitted—for example, medical cases after prolonged absence or those individuals whose working capacity is so lowered by age or by slowly developing debility that they cannot continue their normal occupation. In a new environment, physical and mental capacity is reassessed under gentle conditions but, at the same time, a living wage is paid, and the man is eventually employed again in the factory proper. As soon as workers realize that an alternative to either full work or unemployment is available, they are relieved of much of the anxiety which results from economic insecurity. The worker has a double incentive, (*a*) to earn more than he would on compensation and so would be attracted to work in the shop, and (*b*) to strive towards his pre-disability rate. The man is employed in the shop at the sole discretion of the medical officer, and he returns eventually to his previous work, or to other full work for which he is suitably trained, in other parts of the factory.

The Follow-up of Patients

A follow-up scheme operates in collaboration with shop superintendents. Such a scheme realizes the psychological needs of any incapacitated or handicapped person. It takes him away, early in his treatment, from the hospital atmosphere in which disability and disease are inevitably stressed. It removes financial anxiety and the fear of not being employed again. It alters a man's attitude to his mates, to his manager, to the firm, and to his home, and the change is inevitably for the better, because he lacks reason for grievance. There is less tendency to retain the memory of disabilities. Morale is good and neurotic manifestations and recurrences are minimal. The scheme allows of a day-to-day contact between the medical staff and a section of semi-fit and disabled employees at work. Once the man is told, in simple language, of the immediate and ultimate effects of his disablement, and is reassured about his future employment, he is willing to cease worrying about it, and he transfers his load of anxiety to the shoulders of the doctor.

Absenteeism due to Neurosis

It is common knowledge that much time is lost in factories because of neurotic symptoms. Doubts as to social security, boredom from the monotony of mechanized jobs, fear of unemployment or of inability to work all have a decidedly injurious psychological effect on the workman. In spite of the various efforts made to interest him in his task, including social work of all kinds, incentive schemes, sharing in benefits, paid holidays and national insurance, the fact remains that large numbers of industrial workers have lost joy in their work. In a world which is so insecure it is not surprising that anxiety arising from feelings of instability should plunge into psychoneuroses those workpeople who are so predisposed.

Factors tending to produce neurosis are uncongenial working conditions, mental subnormality, poor placement in which the job requires more skill than the operative possesses, together with extra-factory stresses related to the worker's social and domestic life. Neurosis is as common among skilled workers as among those in less skilled jobs. One characteristic of neurotic disability, considered as an occupational handicap, is its enduring quality.

Incidence of Neurotic Illness

One of the most important studies of the incidence and causation of neurosis in industry was carried out during the Second World War by Russell Fraser (1947) on a sample of light and medium engineering workers in or near Birmingham. The sample consisted of 3,000 workers, and it was found that over a period of six months about 10 per cent of these workers suffered from disabling neurosis, about 20 per cent more from minor neurotic complaints, and, finally, that neurosis was responsible for between one quarter and one third of the total sickness absence. These figures are confirmed by Halliday (1948), who has reported that of 1,000 insured workers who were receiving sickness benefit under certification as unfit for work, 33 per cent were incapacitated as a result of neurosis, and by Wyatt (1945) who found that "nervous debility and fatigue" accounted for 21·2 per cent of sickness absence among 30,000 women workers in munitions factories. In 1966 the Office of Health Economics estimated that neuroses, anxiety states and personality disorders are responsible for the loss of 17 million working days a year.

Assessment of Personality and Morbid Anomalies

Psychiatric handicaps unlike physical disabilities are not limited; they are so often personality handicaps and as such they fluctuate and may greatly interfere with retraining for any job at all. Where the neurotically ill are concerned, a precise diagnosis is less important than assessment of the personality and the morbid anomalies which the worker exhibits. Judgement of the latter is not beyond the competence of the industrial medical officer. It is he who holds the key position in giving psychiatric advice. He sees the workers, he has their confidence and he knows his industry. By his contacts with workers exhibiting maladjustment he can discover where are the trouble spots in his industry (Lewis, 1945).

HUMAN RELATIONSHIPS IN INDUSTRY

In the first half of the twentieth century industrial medicine has made an immense contribution to human health and happiness by its attitude to the group aspect of working life. Labour is more than a mass of individuals collected at random; economists and others have failed to grasp and interpret the importance of the group as an influence on the individual. It is mainly to the medical profession that we owe the concept of labour as a social group whose well-being is as important as that of any other group. Anyone attempting to reorganize factory life must give full consideration to the emotional aspects of human inter-relationships in industry. This is the theme of an excellent book by J. A. C. Brown (1954) entitled *The Social Psychology of Industry*.

Management and the Worker

The study of the reactions of individuals and of groups of individuals to their work, their conditions of work and their working environment, though by no means the prerogative of doctors, nevertheless comes within the scope of occupational health. For this reason the training of the industrial medical officer should be increasingly orientated in this direction because of the practical contribution already made by workers in this field to the contentment and efficiency of occupational groups. Since 1918, the Industrial Health Research Board and the National Institute for Industrial Psychology have carried out research on subjects such as the effects of light, temperature and hours of work on the reactions of individuals; vocational guidance and selection; training methods; the significance of sickness-absence and labour wastage; accident prevention; and human relationships in industry.

Capacity for Working Together

Professor Elton Mayo has said that whereas material efficiency has been increasing for 200 years, the capacity for working together has, in the same period, continually diminished, and this thesis may sum up the vital need for further studies in the field (Mayo, 1945). The practical experience gained by Service psychiatrists and psychologists in the Second World War is of importance to occupational health. The use of psychological methods in the British Army developed in the following main fields: personnel selection; improvement of working methods and conditions; raining methods; morale and incentives (Rees, 1945).

Job Analysis

To be effective the industrial medical officer must know as much as possible about the jobs in his occupational group, whether it be factory, coal mine, shipyard or office. This knowledge is best provided for him by the method of job analysis. This has now developed into a highly technical subject and is normally carried out by specially trained people. It consists in an intensive study of men at work and accurate recording of the observations made there, together with consideration of facts which are relative to the job and which may be obtained from workers, supervisors and technical experts.

Placement of Workers

For medical purposes job analysis can conveniently be divided into two parts—the job description or specification, and an analysis of the demands which the job normally makes upon the worker together with a note of environmental factors which may influence him. The written description should give a vivid picture of what the worker does, how he does it, why he does it and the skill required in doing it. Job analysis is used in industry, however, for purposes other than health or safety; it can form the

basis of the determination of wage-rate systems and may be used in production planning. It is of value to the doctor mainly as an aid to the placement of workers and when interviewing workers who blame their jobs for
causing some health impairment; it is also useful when advice on a suitable
change of occupation is required, or when processes and jobs are potentially
hazardous, or in cases in which excessive fatigue or other harmful results
on health may be produced by inefficient plant design.

Planned Schemes of Selection

The state of the labour market has a bearing upon the selection of
manual workers for jobs. When there is unemployment, industry has a
large choice of workers, a fact which, before the Second World War, retarded the general development of scientific methods of selecting personnel. Today in Great Britain there is an apparent lack of man-power, and the
prospect of redeployment of workers from non-essential jobs, at which they
are skilled, to others in which they may appear as raw material, makes the
time opportune for the introduction of planned schemes of selection with
the aid of job analysis. Results of this will be a reduction in labour wastage
and absenteeism, combined with greater efficiency of the individual and
increased output. The need for improved methods of placing men in industry has been accentuated by the number of disabled and handicapped
persons for whom it is necessary to find employment. A useful step towards
a solution has been taken by the Ministry of Labour, which has introduced
a special form for use in placing disabled people in industry.

Accurate Job Descriptions

There is potential scope for the use of job analysis by hospitals and doctors concerned with rehabilitation, provided that local industries could
supply simple job descriptions. At present, the majority of doctors advise
on employment questions as a direct result of the patient's own description
of the job, and the accuracy of the description is frequently open to doubt.
Job descriptions are probably the best means by which any doctor can
learn about occupation, and written descriptions mean more if accompanied
by a photograph of the man on the job. It must be clearly understood that
job descriptions can only be prepared effectively by persons with special
technical qualifications and experience; this is no amateur task to be
undertaken lightly by a doctor. Here immediate difficulties arise. Who is to
do the descriptions? What will be the cost to the firm? What will be the
eventual benefit to the health of the workers? These questions should be
kept in mind when an approach for help in this matter is made to management, as it must be made, by industrial medical officers with foresight
(Stewart, 1949).

Need for Prolonged Observation and Experience

Assistance in describing certain of the physical and environmental demands of jobs can reasonably be given by doctors with industrial experience. Here, matters such as the amount of lifting, fingering, handling or

stooping have to be assessed, together with factors such as the need for good vision, colour vision, good hearing or the ability to feel. Assessment of the psychological or mental demands of jobs is a matter of much greater difficulty. Factors such as wage incentives, monotony, the potential satisfactions to be found in the job and the opportunity for responsibility and promotion have all to be considered. The psychological characteristics of the individual can be assessed, in part at least, by psychologists and by doctors trained in psychiatric methods. These characteristics include intelligence, aptitudes, personality traits, and social adequacy, as well as educational levels and technical skill; the matching of these against the equivalent demands of the job, however, is a matter the significance of which can only be decided after prolonged observation and experience.

Training within Industry

Training of new entrants to industry, particularly of youths under apprenticeship schemes, is generally accepted in the engineering trades. At Government Training Centres men and women receive simple vocational training designed to fit them for future careers, largely in the semi-skilled occupations. Schemes for the training of foremen and supervisors are sponsored by the Ministry of Labour. These schemes have three phases: methods of job instruction, instruction in human relations and leadership and instruction in efficiency—that is, in the development of simple, time-saving and fatigue-reducing methods of production. Education and experience are equally necessary in industrial management. In Great Britain over 400,000 persons are engaged in managerial work, and an annual intake of some 12,000 recruits is required. The syllabus of training, which is comprehensive in the technical, business and commerical fields, also covers such subjects as industrial psychology, including the psychology of individual differences, measurement of intelligence, attainments and special aptitudes, personality and character, testing of temperament, interview techniques, vocational guidance and selection, psychology of training, of work, of incentives and of work study, and social psychology, including the human factor in industrial relations.

Morale and Incentives in Industry

Efficiency and high productivity depend upon industrial morale no less than on mechanical equipment. Factors influencing morale are, among others, the development of security, discipline and disciplinary action, leadership, individual behaviour, conditions at work, facilities for joint consultation and the development of joint responsibility, and specific incentives. The causes of good or bad morale are not easily determined, but seem to include economic irresponsibility, an attitude derived from the economic structure of an industry and a locality. This attitude is certainly closely related to political and social factors outside industry.

Symptoms of Lowered Morale

Some of the symptoms of lowered morale are indifference to output and to the achievement and fate of the enterprise for which a man works, failure of the individual to understand the significance of his own work to the community, suspicion of the motives of the management, and the belief that the interests of labour and management are diametrically opposed to each other. These points have to be frankly discussed before any formal consultative machinery in industry can be made to work. Habits of mutual trust and consultation before decisions are made are fundamental for democracy in industry. The ultimate function of joint consultation is to get rid of the division of factories into bosses and the rest, which still colours the thoughts of most people. This wrong conception of management is traceable to the fact that some people when given responsibility do not like to consult the people under them.

The Defensive Partisan Approach

Additional evidence of low morale is shown when workers demand security and control of industry but refuse to share the risks of industrial enterprise. They pursue their own sectional claims, regardless of the effect of such behaviour upon the national economy. This is a menace to the national well-being and is incompatible with political responsibility and good citizenship. Yet a change of attitude on the part of labour cannot be expected unless there is a modification of those features in the industrial structure which are incompatible with a democratic way of life. The psychological effect on workpeople of having been consulted is more important as a rule than is the actual contribution of ideas made by them. Many employers are still insufficiently aware that the working group is a miniature society, and that, for its proper functioning, the art of social management is as important as is the technical management of machinery and processes (Stewart, 1949).

The Hawthorne Experiment

The experiment carried out at the Hawthorne Works of the Western Electric Company in the United States of America is perhaps the most significant contribution yet made to the problem of determining morale in industry (Whitehead, 1938). The immediate lesson appears to be that we have to recognize and respect those work-relationships which develop within groups in most organizations, whether large or small. Groups develop an identity of their own which can enable them to take over some of the functions of supervision and to set behaviour standards which are at least as high as most employers would demand. On the other hand, they can develop, among employees, attitudes towards work which are based on misunderstandings due to lack of correct information. From this awkward situations may arise in which groups faithfully believe something to be true which is, in fact, untrue. The experiment showed that improvement in conditions of work, discussed and explained to workers, gave rise to increased output. A more important point, however, was that the increased range of output continued when a return was made to the original imperfect conditions. These results were fully confirmed. The group had obviously developed some inherent force and had unconsciously, but yet effectively, organized itself for the specific task before it (Roethlisberger and Dickson, 1947).

Incentives and Contentment

Probably the strongest motive for working is a man's desire to secure his own livelihood and that of his family. There is the lesser motive of a desire or urge to create. Also, there is the determination of a man to achieve distinction among his fellows. These motives are strengthened and reinforced by schemes and devices, at the place of employment, to which the term incentive is applied. The incentive has the power of awakening, maintaining and strengthening the motive (Hall and Locke, 1938). Satisfying incentive systems will improve morale, and in these the basic incentive is that of finance. There are other incentives, however, and some of these have been outlined by presupposing the existence of certain qualities, such as pride in rendering a service useful to the community, satisfaction in doing a job well, contentment through working in security with a competent and trusted chief, stimulation conditioned by opportunity for promotion, fulfilment arising from the performance of creative or constructive work, responsibility developing from opportunity to take the initiative and a sense of participation arising from being consulted in matters of management (Millward, 1946). The application of these incentives in industry would do much to improve relationships and to encourage mutual trust between management and employees. Opportunities of personal satisfaction for the individual would be regained, and harmony promoted more readily than through the defensive partisan approach of worker groups (Stewart, 1949).

THE NATIONAL INSURANCE (INDUSTRIAL INJURIES) ACT, 1946

The present national schemes for insurance against industrial injury began on 5th July 1948 as the *National Insurance (Industrial Injuries) Act, 1946*, subsequently replaced by a new act in 1965 which was amended in 1967. For twenty years they were the responsibility of the Ministry of Pensions and National Insurance which, in 1966, became the Ministry of Social Security. Of all the post-war social schemes they were probably the most revolutionary. To understand the full implications of this legislation it is necessary to appreciate some of the principles on which the *Workmen's Compensation Acts (1897–1945)* operated. The new Act has of course replaced the Workmen's Compensation Acts. Before 1897 an injured worker could recover damages only at common law or, in certain cases, under the *Employers' Liability Act, 1880*. In either case, the worker was required to establish negligence to succeed in his claim. The Act of 1897, and subsequent amending Acts, established the principle, irrespective of negligence, of the employer's responsibility for the payment of compensation. But claims remained subject to individual litigation and the case law built up made the Workmen's Compensation Acts so complex as to cause many anomalies and much bewilderment. The new scheme of industrial injuries insurance has removed those anomalies.

How the Scheme Works

Everyone employed under a contract of service or apprenticeship is insured under the *National Insurance (Industrial Injuries) Acts* and generally also under the *National Insurance Acts*. The Industrial Injuries Acts insure people against incapacity, disablement or death due to accident at work or to certain industrial diseases. Part of the weekly insurance stamp contribution is earmarked for industrial injuries. The amounts paid are:—

	Men		*Women*	
	18 or over	under 18	18 or over	under 18
Paid by employee	10d.	5d.	7d.	3d.
Paid by employer	11d.	5d.	8d.	4d.
Total	1s. 9d.	10d.	1s. 3d.	7d.

These contributions, plus an exchequer supplement, are paid into a special fund. There are no age limits for the Industrial Injuries Scheme and contributions are compulsory. Benefits do not depend on having paid a certain number of contributions and, save for the special hardship allowance, are not based on loss of earnings, as they partly were under the Workmen's Compensation Acts. They are the same for both men and women, but boys and girls get a lower rate. Benefits are of three kinds: injury benefit, payable for an initial period of incapacity after the accident or development of the disease; disablement benefit, where there is disablement, whether permanent or not; and death benefit.

Industrial Injury and Disablement Benefit

Injury Benefit is payable for incapacity during the first 26 weeks after an accident or development of an industrial disease and so covers in the vast majority of cases the whole period during which the insured man or woman is incapable of work through the injury. This benefit is £7 5s. 0d. a week with £2 16s. 0d. for a wife or other adult dependant, £1 5s. 0d. for the first child under school-leaving age, and 17s. for each younger child. It is paid in addition to family allowances. *Disablement Benefit* is payable if the person suffers through the accident or disease any *loss of physical or mental faculty*, including disfigurement. Disablement pensions range from £7 12s. 0d. a week for 100 per cent disablement to £1 10s. 6d. a week for 20 per cent disablement. For a life award of less than 20 per cent, down to 1 per cent, a gratuity varying from £500 to £50 is paid. For the prescribed diseases, pneumoconiosis and byssinosis, neither injury benefit nor disablement gratuities are payable; where benefit is payable it takes the form of a pension.

Industrial Injuries Medical Boards

The rate of disablement benefit thus depends on the degree of disablement and this is assessed by a medical board consisting of two or more doctors. The first assessment is normally for a limited period and further assessments may follow. On the matter of the assessment there is an appeal to a medical appeal tribunal. Each medical appeal tribunal consists of a legal chairman and two doctors of consultant rank. No allowance for dependants is payable with disablement benefit, except where an unemployability supplement is paid or the beneficiary is in hospital for treatment for his injury. If there is treatment in hospital or of the relevant injury or disease the pension or gratuity is raised to the 100 per cent rate of pension for each day in hospital. Disablement pension is not affected by any earnings of the claimant after the accident, even if they are as much as or more than before. A man getting basic disablement benefit can also get sickness or unemployment benefit. Of course, if no disablement remains when injury benefit ceases, which is the position in most cases, no disablement benefit is payable. On the other hand, if disablement grows worse a man can apply for a review of his case.

Special Allowances payable with Disablement Benefit

If a man has to take work different from that which he was doing before the accident he may get a *special hardship allowance* of up to £3 1s. od. a week unless he could do work of a standard equivalent to his old job. But the disablement pension and special hardship allowance together must not exceed £7 12s. od. What about the man who, because of his disability, will never be able to go back to any work? The Act provides for him a special allowance of £4 10s. od. a week with allowances for dependants, which can be paid in addition to the pension. This allowance is called an *unemployability supplement* and a man entitled to it is one who is never likely to be able to earn more than £104 a year. His average earnings, therefore, could be £2 a week and he could still get the £4 10s. od. allowance. If a man's disablement is assessed at 100 per cent and his injuries are such that he requires the attendance of some person to look after him, a *constant attendance allowance* of up to £3 can be paid even if his own wife is attending him; in cases of exceptionally severe disablement, up to £6 or in exceptional cases up to £9 may be paid. A man with a 100 per cent pension who was entitled to unemployability supplement and constant attendance allowances would therefore be paid £15 2s. od. a week, or in cases of exceptionally severe disablement £15 2s. od. with perhaps further allowances of £4 1s. od. for a wife and child.

The Adjudication Procedure

If a worker suffers an accident at his work, he, or someone for him, should tell his employer at once. In factories, mines, quarries and at larger business premises an accident book is kept for this purpose. Claims are decided, not by the Minister of Social Security, but by authorities independent of the Minister. The claim is considered initially by an Insurance Officer, who decides whether or not benefit is payable. If the claimant is dissatisfied he can appeal to an independent local tribunal or, on the question whether he is suffering from a prescribed disease, to a medical board. In some cases there may be a further appeal to the Commissioner appointed by the Crown, whose decision is final. As already stated, medical questions on industrial disablement benefit are decided by medical boards and on appeal by Medical Appeal Tribunals.

Industrial Death Benefits

In case of death a weekly pension is paid to a widow who was living with her husband or being maintained by him. The amount is £6 7s. od. for the first 26 weeks after widowhood, followed by £5 1s. od. a week if the widow is over 50, or incapable of self-support, or if she has a child. In the latter case, the £5 1s. od. pension will continue after she ceases to have a qualifying child in her family, provided that she is over 40 years of age at that time. There is an addition of £1 5s. od. a week for the first child and 17s. a week for other children, apart from family allowances. Where there is no child, a widow under 50 who is capable of self support will get £2 a week. These pensions are for life, unless the widow remarries, in which case she will get one year's pension as a gratuity. A pension of £5 1s. od. a week is also paid to the widower of a woman who dies from industrial injury, if he was being maintained by her and is not capable of supporting himself. In addition, the present scheme provides pensions, allowances and gratuities for parents certain relatives and a woman having care of a child of the deceased, according to the extent of their dependence on the dead person. All these benefits are called *Industrial Death Benefits*.

Prescribed Industrial Diseases

In Great Britain a worker who develops one of the 44 industrial diseases, as well as pneumoconiosis and byssinosis, prescribed by regulations is entitled to industrial injuries benefit, in the same way as a person who has met with an industrial accident, if he has been insurably employed in a prescribed occupation on or after 5th July 1948, and the disease is due to the nature of his employment. The list of prescribed diseases is extended from time to time as evidence accumulates to justify this. The original schedule of prescribed diseases has been amended from time to time. The question whether a person is suffering from a prescribed industrial disease is a medical one and decisions given by medical boards, usually of two doctors, are final, though boards may review their decision if there is fresh evidence. As under the Workmen's Compensation Acts, special arrangements apply to the industrial lung diseases, pneumoconiosis and byssinosis; the medical questions are for decision by Pneumoconiosis Medical Boards consisting of specially qualified doctors. The Boards are stationed at several centres throughout the country.

Supplementary Schemes

Provision has been made by way of supplementary schemes for the payment out of the Industrial Injuries Fund of certain benefits and allowances for dependants, to persons disabled before 5th July 1948. The *Workmen's Compensation Supplementation Scheme, 1951*, provides for supplementary payments to workmen who are receiving low rates of compensation for accidents which occurred before 1924, and the *Pneumoconiosis and Byssinosis Benefit Scheme* provides benefits for workmen who are disabled by pneumoconiosis or byssinosis, but who are entitled neither to workmen's compensation nor industrial injury benefits. It also provides for the dependants of certain workmen who have died from either disease.

The National Insurance (Industrial Injuries) (Prescribed Diseases) Regulations, 1967

First Schedule, Part 1

Description of disease or injury	Nature of occupation
Poisoning by:	*Any occupation involving:*
1. Lead or a compound of lead .	The use or handling of, or exposure to the fumes, dust or vapour of, lead or a compound of lead, or a substance containing lead.
2. Manganese or a compound of manganese . . .	The use or handling of, or exposure to the fumes, dust or vapour of, manganese or a compound of manganese, or a substance containing manganese.
3. Phosphorus or phosphine or poisoning due to the anti-cholinesterase action of organic phosphorus compounds	The use or handling of, or exposure to the fumes, dust or vapour of, phosphorus or a compound of phosphorus, or a substance containing phosphorus.
4. Arsenic or a compound of arsenic	The use or handling of, or exposure to the fumes, dust or vapour of, arsenic or a compound of arsenic, or a substance containing arsenic.
5. Mercury or a compound of mercury	The use or handling of, or exposure to the fumes, dust or vapour of, mercury or a compound of mercury, or a substance containing mercury.
6. Carbon bisulphide . .	The use or handling of, or exposure to the fumes or vapour of, carbon bisulphide, or a substance containing carbon bisulphide.
7. Benzene or a homologue .	The use or handling of, or exposure to the fumes of, or vapour containing, benzene or any of its homologues.

Description of disease or injury	Nature of occupation
Poisoning by:	*Any occupation involving:*
8. A nitro- or amino- or chloro-derivative of benzene or of a homologue of benzene, or poisoning by nitrochlorbenzene . . .	The use or handling of, or exposure to the fumes of, or vapour containing, a nitro- or amino- or chloroderivative of benzene or of a homologue of benzene or nitrochlorbenzene.
9. Dinitrophenol or a homologue or by substituted dinitrophenols or by the salts of such substances. . .	The use or handling of, or exposure to the fumes of, or vapour containing, dinitrophenol or a homologue or substituted dinitrophenols or the salts of such substances.
10. Tetrachlorethane . .	The use or handling of, or exposure to the fumes of, or vapour containing, tetrachlorethane.
11. Tri-cresyl phosphate . .	The use or handling of, or exposure to the fumes of, or vapour containing, tri-cresyl phosphate.
12. Tri-phenyl phosphate . .	The use or handling of, or exposure to the fumes of, or vapour containing, tri-phenyl phosphate.
13. Diethylene dioxide (dioxan) .	The use or handling of, or exposure to the fumes of, or vapour containing, diethylene dioxide (dioxan).
14. Methyl bromide . .	The use or handling of, or exposure to the fumes of, or vapour containing, methyl bromide.
15. Chlorinated naphthalene .	The use or handling of, or exposure to the fumes of, or dust or vapour containing, chlorinated naphthalene.
16. Nickel carbonyl . . .	Exposure to nickel carbonyl gas.
17. Nitrous fumes . . .	The use or handling of nitric acid or exposure to nitrous fumes.
18. *Gonioma kamassi* (African boxwood)	The manipulation of *Gonioma kamassi* or any process in or incidental to the manufacture of articles therefrom.
19. Anthrax	The handling of wool, hair, bristles, hides or skins or other animal products or residues, or contact with animals infected with anthrax.
20. Glanders	Contact with equine animals or their carcases.

Description of disease or injury	Nature of occupation
	Any occupation involving:
21. (a) Infection by *Leptospira icterohæmorrhagiæ*,	Work in places which are, or are liable to be, infested by rats.
(b) Infection by *Leptospira canicola*.	Work at dog kennels or the care or handling of dogs.
22. Ankylostomiasis . . .	Work in or about a mine.
23. (a) *Dystrophy of the cornea (including ulceration of the corneal surface) of the eye.*	
(b) Localised new growth of the skin, papillomatous or keratotic,	
(c) Squamous-celled carcinoma of the skin, due in any case to arsenic, tar, pitch, bitumen, mineral oil (including paraffin), soot or any compound, product (*including quinone or hydroquinone*), or residue of any of these substances.	The use or handling of, or exposure to, arsenic, tar, pitch, bitumen, mineral oil (including paraffin), soot or any compound, product (*including quinone or hydroquinone*), or residue of any of these substances.
25. Inflammation, ulceration or malignant disease of the skin or subcutaneous tissues or of the bones, or blood dyscrasia, or cataract, due to electro-magnetic radiations (other than radiant heat), or to ionising particles. .	Exposure to electro-magnetic radiations other than radiant heat, or to ionising particles.
26. Heat cataract . . .	Frequent or prolonged exposure to rays from molten or red-hot material.
27. Decompression sickness .	Subjection to compressed or rarefied air.
28. Cramp of the hand or forearm due to repetitive movements.	Prolonged periods of handwriting, typing or other repetitive movements of the fingers, hand or arm.
31. Subcutaneous cellulitis of the hand (Beat hand). . .	Manual labour causing severe or prolonged friction or pressure on the hand.
32. Bursitis or subcutaneous cellulitis arising at or about the knee due to severe or prolonged external friction or pressure at or about the knee (Beat knee). . .	Manual labour causing severe or prolonged external friction or pressure at or about the knee.

Description of disease or injury	Nature of occupation
	Any occupation involving:
33. Bursitis or subcutaneous cellulitis arising at or about the elbow due to severe or prolonged external friction or pressure at or about the elbow (Beat elbow).	Manual labour causing severe or prolonged external friction or pressure at or about the elbow.
34. Traumatic inflammation of the tendons of the hand or forearm, or of the associated tendon sheaths.	Manual labour, or frequent or repeated movements of the hand or wrist.
35. Miner's nystagmus . .	Work in or about a mine.
36. Poisoning by beryllium or a compound of beryllium. .	The use or handling of, or exposure to the fumes, dust or vapour of, beryllium or a compound of beryllium, or a substance containing beryllium.
37. (*a*) Carcinoma of the mucous membrane of the nose or associated air sinuses (*b*) Primary carcinoma of a bronchus or of a lung	Work in a factory where nickel is produced by decomposition of a gaseous nickel compound which necessitates working in or about a building or buildings where that process or any other industrial process ancillary or incidental thereto is carried on.
38. Tuberculosis . . .	Close and frequent contact with a source or sources of tuberculous infection by reason of employment:— (*a*) in the medical treatment or nursing of a person or persons suffering from tuberculosis, or in a service ancillary to such treatment or nursing; (*b*) in attendance upon a person or persons suffering from tuberculosis, where the need for such attendance arises by reason of physical or mental infirmity; (*c*) as a research worker engaged in research in connexion with tuberculosis; (*d*) as a laboratory worker, pathologist or person taking part in or assisting at post-mortem examinations of human re-

Description of disease or injury	Nature of occupation
	Any occupation involving:
38. Tuberculosis (*cont.*) . .	mains where the occupation involves working with material which is a source of tuberculous infection.
39. Primary neoplasm of the epithelial lining of the urinary bladder (Papilloma of the bladder), or of the epithelial lining of the renal pelvis or of the epithelial lining of the ureter.	(*a*) Work in a building in which any of the following substances is produced for commercial purposes:— (i) *alpha*-naphthylamine or *beta*-naphthylamine; (ii) diphenyl substituted by at least one nitro or primary amino group or by at least one nitro and primary amino group; (iii) any of the substances mentioned in sub-paragraph (ii) above if further ring substituted by halogeno, methyl or methoxy groups, but not by other groups; (iv) the salts of any of the substances mentioned in sub-paragraphs (i) to (iii) above; (v) auramine or magenta; (*b*) the use or handling of any of the substances mentioned in sub-paragraphs (i) to (iv) of paragraph (*a*), or work in a process in which any such substance is used or handled or is liberated; (*c*) the maintenance or cleaning of any plant or machinery used in any such process as is mentioned in paragraph (*b*), or the cleaning of clothing used in any such building as is mentioned in paragraph (*a*) if such clothing is cleaned within the works of which the building forms a part or in a laundry maintained and used solely in connexion with such works.

Description of disease or injury	Nature of occupation
	Any occupation involving:
40. Poisoning by cadmium. .	Exposure to cadmium fumes.
41. Inflammation or ulceration of the mucous membrane of the upper respiratory passages or mouth produced by dust, liquid or vapour. .	Exposure to dust, liquid or vapour.
42. Non-infective dermatitis of external origin (including chrome ulceration of the skin but excluding dermatitis due to ionising particles or electro-magnetic radiations other than radiant heat). . . .	Exposure to dust, liquid or vapour or any other external agent capable of irritating the skin (including friction or heat but excluding ionising particles or electro-magnetic radiations other than radiant heat).
43. Pulmonary disease due to the inhalation of the dust of mouldy hay or of other mouldy vegetable produce, and characterized by symptoms and signs attributable to a reaction in the peripheral part of the broncho-pulmonary system, and giving rise to a defect in gas exchange (Farmer's lung).	Exposure to the dust of mouldy hay or other mouldy vegetable produce by reason of employment:— (a) in agriculture, horticulture or forestry; or (b) loading or unloading or handling in storage such hay or other vegetable produce; or (c) handling bagasse.
44. Primary malignant neoplasm of the mesothelium (diffuse mesothelioma) of the pleura or of the peritoneum. .	(a) The working or handling of asbestos or any admixture of asbestos; (b) the manufacture or repair of asbestos textiles or other articles containing or composed of asbestos; (c) the cleaning of any machinery or plant used in any of the foregoing operations and of any chambers, fixtures and appliances for the collection of dust; (d) substantial exposure to the dust arising from any of the foregoing operations.

First Schedule, Part 2

Pneumoconiosis. Fibrosis of the lungs due to silica dust, asbestos dust or other dust, and including the condition of the lungs known as dust-reticulation.

1. Any occupation involving—

(*a*) the mining, quarrying or working of silica rock or the working of dried quartzose sand or any dry deposit or dry residue of silica or any dry admixture containing such materials (including any occupation in which any of the aforesaid operations are carried out incidentally to the mining or quarrying of other minerals or to the manufacture of articles containing crushed or ground silica rock);

(*b*) the handling of any of the materials specified in the foregoing subparagraph in or incidental to any of the operations mentioned therein, or substantial exposure to the dust arising from such operations.

2. Any occupation involving the breaking, crushing or grinding of flint or the working or handling of broken, crushed or ground flint or materials containing such flint, or substantial exposure to the dust arising from any of such operations.

3. Any occupation involving sand blasting by means of compressed air with the use of quartzose sand or crushed silica rock or flint, or substantial exposure to the dust arising from such sand blasting.

4. Any occupation involving work in a foundry or the performance of, or substantial exposure to the dust arising from, any of the following operations:—

(*a*) the freeing of steel castings from adherent siliceous substance ;

(*b*) the freeing of metal castings from adherent siliceous substance:

(i) by blasting with an abrasive propelled by compressed air, by steam or by a wheel; or

(ii) by the use of power-driven tools.

5. Any occupation in or incidental to the manufacture of china or earthenware (including sanitary earthenware, electrical earthenware and earthenware tiles), and any occupation involving substantial exposure to the dust arising therefrom.

6. Any occupation involving the grinding of mineral graphite, or substantial exposure to the dust arising from such grinding.

7. Any occupation involving the dressing of granite or any igneous rock by masons or the crushing of such materials, or substantial exposure to the dust arising from such operations.

8. Any occupation involving the use, or preparation for use, of a grindstone, or substantial exposure to the dust arising therefrom.

9. Any occupation involving—

(*a*) the working or handling of asbestos or any admixture of asbestos;

(*b*) the manufacture or repair of asbestos textiles or other articles containing or composed of asbestos;

(*c*) the cleaning of any machinery or plant used in any of the foregoing operations and of any chambers, fixtures and appliances for the collection of asbestos dust;

(*d*) substantial exposure to the dust arising from any of the foregoing operations.

10. Any occupation involving—

(*a*) work underground in any mine in which one of the objects of the mining operations is the getting of any mineral;

(*b*) the working or handling above ground at any coal or tin mine of any minerals extracted therefrom, or any operation incidental thereto;

(*c*) the trimming of coal in any ship, barge or lighter, or in any dock or harbour or at any wharf or quay;

(*d*) the sawing, splitting or dressing of slate, or any operation incidental thereto.

11. Any occupation in or incidental to the manufacture of carbon electrodes by an industrial undertaking for use in the electrolytic extraction of aluminium from aluminium oxide, and any occupation involving substantial exposure to the dust arising therefrom.

12. Any occupation involving boiler scaling or substantial exposure to the dust arising therefrom.

Byssinosis. Employment for a period or periods amounting in the aggregate to not less than ten years, in any occupation in any room where any process up to and including the carding process is performed in factories in which the spinning or manipulation of raw or waste cotton is carried on.

Health and Welfare of the Miner

In contrast with the early years of the nineteenth century, when it was far from being admitted that the State had either a right or a duty to interfere in any way with underground conditions, the law today enforces the adoption of every endeavour to protect the life, health and welfare of the miner.

The Coal Mines Act, 1911

The law exerts all its force to ensure the proper and safe performance of the most commonplace operations in mining to the extent of specifying such details as the precise signals to be employed in connexion with haulage and winding. It also protects the underground worker from any ill-effects of working conditions on his health by demanding the provision of adequate, clean air, sanitation and bathing facilities. All this and much more is provided for in the *Coal Mines Act, 1911*, with its 127 sections dealing with management, safety, health, accidents, employment and other important aspects of mining operations, and by more than 400 regulations issued subsequently. It is a matter for just pride that, owing to the adoption of protective measures which modern science has rendered available, British coal mining is amongst the safest in the world.

The Mines and Quarries Act, 1954

Legislative policy must always follow practical development, but a study of British Mining Legislation shows that as safety measures have become available there is little delay in enforcing their adoption. This is shown clearly by the growing volume of Regulations relating to safety and health in coal mines which are constantly revised and extended and of which a full edition is published annually. These, together with the Coal Mines Act, constitute an invaluable guide on all matters connected with the safe and healthy conduct of mining operations. They not only prohibit dangerous practices, but, what is more important, they demand safety precautions which, if fully adopted, would further reduce the declining accident rate in our mines. The *Mines and Quarries Act, 1954*, which replaces the *Coal Mines Act, 1911*, tightens up the existing safety law bringing it into line with modern mining practice.

The Mines Inspectorate

In order to ensure compliance with all statutory safety requirements and to foster the best practices in our mines, the Ministry of Fuel and Power maintains a Mines Inspectorate, which is comprised of specially qualified and experienced mining engineers appointed by the State for this purpose. The number of inspectors is continually increasing and the scope of their duties is being extended. Thus in 1921 there were 93 inspectors of mines, whereas in 1953 the establishment was 158 (Table II). There is a Chief Inspector of Mines, with headquarters and staff in London, and a Divisional Inspector in each Division aided by a staff of District Inspectors and Inspectors in various areas. Visits of inspectors are unannounced, and may take place at any time of the day or night. In this way a constant check is kept upon working conditions. Should anything unsatisfactory be found, it is brought to the notice of the manager and measures suggested for putting it right.

Specialist Inspectors

Progress in certain branches of mining practice has made necessary the appointment of Specialist Inspectors devoting attention to particular problems (Statham, 1951). These include Electrical Inspectors, Mechanical Engineering Inspectors, Medical Inspectors, Horse Inspectors and others for dealing with Roof Control and Dust Problems. The establishment for the Medical Inspectorate consists of a Principal Medical Inspector, a Deputy Principal Medical Officer and three Medical Inspectors (Table II). Their services are always at the disposal of the industry, not only to see that the law is obeyed but to offer advice on all matters relating to the safe working of the mines. In addition, inspectors or examiners appointed by the miners themselves make frequent inspections of mines, so that every effort is made in the interests of mine safety.

National Coal Board Medical Service

The National Coal Board provides a comprehensive industrial health service for all its employees. The Medical Service is an independent department of the Board represented at headquarters and in the divisions and areas. It is headed by a medical officer in each case. In the larger areas the area medical officer has an assistant. State-registered nurses are employed at the larger collieries. By 1956 there were 70 medical officers in the Service, including three engaged on medical research, and about 300 nurses. The Medical Service carries out the following functions:—

(i) *Pre-employment Examination of Workers:* All new entrants to the mining industry are examined by the Medical Service. Since the beginning of 1959 a regulation has been in force making radiographic examination of the chest universal throughout the coal mines of Great Britain.

(ii) *Advising Management on the Hygiene of the Working Environment:* It is particularly difficult to secure good hygienic conditions in coal mines. Unlike the factory worker whose working conditions remain much the same from day to day, the miner is continually battling with changing conditions. Lighting, dust and ventilation as well as heat and humidity in deep mines all present challenging environmental problems.

(iii) *Advising Management on the Medical Aspects of Safety:* Careful pre-employment examinations can make an obvious contribution to safety. Further, the study of mining jobs by doctors in the industry, who have special knowledge of the psychological and physiological problems involved, should make for safer working.

(iv) *Organization of First Aid:* Owing to the dangerous nature of mining operations the accident rate in coal mines is higher than in any other major industry. A highly efficient first-aid organization is thus essential if loss of life and disability are to be kept as low as possible. There are some 20,000 volunteer first-aid men in British coal mines and a considerable effort is required to assure that their knowledge of first aid is kept up-to-date.

(v) *Treatment of Injury and Illness:* The first treatment of men sustaining an injury or becoming ill at work is a responsibility of the Medical Service. At the larger pits treatment is given at medical centres staffed by state-registered nurses. The smaller pits have good first-aid rooms staffed by medical-room attendants.

(vi) *Resettlement of Miners after Injury or Illness:* The miners' rehabilitation units provide an excellent rehabilitation service, the importance of which needs no emphasis. The service is extended by a follow-up when the convalescent miner returns to the pit. In addition to cases due to injury men suffering from pneumoconiosis require regular supervision.

(vii) *Research:* Fundamental research on miners' diseases is, generally speaking, carried out by units of the Medical Research Council. Applied research, on the other hand, is the responsibility of the Medical Service.

This research is carried out either directly by the research staff of the Medical Service or indirectly by selected departments in certain medical schools which receive grants of assistance from the Board.

TABLE II

Health Services for Coal Mines

Doctors employed by the National Coal Board	70
State-registered nurses	300
Inspectors of mines	138
Medical inspectors of mines	5
Electrical inspectors of mines	9
Inspectors of horses	7
Inspectors of quarries	9

The Miners' Welfare Fund

The surroundings in which large numbers of coal miners are still compelled to live and work are far from pleasant. The grim aspect of the older mining areas is the legacy of 150 years of uncontrolled building with thoughtless destruction of natural beauty, bad and ill-located housing, dereliction of land, disfigurement by heaps of spoil from the pits, coal dust, smoke and unsightly colliery buildings. Provision for the recreation, health and education of coal miners was made in the *Mining Industry Act, 1920*. The Miners' Welfare Fund which was administered by a Central Miners' Committee, later a Commission, came from the levy of a penny on every ton of coal raised, and the Act provided for this to be applied to

> purposes connected with the social well-being, recreation and conditions of living of the workers in or about coal mines, and with mining education and research.

Between 1920 and 1943 the Fund had enabled roughly 700 institutes and 850 recreation grounds to be provided, an effort which was but a palliative since the great majority of mining people still lived in squalor.

Pithead Baths

A further development took place in 1926 when the income of the Fund was increased by the imposition of a 5 per cent levy on mining royalties. The *Mining Industry Act, 1926*, placed upon the Miners' Welfare Committee on duty

> to secure as far as reasonably practicable the provision at all coal mines of accommodation for workmen taking baths and drying clothes.

On the continent of Europe the advantages of pithead baths were realized much earlier than in Britain; their use was compulsory in Westphalia after 1900 and their provision obligatory in Belgium in 1913. But the Continental installations had the disadvantage that men and clothes begrimed from work came into contact with home clothes and clean men. The British pithead bath was a new departure, providing separate drying-rooms and heated clothes-lockers for home and pit clothes. Facilities are afforded also for brushing and greasing boots and for the parking of bicycles. Colliery canteens, first-aid rooms and medical centres are sometimes incorporated in a complete Pithead Unit. In 1945, when the building of baths was resumed after being virtually suspended since 1942, 345 collieries had already been equipped, but unhappily 500 remained unequipped. By 1950 bathing facilities were available at 390 installations, for nearly 468,000 persons, representing about 67 per cent of the total employed. The daily bath does much to prevent infection of small wounds and the *beat diseases*. Pithead baths benefit not only the miner but also his wife, who is relieved of much drudgery. They inculcate a desire not only for personal cleanliness and tidiness, but for these same features in his work and surroundings generally.

New Development and Reconstruction

While the work of the Miners' Welfare Commission and its successor, the Coal Industry Social Welfare Organization, has enabled some progress to be made towards improving the environment of mining people, the betterment affected is small by comparison with the total need. A satisfactory physical environment is necessary to secure enjoyment of full social life, and neither can result from piecemeal methods. Long before 1946 some colliery owners began to tidy up their pithead premises and even to lay out greensward, flowers, shrubs and trees. Pithead baths, therefore, were not only beginning to make a contribution towards improving the standards of industrial architecture, they were also slowly arousing a new interest on the part of colliery owners and awakening a realization that ugliness, untidiness and grime were not inevitable features of a pithead. When new pits were sunk at Comrie in Fife and Calverton in Nottinghamshire, architects, in consultation with mining engineers, for the first time took a leading part in planning surface layouts and in designing the pithead buildings. The *Coal Industry Nationalization Act, 1946*, and the *Town and Country Planning Act, 1947*, now provide powers which enable mining people to embark upon one of the greatest experiments in the control of their environment ever attempted by a free society. The reorganization of the coal industry is an immense and complicated task, but it presents a splendid opportunity for planning and landscape treatment on a large scale, also for good design and rational building, which are essential to pleasant and healthy environment (Kemp, 1949).

Welfare under Nationalization

When the mining industry was nationalized, the *Coal Industry Nationalization Act, 1946*, confirmed the existence of the Miners' Welfare Commission but it also laid upon the National Coal Board the duty of securing the welfare of persons in their employment. To co-ordinate the activities of the two bodies a National Miners' Welfare Joint Council was established in 1948. The National Coal Board provided additional funds to those derived from the statutory levies to assist in particular the speedy erection of pithead baths and the improvement of pithead canteens. Under the then existing legislation the output levy was due to cease at the end of 1951, and at the suggestion of the Minister of Fuel and Power the National Coal Board and the National Union of Mineworkers opened discussions in 1950 to consider how miners' welfare should in future be organized. On 24th July 1951 an Agreement was signed which provided for the division of welfare in the Coal Industry into two categories—colliery welfare and social welfare. The Board would assume responsibility for colliery welfare as a normal function of management and the responsibility for social welfare would pass to a new body, the Coal Industry Social Welfare Organization. Statutory effect was given to the provisions of this Agreement by the *Miners' Welfare Act, 1952*, and on 30th June 1952 the Miners' Welfare Commission was dissolved.

Achievements of the Miners' Welfare Fund

The establishment of the Miners' Welfare Fund in 1920 was described at the time as an experiment. It was the first and only statutory provision for the social welfare of workers in any industry, a recognition that the conditions under which miners worked and the isolation of many of the colliery villages where they lived, called for special attention to the welfare needs of mineworkers and their families. Over 400 pithead baths were provided, many of them of considerable architectural merit, and canteens were established at over 900 collieries. Institutes and recreation grounds were provided for mining communities which would not otherwise have possessed them. Twenty convalescent homes were made available to mineworkers and their wives.

Present Activity

The provision of pithead baths at all collieries where the life of the colliery seemed to justify it was completed by the end of 1960. The National Coal Board, through the agency of the Coal Industry Housing Association set up in 1952, has carried out a housing programme in those areas where more houses were urgently wanted than the local authorities could provide, and some 20,000 houses have been built in well laid-out estates. The Coal Industry Social Welfare Organization has continued the activities of the Miners' Welfare Commission in the social welfare field, and in addition to the provision of additional community centres and playing fields they have stressed the encouragement of sporting and cultural activities. The Organization has undertaken a survey into the social needs of 550 paraplegic mineworkers and holiday schemes and other amenities have been provided for these men. Consideration is being given to extending a personal welfare service to other mineworkers who are seriously disabled, whether through accident or disease.

Occupational Health Services in Countries Abroad

The early factory legislation of the various European nations induced industry to organize its working places so as to diminish accidents, improve lighting conditions and ventilation, limit working hours and protect the health of workers in general. Some years later, the Workmen's Compensation Acts, first in Europe and then in America, provided strong additional inducements for the adoption of safety measures and also for the establishment of first-aid medical services in factories. Throughout Western Europe, where modern industry had its beginnings, it is the general rule that health and safety in industry comes under the jurisdiction of Ministries of Labour.

Norway illustrates the General Pattern

The situation in Norway illustrates the general pattern. The Norwegian Ministry of Labour has a Directorate of Factory Inspection first organized in 1892. The staff consists of seven Labour Inspectors covering the country on a district basis, together with three inspectors of special problems and three Medical Inspectors. Periodic inspections of factories are made to enforce legislation designed to prevent occupational diseases and accidents. Under the Workers Protection Act of 1936 pre-employment and periodic medical examination are required for young workers of from fifteen to eighteen years of age, and for workers exposed to siliceous dusts and to radioactive substances. In each of 750 communities there is a local Labour Inspection Committee to help enforce the law. An Institute of Occupational Health is maintained by the Ministry of Labour in Oslo, to assist in the diagnosis of cases of occupational disease and to perform relevant laboratory tests (Bruusgaard, 1953).

Factory Inspection in Other European Countries

The other Scandinavian countries have a similar arrangement. In Sweden, Denmark and Finland the Factory Inspectorate is in the Ministry of Social Affairs, but its functions are essentially the same. Being one of the oldest and largest industrial nations with a strong tradition for government control, Germany has a strict system of factory inspection based on the Department of Labour in each state. The social upheaval of the Second World War caused a general extension in the scope of the programme for occupational health. This is best seen in the introduction in Belgium and France of the requirement of a general medical examination of all workers prior to employment. It became clear that it was to the common benefit of industry and the worker not only to prevent accidents and industrial diseases but also to ensure that a man was physically and mentally suited to a particular job.

State Departments of Labor in the United States of America

In the United States of America the assumption by government of responsibility for the health of the workers came later than in Europe. The earliest programme for industrial health was developed in Massachusetts where the first State Labor Bureau was set up in 1869. New Jersey and Wisconsin followed in 1883; State Departments of Labor developed slowly in the early twentieth century and they had little power. The men engaged for the work of factory inspection were rarely trained in engineering or chemistry and in only one state was medical guidance sought. In 1907 in New York State a single Medical Inspector of Factories was appointed, but the idea did not spread.

A Cheap Labour Force of Immigrant Workmen

The lack of any significant social conscience concerning the dangerous trades was part of the *laissez-faire* liberalism of the day. Immigrant workmen from Central Europe and the Mediterranean countries formed a cheap labour force and were scarcely treated as white men, they were only Wops and Hunkies. In a big smelting works in Utah, to take one example, the accidents amongst such men were so terrible and so numerous that a little thing like lead colic attracted no attention. Burns, crushing accidents, amputations of both arms, the loss of eyes and deaths from rupture of the liver or intestines constantly occurred and were not covered by any scheme of compensation.

Pioneer Work of Alice Hamilton

In her autobiography, *Exploring the Dangerous Trades* (1943), Alice Hamilton (fig. 66) describes her visit to Brussels in 1910 to attend the Fourth International Congress on Occupational Accidents and Diseases.

The Brussels Congress was a very interesting experience for me, meeting and hearing the famous authorities I knew so well from their writings: chiefly German and English, but also French, Austrian, Dutch, Belgian, Italian. But for an American it was not an occasion for national pride. There were but two of us on the program, Major Bailey Ashford, with a paper on hookworm infestation in Puerto Rico, and myself with one on the white-lead industry in the United States which revealed only too clearly the lack of such precautions as were a commonplace in the older countries. It was still more mortifying to be unable to answer any of the questions put to us: What was the rate of lead poisoning in such and such an industry? What legal regulations did we have for the dangerous trades? What

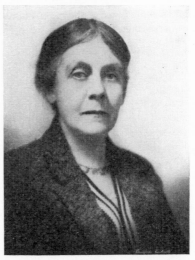

FIG. 66.—Dr. Alice Hamilton of Harvard
(*Photograph by Bradford Bachrach*)

was the system of compensation? Finally Dr. Glibert, of the Belgian Labor Department, dismissed the subject: "It is well known that there is no industrial hygiene in the United States. *Ça n'existe pas.*"

U.S. Office of Industrial Hygiene and Sanitation

In 1914 the United States Public Health Service established the Office of Industrial Hygiene and Sanitation primarily for research purposes. Similar research activities were undertaken in the Departments of Labor of New York and Ohio, but other states and local public health agencies in general were too weak to tackle the problem. The Workmen's Compensation laws, which were initiated only after 1911, stimulated the use of preventive measures against the occurrence of occupational diseases.

U.S. Industrial Hygiene Units

The great industrial depression in 1929 led to the passage of the Social Security Act of 1935. Under this law larger funds were made available for public health services than ever before through the device of federal grants-in-aid to the states. The Public Health Service administered these grants and, having now had twenty years of experience in industrial hygiene research, it used them to help the states develop industrial hygiene units in the State Departments of Health. The idea took hold and grew rapidly, so that by 1953 every state public health agency, except four, and several large city health departments contained specialized staffs for promoting the protection of the health of workers.

Health of the Worker in the Newest Industrial Nations

In the newest of the industrial nations, Soviet Russia, where the entire system of health service was reorganized after the Revolution of 1917–18, industrial health services have been made part of the general responsibility of the Commissariat of Health. And among nations with a new sense of their national destiny, like Egypt and Iran, one sees an interesting sharing of administrative responsibility. On the one hand, influenced by the precedent of the Western European powers, the Ministries of Labour of these countries maintain factory inspection systems, while, on the other hand, with a broad conception of responsibility of government for total health, their Health Ministries assume many responsibilities in carrying out the health and sanitary supervision of working places. The same process is occurring in Latin America (Roemer and Da Costa, 1953).

DISTRIBUTION OF MANPOWER

In Great Britain, twenty-five million men and women earn their daily bread by manual labour or otherwise. There are also about ten million housewives who work hard in the home but are not paid. The twenty-five million workers are scattered through many occupations and include those serving with the armed forces, those in industry, those on

TABLE III

Manpower and Employment, 1966

	Thousands
Total Working Population	25,644
Armed Forces	417
Mining and Quarrying	577
Gas, Electricity, and Water	423
Transport and Communication	1,649
Agriculture and Fishing	799
Manufactures	8,962
Construction	1,849
Distributive Trades	3,504
Professional, Financial, and Miscellaneous Services	5,865
National Government Service	557
Local Government Service	789
Wholly Unemployed	253

the land, those in professions, and the registered unemployed. Table III shows the distribution of the working population of Great Britain in June, 1966.

Basic Industries and Services

The basic industries and services are mining and quarrying; gas, electricity, and water; transport and communications; and agriculture and fishing. On these, the country depends for its food, the rest of its industrial and manufacturing activities, and much of its daily life. Without coal, there would be no steam, gas, or electricity; without water, sanitation and drainage would break down; without fishing and agriculture there would be inadequate food; without quarrying, little building; and without transport and communications our complicated economic life would come to a stop. These industries serve the manufacturing industries. They move the machinery, light the workshops, bring raw materials to the factories, and distribute the finished goods. Although the adult male in the prime of life is generally the most efficient worker, there are certain jobs for which he is not particularly suited and, further, there are insufficient men in their prime to do all the industrial work needed. For these and other reasons, young persons, women, and old people are employed in industry in large numbers. Women form less than one-third of all industrial workers. In the basic industries of mining and quarrying, supply services, transport and communications, where much of the work is heavy and shift work is common, very few women are found. In building there are even fewer, and in the heavy metal and chemical trades they comprise less than one-fifth of the labour force. Half the workers in the distributive trades are women, mostly shop assistants. The textile and clothing industries employ more women than men.

The Working Environment

The health and happiness of the worker in industry depend on circumstances which are as complex as they are numerous. Experts in widely differing fields are constantly at work to secure the best results. *Architects* must be employed so that industrial firms may set out to design factories which are a joy to work in rather than being just tolerable. *Ventilating engineers* are needed to maintain comfort in working and in the case of the dangerous trades to keep the working atmosphere free from poisonous vapour, fume, and dust. *Chemists* will help in this work, and wherever there is a hazard from radioactive substances, *physicists* will be consulted. *Illumination engineers* will be required for innumerable jobs, and of course their contribution to safety is considerable. *Mechanical engineers* will devise machines which are fool-proof against amputating people's fingers, and *electrical engineers* will arrange switching systems making machines fool-proof against electrocution accidents. *Safety officers* will provide protective clothing from plastic helmets to boots with steel toe-caps. The Works Safety Committees will hold discussions on accident prevention and arrange propaganda devices in such forms as posters and competitions. And then *factory inspectors* will come to see that all the regulations are obeyed. They may seek the assistance of *medical inspectors, electrical inspectors,* or *engineering and chemical inspectors. Personnel managers* and *welfare workers* will be responsible for incentive schemes. *Statisticians* will contribute to the study of health in industry by arranging punched-card systems to record sickness absence in groups of employees. In this the London Transport Executive (1956) has led the way by setting up a Central Record of Staff Statistics at its headquarters.

The Works Medical Department

The medical department will be in charge of the *works medical officer* assisted by *nurses* specially trained for the job and perhaps *physiotherapists. Dental surgeons* may attend regularly for the benefit of the workers. The works doctor will supervise the training of squads of *first-aid men* in rescue work and they will keep all the special breathing apparatus and other rescue gear constantly in working order. *Dietitians* may be employed to arrange the menus in the works canteens and they may consult *canteen advisers.* The quality of the medical work which the works doctor has to offer will always be of paramount importance. The actual impetus for improved conditions at work has largely come from doctors and will continue to do so.

TRAINING THE DOCTOR FOR INDUSTRY

Clearly the doctor in training must understand that the factors concerned in keeping the worker healthy are more than medical, they are social, economic, environmental, political, psychological and personal. How is this brought about in our medical schools?

Training the Medical Student

Let us begin by considering some points in the training of students in the medical schools of Great Britain. What they have to learn is difficult and complex and necessitates long concentration on bedside methods in which they are taught how to question and examine patients. In doing this they learn to take an interest in patients as men and women who lead a particular kind of life in a certain kind of way, as persons with family ties and obligations, with anxieties, hopes, and fears. A good doctor takes into account social and economic factors, conditions of work and leisure, standards of housing, clothing, diet, and personal habits. He sees the injured worker as a bread-winner, the woman in childbirth as a wife and mother, the handicapped child as an educational problem and a source of special anxiety for the parents. Hence, from the beginning of his training, the medical student should be led to embrace the notion of a diagnosis which relates both the physical condition and the patient himself to the environment in which he lives, works, and plays. The environment of the patient may be thought of as psychological, occupational, and socio-economic.

Promotion of Positive Health

The social aspects of the doctor's work are today linked very closely with the positive promotion of health and the prevention of disease. The effective treatment of occupational diseases is essentially preventive. Often in undergraduate medical education the role of social and preventive medicine is too little emphasized. In some medical schools the under-graduate receives inadequate instruction in matters upon which health largely depends: nutrition, housing, factory hygiene, personal hygiene, socio-economic status, social security, and organized public health and medical-care services. A medical graduate with nothing but a bedside training might very well practise medicine without ever having asked himself: "How much of this disease is there? In what circumstances is the incidence high or low? How could it be prevented?" He might never have formulated the questions: "What social aids are needed to reinforce medical care? How completely and in what manner are they provided? What is my part as a practising doctor in the medical welfare services maintained by the State and other agencies? What are the wider duties in society of the profession to which I belong?" There can be little doubt about the vocational and educational inadequacy of medical training which does not raise, examine, and point the way to answering these and other questions of like nature. Fortunately the World Health Organization is interested in this subject and has published relevant symposia for the benefit of teachers both of undergraduates and of postgraduates.

Visits to Factories, Docks and Mines

Should the teachers of medicine arrange to take medical students on visits to factories, docks, and mines? Undoubtedly they should, but too often they do not. The pressure of other duties is no doubt their excuse. A visit to sewers is a single example of what may be done. Teachers in any medical school in Great Britain can arrange with the main drainage engineers of the local authority to walk with their students through a section of the sewers of the town in which they work. And when the student becomes a qualified doctor he should take the opportunity to enrich his general knowledge and experience by studying the conditions of work in those industries which fall within the area of his practice. By visiting the places where his patients work not only will he understand their problems better, but also he will be able to help them by making contact with the welfare and medical departments within the factories concerned. No doctor can be expected to be familiar with the details of all occupations and every working environment, but at least he should learn how to obtain the requisite information from libraries.

Training the Industrial Medical Officer

In Great Britain there are fewer than 3,000 medical men and women engaged in one way or another in industrial medicine and only about 250 who give their whole time to it. There are approximately 250,000 factories in the country and of these 230,000 employ fewer than 250 persons each, many as few as 25 persons. Of those factories with 250 employees only 50 per cent employ a doctor, and where there are fewer than 100 workers only 4 per cent have the services of a doctor. To qualify as competent to carry out the duties of full-time industrial medical officer a doctor will follow a prolonged course of study for a special diploma, usually of a university. The details need not be given here, but let it suffice to say that he must be prepared to make himself technically minded to a degree that used to be thought quite foreign to the sphere of practical medicine.

Subjects for Detailed Study

Lighting, heating, ventilation, humidity, dust control, prevention of emission of toxic gas and fume, optimum methods of working, weight lifting, shift systems, ways of avoiding boredom in repetitive work, adjustment of human relations, detection and removal of sources of friction and fear, investigation of processes known or suspected to lead to disease, development of physical and chemical methods to determine the absorption by the worker of dangerous compounds, maintenance of high standards of hygiene and sanitation, control of nutritional standards in canteens, development of the best technique for the treatment of injuries and poisoning—all come within the scope of environmental study, in the factory and in the laboratory. By such detailed study of industrial environment he appreciates the background against which to place new entrants, for rehabilitating the injured and partly disabled, for choosing alternative work for a man who has been sick, and for elucidating possible causes of acute and chronic illness among the workers.

A Proper Regard for Social Values

The full-time industrial doctor of the future must be so well trained that he will be invited to co-operate with managers, workers, engineers, chemists, and architects. He should aim at discovering all possible faults in the working environment with a view to finding proper remedies for them. One of his most interesting duties must be to bring into the effective service of industry the discoveries of the research worker. Only then will he be in a position to make the industrialist understand the risks to which his men are exposed, and that the guiding principle of low costs and large profits retards progress. He should have an aptitude for administration, though in the factory he is best employed in an advisory, not an executive, capacity. He should be responsible to the managing director, and not to any other official of the company, such as the labour manager. He should take charge of all first-aid, medical, and nursing services. He should have had considerable experience in clinical work and should have held resident hospital appointments; he should know something of social problems and should be able to undertake original research in medicine. The factory medical officer should never allow his special technical knowledge to assume greater importance than his knowledge of doctoring in general. He should strive to be a good doctor in the broadest sense of the term, to preserve contacts with academic medicine, to cultivate interests outside his profession, and to follow his various activities with a constant regard for social values.

Assessment of Workers as Emotional Beings

In modern industrial medicine the emphasis is upon people, the conditions in which they live and work, their hopes and fears, their abilities, their attitudes towards their job, their fellow workers, and their employers. Of course, the industrial doctor must have a practical clinical background which will enable him to assess physical factors in health and disease, and detect disease attributable to occupation. Far more difficult is the assessment of men and women as emotional beings, moved by trivial things, overturned by worries and anxieties, torn by conscience, stunned by the inevitable trials of family life, and easily captured by a sense of frustration and persecution. It is the interaction of this complex, an individual and his industrial environment, animate and inanimate, that the industrial doctor tries to analyse, and from the analysis to establish an equilibrium which permits a stable relationship. As social-mindedness develops, a better industrial medical service will be demanded. At present the supply of competent doctors is inadequate to fill the number of posts which already exist in factories. Meanwhile the majority of our medical schools and teaching hospitals are not alive to this need.

THE OCCUPATIONAL CASE HISTORY

SINCE the time of Hippocrates the existence of specific occupational diseases has come to be recognized in our common speech in such expressions as brassfounders' ague, chimney-sweeps' cancer, divers' paralysis, glass-blowers' cataract, grocers' itch, hatters' shakes, housemaids' knee, knife-grinders' phthisis, miners' nystagmus, painters' colic, tailors' callosities, woolsorters' disease and writers' cramp. Less well-known examples are aero-embolism of aviators, apple sorters' disease, apple thinners' disease, aviation deafness, bakers' asthma, bakers' dermatitis, Billingsgate hump, bird-breeders' lung, bird-fanciers' lung, biscuit makers' dermatitis, blacksmiths' deafness, boilermakers' deafness, brass chills, braziers' disease, butchers' tubercle, caisson disease, calico-printers' dermatitis, chain-makers' cataract, cigarette cutters' asthma, coal-miners' phthisis, colour-developers' dermatitis, confectioners' dermatitis, coolie itch, copper fever, cotton-carders' asthma, cotton card-room asthma, cotton-twisters' cramp, cotton weavers' deafness, Covent Garden hummy, dairymen's itch, deal-runners' shoulder, Dogger Bank itch, drysalters' itch, duck fever, dust consumption, dustmen's shoulder, engineers' dermatitis, farmers' lung, feather pickers' disease, file cutters' paralysis, firemen's cataract, firemen's eye, fish handlers' disease, fish porters' bursitis, flour workers' dermatitis, foundry fever, French polishers' dermatitis, galvanizers' poisoning, ganister disease, gold smelters' cataract, grain handlers' asthma, grinders' asthma, grinders' consumption, grinders' rot, grit consumption, hodmen's shoulder, hoppers' gout, humpers' hump, iron puddlers' cataract, labourers' spine, lightermen's bottom, malthouse-workers' cough, metal-fume fever, metal platers' dermatitis, millers' asthma, mill fever, millworkers' asthma, miners' asthma, miners' beat elbow, miners' beat hand, miners' beat knee, miners' bunches, miners' cramp, miners' phthisis, Monday fever, mule-spinners' cancer, nickel refiners' itch, nuns' bursitis, painters' dermatitis, photographers' dermatitis, pigeon-fanciers' lung, pneumatic hammer disease, polymer fume fever, pork finger, potters' asthma, potters' rot, pottery firemen's cataract, poultrymen's itch, printers' asthma, printers' dermatitis, prosectors' wart, radiologists' cancer, railway brain, railway spine, rock tuberculosis, seal finger, silo-fillers' disease, silo-workers' asthma, smelters' cataract, spelter shakes, stokers' cramp, stone cutters' asthma, stone-hewers' phthisis, stonemasons' disease, sugar refiners' dermatitis, tailors' ankle, tar workers' dermatitis, telegraphists' cramp, threshers' lung, tinplate workers' cataract, tunnel-workers' anæmia, washerwomen's itch, weavers' bottom, weavers' cough, weavers' deafness, welders' ague, whale finger, zinc chills and zinc oxide chills. No doctor can be expected to be familiar with the details of all occupations and every working environment, but at least he should take the opportunity to study those industries which fall within the area of his practice.

Intelligent Knowledge of the Patient's Job

There are few surer and quicker means of gaining a patient's confidence than the display of an intelligent knowledge of his job. The workman has his own notions and he may be governed very much in his thinking by the mass opinions of his fellow workers. The London artisan is usually intelligent and co-operative and often a good witness, but what if he be deaf, disconsolate, forgetful or obtuse? He may be either garrulous or monosyllabic, but in spite of these possibilities he is still the best witness to what has happened and should be handled with great patience and understanding (O'Donovan, 1952).

A Chronological List of all the Jobs ever Done

Doctors working in many different branches of medicine know that it is far more difficult to take an adequate history than to make an adequate physical examination. To elicit and assess at its full value all the evidence which can be obtained from interrogating the artisan patient requires a wealth of special knowledge and experience. It follows that a definite technique must be used in recording the occupational history. Further, this must be applied on first seeing the patient. Never should history taking await the direction of evidence subsequently revealed by radiographic or other special tests. It is a wise rule to take the occupational history from the time the patient left school. One should record the dates and items of all subsequent jobs.

A Previous Occupation responsible for the Hazard

Of course, it is most likely that the noxious substance responsible for his ill health is to be found in his present occupation, but this is not to be taken for granted. Thus, a housewife with pulmonary tuberculosis may be suffering from this illness as a complication of asbestosis contracted while she was a single woman working in an asbestos factory years before. The long latent interval which may occur before the appearance of occupational cancer of the skin leads to the same error. Thus, a man describing himself as an ice-cream vendor may have cancer of the skin of the hand due to his having worked in the pitch beds of a gas works twenty years before. Henry (1950) has described the present job of such a man as an *end occupation*. Others are that of caretaker, time-keeper, hotel or lodging-house keeper, gate-keeper, lock-keeper, commissionaire, watchman or even shopkeeper, stationmaster, or agent or manager of a coal mine.

Cancer of the Skin from a Previous Occupation

A man suffering from carcinoma of the skin on the lower limbs or penis may have been a maker of hand-made boots and shoes. This can be accounted for by the ball of soft pitch formerly used for applying to the thread. A worker in the heavy metals industry with a carcinoma of the ear had dipped pipes into coal tar for sixteen years. Carcinoma of the skin due to X-rays has been found in a commissionaire who was previously a qualified male nurse at a radium institute. It is always important in a man employed as a photographer to inquire whether he has had some previous case work with X-rays. Lastly, we should never omit inquiries as to hobbies in addition to occupation, as in the case of a director of a railway who died from a carcinoma on the hand which he himself considered was due to manipulating tarred ropes on his luxurious yacht (Henry, 1950).

Technical Names of Trades

Ask him the name of his trade, the processes employed, the tools used and the substances handled. The name he gives to his job may be an obvious euphemism. If he tells you he's a *salvage officer* he means a *dustman*, if a *street orderly* he means *roadsweeper*, and if he says *vermin exterminator* or *rodent operative* he means *rat catcher*. On occasions it is necessary to remember the transferred epithet as in *reinforced-concrete draughtsman*, *sagger-maker's bottom knocker*, *greasy darner* and *invertebrate physiologist*. The imagination of the interrogator, say of pottery workers, will overcome such terms as *lithographic artist*, *tunnel oven operative* and *insulator turner*, but not *jiggerer*, *dobie girl* and *saggar wad pugman*. In such cases, naturally. the artisan himself will define what the name of his job really means, Whether he be a *fish hobbler*, *getter-up-charger*, *head sinker*, *nobbler*. *mucker-out*, *swadge sawyer*, *teazer*, *trolloper* or *whammeler*, he will respond to your detailed questions if only you are firm and tactful and show appreciation of his skill.

Many Names for One Job

The name of an occupation may mislead you, for different names are used for the same or closely similar processes in different parts of Great Britain. Thus, in foundries a man who cleans metal castings with a compressed-air chisel or a carborundum wheel is variously known as a *fettler*, a *trimmer* or a *steel dresser*. In coal mining the shale or rock between the seams of coal is drilled or blasted by miners who may work in separate shifts from the coal-getters. The man who does this type of work is usually called a *hardheader* in South Wales, a *brancher* in Somerset, a *stoneman* in Durham, a *ripper* in Yorkshire and a *brusher* in Kent (see p. 983). More than sixty names have been given to variants of this job, of which the following are examples: *canchman, concher, crutter, dinter, drifter, kenchman, lipper, rock header, rockman, shifter* and *tunneller* (*Classifications of Occupations*, General Register Office, 1960, H.M.S.O., London).

Name of the Job Misleading

But there is another misleading point, for a man who calls himself an engineer's fitter may do his work on chromium plating vats and thus encounter the hazard of chrome dermatitis. A glass-blower may be exposed to the hazard of mercury poisoning if he does his work in a thermometer factory. A bricklayer is not necessarily employed in building houses. He may demolish, with a compressed-air chisel, furnace linings made of firebricks or of special refractory bricks containing up to 80 per cent of free silica. Sometimes he calls himself a *furnace bricklayer*. In special places, for example in some parts of Derbyshire, a gravedigger does not handle gravel or clay, but excavates sandstone and is therefore liable to silicosis from the siliceous dust he produces (Meiklejohn, 1949).

Popular Names used in Chemistry, Mining and Metallurgy

It often happens that workmen and foremen refer to chemical substances by their popular names and not by their chemical names. This is especially true of small establishments employing no chemist and maintaining no department for research. Examples of such names are *lunar caustic* for silver nitrate, *caustic potash* for potassium hydroxide, *oxymuriate of potash* for potassium chlorate, *saltpetre* or *nitre* for potassium nitrate, *corrosive sublimate* for mercuric chloride, *oil of vitriol* for sulphuric acid, *blue vitriol* for copper sulphate, *green vitriol* for ferrous sulphate, *white vitriol* for zinc sulphate, *butter of antimony* for antimony pentachloride, *butter of zinc* for zinc chloride, *sugar of lead* for lead acetate, *wood spirit* for methyl alcohol and *oil of mirbane* for nitrobenzene. Often such names are older than the present names, for example the term *muriatic acid* was in use long before the elementary nature of chlorine had been established, when the name was changed to hydrochloric acid. The worker may use expressions unfamiliar to you, for example, *I chute chrome yellow into a kibbler*, by which he means that he throws lead chromate down an inclined channel so that it enters a machine which breaks it up. A man who says *I run the liquid sally from the top gantry* means that he runs a solution of *sal ammoniac* (ammonium chloride) from the top barrel. In metalliferous mines the terms *ore body*, *lode* or *vein* refer to ore deposits of differing magnitude. Foundry workers also use popular names which may be misleading. Thus a metal founder bleaching brass by alloying it with 25 per cent nickel may call the alloy *nickel silver* when it is nothing but white brass. Bars of metals and their alloys of various shapes and sizes are referred to by the metallurgist and the foundryman as *pigs, ingots, billets, sticks, slugs* and *skillets*. These names are to some extent interchangeable and may be used with a different connotation in the ferrous and non-ferrous metals industries.

Chemical Nature of Building Stones

In the case of stonemasons it may be difficult to ascertain the chemical nature of the building stones handled. Thus, Portland stone, Bath stone, Casterton stone, Ketton stone, Linby stone and Hopton Wood stone are all composed of limestone—that is, calcium carbonate, the dust of which is harmless. On the other hand, York stone, Robin Hood stone, Longridge stone, Darley Dale stone, Corsehill stone and Pennant stone are sandstones containing a proportion of free silica, the dust of which, if inhaled, is highly dangerous. An additional difficulty arises where building stones are sold under misleading names. Thus, Mendip granite is not granite at all but limestone, and thebaic marble is not marble at all but syenite, a form of granite (p. 975).

Trade Names used in Industry

The materials handled in industry are as much riddled with trade names as those handled in pharmacy. Thus, trichlorethylene is encountered as *benzinol, blanco-solv, chlorylene, cinco-solv, cocolene, crawshawpol, dukeron, flock-flip, gemalgene, lanadin-lap, lith lithurin, Lithuin E, pern-a-chlor, tetraline, trethylene, trielin, triklone, trilene, triol, tripur, vestrol* and *westrosol*. When a man refers to the use of a substance by its trade name it is best to telephone or write to his works manager asking what is the nature of the substance in question. The handling of such inquiries by the staff of the factories concerned is usually both courteous and helpful.

Finding which of Many Substances is Responsible

The man may be ignorant of the nature of the substances he uses or they may be trade secrets. Even when he knows the exact names of the substances he handles it may be difficult to determine which of many is responsible for his symptoms. This is seen in the case of workers employed in the manufacture of synthetic dyes who handle many chemical substances including aniline, *para*-toluidine, xylidines, naphthylamines, fuchsine, benzidine and rosaniline. In the dye industry it is common to have more than one process going on in the same room. Further, over a number of years the workman may have moved from one factory to another or from one department in the same factory to another, each change bringing new compounds into question. Lastly, the same compounds used in different processes may be attended with very different degrees of danger. Thus, in making benzidine there may be greater exposure to aniline vapour than in the manufacture of aniline itself.

Special Questioning to discover Exposure to Lead

Often a man's occupation does not at first sight suggest that he is exposed to compounds of lead. Thus, it is elicited only by special questioning that a man describing himself as a *fitter* may be exposed to dust or fume of lead. The work of a *cooper* becomes dangerous when the barrels on which he works have contained white lead, red lead, litharge or lead chromate. A *moulder* in a foundry pouring a molten alloy into moulds may be exposed to dust and fume of lead if the alloy be leaded bronze. He may likewise trim the resulting castings with a carborundum wheel, thus producing further dust. *Vitreous enamellers* working, for example, on baths may sift a powder containing lead silicate on to the bath which has been heated in a furnace. They sometimes use a compressed-air apparatus which forces the enamel through a sieve. In the electric accumulator trade, *pasters* fill the spaces in accumulator plates with aqueous pastes containing lead, litharge and red lead. *Colour manufacturers* grind colours into a fine powder under edge runners with the production of much dust; they frequently use lead chromate and red lead. A *slate mason* may construct storage tanks by fixing together slabs of slate with putty containing white lead. A *bullion refiner* may use a process in which he adds lead to refinable silver in a furnace and taps off molten litharge. A *rubber compounder* may add oxides of lead to crude rubber in preparation for vulcanization. A *perambulator maker* may be employed in painting the body-work of perambulators with lead paint and then rubbing down the surface with dry sand-paper. An *embroidery worker* sometimes stencils materials by dabbing on the pattern commercial white lead, whereas talc is equally efficacious and quite harmless.

Trades with More than One Hazard

The department of an industry in which a man works may be important. It is inadequate to ascertain that a man is a *rubber worker*, for at least three harmful substances may be handled in the rubber trade—benzene and carbon disulphide as solvents and lead monoxide in vulcanizing. In the painters' trade the hazards may come from lead, benzene, turpentine and even methyl alcohol. In the leather trade the risks are of anthrax and poisoning by carbon dioxide, sulphuretted hydrogen, nitrobenzene and aniline.

Ask if Protective Devices are in Use

Question him as to the general environmental conditions at his place of work. If necessary, ask him to sketch on paper a plan of his workshop, including the apparatus he uses and the protective devices installed. Most of the toxic substances encountered in the dangerous trades enter the body by inhalation. It follows that toxic dust, fume, mist or vapour must be either suppressed or removed from the working environment by means of exhaust ventilation. Ask whether a hood is installed over his bench and, if so, whether air is drawn into it through metal ducts connected to a suction system. Those substances which cause dermatitis by contact, or as systemic poisons are capable of absorption through the skin, must be warded off by means of strict cleanliness and the use of barrier creams or gloves. Ask the workman or technician about the provision of protective clothing at his place of work. If he wears a special suit, gloves or goggles, he will usually know why.

Presence and Cause of Dust or Fume

Is the job dusty and, if so, what tools make the dust? Remember that the very fine dust which causes silicosis is entirely man-made by such deliberate acts as drilling holes in siliceous rock with compressed-air drills, blasting such rock with dynamite, crushing flint, sand-blasting castings, dressing granite stones, freeing steel castings from adherent siliceous substance by means of compressed-air chisels and using sandstone wheels for grinding knives and other objects. Is any fume produced and, if so, by what apparatus? Remember that the fume produced by heating lead is dangerous in proportion to the heat of the flame used (fig. 70). A *Post Office linesman* using a methylated spirit blowlamp (900° C.) and a *domestic plumber* using a paraffin blowlamp (1,100° C.) face a hazard of lead absorption which is slight indeed compared to that encountered by the *lead burner* or *chemical plumber* who uses an oxy-hydrogen blowpipe flame (2,800° C.) or the *shipbreaker* who uses an oxy-acetylene blowpipe flame (3,500° C.).

Similar Illness in a Fellow Workman

Ask whether any similar illness has occurred in a fellow workman. Thus, a dock labourer unloading a cargo of barley, cotton seed, copra, figs or vanilla may exhibit an intensely itching papular eruption all over the body. If all his mates are complaining of the same disability, it is because the cargo is infested with mites which have transferred themselves to the men. Special consideration must be given to the case of a workman exposed to the dusts of compounds of lead, for here individual susceptibility is of major importance. A patient who is unusually susceptible may develop lead colic after ten days' exposure to a concentration of dust which has failed to do harm to his mates although they have been exposed to it for months or years. The works' chemist, with his lack of knowledge of the biological sciences, may fail entirely to appreciate this point. He may then bitterly oppose your assertion that your patient suffers from lead colic on the ground that the other men are so well.

Good Housekeeping in the Factory

Good housekeeping in factories includes cleanliness and tidiness. Some men and women are clean workers, others are by nature dirty and untidy. Doctors and nurses are apt to assume in the sheltered conditions in which they work that others are as fortunate. We can safely handle almost anything because always wherever we work we have at hand running hot water, soap and towels. But we should visualize the plight of thousands of workmen who are exposed not only to the dust of their regular work but also to adventitious dusts, such as cement, fragments of synthetic glue, oily shavings and particles of decomposed vermin and maggots in sacks collected from neglected premises (O'Donovan, 1952).

Primitive Facilities for Washing

The doctor should bear in mind that in many small establishments facilities for washing are likely to be most primitive. Workers supplied with a bucket of hot water may not change it when ten men use it in quick succession. Since washing soda is a good grease solvent it is often added to the water in excess, for the stronger the soda solution the quicker the toilet. And so an outbreak of alkali dermatitis may escape detection. Even where factory premises are constructed with washbasins and running water the basins are often perpetually soiled, soap absent, towels purloined or a single roller towel for twenty workpeople is provided and changed weekly. It certainly is important that all of us should realize these things.

Occupation Not Responsible for Illness

Since today so many chemical poisons are manufactured in factories, handled in various industrial processes and sprayed on to plants in fields, orchards and hothouses, it is important to be able to discover in a given patient when the symptoms and signs are *not* due to the occupation followed.

Thus, a man, fifty-five years of age, was admitted to hospital complaining of headache, giddiness, loss of memory and depression. Papillœdema was present. He had worked many years for a firm engaged in the manufacture of rubber goods used as surgical appliances. Here the rubber is treated by means of a cold-curing process, thin strips of rubber being dipped into a solution of sulphur monochloride in carbon disulphide. All his symptoms and signs could have resulted from repeated inhalation of the vapour of carbon disulphide. Yet a visit to the factory showed that he had never worked anywhere near the rubber-curing process and therefore carbon disulphide poisoning was ruled out. The headache and papillœdema increased, he died, and necropsy showed a cerebral tumour.

A Visit to the Place of Work

In such a case the golden rule is to visit the factory in order to ascertain the conditions of work on the spot. Although the legal right to enter factories is limited to H.M. Inspectors of Factories, a tactful request on the part of the practising doctor to the works manager to be allowed to visit his factory is rarely met by a refusal. Whenever a case supposedly of occupational origin presents difficulties in diagnosis, and in all cases in which new chemical substances are held in suspicion, the practitioner should enlist the help and advice of the Factory Department. His letter should be addressed to: H.M. Senior Medical Inspector of Factories, Ministry of Labour and National Service, Baynards House, Chepstow Place, London, W2 (01-229 3456). The same applies to cases of mine workers when the letter should go to: H.M. Principal Medical Inspector of Mines, Thames House South, Millbank, London, S.W.1 (01-222 7000).

Jobs Unsuitable in Convalescence

There are other aspects of the case history no less important which remain to be considered. A particular illness may render a man temporarily or permanently unfit to do his work. Thus, a tailor's presser who stands ten hours a day wielding a 16-lb. iron must find another job if he is convalescent from pulmonary tuberculosis. The doctor must be aware that conditions peculiar to certain trades may cause disease which predisposes to infection. Thus, silicosis leads to an excessive mortality from pulmonary tuberculosis and also from pneumonia. But diseases other than infections may be involved. Thus, there is a heavy mortality from cirrhosis of the liver as well as from tuberculosis in publicans, cellarmen, barmen, wine waiters, brewers' draymen and others who have ready access to alcohol.

The Worker as a Carrier of Disease

It is important for the doctor to have regard for his patient's work, even when he is suffering from a disease which is non-occupational. Thus, a man who has a chronic duodenal ulcer is better off at a works where he has access to a canteen with facilities to prepare and serve special diets. And then it is important to know whether a man does a job which makes him a danger to others. Thus, a cowman or dairyman with open tuberculosis can contaminate milk with tubercle bacilli by coughing. Cooks and others who handle food can initiate outbreaks of typhoid fever, dysentery and cysticercosis by acting as carriers. The subject is endless. It concerns, of course, a branch of the public health for which the Ministry of Health, and not the Ministry of Labour, is responsible. But Ministers or no Ministers we would do well to remember that, as medicine develops, a more and more bewildering growth of techniques and specialities, the value of good history taking grows rather than lessens in importance.

BIBLIOGRAPHY

ALEXANDER, W., and STREET, A. (1951), *Metals in the Service of Man*, Penguin Books, London.

BROWN, J. A. C. (1954), *The Social Psychology of Industry*, Penguin Books, London.

BRUUSGAARD, A. (1953), Personal communication.

CHARLEY, I. H. (1949), *Proc. Ninth Internat. Congr. Industr. Med., London*, Wright, Bristol, p. 347.

COLE, M. (1961), *The Story of Fabian Socialism*, Heinemann, London.

CRANKSHAW, E. (1967), *The Observer*, London, Suppl., 27 Aug., p. 20.

DAMON, W. A. (1953), Personal communication.

EDWARDS, J. L. (1958), *Internat. Labour Review*, Geneva, **77**, 147.

FRASER, R. (1947), *The Incidence of Neurosis among Factory Workers*, Med. Res. Counc. Industr. Hlth. Res. Bd., No. 90.

GIBBS, F. W. (1961), *Organic Chemistry Today*, Penguin Books, London.

HALL, P., and LOCKE, H. W. (1938), *Incentives and Contentment*, Pitman, London.

HALLIDAY, J. L. (1948), *Psychosocial Medicine*, Heinemann, London.

HAMILTON, A. (1943), *Exploring the Dangerous Trades*, Little, Brown and Co., Boston.

HAMMOND, J. L. (1929), "The Industrial Revolution," *Encyl. Brit.*, **12**, 303, 14th Ed., London.

HENRY, S. A. (1950), *Ann. R. Coll. Surg. Engl.*, **7**, 425.

HUNTER, C. (1954), Personal communication.

KEMP, C. G. (1949), *Proc. Ninth Internat. Congr. Industr. Med., London*, Wright, Bristol, p. 215.

LEWIS, A. (1945), *Brit. J. industr. Med.*, **2**, 41.

MANN, C. (1946), *Industr. Welf.*, **28**, 102.

MAYO, E. (1945), *Social Problems of an Industrial Civilization*, Harvard University Press, Cambridge, Mass.

MEIKLEJOHN, A. (1949), *Lancet*, **2**, 360.

MILLWARD, G. E. (1946), *An Approach to Management*, Macdonald and Evans, London.

O'DONOVAN, W. J. (1952), *Trans. Assoc. industr. med. Off.*, **2**, 34.

PEARSON, J. F. (1954), *Science News, 31*, Penguin Books, London.

REES, J. R. (1945), *Shaping of Psychiatry by War*, Chapman and Hall, London.

ROBINSON, R. (1956), *Endeavour*, **15**, 92.

ROEMER, M. I., and DA COSTA, O. L. (1953), *Arch. Industr. Hyg.*, **7**, 111.

ROETHLISBERGER, F. J., and DICKSON, W. J. (1947), *Management and the Worker*, Harvard University Press, Cambridge, Mass.

SHEARER, A. (1967), *The Guardian*, London, 1 Sept., p. 8.

STEWART, D. (1946), *Proc. R. Soc. Med.*, **39**, 158; (1949), "Occupational Health" in MASSEY, A., *Modern Trends in Public Health*, Butterworth, London.

TAYLOR, W. (1948), *Brit. J. industr. Med.*, **5**, 107.

THOMSON, D. (1950), *England in the Nineteenth Century*, Penguin Books, London.

WHITEHEAD, T. N. (1938), *The Industrial Worker*, Harvard University Press, Cambridge, Mass.

WIENER, N. (1950), *The Human Use of Human Beings*, Eyre and Spottiswoode, London.

WYATT, S. (1945), *A Study of Certified Sickness Absence among Women in Industry*, Med. Res. Counc. Industr. Hlth. Res. Bd., No. 86.

CHAPTER V

THE ANCIENT METALS

THE metals have been arbitrarily distributed among three chapters, *The Ancient Metals*, *The Other Metals* and *The Newer Metals*. Even more arbitrarily, under the second of these headings we have included arsenic, a metalloid, and phosphorus, a non-metal. In the third section two further metalloids are described, namely selenium and tellurium. *The Newer Metals* are those more recently introduced into industry than the others.

THE METALS

The division of elements into metals and non-metals is but a rough classification adopted for convenience. Exact subdivision is not practicable, for some elements have properties characteristic of both metals and non-metals. These hybrids are known as *metalloids* or *half-metals*. They include antimony, arsenic, bismuth, silicon, selenium and tellurium.

Innocent Metals with Poisonous Compounds

A metal may enter the tissues without acting as a poison. Thus, silver produces no toxic symptoms although it can bring about lifelong disfigurement in the form of generalized argyria. Other metals which are themselves harmless nevertheless form certain toxic compounds. Thus, nickel is innocent of toxic effects, yet the inhalation of nickel carbonyl causes destructive lesions in the lungs. Relatively large quantities of tin can be dissolved by acid materials preserved in tin cans without imparting any taste or flavour to food materials and without producing injury on ingestion. Yet tetramethyl tin is intensely poisonous to nervous tissues, and tin tetra-hydride is more toxic than arsine.

Effects of Organo-metallic Compounds

A metal or a compound of a metal may have a different effect according to whether it exists in organic or inorganic form, whether its physical properties are those of a solid, a liquid or a gas, whether the valency of the metal radical is high or low, or whether it falls upon the skin or enters the body through the respiratory or alimentary tract. Thus, arsine acts as a powerful hæmolytic poison whereas the inorganic compounds of arsenic never produce this effect. Men poisoned by tetra-ethyl lead show cerebral symptoms and signs, the well-known symptoms of poisoning by inorganic compounds of lead being absent. Similarly, men poisoned by methyl-mercury compounds do not show the symptoms and signs of poisoning by the metal itself, but they present the picture of a unique disease of the nervous system. A third metal showing a specific selection for certain parts of the brain is manganese. This attacks the globus pallidus, the lenticular nucleus and the caudate nucleus, and the patient shows the corresponding signs of involvement of the extrapyramidal motor system. The white allotrope of phosphorus causes necrosis of the jaw; organic phosphorus compounds are inhibitors of cholinesterase, and as such they attack the nervous system.

Physical Form of Metallic Compound

The physical form in which a metallic compound exists in the atmosphere may determine its toxicity. Thus, zinc oxide produces fever and rigors when inhaled as freshly formed fume and yet it is inert when inhaled as dust. The different effect is probably due to the smaller particle size of the fume. Lead absorption is always greatest amongst those exposed to freshly formed lead fume. Thus, in the occupation of lead burning performed with an oxy-acetylene flame, 100 per cent of men absorb lead, whereas in spray painting only 44 per cent do so. This again is a question of particle size. The effects of a metallic poison may differ according to its portal of entry. Thus, workers exposed to the vapour of mercury may suffer from tremor, whereas this symptom does not occur when mercury is rubbed into the skin.

Distinctive Toxic Effect of each Metal

The behaviour of metals and their compounds is far less predictable than that of great groups of organic compounds. The nitro- or amino-compounds or the halogenated hydrocarbons have many characteristics which permit some evaluation of the toxic qualities of the individual members of the group from what we know of the group in general. One set of metallic compounds is an exception to this rule. Hydrogen arsenide, hydrogen selenide and hydrogen telluride are all gases which act as intense hæmolytic poisons. Fortunately, only the first constitutes an industrial hazard. It follows that in discussing the toxicological action of the metals and their compounds, each one must be considered as a separate entity.

The Ancient Metals

Naturally some metals have been in use much longer than others. It is possible to trace with some accuracy, over a period of at least 2,000 years, the history of the use of lead and mercury and some of their compounds, Hippocrates was probably the first of the ancients to recognize lead as the cause of colic, and Pliny describes mercurialism in writing of the diseases of slaves. But new uses for these ancient metals are constantly found, and some of their compounds, especially the organic derivatives, have been newly introduced into industry.

Lead

Lead poisoning may occur in industry in two forms: (a) from exposure to the inorganic compounds of lead, and (b) from handling organic compounds, especially tetra-ethyl lead. The clinical picture is different in the two forms. Poisoning by the inorganic compounds causes colic, wrist drop, stippling of the red cells and anæmia. In poisoning by tetra-ethyl lead the picture is that of insomnia, mental confusion, delirium and mania.

(a) Lead

Lead, Pb, is a soft bluish-grey metal, heavy, malleable and ductile. It is protected from corrosion by the formation of a thin coating of grey oxide. There is evidence that lead has been used for about 6,000 years, for there is a lead figure in the British Museum that was made before 3800 B.C. It was among the earliest metals used by man and was known to the early Egyptians and Hebrews. The Phœnicians mined it in Spain about 2000 B.C. The Hanging Gardens of Babylon had lead pans to hold plants, and the Romans, to satisfy their great enthusiasm for sanitation and bathing, exploited the lead mines in the Mendips, Shropshire, Derbyshire and Flint. Together with Spain, Britain became the principal source of lead in the Roman Empire. Lead pipes made 2,000 years ago have been excavated in Pompeii, Rome and Bath, and found to be in good condition. In modern times the principal lead-producing countries are the United States of America, Mexico, Australia and Canada. World production of lead for the year 1953 was 2,050,000 tons. The principal lead ore is galena, PbS, and this is usually associated with the sulphides of silver, copper, arsenic, antimony, bismuth and tin. Other common ores of lead are cerussite, $PbCO_3$, and anglesite, $PbSO_4$.

Uses

Lead is so soft that it can easily be rolled into sheet and foil and extruded cold into rods, pipes and tube containers. In building construction it is used for roofing, cornices, tank linings, electrical conduit, water pipes and sewer pipes. Because of its weight and malleability it is utilized in yacht keels, plumb-bobs and sinkers in diving-suits. Alloyed with tin and antimony, lead proved the most satisfactory substance for casting type when movable type was invented in the fifteenth century, for it made a sharp impression and when broken could be easily recast. Antimonial lead is now the chief type-metal. Lead-antimony alloys are also used for accumulator plates, cable coverings, toy soldiers, ornamental castings and the fillings of bullets for small-arms ammunition. Soft solder, used chiefly for soldering tinplate and lead pipes, is an alloy of lead and tin which remains in a plastic state sufficiently long to enable the plumber to wipe the joint. Certain lead-base alloys are used in engineering to make bearing-metals. Lead is now encountered in more than 200 industries. The annual world production of pig lead exceeds two million tons, and in Great Britain alone more than 25,000 tons of white lead and 20,000 tons of red lead and litharge are manufactured annually. In 1951 in Great Britain there were more than 1,500 workers in the lead industries and 150,000 painters.

History

White lead, $Pb(OH)_2.2PbCO_3$, and red lead, Pb_3O_4, are amongst the oldest pigments known, and it is possible to trace their history with some accuracy over a period of at least two thousand years (Klein, 1913). The earliest prototype of white lead was the native carbonate of lead, $PbCO_3$, known as cerussite. The Egyptians used this as an ingredient of a pottery glaze before 500 B.C. Xenophon (400 B.C.) makes one of the earliest references to this material, which he describes as cerussa and records that it was used as a cosmetic. Vitruvius (15 B.C.), referring to red lead as sandaraca, states that it was discovered by accident in a cosmetic jar of white lead which had been exposed to heat in the burning of a house at the Piræus. Early in the Christian era it was made by roasting ceruse. It was not until much later that the method of manufacture from lead or litharge, PbO, was discovered.

The many symptoms of plumbism were noted long before they were ascribed to the action of lead. Gradually, however, physicians came to appreciate the cause of these disturbances and the syndrome was designated saturnism, for lead was called saturn by the alchemists because it absorbs and devours, so to speak, all other imperfect metals. Certain of the toxic effects of lead were familiar to Greek, Roman and Arabian physicians before the Christian era. Hippocrates (370 B.C.) described a severe attack of colic in a man who extracted metals, and was probably the first of the ancients to recognize lead as the cause of the symptoms.

The relationship of constipation, colic, pallor, paralysis and ocular disturbances to the action of lead on the body was observed by Nicander in the second century B.C. Pliny (A.D. 23–79) states that the ancients painted their ships with native ceruse, that lead poisoning was known in his day and that the workers in lead products tied up their faces in loose bags lest they should inhale the pernicious dust.

Dioscorides (A.D. 100) knew that ingestion of lead compounds caused colic, paralysis and delirium. It is known that white lead was used in England in the thirteenth century, and the fact that it poisoned workmen who handled it was recorded in the seventeenth century. In 1713 Ramazzini noted that potters who worked with lead often showed its noxious effects, "at first tremors appear in the hands, soon they are paralysed."

Nineteenth-century Legislation

In 1839 Tanquerel des Planches published in Paris his work on 1,200 cases of lead poisoning. His studies were so complete that later investigators have added little to our knowledge of the symptoms and signs of the disease. In England during the last thirty years of the nineteenth century, factory inspectors and other people became increasingly disturbed over the problem of specific industrial diseases, and of these lead poisoning was one of the most widespread. Women and children were employed indiscriminately in all lead processes, including the highly dangerous jobs of pottery glazing, the smelting of lead ores and the manufacture of lead compounds, particularly the basic carbonate or white lead. Since 1864 they had been forbidden to take their meals in dipping houses or dippers' drying-rooms in potteries, and under the Consolidating Act of 1878 children and young persons were excluded from the manufacture of white lead. Mr. Alexander Redgrave, the Chief Inspector of Factories, in 1882 submitted a report to the Secretary of State on the need for further protection of persons employed in white-lead works, in which he specifically advised against the exclusion of women on the ground that women workers would have difficulty in finding alternative employment, but he did demand certain definite measures of protection and these were included in the *Factories (Prevention of Lead Poisoning) Act, 1883*, which required all white-lead factories to conform to prescribed standards with regard to ventilation, lavatory accommodation, baths for women, mealrooms, protective clothing and respirators. This was the first Act of Parliament to be directed against a specific occupational disease.

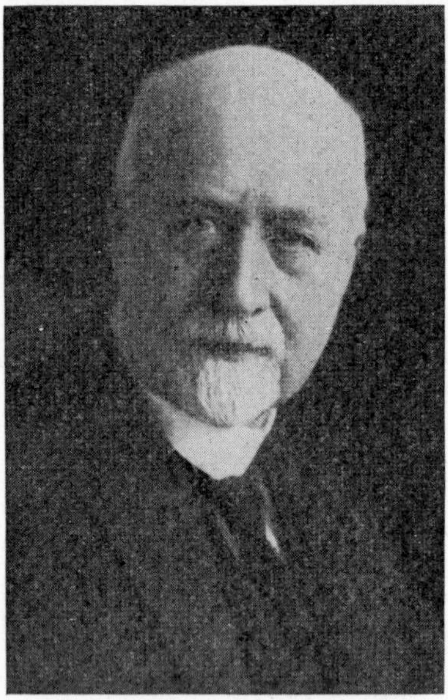

First Medical Inspector of Factories

After 1900 intensive studies of industrial hygienic conditions in the lead trades were carried out by such pioneers as Oliver (fig. 67), Legge and Goadby in England, Meillère in France, Teleky in Germany and Alice Hamilton in the United States of America. As a result, many regulations were introduced in these countries to safeguard workers and compensate them for disability. In Great Britain, although factory inspectors were appointed in 1833 to administer the provisions of the Factory and Workshops Acts, it was not until 1898 that the importance of the medical aspect of the work of a factory inspector was appreciated.

FIG. 67.—Sir Thomas Oliver, 1853–1942

This resulted in the appointment of Dr. T. M. Legge (afterwards Sir Thomas Legge) as the first medical inspector of factories. In Great Britain the question of industrial lead poisoning was actively investigated from 1891 onwards, and as a result of Legge's work it was made notifiable in 1899. Since then a satisfactory decline has occurred in the incidence of the disease. Thus, 55 cases of lead poisoning were notified in 1960 as compared with 1,058 in 1900. The effect of notification in controlling the lead hazard is illustrated in fig. 68, which shows that, despite a steady increase in the consumption of lead, the incidence of lead poisoning in Great Britain has fallen steadily throughout the first half of the twentieth century.

Aphorisms of Sir Thomas Legge

The grasp gained by Sir Thomas Legge of the nature of the hazards in the dangerous trades can be judged from his aphorisms (Legge, 1934).

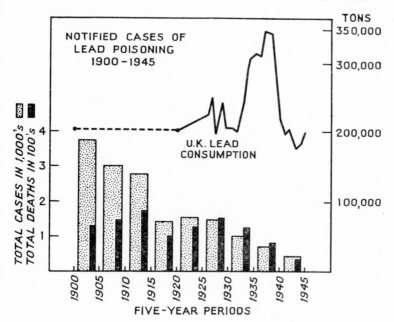

FIG. 68.—Control of the Lead Hazard as a Result of Notification
(After Professor R. E. Lane, Milroy Lectures, 1947)

1. I shall lay stress on some axioms which experience has led me to enunciate: Unless and until the employer has done everything—and everything means a good deal—the workman can do next to nothing to protect himself, although he is naturally willing enough to do his share.

2. If you can bring an influence to bear external to the workman (that is, one over which he can exercise no control), you will be successful; and if you cannot or do not, you will never be wholly successful.

3. Practically all industrial lead poisoning is due to the inhalation of dust and fume; and if you stop their inhalation you will stop the poisoning.

4. All workmen should be told something of the danger of the material with which they come into contact and not be left to find it out for themselves—sometimes at the cost of their lives.

5. Examples of influences—useful up to a point, but not completely

effective—which are not external, but depend on the will or whim of
the worker to use them, are respirators, gloves, goggles, washing conveniences and waterproof sand-paper.

Exposure Hazards

In lead mines the incidence of lead poisoning depends upon the type of
ore. Blasting and shovelling galena rarely gives rise to plumbism, but

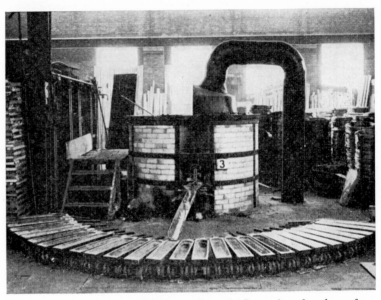

FIG. 69.—Molten Lead running from a Furnace. Protection of workmen from
the inhalation of Lead Fume at Furnaces is a Difficult Problem

there is usually a hazard of silicosis from the free silica in the associated
rocks. Thus in some of the lead mines in Spain the mother rock is quartzite and silicosis is prevalent amongst the miners. When the Broken Hill
Mines of Australia were first worked, cerussite, $PbCO_3$, was encountered
and the fine dust inhaled led to plumbism, including some cases of encephalopathy. Happily, the cerussite was soon worked out and the subjacent
galena, PbS, caused no trouble (Oliver, 1925). The low incidence of lead
poisoning in men mining galena is probably due to the insolubility of lead
sulphide in the tissue fluid of the lungs (Fairhall, 1949). Men are exposed
to danger in the milling of lead ores. Lead smelters are exposed to the fume
and dust of furnaces and flues (fig. 69). Lead burners, chemical plumbers
and shipbreakers use oxy-acetylene (3,500° C.), oxy-hydrogen (2,800° C.)
or oxy-coal-gas (2,200° C.) blowpipes in their work (fig. 70). The very
high temperature of such flames constitutes a much greater risk than that
faced by the domestic plumber who uses a paraffin blow-lamp (1,100° C.)

for water pipes, or the telephone linesman who uses a spirit blow-lamp (900° C.) for cable sheathing. There is some risk in the casting of lead and its alloys, including lead shot (fig. 71), and metal bearings for machinery. The function of lead in a bearing alloy is to act as a sort of metallic lubricant when at very high speeds and pressures the oil film breaks down. In bearings for aeroplane and motor-car engines, the alloy used is leaded bronze consisting of copper with about 30 per cent of lead and sometimes up to 5 per cent of zinc, nickel or tin. A bearing alloy called *Bahn-metal* developed in Germany contains 98 per cent lead with small quantities of lithium, sodium and calcium. Men are exposed to danger in vitreous

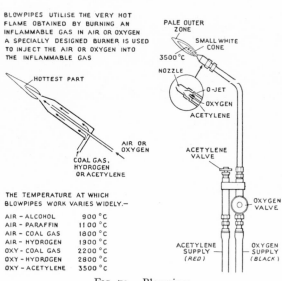

BLOWPIPES

BLOWPIPES UTILISE THE VERY HOT FLAME OBTAINED BY BURNING AN INFLAMMABLE GAS IN AIR OR OXYGEN A SPECIALLY DESIGNED BURNER IS USED TO INJECT THE AIR OR OXYGEN INTO THE INFLAMMABLE GAS

PALE OUTER ZONE

SMALL WHITE CONE

3500°C

NOZZLE

HOTTEST PART

O-JET

OXYGEN

ACETYLENE

AIR OR OXYGEN

ACETYLENE VALVE

COAL GAS, HYDROGEN OR ACETYLENE

THE TEMPERATURE AT WHICH BLOWPIPES WORK VARIES WIDELY.—

AIR – ALCOHOL	900 °C
AIR – PARAFFIN	1100 °C
AIR – COAL GAS	1800 °C
AIR – HYDROGEN	1900 °C
OXY – COAL GAS	2200 °C
OXY – HYDROGEN	2800 °C
OXY – ACETYLENE	3500 °C

OXYGEN VALVE

ACETYLENE SUPPLY (RED)

OXYGEN SUPPLY (BLACK)

Fig. 70.—Blowpipes
(*After R. Coles, 1948*)

enamelling, pottery glazing, shipbuilding, coach painting, motor-car body building, soldering and house painting, and in the manufacture of white lead, red lead, litharge, lead chromate and other coloured pigments, electric accumulators, rubber, glass, cement, varnish and linoleum. There is some risk to gasfitters who use red and white lead.

Composition of Paints

White lead and red lead are manufactured mainly for use in paint. When suspended in linseed oil and applied as a thin coating, these pigments form an elastic film which, when dry, is impervious to water. This is the principle upon which the use of lead paint is based. White lead has great covering power and durability. Nevertheless, white lead is not the only white paint pigment; zinc oxide, ZnO, lithopone and titanium oxide are also used, especially for interior decorating. Lithopone consists of 70

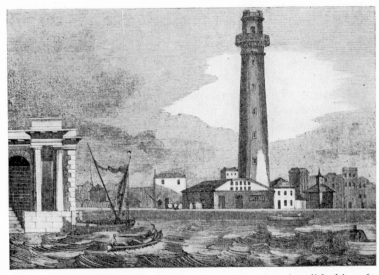

Fig. 71.—The Shot Mill, near Waterloo Bridge, London, demolished in 1962

per cent barium sulphate, BaSO$_4$, and 30 per cent zinc sulphide, ZnS. Its cost is about half that of white lead or zinc oxide, and it is non-poisonous. The use of titanium oxide, TiO$_2$, as a white pigment in paints, varnishes and lacquers is increasing at the expense of both lithopone and white lead, because of its exceptionally high hiding power, its extreme whiteness, cheapness, inertness, durability and non-toxic qualities. It is estimated that titanium pigment has three times the opacity of white lead, and twice that of zinc oxide.

White lead has certain other uses than for painting—for example, pottery glazing and the manufacture of putty and coloured pigments. But it is estimated that only 15 per cent of white lead is used for purposes other than paint making. Red lead is used for the protection of iron and steel structures, and for the manufacture of electric accumulators, glass, glazes, cement, varnish and linoleum. Litharge is used for the manufacture of electric accumulators, rubber, varnish and lead colours.

Red-lead Paints

As a coating for metals exposed to the weather, and especially to sea water, red lead remains indispensable. The protective action of red-lead paint on metals is partly physical and partly chemical in nature. In the first place, the metal surfaces are protected mechanically by the paint layer from contact with corrosive agents. Lead paint forms a thick, heavy, tough, elastic, waterproof film of great strength, which does not crack through wear or variations in temperature, because the film expands and contracts in unison with the surface of the metal to which it is attached.

Red lead is almost unique amongst pigments in that although it is comparatively stable it exerts a retarding and inhibiting effect on corrosion by reason of its chemically basic character. It neutralizes traces of acid which occur in the atmosphere or dissolved in rain water, especially in large towns. In addition, it inhibits the rusting and corrosion of iron and steel, because owing to its oxidizing properties it causes the formation over the surface of iron and steel of a passive film of iron oxide which is strongly resistant to corrosion.

The rusting and corrosion of iron and steel is a phenomenon of great economic significance, resulting as it does in the financial loss throughout the world of many hundreds of millions of pounds per annum. The authorities responsible for ships, lighthouses, bridges, railways and other iron and steel structures are particularly alive to the value of lead paint as a protection against atmospheric attack. For example, in London squads of men are continuously on duty painting the Tower Bridge, and for this purpose they use 25 tons of lead paint every year. Similarly, in Australia thirty painters are continuously employed on Sydney Harbour Bridge. It takes five years to paint the bridge, and when they have finished they start again. The bridge is made up of 51,300 tons of steel. In each painting cycle 90 tons of red-lead paint and 250 tons of battleship grey are used.

Manufacture of Litharge

In the manufacture of litharge, PbO, and red lead, Pb_3O_4, it is impracticable to use wet methods. In the old days when litharge was made by roasting metallic lead in a furnace, the man who fed and raked the furnace was necessarily exposed to dust and fume (fig. 72). In the modern process lead is fed mechanically into a pot, and there is an automatic mixer working under a current of compressed air. Since the litharge produced is blown over into a closed-in collecting chamber, the hazard of lead poisoning no longer exists. When litharge is further heated in contact with air at carefully controlled temperatures, it combines with more oxygen and red lead is formed. Again, in the modern process, covered conveyers, mechanical mixers, closed-in furnaces and automatic packing machinery operated under exhaust ventilation are employed.

Manufacture of White Lead

Theophrastus (300 B.C.) states that in his time white lead was made artificially from lead and vinegar. After the metal was corroded the white lead was scraped off, boiled with water and allowed to settle. This is probably the earliest record of the manufacture of white lead. Other Greeks, notably Plautus (200 B.C.) and Ovid (10 B.C.), also referred to artificial white lead in their writings. From the Romans the manufacture spread gradually to France and Belgium. The first reference to its use in England is found in 1274 in the Close Rolls of Edward I, where an account is rendered for painting materials supplied for the decoration of the Painted Chamber. It was not until the seventeenth century that white lead was

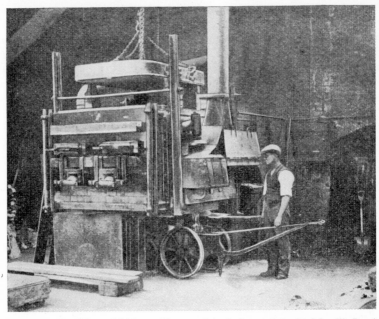

FIG. 72.—Old Type of Litharge Furnace (1915). It was fed with Metallic Lead through the Doors seen in front, and the Litharge was raked out into the Bogie underneath

made in large batches and that animal manure was regularly used to furnish heat and carbon dioxide in the process. Until the seventeenth century the Venetians appear to have been the principal manufacturers of white lead, and after that date the process was largely developed in Holland. Although this process became known as the Dutch process, it was adopted in England, France and Germany. Probably the earliest record of lead poisoning amongst white-lead workers in England is that of Vernatti (1678):

> The Accidents to the workmen are, immediate pain in the Stomack, with exceeding contortions in the Guts, and Costiveness that yields not to Catharticks, hardly to often repeated Clysters. . . . And these we find effected principally by the mineral steams in the casting of the plates of lead, and by the dust of the flakes. . . . Next, a vertigo, or dizziness in the head, with continual great pain in the brows, blindness, stupidity, and paralytick affections, loss of appetite, sickness, and frequent vomitings. . . . And these chiefly that have the charge of grinding, and over the drying place.

It was not until the end of the eighteenth century that tan bark was substituted for manure as a source of heat and carbon dioxide in the manufacture of white lead.

The Old Dutch or Stack Process

In the Old Dutch or Stack process, lead of special purity was cast in perforated strips. It was then taken to the stack or corroding house, which

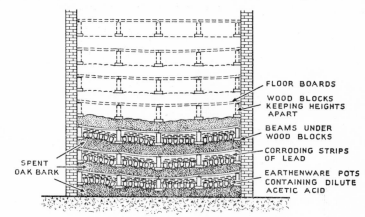

FIG. 73.—Diagrammatic Section of White Lead Stack in Course of Erection
(*By courtesy of Goodlass Wall and Lead Industries, Ltd.*)

might ultimately contain 100 tons of lead. Such a house was a four-sided brick construction about 20 by 16 by 13 feet (fig. 73). The floor was covered to a depth of 3 feet with tan bark. Earthenware pots were placed side by side so as to cover the floor, leaving a clear space round the edges which was filled with tan bark. The pots were partly filled with 3 per cent acetic acid. The perforated strips of lead were laid over the pots in three or more layers, and a double layer of boards was placed on top supported by wooden blocks and arranged to carry the weight. This plan was followed until the building was full. Arrangements were made for the ventilation of the stack (fig. 74), which was then left for some hundred days for corrosion to be effected. Fermentation of the tan bark was due to micro-organisms. There was evolution of heat and carbon dioxide, which caused evaporation of the water and acetic acid. A chemical reaction then converted metallic lead

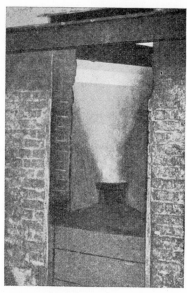

FIG. 74.—Top of White Lead Stack showing Water Vapour produced during Corrosion

into the basic carbonate, white lead, $Pb(OH)_2.2PbCO_3$. When the process was nearly finished the stack was dismantled, and most of the metallic lead originally present was found to be converted into white lead. Corrosion was not complete, for about 25 per cent of the metal remained as a thin unaltered core in each strip. The stack was then broken down, but before the perforated strips were carted away, each layer of the stack was hosed freely with water to prevent the raising of dust (fig. 75). In some countries stack breaking was performed in the dry state by workmen who emptied the flaky white lead into trucks. In these circumstances the process was a potent source of lead poisoning. The strips removed from the stack were passed through rollers in order to crush the white lead, whilst the unchanged metal was merely flattened out. Grinding and sieving in water yielded a pulp of white lead and water, which was then freed of lead acetate by washing with water either in filter presses (fig. 76) or by decantation. White lead is sold either as a dry powder or as an oil paste, containing from 6 to 9 per cent of linseed oil. The drying of white lead was carried out in driers of various types, including vacuum driers, continuous band driers, stoves, or in simple drying pots on shelves. The preparation and handling of dry white lead was far from being a salutary occupation, and hygienists hoped for a decline in this branch of the industry. Fortunately, it is possible to avoid handling white lead in the dry state. It can be taken as an aqueous paste direct from the filter presses and mixed with a predetermined quantity of linseed oil in a mechanical mixer. After about half an hour's mixing the mass suddenly changes in appearance, and it is found that the linseed oil has displaced the water in the paste, so producing a white-lead oil paste from which the water can readily be drained. The hygienic value of this process whereby pulp white lead is converted into oil paste in automatic closed-in machines and without dry grinding will be realized (fig. 77).

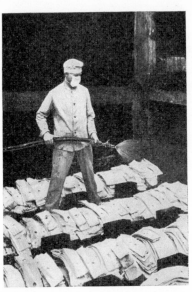

FIG. 75.—White Lead Stack Breaking by the Wet Method. The workman is hosing with Water the Corroded Lead Strips in order to suppress the Dust of White Lead

In *The Uncommercial Traveller* (1867), Charles Dickens describes a visit he made to a white-lead works near Limehouse Church, London. Two intelligent managers of the works, brothers and partners with their father in the concern, showed him everything quite freely.

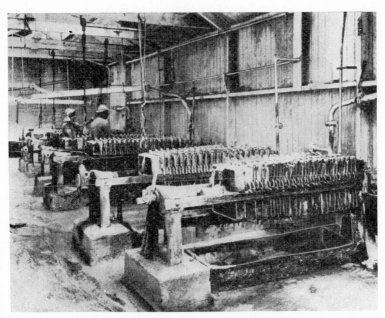

FIG. 76.—White Lead Filter Presses. The Presence of the Dust of White Lead on the Floor is dangerous to workmen who may inhale it

The purport of such works is the conversion of pig-lead into white-lead. This conversion is brought about by the slow and gradual effecting of certain successive chemical changes in the lead itself. The processes are picturesque and interesting,—the most so, being the burying of the lead, at a certain stage of preparation, in pots, each pot containing a certain quantity of acid besides, and all the pots being buried in vast numbers, in layers, under tan, for some ten weeks.

Hopping up ladders, and across planks, and on elevated perches, until I was uncertain whether to liken myself to a bird or a bricklayer, I became conscious of standing on nothing particular, looking down into one of a series of large cocklofts, with the outer day peeping in through the chinks in the tiled roof above. A number of women were ascending to, and descending from, this cockloft, each carrying on the upward journey a pot of prepared lead and acid, for deposition under the smoking tan. When one layer of pots was completely filled, it was carefully covered in with planks, and those were carefully covered with tan again, and then another layer of pots was begun above; sufficient means of ventilation being preserved through wooden tubes. Going down into the cockloft then filling, I found the heat of the tan to be surprisingly great, and also the odour of the lead and acid to be not absolutely exquisite, though I believe not noxious at

D.O.—9*

that stage. In other cocklofts, where the pots were being exhumed, the heat of the steaming tan was much greater, and the smell was penetrating and peculiar. There were cocklofts in all stages; full and empty, half filled and half emptied; strong, active women were clambering about them busily; and the whole thing had rather the air of the upper part of the house of some immensely rich old Turk, whose faithful seraglio were hiding his money because the sultan or the pasha was coming.

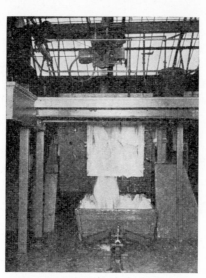

FIG. 77.—White Lead Oil Paste being discharged from an Automatic Closed-in Pulping Machine

As is the case with most pulps or pigments, so in the instance of this white-lead, processes of stirring, separating, washing, grinding, rolling, and pressing succeed. Some of these are unquestionably inimical to health, the danger arising from inhalation of particles of lead, or from contact between the lead and the touch, or both. Against these dangers, I found good respirators provided (simply made of flannel and muslin, so as to be inexpensively renewed, and in some instances washed with scented soap), and gauntlet gloves, and loose gowns. Everywhere, there was as much fresh air as windows, well placed and opened, could possibly admit. And it was explained that the precaution of frequently changing the women employed in the worst parts of the work (a precaution originating in their own experience or apprehension of its ill effects) was found salutary. They had a mysterious and singular appearance, with the mouth and nose covered, and the loose gown on, and yet bore out the simile of the old Turk and the seraglio all the better for the disguise.

At last this vexed white-lead, having been buried and resuscitated, and heated and cooled and stirred, and separated and washed and ground, and rolled and pressed, is subjected to the action of intense fiery heat. A row of women, dressed as above described, stood, let us say, in a large stone bakehouse, passing on the baking-dishes as they were given out by the cooks, from hand to hand, into the ovens. The oven, or stove, cold as yet, looked as high as an ordinary house, and was full of men and women on temporary footholds, briskly passing up and stowing away the dishes. The door of another oven, or stove, about to be cooled and emptied, was opened from above, for the uncommercial countenance to peer down into. The uncommercial countenance withdrew itself, with expedition and a sense of suffocation, from the dull-glowing heat and the overpowering smell. On the whole, perhaps the going into these stoves to work, when they are freshly opened, may be the whole part of the occupation.

But I made it out to be indubitable that the owners of these lead-mills honestly and sedulously try to reduce the dangers of the occupation to the lowest point.

A washing-place is provided for the women (I thought there might have been more towels), and a room in which they hang their clothes, and take their meals, and where they have a good fire-range and fire, and a female attendant to help them, and to watch that they do not neglect the cleansing of their hands before touching their food. An experienced medical attendant is provided for them, and any premonitory symptoms of lead-poisoning are carefully treated. Their tea-pots and such things were set out on tables ready for their afternoon meal, when I saw their room; and it had a homely look. It is found that they bear the work much better than men; some few of them have been at it for years, and the great majority of those I observed were strong and active. On the other hand, it should be remembered that most of them are very capricious and irregular in their attendance.

American inventiveness would seem to indicate that before very long white-lead may be made entirely by machinery. The sooner, the better. In the meantime, I parted from my two frank conductors over the mills, by telling them that they had nothing there to be concealed, and nothing to be blamed for. As to the rest, the philosophy of the matter of lead-poisoning and workpeople seems to me to have been pretty fairly summed up by the Irishwoman whom I quoted in my former paper: "Some of them gets lead-pisoned soon, and some of them gets lead-pisoned later, and some, but not many, niver; and 'tis all according to the constitooshun, sur; and some constitooshuns is strong and some is weak."

Retracing my footsteps over my beat, I went off duty.

This factory has been identified as the Burdett Road works of W. W. and R. Johnson and Sons, Ltd., and it is still producing white lead. Nobody would quarrel with the novelist's description of the stack process he saw in operation. Charles Dickens was so keen in his questions and observations as to discover that the workpeople of his time possessed full knowledge of constitutional susceptibility. Happily, his prediction that American inventiveness would result in white lead being made entirely by machinery has been fulfilled. Under the management of Associated Lead Manufacturers Limited the Burdett Road works and all other factories in Great Britain have scrapped the stack process, replacing it by an entirely mechanized plant which converts pig lead into white lead in twenty-four hours. Credit for the achievement of such quick processes is every bit as much English as American, a point which might have pleased the distinguished novelist. It is interesting to reflect that between 1930 and 1950 Great Britain discarded a process for the manufacture of white lead which had been devised more than 2,000 years before and which in spite of many modifications was never entirely without hazard to the health of the workpeople.

The Euston Process

The best-known of the quick processes is the Euston process, certain steps of which were patented by Edwin Euston of Philadelphia at the end of the nineteenth century. Refined metallic lead is melted and run into water, where it solidifies as a feathery mass. The feathered lead is placed in large tanks, where it is exposed to surface oxidation by the action of air. The lead oxide is dissolved off by means of normal lead acetate solution and basic lead acetate is formed. This is run into carbonaters, where it is treated with carbon dioxide to form white lead which settles as a thick slurry. This is pumped to the filters, where it is filtered and thoroughly washed to remove all mother liquor. The plant is completely enclosed, so that the white lead is not seen from the time the pig lead enters the process until it appears as the finished product—namely, ground white lead in linseed oil. The increasing use in paint technology of media which are not simple oils creates a demand for 50 per cent of all the white lead produced to be in the dry form. Since in the modern plant all the processes are completely enclosed, this creates no hazard to health. The dry white lead is seen in the intermediate stage only on a rotary filter, where it is in the form of water pulp. From this filter it again goes under cover to steam-heated dryers and does not reappear until it has been packed in containers for sale (Mattiello, 1942).

Changes in Method

It frequently happens that changes in methods or the appearance of new industries provide new causes of lead poisoning. This was the case with shipbreaking following on the scrapping of warships after 1918. In this industry the volatilization of lead from the paint and red-lead stopping on the armour plating occurs in the great heat (3,500° C.) of the oxy-acetylene blowpipe flames used for cutting purposes. Between 1922 and 1924 a rapid increase in the use of wireless-receiving apparatus and motor cars led to the occurrence of a greater number of cases of lead poisoning in electric accumulator factories. Such expansion of an industry makes great demands on those responsible for the prevention of disease in the factories concerned, and special regulations may be necessary to ensure added protection to the workman (fig. 78).

Mass-production methods in the motor-car industry have provided at least two new lead hazards. In the occupation of metallizing with wire there is significant exposure to lead fume. In Detroit in 1934 in the building of motor-car bodies the biggest known outbreak of lead poisoning occurred from the inhalation of the dust of a solder of tin and lead. A new stream-

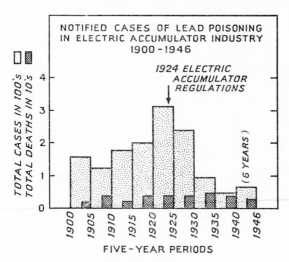

FIG. 78.—Effect of Special Regulations applied to the Electric Accumulator Industry in 1924
(*After Professor R. E. Lane, Milroy Lectures, 1947*)

lined motor car was produced in which some of the welds of the steel body work were rendered smooth by the use of 80 lb. of the solder. In the works of three manufacturers, McCord (1945) investigated 2,700 cases of lead poisoning and estimated that there were 4,000 cases in the whole district. The outbreak arose because a final treatment of the body surface, and especially of the soldered parts, by a portable grinding disc gave rise to large amounts of dust containing lead. This was inhaled not only by the metal finishers engaged on the actual process but also by others in the vicinity. The men affected had stippled red cells and there were many cases of colic. At least twelve men suffered from lead encephalopathy and died in consequence, some of them by suicide. The outbreak ceased when McCord forbade the discing, replaced it by metal shaving with milling files, and at the same time reduced the amount of solder used to 5 lb. per car body.

Streamlining of motor-car bodies is now universal, and in many countries the trade has installed precautions which are both complicated and expensive, in an attempt to protect their workmen from the inhalation of lead dust (fig. 79). But this is the wrong way to tackle the problem. Since 1934 the British motor-car industry has been aware of the hazard of lead poisoning which this method presents to its workmen. Yet it continues to express the vague hope one day to abolish the hazard by producing cars made to well-known bodywork designs in which no lead solder is

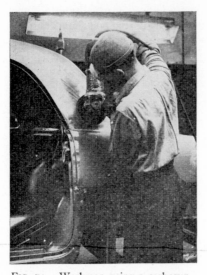

Fig. 79.—Workman using a carborundum grinding disc to smooth lead-tin soldered welds in a motor-car body

used. But nothing further happens. Why not? It is the duty not only of designers, engineers and managing directors in the motor-car industry but indeed of all men and women of goodwill to heed the slogan of the World Health Organization—*Health is a fundamental right, but it must be won.*

Sometimes the converse is true, and lead poisoning is found to show a remarkable diminution in a given industry. Thus, the substitution of machine methods for hand labour has abolished the disease among file cutters (fig. 80). The fall in the incidence of lead poisoning in the coach painting of motor cars is due to the adoption of primers which consist of ferric oxide in place of red lead. They are covered by leadless cellulose lacquers applied by the method of spray painting.

Details of Occupation

The past occupations of the patient should be inquired into, for *latent lead poisoning* is well known to occur. The present occupation is of great importance and the details of the work which he does should be elicited from the patient (see p. 226). Where a man describes himself as a vitreous enameller, colour manufacturer or accumulator paster, the association of his work with compounds of lead may well be imagined. However, it may not occur to the interrogator that a fitter, cooper, rubber compounder or foundry worker can be exposed in a similar way. At one time *police officers* engaged in detecting latent finger-prints at the site of crime were exposed to a lead hazard. For purposes of photography they dusted articles of furniture with white lead and then brushed the excess of the powder away (Nyfeldt, 1937).

Diagnostic Criteria

Individual opinion differs widely as to what is necessary for the diagnosis of lead poisoning. Constipation and slight stippling of red cells are insufficient; neither a blue line on the gums nor detection of lead in the urine can be taken as proof of poisoning, for the patient may be insusceptible. Where a worker is exposed to risk, a diagnosis of lead poisoning can be made before the occurrence of a toxic crisis. A falling hæmoglobin percentage, with or without a rising punctate count, raises a suspicion that absorption is passing into poisoning. This suspicion becomes a certainty when these changes are marked or progressive. The diagnosis offers no difficulty in the presence of colic, palsy, anæmia or encephalopathy.

Lead Colic

Intestinal colic is the commonest manifestation of plumbism. It is ten times as common as lead palsy. An attack of colic is preceded by several days of constipation. The pain is situated around or below the umbilicus. The patient indicates where it is by spreading both hands widely over the abdomen. He becomes cold, pale and drenched with perspiration, and may bend over or writhe in bed in intense pain. Examination reveals a scaphoid abdomen, held tensely, but showing no rigidity. Vomiting frequently occurs at the onset of the pain.

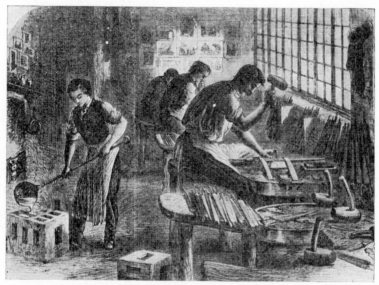

Fig. 80.—Old Method of File Cutting in Sheffield (1866). In cutting the Serrations in the File the workman held the Tool in his Left Hand. The File was supported on a Block of Lead which was slowly pulverized. Note the Employment of a boy who used to run Molten Lead into Moulds without Protection from Fume

(*By courtesy of The Illustrated London News*)

Lead Encephalopathy

Saturnine encephalopathy is the most dramatic manifestation of lead poisoning and is always of serious prognostic significance. It is a cumbrous term, vague and non-specific; it includes attacks of coma, delirium, convulsions, toxic psychosis resembling the Korsakow type, transient pareses, aphasias and anæsthesias. On occasion one or other cranial nerve is affected singly or in a group. Aphonia due to laryngeal palsy was known to Tanquerel; the facial and oculo-motor nerves are sometimes involved. The frequent occurrence of convulsions in lead poisoning is recorded by ancient writers, but with the improvement of industrial conditions the incidence of lead encephalopathy has progressively decreased, and today cases are rarely seen.

Acute and Chronic Forms

The acute form begins suddenly with epileptiform convulsions. Grisolle (1836) studied twenty-nine such cases and divided them into three groups —the convulsive, comatose and delirious. The convulsive crises seem to be due to toxic meningo-encephalopathy and not to hypertension, for lumbar puncture shows that though the cerebrospinal fluid is under increased pressure it contains an excess of cells, usually 100 small lymphocytes per c.mm. (Mosny and Malloizel, 1907). Furthermore, in one case of lead encephalopathy 0·08 mg. of lead was recovered from 80 ml. of cerebrospinal fluid (Aub, Fairhall, Minot and Reznikoff, 1925). Chronic cases may show mental dullness, inability to concentrate, poor memory, headache, head retraction, trembling, deafness, transitory aphasia and hemianopia, and amaurosis without fundus changes.

Visual Changes

Amaurosis on one or both sides and concentric diminution of the visual fields can occur without fundus change. Writers of long ago described cases of blindness from optic atrophy, but it is not clear whether this was primary or secondary (Hutchinson, 1873). Papilloedema, secondary atrophy and post-neuritic atrophy of the disc, sometimes with permanent blindness, frequently complicate the cerebral forms of plumbism. In comparison with that of other toxic substances lead amblyopia among adults is decidedly rare. Whether the optic nerve lesion is due to papilloedema or is post-neuritic or indeed both cannot always be determined.

Encephalopathy in Children

Children with lead poisoning are more apt to suffer from papilloedema than adults. In Queensland, Australia, a special type of encephalopathy occurs among children. It is distinguished by headache, vomiting, occasional convulsions, intense papilloedema and paralysis of the external rectus oculi. Among 200 cases of lead poisoning admitted to the Brisbane Children's Hospital, 54 examples of papilloedema were found, the swelling sometimes measuring up to 6 dioptres (Gibson, 1922).

Wrist-drop, the Common Lead Palsy

We owe our knowledge of the clinical types of lead palsy to Duchenne (1872). The commonest form is wrist-drop which begins on the right side in right-handed persons and later becomes bilateral. Paralysis does not appear to be related to the length of exposure. It may develop during the first month of work or only after many years' exposure. The palsy first appears in the long extensors of the middle and ring fingers. It spreads to the other fingers, and then to the long extensors of the wrist (fig. 81). The supinator longus and usually the long abductor escape. The wrist-drop causes the flexors of the fingers to work at a mechanical disadvantage, which can be at once overcome by passive fixation of the wrist joint. Wasting flattens the posterior aspect of the forearm, throwing into relief the integrity of the supinator longus. On the back of the wrist a synovial swelling known as *Gubler's tumour* induced by slight displacement may be observed. A further motor symptom is *tremor saturninus*, a fine irregular movement of interossei and flexors, sometimes also of the lips, not distinguishable from that seen in mercurialism (p. 296).

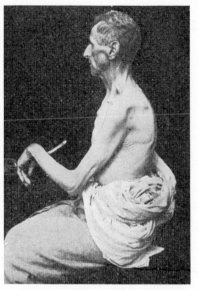

FIG. 81.—Chronic Lead Poisoning in an American House Painter. J. C. P., man aged 60. 5 years: Repeated Attacks of Lead Colic. 18 months: Bilateral Wrist-drop. 3 weeks: Symmetrical Paralysis and Wasting of Shoulder-girdle Muscles. After treatment with Ammonium Chloride the Shoulder-girdle Paralysis largely recovered but Complete Bilateral Wrist-drop persisted

Types of Palsy distinct from Wrist-drop

A type of atrophic palsy of the hands and fingers resembling in distribution the *Aran-Duchenne* form of progressive muscular atrophy may occur. The brachial type of paralysis involves the deltoid, biceps and triceps, but rarely occurs without wrist-drop. A third form of lead palsy used to occur in the left hand of file cutters who were exposed to the dust and fume of lead. In *file-cutters' paralysis* there was progressive atrophy of the thenar and hypothenar eminences and of the interossei. Since fatigue plays an important part in determining the site of lead paralysis, this type of palsy is of great interest, because file cutters not only used the muscles mentioned, but placed a greater strain upon the left hand than upon the right (fig. 80). The substitution of machine methods for hand labour has abolished lead poisoning amongst file makers.

Involvement of the Lower Limbs

Lead palsy rarely occurs in the lower limbs, but when it does it affects the extensors of the toes, giving rise to foot-drop. In the days of prohibition in the United States of America this form of palsy was seen in cabaret dancers who had partaken of alcohol distilled with the aid of a coil of lead pipe. Apart from this, leg paralyses in adults are exceptional. The converse is true of children, as can be seen in the Australian cases. Peronei, extensor longus digitorum and tibialis anticus are affected in varying degree. An upper-leg type may begin with the ilio-psoas and quadriceps extensor cruris. Typical wrist-drop is sometimes followed by cramps, fibrillation and wasting of the arms and shoulders (fig. 81), together with spasticity of the legs, increased tendon reflexes, ankle clonus and extensor plantar responses. When pyramidal signs supervene, the condition becomes clinically inseparable from amyotrophic lateral sclerosis.

A Disorder which begins in Muscle

The paralysis is in the first instance a muscle disease. Fatigue plays an important part in determining the sites attacked. Experimental evidence supports the clinical view that the lesion begins in muscle. Thus Aub and Reznikoff (1924) devised experiments which showed that the diffusion of inorganic phosphates from isolated frog's skeletal muscle immersed in Ringer's solution is greatly increased when lead salts are added to the solution. These observations, which indicate that lead may readily alter the chemical relationships in muscle, were followed by others which showed that leaded muscles tire more readily than their normal fellows, and that phosphate diffusion is extremely rapid in fatigued leaded muscles. Lactic acid, which forms in muscle cells as the result of activity, combines with the lead phosphate in the blood to form lead lactate. As this soluble lactate comes into contact with inorganic phosphate at the surface of the muscle cells, the lead is re-precipitated as insoluble phosphate, causing alteration in the surface permeability. Efforts to show that reasonable concentrations of lead affect the conductivity of nerve were unsuccessful.

Experiments inducing Fatigue in Leaded Cats

On this basis further experiments were made on intact animals. Cats were exercised in a revolving drum and the fatigue produced was increased locally by attaching a weight to the right fore-paw. It soon became apparent that if the animals were given lead the limb most affected was the one raising the weight (fig. 82). In other words,

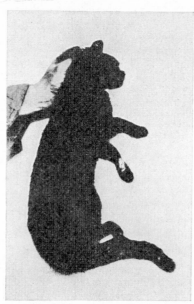

FIG. 82 —Lead Palsy affecting the Right Forepaw of a Cat
(By courtesy of Professor J. C. Aub and the Williams and Wilkins Co., Baltimore)

lead attacked the site of greatest fatigue. The weighted foot showed signs
of weakness after about two weeks of exercise. The threshold of the
weighted muscle to stimulation through nerve was higher than that of
the opposite foot, and a similar difference was apparent with direct
muscular stimulation in most of the cases tested.

Blue Line on the Gums

The well-known blue line on the gums, sometimes called the Burtonian
line, was described by Grisolle in 1836 and by Burton in 1840. It consists
of fine granules of pigment, arranged in the form of a dark blue stippled
line, within the tissue of the gum and about a millimetre from the gingival
margin (fig. 83). It is more marked round teeth having infected gingival

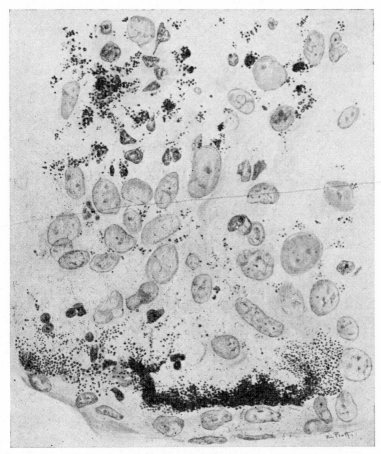

FIG. 83.—-Microscope Drawing showing Sub-epithelial Position of Lead
Line in Gum
(*By courtesy of Professor J. C. Aub and the Williams and Wilkins Co., Baltimore*)

troughs and occasionally may be found on the mucosa of the cheek opposite such teeth. The line is more frequently seen on the mandibular gums than on the maxillary, and in the incisor region than in the molar. If there are no teeth it does not occur. It is a precipitate of lead sulphide caused by the action of hydrogen sulphide upon the lead salts in the circulation. The gas is formed by micro-organisms in infected gingival troughs. Despite the pigment lying within the tissues, careful cleansing of the mouth and teeth often causes it to disappear. It is significant of absorption and not of intoxication. Its intensity and size provide a rough guide to the duration and severity of exposure to lead. At necropsy a broad blue line of lead sulphide may be found in the mucosa of the rectum near the anal margin.

Lead Anæmia

As early as 1831 Laennec described pallor of the tissues and thinness of the blood in cases of plumbism. The red-cell count was first found to be low in lead poisoning in the year 1840. Studies of lead anæmia are important, not only because of its clinical significance, but also because a clear understanding of the action of lead on the red blood corpuscle as an isolated cell throws considerable light on the mechanism of its reaction with other cells in the body. Chronic lead poisoning may give rise to a mild low colour-index anæmia. It is therefore of value to estimate the hæmoglobin figure in persons exposed. In differential diagnosis it is important to remember that in any case of industrial plumbism it is rare to find less than 3,000,000 red cells per c.mm.

Punctate Basophilia

Examination of the blood for punctate basophilia is of value in the prophylaxis of plumbism and, indeed, essential in the hygienic control of lead processes if the occurrence of manifest plumbism is to be avoided. The presence of basophilic stippling in the blood is not a specific sign of lead poisoning. It is seen in pernicious anæmia, leukæmia, the anæmias of carcinomatosis, in pneumonia in infants and sometimes in normal persons. However, its occurrence in these conditions is rare and slight as compared with the frequency and intensity of its appearance during plumbism. Ehrlich believed the stippling to be of cytoplasmic origin, and this view is undoubtedly correct. The basophilic granules are independent of the nuclear substance and have origin in the reticulum. Direct transition between nuclear fragments and stippling has never been observed.

Cytoplasmic Origin of Basophilic Granules

Furthermore, in marrow preparations made by sternal puncture the granules are frequently seen in erythroblasts with intact nuclei. The granules show none of the photographic or staining properties of nuclear substance. There is much evidence of the close alliance of basophil punctation with polychromatophilia and reticulation. The same fixatives and the same differential stains are effective for all three conditions. Blood films can be

prepared showing all stages between polychromatophilia, stippled fragments and typical reticulum. This action of lead on the reticulated red cell
is analogous to its effect on other young tissues, such as the chorion epithelium, and the sarcoma cell. Circulating lead singles out the youngest
tissues for its attack, and in the case of peripheral blood the youngest cells
are the reticulocytes (Key, 1924).

Methods of Staining and of Microscopy

Thin blood films are fixed with methyl alcohol and stained with alkaline methylene-blue (methylene-blue 2 parts, sodium bicarbonate 12
parts, distilled water 400 parts). They are examined with a 1/12th-inch oil-
immersion lens by dark-ground illumination. When employing this method,
the red cells are seen as circles of light and the stippling appears as golden
dots within the circle (fig. 84). Large granules have a greater significance
than small ones and denote excessive absorption or mobilization of lead

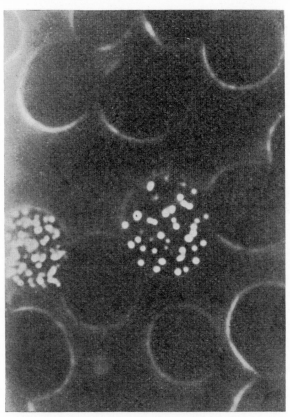

FIG. 84.—Erythrocytes showing Punctate Basophilia as seen
by Dark-ground Illumination
(After Professor R. E. Lane, Milroy Lectures, 1947

(Lane, 1931). If more than one stippled cell is present per field, excessive lead absorption may be suspected. The danger level is 3,000 stippled cells per million erythrocytes. It must be understood that different figures will be obtained if other staining methods and other methods of microscopy are used. The method of dark-ground illumination gives figures approximately twice as great as those obtained with transmitted light.

Basophilic Aggregation Test

Another method which has sometimes been applied in the supervision of lead workers is the basophilic aggregation test, which depends on the vital staining of hæmolysed red cells. In normal adults these aggregates rarely exceed 1 per cent of the total number of red cells. A figure of 2 per cent suggests early lead poisoning. Since in chronic cases the test is not always positive, it is not generally used in industry (McCord and others, 1924).

Coproporphyrinuria

In chronic plumbism the urine contains large amounts of coproporphyrin III. In severe cases increased urinary coproporphyrin I has also been observed (Kench and others, 1952). The laboratory estimating the amount of these substances should be careful to use normal urines as controls for the particular method used. The coproporphyrinuria is much more marked in plumbism than in other disorders and is often found before basophilic stippling is demonstrable (Maloof, 1950). Increased urinary coproporphyrin III is found also in porphyria including that caused by hexachlorobenzene poisoning (see p. 521), in some types of liver disease and in patients with a high reticulocyte count.

Cause of the Anæmia

The work of Aub and Reznikoff (1924) suggested that anæmia in lead poisoning was due to physical changes in the red-cell envelope. They exposed washed human red cells to a concentration of only two parts of lead chloride per million (1 ml. of corpuscles per 0·001 mg. of lead). The surface of the cell became hard, brittle and inelastic; it shrank, lost its power of agglutination and showed increased resistance to osmotic surroundings. It seemed that when the leaded cells circulate in the body, with the trauma attendant on passage through the capillaries, they break up rapidly in the peripheral circulation. Subsequent work, however, points to inhibition of hæmoglobin synthesis as the chief mechanism whereby anæmia develops in chronic lead poisoning. The work of Rimington (1938) suggests that the synthesis is inhibited at the point where iron should be incorporated into the porphyrin molecule.

Interference with Enzyme Systems

Lead may also act by interfering with the enzyme systems concerned in the biosynthesis of protoporphyrin (Kench, Gillam and Lane, 1942; Watson, 1950). This view gains support from the *in vitro* studies of

Eriksen (1955), in porphyrin and hæm synthesis in duck and rabbit erythrocytes. Lead ions inhibited hæm biosynthesis very strongly by reducing the formation of porphyrin prior to the coproporphyrin stage. No effect of lead on the incorporation of iron into protoporphyrin was observed. Coproporphyrin III in the urine is probably newly formed as the result of the action of lead and is not a product of hæmoglobin break-down (Grinstein and others, 1950). The intensity of stippling is invariably higher in the bone marrow than in the peripheral blood and it has been postulated that the action of lead is primarily upon the nucleated red-cell precursors in the bone marrow. In experimental studies it was observed that splenectomy results in a very considerable increase in the frequency of stippling in the peripheral blood as well as amelioration of the anæmia (McFadzean and Davis, 1949). It seems likely, therefore, that lead intoxi-cation, in addition to inhibiting hæmoglobin synthesis, also results in the producton of defective erythrocytes, which are removed from the circula-tion by the spleen and other parts of the reticulo-endothelial system. For a stimulating and comprehensive review of the effects of enzyme poisons see Goldblatt and Goldblatt (1956).

Other Symptoms and Signs

Transitory pains in muscles and joints are commonly associated with plumbism, and temporary effusions of fluid into bursæ and tendon sheaths may occur. In 1854 Garrod pointed out that gout was common among lead workers in Great Britain, but there is nothing to show that the occurrence of these two conditions in one patient is other than fortuitous. Abortion was common among women who worked in the potteries in the days before protective measures were in operation. Neglected cases of plumbism are likely to show generalized wasting; this has been referred to both as *lead cachexia* and *lead tabes*.

Chronic Nephritis

Conflicting statements have been made as to whether or not prolonged absorption of lead causes hypertension or chronic nephritis. The exposure to lead of young children in the tropical parts of Australia provides sugges-tive evidence. In Queensland, the paint on exposed surfaces readily turns to powder, producing an abundance of lead carbonate which rubs off fences and verandah railings like chalk. Numbers of children living in these houses develop lead palsy in childhood and die at an early age from chronic nephritis; sometimes several members of one family are affected. Nye (1933) studied a series of thirty-four patients with nephritis who had suffered from lead palsy in childhood. Inquiry showed that they had all spent their childhood in wooden houses; thirty were nail-biters or thumb suckers, all but seven had albuminuria, and twenty-nine had well-estab-lished renal insufficiency. Some had renal dwarfism, hypertension, marked urea retention and low urinary concentration. The death-rate was corre-spondingly high. Since 1955 the use of lead paint on the exterior parts of houses in Queensland has been forbidden by law. In adults it seems that ischæmic nephritis may occur after prolonged exposure to lead dust or fume, but that it is unusual.

The Blood-pressure in Lead Workers

Vigdortchik (1935) found an association between lead absorption and hypertension, but he based this on single observations of the blood-pressure of 2,769 workers in whom only the systolic pressure was recorded. He gave no serial figures of individual cases and he omitted to state the amount of lead absorption in each worker. Belknap (1936) reported 2,600 serial blood-pressure readings made month by month for over a year in workers who had absorbed large amounts of lead. Of eighty-one men observed all were heavily exposed either to fume of molten lead or to dusts of lead oxides, and all showed either a blue line on the gums, punctate basophilia or high lead excretion in the urine. Fifty-eight per cent of them had been exposed for periods varying from five to nine years. The cases were studied by age-groups. The writer concluded that there was no variation from normal in the blood-pressure. Teleky (1937) disputed the validity of these results on the ground that the men had not worked long enough in the lead industries to develop high blood-pressure. He stated that he would have expected, from his experience, only sporadic cases of high blood-pressure in men exposed for such relatively short periods.

Standard Mortality in Paperhangers and Painters

Fouts and Page (1942) failed to produce hypertension in dogs treated with lead for a long time. One animal received large amounts of lead for three years, a third of its life-span. Dreessen (1943) showed that among 776 workmen, albuminuria and symptoms of early plumbism were most common in those exposed to the highest atmospheric lead concentration, but the prevalence of arterial hypertension among these employees was not significantly different from that observed in other industrial workers. The figures of the Registrar-General for 1931 show there were then 178,170 paperhangers and painters in Great Britain and that deaths from cerebral vascular lesions numbered 398, arteriosclerosis 40, and Bright's disease 265. The standard mortality for the same diseases was 263, 33, and 202. There seems little evidence, therefore, that lead significantly predisposes to hypertension or Bright's disease, except perhaps in children.

Differential Diagnosis

In diagnosis there is a danger of wrongly attributing to lead poisoning any symptoms which may occur in persons exposed to lead. Acute appendicitis, chronic gastric or duodenal ulcer, and carcinoma of the stomach occur in lead workers just as they do in others. They must be carefully differentiated from colic. A lead worker can suffer from pernicious anæmia or secondary anæmia due to piles, melæna or hæmatemesis. It is important to remember that lead poisoning has to be severe before the red-cell count drops below 3,000,000 per c.mm. In industrial cases the blue line is unlikely to give rise to confusion. A similar phenomenon is commonly seen in patients under treatment with bismuth preparations given intramuscularly. The differential diagnosis of lead palsy should give rise to no difficulty, since the changes are entirely motor. Litigation hysteria is all too common in the lead worker. The manifestations include hysterical spasm of the hand and arm, weakness of various movements, including the flexors of the wrists and fingers, glove and stocking anæsthesia, complete hemi-anæsthesia, and hysterical aphonia. Such symptoms and signs indicate a *compensation neurosis* (p. 1105) and as such they are rarely alleviated until legal proceedings are completed.

Absorption of Lead

In 1839 Tanquerel des Planches wrote:

> All the characteristic traits of the primary effects of plumbism may be quickly observed in workmen who are habitually in an atmosphere of lead dust and fume. None of the primary effects are found in workmen who handle lead in a fixed state.

Other clinical observers have since come to the same conclusion. For example, Legge and Goadby (1912) stated that in industry absorption through the respiratory tract is a hundred times more important than by the gastro-intestinal tract. Until the work of Aub, Fairhall, Minot and Reznikoff (1925), observations of a quantitative nature on lead absorption were lacking (fig. 85). These workers realized that the majority of the fundamental physiological problems concerning plumbism were still unsolved, and that the results of previous experiments were for the most part contradictory, inaccurate or incomplete. Their work threw light on the puzzling problems of lead absorption, storage and elimination, and on the mechanism of its action on blood, muscle and nerve. Accurate methods for the detection and quantitative estimation of small amounts of lead in biological material were devised, the titrimetric chromate method by Fairhall (1924) and the diphenyl thiocarbazone (dithizone) method by Fairhall and Keenan (1941).

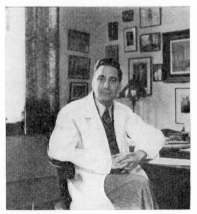

FIG. 85.—Dr. Joseph C. Aub, of Harvard

Importance of Inhaled Lead

Studies made by Minot in cats showed how readily absorption

occurs from the respiratory tract. She analysed all the organs quantitatively and found that as much lead may be absorbed in one day from a single injection into the respiratory tract as from gastrointestinal exposure lasting for months. When lead was given by stomach tube in cats, most of it could be promptly recovered in the fæces. This occurs partly because most of the ingested lead is not absorbed, and partly because a great proportion of the fraction which is absorbed is taken up by the liver and excreted into the intestinal tract by way of the bile. Very large doses (50 mg. per kilogram three times a week) are required to poison a cat when given orally, and they must be continued for weeks before symptoms of intoxication appear. Thus the experimental method confirmed the truth of the clinical view that dust and fume should be minimized in order to prevent lead poisoning.

Physico-chemical Behaviour of Lead

The problem of the physico-chemical behaviour of lead in the animal body has been approached experimentally. Fairhall (1924) determined the solubility of various lead compounds in serum, studied the reactions and equilibria involved in the formation of the phosphates of lead, and carried out electrometric measurements in which lead salts were added to serum. His experiments suggest that lead is transported in the blood-plasma as the insoluble tertiary phosphate in the highly dispersed or colloidal form.

Storage of Lead in Bone

Since lead is a cumulative poison, there must be some place in the body where it can be retained in fairly large quantities. The work of Gusserow in 1861, followed by that of Heubel in 1871, suggested that this storehouse was the skeleton (fig. 86). Minot and Aub (1924) showed quantitatively that in animals and man nearly all the lead is stored in the bones (fig. 87). Fairhall studied such bones, and the results of his experiments suggest that the lead is present as the very insoluble tertiary phosphate. Various experiments showed that it is deposited in the calcareous portion of the bone and not in the marrow. Minot obtained proof of this by producing lead poisoning in chickens and examining the respiratory bone of the wings, which consists of a shaft without marrow. She showed that these bones contained relatively as much lead as did the other bones of the chicken. The lead must therefore have been stored in bone and not marrow.

Migration of Lead from Trabeculæ to Cortex

In 1932 Aub, Robb and Rossmeisl found by analysis that for as long as four months after intratracheal injection adult cats had about twice the concentration of lead in the trabeculæ as was present in the cortex of bone (fig. 88). In 1954 McLean, Calhoun and Aub studied the migration of lead within the bones of animals by using radioactive lead. They gave to dogs intravenous injections either of inert lead or of lead tagged with radium D. Comparison of total lead in the humerus of dogs which received

STORAGE AND ELIMINATION OF LEAD

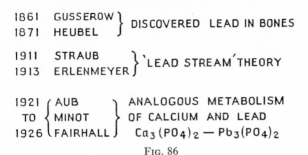

1861 GUSSEROW ⎫
1871 HEUBEL   ⎬ DISCOVERED LEAD IN BONES

1911 STRAUB   ⎫ 'LEAD STREAM' THEORY
1913 ERLENMEYER ⎭

1921 ⎧ AUB   ⎫ ANALOGOUS METABOLISM
TO   ⎨ MINOT   ⎬ OF CALCIUM AND LEAD
1926 ⎩ FAIRHALL⎭ $Ca_3(PO_4)_2 - Pb_3(PO_4)_2$

FIG. 86

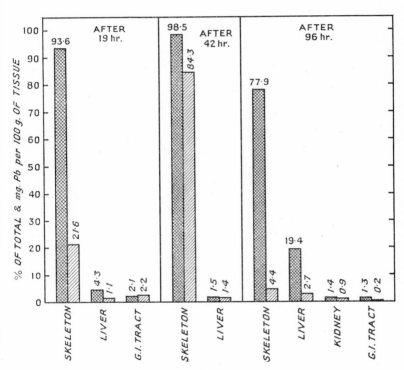

FIG. 87.—Storage of Lead in the Tissues of Cats after Absorption by the Respiratory Tract. In each Animal the Œsophagus was Ligated and Approximately 250 mg. of Lead Carbonate were introduced into the Trachea. Of the Total Amount of Lead held in the Body, note the High Percentage retained in the Skeleton

(*By courtesy of Professor J. C. Aub and the Williams and Wilkins Co., Baltimore*)

inert lead with one which received tagged lead showed no real difference in the total lead stored. The concentration of tagged lead in the trabeculæ of long bone was found to be from five to sixteen times that of the cortex, but the mass of cortex is much greater. The migration of lead from trabeculæ to cortex of long bones appeared to be very slow when measured by increase in concentration in cortex with time.

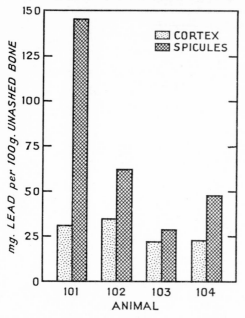

FIG. 88.—Migration of Lead from Trabeculæ to Cortex of Bone. For as long as Four Months after Intratracheal Injection of Lead Carbonate Adult Cats had about Twice the Concentration of Lead in the Spicules of the Spongiosa as was present in the Cortex of Bone

(*Aub, J. C., Robb, G. P., and Rossmeisl, E., J. Publ. Hlth.,* *1932,* **22,** *825*)

Distribution of Lead in the Tissues

During different stages of intoxication the distribution of lead within the body varies. When absorption is slow during the chronic stage of plumbism, about 95 per cent is held harmlessly in the skeleton. On the other hand, if lead is being absorbed in large quantity it is distributed more evenly throughout the tissues. Under these conditions, acute symptoms of poisoning occur. Analysis of bone obtained at necropsy from lead workers has shown that the total amount of lead stored in the skeleton varies from 0·2 to 0·8 g. Since calcium and lead are stored in the skeleton in the form of phosphate, the discovery that the excretion of these two substances runs parallel is of great interest. Repeated observations have shown that conditions which favour storage of calcium in the body also favour storage of lead. When conditions are unfavourable for the retention of calcium, the excretion of stored lead increases.

Excretion of Lead

In studies of lead excretion it is to be noted that no satisfactory figures can be obtained unless specimens of stools and urine are collected for at least three days. Normal persons with no occupational exposure to lead may excrete lead in the fæces and urine. This happens because lead is frequently present in the soil and hence in vegetation and animal food. Cholak and Bambach (1943) found that in 1,052 normal persons with no occupational lead hazard, the mean lead concentrations were 0·03 mg. per 100 ml. of blood, 0·027 mg. per litre of urine and 0·28 mg. per 24 hours' sample of fæces. Exposure to lead in industry raises these values, and the corresponding figures for eighty-six men engaged in making white lead were 0·086, 0·241 and 3·76.

Lead in the Blood

The absence of a direct relationship between blood lead and the appearance or severity of symptoms of lead poisoning has been frequently noted (Cantarow and Trumper, 1944). Although it has been shown repeatedly that the blood lead values of groups of lead workers are greater than normal, yet changes in lead absorption are not so quickly reflected in these figures as they are in the figures for urinary excretion. Sometimes in a case of chronic plumbism the blood lead repeatedly shows normal figures 30 to 80 micrograms per 100 ml.), whereas occasionally a healthy lead worker shows values as high as 160 micrograms per 100 ml. Therefore too much reliance must not be placed on the figures for blood lead. Attempts to establish critical values above which poisoning occurs and below which safety may be presumed must needs break down (Lane, 1949). Nevertheless blood lead figures which are higher than normal do indicate excessive absorption and therefore point to the need for re-assessment of the efficacy of precautionary measures against dust and fume in the workshop concerned. In most lead works it is the practice to consider blood lead figures below 60 micrograms per 100 ml. to be normal. Between 60 and 80 micrograms a closer watch is kept over both workshop and employees, and above 80 micrograms workers are transferred temporarily to jobs where no further exposure is involved.

Lead in the Stools

A man working in a dusty lead industry, in addition to inhaling lead, may swallow repeated small amounts and pass lead unabsorbed in the fæces. Therefore to prove the absorption of lead, it is necessary to find excess in the urine. Lead has been found in the stools of persons who have been removed from exposure for more than two years, and Oliver (1914) found it in the urine of a woman eleven years after exposure. Thus, as suggested by Straub (1911) and Erlenmeyer (1913), there may be an intermittent stream of lead entering the circulation which is only gradually excreted.

Control of Lead Risk in Industry

In industry control of a lead risk must be based upon the concept of lead absorption rather than on that of lead poisoning. Because of variations of susceptibility in workmen, some men show signs of poisoning at levels of absorption at which other men show no abnormality. Thus control must be based upon an accepted level of lead absorption low enough to protect all but the very susceptible individual, who may be detected clinically at an early stage and removed from risk. Combinations of laboratory tests such as lead in the blood, lead in the urine, coproporphyrin excretion,

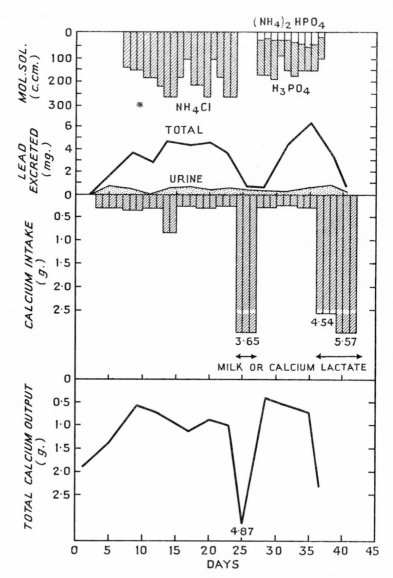

Fig. 89.—Effect of Ammonium Chloride, Phosphoric Acid and Diet upon Lead Excretion in Man. The Doses are shown in Blocks representing Millilitres of Molar Solution taken per Day. In the Middle Section of the Chart is shown the Calcium Intake in Blocks of Three Days. In the Lowest Section is shown the Total Calcium Output in Urine and Fæces in Three-day Periods

(By courtesy of Professor J. C. Aub and the Williams and Wilkins Co., Baltimore)

punctate basophilia and hæmoglobin may be used successfully provided the doctor understands the limitations of these tests, particularly those on spot specimens of urine, and the wide range of any one with respect to the others which may be observed. This aspect was investigated by King and Thompson (1961) and their results show the varying relationships between the biochemical tests and clinical observations on 540 workmen in the motor-car-body industry. They suggest that although there is no complete single answer to the problem of which test to use, the intelligent use of any of the tests or combinations of tests used today, if combined with engineering action to remedy failings in equipment or in housekeeping responsible for increased absorption, will give adequate protection to the workmen. Full control of a lead risk must be based upon lead absorption, and it must be accepted that in the absence of other evidence failure to find cases of lead poisoning in a group of workmen may merely indicate a fortunate choice of workmen rather than safe conditions.

Liberation of Lead from the Tissues

The conditions favouring liberation of lead from the bones have been studied experimentally in cats poisoned with lead. During starvation, acute symptoms may develop suggesting that there is something unusual in the metabolism of the body which sets lead free from the bones. Acidosis seems the most probable explanation for the change (Aub, Fairhall, Minot and Reznikoff, 1925). Acidosis has been produced in men exposed for long periods in lead industries. They were given either hydrochloric acid, phosphoric acid or ammonium chloride, in combination with a known low calcium diet containing no milk, eggs, green vegetables or fruit. Under this régime the excretion of lead in the fæces rose to about 2 mg. in each twenty-four hours (fig. 89). Fairhall (1924) showed that the tertiary phosphate of lead has an extremely low solubility at the normal pH of the body, but under slightly more acid conditions it is converted into the secondary phosphate, which is a hundred times more soluble. Hence the ingestion of acid serves to liberate lead from the skeletal stores by converting it into a more soluble salt.

Effect of Parathyroid Extract

When, in 1925, Collip prepared parathyroid extract, it was possible to confirm the hypothesis that the metabolism of lead runs parallel to that of calcium. He showed that the extract, administered to parathyroidectomized dogs, prevented tetany by restoring the level of the serum-calcium to normal, and that elevations in that level could be produced in normal dogs. In 1926 Hunter and Aub studied the effect of repeated injections in six patients with chronic lead poisoning. They were given a diet of known calcium content, routine daily estimations of the serum-calcium were made and all the fæces and urine were collected for the quantitative estimation of lead and calcium. These analyses showed increased excretion of calcium and lead from the bones; the extract caused elevation in the serum-calcium, an effect observed even on a diet deficient in cal-

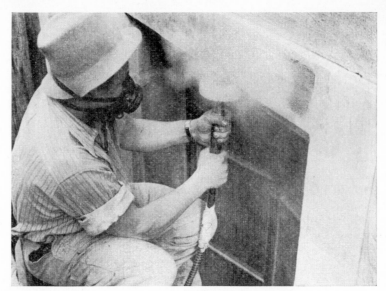

FIG. 90.—A Workman in Geneva re-facing with a Grinding Disc Stone previously painted with a White Lead Paint

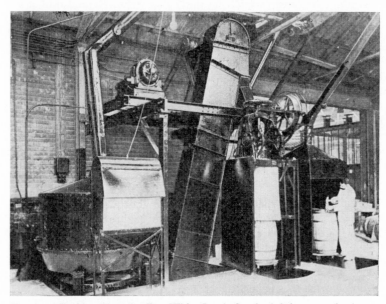

FIG. 91.—Packing Plant for Dry White Lead. On the left is a completely enclosed Grinding Mill electrically illuminated from within. On the right are Steel Packing Chambers used for Heading Up Casks. Clean Air flows past the Operator into the Hood above the Cask. The Hood is connected to the System for Exhaust Ventilation. Note that the Floor is kept Wet

(By courtesy of Associated Lead Manufacturers, Ltd.)

cium. When parathyroid extract was first given it greatly increased the excretion of lead from trabecular bone. However, if it were given a second time after an interval, it failed to mobilize the remaining lead stored in a less available form in cortical bone. This action confirms the striking parallelism between the storage and excretion of calcium and of lead. No ill effects were produced, but it is a drastic procedure and has little value in practical therapeutics. It might produce acute episodes of lead poisoning or the symptoms of prolonged hypercalcæmia.

Preventive Measures

In Great Britain, preventive measures are carried out with striking success. Lead encephalopathy has disappeared from industry. It is unusual today to meet with a case either of severe colic or of extensive palsy. Few cases of lead poisoning are seen and these are mild. The effect of notification in controlling the lead hazard is seen in fig. 68, p. 237.

Prevention of Dust and Fume

Nearly all lead hazards can be controlled by engineering devices; the most important single measure of prophylaxis is the prevention of dust and fume (fig. 90). As advocated by Legge (1934), success has been achieved by the institution of protective measures over which the worker concerned can exercise no control. One such method is exhaust ventilation applied through hoods at the source of origin of dust or fume.

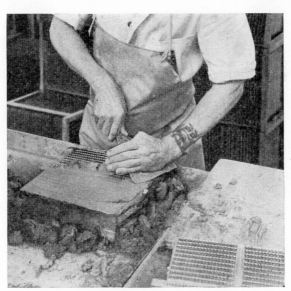

FIG. 92.—Accumulator Paster at Work
(By courtesy of Pritchett & Gold and E.P.S. Co., Ltd.)

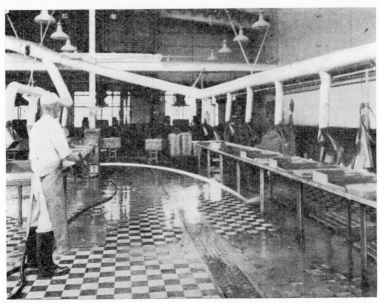

FIG. 93.—Hosing down with Water an Accumulator Pasting Shop at the Close of Work

(*By courtesy of Pritchett & Gold and E.P.S. Co., Ltd.*)

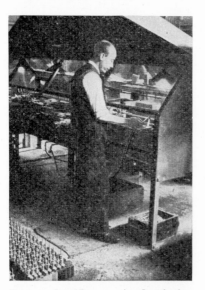

FIG. 94.—Lead Burner using Oxy-hydrogen Flame to weld Terminals on to Accumulator Plates. Exhaust Ventilation operates behind a Plate-glass Screen

By courtesy of Pritchett & Gold and E.P.S. Co. Ltd.)

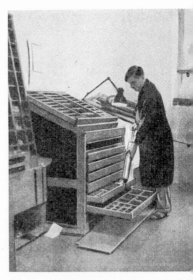

FIG. 95.—A Printer in Croatia blowing Dust from Cases of Type

(*By courtesy of Prof. B. Kesić*)

Hygiene of the Workshop

The hygiene of the workshop and cleanliness of the worker are both important. Benches, tools, floors and walls must be spotless, often at the expense of the constant vigilance of several good foremen. No scrap lead or dry white lead should be handled unless it has been thoroughly soaked by the use of a hose. Mechanical means, such as cranes, rails, hoists, covered conveyers and hoppers, and automatic packing machinery, should be substituted for hand carriage (fig. 91). Between 1899 and 1939 the lead manufacturers in Great Britain spent over £200,000 on alterations and dust-removal plant in order to render the conditions of employment more healthy. Between 1930 and 1950 more than £250,000 was spent in changing over entirely from the old stack process to the quick process in the manufacture of white lead.

Electric Accumulators

In the manufacture of electric accumulators, suppression of dust in the pasting shops is effectively carried out by the use of exhaust ventilation over the benches combined with repeated hosing with water of the benches and floors (figs. 92 and 93). The lead burner and the chemical plumber must receive special protection, for it has been shown that lead absorption is always greatest among those exposed to freshly formed lead fume. Thus, when lead burning is performed with an oxy-acetylene flame 100 per cent of men absorb lead, whereas in spray painting only 44 per cent do so (Fairhall, 1936). The lead burner must therefore be rigidly protected by a system of exhaust ventilation. In the electric accumulator trade this is arranged to operate behind a plate-glass screen so that his nose and mouth are safely protected from lead fume; meanwhile, he is able to see to do his work through the glass (fig. 94).

Printing

In the printing trade the compositor keeps his type in cases. From time to time he removes the dust containing lead oxide from the surface of the type by the use of a vacuum cleaner. At one time it was customary for him to blow off this dust, and there was then a risk that he would inhale some of it (fig. 95). The hazard in the case of linotype workers is slight only. Linotype metal is an alloy of 85 per cent lead, 12 per cent antimony and 3 per cent tin. This is kept in the molten state in a container on the machine, but the temperature is low (350° C.) and the total quantity is only one gallon.

Painting

Since 1927 it has been illegal for a painter to rub down by dry methods any indoor structure previously treated with lead paint. Dust can be avoided by using a damp rubbing-down process for lead-painted surfaces. Waxed sandpaper, which the workman dips repeatedly in a bucket of water, has made this possible (Klein, 1923). This material is

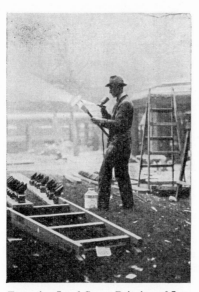

FIG. 96.—Lead Spray Painting of Iron Drain Pipes, a process strictly forbidden

impervious to water, and it has been found possible to immerse it for six months without deterioration in the quality of the paper or loosening of the abrasive. The paper has a much longer working life than ordinary paper applied in the dry method, and this adds to its efficacy. Master painters agree that the damp process can be applied efficiently to all types of work, including the rubbing down of curved surfaces. Spray painting where the paint contains compounds of lead must be strictly forbidden (fig. 96).

Lid Labels for Lead Paint

The hazard of lead poisoning in children from ingestion of compounds of lead is serious especially during the age of teething. In Baltimore, U.S.A between 1931 and 1959 a total of 744 such children were poisoned, and of these 123 died. A special ordinance (No. 1504) for the City of Baltimore was adopted as a regulation on 27th April, 1959. The text of the regulation is as follows: "Lid Labels. No lid label bearing the warning as required by this ordinance shall be less than three inches in diameter for pint and larger size containers or less than one and one-half inches in diameter for cans smaller than pint size. In addition to the warning statement the lid label shall contain the name and address of the manufacturer. The word WARNING preceding the warning statement shall be of larger letters than the name and address of the manufacturer. The warning statement shall be as large as the lid will permit. The lid label shall adhere firmly to the lid of the container." The text of the label warning required by the Baltimore ordinance for all paint containing more than one per cent of lead reads as follows: "WARNING—*Contains lead. Harmful if eaten. Do not apply on any interior surfaces of a dwelling, or of a place used for the care of children, or on window sills, toys, cribs, or other furniture.*"

Non-setting Red Lead

In mixing paint a painter is rarely exposed to dry white lead since it comes to him already mixed in oil. Paint technologists have invented a non-setting red lead, which is issued to the painter of metals already mixed in oil. He is therefore protected from exposure to the dust of red lead, for he no longer mixes the materials himself. The setting properties of red-lead paints depend upon the proportions of true red lead and lead monoxide present, the latter being more active chemically towards linseed oil. It is now technically possible to produce commercial red lead having so little immediate action on the paint media that it can be ground with linseed oil into a paste which remains soft for many months. Originally, dry red lead as obtained by the painter contained such high proportions of the monoxide that it had to be mixed with linseed oil immediately before it was required for use, as otherwise it would set hard.

Litharge Rubber

The use of litharge rubber—that is, rubber in which litharge has been incorporated in excess in a mother batch even to the extent of 90 per cent—has abolished lead poisoning in men who vulcanize rubber (Klein, 1922). The litharge rubber is manufactured in a central factory and is sent to scores of other factories where vulcanizers throw it in solid pieces into batches of crude rubber. Prior to the invention of litharge rubber they used powdered litharge, some of which inevitably they inhaled.

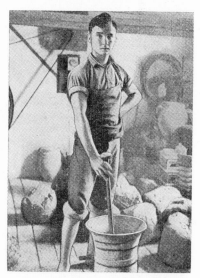

Lead Glazes

At one time the occupation of pottery glazing exposed men to the hazard of lead poisoning. The potter glazes his ware with vitreous materials of various types. The glazes always contain silica, alumina and at least one alkali or alkaline earth metal, and many contain up to 70 per cent of lead oxide (fig. 97). In pottery glazing, removal of dust by locally applied exhaust ventilation has accomplished much in the diminution of poisoning. So also has the use of low-solubility glaze or frit, a substance introduced by Thorpe (1901). It is a product in which oxides of lead have been

FIG. 97.—A workman crushing Lead Silicate Glaze in a Pottery in Eastern Croatia
(*By courtesy of Prof. B. Kesić*)

fused with the raw constituents of the glaze, thus converting them into the insoluble lead bisilicate. Up to 1900, red lead or white lead had been almost universally used for pottery glazing, and the good effect of using a non-dusty, highly insoluble substitute can readily be imagined.

Leadless Glazes

Chemically considered, glazes must be regarded as being closely related to glasses, but they differ from the ordinary varieties of glass in containing in addition to silica another acidic oxide such as boric oxide, which renders the glaze more fusible than glass and confers hardness and brilliancy. Both borax and boric acid are excellent fluxes and their introduction into the ceramics industries made possible the production of leadless glazes. It is claimed that glazes containing complex boro-silicates have a greater covering power than the older lead glazes. In combination with feldspar, boric acid is being used in increasing quantities for the manufacture of highly resistant glazes. A typical frit for glazing English porcelain would have the following composition: feldspar 56, quartz 20, sodium carbonate 8, borax 8, and zinc oxide 8.

Pottery Glazing

The observations of Alice Hamilton (1925), contrasting the state of affairs in the potteries of England and the United States of America, may be quoted to show what can be achieved by the suppression of dust.

Of Trenton, New Jersey, she states that the dipping or glaze room is almost always full of glaze dust (fig. 98). The floor is of wood, rough, worn out and deeply impregnated with dried glaze, and there are accumulations of glaze dust on ware boards and racks. Handling these boards, dropping them frequently down on end, and sweeping the floor all keep the dust

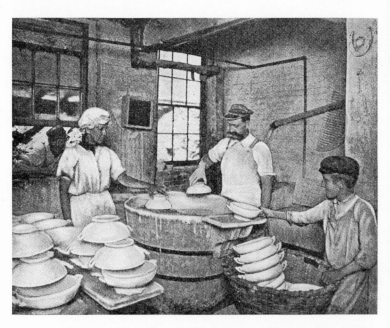

FIG. 98.—A Glaze-dipping Room in the Potteries of Trenton, New Jersey, U.S.A., in 1912. The Conditions of Work are bad, Glaze having dripped and spattered over the Walls and Elsewhere. Note the Employment of a Woman and a Boy

stirred. Finishing tiles is very dangerous work. The glaze that runs down over the sides must be scraped or brushed off. The tiles are often kept overnight before they are finished, and girls and boys scrape and blow away a fine powdery glaze containing sometimes as much as 60 per cent of white lead. The powder can be seen on their clothes and hair, and even in their nostrils.

Of the Staffordshire potteries she states that the factory is obliged to employ a physician to examine once a month all men and women exposed in any way to lead. The employer provides, mends and launders full suits of washable working clothes, one clean suit a week. The workers are required to take off their working clothes and wash their hands and faces before leaving work or going to the lunch room, the only place where they are permitted to eat or to keep food. The floors of the dipping rooms are of cement, sloping to a drain, and some have white tiled walls (fig. 99). The floors are never swept dry, but are flushed with a hose every evening. The boards on which the glazed ware is placed are beautifully clean, for they are washed every evening. Finishing, if dry, is done over a large vessel of

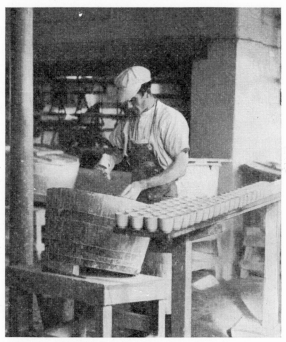

Fig. 99.—A Dipping House in the Potteries of Stoke-on-Trent. The Walls are covered with White Tiles and the Floor slopes to a Central Gutter. The Floors are flushed with a Hose every Evening and the Boards on which the Glazed Ware is placed are washed clean

(By courtesy of Messrs. Doulton, Ltd.)

water to catch the heavier particles of glaze, and in front of an air exhaust which carries off the lighter particles.

Striking figures can be quoted to show the effects of these very different methods. In 1921 the United States Public Health Service examined 1,809 men and women potters and found an incidence of plumbism of at least 13·5 per hundred employed, whereas the rate in the English potteries in 1913 was only 0·9 per hundred, one-fifteenth of the American rate (Newman and others, 1922).

Vitreous Enamelling

In the manufacture of porcelain-enamelled sanitary ware, both lead poisoning and silicosis must be prevented. In the United States of America between 1912 and 1929 great progress was made in protecting bath enamellers from these two risks. This is described by Alice Hamilton in *Exploring the Dangerous Trades* (1943).

> Because enameling tubs was notoriously hard, hot, and dangerous, most American men shunned it and I found in 1912 in Pittsburgh and the surrounding towns, in Trenton and in Chicago, foreign-born workmen, Russians, Bohemians, Slovaks, Croatians, Poles. I remember a foreman saying to me, as we watched the enamelers at work, "They don't last long at it. Four years at the most, I should say, then they quit and go home to the Old Country." "To die?" I asked. "Well, I suppose that is about the size of it," he answered. It was not the lead, as I discovered then, that did the greatest harm, but the silica dust. Many of the doctors I talked to told me that there was where my attention should be turned, to the pulmonary consumption; lead poisoning was a minor evil. But lead dust was my job, not silica.
>
> The lead dust was bad. In the enameling rooms of the plants, this would be the picture. In front of the great furnaces stood the enameler and his helper. The door swung open and, with the aid of a mechanism which required strength to operate, a red-hot bathtub was lifted out. The enameler then dredged as quickly as possible powdered enamel over the hot surface, where it melted and flowed to form an even coating. His helper stood beside him working the turntable on which the tub stood so as to present all its inner surface to the enameler. The dredge was big and so heavy that part of its weight had to be taken by a chain from the roof. The men during this procedure were in a thick cloud of enamel dust, and were breathing rapidly and deeply because of the exertion and the extreme heat. I found that I could not stand the heat any nearer than twelve feet but the workmen had to come much closer. They protected their faces and eyes by various devices, a light tin pan with eye-holes and a hoop to go around the head, or a piece of wood with eye-holes and a stick nailed at a right angle so that it could be held between the teeth.
>
> When the coat had been applied, the tub was swung back into the

furnace and then usually there would be a few minutes of respite, for the men to relax, to go to the window for a breath of air or to take a bite of lunch. There was never any break in the eight- or six-hour shift, so the man had the choice between fasting (and an empty stomach favors lead poisoning) and eating his lunch with lead-covered hands in a lead-laden atmosphere. I saw plenty of sandwiches lying on dusty window sills and plenty of hasty lunches taken between two bouts at the furnace. Women told me of finding white powder in their husband's lunch boxes.

I visited many of the homes of these workers. The enamelers are skilled men and the homes I saw were pleasant, the standard of living comfortable, yet they stayed only a few years in their well-paid jobs. I secured full histories of 186 cases of lead poisoning; 38 men had worked less than a year, 137 less than ten years. Lead poisoning and consumption both were notorious in those neighborhoods; I heard of them not only from the men but from doctors, priests, apothecaries, shopkeepers. And I found an unusually high proportion of severe forms among these cases, men who had had four, six, even eight attacks of colic. There were tragic stories of men who had gone back to their old homes in Austria-Hungary broken in health, paralyzed or dying. Sometimes the tales came from trustworthy sources but I could not add them to my records unless I had a doctor's diagnosis. I did, however, gain from doctors and from hospitals the details of 177 cases, and of these 28 had palsy, eight had the brain form of plumbism, and seven were fatal.

Seventeen years later, in 1929, I made a second survey of this industry, this time with special regard to the dust hazard. The risk of lead poisoning had been moderated; silicosis had by then become the most important of the industrial diseases and I knew that in making porcelain-enameled sanitary ware not only the enamelers but many other workmen were exposed to silica dust. I found the work of the enamelers not nearly so bad as it had been. In the first place no plant was using as much lead as it had in 1912 and three out of ten used none at all for ordinary enamel. Then there was far less dust both in the grinding room and in enameling. The enamelers' work was much less heavy, mechanical devices had been introduced for opening and closing furnaces, lifting ware, and controlling the turntable. The heat was still as great as ever, the workday still unbroken for lunch or rest, and now there are many double furnaces, which means that the men must work without even the few moments' break while the ware is heating. Even when the day is cut from eight to six hours, the work is more exhausting than on the single furnaces.

But the department that interested me most in this second study was the one where the ironware is prepared for coating with enamel. As the tubs come from the foundry their surface is smooth and enamel will not stick to it, so in order to roughen it a blast of fine sand is turned on and the million particles of sand make millions of tiny dents in the metal so that it is frosted all over. This, every industrial physician knew to be one of the most dangerous jobs in all industry and the National Safety Council had appointed a committee, of which I was a member, to study sandblasting and suggest how the danger might be controlled. So I had seen a good deal of this process in other industries but never anything approaching what I saw in sanitary-ware manufacture.

Imagine a great room filled with men cleaning mold sand off the tubs from the foundry. At one end through a thick fog of dust can dimly be seen eight lamplit little rooms open to the big room, in each of which a grotesque figure is manipulating a sandblast which with a deafening roar, shoots sand at something, one cannot see what. Great clouds of sand come eddying out into the room and filling the air the cleaners must breathe. Some attempt is made to protect the sand-blaster, none at all to protect the cleaner.

This was the worst plant I saw, but three others were almost as bad, all in states where no compensation law for occupational diseases existed. The others were all much less dangerous and one was excellent in every respect. This was the Kohler plant in Sheboygan, Wisconsin, or rather in the charming village of Kohler. I remembered it from 1912, for Walter Kohler was the only employer I met then who was seriously concerned with the problems of lead poisoning and of dust. In the intervening years he had done away with the lead and now he had brought the dust under control. In some of the other plants I saw excellent conditions, but Kohler's stood at the head in 1929. What Mr. Kohler had done was to make the sandblast chambers dust-proof, so that no man outside was endangered, and to provide the sandblaster with pure, dust-free air, fed to him through a pipe which led to his respirator. And of course a physician kept close watch on all these men.

Enameling sanitary ware is still a dangerous trade, for only the greatest precautions can prevent silicosis in sandblasters and enamel-ers, and even if there is no lead in the enamel the excessive heat is harmful. But compared with the situation in 1912 the trade has made enormous progress, aided, no doubt, by the passage in 1939 of a law in Pennsylvania awarding compensation for occupational disease.

Personal Hygiene

In addition to cleanliness in the work-places, personal cleanliness is of the first importance. Cloak-rooms, washing-rooms, mess-rooms, baths, nailbrushes, towels and soap must be provided. The hands should always be washed before eating, and the work-people urged to take a warm bath frequently. Food and drink must not be brought into the workrooms and smoking at work must not be allowed.

Periodic Medical Examination

Medical examination of the workers exposed must be carried out periodically. At present we have no biological test by which to select workmen who are immune to the toxic effects of lead. Since they have been found unduly susceptible, it is necessary to forbid the employment in the potteries and other lead trades of pregnant women and of all persons under eighteen years of age.

Education of the Worker

The importance of education of the worker himself must be stressed. He must understand fully in what way his work is dangerous. No attempt must be made to hide this or to minimize it, but he must at the same time be shown his own responsibilities in any safety programme. This needs patience and hard work on the part of the doctor. He must inspire employers and workers alike with enthusiasm for safe working conditions. The employer can, and must, do a great deal, but final and complete success will be impossible without the co-operation of the workman. This co-operation is forthcoming if the approach is the right one; the responsibility for procuring it lies with the doctor (Lane, 1949).

Issue of Free Milk

In the prevention of lead poisoning a diet of high calcium content plays its part. In lead works in Great Britain it has for many years been customary to provide the workmen with a glass of milk each morning free of cost. This is empirical treatment of considerable merit, anticipating as it did by many years the discovery that a high calcium intake assists the storage of lead in a harmless form in the bones. Workers should drink plenty of water which will help to avert constipation and often render the use of aperients unnecessary.

Suspension from Work

Any worker who shows evidence of abnormal absorption, such as pallor, a drop in the hæmoglobin or a continued rise in the punctate count, must receive treatment. This means stopping lead absorption by suspending him from work in contact with lead and giving him a high calcium diet. Such suspension should not involve financial hardship, and should last for about three months. Any question of return to the old work must receive careful consideration. If it has been possible to modify the operation or conditions of work, including hours, which were responsible for the trouble, the man may be allowed to return. If no such modification is possible, he should be considered unsuitable for that particular job. Workmen should not be allowed to go back to a lead hazard immediately on their return to work after a febrile infection; there is ample evidence that infection is likely to precipitate lead mobilization.

Curative Treatment

Treatment which aims at the cure or amelioration of lead poisoning should never be made the excuse for negligence in enforcing all the known measures for the prevention of exposure and absorption. Since a high calcium intake causes lead excretion rapidly to diminish it follows that a high calcium diet is useful in treatment. In mild cases of lead poisoning a diet containing two pints of milk a day or a daily dose of 10 gm. of calcium lactate is all that is necessary to store lead in the bones so that it will not be free in the circulation to cause harm. In cases of lead poisoning showing toxic symptoms the diet should contain four pints of milk daily and include milk puddings, junket and ice-cream, together with butter, cheese and eggs. Large quantities of calcium lactate, 5 gm. (75 gr.) three times a day, should be given. In the presence of acute symptoms the patient should be admitted to hospital for treatment by intravenous injections of calcium EDTA (p. 281).

Methods used to increase the Excretion of Lead

The ideal method to increase the excretion of lead from the tissues is still being sought. Many nations have contributed to this problem. In 1844 France gave us potassium iodide, then the United States of America gave us first the use of acid salts with a low calcium diet (1925) and then sodium citrate (1943), Switzerland gave us the use of versene compounds (1948) and finally Sweden gave us penicillamine.

(i) Potassium Iodide

Potassium iodide was first used in the treatment of lead poisoning by Guillot and Melsens in 1844. The dose should be increased from 5 gr. three times a day to 15 gr. three times a day. Its physiological effectiveness appears to diminish progressively after the first few days of treatment. It has been known to precipitate an acute attack of lead poisoning in an apparently healthy subject as long as sixteen years after exposure to lead has ceased. Oliver (1914) quoted such a case in which administration of potassium iodide was promptly followed by the appearance of a blue line on the gums and wrist-drop, although previously there had been no evidence of lead intoxication. The condition has been referred to as *latent lead poisoning*.

(ii) Ammonium Chloride with a Low Calcium Diet

A few weeks after the acute toxic episodes have passed, the elimination of lead may be accelerated by the use of a low calcium diet, together with ammonium chloride to facilitate the release of lead from the bones. All milk, milk products, green vegetables and eggs are omitted from the diet, which may, however, contain meat, liver, chicken, potato, peas, rice, tomato, banana, apple, lemon, tea, coffee, sugar, honey, salt and pepper. In those places where the water supply is hard, vegetables should be cooked in distilled water and all drinks made up with it. Ammonium chloride is given cautiously in doses of 1 gm. (15 gr.) in a glass of water eight or ten times daily for three weeks at a time. The dose should be reduced if loss of appetite and headache appear, for these symptoms indicate the limit of tolerance to such treatment. Since it would doubtless require several years, it is useless to attempt the elimination of all the lead stored in the body. It is desirable to eliminate only the most readily mobilized lead. Thus, after three weeks' treatment by a low calcium diet and ammonium chloride, there should be a rest period of a week with normal diet and abundance of milk to correct the calcium deficiency. Treatment to accelerate elimination should then begin again. Neither ammonium chloride nor potassium iodide should be used in the presence of nephritis or of toxic symptoms. Should any toxic episode appear during the use of ammonium chloride or potassium iodide, these drugs must be stopped and a high calcium diet at once used to favour the storage of lead.

(iii) Sodium Citrate

Because all previous methods used to eliminate lead from the body involved the risk of making the symptoms worse, attempts were made to render the mobilized lead harmless by converting it into a more complex chemical substance. Since in dilute solutions sodium citrate dissolves tertiary lead phosphate, and since the soluble complex of lead citrate so formed has an extremely low dissociation constant, Kety and Letonoff (1943) suggested that this might prove to be a safe and effective way to rid the body of lead. They reported favourable results from treatment by sodium citrate.

(iv) Calcium di-sodium Versenate

In 1948 Schwarzenbach and Ackermann showed that sodium ethylene-diamine tetra-acetate (sodium EDTA; sodium versenate) is a powerful chelating agent having a strong avidity for calcium and heavy metals. This property has been utilized in the treatment of acute and chronic lead poisoning. When calcium di-sodium EDTA (calcium EDTA; calcium versenate) is administered parenterally the lead displaces the calcium and the resulting lead chelate is excreted by the kidney. Not only is the rate of excretion of the metal thus increased, but the circulating un-ionized chelate is much less toxic than would be a similar quantity of ionized metal. Three patients with chronic lead poisoning were treated with from four to seven daily intravenous injections of 3 grams of calcium EDTA in 600 ml. of 5 per cent dextrose in distilled water given over a two-hour period. Striking increases in the urinary excretion of lead as high as from 8 to 13 milligrams per day occurred, and the urinary coproporphyrin levels fell (Hardy and others, 1954). Judged by measurements of the excretion of lead in the urine and fæces of patients with lead poisoning oral calcium EDTA elicits two-thirds as much response as does therapy by the intravenous route (Bell and others, 1956). Large doses either by the intravenous route or by mouth must be avoided. Several cases of renal damage, some of them fatal, have occurred after excessive dosage (Ohlsson, 1962). Calcium EDTA may be lethal in animals. In man large doses of sodium EDTA cause severe tetany by removing calcium salts from the tissues; they may even result in death from renal tubular necrosis.

Treatment of Colic

In his study of untreated lead colic, Tanquerel des Planches (1839) found that it may persist for from four to twelve days or more. Brouardel (1904) stated that colic usually yields to treatment within eight days, but that if neglected it may continue for two, five or even six weeks. Treatment with a high calcium diet almost invariably brings relief within two days (Aub and others, 1925). The relief of lead colic by calcium therapy involves more than the ability of calcium to favour storage of lead. Since the pain is due to violent peristalsis behind a contracted tonic ring of intestine, the antispasmodic effect of calcium salts on involuntary muscle is beneficial. In severe cases it is possible, by the slow intravenous injection of 15 ml. of a 20 per cent solution of calcium gluconate, or of 10 ml. of a 5 per cent solution of calcium chloride, to relieve the pain by the time the injection is over. The patient feels hot and flushed and may vomit. If necessary, the injection may be repeated in two hours. Should such treatment not be available, a hypodermic injection of atropine sulphate gr. $\frac{1}{60}$ may be given. Enemata of olive oil and mild aperients may be used. Sidbury (1955) has shown that where colic is unrelieved by intravenous calcium gluconate, or even morphine, the use of calcium EDTA may be effective. In one of his patients, a man of 38 who had worked for 12 years casting lead battery plates, this treatment relieved the pain at once and abolished it by the end of the third day.

Treatment of Encephalopathy

Lead encephalopathy should be treated by lumbar puncture and a high calcium diet. Of six cases observed in the United States of America three occurred before this treatment was in use and all died. The other three were given large quantities of milk and calcium lactate and promptly recovered (Aub and others, 1925). The control of lead encephalopathy by the use of calcium EDTA both in children and in adults is life saving. Sidbury (1955) treated a Negro baby 18 months old who had been exposed to lead fume from the burning of storage battery casings over a period of eight months. The baby was in coma and remained so for 24 hours after treatment began. During the second day he remained irritable but he recognized relatives on the third day. Subsequently his recovery was complete.

Treatment of Palsy

During the development of lead palsy a high calcium diet should be used to favour the storage of lead. Massage and electrical treatment are also useful. In the early stages the hands, when affected by wrist-drop, should be supported on splints.

(b) Tetra-ethyl Lead

Tetra-ethyl lead is an organic lipoid-soluble compound readily absorbed through the skin and respiratory tract. It is a clear, heavy, oily liquid with a peculiar sweetish odour, and is somewhat volatile at ordinary temperatures. It was found to have anti-detonant properties by Thomas Midgley in 1921 during a programme in which several hundreds of compounds were tested. It was first added to motor spirit in 1923 in proportions up to 1 in 1,260 (Kehoe, 1925). Twelve per cent of the annual consumption of refined lead is used in its manufacture.

Historical Summary

In 1923, when it was first manufactured in the United States of America, cases of encephalopathy began to occur in men employed on three separate plants. The victims were not only workmen engaged in blending and quite ignorant of any danger, but also chemists who handled the liquid recklessly, for there was general ignorance of its extreme toxicity and the ease with which it enters the body. Within seventeen months 139 cases with 13 deaths were reported. Much excitement and alarm were caused, and this led at first to the prohibition of the manufacture. The men affected suffered from restlessness, talkativeness, ataxia, insomnia and delusions. There were no paralyses or convulsions, but the condition terminated with violent mania, the patient shouting, leaping from bed and smashing furniture. By attention to plant design, further castastrophies of this sort were avoided. In the U.S.A. it was proved that the lead exposure associated with the handling and dispensing of gasolene containing tetra-ethyl lead at service stations is negligible (Kehoe, 1953). Apprehension as to the possibility of the poisoning of garage and aircraft workers by lead from the exhaust gases of petrol engines has proved to be without foundation.

Exposure Hazards

In the Second World War a new hazard arose in the process of cleaning storage tanks which had held ethyl-petrol. In England some of these tanks were underground and were of 4,000 tons capacity. After the petrol had been pumped out and the air rendered gas-free by ventilation, the floors, walls and supporting pillars were scraped clean. Men engaged in the work were required to wear an air-line mask and were supplied with a complete outfit of clothing including boots, gloves and headgear. The protection afforded was satisfactory, but there were occasional instances of failure to obey the regulations, with the result that twenty-five cases of poisoning by tetra-ethyl lead occurred, two of them fatal (Cassells and Dodds, 1946). War conditions in countries of the Middle East and Far

East made the cleaning of tanks difficult to supervise, and there were 200 cases of poisoning, with forty deaths. Unhappily many of these cases were not recognized soon enough. Mistaken for drunkards and lunatics, sometimes they were starved and beaten instead of being treated properly. To prevent such unnecessary exposures, adequate supervision of the cleaning of tanks has now been instituted all over the world (Kehoe, 1953).

Symptoms and Signs

The early symptoms include insomnia, loss of weight, anorexia and morning nausea, but there is no colic. Mental manifestations dominate the clinical picture, and in severe cases restlessness, bad dreams, hallucinations and delusions are common. Several symptom-complexes have been distinguished—the delirious, manic, confused, and schizophrenic (Machle, 1935). With severe exposure there may be the abrupt onset of acute maniacal symptoms with suicidal tendencies or the occurrence of a convulsion. Less severe cases begin with insomnia, sleep being difficult, broken and restless, sometimes with wild and terrifying dreams. By day, mental excitement may be marked, headache is usual and often severe, and vertigo is frequent. Blurred vision and diplopia owing to weakness of the extrinsic ocular muscles are occasional complaints. Evidences of meningeal irritation are absent; the cerebrospinal fluid may at times be under increased pressure, but it is not otherwise abnormal.

Colic, Palsy and Stippling are absent

Punctate basophilia is absent or slight, and the test for its presence in the blood therefore has little significance. Anorexia, nausea and vomiting are constant, but colic does not occur. Many patients complain of a metallic taste in the mouth, and diarrhœa sometimes occurs. Weakness, tremor, muscular pains and ease of fatigue are frequent complaints. The tremors affect the extremities, lips and tongue, and are coarse and jerky, and aggravated both by effort and by attempts at control. In the patients who recover, all symptoms disappear in from six to ten weeks. Occasionally an anxiety state persists for a time.

Fatalities from Dry Cleaning

In 1947 Bini and Bollea described two fatal cases of poisoning, where ethyl-petrol intended for use as aviation fuel was used for the dry cleaning of clothes. The patients were Italians, a man of twenty and a woman of thirty, who cleaned and pressed the uniforms of American airmen stationed in Italy. They worked in a room which was small, closed and poorly ventilated, and they ironed the clothes while they were still wet with the leaded petrol. After a few days' exposure they suffered from anorexia, vertigo, general weakness and insomnia. About a week later there was psychomotor agitation, with a rapid stream of disconnected talking and mental confusion in the nature of a toxic confusional delirium with visual and auditory hallucinations occurring together, tremors affecting all muscles, myoclonus and choreiform movements. Two days later they became comatose and died with a temperature of 105° F.

Conjugation and Pathology

Tetra-ethyl lead is insoluble in water so that if it is inhaled it must be made water-soluble before it can be excreted. It does not concentrate in the brain as is sometimes supposed but is metabolized in the liver, where one of the ethyl groups is removed to form the water-soluble tri-ethyl lead ion (Cremer, 1959). This gets into the circulation, and by its interference with cellular metabolism in the brain it produces serious and often fatal effects. At necropsy the brain shows diffuse hyperæmia of the cortical grey matter and the basal ganglia. Histologically there are both diffuse and focal changes. Throughout the cerebral and cerebellar cortex there are diffuse acute degenerative changes in almost all the nerve cells. In places, groups of nerve cells show severe degenerative changes with complete disintegration of the cell bodies. Focal lesions are found especially in the mamillary bodies and to a lesser degree in the floor of the fourth ventricle and in the corpora quadrigemina. The nerve cells in the mamillary bodies appear to be severely injured and in some areas they completely disappear. In addition there is intense proliferation of the glia with predominance of microglia cells. Where this occurs, there is also new formation of capillaries and perivascular infiltration with small round cells including mast cells.

Treatment

In mild cases removal from exposure, a normal diet with extra fluids and the relief of insomnia by the proper choice of barbiturates are all that is required. Severe cases call for strict supervision and skilled nursing because of hallucinations and impulsive suicidal tendencies. Morphine is contra-indicated; the sedative action of repeated doses of barbiturates together with adequate fluid intake are the essentials in treatment (Kehoe, 1953). Pentobarbitone sodium may be given in repeated full doses to obtain rest. Glucose, 5 per cent in saline, may be given intravenously up to 3 litres a day, and if it is given as a drip, hexobarbitone may be added. Machle (1935) recommends the intravenous administration of from 2 to 4 grams of magnesium sulphate in 2 per cent aqueous solution, accompanied by doses of pentobarbitone sodium up to 15 gr. daily by mouth. Cassells and Dodds (1946) found that enemata of 6 ounces of a saturated solution of magnesium sulphate often had a sedative effect when they could be retained. Neither EDTA nor BAL is of any value in treatment; this is to be expected since it has been shown (Cremer, 1959) that tri-ethyl lead, the toxic metabolite formed in the liver in these patients, does not combine with either EDTA or BAL.

Preventive Measures

By meticulous attention to detail, it is possible to manufacture tetra-ethyl lead and to blend it with petrol without risk to the workers. Both manufacture and blending are carried out in closed systems. Elaborate precautions are taken in transport, storage and handling of the fluid, and great care is exercised to avoid leakage or spilling (Kehoe, 1935). In blending and laboratory work, impervious gloves and respirators are used (fig. 100). Strict regulations must be laid down for the cleaning of tanks which have contained leaded petrol. Those responsible should make it quite clear that such work is never to begin without reference to some authorized person. This makes it possible to do the work under supervision and to use trained workmen properly equipped with protective clothing (Kehoe, 1953). Although ethyl-petrol contains less than one part in a thousand of tetra-ethyl lead it should not be used for cleansing the skin, and to prevent this it is coloured by a dye. While decarbonizing engines which have burned leaded petrols, mechanics must wear dust masks. Routine medical examinations should be carried out wherever possible.

Case 1. Bullion refiner—exposure to lead fume for four years—lead colic and anæmia.

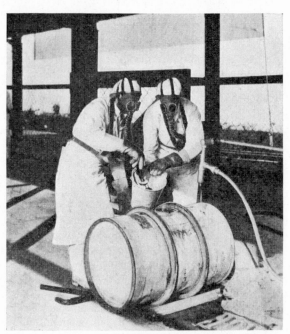

Fig. 100.—Men in Protective Clothing opening a Drum containing Tetra-ethyl Lead. The man on the left has removed the Bung with Tongs and is about to immerse it in Kerosene

(By courtesy of the Ethyl Export Corporation

F. M., a man aged 23, L.H. Reg. No. 31757/1934. He had been employed for four years in silver refining by the cupellation process, usually working twelve hours a day for five days a week. His work was to heat refinable silver containing copper and other metals, on a shallow hearth in a bricked-up oil furnace, to add from time to time bars of lead through a door in the furnace, and to tap off continuously for four hours out of twelve molten litharge containing small amounts of other metallic oxides. During the whole operation a current of air is blown mechanically on to the molten surface of the metals. The process depends on the fact that all metals except the noble metals are oxidized by heating in air. The function of the added lead is to facilitate removal of other metallic oxides, and its action is probably partly physical and partly chemical. *Eighteen months ago:* he had attacks of abdominal pain and was admitted for observation to a surgical ward of a hospital in London. *Seventeen weeks:* President Roosevelt having announced that the U.S.A. would buy large quantities of silver, London as a centre for commodities had to face a large increase in silver refining to meet the demands of speculators. Consequently the patient had had to work twelve hours a day for seven days a week. *Seven weeks:* constipation, loss of appetite, nausea. *Eight days:* several attacks of cramp-like abdominal pain, sometimes with vomiting.

On examination: muscular man, mucous membranes somewhat pale, blue line on gums, extensive faint grey-blue callosities on palms of hands, grey-blue spot 2 mm. diameter in skin over left side of manubrium sterni. Blood count: red cells 4,000,000 per c.mm., hæmoglobin 74 per cent, colour index 0·92, white cells 7,600 per c.mm., considerable punctate basophilia. Stools and urine: no lead detected. He was treated with a high calcium diet, and given calcium lactate 10 grams a day by mouth. No further colic or vomiting occurred.

Case 2. Perambulator painter—exposure to dust of lead paint for one year— lead colic and anæmia.

A. S., a single woman aged 22, L.H. Reg. No. 40274/1930. She gave her occupation as that of pram maker. On further inquiry she stated that for one year her work had consisted of painting the body work of perambulators, and then sandpapering the painted surface next day. Dry sandpaper was used, and the work was dusty. Ten months ago: she began to have generalized abdominal pain, colicky in character; it often doubled her up, and sometimes occurred with vomiting. She had been twice admitted to a hospital in London and was thought to suffer from appendicitis. Later on two occasions radiographs were taken of the spine and pelvis. The menstrual history was normal.

On examination: pale skin and mucous membranes; blue line on gums; no weakness of wrists. Blood count: red cells 2,200,000 per c.mm., hæmoglobin 44 per cent, colour index 1·0, white cells 6,600 per c.mm., considerable punctate basophilia and polychromatophilia. Urine contained lead. She was removed from exposure, and treated as an out-patient with a high calcium diet and calcium lactate. Ten weeks later she was admitted to hospital. Blood count: red cells 4,900,000 per c.mm., hæmoglobin 70 per cent, colour index 0·71, white cells 7,600 per c.mm., no punctate basophilia seen. She was treated with a low calcium diet, and one gram of ammonium chloride four times daily. After twelve days she developed severe abdominal pain, which was promptly relieved by a high calcium diet and large doses of calcium lactate. She was then treated as an out-patient, taking diminishing doses of ammonium chloride, together with a low calcium diet for four months. No further colic occurred, and the blood count became normal. An investigation revealed that the paint in use, though described as leadless, was an ordinary lead paint. Of four other workers examined, two showed symptoms suspicious of lead absorption, and punctate basophilia was demonstrated in blood films. Notification was followed by considerable improvement in the conditions of work and ventilation at this factory.

Case 3. Embroidery stenciller—exposure to dust of white lead for 3 months—anæmia of lead poisoning.

W. H., a man aged 26, seen in 1934. He had been employed for eleven years as an embroidery stenciller. The work consists of stencilling coat materials and embroidery by dabbing on the pattern a white powder. The powder used was usually chalk, or chalk and resin. About three months before a flake white was substituted for the chalk, and of this, a 5-lb. tin lasted six weeks. *Six years:* attacks of abdominal pain with transient jaundice, occurring at intervals and diagnosed as biliary colic. *Seven weeks:* pain and stiffness in many joints; constipation, no abdominal pain.

On examination: skin and mucous membranes pale. Blue line on gums. Blood count: red cells 4,730,000 per c.mm., hæmoglobin 68 per cent, colour index 0·71, white cells 10,000 per c.mm., considerable punctate basophilia. Urine contained lead. A sample of the flake white was analysed, and found to contain 77 per cent of lead. It was therefore probably commercial white lead. Of seven other workers examined, two showed a blue line on the gums and large numbers of stippled red cells. As a result of this investigation, the firm arranged to give up the use of flake white.

MERCURY

Mercurial poisoning may occur in industry in three forms: (*a*) from exposure to metallic mercury or its vapour; (*b*) from contact of the skin with mercury fulminate, and (c) from exposure to organic mercury compounds. The clinical picture is different in each of these three types. Poisoning by metallic mercury leads to stomatitis, erethism and tremor. Contact with mercury fulminate leads to dermatitis, and methyl and ethyl mercury compounds attack the nervous system, causing severe ataxia, dysarthria and gross constriction of the visual fields. The subject of mercury poisoning in all its aspects has been ably reviewed by Bidstrup (1964).

(a) Mercury

Mercury (Hg) is a silvery-white metal which is peculiar in being liquid at ordinary temperatures. It was first called quicksilver about 350 B.C. by Aristotle. About A.D. 50 Dioscorides called it ὕδωράργυρος, liquid silver, while Pliny called it *hydrargyrum*, hence the symbol Hg. The poisonous properties of mercury were known to the Romans. Its truly metallic character does not seem to have been definitely admitted until it was frozen to a malleable solid (melting point $-38.9°$ C.) in 1759, although the freezing of mercury in a thermometer was noticed in Siberia in 1736. It vaporizes at room temperature, a fact of much importance since it seeps into crevices, mixes with dust and readily penetrates substances such as wood, tile, iron pipe and firebrick. In reduction plants for obtaining the metal from the ore, mercury has been recovered from the ground as much as 30 feet beneath an old furnace.

Uses

Mercury is widely used in physical apparatus such as thermometers, barometers and vacuum pumps. In the electrical industry it is used for mercury-arc rectifiers, contact breakers, automatic switches for refrigerators and for direct-current meters. Of the world's total production of mercury, approximately a third is employed in the metallic state, the remaining two-thirds being used as mercury compounds. These include mercury fulminate for use as a detonator, tolyl and phenyl mercury acetate for use as fungicides, and a great number of pharmaceutical compounds and surgical dressings. The sulphide of mercury, vermilion, has been used by the Chinese for over a thousand years and is still considered indispensable as a red pigment. The red oxide of mercury is used in the manufacture of anti-fouling paints for application to ships' bottoms. When acted upon by the chlorides in sea water, such paints become poisonous to barnacles.

Mercury Amalgams

Mercury is a good solvent for some of the metals, and the solutions are called amalgams. Their properties differ from those of alloys. Tin amalgam was formerly employed for making mirrors, and gold amalgam is still used for gilding brass buttons. Silver-tin amalgam is used as a dental filling. It is made by mixing mercury with an alloy of silver and tin. When first prepared it is plastic, but after a few hours it sets to a hard mass.

Exposure Hazards

Occupations giving rise to the risk of exposure to metallic mercury include mercury mining, recovery of the metal from the ore (fig. 101), separation of gold and silver from their ores by means of an amalgam with mercury, manufacture of barometers and thermometers, and direct-current electric meters, electric lamps and radio valves, manufacture of tungsten-molybdenum rod and wire, fire gilding by means of a gold-mercury amalgam, manufacture of pharmaceutical compounds and surgical dressings containing mercury salts, bronzing of field-glasses and photo-engraving, the felting of fur and the manufacture of felt hats, the identification of fingerprints by dusting with a powder of mercury and chalk, and the filling of cavities in teeth with silver-tin amalgam, the dental surgeon affected being the one who repeatedly shapes the fillings with his bare finger and thumb. Since 1920 the average number of cases of mercurial poisoning notified annually in Great Britain has been less than five.

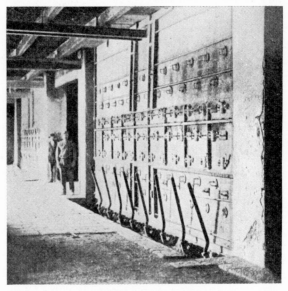

FIG. 101.—Cermak-Spirek Mercury-smelting Furnaces
at Monte Amiata, Italy

According to Bloomfield and his colleagues there were 32,855 persons exposed to a mercury hazard in the United States of America in 1940.

Sources

The red sulphide cinnabar (HgS) is the chief ore of mercury. It is mined in Spain, Italy, Yugoslavia, Russia, China, Japan, Mexico, California and British Columbia. A certain amount of native mercury occurs in shales wherever cinnabar is found. Even where it cannot be seen as globules, it may be detected under the microscope. Quicksilver has been mined in Almaden in Spain since at least as far back as 415 B.C., and for many centuries the work was carried on by slaves and convicts. We know that the Romans obtained cinnabar from these mines; they also recognized mercury poisoning, for Pliny mentions it in writing of the diseases of slaves. The existence of mercury in Idria was discovered in 1490 by a cooper, who found mercury droplets when filling his container from a well. He established a mining company, but after 1580 the mines became the property of the prince of the province and later of the Austro-Hungarian emperors. After the First World War the mines were ceded to Italy, and after the second to Yugoslavia.

Danger in mining Native Mercury

Although the main source of mercury in the Idria mines is cinnabar, there are places where the quicksilver runs free. Mining this native mercury is one of the most dangerous of occupations and it is therefore not surprising that as early as 1553 Paracelsus described mercury poisoning in the miners of Idria. In 1665 tremors affecting the hands of these miners led to the shortening of the working day to six hours; this is said to be the first legislative measure of industrial hygiene known to history (Hamilton, 1922). In 1713 Ramazzini wrote: "It is from mercury mines that there issues the most cruel bane of all that deals death and destruction to miners." In 1721 Antoine de Jussieu described the symptoms of salivation, ulceration of the gums and tremor which affected the quicksilver miners of Almaden. In 1923 Alice Hamilton found that both native mercury and cinnabar were mined at New Almaden, California. She noticed that drilling for the charge produced a fine dust laden with tiny droplets of mercury. The quicksilver released by blasting coalesced into large drops which collected under the rock and dust and had to be scooped up. Even working the men in two-hour shifts with two hours off and urging them not to exert themselves too much was not enough to prevent sore mouth, ulcerated gums, ptyalism, tremor, nervousness, irritability, depression, insomnia or drowsiness. Sometimes these symptoms developed with great rapidity so that men were known to become affected within two weeks of starting work in the mine.

Hazards in recovery of Mercury from Cinnabar

In reduction plants for obtaining the metal from the ore, volatilized mercury was encountered in cleaning out the condensers, in work at the steam tables and in charging, raking and discharging the retorts. The dust from the furnaces was partly composed of what the miners called quicksilver flour, which was a suspension of mercury in a state of fine subdivision. The California miners were familiar with the symptoms of mercurialism, and most of them had at some time suffered from at least one attack of what they called salivation, although it was plain that they used that term to cover mercurial poisoning in any form whether or not there was increased secretion of saliva. The mouth and lips usually became swollen so that the man could hardly speak and could take only liquid food. The teeth became loose, there were ulcers in the mouth, with ptyalism and a fetid breath. Often there was diarrhœa, sometimes with blood. These symptoms were followed by tremor which lasted weeks or months. In the more slowly developing cases the lesions in the mouth were milder and sometimes absent, while tremor was the most conspicuous symptom. Some men with marked tremor had never had more than a metallic taste in the mouth and a slight redness of the gums. Others had had only tremor, headache, insomnia and irritability (Hamilton, 1925, 1943).

A Quicksilver Mine on Fire

In 1803 there was a fire in a quicksilver mine in Idria and mercury vapour escaped into the air and spread over the countryside; 900 persons in the neighbourhood had mercurial tremor and many cows suffered from salivation, cachexia and abortion. But poisoning can occur from exposure to mercury at ordinary temperatures. In 1810 the British sloop *Triumph* had some mercury containers broken in the hold. As a result, all the birds and cattle on board died, 200 sailors in the ship had symptoms of mercury poisoning, and three of them died.

Vaporization of Mercury at Air Temperature

Since mercury evaporates even at ordinary temperatures it contaminates the air wherever it is exposed. The concentration reached by the vapour in the air depends upon the temperature, the extent of surface exposed and the rate of air exchange in ventilation. Thus, in workshops where direct-current electric meters were repaired, Bidstrup and others (1951) in estimations made in August and September 1950 found the concentration in the general atmosphere to vary between 10 and 200 micrograms per cubic metre. But near the work-benches, a lathe and a still, values as high as 1,700 micrograms of mercury per cubic metre were recorded. Although there is no doubt that it can be absorbed through the unbroken skin, the use of the metal in industrial processes gives rise to poisoning mainly through the respiratory tract.

Danger to Goldsmiths in the Middle Ages

Describing the diseases of gilders, Ramazzini said:

> We all know what terrible maladies are contracted from mercury by goldsmiths, especially by those employed in gilding silver and copper objects. This work cannot be done without the use of amalgam, and when they later drive off the mercury by fire they cannot avoid receiving the poisonous fumes into their mouths, even though they

turn away their faces. Hence craftsmen of this sort very soon become subject to vertigo, asthma and paralysis. Very few of them reach old age, and even when they do not die young their health is so terribly undermined that they pray for death. I had lately under observation a young gilder who finally died after keeping his bed for two months. He had not been careful to protect himself from the fumes of mercury and first contracted general cachexy, then his face became wan and cadaverous, his eyes bloodshot, his breathing difficult, with mental stupor and torpor of the whole body; fetid ulcers developed in his mouth, and from them a great quantity of the foulest sanies dripped continually. However, he died without having had the least sign of fever.

Fire Gilding practised since Ancient Times

In the ancient process known as amalgam plating, fire gilding or hot gilding, mercury was volatilized from an amalgam by heat over a fire. This process was known to the Inca empire in South America. It was practised, for example, for the gold plating of silver objects. For certain purposes, gold electroplating has not taken the place of amalgam plating Thus in the centre of London this ancient method is still used for plating military, naval, sporting and livery buttons. The reason for this is that the resulting coating of gold is more durable than that produced by electroplating. This is a property of special value in the case of uniforms for officers of the Royal Navy and the merchant marine.

Amalgam Plating of Brass Buttons

An amalgam is made by heating in a crucible one part of gold with about ten parts of mercury. After cooling in water the amalgam is squeezed through chamois leather to remove excess of mercury. The brass buttons are coated with the mercury-gold amalgam by agitating them in a bucket. They are then transferred to a cylindrical wire cage which is inserted into a gas-heated furnace and slowly rotated. The heat of the furnace drives off the mercury, causing the gold to be deposited on the base metal of the buttons. The furnace is constructed in such a way as to obviate any hazard to the workmen. Nevertheless, 20 per cent of the mercury used is lost to the atmosphere through the chimney, and cases of mercury poisoning have been reported in chimney sweeps who have cleaned the chimneys of gilding establishments. Mercury is still used for the extraction of gold and of silver from the crushed ore containing these metals. When they are brought into contact with mercury they form pasty amalgams. These are heated in retorts where the mercury is driven off as vapour and recovered, leaving the gold or silver as a spongy mass in a state almost pure.

Danger to Surgeons in the Seventeenth Century

Ramazzini described the ill effects on surgeons of giving their patients mercurial inunctions for syphilis. He said that these persons—

belong to the lowest class of surgeons who carry on the business for the money to be made; for the better sort of surgeons avoid a service so disagreeable and a task so full of danger and hazard. Though they wear a glove when so engaged, it is impossible for them to prevent the mercurial atoms from penetrating the leather and so reaching the hand of him who applies the ointment; in fact, for other purposes it is leather that we use for straining and clarifying mercury. For those who rub in this ointment I can suggest no sounder precaution than that employed by a surgeon of our day who had learned to his cost that his fee did not compensate for his own loss, since he found that the process of anointing did more harm to him that to those he treated; for he was terribly afflicted by diarrhœa, colic, and profuse salivation. So he now prepares the mercurial ointment and stays by the patients who are to be treated, but he orders them to rub in the ointment themselves with their own hands and declares that this is better for him and for them.

The Mirror Makers of Venice, Fürth and Nuremberg

Of mirror makers, Ramazzini says—

they learn by experience just like gilders how malignant is mercury when, as is the custom, they coat with quicksilver huge sheets of glass so that the other side may give a clearer reflection. Those who make mirrors become palsied and asthmatic from handling mercury. At Venice on the island called Murano, where huge mirrors are made, you may see these workmen gazing with reluctance and scowling at the reflection of their own sufferings in their mirrors and cursing the trade they have adopted.

In 1861 Adolf Kussmaul, professor of medicine in Erlangen, wrote his classic work on the subject of chronic industrial mercury poisoning based on his experience among the silverers of mirrors in Fürth and Nuremberg. At that time mirrors were tinned with an amalgam of tin and mercury. The glass was first bevelled, and then smoothed with emery powder and polished with jewellers' rouge. Tin leaf the size of the mirror was then spread on a marble table and the area framed on three sides with wood. Mercury was slowly poured over it and spread with a piece of flannel to make the amalgam. The glass, cleaned and dried, was then slipped carefully into the frame to avoid air bubbles and weighted down on to the amalgam. A slight inclination of the table favoured the expulsion of any excess of mercury. After three or four weeks the mirror was ready for use.

Kussmaul finds all Male Adults Toothless

The workmen not only inhaled mercury vapour and amalgam dust but also their clothes were found to contain up to 2·5 grams of mercury. There was a further hazard from scraping the amalgam from old mirrors, and this can still occur today. The working conditions were so bad that Kussmaul found almost every male adult in Fürth and Nuremberg to be without a single tooth. Besides salivation and stomatitis he described reddening of the pharynx (Kussmaul's sign) and stomatitis ulcerosa of the buccal mucosa and palate. He described how the disability advanced in three clinical stages—erethism, tremor and cachexia. The publication in detail of his observations led to stringent regulations which have since caused the mercury process in mirror making to be abandoned in favour of the silver nitrate process which is harmless.

The Felt-hat Industry

In the felt-hat industry the occurrence of mercurialism has been notorious for centuries. Among hatters and hatters' furriers the onset of poisoning has usually been slow and the symptoms mild. In this industry the

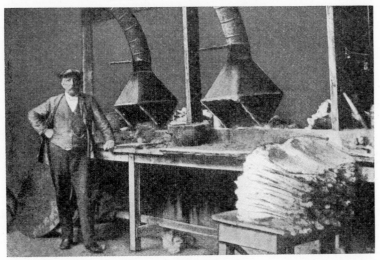

FIG. 102.—Hatters'-furriers' Workshop. The Bench is provided with Exhaust Ventilation operating through Hoods

danger arises from the presence in the air of the workshops of fine fur which has been treated with mercuric nitrate in the process of felting (fig. 102). The fine hairs which form the fur of rabbits, hares, muskrats and beavers are smooth, resilient and straight. Treatment with some chemical substance which makes them limp, twisted and rough greatly aids the felting process, and many substances have been shown to produce such an effect. Among them is an acid solution of mercuric nitrate, which is used in the preparation of hatters' fur in some countries (fig. 103).

Hazards of the Hatters'-furriers' Workshops

Neal and his colleagues (1941) examined 544 hatters employed in five representative felt-hat factories in the United States of America. He

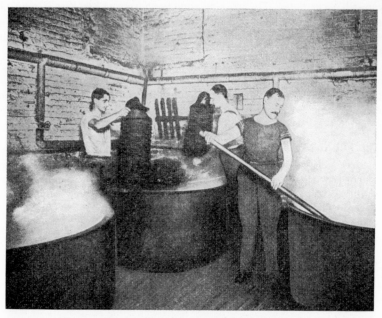

FIG. 103.—Workmen dipping Felt Hats in an Acid Solution of Mercuric Nitrate
(*The Occupational Diseases, W. Gilman Thompson, D. Appleton & Co., New York, 1914*)

showed that 59 of these workers had signs of chronic mercurialism. Four of the 21 men engaged in mixing and blowing, 8 of the 34 coners, 6 of the 29 hardeners, and 33 of the 179 starters, wetters-down, and sizers were so diagnosed. Mixers and blowers were exposed to 5 milligrams of mercury per 10 cubic metres of air, hardeners to 2·7 milligrams, and starters, wetters-down and sizers to 2·1 milligrams. In any range of exposure above 100 micrograms of mercury per cubic metre of air the incidence of mercurialism increases with increasing duration of employment. No cases were found among hatters exposed to less than 100 micrograms per cubic metre of air as measured by the Nordlander instrument.

Chronic Mercury Poisoning

Salivation and tenderness of the gums and mouth are usually early symptoms. The gums are swollen and bleed readily, but it is not easy to distinguish an early mercurial gingivitis from the pyorrhœa of a neglected mouth. Rarely a mercurial line is seen on the gums. It usually resembles the blue line due to absorption of lead, but sometimes is dark brown. In a few cases mercury causes dermatitis when it is constantly in contact with the skin, as in men who fill the standard 76-lb. iron flasks and spill mercury on their hands and feet. It is a papular erythema with slight hyperkeratosis which affects the dorsum of the hand and foot and spreads to some extent up the leg. With change of work the prognosis is always good.

The symptoms of mercury poisoning arising in industry are as a rule slower in onset and more insidious in character than those which result from the continued internal administration of mercury. In chronic cases, as, for example, in mercury miners and thermometer makers, two characteristic sets of symptoms which are but rarely seen in medical cases occur, namely tremor and erethism.

The Hatters' Shakes

The most characteristic symptom, though it is seldom the first to appear, is mercurial tremor (fig. 104). It is neither so fine nor so regular as that of hyperthyroidism. It may be interrupted every few minutes by coarse jerky movements. It usually begins in the fingers, but the eyelids, lips and tongue

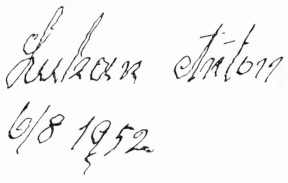

FIG. 104.—Tremor in a Mercury Miner of Idria, Yugoslavia
(By courtesy of Dr. Ivan Hribernik)

are affected early. It may become less severe when familiar tasks are performed. As it progresses it passes to the arms and then to the legs so that it becomes very difficult for a man to walk about the workshop, and often he has to be guided to his bench. At this stage the condition is so obvious that it is known to the layman as the *hatters' shakes*, and in the United States of America as the *Danbury shakes*. The tremor often passes away if the patient gives up his work before it has reached a serious stage. Alcoholism greatly favours its development and it is claimed that no total abstainer has ever suffered from tremor in severe form (Hamilton, 1925).

Mercurial Erethism

The symptoms known as *erethism* have been rare since silver took the place of mercury in mirror making. The man affected is easily upset and embarrassed, loses all joy of life and lives in constant fear of being dismissed from his job. Sometimes he is quarrelsome and neglects his work and his family. He has a sense of timidity and may lose self-control before strangers. Thus if a visitor stops to watch such a man in the factory, he will sometimes throw down his tools in anger and turn on the intruder, saying that he cannot work if watched. Occasionally a man is obliged to give up work because he can no longer take orders without losing his temper, or if he is a foreman because he has no patience with the men under him. Drowsiness by day, depression, loss of memory and insomnia may occur, but hallucinations, delusions and mania are now rare. That this has not always been the case may be judged from the expression *as mad as a hatter*.

Mercurialentis

In 1943 Atkinson added a new physical sign to the picture of chronic mercurial poisoning. This was *mercurialentis*, detected by examination with the slit-lamp microscope. His patient had inhaled mercury vapour for less than five years while making thermometers. The change in the lens consists of a discoloration of the anterior capsule showing as a reflex varying in intensity from light brown to coffee brown. The change is bilateral and symmetrical, and is usually accompanied by fine punctate opacities in each lens, especially in the anterior cortex. Visual acuity is unaffected by the changes. The discoloration of the lens capsule appears a long time before the onset of general signs of mercury poisoning and is therefore of value in the early detection of exposure to atmospheric mercury (Hunter and Lister, 1953). Mercurialentis has been described by Locket and Nazroo (1952) in twelve out of fifty-one men exposed to mercury vapour and dust in repairing direct-current electric meters. It has also been seen as the earliest sign of absorption of mercury in hatters' furriers (Rosen, 1950).

Policemen poisoned from Fingerprint Photography

In photographing fingerprints at the site of housebreaking and other crimes, a light-coloured powder is applied to a dark background. We have seen (p. 250) how lead poisoning arose in Denmark in 1937 from the use of white lead for this purpose. But the powder most commonly used is mercury-with-chalk or grey powder (hydrargyrum cum creta, B.P.) prepared in the usual way by triturating one part by weight of metallic mercury with two parts of chalk in a mortar. The powder is dry and finely divided. It is applied liberally with a well-loaded, flat squirrel-hair or camel-hair brush and the excess is brushed or blown off. The brush itself is often cleaned by rubbing against a convenient door-post, and powder rises in a cloud. The Lancashire Constabulary sets particular value in such techniques, and in 1949 Agate and Buckell found that of thirty-two men engaged regularly on such work, four exhibited tremor and erethism and three tremor alone. Exposures in excess of 250 hours per year were considered to constitute a definite risk. Urinary mercury estimations were of no assistance in diagnosing individual cases or estimating exposures, but the average excretion of the group was abnormally high.

Subacute Mercury Poisoning

Subacute poisoning occurs, for example, in the men who clean the flues of the recovery plant. At the Idria mines this is done once a year; it takes three weeks and no man works more than one day at the job (Koželj, 1953). As the workmen scrape the soot from ledges, walls and floors, mercury globules are visible everywhere in the soot. They wear canister masks because the flues are 100 per cent saturated with mercury vapour at a concentration of 14 milligrams per cubic metre of air (fig. 105). Unless they are protected in this way they develop a type of poisoning in which there is accentuation of the gastro-intestinal symptoms. Salivation is uncommon, but sore gums occur. In addition to the gingivitis, the pharynx may be mildly inflamed and shallow ulcers may occur on the buccal mucosa and palate. Vomiting and mild diarrhœa with perhaps four stools a day may be seen.

Excretion of Mercury

In their investigation of poisoning in men repairing direct-current meters, Bidstrup and others (1951) estimated the urinary excretion of mercury in twenty-four hours in 126 cases. To lessen the risk of contamination from clothing and atmosphere the men were asked to collect the specimen away from the workshop, preferably at week-ends. Of the twenty-seven who showed clinical evidence of chronic mercury poisoning, twenty-one excreted more than 300 micrograms of mercury in twenty-four hours. On the other hand, sixteen of 101 men with no clinical evidence of poisoning excreted more than 300 micrograms of mercury in twenty-four hours. When the results of urine examinations were known in these cases, six of the men were recalled for further clinical examination. No symptoms or signs of poisoning were detected at the second interview, nor was any past history of mercury poisoning elicited. They therefore suggested that a high urinary excretion of mercury is of diagnostic significance only when symptoms and signs of poisoning can be demonstrated. The urinary excretion of more than 300 micrograms of mercury in twenty-four

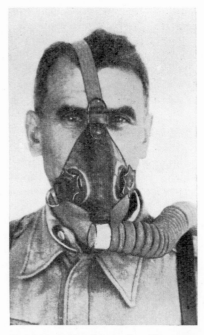

Fig. 105.—Respirator for Protection against Mercury Vapour. The Canister contains Iodized Carbon. Two Exhaling Valves seen on the Facepiece are designed to reduce the Breathing Resistance as much as possible

(Photo by Gerasimov, A. Photographic Laboratory, School of Public Health, Zagreb, from Vouk, V. B., Topolnik, Z., and Fugaš, M., Brit. J. Industr. Med., 1953, 10, 69)

hours is likely to be accompanied by clinical manifestations of chronic mercury poisoning. In a group of men who had no contact with mercury in their work Buckell and others (1946) found that the urinary excretion of mercury in twenty-four hours was not more than 100 micrograms in any case.

Renal Lesions occurring in Mercury Poisoning

The kidney is the organ in which the highest concentrations of mercury are localized following absorption. Although albuminuria among workers exposed to mercury has been reported on many occasions, and despite the role of the kidney in the storage and elimination of mercury, there has been some uncertainty in the past as to whether renal damage occurs as a manifestation of mercury poisoning of occupational origin. A number of reports are available now which indicate that the nephrotic syndrome develops in certain persons exposed to mercury. The same is true of some cases of chronic nephritis. On the evidence provided by these cases there can be no doubt that occupational exposure to mercury can cause renal damage. The nephrotic syndrome accompanied by an abnormally high output of mercury in the urine is the usual manifestation, and recovery follows removal from contact in most cases. It is of interest that in most of the cases reported other symptoms and signs of mercury poisoning have been absent. The condition of the patient is not necessarily related to the duration of exposure.

Distribution of Mercury in Rat Tissue

Rothstein and Hayes (1960) studied the metabolism of mercury in the rat using intravenous and intramuscular injections of mercuric nitrate in which the isotope ^{203}Hg was present. They demonstrated that the liver acts as a reservoir for mercury for a few days after intravenous injection, but that after about two weeks 85 per cent or more of a given dose is found in the kidney and 66 per cent is subsequently excreted in the urine. In animals given labelled mercuric nitrate by intramuscular injection, the site of the injection acts as a reservoir from which clearance to the kidneys occurs in about two weeks. The mercury accumulates in the collecting tubules, the distal parts of the proximal convoluted tubules, and the wide parts of Henle's loops, but not in the glomeruli (Bergstrand and others, 1958).

Nephrosis in Workers making Chlorine from Brine

Benning (1958) refers to two cases of kidney disease among women using a tamping compound containing 22 per cent mercury amalgamated with copper in the manufacture of carbon brushes for generators. Friberg and others (1953) review the relevant literature and refer to two cases of nephrosis reported by Riva (1945) in men exposed for five months and three years respectively in an ammunition factory, and to eight cases of nephrosis reported by Lederberger (1949). Friberg and his colleagues describe two cases of nephrotic syndrome in men employed for less than one year in the production of chlorine by an electrochemical process. In this process, chlorine is formed from brine by electrolysis using mercury contained in a rubber-lined trough as the cathode and anodes of graphite which are horizontal plates suspended from the cell cover by vertical graphite stubs which protrude through the cover. The electrical connection to the mercury is by means of iron structures shaped like mushrooms set in the rubber lining of the trough. Chlorine is discharged at the anode and an amalgam of sodium and mercury forms at the cathode. The cells are sloped to allow the mercury amalgam to flow continuously to a decomposer where it reacts with water to form caustic soda and hydrogen, and the mercury is freed and recirculated. Hazards to operators exist during maintenance procedures on the cell and from spills and leakage at the pump end. Air analyses in the factory in which the two men who developed nephrosis worked revealed mercury concentrations of 0·02–0·45 mg. Hg/m³. Before clinical evidence of renal involvement was apparent the excretion of mercury in the urine on two occasions was, in one case, 0·90 and 0·68 mg/l. and in the other 0·60 and 0·16 mg/l. Significantly large amounts of mercury continued to be excreted in the urine for at least two months after removal from exposure. Fatigue, irritability and œdema of the face and ankles, and the presence of protein and hyaline casts in the urine were the significant features of the illness. Both men recovered completely several months after removal from exposure to mercury.

Nephrosis in other Workers handling Mercury

Kazantzis and others (1962) report on four men with albuminuria who had worked with mercury and its compounds in two different factories. In one, men were exposed to metallic mercury, oxides of mercury, mercurous and mercuric chloride, and phenyl mercury acetate, and in the other to mercuric oxide; three of the four men developed symptoms and signs characteristic of the nephrotic syndrome and all recovered completely on removal from exposure to mercury and its compounds. Clinical recovery coincided with disappearance of mercury from the urine, and there was no evidence that the nephrotic syndrome in these cases was due to any of the commonly-recognized underlying causes of this condition. Estimation of the excretion of mercury in the urine revealed that all four men were excreting more than 1000 μg./l. at the onset of their illness, but a survey made in the factories concerned demonstrated that a number of men who had no symptoms nor signs of mercury poisoning were excreting equally large, or larger, amounts of mercury in the urine. Kazantzis and his colleagues suggest, therefore, that the occurrence of the nephrotic syndrome in persons exposed to mercury results from an idiosyncrasy. Friberg and his colleagues (1953) were unable to demonstrate hypersensitivity to mercury by means of skin tests, and conclude that the exact mechanism for the origin of the kidney injury is not known. Although complete recovery from the nephrotic syndrome following exposure to mercury is the usual outcome, death attributed to damage to the kidney caused by mercury has been reported (Lederberger, 1949).

Electrophoretic Pattern of the Urinary Protein

By electrophoresis and ultra-centrifuging Smith and Wells (1960) investigated protein in the urine of two of three men exposed to metallic mercury. Neither of these had had proteinuria before working with mercury. One of them continued to pass protein in the urine in small amounts for three months after removal from contact with mercury, and the other for an indefinite time. In the latter case the electrophoretic pattern of the protein was different during and after exposure. The protein attributed to the effect of mercury on the kidney was separable on electrophoretic analysis into five components, the first three of which corresponded to albumen, α_2-globulin, and β-globulin, but the remaining two, present only in small amounts, were not identified. The results of analysis by ultra-centrifuging and amino-acid identification led the authors to conclude that the proteins which appeared in the urine were serum proteins which had been eliminated by the kidney by an undetermined mechanism. Since the proteinuria ceased in two cases after removal from the mercury hazard, it is assumed that the renal damage in these cases was reversible. In the case in which the proteinuria persisted, the diagnosis of chronic nephritis was made and supported by the results of biochemical investigations; it was not possible to decide whether the chronic nephritis was the result of the preceding exposure to mercury.

Safe Substitutes for Mercury

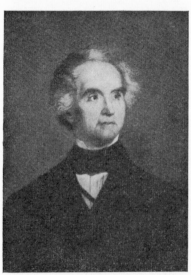

FIG. 106.—Justus von Liebig, 1803–73

The work of chemists leading up to the discovery of safe substitutes for mercury dates back more than a hundred years. Mercury poisoning was common in the mirror-making industry until silvering was introduced. In 1835, working on the oxidation of alcohols, Justus von Liebig isolated acetaldehyde (fig. 106). Seeking a test for aldehydes he observed that a test tube becomes coated with silver if an ammoniacal solution of silver nitrate is warmed with an aldehyde. The mirror so formed provided a more perfect reflecting surface than one made with tin amalgam, and mercury poisoning disappeared in the trade. Similarly, powders containing mercury or its compounds used for the identification of fingerprints must also disappear. Salts of calcium, bismuth, barium, zinc or titanium should be used instead (Agate and Buckell, 1949).

Invention of Electroplating

The introduction into commerce of electrolytic gold plating in 1840 also led to a great reduction of mercury poisoning because this process largely replaced amalgam plating. *Animal electricity* was discovered in Bologna in 1790 by the anatomist Luigi Galvani who made experiments on the muscular contractions of the legs of frogs which were brought in contact with rods of different metals. In 1800 the invention of the voltaic pile by the physicist Alessandro Volta of Pavia led to the experiment in which two copper wires connected to the pile were immersed in one per cent hydrochloric acid and the copper from one wire was seen to be deposited on the other. This discovery of electrolysis paved the way for the electro-chemistry of modern industry. In England the commercial use of electroplating was advanced by the invention of an improved battery by John Frederic Daniell in 1836. In Birmingham G. R. and H. Elkington were pioneers in this work. John Wright, a surgeon of Bordesley Green, perfected solutions of silver and potassium cyanides and disposed of his discovery to Elkingtons at a royalty of one shilling per ounce of silver deposited. In 1845 Michael Faraday saw this application of his invention of the magneto-electric machine applied to the deposition of silver at a works in Northwood Street, Birmingham.

Exhaust Ventilation and Avoidance of Contact with the Skin

The mistake of forcibly ventilating open workshops must be avoided, since it increases the vaporization of mercury. Exhausts should be placed to draw off the air from apparatus where mercury is used, and the work space supplied with fresh air from an outside source. Concentrations of mercury should never rise above 75 micrograms per cubic metre whatever the weather conditions. Where fire gilding is employed for gold plating of metal objects, adequate ventilation must be provided. A water trap must be built into the flue of the furnace used in order that the mercury vapour driven off will condense, collect under the water and remain harmless. The necessity to avoid contact of mercury with the skin is seen from the fact that men in a thermometer shop may excrete more mercury than they can absorb from the air (Buckell, Hunter, Milton and Perry, 1946).

Cleanliness of Hatters'-furriers' Workshops

In the furriers' workshops of the hat trade the technical processes of carroting, drying, brushing, sorting and packing are carried out; if the fur-cutting shops are small, cheaply built and badly managed, poisoning will readily arise. Exhaust ventilation and spotless cleanliness must be introduced in such shops. These measures may not eliminate all risk, for after the carroted fur has left the furriers' workshops it goes through further processes known as blowing, forming, hardening, sizing, blocking, shaping, crown and brim ironing, planking, proofing, stoving and pressing.

Substitution of Potash for Mercury Salts

Neal and his colleagues (1941) have shown that poisoning does not occur among hatters' furriers if the concentration of mercury in the atmosphere is less than 100 micrograms per cubic metre. In Great Britain preventive measures have reduced the number of cases of poisoning to negligible proportions, but there are still many in Italy. Russia has abolished the use of mercury compounds and substituted a potash method for the felting of fur, but this produces felt of inferior quality. A harmless substitute for nitrate of mercury has been introduced into the industry in the United States of America (Beal, McGregor and Harvey, 1941).

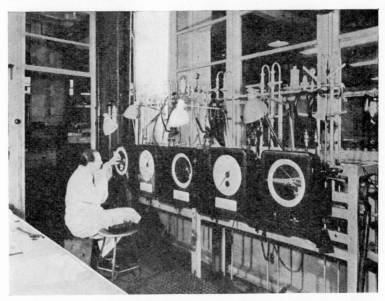

FIG. 107.—Test Room for calibrating Pressure Gauges. Mercury spilt on the Floor falls through an Iron Grill into a Trough containing Water
(*Stocker, F., Brit. J. industr. Med., 1951, 8, 271*)

Impervious Floors and Water Traps

In all processes in which mercury is handled it is necessary to observe strict cleanliness. Mercury can seep into crevices, collect in interstices and penetrate wooden floors. Since it vaporizes at room temperature, harmful concentrations may occur in the atmosphere from what may seem negligible spillage. Construction in wood should be avoided; floors of concrete should be maintained without cracks or open interstices. More attention should be paid to the risk of poisoning in the filling, emptying and repairing of apparatus such as vacuum pumps, mercury rectifiers and electromedical apparatus. Here it is difficult to prevent drops of mercury from falling on the floor, and a safety device incorporating a water trap must be built into the floor of the workshop (Stocker, 1951). This consists of a

large flat trough full of water beneath the working-point (fig. 107) covered
by an iron grill. When mercury is spilt on the floor it falls through the grill
into the trough containing water. A quantity of mercury which has fallen
into the trough during a short working period is shown in fig. 108. The
water is syphoned off through the plug in the centre of the gutter in which
the mercury collects. The mercury is then easily removed and purified for

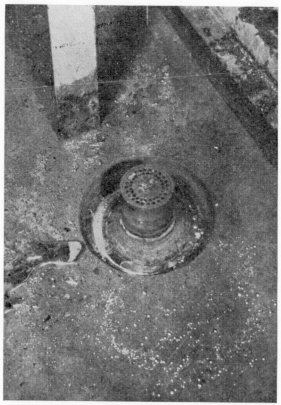

FIG. 108.—Mercury has fallen into the Water Trough and
Gutter. The Perforated Plug syphons off the Water from
the Trap
(*Stocker, F., Brit. J. industr. Med., 1951, 8, 271*)

further use. Benches should be covered with a smooth and impervious
surface tilted in such a way that mercury can be drained and collected,
thus preventing vaporization and contact with the skin. Wherever
possible, mercury should be handled in enclosed apparatus.

Dental Supervision

Overalls, mess-rooms and adequate washing facilities must be provided,
and there must be strict supervision to ensure that the workers wash their

hands after each shift and before all meals. The mouth and pharynx should be frequently rinsed with a mouth-wash and the teeth cleaned with a soft tooth-brush and a dentifrice. Periodical medical and dental examination can achieve a great deal, especially by emphasis on the proper hygiene of the mouth. Cavities in carious teeth should be filled, sharp angles smoothed and useless teeth extracted (Legge, 1934).

Concentration of Mercury in the Idria Mines

Vouk and his colleagues (1950) measured the average concentration of mercury in the air breathed by the miners of Idria. The mercury occurred in the atmosphere in three forms—as mercury vapour, as mercury aerosol and as mineral dust contaminated with metallic mercury. Where only cinnabar was won and no toxic hazard existed, the concentration varied between 0·05 and 0·08 mg. of mercury per cubic metre of air. Where native mercury was mined in shale, the work was known to be very dangerous and the atmosphere concentration was found to vary between 2·0 and 5·9 milligrams of mercury per cubic metre of air.

Protection of the Mercury Miner

Protective measures in mining must include good ventilation, wet methods in drilling and the use of canister respirators containing both iodized carbon and activated charcoal (Vouk and others, 1953). Periodical medical examination should aim at the frequent alternation of workers at danger points and should pick out all men showing any symptoms of mercury poisoning. These must either be withdrawn immediately or given other jobs presenting no mercury hazard. In smelting plants, especially dangerous operations are the charging of furnaces, the processing of soot containing up to 80 per cent of metallic mercury, the filling of iron bottles and the cleaning of condensation pipes and chimneys. Men doing these jobs must wear respirators or hose masks. Measures for general hygiene should include washing facilities, shower baths and lockers.

Inefficacy of BAL

Mercuric chloride, mercury perchloride, $HgCl_2$, or some other soluble compound of mercury may be swallowed by accident or for purposes of suicide or homicide. If used in time, certain monothiols and dithiols reverse the toxic action of mercuric chloride. Thus animal experiments show that therapy with 2:3-dimercaptopropanol (British Anti-Lewisite or BAL) can prevent completely the necrotizing action of soluble mercury compounds on renal tubules. Where treatment has been carried out within three hours of swallowing the poison the patient will be free from symptoms in forty-eight hours, and will have recovered entirely within from three to seven days. Treatment by injections of BAL has reduced the mortality rate of acute mercurial poisoning from 32 per cent to 4 per cent (Longcope and Luetscher, 1946). It is therefore disappointing that the slow absorption of mercury vapour in the victims of industrial poisoning denies them the benefit of this treatment. Indeed, it is not yet clear whether in chronic mercury poisoning the mercury-BAL complex may not be more harmful than the mercury itself.

Case 4. Thermometer filler—exposure to mercury vapour for 13 years— salivation, stomatitis and tremor

H. T., a man aged 26, L.H. Reg. No. 30939/1939. He had been employed as a thermometer filler for thirteen years, exposed to an open tray of mercury about 9 inches in diameter, in a workshop where other men used similar trays. He heated the thermometer bulbs in a bunsen flame and filled them by dipping the open ends of the thermometer tubes under the surface of the mercury. For eight weeks his hands had trembled so that he found it difficult to perform the finer movements necessary in his work. Two weeks before admission he suffered from excessive salivation, unpleasant breath and tooth-ache. His doctor told him his gums were diseased and that he must have all his teeth removed. There was no depression, drowsiness, loss of memory nor insomnia.

On examination: a man of feeble physique; mucous membranes of normal colour; halitosis, extensive red swelling of gums with purulent exudate in places, no blue line; slight enlargement of right sub-maxillary lymph nodes; no mental abnormality; no tremor of eyelids, lips, tongue, neck or head; moderately fine, slightly jerky tremor of outstretched hands affecting the writing; no alteration in tone, power, sensation or reflexes in limbs. Blood count normal; Wassermann re-action negative in blood and c.s.f.; urine, no albumin or sugar, mer-cury detected; fæces, mercury detected. During five weeks in hospital he was treated with mouth-washes, and no dental extractions were necessary. He gained weight. The tremor improved but did not disappear.

Case 5. Police detective—exposure to mercury for 13 years—tremor and erethism.

(Agate and Buckell, 1949.) A. B., a detective sergeant, aged 45, had joined the police at the age of 21 and spent the first eleven years of his service on foot-patrol duties. In 1936 he was trained at the finger-print department, and, after a few months, he was sent out to a division where he had to investigate about 300 crimes a year for three years. During this time he became "a nervous wreck" and gave up smoking to try to cure himself, without success. He was then unable to hold a glass of water without spilling it, and even his ten-year-old child remarked on his tremor. Before long he found that giving evi-dence in court was "becoming a nightmare"; he could not stand still or answer questions without embarrassment.

Between 1939 and 1942 crime diminished in his division, and his symptoms seemed to become less pronounced. In 1946 and 1947 they became worse again, reflecting a recrudescence of breaking-in offences. Of late his exposure and his symptoms had lessened, because more men had been able to help him. At various times his gums had been very tender, but they seldom bled. He did not complain of excessive salivation.

On examination: five of his teeth were loose, and tremor was present in his hands, tongue, eyelids and rectus abdominis muscles. The tremor was coarse and irregular, being of intention type; it was so severe that he could not lift a full cup to his lips without spilling it. His speech sounded tremulous and somewhat halting. His gait was normal, but his handwriting was slightly irregular compared with a specimen of seventeen years before, and the act of writing required great concentration. His mental state appeared normal. The tendon-reflexes were brisk.

The history of this case is remarkable in that the severity of the man's symptoms had a direct relationship to the intensity of his exposure, even though at the interview he did not attribute the symptoms to his work. When his tremor had been at its worst he had been a moderate drinker of beer, but now he took less and felt better for it. His embarrassment in the courts doubtless indicates mercurial erethism, and the periodic tenderness of the gums can also be considered a specific symptom.

Case 6. Repairer of direct-current meters—exposure to mercury for 20 years —chronic mercurial poisoning.

(Bidstrup and others, 1951.) W. F., a man aged 47, L.H. Reg. No. 52092/1949, had been employed as a direct-current meter repairer for twenty years. He attended hospital on 15th December 1949, complaining of tremor for twelve months.

In January 1949 he first noticed tremor of the hands and arms, particularly when he was nervous. From that time onwards he became irritable and short-tempered, shy and easily embarrassed. He stammered for the first time in his life. The tremor of the hands and arms gradually became more noticeable and after two months affected his legs so that he became unsteady on his feet. His whole body shook as though he was shivering from cold.

At this time he was told he was "suffering from nerves" and advised to rest. In February 1949 the condition was diagnosed as disseminated sclerosis. The patient continued at work until June 1949, when he went away for a holiday. The tremor was now so marked that his handwriting had become almost illegible and his signature was queried by a Post Office clerk, who refused to let him withdraw money from his savings account. While he was on holiday he noticed a tingling and numbness of his hands and feet, and could not distinguish different coins by touch.

In August 1949 he read about men poisoned by mercury as a result of their work, and told his family doctor that he handled mercury in his job (fig. 109). As a result of this information chronic mercury

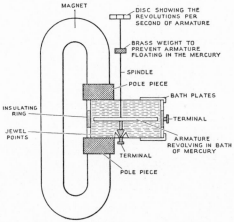

FIG. 109.—The Direct-current Meter

poisoning was considered as a likely cause of his symptoms for the first time in his illness.

On examination he was an intelligent healthy-looking middle-aged man, but appeared tense and apprehensive. There was no blue line on the gums and the buccal cavity was quite normal. No abnormality was detected in the lungs or cardiovascular system. There were coarse irregular tremors affecting mainly the upper limbs but present also in the lower limbs. The tremor was much worse when the patient was under observation.

Investigations

January 1950	Excretion of mercury in 24-hour specimen of urine	1,500 µg.
March 1950	Excretion of mercury in 24-hour specimen of urine	960 µg.
November 1951	Excretion of mercury in 24-hour specimen of urine	90 µg.

Follow-up. The patient returned to work in March 1950 and was transferred to the repair of A.C. meters where the exposure to mercury is negligible. The tremor was already less severe, and he was able to shave himself for the first time in twelve months. In July 1950, six months after the diagnosis of chronic mercury poisoning had been made and with no treatment other than removal from exposure to mercury, he had no tremor and co-ordination of movements was normal.

Past Medical History. In April 1947 he had suffered a transient partial blindness of his right eye, lasting seven months. While under observation because of chronic mercury poisoning he had a recurrence of his eye symptoms in August 1950. An amber-coloured haze appeared with a peripheral dark spot in the temporal field; there was a wedge-shaped defect in his right temporal visual field. He was seen by an ophthalmic surgeon who reported that "near the right macula there

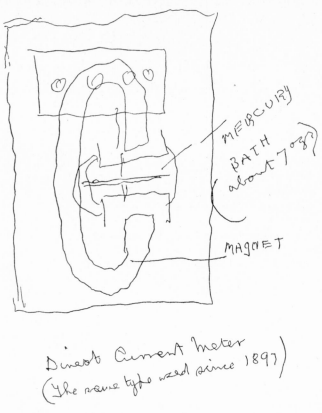

FIG. 110.—Sketch by Patient on Admission to Hospital

is a patch of pigmentary disturbance and neighbouring retinal œdema and this is the cause of the deterioration of the right vision and his positive scotoma. . . . I think that his eye symptoms are entirely due to this retinal lesion and not to retrobulbar neuritis, and a point against it being toxic is the fact that the condition is not bilateral. . . . I feel that it is probably inflammatory and that he has had a recent recrudescence." The condition settled down, and in December 1950 the vision in the right eye had almost completely cleared.

Figs. 110 and 111 illustrate the disappearance of tremor in this patient. Fig. 110 represents an attempt to draw a mercury meter at the time of his first attendance at hospital. Fig. 111 is an exact repetition twelve months after removal from exposure to mercury.

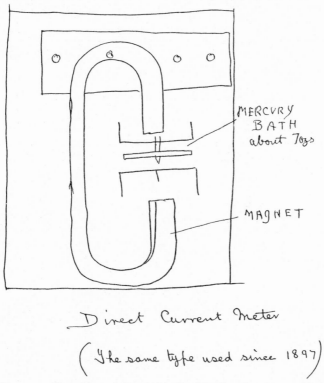

FIG. 111.—Repetition of Sketch Twelve Months after Removal from Exposure to Mercury

(b) Mercury Fulminate

Mercury fulminate has the spectacular property of exploding on percussion (fig. 112). It has been used as a primer in percussion caps since 1814. It is handled in explosives factories where detonators and percussion caps are made. It is obtained by the reaction on alcohol of a solution of mercuric nitrate in excess of nitric acid.

Exposure Hazards

The following workers are exposed to risk—fillers, packers, cleaners, cap loaders, pressers, dryers, sievers, mixers, decanters and inspectors. In one process wet fulminate of mercury is spread out by hand on cloths placed on a hot table. One end of the cloth is then raised, and the powder tilted to the other end. In a later process the fulminate is passed through sieves of horsehair to obtain the fine powder necessary for the caps. The

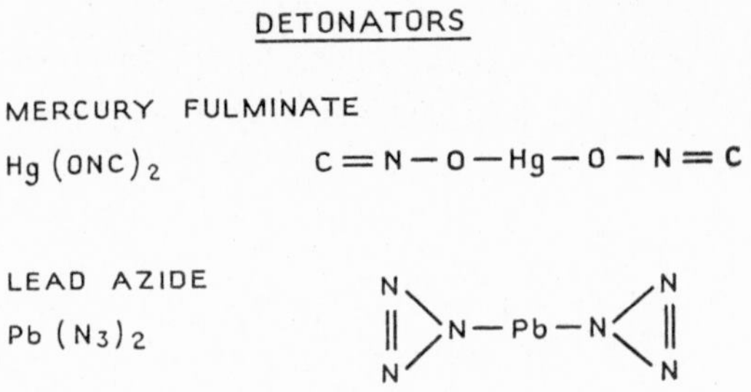

DETONATORS

MERCURY FULMINATE

$Hg(ONC)_2$ $\qquad C = N - O - Hg - O - N = C$

LEAD AZIDE

$Pb(N_3)_2$

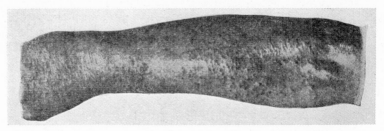

Fig. 112

fine dust falls upon the skin and dermatitis follows. In one department operatives moisten the material with methylated spirit, work it with the fingers and then press it into moulds.

Fulminate Itch

The skin of most of those employed in mixing, drying, filling and preparing the composition shows characteristic lesions. The susceptibility of some individuals is such that they cannot stand it for a day, whereas others suffer only in warm weather. As a rule the cases of *fulminate itch*, as they are called in the trade, are slight. Generally the uncovered parts of the body

Fig. 113.—Papular Dermatitis of Forearm caused by Mercury Fulminate
(*By courtesy of Dr. J. M. H. Macleod*)

are attacked by an erythema accompanied by intense itching, swelling and œdema, particularly on the face, eyelids, neck, behind the ears and on the forearms (fig. 113). Erythematous papules break out on the inflamed areas and may become vesicles, bullæ and pustules. A pustular folliculitis often develops on the hairy parts of the skin (Koelsch, 1930).

Powder Holes

The fulminate may lodge in a crack or abrasion of the skin and act as a corrosive, causing small painful necrotic lesions on the hands, especially the tips of the fingers, which last about a fortnight (MacLeod, 1916). The operatives call them *powder holes*. If the fulminate attacks the knuckles or the roots of the nails, ulceration may penetrate to the joint and bone.

Exceptionally the whole body is affected. Recovery takes place in from one to two weeks and is accompanied by desquamation.

Perforation of the Nasal Septum

The superficial mucous membranes also are irritated in persons carrying out sieving operations. After staying a short time in the rooms where this work is done, slight pricking of the eyes and nose is felt, with an inclination to sneeze, and irritation of the throat. The conjunctivæ, nose, and larynx may become inflamed. Perforation of the nasal septum has been observed (Marr, 1945). The majority of workers are careless of their dental toilet and their teeth become blackened owing to the formation of mercury sulphide.

Exhaust Ventilation and Protective Clothing

In the manufacture of mercury fulminate, meticulous attention should be paid to detail in all matters of cleanliness in the plant. The gases formed in the preliminary processes should be either condensed or removed to the outer air well above the heads of the workers. Substitution of machinery for hand labour is impossible on technical grounds. In the rooms where the detonators are filled with the composition, the fume resulting from the numerous small explosions should be removed by means of mechanical ventilation. All persons employed should be provided with well-fitting overalls, caps and rubber gloves, and, if necessary, respirators. The face and other parts of the body should not be rubbed with soiled hands. Washing accommodation should be provided close to the workroom, and a separate towel provided for each worker. The hands and arms should be washed in a 10 per cent aqueous solution of sodium thiosulphate before meals and before leaving work.

Hygiene of the Skin and Mouth

In some factories work-people coming into contact with mercury fulminate are given ointment wherewith to restore softness to the skin after washing. Such ointments contain lanolin, and either sodium carbonate, balsam of Peru or phenol (White, 1934). Periodical medical examination is important, and in the first instance persons with delicate skins and those who have suffered from skin diseases must be rejected. Regular dental examination can achieve much, especially by emphasis on the hygiene of the mouth. Whenever powder penetrates the skin through an abrasion or cut, it must be washed in a 10 per cent aqueous solution of sodium thiosulphate. For the conjunctivitis a 2 per cent solution of this substance as an eyewash has been beneficial (Legge, 1934).

(c) Organic Mercury Compounds

Since about 1930 both aryl and alkyl mercury compounds have been produced on a commercial scale. Of the aryl derivatives salts of phenyl mercury hydroxide (C_6H_5-Hg-OH) and various acids are used as anti-septics, seed disinfectants, fungicides and weed-killers. Of the alkyl derivatives various methyl, ethyl and di-ethyl compounds are used as seed fungicides. The organic compounds of mercury with hydrocarbon groups of low molecular weight have been found the most toxic, and the only cases of systemic poisoning recorded in man have been due to methyl and ethyl derivatives.

History

Organic compounds of mercury were first used in chemical research in 1863 with the result that in 1866 two London laboratory technicians died of di-methyl mercury poisoning. Introduced into therapeutics in Germany in 1887 in the form of hypodermic injections of di-ethyl mercury for syphilis this compound was at once abandoned as being too highly toxic. The value of organic mercury compounds as fungicidal seed dressings for cereals was established in 1914. The first cases of poisoning in industry occurred in the manufacture of methyl mercury iodide in a factory in London in 1937. An outbreak of poisoning by organic mercury compounds occurred in 1953 in a scattered community of fishermen along the shores of Minamata Bay in Japan. The cause was traced to the poisoning of fish from the effluent into the bay of a factory making vinyl chloride and using mercuric chloride as a catalyst. It is possible that deactivation of the catalyst involved the formation of stable organic mercury compounds although these were not identified. In 1956 and 1960 in Iraq mass poisoning of peasants and their families occurred when they used dressed seed wheat in the preparation of home-made bread. The seed dressing was ethyl mercury *para*-toluene sulphonanilide.

Deadly Effects of Di-methyl Mercury

Frankland and Duppa (1863) used di-methyl mercury in the course of some research work undertaken at St. Bartholomew's Hospital to determine the valency of metals and metallic compounds, and two laboratory technicians engaged in this work developed symptoms of poisoning and died (Edwards, 1865, 1866). One of them was a German aged thirty years who had been exposed to di-methyl mercury for three months. He complained of numbness of the hands, deafness, poor vision and sore gums. He was found to be slow and dull in manner, unsteady in gait and unable to stand without support. There was no motor palsy and the fundi were normal. Within a week he became rapidly worse, restless, unable to answer questions, incontinent of urine and comatose. He died two weeks after the onset of symptoms.

Death of Laboratory Technicians

A second technician, aged twenty-three years, had worked in the laboratory for twelve months and had handled di-methyl mercury for a period of two weeks only. The record does not state how soon after exposure he became ill. It could have been from 2 days to 2 months. He complained of sore gums, salivation, numbness of the feet, hands and tongue, deafness and dimness of vision. He answered questions only very slowly and with indistinct speech. There was ataxia, but no weakness of the upper limbs. Three weeks later he had difficulty in swallowing, was unable to speak, had incontinence of urine and fæces, and was often restless and violent. He remained in a confused state and died of pneumonia twelve months after the onset of symptoms. A third technician was affected with symptoms similar in character but less severe. He eventually recovered. The story of these deaths has been handed down verbally from one generation of chemists to another.

Effects of Di-ethyl Mercury on Animals

In 1887 Hepp used hypodermic injections of di-ethyl mercury in the treatment of syphilis. He gave doses ranging from 0·1 to 1·0 ml. of a 1 per cent solution of this substance. No patient received more than two injections, for in the meantime animal experiments had been carried out which suggested that the substance was highly toxic. The picture of di-ethyl mercury poisoning in animals was found to differ from that of poisoning by inorganic mercury compounds. There was only moderate inflammation of the intestinal tract, but the nervous system was constantly involved. An ascending paralysis was combined in some animals with ataxia. Inco-ordination of movement was noticed especially in rabbits, and motor paralysis in dogs and cats. Tremor, blindness, loss of the sense of smell, transient deafness and attacks of wrath on the slightest provocation were also noticed in many of the dogs.

Seed-borne Diseases of Cereals

Seed-borne diseases of cereals and of flax are often treated by organic compounds of mercury including both alkyl and aryl derivatives. The alkyl compounds include methyl mercury benzoate, dicyandiamide, hydroxide, iodide, nitrate and phosphate, together with ethyl mercury chloride, ethyl mercury *para*-toluene sulphonanilide and di-ethyl mercury phosphate. The aryl compounds used are phenyl and tolyl mercury acetates. They have been used in the prevention of such diseases as bunt of wheat (*Tilletia tritici*) (fig. 114), covered smut of barley (*Ustilago hordei*), leaf stripe of oats (*Helminthosporium avenæ*), leaf stripe of barley (*Helminthosporium gramineum*), foot rot of flax (*Phoma*), stem break of flax (*Polyspora lini*), seedling blight of flax (*Colletotrichum lini*) and flax wilt (*Fusarium lini*) (Martin, 1936; Muskett and Colhoun, 1947).

Studies in the Inhibition of Germination

The relationship between the molecular structure and the fungicidal activity of organic compounds of mercury has been investigated. Riehm (1923) determined the minimum concentration of different compounds necessary to inhibit germination of bunt spores under standard conditions. Gassner and Esdorn (1923) used a similar method and were able to demonstrate the importance of molecular structure in determining the fungicidal properties of these compounds. Thus, inhibition of germination

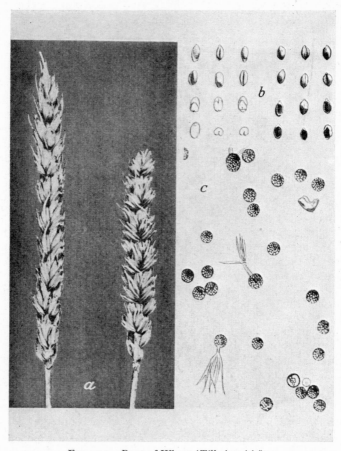

FIG. 114.—Bunt of Wheat (*Tilletia tritici*)

(*a*) Healthy wheat ear on the left, bunted ear on the right. The chaffy scales are pushed apart, but otherwise the external appearance is little altered.

(*b*) Clean grain on the left, bunted grain on the right. Each bunt ball is a black mass of from 4 to 9 million spores.

(*c*) Photomicrograph of germinating spores, each about 0·02 mm. in diameter.

under standard conditions was produced by different compounds in the following proportion—mercuric chloride 0·025, chlor-phenol mercury 0·07, and methyl mercury iodide 0·001. Methyl mercury iodide was thus the most active of the compounds tested, but was discarded by these authors on the score of its highly poisonous character. Weston and Booer (1935), employing tolyl, phenyl, ethyl and methyl mercury compounds against a large number of seed-borne diseases of cereals, confirmed the view that the fungicidal properties decrease with increase of the molecular weight of the hydrocarbon group.

Manufacture of Phenyl and Tolyl Derivatives

The manufacture of phenyl and tolyl mercury acetates in large quantities by the chemical industry in this country and in Germany has been carried on by automatic methods in enclosed apparatus. The products are used mainly in the form of dusts, though sometimes they are employed in solution. So far as is known, no mishap worse than an occasional burn on the skin has occurred in handling them. If an organic mercury compound comes in contact with the skin, warmth and redness occur after six hours, and blistering after eighteen to twenty-four hours. The blister contains serous fluid, and the lesion remaining after it bursts may take three weeks to heal.

Vesication of the Skin in Lumbermen

In 1940 Vintinner described forty-two cases of dermatitis among lumbermen who were applying a fungicide to newly cut timber in order to combat stain-producing fungi. The substance used was an aqueous spray containing one part in 6,600 of ethyl mercury phosphate. The hands and forearms of all but a small percentage of the men exposed became red and swollen, and then covered with blebs more than an inch across, simulating burns. The disability lasted from five to thirty days.

Symptoms and Signs of Poisoning by Methyl Mercury Compounds

In 1940 Hunter, Bomford and Russell recorded four cases of poisoning by inhalation of methyl mercury compounds in a factory where fungicidal dusts were manufactured without the use of enclosed apparatus. The cases occurred in the only factory in England where these substances had ever been made. With the exception of tremor, the symptoms of poisoning by metallic mercury—namely, salivation, stomatitis and erethism—were absent, and the nervous system alone was involved. There was severe generalized ataxia, dysarthria and gross constriction of the visual fields, while memory and intelligence were unaffected. One of these men was still disabled thirty years after exposure had ceased (see p. 320).

Morbid Anatomy and Histology

Experiments on rats and a monkey confirmed the selective effect of methyl mercury iodide and nitrate on the nervous system. There was an intense and widespread degeneration of certain sensory paths of the nervous system, the peripheral nerves and posterior spinal roots being affected first, the posterior columns and the granular layer of the middle lobe of the cerebellum later. The worst of our four patients died 15 years after exposure had ceased. At necropsy the generalized ataxia was referable to cerebellar cortical atrophy, selectively involving the granule-cell layer of the neocerebellum, while the concentric constriction of the visual fields was correlated with bilateral cortical atrophy around the calcarine fissures, that is in the area striata which constitutes the visual cortex (Hunter and Russell, 1954).

Fatalities in Canada from Di-ethyl Mercury

In 1943 Hill reported the death, in Canada, of two girls who were stenographers in a warehouse which stored di-ethyl mercury for use as a fungicide. Their desks were about 15 feet from a stock pile of 20,000 lb. of the fungicide, and at a point 3 feet from the di-ethyl mercury and 30 feet from the floor the atmosphere contained 2·7 mg. of mercury per cubic foot of air. Exposure had occurred for six months, but no clinical details were given.

Poisoning in Russia from Ethyl Mercury Chloride

In 1944 Drogichina and Karimova described six cases which had occurred in Russia of chronic poisoning from the use in the preparation of food of seed grain treated with Granozan, a product containing ethyl mercury chloride. The average time of exposure was 14 weeks, the illness was chronic, the principal symptoms were ataxia and loss of memory and the outcome was recovery.

Deaths in Sweden from Methyl Mercury Hydroxide

In 1948 Ahlmark described five cases of poisoning by methyl mercury compounds in Sweden, including two deaths. Of these, one handled methyl mercury iodide in a factory, and he was affected in spite of observing all the protective precautions in detail. Three of the men packed a seed dressing containing methyl mercury hydroxide and one of these died. The fifth man died after repeatedly impregnating wood by spraying it with a 0·25 per cent solution of methyl mercury hydroxide. In all cases the illness began with tinglings and numbness of the fingers and lips, and when it progressed further the patient developed gross inco-ordination of movement which ultimately interfered with both gait and speech. One of the men developed concentric scotomata of the fields of vision and later became completely blind.

A Death in England from Ethyl Mercury Phosphate

Death due to poisoning by ethyl mercury phosphate was reported in 1955 in a nursery foreman who had used it to treat *Didymella lycopersici* infestation of tomato plants in greenhouses. In April 1954 he had made up dilute solutions of ethyl mercury phosphate in water and applied the fungicide by hose. The first symptoms occurred in December 1954, and consisted of headache, nausea and vomiting; ataxia of the lower limbs had developed by May 1955 and he died in July 1955. At necropsy the anatomical and histological changes in the cerebral hemispheres and cerebellum were identical with those found by Hunter and Russell in 1954 in the case of poisoning by methyl mercury compounds described above (Russell, 1956).

Mass Poisoning of Peasants in Iraq

In a rural district in the north of Iraq in 1956, after the distribution of seed wheat dusted with ethyl mercury *para*-toluene sulphonanilide as a fungicide, more than 100 patients suffering from organic mercury poisoning were admitted to hospital in Mosul, and of these fourteen died. In 1960 many farmers and members of their families from the central part of Iraq were affected, and 221 patients were admitted to one hospital in Baghdad. Other patients went into other hospitals. There were at least twenty-two deaths, and patients usually spoke of deaths in their own families and locality (Jalili and Abbasi, 1961). In spite of warnings not to eat the seed wheat they had used it in the preparation of home-made bread. Symptoms usually appeared within one or two months of eating the bread. If large amounts had been consumed there were symptoms of gastro-enteritis sometimes with melæna and also oliguria and albuminuria. The main symptoms and signs arose in the nervous system and were identical with those found in poisoning by inhalation of methyl mercury iodide (p. 317). But additional symptoms and signs were observed. Thus as well as gross constriction of the fields of vision optic atrophy was sometimes found and in one instance it affected three brothers. In addition to gross ataxia and dysarthria there was occasionally paraplegia. Muscular twitching, skeletal pain, polyuria, and pruritus of the palms, soles and genitalia were often seen. In severe cases the pulse was irregular, sometimes with bradycardia. In such cases electrocardiograms showed frequent ventricular ectopic beats, prolongation of the Q-T interval, depression of the S-T segment and T inversion. At necropsy mercury was found in certain organs; in some cases the level in the liver exceeded 8 mg. per 100 grams.

Preventive Measures

Work published in 1940 made it clear that methyl and ethyl mercury compounds are so dangerous that they should never be manufactured again. The warning remains unheeded and the grim record of deaths still occurring in many countries is a sad monument to the greed and stupidity of men. Since the phenyl and tolyl compounds of mercury are effective fungicides and since they are less dangerous and can be handled with safety, *only these* should be manufactured. In the factory adequate precautions must be taken to ensure that dusts and vapours of these compounds do not come in contact with the skin and are not inhaled. The use of gloves and respirators is inadequate as a means of protection; the whole process of manufacture, including the final packing of the dust, should be carried out mechanically. The farmer should be warned that mercurial dressings are poisonous, and should obtain seed which has already been dressed in an enclosed apparatus (fig. 115). There is considerable hazard to men spraying crops in fields and greenhouses. For such men the use of protective clothing and other preventive measures are enforced by the provisions of *The Agriculture (Poisonous Substances) (Organo-mercury Compounds) Order, 1956*. Every available means must be used to educate people not to use dressed seed wheat for making bread. All dressed seed grain should be distributed immediately before the sowing season and clearly labelled that it is to be used for this purpose only. In countries where peasant populations are illiterate this precaution will usually fail.

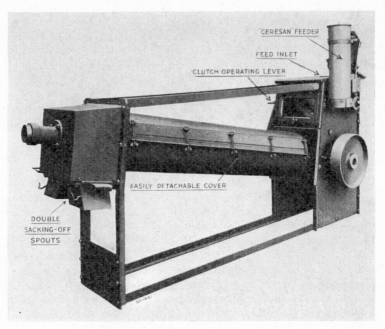

FIG. 115.—Apparatus for Dressing Seed with Fungicidal Dusts containing
Organic Mercury Compounds
(*By courtesy of E. R. and F. Turner ,Ltd. ,Ipswich*)

It has been suggested (Jalili and Abbasi, 1961) that a dye or a substance with an unpleasant taste be added to the fungicidal dust to make it almost impossible to use the dressed grain as food.

Treatment of Patients

The ataxia and dysarthria of methyl mercury poisoning must be treated by re-educative movements such as teaching the patient to walk on chalked lines. An expert in charge of a speech clinic with patience and the use of a mirror may teach him to speak; and with perseverance in some cases the patient may be taught to use knife, fork, pencil and even a typewriter.

Case 7. Works' laboratory technician—exposure to methyl mercury compounds for four months—severe generalized ataxia, dysarthria, gross constriction of fields of vision and tremor.

(Hunter, Bomford and Russell, 1940.) A. H., a boy aged 16, L.H. Reg. No. 30569/1937. *Four months* before admission the patient left a technical school with distinctions to his credit to work as a technical assistant in a laboratory attached to a plant for the manufacture of mercury compounds, including seed dressings. He handled methyl iodide, methyl mercury iodide, nitrate and phosphate, as well as ordinary laboratory reagents. No special ventilation was provided, but he wore a mask and gloves while at work. *Five weeks* before admission he first noticed numbness starting in the tips of his fingers and toes and spreading to his hands and feet. This feeling increased, and he began to have difficulty in performing such complicated movements as buttoning and unbuttoning his clothes. *Three weeks* before admission he appeared irritable and began to use abusive language. *Two weeks* before admission his speech became slow and difficult, and he noticed difficulty in understanding what was said to him. At the same time he noticed that he could not see certain objects in his field of vision, especially moving ones, and was therefore nearly run over by approaching motor cars. His speed of reading was much reduced. *Two days later* he began to be unsteady on his legs, and was seen to stagger as he walked. He was also becoming increasingly irritable and morose. *Four days* before admission he became obviously clumsy, and had difficulty in handling a knife and fork and in inserting food into his mouth, though his appetite remained normal.

On examination: A boy of spare build but healthy appearance. He sleeps a great part of the day, lying curled up on his right side. When roused, he appears to take less than a normal amount of interest in his surroundings, but when allowance has been made for his difficulties in speech and hearing it appears that his memory and intellectual faculties are unimpaired. Orientation normal. Speech dysarthric, slow and slurred. Hearing: able to hear quite well even a low voice if spoken to slowly. He cannot understand quick speech however loud. Vision: can read small print. Gross peripheral constriction of visual fields (fig. 116). Fundi normal. Loss of sense of position in tongue, nose and lips; cranial nerves otherwise normal. Upper limbs: marked inco-ordination, especially for fine movements; takes two minutes to fasten four buttons; outstretched hands wander if eyes closed, and left hand tends to drop; finger-nose test very clumsily performed; rapidly alternating movements poorly performed. Lower limbs: marked inco-ordination; reflexes all present and equal; knee- and ankle-jerks exaggerated; plantar responses, right flexor, left extensor. Sensation: gross postural loss in fingers, toes and face; two-point discrimination grossly impaired at finger-tips; astereognosis so severe in hands that he cannot tell with his eyes shut the difference between a coin and a key; vibration and other forms of sensation normal. Gait very ataxic, walks on wide base, Romberg's sign positive. Blood count normal. Wassermann reaction negative in blood and c.s.f. Blood urea 28 mg. per 100 ml. Urine: no albumin or sugar; mercury detected by spectrophotometric test.

Progress: After admission the patient's condition became steadily worse. He slept for increasing periods, and his speech, hearing and general condition all deteriorated. *Eight weeks* after the onset of his symptoms his condition was at its worst. He was completely helpless and apathetic. His ataxia was so severe that he could not perform even the simplest movements for himself. Saliva dribbled from his mouth, and he choked and spluttered when fed. He scarcely attempted to speak, and when he did so produced explosive vowel sounds whose meaning could rarely be recognized. He could understand only the simplest statements spoken very slowly. He was severely constipated,

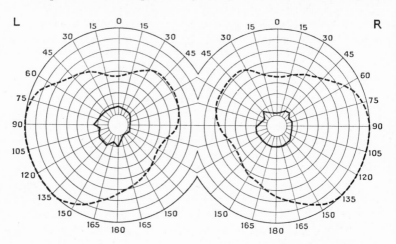

Fig. 116.—Case 7. Poisoning by Methyl Mercury Compounds. The visual fields (object, 2° white) 5 weeks after onset of first symptoms

but was never incontinent at any time. He became emaciated. *Nine weeks* after the onset of symptoms signs of slight improvement were noticed, and he began to take more interest in his surroundings. At the same time it became easier to feed him, and he was first made to walk up and down the ward with support on each side. He responded so much better to written than to spoken questions and requests, that this method was used for communication. *Thirteen weeks* after the onset of symptoms he began to have massage and re-educative movements. By this time he could just hold a tumbler and put it to his mouth almost unaided, though ataxia was still very obvious. *Seventeen weeks* after the onset of symptoms he could still produce no articulate sounds. He learned to communicate by spelling out words and sentences on a printed alphabet which he carried with him. His walking was improving, but his gait was still ataxic. *Two weeks later* he began to perform simple movements for himself, and for the first time walked a few paces unaided. *After sixteen weeks* he first began to produce vowel sounds, and was treated in a speech clinic. After much patient practice in front of a mirror, the explosive consonants were gradually mastered. The lips, the tongue and later the soft palate responded to voluntary effort, and occasionally the alveolar consonants were successfully pronounced. From then onwards his speech slowly but steadily improved. *Six months* after admission he could walk unaided on the level. *A month later* he began to use a typewriter, chiefly with

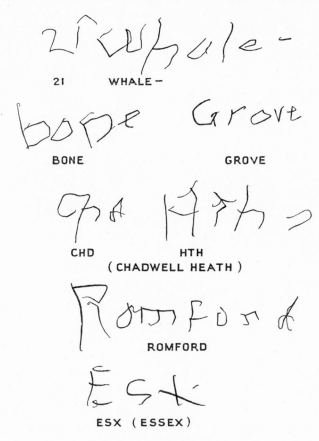

21   WHALE –

BONE   GROVE

CHD   HTH
(CHADWELL HEATH)

ROMFORD

ESX (ESSEX)

FIG. 117.—Case 7. Poisoning by Methyl Mercury Compounds. Handwriting 8 months after onset of first symptoms

his left hand, and at first slowly and laboriously. For another month he made no attempt to speak spontaneously. His general condition throughout this time continued to improve; he gained weight, became more responsive, interested in his appearance and gradually able to do more for himself. *Eight months* after the onset of symptoms he walked round the hospital garden unaided and began to write (fig. 117). He was keenly interested in everything around him, able to remember all that had happened, and to discuss accurately and intelligibly technical problems connected with his occupation before he was ill. From his own accounts it was apparent that even at his worst his memory and intellectual functions were little clouded, though he was quite unable to express himself. From then onwards improvement was maintained. *After nine months* it was possible to understand about half what he said, and he gradually gave up the use of his alphabet. *Two years* after

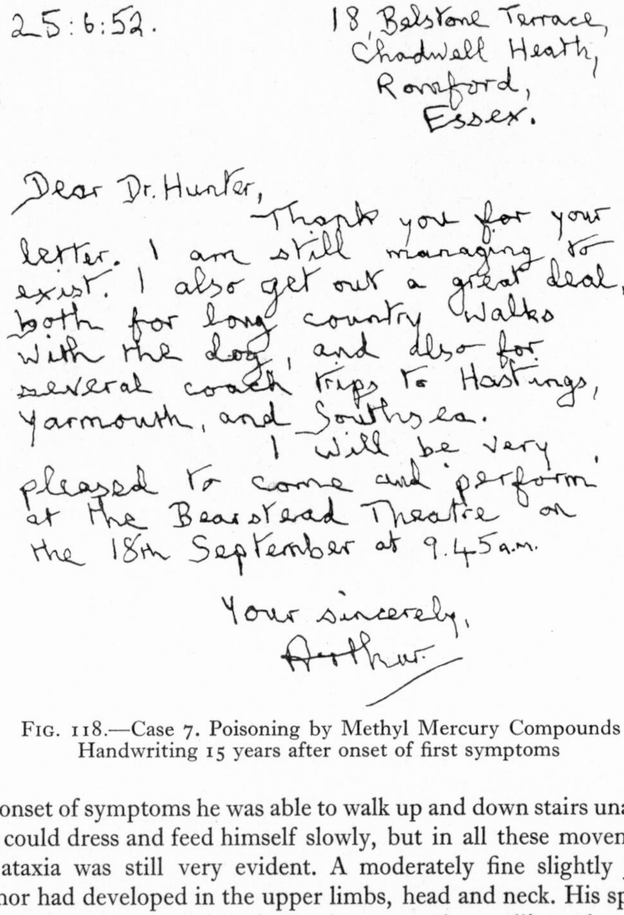

25:6:52.

18, Belstone Terrace,
Chadwell Heath,
Romford,
Essex.

Dear Dr. Hunter,
Thank you for your letter. I am still managing to exist. I also get out a great deal, both for long country walks with the dog, and also for several coach trips to Hastings, Yarmouth, and Southsea.
I will be very pleased to come and 'perform' at the Bearstead Theatre on the 18th September at 9.45 a.m.

Your sincerely,
Arthur.

FIG. 118.—Case 7. Poisoning by Methyl Mercury Compounds
Handwriting 15 years after onset of first symptoms

the onset of symptoms he was able to walk up and down stairs unaided and could dress and feed himself slowly, but in all these movements his ataxia was still very evident. A moderately fine slightly jerky tremor had developed in the upper limbs, head and neck. His speech remained hesitating and explosive, but was quite readily understood. Hearing was practically normal. He could hold a pencil and a pen, and write a letter slowly in scrawling and unsteady letters. *Fifteen years* after the onset of symptoms the ataxia was still gross, and the tremor persisted. Astereognosis was well marked, and his attempts to recognize with his eyes shut objects placed in his hands were still exceedingly poor. The visual fields were unaltered and the optic discs remained normal. He was able to take long walks alone and to travel by train and motor 'bus. His memory and intelligence remained unimpaired and he continued to show a ready sense of humour and considerable personal charm. The ataxia made it impossible for him to take up work of any sort. His writing had greatly improved (fig. 118). *Twenty-five years* after the onset of symptoms the physical signs remained as before.

In order to prevent any recurrence of this disaster among their employees, the firm concerned devised a closed system for the manufacture of organic mercury compounds. Further, they gave up altogether the manufacture of the methyl derivatives, concerning themselves only with the less toxic compounds having hydrocarbon groups of higher molecular weight.

Minamata Disease

From the end of 1953 an unusual neurological disorder began to affect the villagers, mainly poor fishermen and their families, along Minamata Bay on the south-west coast of Kyushu, the most southerly of the main

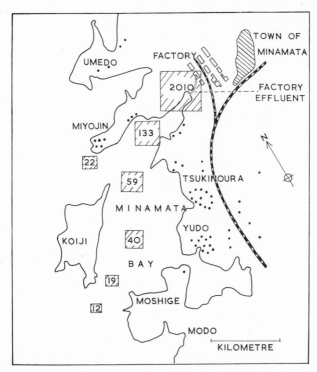

FIG. 119.—Mercury concentrations in silt (p.p.m.) of Minamata Bay. The black circles represent the distribution of clinical cases
(*After Kitamura*, 1960)

islands of Japan. It is commonly referred to in the locality as *kibyo*, the mystery illness. Most of the affected families every day ate fish or shellfish which came from the bay. The illness occurred in people of both sexes and all ages. The symptoms and signs were those of polyneuritis with cerebellar ataxia, dysarthria, deafness and disturbance of vision. By 1956 the outbreak had assumed epidemic proportions. Up to July 1961 the disease had occurred in eighty-eight patients, of whom thirty-five had died. The disease also occurred in animals which had fed upon fish or shellfish caught in the bay. Cats were the most frequently affected; they showed ataxic gait, slow, unsteady movements and frequent convulsions. Sometimes they dashed round in circles, rarely they became blind. Forced running appears to have caused some of them to enter the sea and be drowned. In forty affected families there were sixty-one cats, and fifty of these died between 1953 and 1956, sometimes in as little as two days. In sixty-eight unaffected families there were sixty cats, and of these twenty-four died. In addition five pigs and one dog died (McAlpine and Araki, 1958). Crows and certain sea birds in the bay area showed unsteadiness with frequent abnormal movements, especially falling.

Clinical Features of Minamata Disease

The onset of illness was acute or subacute and usually unattended by fever or constitutional symptoms. In all the adults numbness developed in the extremities and sometimes around the mouth, often accompanied or followed by slurred speech, unsteady gait and increasing disability. Most of the patients complained of deafness and disturbance of vision, the latter being associated with generalized constriction of the fields. Dysphagia and increased salivation were less commonly observed. In some cases insomnia was a striking feature. It was common to find emotional lability in the form of euphoria or depression. The seriously ill patients were mentally confused; drowsiness and stupor alternated with periods of restlessness and shouting often followed by coma and death within about two months (Tokuomi and others, 1961). Cerebellar ataxia and dysarthria were always present, but nystagmus was rarely found. Choreiform or athetotic movements were sometimes observed; hemiballismus was rare. Usually the deep reflexes were exaggerated; an extensor plantar response was occasionally found. Distal hypæsthesia was found in the limbs, but in reports no mention was made of vibration or postural senses or of stereognostic sense. Epileptiform attacks were not unusual. Improvement in hospital was occasionally followed by relapse on returning home. The prognosis was exceedingly poor, many patients being disabled from work and others bedridden. The death rate reached 40 per cent.

Pathology of Minamata Disease

Japanese doctors worked hard to discover the cause of this outbreak. In the absence of fever, encephalitis due to a virus was considered unlikely. Since cats died of the disease it was assumed that poisoned fish might be the cause. In 1957 the disease was produced experimentally in cats by feeding them with fish and shellfish obtained from Minamata Bay. In one of the fishermen who died a focus of destruction was found at necropsy in the lenticular nucleus of the brain and this suggested manganese as a cause. However, feeding experiments with a manganese salt in cats failed to produce the expected illness. Thallium and selenium also were suspected but no proof could be found of their presence. In 1958 while on a visit to Kumamoto University Dr. Douglas McAlpine suggested that the clinical picture in which polyneuritis, cerebellar ataxia and cortical blindness were combined was characteristic of poisoning by alkyl mercury compounds and that a source of organic mercury compounds should be sought. Meanwhile the pathology of Minamata disease had been studied by Takeuchi (1961), who found in eighteen necropsies a toxic encephalopathy with atrophy of the granular layer of the cerebellum and of various cortical neurones, especially around the calcarine fissures, that is in the area striata which constitutes the visual cortex. In affected cats and crows the brain showed these same changes. Affected fish were shown to have an equivalent lesion, namely loss of granule cells in the small brain. It is of course of great significance that these are the lesions in the nervous system which had been found by Hunter and Russell (1954) in a man and in experimental rats poisoned by methyl mercury iodide (p. 317). It therefore became necessary to look for a source of organic mercury compounds to which the fish and shellfish of the bay had access.

Experimental Minamata Disease

But Takeuchi (1961) went further and produced experimental Minamata disease in cats, rats and mice fed with fish and shellfish from the bay. In these animals the clinical and pathological findings were identical with those found in animals spontaneously affected. The clinical and pathological features of Minamata disease were reproduced in cats poisoned by a number of organic mercury compounds (Morikawa, 1961). These were alkyl compounds such as diethyl mercury, ethyl mercuric chloride, diethyl mercuric phosphate and diethyl mercuric sulphide. The cats developed clumsiness in walking, unsteady movement, ataxic gait, tremor, generalized convulsions and other abnormal movements. These symptoms appeared two weeks or more after the oral administration of the mercury compounds. Some of these compounds caused disintegration and loss of granule cells in the cerebellum and of the nerve cells in the cerebral cortices. Of these compounds it was diethyl mercuric sulphide which produced clinical symptoms and pathological changes most closely resembling those of Minamata disease. When pregnant cats were poisoned with this substance some of their kittens were found to be affected.

Mercury Catalyst in Factory Effluent

It was known that a factory discharged its effluent into Minamata Bay and inquiry revealed that it made vinyl chloride using mercuric chloride as a catalyst. The vinyl chloride output increased from 60 tons in 1949 to

18,000 tons per year in 1959. Until fishing in the bay was prohibited the number of new cases of Minamata disease increased in proportion to these figures (Kurland and others, 1960). The mercuric chloride catalyst becomes deactivated after a time and it is possible that the deactivation is caused by the formation of stable organic mercury compounds. Kitamura (1960) analysed the mercury content of various samples of the silt of the bay and found 2,010 p.p.m. of mercury at the factory effluent and 133, 59, 40, 19 and 12 p.p.m. respectively at distances farther out (fig. 119). He also found mercury in considerable amounts in fish and shellfish from the bay and in the brain, liver, kidney and urine of the patients affected. On the basis of these findings the conclusion was reached that Minamata disease is due to poisoning by some form of organic mercury compound. In November 1956 a ban was imposed on fishing in the bay and no further cases occurred in the following nineteen months. The factory has introduced a rust-settling basin and a cyclator, which have reduced the loss of mercury in the wash water from 300 gm. to 10 gm. daily. In the spring of 1958 the factory closed the effluent into Minamata Bay and opened a new one into the Minamata River near the point where it reaches the open sea.

BIBLIOGRAPHY

Lead

(a) Lead

AUB, J. C. (1927), *Arch. Neurol. Psychiat.*, **17**, 444.

AUB, J. C., and REZNIKOFF, P. (1924), *J. exp. Med.*, **40**, 189.

AUB, J. C., FAIRHALL, L. T., MINOT, A. S., and REZNIKOFF, P. (1925), *Medicine*, **4**, 1.

AUB, J. C., ROBB, G. P., and ROSSMEISL, E. (1932), *J. publ. Hlth.*, **22**, 825.

BELKNAP, E. L. (1936), *J. industr. Hyg.*, **18**, 380.

BELL, R. F., GILLILAND, J. C., BOLAND, J. R., and SULLIVAN, B. R. (1956), *Arch. industr. health*, **13**, 366.

BROUARDEL, P. (1904), *Ann. Hyg. publ.*, **1**, 132.

BURTON, H. (1839–40), *Lancet*, **1**, 661.

CANTAROW, A., and TRUMPER, M. (1944), *Lead Poisoning*, Williams and Wilkins, Baltimore.

CHOLAK, J., and BAMBACH, K. (1943), *J. industr. Hyg.*, **25**, 47.

COLLIP, J. B. (1925), *J. biol. Chem.*, **63**, 395.

COLLIS, E. L., and HILDITCH, J. (1912), *Rpt. on the Conditions of Employment in the Manufacture of Tinplate*, Cmd. 6394, H.M.S.O., London.

CREMER, J. E. (1959), *Brit. J. industr. Med.*, **16**, 191.

DREESSEN, W. C. (1943), *J. industr. Hyg.*, **25**, 60.

DUCHENNE, G. B. A. (1872), *De l'électrisation localisée, et de son application à la pathologie et à la thérapeutique*, 3rd ed., Baillière, Paris.

ERICSEN, L. (1955), *Scand. J. clin. lab. invest.*, **7**, 80.

ERLENMEYER, E. (1913), *Z. exp. Path. Ther.*, **14**, 310.

FAIRHALL, L. T. (1924), *J. Amer. chem. Soc.*, **46**, 1593; (1936), *J. industr. Hyg.*, **18**, 668; (1957), *Industrial Toxicology*, 2nd ed., Williams and Wilkins, Baltimore.

FAIRHALL, L. T., and KEENAN, R. G. (1941), *J. Amer. chem. Soc.*, **63**, 3076.

FOUTS, P. J., and PAGE, I. H. (1942), *Amer. Heart J.*, **24**, 329.

GARROD, A. B. (1854), *Med.-chir. Trans. Lond.*, **37**, 181.

GIBSON, J. L. (1922), *Ocular Neuritis due to Lead*, Sydney.

GOLDBLATT, M. W., and GOLDBLATT, J. (1956), *Some Aspects of Industrial Toxicology*, in Merewether, E.R.A., *Industrial Medicine and Hygiene*, Butterworth, London, **3**, 437.

GRINSTEIN, M., WIKOFF, H. M., de MELLO, R. P., and WATSON, C. J. (1950), *J. biol. chem.* **182**, 723.

GRISOLLE, A. (1836), *Recherches sur quelques-uns des accidents cérébraux produits par les préparations saturnines*, Paris.

GUILLOT, N., and MELSENS, L. (1844), *C. R. Acad. Sci. Paris*, **18**, 532.

GUSSEROW, A. (1861), *Virchows Arch.*, **21**, 443.

HAMILTON, A. (1925), *Industrial Poisons in the United States*, Macmillan, New York.

HARDY, H. L., ELKINS, H. B., RUOTOLO, B. P. W., QUINBY, J., and BAKER, W. H. (1954), *Journ. Amer. med. assoc.*, **154**, 1171.

HEUBEL, E. (1871), *Pathogenese und Symptome der chronischen Bleivergiftung*, Berlin.

HUNTER, D., and AUB, J. C. (1926-7), *Quart. J. Med.*, **20**, 123.

HUTCHINSON, J. (1873), *Ophthal. Hosp. Rept., Lond.*, **7**, 6.

KENCH, J. E., GILLAM, A. E., and LANE, R. E. (1942), *Biochem. J.*, **36**, 384.

KENCH, J. E., LANE, R. E., and VARLEY, H. (1952), *Brit. J. industr. Med.*, **9**, 133.

KETY, S. S., and LETONOFF, T. V. (1943), *Amer. Journ. med. Sci.*, **205**, 406.

KEY, J. A. (1924), *Amer. J. Physiol.*, **70**, 86.

KING, E., and THOMPSON, A. R. (1961), *Ann. occup. Hyg.*, **3**, 247.

KINNIER WILSON, S. A. (1947), *Neurology*, **1**, 728, Arnold, London.

KLEIN, C. A. (1913), *Oil and Colour Trades Journ.*, **44**, 1973; (1922), *J. Soc. chem. Ind. Lond.*, **41** (Review, vol. 5), 325; (1922-3), *J. R. Soc. Arts*, **71**, 240.

LANE, R. E. (1931), *J. industr. Hyg.*, **13**, 276; (1949), *Brit. J. industr. Med.* **6**, 125.

LEGGE, Sir T. (1934), *Industrial Maladies*, Oxford University Press, London.

LEGGE, Sir T., and GOADBY, K. W. (1912), *Lead Poisoning and Lead Absorption*, Arnold, London.

McCORD, C. P. (1945), Personal communication.

McCORD, C. P., MINSTER, D. K., and REHM (1924), *J. Amer. med. Ass.*, **24**, 1795.

McFADZEAN, A. J. S., and DAVIS, L. J. (1949), *Quart. J. Med.*, **18**, 57.

McLEAN, R., CALHOUN, J. A., and AUB, J. C. (1954), *Arch. Industr. Hyg.*, **9**, 113.

MALOOF, C. C. (1950), *Arch. Industr. Hyg.*, **1**, 296.

MATTIELLO, J. J. (1942), *Protective and Decorative Coatings*, Chapman and Hall, London, vol. ii, p. 343.

MINOT, A. S., and AUB, J. C. (1924), *J. industr. Hyg.*, **6**, 149.

MOSNY, E., and MALLOIZEL, L. (1907), *Rev. Médecine*, **27**, 505.

NEWMAN, B. J., McCONNELL, W. J., SPENCER, O. M., and PHILLIPS, F. M. (1922), *J. industr. Hyg.*, **3**, 390.

NYE, L. J. J. (1933), *Chronic Nephritis and Lead Poisoning*, Angus and Robertson, Sydney.

NYFELDT, A. (1937), *Ugeskr. Laeg.*, **99**, 283.

OHLSSON, W. T. L. (1962), *Brit. med. J.*, **1**, 1454.

OLIVER, Sir T. (1914), *Lead Poisoning*, London; (1925), *Lancet*, **2**, 630.

RAMAZZINI, B. (1713), *De Morbis Artificum Diatriba*, translation by W. C. Wright, University of Chicago Press, Chicago, 1940.

REGISTRAR-GENERAL'S *Decennial Supplement to the Census, Tables of Occupational Mortality* (1931).

RIMINGTON, C. (1938), *C. R. Lab. Carlsberg, sér. chim.*, **22**, 463.

SCHWARZENBACH, G., and ACKERMANN, H. (1948), *Helvet. Chim. Acta*, **31**, 1029.

STRAUB, W. (1911), *Dtsch. med. Wschr.*, **37**, 1469.

TANQUEREL DES PLANCHES, L. (1839), *Traité des maladies de plomb, ou saturnines*, Paris.

TELEKY, L. (1937), *J. industr. Hyg.*, **19**, 1.

THORPE, T. E. (1901), *Work of the Government Laboratory on the question of the Employment of Lead Compounds in Pottery*, Cmd. 679, H.M.S.O., London.

VERNATTI, P. (1678), *Phil. Trans.*, **12**, 935.

VIGDORTCHIK, N. A. (1935), *J. industr. Hyg.*, **17**, 1.

WATSON, C. J. (1950), *Arch. intern. Med.*, **86**, 797.

(b) Tetra-ethyl Lead

BINI, L., and BOLLEA, G. (1947), *J. Neuropath.*, **6**, 271.

CASSELLS, D. A. K., and DODDS, E. C. (1946), *Brit. med. J.*, **2**, 681.

KEHOE, R. A. (1925), *J. Amer. med. Ass.*, **85**, 108; (1935), *J. Med. Cincinnati*, **16**, 527; (1953), Personal communication.

MACHLE, W. E. (1935), *J. Amer. med. Ass.*, **105**, 578.

Mercury

BIDSTRUP, P. L. (1964), *Toxicity of Mercury and its Compounds*, Elsevier, Amsterdam.

(a) Mercury

AGATE, J. N., and BUCKELL, M. (1949), *Lancet*, **2**, 451.

ATKINSON, W. S. (1943), *Amer. J. Ophthal.*, **26**, 685.

BEAL, G. D., McGREGOR, R. R., and HARVEY, A. W. (1941), *Industr. Engng. Chem. (News)*, **19**, 1239.

BENNING, D. (1958), *Indust. Med. Surg.*, **27**, 354.

BERGSTRAND, A., FRIBERG, L. and ODEBLAD, E. (1958), *A.M.A. Arch. Ind. Health*, **17**, 253.

BIDSTRUP, P. L., BONNELL, J. A., HARVEY, D. G., and LOCKET, S. (1951), *Lancet*, **2**, 856.

BLOOMFIELD, J. J., TRASKO, V. N., SAYERS, R. R., PAGE, R. T., and PEYTON, M. F. (1940), *U.S. Publ. Hlth. Bull.*, No. 259, p. 199.

BUCKELL, M., HUNTER, D., MILTON, R., and PERRY, K. M. A. (1946), *Brit. J. industr. Med.*, **3**, 55.

FRIBERG, L., HAMMARSTRÖM, S. and NYSTRÖM, A. (1953), *A.M.A. Arch. Ind. Hyg. Occup. Med.*, **8**, 149.

HAMILTON, A. (1922), *J. industr. Hyg.*, **4**, 219; (1925), *Industrial Poisons in the United States*, Macmillan, New York; (1943), *Exploring the Dangerous Trades*, Little, Brown and Co., Boston.

HUNTER, D., and LISTER, A. (1953), *Brit. J. Ophthal.*, **37**, 234.

DE JUSSIEU, A. (1721), *Histoire de l'Académie royale des Sciences pour l'année* 1719, Paris, p. 359.

KAZANTZIS, G., SCHILLER, K. F. R., ASSCHER, A. W. and DREW, R. G. (1962), *Quart. J. Med.*, **29**, 1.

KOŽELJ, A. (1953), Personal communication.

KUSSMAUL, A. (1861), *Untersuchungen über dem constitutionellen Mercurialismus*, Würzburg.

LEDERBERGER, E. (1949), *Schweiz. med. Wschr.*, **79**, 263.

LEGGE, Sir T. (1934), *Industrial Maladies*, Oxford University Press, London, p. 72.

VON LIEBIG, J. (1835), *Annalen der Pharmacie*, **14**, 133.

LOCKET, S., and NAZROO, I. A. (1952), *Lancet*, **1**, 528.

LONGCOPE, W. T., and LUETSCHER, J. A. (1946), *J. clin. Invest.*, **25**, 557.

NEAL, P. A., FLINER, R. H., EDWARDS, T. I., REINHART, W. H., HOUGH, J. W., DALLAVALLE, J. M., GOLDRAM, F. H., ARMSTRONG, D. W., GRAY, A. S., COLEMAN, A. L., and POSYMAN, B. F. (1941), *U.S. Publ. Hlth. Bull.*, No. 263.

RAMAZZINI, B. (1713), *De Morbis Artificum Diatriba*, translation by W. C. Wright, University of Chicago Press, Chicago, 1940.

RIVA, G. (1945), *Helv. med. Acta.*, **12**, 539.

ROSEN, E. (1950), *Amer. J. Ophthal.*, **33**, 797.

ROTHSTEIN, A. and HAYES, A. D. (1960), *J. Pharmacol. exp. Ther.*, **130**, 166.

SMITH, J. C. and WELLS, A. R. (1960), *Brit. J. indust. Med.*, **17**, 205.

STOCKER, F. (1951), *Brit. J. industr. Med.*, **8**, 271.

VOUK, V. B., FUGAS, M., and TOPOLNIK, Z. (1950), *Brit. J. indust. Med.*, **7**, 168 ; (1953), *Ibid.*, **10**, 69.

(b) Mercury Fulminate

KOELSCH, F. (1930), *Occupation and Health*, I.L.O., Geneva, **1**, 811.

LEGGE, Sir T. (1934), *Industrial Maladies*, Oxford University Press, London.

MACLEOD, J. M. H. (1916), *Brit. J. Derm.*, **28**, 135.

MARR, N. G. (1945), Personal communication.

WHITE, R. P. (1934), *The Dermatergoses or Occupational Affections of the Skin*, 4th ed., Lewis, London, p. 134.

(c) Organic Mercury Compounds

AHLMARK, A. (1948), *Brit. J. industr. Med.*, **5**, 117.

EDWARDS, G. N. (1865), *St. Bart's Hosp. Rept.*, **1**, 141 ; (1866), *Ibid.*, **2**, 211.

FRANKLAND, E., and DUPPA, B. F. (1863), *J. chem. Soc.*, N. S., **1**, 415.

GASSNER, G., and ESDORN, I. (1923), *Arbeiten aus der Biologischen Reichsanstalt*, **11**, 373.

HEPP, P. (1887), *Arch. exp. Path. Pharmak.*, **23**, 91.

HILL, W. H. (1943), *Canad. Publ. Hlth. J.*, **34**, 158.

HUNTER, D., BOMFORD, R. R., and RUSSELL, D. S. (1940), *Quart. J. Med.*, **9**, 193.

HUNTER, D., and RUSSELL, D. S. (1954), *J. Neurol. Neurosurg, Psychiat.*, **17**, 235.

JALILI, M. A., and ABBASI, A. H. (1961), *Brit. J. industr. Med.*, **18**, 303.

KITAMURA, M., UEDA, K., NIINO, J., UJIOKA, T., MISUMI, H., and KAKITA, T. (1960), *J. Kumamoto Med. Soc.*, **34**, Suppl., 593.

KURLAND, L. T., FARO, S. N., and SIEDLER, H. (1960), World Neurology, **1**, 370.

MCALPINE, D. and ARAKI, S. (1958), *Lancet*, **2**, 629.

MARTIN, H. (1936), *The Scientific Principles of Plant Protection*, London.

MORIKAWA, N. (1961), *Kumamoto Med. J.*, **14**, 2.

MUSKETT, A. E., and COLHOUN, J. (1947), *Diseases of the Flax Plant*, Belfast

RIEHM, E. (1923), *Z. angew. Chem.*, **36**, 3.

RUSSELL, D. S. (1956), Personal communication.

TAKEUCHI, T. (1961), *Proc. VII Internat. Congr. Neurol.*, Rome.

TOKUOMI, H., and others (1961), *Kumamoto Med. J.*, **14**, 47.

VINTINNER, F. J. (1940), *J. industr. Hyg.*, **22**, 297.

WESTON, W. A. R. D., and BOOER, J. R. (1935), *J. agric. Sci.*, **25**, 628.

CHAPTER VI

THE OTHER METALS

THE effects of antimony, arsenic, calcium, phosphorus, silver and zinc have been studied for many years. Some of their compounds, especially the organic derivatives of arsenic and phosphorus, have been newly introduced and the study of their effects is still incomplete.

ARSENIC

Arsenical poisoning may occur in industry in three forms: (a) from inhalation of or contact with the dusts of inorganic compounds of arsenic; (b) from inhalation of arseniuretted hydrogen gas, and (c) from contact with organic arsenic compounds. The symptoms and signs in the three groups are distinct. The inorganic compounds of arsenic act as local irritants to the skin and mucous membranes, and may have a carcinogenic effect. Arseniuretted hydrogen acts as a hæmolytic agent, causing hæmoglobinuria, anæmia and hæmolytic icterus. The organic arsenic compounds have a vesicant effect on the skin and the mucous membranes as well as powerful systemic effects.

(a) Arsenic

Arsenic, As, was known to the ancients through its sulphides, and the Greek alchemist Olympiodorus obtained white arsenic by roasting one of these. In the sixteenth century the miners of Saxony were puzzled and disappointed when they smelted smaltite, $CoAs_2$, because it gave off poisonous arsenical fumes and yielded no silver in spite of its metallic silver-white appearance. They thought there was a *kobold* or *goblin* in the ore which accounted for its unreasonable behaviour, and this, of course, is the origin of the word cobalt (see p. 477). In 1556, in his *De Re Metallica*, Agricola described the baneful action of this arsenical cobalt, at that time called *cadmia*, which he said ate away the skin of the hands of workmen and necessitated the wearing of long gloves as a protection in handling it. Our understanding of arsenic compounds began in 1733 when Brandt showed that white arsenic was the calx or oxide of the element arsenic.

Sources

The other minerals containing arsenic are cobaltite, CoAsS, enargite, Cu_3AsS_4, the more spectacular orange-red sulphide, realgar, AsS, and the lemon-yellow orpiment, As_2S_3, two substances used as pigments especially in lacquer work. But arsenopyrite, also called mispickel and arsenical pyrites, FeAsS, is the most abundant ore mineral, frequently proving a nuisance in the mining of gold, copper, tin, tungsten, lead and zinc.

Allotropes and Oxides

Arsenic exists in a number of allotropic forms. Yellow arsenic, which volatilizes readily, is extremely poisonous and phosphoresces in air at room temperature. The semi-metallic form of arsenic is a brittle, steel-grey solid with a bright lustre. Arsenic forms three oxides—namely, arsenious oxide, arsenic trioxide or white arsenic, As_2O_3, but only one of these is important. White arsenic is the most abundant commercial arsenical compound and from it practically all manufactured arsenical compounds are derived. Arsenic can be obtained either by the reduction of white arsenic with carbon or by heating arsenical pyrites out of contact with air. Almost all the world's arsenic is obtained as a by-product in the flue dust of smelters treating arsenical ores for the recovery of the gold, copper or other metals that may be present. From the soot of the flues arsenic trioxide is separated, purified and marketed in the form of a white powder.

Arsenical Pigments

The inorganic compounds of arsenic include sodium arsenite, Na_2HAsO_3, lead diarsenate, $PbHAsO_4$, Scheele's green, cupric arsenite, $CuHAsO_3$, and Paris green, cupric aceto-arsenite, $3Cu(AsO_2)_2.Cu(CH_3COO)_2$. This last pigment was much in vogue in the early part of the nineteenth century. It was prepared by mixing the correct proportions of a copper salt, arsenious oxide and acetic acid, but the exact method was kept secret until 1822 when it was published by Liebig. Owing to its poisonous nature the makers in various countries kept giving the pigment different names in the hope that they could sell it as an innocuous substance. As a further disguise they mixed it with baryta and gypsum to lighten the colour. This plains the multitude of names for what was virtually the same substance; Paris, French, Parrot, Vienna, Mitis, Schweinfurt, Imperial and emerald green. There are several versions as to the origin of the pigment. One says that Russ and Sattler made it first in Schweinfurt and another that Mitis of Vienna first made it.

A Hazard of the Nineteenth Century

In the middle of the nineteenth century the use of Scheele's green and Paris green became so extensive that chronic arsenical poisoning from the dusts of these substances was widespread. The symptoms caused were coryza, vomiting, conjunctivitis, laryngitis and dermatitis. About 1880 a committee of the Medical Society of London collected information on the subject and issued the following list of articles in the manufacture of which arsenical pigments were used.

> Paper, fancy and surface coloured, in sheets for covering cardboard boxes; for labels of all kinds; for advertisement cards, playing cards, wrappers for sweetmeats, cosaques, etc.; for the ornamentation

of children's toys; for covering children's and other books; for lamp shades, paperhangings for walls and other purposes; artificial leaves and flowers; wax ornaments for Christmas trees and other purposes; printed or woven fabrics intended for use as garments; printed or woven fabrics intended for use as curtains or coverings for furniture; children's toys, particularly inflated indiarubber balls with dry colour inside, painted indiarubber dolls, stands and rockers of rocking-horses and the like, glass balls (hollow); distemper colour for decorative purposes; oil paint for the same; lithographers' colour printing; decorated tin plates, including painted labels used by butchers and others to advertise the price of provisions; japanned goods generally; Venetian and other blinds; American or leather cloth; printed table baizes; carpets, floorcloth, linoleum, book cloth and fancy bindings. To this list may be added coloured soaps, wafers, sweetmeats and false malachite. Arsenic is also used in the preparation of skins for stuffing and of some preservatives used by anatomists.

The green arsenites of copper were incorporated so loosely into paper and textiles that a considerable dust hazard was present in the workrooms. Thus in the preparation of artificial flowers Scheele's green was powdered over the leaves with the production of much dust. The Committee recognized that for colouring purposes arsenical compounds are unnecessary and should be prohibited, thus anticipating what was soon to come about (Morris, 1902).

Uses

In industry, arsenical compounds are met with in the smelting and refining of ores, in the subliming of white arsenic and in the manufacture of insecticides and weed killers. White arsenic is used as a preservative of hides, skins, furs and wood. In the manufacture of glass it is used to remove the unpleasant greenish tint produced by iron oxide. Paris green is used as a horticultural spray to kill the codling moth and the gypsy moth on fruit trees. Impregnated on vermiculite it is used as a mosquito larvicide. Lead arsenate spray or dust is used to kill the cotton-boll weevil, and cupric arsenite to kill the potato bug. Other insecticidal sprays and dusts contain London purple (calcium arsenite and arsenate), magnesium arsenate, manganese arsenate and zinc arsenite. Sheep dips, cattle dips and powders to kill flies and ants may contain sodium or potassium arsenite, arsenious oxide, arsenic sulphides and thioarsenates. Arsenic compounds are used in anti-fouling paints for ships' bottoms, in dyes and soaps, in calico printing and in the manufacture of pharmaceutical substances. Very little use is made of arsenic in metallic form. About 0·4 per cent of the metal added to molten lead yields harder lead shot and facilitates also the formation of truly spherical pellets when the melt is poured down the shot tower.

Exposure Hazards

The dusts of the arsenical compounds manufactured in industry are light, so that, unless the processes of sifting and packing are carried out in closed apparatus from start to finish, the dust is likely to alight on the skin and remain there. The increasing use in horticulture, and especially in viticulture, of arsenic compounds as insecticides has given rise to cases of arsenical poisoning in vine-dressers, agricultural labourers, gardeners and nurserymen. In 1941 in an apple-growing district of the U.S.A. after extensive spraying by lead arsenate 546 orchardists were examined and of these seven showed clinical signs of arsenical poisoning together with arsenic in the urine. Similarly, cases of arsenical poisoning among vine-dressers have been found in almost every vine-growing district of Germany. The signs were hyperkeratosis of the palms and soles, polyneuritis and sometimes pigmentation of the skin. Only rarely did cancer of the skin supervene (Butzengeiger, 1940). Unhappily it is impossible to prove that the disability was solely of occupational origin because many of these men in addition to spraying also drank large quantities of home-made wine prepared from the skins of grapes which had been treated with the arsenical sprays.

Symptoms and Signs

The skin is affected especially where there are folds, as around the nose and mouth, or around the edges of a respirator, or where surfaces are moist, as in the axillæ or on the scrotum. A dermatitis is set up in these areas. It consists of eczema, sometimes with œdema and the formation of bullæ, and folliculitis in varying degree (Holmquist, 1951). If untreated it leads to ulceration, which may be extensive. Associated with the skin eruption are conjunctivitis, with œdema of the eyelids, coryza, dryness of the throat and hoarseness. In severe cases vomiting occurs, but colic is rare. Headache and paræsthesiæ in the limbs may occur, but widespread polyneuritis is rare and motor involvement is practically never seen. Finely mottled brown pigmentation of the skin, the so-called raindrop pigmentation, usually on the temples, eyelids and neck, is present in those who have worked for years in contact with arsenical dusts. In severe cases there may be intense bronzing of the chest, abdomen and back. The most characteristic lesion produced in the upper air-passages is perforation of the nasal septum, which is painless and may be complete in a month from the time of starting work. On the other hand, by the faithful use of a dust mask, men have worked

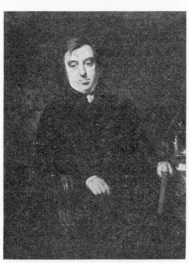

Fig. 120.—John Ayrton Paris, 1785–1856

for years without developing such a lesion. Once the perforation is complete there is no further extension of the erosion and the worker may be unaware of the existence of the condition.

Arsenic Cancer

The widespread use of arsenic and its compounds in industry has led to a prevalent belief that it is responsible for industrial cancer in many occupations. All the available evidence is contrary to such a view, and, apart from that occasionally seen to follow long-continued therapeutic administration of potassium arsenite (Fowler's solution), skin cancer due to arsenic is rare.

Alleged Scrotal Cancer in Tin Smelters

In 1820, John Ayrton Paris (fig. 120), a Cornish physician, alleged, during the period of his practice in Penzance (1813–17), that arsenical fumes from the smelting works occasionally caused scrotal cancer in tin smelters. Later investigation disclosed no definite evidence in favour of his claim. His statement that animals may also be affected has never been substantiated either.

It may, however, be interesting and useful to record an account of the pernicious influence of arsenical fumes upon organized beings, as I have been enabled to ascertain in the copper smelting works of Cornwall and Wales; this influence is very apparent in the condition both of the animals and vegetables in the vicinity; horses and cows commonly lose their hoofs, and the latter are often to be seen in the neighbouring pastures crawling on their knees and not infrequently suffering from cancerous infection in their rumps. . . . It deserves notice that the smelters are occasionally affected with a cancerous disease in the scrotum similar to that which infests chimney-sweepers.

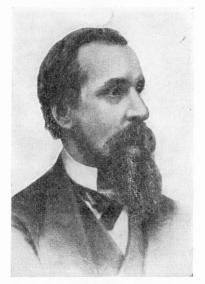

FIG. 121.—Sir Jonathan Hutchinson, 1828–1913

Cancer of the Lung in Schneeberg Miners

In 1879, Haerting and Hesse, discussing the lung disease of the Schneeberg miners, implicated the inhalation of arsenical dust as the major cause of the condition. Many other Continental investigators of this problem have since inclined to the same view, although radon has been detected in the air of the mines. The subject is discussed further on pp. 815–17.

Effect of Prolonged Medication

In 1888 Jonathan Hutchinson (fig. 121) first drew attention to the carcinogenic properties of arsenic. He described cases of carcinoma of the skin in patients treated with arsenical mixtures for psoriasis and other skin conditions. His first recorded case was that of a clerk, aged thirty-four, whom he saw in 1872. He had received prolonged treatment for psoriasis with inorganic arsenic compounds. He developed a wart, which later became a hard-edged sore on the hand (fig. 122). Pye-Smith

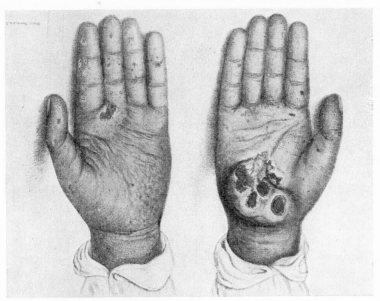

FIG. 122.—Jonathan Hutchinson's Case (1872) of Cancer of the Skin in a man aged 34 who had taken Inorganic Arsenic Compounds by Mouth over many years for Psoriasis

(1913) collected the records of thirty-one cases of cancer, mostly amongst patients receiving prolonged arsenical medication for psoriasis. Two cases involving the skin occurred in sheep-dip workers.

Cancer of the Skin

A similar effect is found in factories where arsenic is handled. The fine powder of arsenical compounds which settles on the skin of the industrial worker may give rise to warts on the nostrils, eyelids, lips, ears and wrinkles of the neck, and, since these compounds of arsenic are carcinogenic, the warts may become malignant. Cases of cancer of the skin due to occupational exposure to arsenic are seen in hospitals from time to time, but they are rare. In forty years only three have been seen at the London Hospital, two in 1910 and one in 1924 (O'Donovan, 1928). Each of these patients had been employed for twenty years or more in the sheep-dip industry, and each developed a squamous-celled carcinoma. The clinical picture of all was made up of pigmentation, keratosis and single or multiple malignant growths. There were no special sites. Face, abdomen, scrotum, buttocks, clavicle and lower chest were affected (figs. 123, 124 and 125).

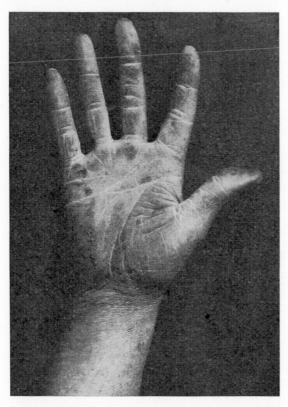

FIG. 123.—Arsenical Hyperkeratosis of the Skin of the Hand in a man exposed for 20 years to the Dust of Sheep Dip

Sheep Dip and Cupric Aceto-arsenite

During the period 1924–30, six cases of skin cancer (three fatal) associated with contact with arsenical dust came to the notice of the Factory Department. In two of these cases exposure was to copper aceto-arsenite, and in the other to arsenical sheep-dip powder. No case of skin cancer has been reported since 1930. Post-mortem examination in one of the fatal cases (cupric aceto-arsenite) disclosed a second primary squamous-

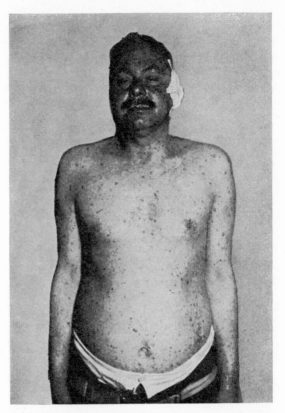

FIG. 124.—Pigmentation of the Skin, Hyperkeratosis and Multiple Warts in a man aged 44 following exposure for 27 years to the Dusts of Inorganic Arsenic Compounds in the manufacture of sheep dip. See also fig. 125

celled carcinoma below the left knee with secondary deposits in the liver and left kidney. The first primary occurred some years previously in the left axilla. The period of exposure to arsenical dust was nineteen years.

Cancer of the Lung in Sheep-dip Workers

Since the trachea and bronchi must be exposed to the same dust as the skin, and since they are lined by a modified squamous epithelium, it is only natural to expect that carcinoma of the bronchus will sometimes occur in men exposed to prolonged inhalation of the dust of arsenical compounds. The total number of workers in Great Britain exposed in this way is small and deaths have usually gone unchecked by necropsy. Legge (1903) gave the first hint in Britain that arsenical dust might possibly damage the lung when he described a condition of irritation of the upper air passages coincident with keratosis of the skin and pigmentation. The affected persons were sheep-dip workers processing white arsenic and sulphur. Henry (1934), on examination of eight men employed in sheep-dip manufacture, found three with warty growths accompanied by keratoses and pigmentation of the skin, and put forward the view that one or two cases of cancer of the lung in sheep-dip workers may have been caused by arsenic.

Necropsy Findings

The first fatal case of lung cancer associated with arsenical dust came to the notice of the Factory Department in 1939, and, since then, two cases (fatal) were reported in 1940 and one case (fatal) in 1943. In the 1939 case the skin of the trunk and limbs was pigmented, with numerous small, flat, warty growths. There was perforation of the nasal septum. At the apex of the right lung there was a hard mass of cancer, and the glands in its neighbourhood showed evidence of metastases. The period of exposure to sheep-dip powder was thirty-seven years. In one of the 1940 cases, post-mortem examination established the cause of death as primary oat-celled carcinoma of the lung. In the 1943 case, the period of exposure to sheep-dip dust was forty-three years, and post-mortem examination revealed a columnar-celled adeno-carcinoma of the upper lobe of the right lung.

Statistical Inquiry in Sheep-dip Workers

In 1948, Hill and Faning analysed the mortality experience in a factory where inorganic arsenic compounds were manufactured. The records for the period 1910–43 showed a proportional and significant excess of deaths attributed to cancer when compared with three other occupational groups living in the same area. The deaths of the former included 29 per cent attributed to cancer, and the latter 13 per cent. The proportional excess was confined to workers in the chemical processes, including engineers and packers, and was entirely absent from printers and

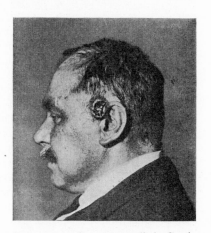

FIG. 125. — Squamous-celled Carcinoma of the Skin in the man seen in fig. 124

box-makers who were unlikely to have been exposed. The numbers were small when subdivided by the site of growth, but there was a suggestion in the figures that the factory workers had been especially affected in the lung and skin. The world literature on arsenic in relation to cancer has been reviewed by Neubauer (1947).

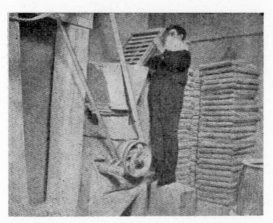

FIG. 126.—Workman sifting Paris Green in an old type of Bolter producing much Dust
(*By courtesy of American Labor Legislation Review, 1912*)

Preventive Treatment

In the prevention of arsenical poisoning in industry, dust must be suppressed (fig. 126). The floors of workrooms and passage-ways should be of impermeable material, and they should be frequently flushed with water. Workrooms should be well ventilated, and hoods connected with a good draught placed over apparatus emitting dust. All poisonous fume should be condensed and any dust caught removed. Hot processes should be carried out under glass hoods and manipulation of powders in closed glass cabinets. When possible, mechanical methods should take the place of hand labour. Apparatus and receptacles must be strong, to avoid breakage. In all processes in which arsenical dust is likely to arise, tables should be provided with downward exhaust ventilation. Since the dust of Scheele's green is light, it is difficult to protect the workers. Automatic packing is not possible, and the ordinary means of protection by respirators favours sweating and consequent ulceration of the skin. Persons with moist skin and those who sweat readily are unsuitable for the work and should be excluded. Special working clothes and head-gear, washing accommodation and towels should be provided (fig. 127). Neither food nor drink should be taken in the workroom, and smoking and the taking of snuff should be prohibited (Balthazard, 1930). Fortunately acaricides based on DDT instead of on arsenic compounds are now being manufactured as sheep dips. Such a safe substitute is very welcome. However in the attack upon the codling moth and the gypsy moth on fruit trees as well as that on the cotton boll weevil Paris green is disappearing from use because parathion has been found more efficient. This is very far from being a safe substitute (p. 397).

Curative Treatment

Deep intramuscular injections of 300 mg. of 10 per cent oily suspension of 2,3-dimercaptopropanol (BAL) repeated every six hours have a specific effect upon the dermatitis, conjunctivitis and pharyngitis of workers in arsenic compounds. Itching, pain and swelling begin to disappear after the first dose. Subsequently, daily injections of 150 mg. should be given for two or three days (Pinto and McGill, 1953).

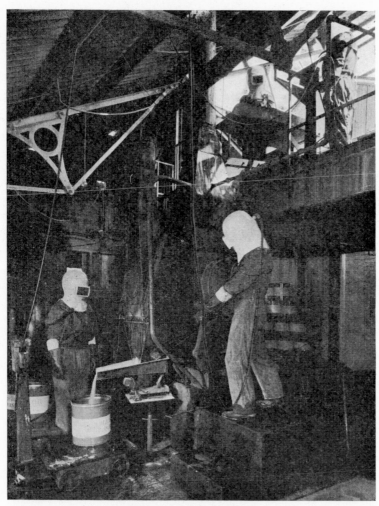

FIG. 127.—Sodium Arsenite Plant showing Protective Clothing and Air-line
Helmets worn by the workmen
(*By courtesy of Hemingway & Co., Ltd.*)

*Case 8. Chemical works' labourer—exposure to dust of white arsenic for ten
years—perforation of nasal septum.*

W. M., a man aged 30, seen in 1947. He had worked for the same
firm for ten years. For the first nine years he had made lead arsenate
and, for the last twelve months, arsenic for the bronzing of gun barrels. Working ten hours a day with three fellow workmen, he charged
and operated a furnace. Between them they handled two tons of white
arsenic a day. They shovelled this, together with charcoal, into cru-

cibles 6 feet high, each total charge being 280 lb. There was no exhaust ventilation and the men tried to protect themselves by tying a handkerchief over the mouth and nose. During the last eight months he had four attacks of hoarseness of the voice, each lasting up to a week. Two weeks: epigastric discomfort and nausea immediately after meals; no vomiting.

On examination: voice, larynx and conjunctivæ normal; clean perforation 1 cm. in diameter in anterior part of nasal septum; necrosis of vomer, which is partly covered by a crust but shows no signs of neoplasm; the skin shows no eruption, pigmentation, hyperkeratosis, papilloma nor carcinoma; nervous system normal. Wassermann reaction in blood: negative.

(b) Arseniuretted Hydrogen

Arseniuretted hydrogen, AsH_3, known also as hydrogen arsenide and arsine, is a colourless gas with a strong odour resembling garlic. It is formed whenever nascent hydrogen is produced in the presence of arsenic or arsenic-bearing substances. It was discovered in 1775 by Scheele. Its toxicity remained unknown until 1815, when Gehlen, a Munich chemist, in the course of some researches "inspired a small portion, and at the termination of one hour was seized with continued vomiting, shivering, and weakness which increased until the ninth day, when he died." Unfortunately, this tragic accident is repeated from time to time.

Laboratory Hazard

In 1920, Schierbeck, of Copenhagen, died from arseniuretted hydrogen poisoning during studies made in collaboration with Lundsgaard on the mixture of air in the lungs with hydrogen. Usually the hydrogen was prepared from hydrochloric acid and zinc, which were both free from arsenic. As a further precaution the gas was washed by passing it through potassium permanganate solution and a sample was tested for arsenic by Marsh's method (Lundsgaard and Schierbeck, 1923). Towards the end of the experiment the workers ran short of arsenic-free hydrochloric acid, and Schierbeck was imprudent enough not only to make use of ordinary laboratory hydrochloric acid in the preparation of the hydrogen, but also to neglect to wash the gas and to test a sample for arsenic. The evening on which the experiments were made he had fever, diarrhœa and copper-coloured jaundice. The urine was red-brown and contained albumin and hæmoglobin. The jaundice persisted and within a few days vomiting occurred, the liver became palpable and the hæmoglobin fell from 46 to 31 per cent. His general condition became rapidly worse, dyspnœa was noticed, suppression of urine supervened and he died on the ninth day after the accident.

Arsenic contaminating Acids and Metals

The first cases to be reported in industry occurred in 1873 in Germany, in men engaged in recovering silver from lead and zinc ores. In a monograph on the subject published in 1908, Glaister, of Glasgow, summarized all the 120 cases which had been reported up to that time. His work remains the best general account of the subject in English. Since 1908 the number of cases recorded has been more than doubled. The majority of cases have been due to the use of acids and alloys or ores contaminated with arsenic. The occupations concerned are the roasting and extraction of mineral ores, the handling by ladlemen in steelworks of silicon-steel slag, lead smelting, the cyanide extraction of gold, the pickling and galvanizing of metals (fig. 128), cleaning of acid tanks, the manufacture of

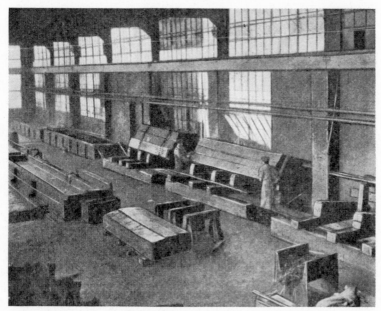

FIG. 128.—Arseniuretted Hydrogen may be evolved when Sheets of Steel are lowered into a Bath of 5 per cent Sulphuric Acid in a Metal-pickling Workshop

bleaching powder, zinc chloride, zinc sulphate and arsenious acid, the manufacture of hydrogen and its use in ballooning, and lastly the making, charging and using of accumulators. It follows that the workman may absorb the poison in operations in which the possibility of poisoning is not so much as imagined.

Action of Water on Metallic Arsenides

The possibility that poisoning might arise from the action of water on the arsenides of alkali metals was recognized by Jones (1907) and Glaister (1908). In 1923 Legge reported two cases of arseniuretted hydrogen poisoning (one of them fatal) from a dross-refining factory in England. A thunderstorm flooded a floor on which bags containing residues from certain refining operations were stored. Two men were employed packing dross at a distance of 10 feet from these bags. One was quite unaffected, but the other suffered from vomiting, intense coppery jaundice and suppression of urine, and died. A third man in charge of a drossing furnace some 20 feet away was slightly affected. A sample of a fresh portion of the contents of the bags was found to contain 1·6 per cent of arsenic, together with lead, tin, antimony, copper and aluminium. It smelt of sulphuretted hydrogen and when moistened gave off large quantities of arseniuretted hydrogen.

Hazard in Tin Refining

In 1932, Bridge gave an account of six cases with two fatalities caused by the damping down to lay the dust of a residue containing a metallic arsenide. He also mentioned three cases which occurred at the same factory earlier in the year and were not reported. In one of the fatal cases traces of arsenic were found in the bones. In 1931, Löning reported eleven cases (with four deaths) which occurred in a tin-refining works at Wilhelmsberg. The patients had been engaged in the process of tin refining described above and had sprinkled water over the dross to avoid the raising of dust. In 1932, Bomford and Hunter described two cases occurring in London from a similar cause. In the process of tin refining a dross containing aluminium arsenide was watered down with several canfuls of water while still hot. Two workmen were affected, and both suffered from hæmoglobinuria and hæmolytic jaundice with anæmia. Both recovered completely.

Rate of Susceptibility and Mortality

Among a group of men at risk there is often great variation in susceptibility. Dudley (1919) described a striking instance of this in a submarine crew during the First World War. While the submarine was submerged there was an escape of arsine from the storage batteries, and the crew of thirty men, all selected for physical soundness, were exposed to the same concentration of the gas for the same length of time, yet they differed considerably in their response to it. One was not affected at all; seven had anæmia and jaundice (the severest case had a count of 1,980,000 red cells); the rest had symptoms of anoxæmia, though not severe enough to need hospital treatment. Twenty-five cases of arseniuretted hydrogen poisoning have been reported in the tin-refining industry, seven of them fatal. The mortality rate of this small series is therefore 28 per cent. It should be noted that this is one of the few industrial poisons which may kill outright.

Symptoms and Signs

Arsine has a specific affinity for the hæmoglobin of the red blood cells, and the symptoms of acute arsine poisoning result from hæmolysis of the red cells with anæmia and hæmolytic jaundice, together with hæmoglobinuria in severe cases. It has been suggested that arsine is carried unchanged to the various tissues by loosely combining with the erythrocytes (Levvy, 1947). In severe cases the first effects of hæmolysis occur within

six hours, when hæmoglobinuria appears. Within twenty-four hours there
is jaundice, and by the third day anæmia in which the red-cell count may
fall below 1,000,000 per c.mm.

Danger of Anuria

Death may occur from anuria in those cases in which the products of
hæmolysis lead to severe damage to the kidneys. Mild cases are often mistaken for food poisoning, and are accompanied by nausea, headache,
shivering, exhaustion, giddiness and vomiting. Reports of series of cases
have often mentioned that a number of other men were affected, but not so
severely as to require admission to
hospital. It therefore seems possible
that a number of cases too mild to
present the classical picture of this
form of poisoning may be occurring
in industry and escaping detection.

Preventive Treatment

The first essential in the prevention of this accident in industry
is that all concerned, particularly
works' managers and appointed
factory doctors, should be fully
alive to the danger of the processes
involved and to the signs of early
and slight poisoning. The workrooms should be ventilated, and in
confined spaces hazardous processes
should be forbidden. Sometimes
a breathing apparatus suitable for
use in irrespirable atmospheres
must be employed. Such an apparatus consists of an oro-nasal mask
with tube connexion to the outer

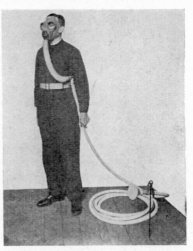

FIG. 129.—Hose Mask Apparatus for
use in Irrespirable Atmospheres. It
consists of an Oro-nasal Mask connected to a Hose, the free end of
which is led out into uncontaminated
air
(*By courtesy of Siebe, Gorman & Co., Ltd.*)

atmosphere. The wearer draws fresh air through the tube by his inspiratory
efforts and expels the expired air through a valve in the mask (fig. 129).
Further, as suggested by Koelsch (1920), a number of bird-cages containing small birds should be hung as near as possible to the work, since
it is known from experience that the gas affects them before it affects man.

*Case 9. Metallurgical worker—exposure to arseniuretted hydrogen—hæmo-
globinuria and hæmolytic jaundice with anæmia.*

(Bomford and Hunter, 1932.) T. R., a man aged 31, L.H. Reg.
No. 30791/1932. This man had been employed continuously by the
same firm for nine years. For seven years he had worked on a wharf
loading barges with pig lead, lead alloys and lead slag. For the last two

years he had been melting and casting alloys of lead, tin and antimony. He had never had any illness, nor a blue line on the gums, nor had his mates.

On 24th June 1932, shortly before noon, he inhaled for about eight minutes fume given off from dross containing aluminium arsenide watered down while still hot. He left work at 2.30 p.m., and went home feeling "well but not lively." Later in the day he felt drowsy and went to bed early. On the following day, 25th June, he rose at 5 a.m. feeling drowsy, and passed a quantity of urine the colour of port wine. During the afternoon he noticed that he looked yellow, and complained of a slight headache and a feeling of weakness. On 26th June he vomited once, and complained of thirst and dryness of the mouth. On 27th June the urine appeared normal. The headache was more severe. He was admitted to hospital at 6 p.m.

Clinical examination on the third day after exposure: temperature 98° F.; pulse rate 96; respiration 24; a well-built man, cheerful, and in no way distressed; moderate jaundice (subicteric tint) of the whole body; mucous membranes pale; teeth dirty, with many carious stumps; no blue line on gums; heart and lungs normal; blood-pressure 130–70; abdomen—liver not palpable and liver dullness normal; spleen not palpable; no abnormality in nervous system. Blood count: red cells 2,800,000 per c.mm., hæmoglobin 44 per cent, colour index 0·78, reticulocytes 12·2 per cent, white cells 7,500 per c.mm., neutrophilic myelocytes 1·5 per cent, proleucocytes 0·5 per cent, polymorphs 48·5 per cent, lymphocytes 46 per cent, eosinophils 2 per cent, large mononuclears 1 per cent, basophils 0·5 per cent, fragility of red cells normal, indirect van den Bergh 1·9 mg. per 100 ml. Urine: hæmoglobin absent; a cloud of albumin; epithelial cells; a few red cells; a few blood casts; occasional hyaline casts; arsenic present, lead and antimony absent; blood urea 0·037 per cent. Wassermann reaction negative.

Progress: the patient continued to complain of headache, but of diminishing severity, until the eighth day after exposure. Slight jaundice of the conjunctivæ only was noticed on that day. On the tenth day he stated that he felt quite well and there was no jaundice; some degree of pallor alone remained. No treatment was given for the anæmia. On the twentieth day the figure for the indirect van den Bergh test was 0·66 mg. per 100 ml. He was discharged from hospital on the twenty-fourth day feeling quite well, and seen again on the forty-fourth day on his return from a holiday. A blood count taken on that day showed normal figures: red cells 5,500,000 per c.mm., hæmoglobin 90 per cent, colour index 0·81, reticulocytes 2·8 per cent, white cells 6,600 per c.mm., polymorphs 60·5 per cent, lymphocytes 33 per cent, eosinophils 3 per cent, large mononuclears 2·5 per cent, basophils 1 per cent. The firm of metallurgists concerned in this case agreed to abandon the process as too dangerous. They adopted a method in which the arsenides in the dross are further oxidized to innocuous arsenates as they are formed, this reaction taking place in a closed apparatus.

(c) Organic Arsenic Compounds

Studies directed to chemical warfare, chemotherapy and the growth of moulds have drawn close attention to the chemistry of organic arsenic compounds. Most of the aliphatic and aromatic arsines employed during the First World War were substances which had been known for some time. The chlorovinyl arsines, and phenarsazine chloride have been studied since 1918. In the Second World War the arsenical smokes received a good deal of attention, in particular the aromatic arsenical cyanides (Sartori, 1940). The organic derivatives of arsine can be divided into three groups as follows:

(i) Aliphatic Arsines

The aliphatic arsines are powerful poisons. Dimethylarsine is not encountered in manufacturing operations but occurs as an accidental poison. The aliphatic chlorarsine derivatives are highly lethal war gases, although in the military sense their aggressive properties are inferior to those of the aromatic arsines. The initial letters following the names of the gases are abbreviations used as military labels.

Dimethylarsine. The use of Scheele's green, emerald green (cupric arsenite), in the preparation of artificial flowers and wallpapers has now only historical interest, because aniline colours have almost entirely taken the place of arsenic in these processes. When arsenical colours were used, as much as 60 grains per square foot were found in samples of wallpapers examined; and such symptoms as coryza, conjunctivitis, gastro-enteritis and tinglings in the extremities were sometimes found to be associated with residence in rooms papered with arsenical wallpapers. The mould *Scopulariopsis brevicaulis* while growing in the paste splits up the arsenic compounds, liberating from them a gas originally thought to be diethylarsine (Biginelli, 1901) but since identified as dimethylarsine (Challenger, 1935). In 1931 in the Forest of Dean a child died owing to inhalation of dimethylarsine from mouldy walls in a damp house. The source of the arsenic in this case was coke breeze, a constituent of the plaster of the walls. The use of concrete blocks containing this substance and the addition of arsenious oxide to cements to increase their rate of hardening are undesirable.

Methyl dichlorarsine (MD) is a colourless liquid with a characteristic odour. Both the liquid and its vapour are lethal substances acting as lung irritants and as vesicants. It is neutralized by chloride of lime and alkalis.

Ethyl dichlorarsine (ED) is a colourless liquid becoming slightly yellow on exposure to air and light. It has a characteristic odour which when highly diluted is reminiscent of fruit. It is a lethal poison acting as a lung irritant and as a vesicant. It is neutralized by chloride of lime.

Chlorovinyl dichlorarsine (Lewisite) is a colourless liquid with a faint odour recalling that of geraniums. It is a very powerful war gas having vesicant, lachrymatory and lung irritant effects. It is neutralized by water and alkalis.

(ii) Aromatic Arsines

These arsines differ from those of the aliphatic series both in their physical and chemical properties and in their biological action. Although they have a lower toxicity, they are more effective as war gases acting as energetic sternutators and lung irritants even at very low concentrations. Their aggressive action is provoked by finely divided solid particles, which on liberation in the air form highly lethal smokes.

Phenyl dichlorarsine (MA) is a colourless viscous liquid with a pungent odour. In air it gradually turns yellow. It has lung irritant, vesicant and lachrymatory effects. In chemical warfare it is employed not as a toxic smoke but as a solvent for other gases.

Development of Skin Lesions

Goldblatt (1945) recorded severe vesication of the skin which occurred in a research chemist aged twenty-six who was working on the preparation of phenyldichlorarsine. A small liquid contamination occurred on the right forearm, and this led in a short time to erythema and later to a few small vesicles on a finger of the left hand and others on the right temple. In order to observe the development of these lesions, no treatment was given and he continued at work with, however, added precautions.

Spread of the Vesicles

On the fifth day from the first contamination a crop of vesicles on a red base was present on the forehead and nose, and erythema had spread to the flexure of the right arm, with multiple vesicles on the forearm. The site of the original contamination on the right forearm now showed a puckered central zone surrounded by a red area sown with minute vesicles. Local irritation was slight but it was greatly aggravated in bed. On the following day there was a spread of vesication round the site of the original con-tamination and of erythema to the back of the neck. He was then removed from contact, but during the next twelve days there was further erythema and a spread of vesication.

Healing by Desquamation

On the nineteenth day the lesions had almost recovered, but a fine desquamation of most areas continued for some days. In the later stages, dressings of oil and calamine were used. The vesication rapidly following the original contamination, and the spread that took place were considered to be due to the fact that he continued to work in low concentrations of vapour. The occurrence of new crops of vesicles after removal from ex-posure was taken to indicate a measure of generalized sensitization.

Diphenyl chlorarsine (DA) is a colourless crystalline solid only slightly

soluble in water. It is readily soluble in phosgene and in henyl dichlorp-
arsine. As a toxic smoke it has lung irritant, vesicant and sternutatory
effects. In the solid state, in solution and as vapour it readily produces
vesicles on the skin. Goldblatt (1945) described vesication of the skin in the
same patient as in the previous paragraph. A month after the first incident
this man was working with a solution of diphenyl chlorarsine when
he splashed it on to his left forearm.

Rapidity of Penetration

It was immediately treated with sodium hypochlorite but, nevertheless,
in fifteen minutes irritation began and a flare of erythema appeared from
elbow to wrist on the ulnar aspect of the limb. Itching and erythema continued for four days, when vesicles began to develop on the reddened area.
On the fifth day the erythema had been replaced by groups of small
vesicles located mainly around the hair follicles. There was no irritation at
this stage and recovery took place after about twelve days. Considering that
inactivation by hypochlorite was immediate, it is evident that the speed
of penetration was very great and that diphenyl chlorarsine, left *in situ*,
would produce severe results.

Diphenyl cyanoarsine (DC) is a colourless crystalline, solid, with a slight
garlic odour. It has such a low vapour pressure that for purposes of war it
must be diffused in the air as a particulate smoke. It is very effective as a
lung irritant, a vesicant and a sternutatory substance.

(iii) Heterocyclic Arsines

The study of the heterocyclic arsines—that is, those containing the
atom of arsenic in the nucleus—led to the discovery of substances, the
effects of which as war gases are even more highly lethal than those of
the aromatic arsines.

Phenarsazine chloride (Adamsite or DM), also known as diphenylamine
chlorarsine, is a yellow crystalline, solid, almost insoluble in water. Used
as a toxic smoke it is a powerful war gas, having both lung irritant and
sternutatory effects.

In Baltimore in 1946 a number of workers exposed to the dust of
Adamsite developed intractable dermatitis involving the exposed areas of
the face, neck and arms. An itching, burning, erythematous papular eruption proved resistant to ordinary forms of treatment. In six of the seven
patients, the dermatitis had persisted for from eighteen to fifty days before
admission to hospital.

Action of British Anti-Lewisite (BAL)

BAL was applied daily as an ointment. It caused intense burning of
the affected areas which lasted for less than an hour, after which the patients
were greatly relieved from the previous itching and discomfort. After the
first day the dose was increased from 100 mg. to 500 mg. The dermatitis cleared completely in from two to eight days with an average of a little

over five days. In these studies the patients served as their own controls, since the eruption had been present for different lengths of time before treatment and had failed to respond to other forms of therapy prior to the use of BAL.

Systemic Effect

It is probable that the effect here was due to the systemic action of BAL as well as to its local effect. Later, BAL was applied to unaffected portions of the skin. These inunctions caused no discomfort and therefore comparatively large amounts of ointment could be employed. The results were highly satisfactory and the dermatitis cleared under this method of application as rapidly as when the inunction had been made to the eruption itself. The fact that arsenic excretion in the urine increased during treatment suggested that it had been released from combination with the cells (Longcope and others, 1946).

The Pyruvate Oxidase System

In the search for antidotes to combat the arsenical blister gases, full use was made of the progress of knowledge of the intermediary metabolism of carbohydrates in tissue cells. Each step in the breakdown of glucose and glycogen to carbon dioxide and water is controlled by a definite enzyme, and one of the penultimate stages of this degradation is pyruvic acid, a three-carbon keto-acid. The enzyme system responsible for the oxidation of pyruvic acid is usually called the pyruvate oxidase system. This system has protein and other components, and interruption of tissue metabolism can occur by active interference with the functioning of any of these components by poisons.

Sensitivity to Arsenite

It is known that the pyruvate oxidase system contains a component sensitive to very small concentrations of arsenite. It follows that the metabolism of carbohydrate may be poisoned at an important stage by traces of an arsenical substance. This is the predominant way in which arsenic compounds can cause biochemical lesions, and any antidote must be capable of reversing this biochemical damage. On the basis of these facts, it was logical to use the pyruvate oxidase system as well as the more classical method of *in vivo* injection as a test for new antidotes against arsenic, and during the Second World War a research upon these lines was initiated and pursued by a team in Oxford (Peters and others, 1945).

Affinity of Arsenic for Sulphydryl Groups

Ehrlich (1909) had already shown that arsenical substances had a strong affinity for sulphydryl groups, and his work led to the observation that when such substances combined with tissue proteins the active sulphydryl group of the latter spontaneously disappeared. The next step was the discovery that when Lewisite reacted with keratin, approximately 75 per cent of the bound arsenic was in combination with two thiol groups. Thus it seemed possible that the high toxicity of trivalent arsenic compounds might be due to their ability to combine with essential sulphydryl groups in certain tissue proteins to form stable arsenical rings. Conversely, in a search for antidotes, it was argued that simple dithiol compounds might form relatively stable ring compounds with Lewisite and might consequently compete effectively with the dithiol proteins in the tissues.

Antidotal Action of 1,2-Dithiols

As a result of the systematic attack made on this problem, it was found that simple 1,2-dithiols are capable both of exerting a marked antidotal action against the poisoning of the pyruvate oxidase system by trivalent arsenic compounds and, more important still, of reversing this poisoning when once established. Of the numerous dithiol compounds prepared and tested, one in particular, the 2,3-dimercaptopropanol recommended itself as a local decontaminant in combating the arsenical blister gases. This compound, generally known as BAL (British Anti-Lewisite), was compounded in ointment form for use on the skin and eyes, and the value of such preparations was abundantly demonstrated in numerous experimental studies (fig. 130).

Preventive Treatment

In the manufacture and handling of all these substances, strict precautions must be observed in the factory, laboratory and practice field. Plant design must be such as to enclose completely the processes of manufacture and to remove toxic vapours by means of adequate exhaust ventilation. Protective clothing is important, and it may include rubber gloves, rubber aprons and canister gas masks. Solutions of neutralizing agents in suitable containers should be ready for immediate application to the skin in case of splashing (Goldblatt, 1945).

Curative Treatment

Where a research chemist, workman or soldier at practice is splashed or otherwise exposed to any of these compounds, he should be kept warm and put to bed in uncontaminated clothing. Where the skin has been contaminated, an ointment containing 5 per cent BAL may be applied, using 500 mg. of BAL daily until healing is complete. If application of the ointment causes pain, BAL should be given intramuscularly instead, using 300 mg. of a 10 per cent solution in benzyl benzoate and arachis oil. Subsequently, daily injections of 150 mg. should be given for two or three days (Longcope and others, 1946). Should the vapour or smoke cause the lung irritant effect, the administration of oxygen may be required as in the case of phosgene poisoning (see p. 680).

Case 10. Research chemist—exposure to organic arsenical compounds for chemical warfare—vesication of right hand by phenyl dichlorarsine— papilloma of bladder.

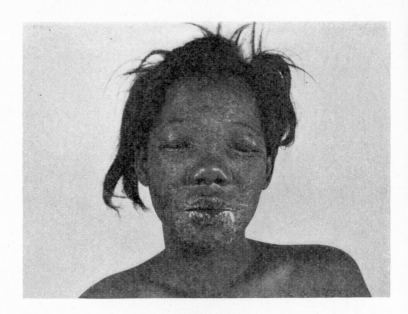

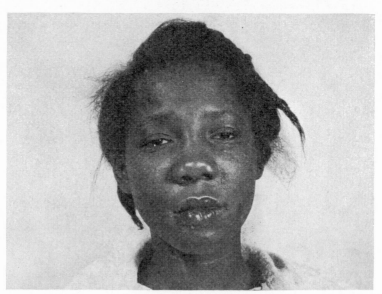

FIG. 130.—Arsenical Dermatitis in a woman of 20 following an injection of
0·3 gram of Diarsenol in the treatment of Syphilis. The lower picture shows
the condition four days later after the application of 1 gram of BAL as
Ointment

(*Longcope, W. T., Luetscher, J. A., Wintrobe, M. M., Jager, B. V., J. Clin. Invest., 1946, 25, 528*)

K. T.-T., a man aged 39, L.H. Reg. No. 16081/1951, had been put to work on 21st August 1940 on a bulk supply of liquid arsenical vesicant containing mainly phenyl dichlorarsine. By mistake he was wearing rubber gloves which had been condemned as too thin to give adequate protection. He had spilled some of the liquid over the back of his right-hand glove, had wiped the glove and, thinking it impervious to

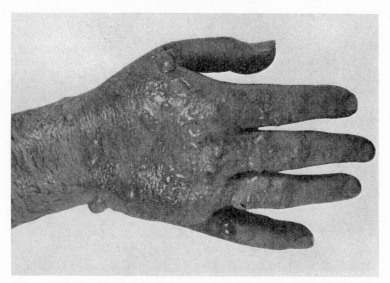

FIG. 131.—Case 10. Vesication of the Skin of the Hand of a Research Chemist photographed after exposure to Phenyl Dichlorarsine

the liquid, had gone on wearing it for two hours longer. That night the dorsum of the right hand was red and painful. By the next morning it was severely blistered from the middle of the fingers to three inches above the wrist (fig. 131). The palm was unaffected. His wife, who handled a towel soiled by the blister fluid, suffered later from minor burns on the skin of her hands. Two days later he had to go to bed because of severe diarrhœa, vomiting and slight jaundice. For about a week he vomited up to four times a day, and for twelve days he had diarrhœa in which he passed on an average six fluid stools daily without blood. The skin of the hand was healed by the tenth day. The jaundice disappeared after three weeks. Minor attacks of diarrhœa had occurred subsequently over a period of three years.

Two years ago: painless hæmaturia at beginning and end of stream. *One year:* three further attacks of hæmaturia. *Four months ago:* the last and most severe attack of hæmaturia. On 10th May 1951 cystoscopy showed a papilloma of the bladder above the right ureteric orifice. This was coagulated by diathermy. The disease of the bladder was considered to be unrelated to his occupation.

Calcium

Calcium, Ca, is a soft silver-white lustrous metal so reactive that it does not occur free in nature. With the exception of lime, which is corrosive, its compounds are non-poisonous. The dusts produced in mining, quarrying and shaping calcium carbonate rocks cause no disease of the lungs. Many different calcium compounds are deposited in the surface of the earth.

Mineral Sources

Impure forms of calcium carbonate, $CaCO_3$, are found as limestone, marble and chalk in huge masses which may form whole mountain ranges. Many limestones are of organic origin containing the calcareous remains of molluscs, crinoids, corals and foraminifera. Mixtures of calcium carbonate with varying proportions of magnesium carbonate form magnesian limestones. The double salt of calcium and magnesium carbonate, $CaCO_3$. $MgCO_3$, is called dolomite, after the French geologist, D. G. Dolomieu, who described it in 1791. Crystalline calcium carbonate is found in nature as aragonite, calcite and Iceland spar. Calcium sulphate occurs in three forms—gypsum, $CaSO_4.2H_2O$, and its granular variety, alabaster, and also anhydrite, $CaSO_4$. Native phosphate rock is impure calcium phosphate, $Ca_3(PO_4)_2$. It also occurs as apatite in the two forms chlor-apatite, $3Ca_3(PO_4)_2.CaCl_2$, and fluor-apatite, $3Ca_3(PO_4)_2.CaF_2$. Another important mineral is fluorspar, calcium fluoride, CaF_2.

Chemical Derivatives

Lime is handled in two forms: quicklime, which is calcium oxide, CaO, and slaked lime, which is calcium hydroxide, $Ca(OH)_2$. Calcium carbide, CaC_2, is made from quicklime, and calcium cyanamide, $CaCN_2$, is made from calcium carbide. Calcium sulphide, CaS, is made from slaked lime. Calcium chloride, $CaCl_2$, is obtained as a by-product in several manufacturing processes—for example, the ammonia-soda process.

(a) Limestone

The limestone of the Mediterranean basin was used to build the pyramids of Egypt, and builders and sculptors in stone have made use of it ever since. The chief sources of ornamental limestones and dolomites in Great Britain lie in a belt which crosses England obliquely from the Dorset coast, through Somerset, Gloucester, Northamptonshire, Rutland, Nottingham and Lincolnshire, to the coast of Yorkshire.

Limestone for Building

In colour these limestones vary from pale cream to buff, according to the amount of iron oxide present. The mellow Bath stone is to be seen in churches and public buildings in Southern England. Cotswold stone has been used to build the lovely Cotswold villages, and Headington stone the Oxford colleges. Ancaster stone is to be seen in most of the great churches and homes of the East Midlands, including Lincoln Cathedral.

Ancaster Stone

Ancaster in Lincolnshire was a Roman station on Ermine Street and has possessed for centuries some of the most notable quarries in the oolitic limestone. But all along this limestone belt there were famous quarries, especially those at Barnack which provided the stone to build Peterborough Cathedral. Cambridge colleges built in the fifteenth century often obtained limestone from Weldon in Northamptonshire. Most of these quarries became so well worked that they were exhausted early in the sixteenth century.

Clipsham Stone

Limestone from Clipsham has been used for nearly a century to repair not only cathedrals such as Canterbury and Salisbury, but also the incomparable pinnacles and parapets which make up the beautiful skyline of the colleges of Oxford. In our day the quarries of Ketton, Casterton and Clipsham have sent stone to repair the colleges of Cambridge and also St. George's Chapel, Windsor, and to rebuild the bombed House of Commons in London.

Limestone Buildings all over the World

Limestone suitable for use as building stone is found all over the world; in the United States of America it has been used in buildings such as the Grand Central Terminal in New York City and the City Hall in Chicago. Sometimes limestone is rejected as a building material because of its unsuitable colour. This is the case in South Africa, where enormous quantities of black dolomite exist in the Western Witwatersrand.

Dolomite for Building

From Nottingham, running almost due north into Yorkshire, the belt is of dolomite. This magnesian limestone is quarried at Mansfield and Tadcaster. It is notoriously easy to carve and is responsible for the carved heads, leaves and flowers of incomparable beauty to be seen in York Minster. The chapter-house of Southwell Minster, Nottinghamshire, likewise shows a profusion of late thirteenth-century sculptured ornament of a quality unique in Britain. Other typical examples of dolomite are Kentish rag and Portland stone.

White Portland Dolomite used by Inigo Jones

One advantage of the use of Portland stone for building is the beauty of its being almost pure white in colour. The quarries on the Portland peninsula had existed from early times, but it was only in the Stuart period that Portland stone began to be used extensively. It was Inigo Jones (1573–1651) who was responsible for introducing brick and stone as building materials to London. He was appointed by James the First Surveyor-General of Royal Buildings. The dignified simplicity of his work in Portland stone in the Queen's House, Greenwich (1617–35) is today still a delight. He prepared designs for a new palace at Whitehall and built in Portland stone the lovely banqueting-hall (1619–22) which remains to the present day a monument alike to the genius of the architect and to the lavish expenditure of the Stuart court.

Sir Christopher Wren builds St. Paul's Cathedral

In the next generation when the First Great Fire of London (1666) destroyed eighty-nine city churches, including the old Gothic St. Paul's Cathedral, Christopher Wren (1632–1723) was at the height of his powers and quickly stamped his genius on the ecclesiastical architecture of the new London. The needs of his colossal work gave a new life to the Portland peninsula, for the new St. Paul's was built of the white Portland dolomite. Vast quarries were opened and roads and piers built so that the stone could be fetched by sea and landed by way of the Thames. The layout of the greatest city in the world continued to be the worst, but Wren's churches, though largely obscured in the rabbit-warren of streets, stood to testify to the grace and dignity of the age and, indeed, of their architect. The rebuilding of St. Paul's was a communal effort worthy of a great nation. A tax on the coal entering the Port of London was voted by Parliament for the purpose. The great work went steadily forward year by year until in 1710 it was completed in the height of Queen Anne's glory.

Portland Stone remains a Fashion in Building

But at the end of the eighteenth century the ancient and noble English industries of stone-quarrying, building and carving began to decline, and today they are mostly in the hands of old men. Unhappily, as these men die out it becomes increasingly difficult to persuade younger men to take up the trade. This intensifies the tragedy of the Second Great Fire of London (1941), which destroyed nearly all the Wren churches. In our time the facings of a new Waterloo Bridge have been fashioned in Portland stone. Happily other cities have taken up the fashion; in 1905 Cardiff began to build what is now a civic centre of great dignity entirely in the beautiful white Portland dolomite. It is of interest that an architectural style set up in Stuart times not only continues to beautify London and other cities but also has been the means of saving hundreds of stonemasons from the risk of silicosis.

Roofing Slats of Laminated Stone

Certain types of limestone develop lamination by weathering. This is true of Collyweston, Stonesfield and Cotswold stone. In these areas there are a few local stone-builders who make roofing slats of this laminated stone. Collyweston stone and roofing slats were largely used to build certain towns and villages in Northamptonshire (Oundle) and Lincolnshire (Stamford). In his *British Craftsmen* (1946), T. Hennell writes:

> These are worked in a succession of sizes—a V-shaped "crest" on the ridge, the smallest and lightest next beneath it; the largest at the eaves. They are known by queer names: cocks, cuttings, mobbities;

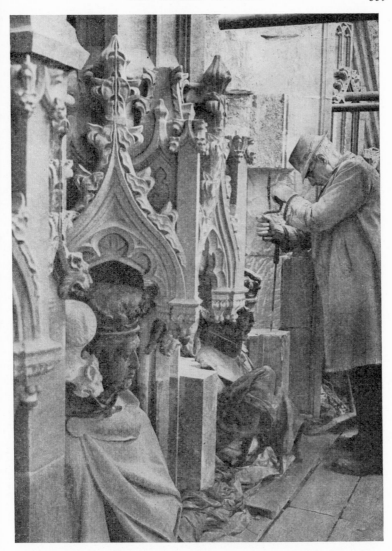

FIG. 132.—Workman in 1948 replacing limestone figures which had crumbled away on the Victoria tower of the Houses of Parliament. Before the *Clean Air Act, 1956* atmospheric pollution hastened the weathering of the stone.
(Photograph by Central Press Photos., Ltd.)

becks, bachelors, nines and wibbuts; elevens to sixteens, follows and eaves. The making and use of such slats has not been carried on for a thousand years and more without developing a truly scientific perfection. And yet reputable modern architects ignore the tradition and order their slats all of one size. Those stone roofs are not only strong and durable against storm and weather; they are organic form like the covering of creatures. They are as much part of the landscape as shepherd and flock, fields and ploughman.

Other Uses of Limestone

Limestone is used also for crushed stone in road and railway construction, for the manufacture of lime, cement and concrete, as furnace flux in the preparation of steel, and for glass, fertilizers, paper and chemicals. On account of its refractoriness to heat, granular dolomite is used for lining the hearths of steel furnaces.

Absence of Hazard to Lungs

The drilling, blasting, shaping, carving and crushing of limestone and dolomite are all harmless occupations. There is no dust hazard to men at work in limestone quarries, to stonemasons handling only limestone and dolomite, nor to men who crush these materials to make stones. It follows that if more of our stone buildings were of limestone or dolomite instead of sandstone or granite, a lot of suffering from silicosis would be avoided. It is essential that the *Clean Air Act, 1956* be implemented not only for reasons of health but also to lessen the weathering of limestone buildings from atmospheric pollution (fig. 132).

Mining of Ores found in Dolomite

In mining, when the ore of a metal occurs in limestone or dolomite, the dust produced in drilling and blasting is harmless. Thus, in most mercury mines, including those of Idria in Yugoslavia, the cinnabar, HgS, is found in dolomite which gives rise to a harmless dust. But in the mines of New Almaden in California the cinnabar is found in sandstone with the corresponding risk to the miners of silicosis.

(b) Marble

Marble (Latin, *marmor*, shining stone) is crystalline impervious limestone or dolomite sufficiently close in texture to admit of being polished. The beautiful lustre of polished statuary marble is due to the light penetrating for a short distance into the rock and then being reflected at the surfaces of the deeper-lying crystals.

Greek Temples and Statues

Ancient Greece had vast supplies of marble, both on the mainland and on the Ægean islands of Naxos and Paros, next to Delos and Melos. This was used by architects to build temples (fig. 133), as well as by sculptors. The lovely marble statue of Asklepios in the British Museum was found on the island of Melos. Parian marble was used by Praxiteles and others for the finest statuary. The Parthenon and therefore the Elgin marbles are built of Pentelic marble which was quarried from Mount Pentelicus near Athens. The Greek marbles have a slight intermixture of iron salts, giving them a beautiful, warm, faint apricot glow in the sun.

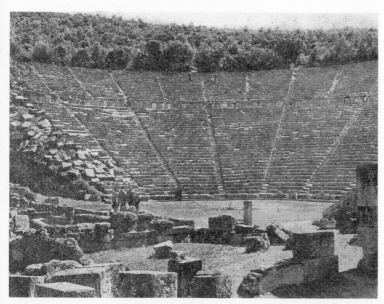

FIG. 133.—Open-air Theatre at Epidauros in Greece built by Polycleitus the Younger about 325 B.C. It was part of the most important of all the Temples of Healing, for it included the Central Shrine of Asklepios himself. The Circular Orchestra 66 feet in diameter has a surrounding Auditorium occupying three-fifths of its Circumference and made up of 55 rows of Marble Seats to hold 14,000 people. It is such a Masterpiece of Theatrical Architecture that in its ruined state it still has perfect acoustics

(Photograph by Sir William Lister)

Rome, a City of Marble

The Romans obtained marble from Carrara in the Apuan Alps, an offshoot of the Apennines, mid-way between Genoa and Florence. It is dispatched by sea from the port of Avenza-Marina, three miles away on the Gulf of Genoa. Carrara marble, with fine grain and exquisitely white, has been quarried for 2,000 years. About 50 B.C. the Emperor Augustus said that he had found Rome a city of brick and left it marble. In 1508 blocks of it were sent to Michelangelo in Rome, and out of this he carved the famous statue of David (fig. 134). In 1518 he went to Carrara so that he could supervise the extraction from the quarries of the blocks he wanted to use for buildings in Florence.

The Carrara Quarries

There are 400 quarries at Carrara, and more than a million tons of marble are blasted from the mountainside every year. The quarrying methods are so wasteful that in 1926, for instance, only 600,000 tons were available for use, and this in spite of the fact that a special blasting powder is used which does not splinter the marble (figs. 135, 136 and 137).

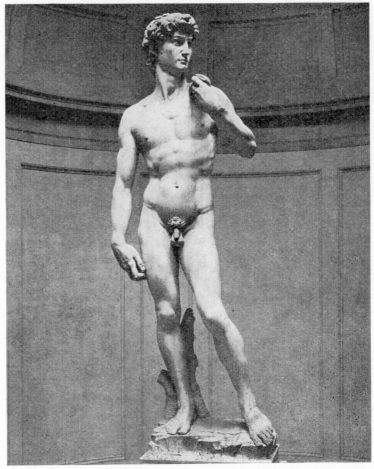

FIG. 134.—Statue of David modelled in Florence in 1508 by the youthful Michelangelo from a gigantic block of Carrara Marble which had been abandoned as spoiled

(*Photograph by Giacomo Brogi*)

Marble for Building and for Lime

In 1828 John Nash designed the Marble Arch and had it erected as a gate to the garden of Buckingham Palace. By order of King George I it was built of Carrara marble. In 1851 the Palace had to be enlarged because Queen Victoria had such a large family and the Arch was moved to become the Cumberland Gate of Hyde Park. And then, widening of the road left it isolated in its present position amid a surge of traffic. But marble is found all over the world; in India the Taj Mahal is built of it and in the United States of America the Harvard Medical School, the New York Public

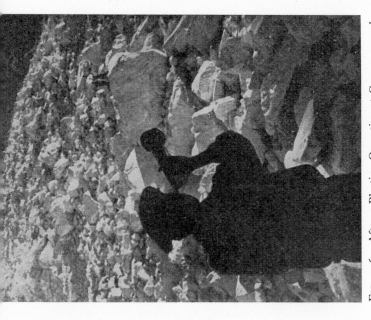

Fig. 136.—After a Blasting Operation at Carrara a workman sounds the All-clear on a Trumpet
(Photograph by Camera Talks)

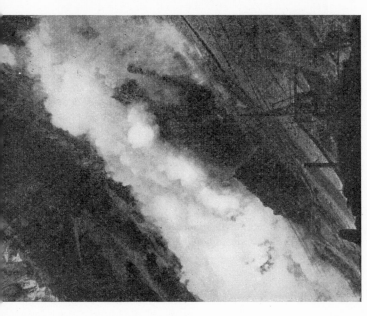

Fig. 135.—White Smoke produced by blasting at Carrara
(Photograph by Camera Talks)

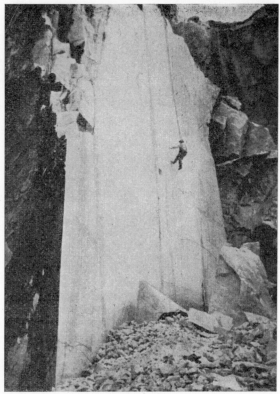

FIG. 137.—A man working half-way up a Quarry Face
at Carrara
(*Photograph by Camera Talks*)

Library and the Lincoln Memorial. Like limestone, it is also used in
making lime and cement and for metallurgical and chemical purposes.

Absence of Hazard to Lungs

The drilling, blasting, shaping, carving and crushing of marble are
all harmless occupations. Therefore in carving statues in marble Michelangelo and his pupils ran no risk of lung disease, nor would compressed-
air chisels have introduced this risk. Statistical inquiry, clinical survey,
studies in morbid anatomy and animal experiments all point to the
changes in the lungs in men exposed to marble dust being minimal. In
1930, Turano examined clinically and radiologically 105 marble workers
of Carrara. There was little evidence of lung disease, although in 28 per
cent he found arborescent markings in the X-ray shadows of the lungs.
In 1934, Dreessen examined clinically and radiologically eighty marble
finishers from a typical plant in Vermont. There was no disability even
after many years of exposure. Radiographs of the lungs showed harmless
arborescent markings just as in the case of the Italian workers.

(c) Chalk

Chalk is a soft white or grey porous limestone which still bears evidence of its organic derivation from minute marine organisms and shells of former ocean deposits. Large quantities of chalk are quarried in England, especially in Kent, but also in Surrey, Sussex, Hampshire, Cambridgeshire and Lincolnshire. It is calcium carbonate in impure form, for it contains magnesium carbonate, clay and silica. With the admixture of clay there may be an insensible gradation from pure chalk to chalk-marl. Egg-shells, sea-shells, pearls and corals contain a large percentage of calcium carbonate.

Uses

Chalk is used in the manufacture of quicklime, and hence of slaked lime, plaster, mortar and cement. It is employed as a writing material, in the manufacture of sodium carbonate and as a flux in the smelting of iron and in metallurgy generally. Whiting is chalk ground to powder and freed from sandy impurities by levigation in water; it is used for polishing and in making putty. Under the name *Paris white*, chalk is used in the manufacture of rubber goods, oilcloth and wallpaper. In the precipitated form, calcium carbonate is employed in pharmacy and in the preparation of tooth pastes. *Nitrochalk*, used as a fertilizer, is a mixture of ammonium nitrate and powdered chalk.

(d) Lime

Calcium forms three different oxides, of which calcium oxide or quicklime, CaO, is the only important one. Quicklime, or caustic lime, is made on a large scale by heating limestone or chalk in a lime kiln. It is obtained in the form of hard white lumps. If a few drops of water be allowed to fall on a cold lump of freshly burnt lime, a hissing noise is produced and clouds of steam are formed. The lump of lime disintegrates to a fine white powder of slaked lime or calcium hydroxide, $Ca(OH)_2$, and the process is known as the slaking of lime.

Uses

Lime is employed in the manufacture of bleaching powder and of caustic soda, in the purification of sugar, in glass making and for making mortar and plaster. The Greeks used lime in their buildings at a very early period. Often their houses were finished in plaster that compared favourably in whiteness to Parian marble. The Romans learned the art of plastering from the Greeks and spread it to their colonies.

Lime Mortar

While the use of adhesive clay and burnt gypsum for cementing together building stones dates back to ancient Egypt, the use of lime mortar for this purpose can be traced only as far back as the seventh century B.C. Lime mortar was made by slaking quicklime with excess of water, the resulting porridge-like mass being used to join bricks together. On exposure to the atmosphere, the excess of moisture gradually evaporated and the calcium hydroxide combined slowly with atmospheric carbon dioxide to form calcium carbonate, which was often deposited in the mortar in crystalline form. It is to this chemical change that the setting of mortar is due.

Accidents at Lime Kilns

Severe caustic burns have been described in workmen who had fallen into a lime pit. Death has then resulted from extension of the lesions. A lime kiln is often built into a mound or cutting with its upper rim open to

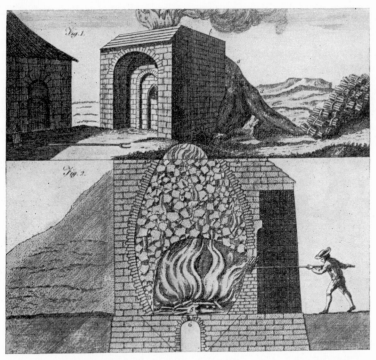

FIG. 138.—Old Print of Lime Kiln built into a Mound. The Limestone is seen above the Fire which the workman is feeding with Wood

the air (fig. 138). It is filled from above with thin layers of coal and heavy layers of broken limestone laid alternately. As the mass burns, the lime and ashes work through, are carried out below, sifted and carted away, and more coal and limestone added above. A cart-track leads from the top opening to the quarry. Cases, often fatal, from poisoning by carbon monoxide are described among workmen who have gone to sleep on the top of lime kilns.

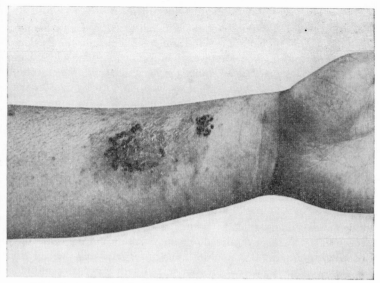

FIG. 139.—Dermatitis in a House Decorator using Lime Distemper
(*By courtesy of Dr. Brian Russell*)

Hazard to the Skin and Eyes

Builders, plasterers, paperhangers, whitewashers, lime burners and slakers, agricultural labourers and others handling lime are exposed to the risk of dermatitis (fig. 139) and ulceration of the skin (*lime hole*). Lime can injure the conjunctiva and the cornea. Frequent thorough irrigations of the eye with saline or 5 per cent ammonium chloride solution should be followed by the use of penicillin drops and ointment. If the cornea shows extensive ulceration, surgical treatment may be necessary. Symblepharon may be a late complication of lime burns, and should be prevented by packing the fornices with penicillin ointment (Minton, 1949).

(e) Calcium Carbide

Since 1894 calcium carbide has been made in quantity by heating a powdered mixture of quicklime and coke to a temperature of 2,000° C. in an electric furnace. The carbide formed is molten at the temperature of the furnace and so can be tapped off. Occupational dermatitis due to carbide was first reported in Vienna in 1913. Men handling the dry product may develop on the pads of the fingers necrotic ulcers with clearly marked edges. The caustic effect may involve also the mucous membrane of the lips and nose as well as the conjunctiva. The workers should wear gloves of sailcloth and goggles with dark glass. Receptacles containing carbide should be stored in dry, well-ventilated places. When proper equipment is installed and adequate precautions carried out, the carbide industry is no more dangerous than other industries (Koelsch, 1930).

(f) Calcium Cyanamide

When heated in an atmosphere of nitrogen to 1,100° C., calcium carbide forms calcium cyanamide and so furnishes a means for the fixation of atmospheric nitrogen. The mixture of quicklime, carbon and calcium cyanamide is sold as a fertilizer under the name *nitrolime*. When coming in contact with sweat or other moisture, nitrolime causes a pasty mass which sticks to the skin. This leads to a papular dermatitis followed by vesicles and weeping excoriations. Itching may be troublesome, and scratching often leads to secondary infection. Small ulcers on the mucous membrane of the mouth, as well as rhinitis, gingivitis and conjunctivitis, may occur. Good housekeeping in the factory and especially exhaust ventilation locally applied goes a long way to prevent these troubles (Koelsch, 1930).

(g) Calcium Sulphide

Calcium sulphide is made by heating slaked lime in an atmosphere of hydrogen sulphide. It is hydrolysed by water forming a mixture of hydroxide and hydrosulphide. It is used in industry for removing the hair from hides. Either in the powdered form or mixed with water, this substance has a corrosive action on the skin, mucous membranes or conjunctiva.

(h) Cement

When an argillaceous limestone or a chalk marl is calcined in a kiln, the lime produced is no longer pure calcium oxide and is sometimes referred to as a lean lime or a hydraulic lime because it slakes with only a feeble heat of hydration and has the property of setting under water. This lime contains a complex system of calcium oxide, alumina and silica, and combination occurs between these three oxides, giving rise to calcium aluminate and calcium silicate. These combinations occur independently of atmospheric carbon dioxide.

History of Cement Manufacture

The fact that marls on heating are converted into cement-like material which set when mixed with water was known to the Romans, who were probably the first to utilize hydraulic cement. Throughout the Middle Ages mortars and hydraulic cements were produced adventitiously. No fundamental knowledge of the essential setting materials was forthcoming until the middle of the eighteenth century, when John Smeaton was engaged in the rebuilding of the Eddystone lighthouse in 1756. He investigated several hydraulic limestones and showed by their composition why they made good cements.

Early Portland Cement

The Medway-Thames district of Kent is the historic home of cement, the essential ingredients of which, chalk and clay, occur locally in the North Downs and in Cliffe marshes. Clays originate from the weathering of feldspars, which are constituents of granite. The feldspar is more readily attacked by water and carbon dioxide than the other ingredients, quartz and mica. Natural cement rocks and marls occur in various parts of the world—for example, at Tring in the Chiltern Hills. Until it was all used up, there was at Snodland in Kent a Medway marl in which clay and chalk were of exactly the right proportions for cement—namely, 77 per cent of calcium carbonate. In 1824 in Northfleet, Kent, Joseph Aspden devised what he called Portland cement. He invented this name because the colour and properties of concrete made from the cement reminded him of Portland stone, a variety of dolomite. What he made was only a calcined and

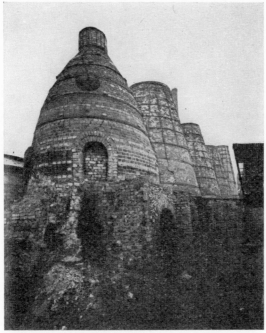

FIG. 140.—Cement Kiln used by Joseph Aspden in 1824 in Northfleet, Kent. It was destroyed by Enemy Action in 1943
(*By courtesy of Associated Portland Cement Manufacturers, Ltd.*)

not a clinkered mixture. The kiln which he used (fig. 140) was still to be seen in Northfleet until 1943, when it was destroyed by air warfare.

Modern Portland Cement

Modern Portland cement was first made in 1845 in Swanscombe, Kent, by burning the raw materials at a temperature sufficiently high to vitrify or clinker the mass. The raw materials are transported from quarries to a crusher house, where they are broken into sizes convenient for grinding. Proper proportions are passed through wash mills and pulverized to form a slurry, which is stored. For calcining this material the rotary kiln patented

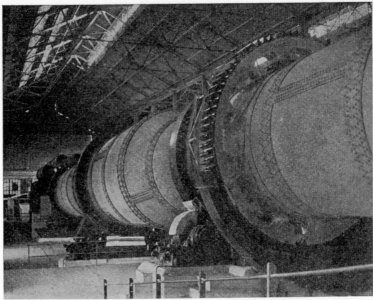

Fig. 141.—Modern Rotary Kiln, a huge steel Cylinder lined with Firebrick, used to make Cement
(*By courtesy of Associated Portland Cement Manufacturers, Ltd.*)

in 1885 by Ransome has superseded the stationary kiln. The original rotary kiln was 25 feet long. The most recent kiln is a steel cylinder lined with firebrick 405 feet long, 10 feet in diameter and set at an inclination of 1 in 25 (fig. 141).

Calcining the Slurry

The slurry is fed by gravity into the kiln at the upper and cooler end, where a system of moving chains dips into the wet material to expose a larger surface of the slurry to the hot gases issuing from the lower calcining region. These gases dry the incoming slurry, and as it descends to the hotter zone (1,540° C.) the clay and limestone react, evolving carbon dioxide and sulphur dioxide, the silica meantime fusing into a flux. In the hottest part of the kiln, calcination takes place and the lime, alumina and silica combine to form a cement clinker which is hard and bluish-black. It consists essentially of tricalcium silicate and aluminate. The clinker is cooled, mixed with 5 per cent gypsum to control the rate of setting and ground into powder in ball mills. Vertical storage is found most convenient, and modern cement silos hold as much as 28,000 tons.

Significance of Exposure to Dust

The manufacture of Portland cement is carried on all over the world. Employees at different parts of the works are frequently exposed to heavy concentrations of dust. Both the nature of the dust and the extent of exposure have forced upon doctors the need to investigate the state of health of workers in the industry. Gardner and others (1939) made a survey of seventeen cement works employing 2,278 men. While their work showed the presence of a high concentration of dust in the atmosphere of the finishing mills and packing departments, the dust was found to contain but very little free silica.

Absence of the Hazard of Silicosis

In the department where the raw materials were crushed by a dry process, the dust was found to contain from 1 to 30 per cent of silica. In spite of this, X-rays of the chest showed nodular silicosis in only eight out of the 2,278 employees, and in six of these previous exposure to silica dust in other jobs was evidently responsible. The incidence of tuberculosis and other chronic affections of the lung was found to be less than in the general population and it was concluded that prolonged inhalation of cement dust does not predispose to tuberculosis. In general, Gardner considered that, compared with the dust hazards in the mining and cutting of siliceous rock and other silica industries, the problem of dust disease of the lungs in the cement industry is trivial.

Hazard to Skin, Nose and Eyes

Cement workers, builders, labourers and others handling cement may suffer from dermatitis, conjunctivitis and injuries to the cornea. Marchand (1945) described symptomless perforation of the nasal septum as among the occupational disabilities of cement workers.

(j) Calcium Sulphate

Calcium sulphate occurs native as anhydrite, $CaSO_4$, and as gypsum, $CaSO_4.2H_2O$. If the gypsum occurs in clean, fine-grained masses it is called alabaster, if in colourless translucent crystals it is known as selenite, the σεληνίτης of Dioscorides, so named from σελήνη, the moon, probably in allusion to the soft moon-like reflection of light from some of its faces. Selenite must not be confused with compounds of selenium (see p. 484).

Permanent Hardness of Water

Deposits of gypsum are found in many parts of the world; in England it is quarried in Nottinghamshire, Staffordshire, Derbyshire, Cumberland and Sussex. It is a white substance so soft as to be scratched even by the finger-nail (hardness 1·5–2). It is slightly soluble in water, and waters percolating through gypseous strata dissolve the calcium sulphate and thus become permanently hard or selenitic. The scale formed in boilers by selenitic water is very hard. Water such as this has special value for brewing pale ale, and the water used by the Burton breweries is of this character; hence the addition of gypsum to water for purposes of brewing is known as *burtonization*.

Uses of Gypsum

Gypsum is used for making plaster of Paris and Keene's cement, whence it is sometimes known as *plaster stone*, and since much is sent to the Potteries for making moulds it is also termed *potter's stone*. It is employed in making mineral white or *terra alba*, in foundry cores, in paints, as a filler in paper and cotton, for dusting underground passages in collieries and in Portland cement to retard the time of setting. Gypsum is used as a soil fertilizer, as insulating material in building, for fireproof building blocks and for acoustical plaster in auditoriums.

Uses of Anhydrite

The anhydrite deposits at Billingham, County Durham, are treated with synthetic ammonia to form ammonium sulphate for use as a fertilizer. Much of the anhydrite is reduced with coke to form sulphur dioxide for the manufacture of sulphuric acid. The calcium carbonate formed during one of the processes is treated with nitrogen to form the fertilizer nitro-chalk.

Uses of Alabaster

Alabaster is a granular marble-like form of gypsum. It is usually white, pink or yellowish in colour, often with darker streaks and patches. In ancient Egypt, beautiful ornaments were carved in alabaster. Flower vases and lamps in this material found in the tomb of Tutankhamen have been preserved in the Cairo Museum. In the fourteenth and fifteenth centuries the gypsum quarries of Derbyshire and Nottinghamshire provided the material for schools of carvers who made alabaster reliefs for use as altar-pieces, not only throughout England but all over the Western world from Iceland to Portugal. Many fine alabaster tombs, effigies and monuments also were produced by these sculptors. On the continent of Europe the centre of the alabaster trade is Florence, but it is also mined in Greece and Germany.

Uses of Plaster of Paris

When gypsum is heated to 120° C. it loses more than half of its water of crystallization and forms the so-called hemi-hydrate, $(CaSO_4)_2H_2O$. This substance is known as plaster of Paris, having first been made from the gypsum of Montmartre. When water is added to plaster of Paris it forms a plastic mass which sets in ten minutes to a white, porous, hard mass. A slight expansion occurs during the setting so that it will take a sharp impression of a mould. It is therefore used by potters, modellers, marble workers, lithographers, orthopædic surgeons and dental surgeons. Plaster of Paris is extensively employed in the building trade in the form of wall plasters, sheets, plasterboard and wallboard, for stucco work and for temporary buildings at exhibitions such as the White City at Shepherd's Bush, London. Admixture of alum with plaster of Paris produces hard quick-setting cements such as *Keene's cement* and *parian*.

Exposure Hazards

The abundant white dust which covers from head to foot the miners of alabaster, gypsum and anhydrite, making them resemble millers, sets up only the slightest irritation of the eyes, nose and pharynx. There may be muco-purulent expectoration rich in dust particles, but diseases of the respiratory tract are not in excess of those for the general population. In the mines of Tuscany at Volterra, Pisa and Leghorn, rough shaping of the alabaster block is practised at the rock face and the miner carries each block out of the mine. This is a heavy task and many men develop scoliosis, with the concavity directed to the side opposite to that on which the block is habitually carried. On the shoulder, either on the right or left side, is a callosity, a fibro-lipoma with pronounced hypertrichosis, produced by the pressure of the alabaster block. Callosities caused by hammer and chisel are found on the hands (Pieraccini, 1906). Occasionally hydrogen sulphide is encountered as a hazard in gypsum mines.

(k) Calcium Chloride

In experimental pathology, calcium chloride is often chosen as a necrosing agent for various animal studies. In 1935 Oppenheimer described sloughing ulcers on the skin of an ice-cream maker who spilt drops of a concentrated solution of calcium chloride used as freezing salt on to the dorsa of his feet. Similar cases have been caused by the use of a method of dust suppression in the South Wales coal mines. The method depends upon the hygroscopic properties of calcium chloride used as a 40 per cent aqueous solution mixed with a wetting agent.

Indolent Ulceration of the Skin

Heppleston (1946) described the case of a man who sprayed the road-ways of a mine for eight hours with this solution, allowing some of it to contaminate his skin and his clothing. Burning pain in the areas of skin affected was followed by the appearance of pearly yellow nodules, especially on the legs where friction occurred from the tops of his rubber boots. Eleven days later the lesions on the legs and hands broke down, leaving large sloughing ulcers with raised, dark-red edges. The ulcers were so indolent that epithelialization was not completed until after thirteen weeks. The delayed resolution of the lesions must be attributed to the persistence of calcium-necrosed tissues.

Focal Necrosis of the Dermis only

Histological examination of one of these showed focal necrosis of the dermis without evidence of any kind of inflammatory reaction and without any change in the epidermis. The fact that the epithelium over the non-ulcerated lesion was normal suggests that strong aqueous solutions of calcium chloride can penetrate the epidermis, leaving it intact. The use of such solutions for industrial purposes demands adequate protection of the skin and especially of the eyes.

PHOSPHORUS

Phosphorus and its compounds give rise to poisoning in industry in four forms: (a) from handling yellow phosphorus; (b) from the inhalation of phosphoretted hydrogen; (c) from handling tri-*ortho*-cresyl phosphate, and (d) from the manufacture and use of organic phosphorus insecticides. Although yellow phosphorus is no longer used in the manufacture of matches, it is made on a large scale for military purposes. In order to prevent phossy jaw, strict precautions are necessary in handling it. Phosphine is a by-product of many processes, and wherever the hazard of poisoning exists the worker must wear appropriate breathing apparatus. Tri-*ortho*-cresyl phosphate is manufactured for use as a plasticizer. It inhibits the action of the enzyme acetylcholine esterase, or α-cholinesterase usually called cholinesterase. It particularly inhibits the pseudo-cholinesterase in the peripheral nerves and the white matter of the spinal cord. The organic phosphorus insecticides are also inhibitors of cholinesterase. Both the true and pseudo-enzyme activity may be greatly reduced by these compounds or, as in the case of tri-*ortho*-cresyl phosphate, there may be selective inhibition of pseudo-cholinesterase. Very great care is necessary in handling these substances both in the factory and in the field.

(a) Phosphorus

Phosphorus, P_4, does not occur free in nature because it is so very readily oxidized in contact with air. It is widely distributed in the form of phosphate rock which is impure calcium phosphate, $Ca_3(PO_4)_2$, and also as chlor-apatite, $3Ca_3(PO_4)_2.CaCl_2$, and fluor-apatite, $3Ca_3(PO_4)_2.CaF_2$. There are three allotropes of phosphorus: white (or yellow), red and black.

Properties of White Phosphorus

Pure white phosphorus is a transparent waxy solid soft enough to be cut with a knife. If exposed to light it undergoes yellow discoloration. It is highly inflammable, taking fire in the air at $30°$ C., burning with a bright white flame and forming dense white clouds of phosphorus pentoxide, P_2O_5. The heat of the body suffices to raise the temperature of phosphorus above its kindling temperature, hence it should always be picked up with forceps and never with bare fingers unless under water. Burns produced by phosphorus are very painful and heal only slowly. Yellow phosphorus is volatile at room temperature and its vapour is poisonous. In contact with air it is readily oxidized, giving off fumes of phosphorus trioxide, P_2O_3, which smell like garlic and are poisonous. When yellow phosphorus is exposed to air in the dark it emits a pale greenish light. This glow is associated with oxidation but is not completely understood.

Properties of Red Phosphorus

Red phosphorus, sometimes wrongly called amorphous phosphorus, is the stable form of phosphorus at ordinary temperatures. It is a reddish-violet powder which volatilizes only very slightly at $280°$ C. and does not glow in the dark. It is tasteless, odourless and non-poisonous. The difference between the molecules of red and yellow phosphorus is not known.

History

Phosphorus was discovered in 1674 by Hennig Brandt, a German alchemist and physician who worked in Hamburg. Envious opponents referred to him as an "uncouth physician who knew not a word of Latin." He was engaged in research and expected to make gold from human urine, or at least convert silver to gold. Instead, he produced a soft, white, waxy substance which glowed in the dark even when cold. Phosphorus was the first chemical element to be isolated by research methods. Although Brandt may have been disappointed at his failure to make gold, he earned his living afterwards by demonstrating the glow of phosphorus in dark rooms and advertising it as a valuable therapeutic agent. The risks of such therapy are illustrated in a story of later date. A doctor prescribed for a patient tonic pills containing strychnine and phosphorus, telling him to stop taking the pills should the strychnine make him twitch. The patient returned twenty-seven years later, and although he had not suffered from twitching he nevertheless had advanced phossy jaw (Coltart, 1931). At first Brandt kept his method of making phosphorus secret, but in 1676 he sold it to Krafft of Dresden who promised not to give it away. Krafft came to England and was rewarded for showing the glowing substance to King Charles II and his Court. During this visit in 1677 he hinted to Robert Boyle that phosphorus was prepared from "somewhat that belonged to the body of a man." In 1680 Boyle succeeded in making phosphorus by heating the residue from evaporated urine to a temperature high enough to reduce the sodium ammonium phosphate, with carbon already present or with added sand, and distilling over the free phosphorus into water.

Manufacture of Yellow Phosphorus

In 1771 Scheele showed that phosphorus could be prepared from bones heated with sand, and later devised the even better method of treating them with nitric acid. It is uneconomical to collect animal bones as a source of phosphorus, and in modern industry phosphate-bearing rocks and to some extent basic slag replace them. The process used is electrothermal. Phosphate rock, $Ca_3(PO_4)_2$, is mixed with anthracite and silica chippings and heated to 1,450° C. in the electric-arc furnace. The final products are carbon monoxide, which is used as fuel in the process, and phosphorus vapour. This is liquefied under water, and the crude phosphorus is stored and transported without exposure to air.

Manufacture of Red Phosphorus

Red phosphorus is made commercially by heating yellow phosphorus in an iron pot, having a cover through which passes a long narrow upright iron tube to prevent the development of pressure. The pot is heated to 240° C., the temperature being carefully controlled. A little of the phosphorus burns, removing the oxygen from the air initially present. When the conversion to the red form appears to be complete, the product is ground with water and boiled with sodium hydroxide solution to remove any unchanged yellow phosphorus. The red phosphorus is then washed with water and dried.

Uses

The use of phosphorus in the manufacture of matches, fireworks and for purposes of incendiary warfare is well-known. Although the use of white phosphorus is prohibited in the manufacture of fireworks, it is still used in making smoke screens, marker shells, tracer bullets, incendiary bombs, hand grenades, markers for air-sea rescue work and coloured flares for bombing. Phosphorus acts as a catalyst in the refining of petroleum, and is a constituent of alloys such as phosphor-tin which is used to make phosphor-bronze. Occasionally pastes containing from one to five per cent of yellow phosphorous are used to destroy rats and cockroaches. Unfortunately, too, (p. 374) zinc phosphide is used as a rodenticide and aluminium phosphide (p. 375) as an insecticide.

Compounds of phosphorus are necessary in the manufacture of detergents, in brewing, food processing and in the soft-drinks industry. Baking-powder contains calcium or sodium phosphate, which must be free from arsenic and fluorine compounds and is therefore made from pure phosphoric acid. In paper-making, printing and the manufacture of cellulose, dyes and soaps, phosphorus compounds are used in one form or another. Phosphoric acid is used in the rust-proofing of steel prior to painting.

Calcium phosphate is an important fertilizer, but its action is slow on account of its poor solubility. To convert it into a more soluble acid salt, it is treated with sulphuric acid in order to turn it into monocalcium phosphate, $Ca(H_2PO_4)_2$. This results in a mixture of the acid phosphate which has become $Ca(H_2PO_4)_2.H_2O$ and the sulphate, $CaSO_4.2H_2O$. This mixture, which is called superphosphate, usually contains a little undecomposed normal phosphate. Millions of tons of superphosphates are added to the soil in all parts of the world every year to provide phosphorus, which is essential for plant growth. Basic slag obtained in the manufacture of steel is another important fertilizer. It contains mainly calcium silico-phosphate, $Ca_3(PO_4)_2.CaSiO_3$.

The metaphosphates are of importance in the manufacture of detergents and in the processing of fibre. Sodium hexametaphosphate, $Na_2[Na_4(PO_3)_6]$, known commercially as *calgon*, is used for softening water on a small scale. This does not precipitate the calcium, but forms with it a complex ion which does not react with soap. Organic phosphorus compounds are used as plasticizers and insecticides.

The Lucifer Match

The first friction match contained potassium chlorate but no phosphorus. It was invented in 1826 by John Walker, a chemist of Stockton-on-Tees, and it took the form of a wooden splint, one end of which had been dipped into a paste containing potassium chlorate, antimony sulphide and gum arabic. The mat was ignited by folding a piece of sandpaper over the head and then drawing out the splint suddenly and forcibly. This match was copied in London by Samuel Jones and sold by him in 1829 under the name lucifer match.

The Congreve Match

It was soon found that a more readily ignitable match could be made with white phosphorus, and such matches became quickly popular. They were first manufactured in 1832 by J. Siegel in Austria and J. C. Kammerer in Germany, and they became known as congreves after Sir William Congreve who had died four years previously. A frictional surface was provided by sanding the side of the matchbox, but, of course, rubbing the match upon any hard substance was sufficient to ignite it. Although only a very small amount of the inflaming composition was placed on the tip of the match, all early forms of the phosphoric friction match were dangerous in the extreme, owing to their too-ready ignition. Houses were set on fire by boxes left on shelves and especially on window-sills exposed to the sun. A box of such matches receiving a sharp jar was likely to become ignited; and the destruction by fire of carriers' carts passing over rough roads was frequently caused by the ignition of boxes of matches included in their lading. Protective metal boxes were devised, but the fire hazard was not eliminated. Before 1840 the congreve match had driven the lucifer out of use, but the name lucifer remained and became used vulgarly to designate many kinds of match, none of which had any but a general resemblance to the original lucifer of Jones. The congreve match remained in use in Great Britain until about 1870.

Phossy Jaw

Meanwhile the stage had been set for the greatest tragedy in the whole story of occupational disease. Unhappily, white phosphorus is a deadly poison. In 1844, twelve years after phosphorus matches were first manufactured, phosphorus necrosis of the jaw was identified and twenty-two cases were reported from match factories near Vienna. Within a few years practically every civilized country had discovered this new occupational disease. The poisoning was slow to occur, the average time of onset after the man was first exposed being five years (Oliver, 1902). Less than 5 per cent of those exposed acquired the disease. Some extremely susceptible patients were found who succumbed to the effects of the poison within a few months.

Early Symptoms

The first symptom is toothache, which usually begins in a tooth already affected with caries. At first the pain is slight, amounting to little more than discomfort, and it may be intermittent. A dull red spot on the buccal mucosa is present at this stage and is pathognomonic of phosphorus necrosis of the jaw (Kennon and Hallam, 1944). At a later stage it is common to find a sinus surrounded by dull red mucosa leading to a cavity beneath. Sequestra up to one centimetre in diameter may be found. They are both osteoporotic and carious, and have been likened to pumice stone.

Abscesses and Sequestra

In the middle of the nineteenth century the hazard was not fully understood. Many cases occurred in which pain, increasing in severity, followed the early symptoms, and swelling of the gum and jaw soon appeared. Suppuration occurred spontaneously, or more commonly, after dental extraction. If the worker returned to work too soon and was again exposed to phosphorus, the inflammation spread rapidly. Chronic abscesses were formed, and sequestra continued to separate over many years and would sometimes involve the whole jaw. It was the most distressing of all the occupational diseases because it was very painful and was accompanied by a fetid discharge which made its victims almost unendurable to others.

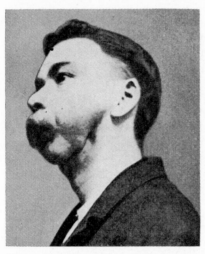

Disfigurement

It was obstinate and chronic, the treatment was agonizing, and the final result was a distressing disfigurement (fig. 142). It was this disfiguring effect plain to every observer that made phosphorus poisoning so notorious and led to determined efforts for its abolition in all countries. Sometimes extension of the suppuration to the orbit or meninges caused death, but more often this was brought about by septicæmia.

FIG. 142.—Deformity resulting from Excision of Entire Lower Jaw in a Case of Phosphorus Necrosis
(*Case of Dr. J. P. Andrews. "The Occupational Diseases," W. Gilman Thompson, D. Appleton Co., New York, 1914*)

The mortality rate was about 20 per cent. Involvement of bones other than the jaw leading to multiple spontaneous fractures was recorded in many countries (Dearden, 1899). The case here recorded from the records of the London Hospital will serve to point out the horrors of phosphorus necrosis of the jaw.

Case 11. Match dipper—exposure to white phosphorus for twelve years— phosphorus necrosis of jaws—excision of entire lower jaw.

A. R., a man aged 30, L.H. Reg. No. 597/1879. Admitted to the London Hospital under the care of Dr. Hughlings Jackson. *Twelve years:* employed as a match dipper using white phosphorus. *Twelve weeks:* pain in gums and teeth of left upper jaw. Three teeth extracted without relief, the pain subsequently extending to the left eyebrow and orbit.

On examination: prominence of left cheek with swelling and tenderness of gums in left upper jaw. Many teeth loose and surrounded by purulent sinuses. In August and September 1879 three operations were performed by Mr. Rivington and Mr. Reeves for removal of teeth and necrosed bone in the left superior maxilla. In September

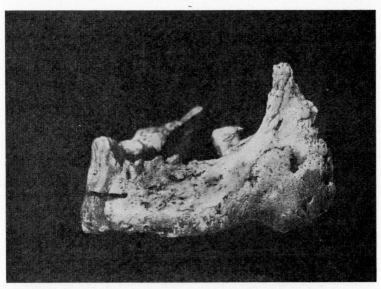

FIG. 143.—Case 11. Entire Lower Jaw excised by Mr. Jeremiah McCarthy in 1884 in the case of a man who had been employed for 12 years as a Match Dipper using Yellow Phosphorus
(*London Hospital Medical College Museum*)

1879 pain and swelling occurred in the right side of the face and mouth, and necrosed bone was removed from the right superior maxilla. He then remained ill with a fetid discharge from the upper jaw, until in 1884 great pain and swelling occurred in the left side of the lower jaw. Between June and August 1884 four operations were performed on the lower jaw by Mr. Waren Tay for removal of necrosed bone. Improvement was only temporary, and in November 1884 Mr. McCarthy excised the whole of the lower jaw, which showed extensive necrosis (fig. 143). No further account of this case is to be found in the records, but the fate of the patient may readily be imagined.

Secondary Infection

The way in which phosphorus acts to produce necrosis of the jaw is unknown. It seems likely that it is absorbed into the blood stream and deposited in bone, particularly in the lower jaw. Infection occurs later from a dental source. This theory is supported by the analogous condition, delayed necrosis of the jaw following exposure to radium. In both there is commonly a latent interval, sequestra separate slowly and incompletely, and exacerbation of symptoms frequently follows upon extraction of a tooth (Kennon, 1944). The radiographic and histological changes in early cases indicate that the periosteal reaction is secondary to infection. The early changes are osteoporosis, decalcification and rarefaction of both sequestrum and surrounding bone. The sequestra of osteomyelitis are, by contrast, dense and well calcified (Kennon and Hallam, 1944).

The Salvation Army investigates Phossy Jaw

About 1890 General Booth discovered that some of Britain's most important match-manufacturers treated their 4,000 employees very badly and he set out to stir the nation's conscience. His chief investigator, Colonel James Barker soon came up with a burden of appalling proof. In one case a mother and two children aged under nine were slaving in a factory sixteen hours a day to make approximately 1,000 match-boxes for a pay of 1s. 3¾d. Unable to pause even for meals, they gobbled dry bread as they pasted and cut. But there were worse evils than sweating. Though many countries compelled their match manufacturers to paste harmless red phosphorus on the side of the match-box, Britain lagged behind. To flood the market with vast quantities of cheap wax-vestas, manufacturers dipped their match-heads in yellow phosphorus. At the rock bottom price of a penny per dozen boxes, these strike-anywhere matches were a tempting bargain. For these excessive profits others paid with their lives. So toxic were the fumes of yellow phosphorus that Barker found scores of women workers plagued by severe pain in the jaw resulting from phosphorus necrosis.

General Booth's model Match Factory

The Salvation Army was swift to act. As early as May, 1891, Booth's airy, well-lit model match-factory for 120 workers opened in East London at Lamprell Street, Old Ford. From the first his *Lights in Darkest England* match-boxes held only safety matches tipped with harmless red phosphorus. At peak this factory was turning out six million boxes a year. But Booth was not in business for its own sake: he was out to reform the industry from top to bottom. Soon James Barker was piloting conducted tours of newsmen and members of Parliament round the factory-workers' homes to demonstrate the grim price of matches at twopence farthing a gross as against The Salvation Army's regulation fourpence. At the climax of each visit, Barker would lean forward to turn out the gaslight and a low gasp of horror stirred in the room. In the darkness the victim's jaw as well as hands and blouse glowed greenish-white like a spectre's. The campaign was no overnight success for conservative Britons still prized strike-anywhere matches above the new Swedish safety-matches. And so not for the first time, Booth had pointed the Victorians towards recognition of the need for modified State intervention. Gilbert Bartholomew, managing director of Bryant and May's match factory gave promising evidence to the Home Office Lucifer Match Committee, namely that his firm had totally banned the use of yellow phosphorus for ten months. But Booth, a year earlier, had closed down his own factory, aware that *Darkest England* had scored its first victory (Collier, 1965).

Berne Convention of 1906

Abolition did not come easily. All sorts of preventive measures were first tried, the British and German regulations being very elaborate and detailed. In Great Britain, not only were the factories constructed according to Government requirements and special machinery introduced, but a limit was imposed as to the proportion of phosphorus in the paste, and the employer was required to furnish tooth-brushes, mouth-washes and free dental service. These requirements were financially burdensome to the manufacturer and irksome to the workers; furthermore, they failed in their purpose. Abolition began to exercise the minds of men in the Governments of the chief match-producing countries in the world. Finland took the first step, abolishing the use of white phosphorus in 1872, and Denmark followed her example in 1874, Switzerland in 1898 and the Netherlands in 1901. In 1906 all the important countries of Europe agreed by the Berne Convention to forbid the manufacture and import of white phosphorus matches. In 1910 in England the use of white phosphorus in the manufacture of matches was prohibited by law. Thus for the first time, and as yet for the last, by agreement amongst the nations of Europe, a notorious danger in industry was legislated out of existence. In 1919 India and Japan agreed to abolish the use of white phosphorus in the manufacture of matches, and the League of Nations induced China to do likewise in 1925.

America Disillusioned

In the United States of America the belief was held by medical men and by the general public that phossy jaw never occurred in American match manufacture because the factories were so much cleaner and superior in every way to European ones and the employees so much better paid and better fed. America was disillusioned in 1902, and within a few years of this date 150 cases, including four deaths, were recorded (Andrews, 1910). In 1931 the United States Federal Government, which could not on constitutional grounds sign the Berne Convention, passed a law placing a prohibitive tax on white phosphorus matches and forbidding their import and export.

Failure of Hygienic Methods

The history of phosphorus poisoning shows that a very serious disease can exist in an industry without medical men knowing anything about it;

that all possible hygienic measures may prove to be unavailing in the prevention of further cases; that when this proves to be the case the only thing to do is to work for abolition of the poisonous substance in question; and that it is possible by arousing public opinion to bring about such abolition in all civilized lands, although the industry involved is large, important and influential, and even, as in the case of France, a lucrative Government monopoly.

Harmless Derivatives of Phosphorus

Two discoveries by chemists have been responsible for rendering harmless the processes in the manufacture of matches. In 1844 a Swedish professor of chemistry, Gustaf E. Pasch, stated the principle of the safety match.

Red Phosphorus

In 1845 Professor Anton Schrötter of Vienna discovered the allotrope red phosphorus, which was found to be harmless. By 1851 this was produced in a pure state and on a commercial scale in England. In 1855 the Swede J. E. Lundström, using English red phosphorus, succeeded in making a satisfactory safety match and he may be regarded as the actual inventor. The match-head contains the oxidizing ingredients potassium chlorate and antimony sulphide, and these are separated from the inflaming ingredients red phosphorus and sand, which are spread on the outside edges of the box. Since the match can be ignited only on this specially prepared surface, security against accidental fires is obtained. What is even more important is that red phosphorus cannot produce phossy jaw nor, indeed, any other harmful effect on the worker.

Phosphorus Sesquisulphide

Unhappily, for forty-three more years strike-anywhere matches continued to be made with the noxious white phosphorus. Then in 1898 two French Government chemists, H. Sévène and E. D. Cahen, discovered the harmless phosphorus sesquisulphide, P_4S_3, and used it as a satisfactory substitute for white phosphorus. Since 1900 strike-anywhere matches have been made with this substance in all industrial countries and no harm has ever come to the worker who handles it.

Phossy Jaw in Modern Times

In a phosphor-bronze works in Austria a case of phossy jaw occurred, although the proportion of phosphorus in the bronze was only 0·76 per cent (Hamilton, 1925). In 1923 Pickerill described a case in a man aged sixty who had been engaged for many years in mixing rabbit poison containing white phosphorus. In 1928 Ward reported fourteen cases of phosphorus necrosis of the jaw in workers in the fireworks industry. Thirteen of these patients were women. Acute phosphorus poisoning occurred among children who put such fireworks into their mouths (Heimann, 1946). The occurrence of phosphorus caries and necrosis in modern times is illustrated in eight cases reported by Kennon and Hallam (1944). These occurred in an up-to-date factory manufacturing white phosphorus for military purposes.

Preventive Treatment

Successful supervision of the worker handling white phosphorus demands elaborate and continuous care of the teeth and jaws. A dental clinic with X-ray equipment and the services of dental surgeons is essential. Records must be kept of all those exposed to the hazard, and it should be known which workers have been excluded permanently or temporarily from exposure. Employees must be carefully selected. Not only must they have good general health, but also their teeth must be normal both clinically and radiologically. X-ray examination of both jaws should be made before work begins, and it must be repeated annually. The X-ray films must be searched in detail for areas of decalcification indicating caries of bone. This is of special importance in the third to fifth years of employment. Repeated routine dental examination must be carried out in every worker showing symptoms.

Surgical Treatment

Where a sequestrum is found and surgical treatment undertaken for its removal, rapid and complete recovery follows. The dreadful sequelæ of the neglected disease need never occur. Indeed, in Great Britain, during the Second World War when the amount of white phosphorus manufactured for use in incendiary warfare exceeded all previous record, no case of advanced phossy jaw developed. This was entirely due to the provision of efficient dental units. All workers at risk were examined at regular intervals, and at the earliest signs of necrosis of the jaw were treated and removed from further exposure (fig. 144). No patient who has ever had a jaw lesion should be allowed to return to work involving exposure to phosphorus (Baron, 1944). Many cases are known where the disease has revealed itself up to two years after a worker has left the industry concerned.

(b) Phosphoretted Hydrogen

Phosphoretted hydrogen or phosphine, PH_3, is a colourless gas with a distinctive and most disagreeable odour like decaying fish. It has a specific gravity 1·53 times that of air. Even 2 parts per 100,000 in the atmosphere is perceptible and 20 parts per 100,000 will quickly cause death. It is not a substance of any great commercial importance, and cases of poisoning are usually accidental rather than due to exposure to phosphine evolved continuously from manufacturing operations.

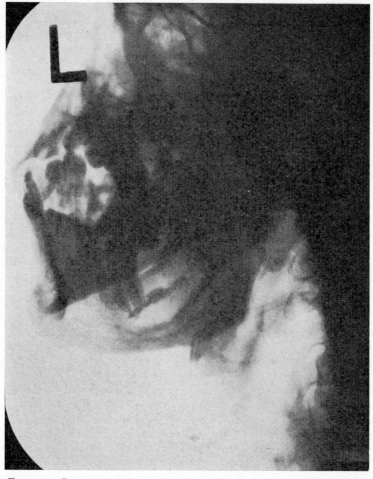

FIG. 144.—Sequestrum in Lower Jaw detected by Routine Radiographic Examination and removed surgically in a man making White Phosphorus for
Incendiary Warfare

(*By courtesy of Dr. A. Thelwall Jones*)

Uses

Phosphine is carried about in steel cylinders, and these must be labelled
clearly as dangerous and poisonous. Poisoning may arise in the preparation
and use of calcium phosphide for filling certain kinds of flare mines, in the
manufacture of acetylene with impure calcium carbide, in the quenching
of metal alloys with water, in the accidental wetting of zinc phosphide for
use as a rodenticide and of aluminium phosphide in fumigating grain,
and even in the chemical preparation and handling of phosphoretted
hydrogen in the laboratory. Gessner (1937) reported twelve cases of illness
beginning with nausea and including one death in a house adjacent to a

warehouse in which bags of aluminium phosphide were stored and had become damp. The atmospheric moisture had caused the liberation of phosphine in dangerous concentrations. In Sydney, Australia, Bell (1961) saw fifty cases of mild poisoning in men fumigating grain to kill insects by means of tablets of aluminium phosphide wetted with water. The men were young; most of them had mild respiratory symptoms and a few had angina and quickly recovered. One man, in spite of strict instructions to the contrary, removed his canister gas-mask while in the grain store and instantly died. Many of the cases of poisoning recorded have resulted from the carriage of ferro-silicon as badly ventilated cargoes when the persons responsible were ignorant of the nature of the poison evolved.

Cargoes of Ferro-Silicon

Between 1905 and 1908 a number of cases of mysterious illness, often with dramatically fatal outcome, occurred in ships and canal boats carrying cargoes of ferro-silicon. The matter was investigated by Copeman (1909) and by Hake (1910). They concluded that grades of ferro-silicon containing from 40 to 60 per cent of silica were the most dangerous. Their work showed that the poisonous substances evolved from ferro-silicon consisted mainly of phosphoretted hydrogen, sometimes accompanied by small proportions of arseniuretted hydrogen and acetylene. They attributed the evolution of these gases to the action of water on calcium phosphide, arsenide and carbide respectively. They did not make it clear which of the gases they held responsible for the symptoms of poisoning. Subsequent writers have also evaded this question and the cases are often referred to under the heading of arseniuretted hydrogen poisoning.

Symptoms and Signs

The chief symptoms are abdominal pain, nausea, vomiting and severe diarrhœa, often followed by staggering gait, convulsions, coma and death within twenty-four hours. Neither jaundice nor anæmia appears to have been described in any of the reports. In rabbits and guinea-pigs, phosphine, unlike arsine, does not affect the blood picture (Muller, 1940). In one series of cases, Bruylants and Druyts (1909) found traces of arsenic present in the bodies of all of four cases. It seems probable that phosphoretted hydrogen was responsible for the symptoms observed in most of these cases, if not in all. Indeed, very often phosphoretted hydrogen alone has been obtained from samples of the ferro-silicon concerned (Thiele, 1921).

Preventive Measures

Where exhaust ventilation is installed, it should work in a downward direction since the gas is heavier than air. A breathing apparatus should be used which enables the worker to breathe the outside air. Such an apparatus has been worn with success by girls engaged in filling mines with calcium phosphide. The following recommendations suggested by Copeman should be adopted in handling ferro-silicon: it must be broken up into pieces of the size required at the place where it is used; it must be exposed to the air in a sheltered place for a month at least before being loaded into ships; prohibition of transport in passenger ships or on the top of the cargo must be enforced—it should be carried on deck or, if this cannot be managed, in holds carefully ventilated and separated by airtight doors from living quarters; these measures must apply to barges in inland waters: packing-cases containing ferro-silicon should have inscribed on them clear particulars concerning the materials, such as the percentage of silicon, the date of manufacture and the place of origin. Where ferro-silicon is stored, work should never begin until the room has been ventilated. Zangger (1930) recommended that such storerooms should be under lock and key and that no one should be allowed inside without a permit from the person responsible for effective renewal of the air. Masters of ships carrying ferro-silicon should not only take all necessary measures of safety but should also instruct all persons handling the product as to the risk.

(c) Tri-*ortho*-cresyl Phosphate

Tri-*ortho*-cresyl phosphate is sometimes known in industry as *lindol*. It is used in the recovery of phenol residues from gas-plant effluents, and as a grinding medium for pigments, and it is added to petrol to make for smoother running of motor-car engines by controlling pre-ignition. It is added as a plasticizer to cable sheaths, lacquers, textile coatings, polyvinyl chloride sheeting and other plastics.

The Action of Plasticizers

A plasticizer is a substance used to render a plastic material more pliable. By alteration of the amount of the plasticizer added, such characteristics as flexibility, hardness, water-resistance and inflammability can be varied between wide limits. In the plastics industry TOCP is used in large quantities—for example, as much as 50 per cent is sometimes added to polyvinyl chloride. Tricresyl phosphate used in industry is an oil with a slightly pungent odour; of the three isomerides, the *ortho*- and *meta*- are liquids and the *para*- is a crystalline solid. Industrial tricresyl phosphate is prepared by treating cresols with phosphorus oxychloride in the presence of an aluminium catalyst.

Effect upon Pseudo-cholinesterase

TOCP inhibits the action of pseudo-cholinesterase, an enzyme present in the blood-serum, the peripheral nerves and the white matter of the spinal cord, and distinct from the true cholinesterase present at the motor end-plates and in the red blood cells. Bloch (1941) showed that the cholinesterase of horse serum was inhibited by low concentrations of TOCP. Two years later Hottinger and Bloch (1943) demonstrated that the hydrolysis of acetylcholine by human and rabbit serum, liver and brain was also inhibited by TOCP; in addition, the splitting of tributyrin by serum and liver was found to be diminished by this compound, although serum phosphatase and pancreatic lipase were unaffected. No attempt was made at that time to study the different types of cholinesterase by means of selective substrates.

Maintenance of the Myelin Sheaths of Nerve

Earl and Thompson (1952) studied the action of TOCP on the true and pseudo-cholinesterases of a number of tissues of man, the rabbit, the chicken and the rat. With human tissues TOCP was found to be a selective inhibitor of the pseudo-cholinesterase, concentrations which caused 75–99 per cent inhibition of this enzyme in cerebrum, spinal cord, sciatic nerve and serum causing only 7–10 per cent inhibition of the true cholinesterase in cerebrum, spinal cord, striated muscle and erythrocytes. With rabbit and chicken tissues a selective inhibition of the pseudo-cholinesterase was also observed, although tissues from these species were rather less sensitive to TOCP than those from man. The pseudo-cholinesterase of the albino rat, an animal apparently insensitive to poisoning by TOCP, was only partially inhibited even by very high concentrations; the true cholinesterase in this species was also insensitive. The possibility must therefore be considered that the pseudo-cholinesterase of nerve tissue may be connected in some way with the maintenance of the myelin sheaths of nerve fibres, and that inhibition of this enzyme by TOCP may play a part in the production of the demyelination and consequent paralysis.

Multiple Neuritis from Phospho-creosote in 1899

In TOCP poisoning the clinical picture is that of a polyneuritis with flaccid paralysis of the distal muscles of the upper and lower extremities. Slow but complete recovery usually occurs. Opportunities to study this clinical picture occurred during a period of forty years prior to the discovery of the first victim of industrial poisoning. It was encountered in patients treated for pulmonary tuberculosis with phospho-creosote, in people who had partaken of a beverage known as *Jamaica ginger* or *jake*, in women who had taken apiol as an abortifacient, and in certain victims fed on a soya bean cooking oil adulterated by accident. In 1899 Lorot reported six cases of multiple neuritis out of forty-one cases of pulmonary tuberculosis treated with phospho-creosote. This substance was discovered in 1894. Later, it was shown to contain 15 per cent of TOCP. In the next thirty-five years fifty-three additional cases were recorded in various parts of continental Europe (Roger and Recordier, 1934).

Jamaica Ginger Paralysis in 1930

In the spring of 1930 there appeared suddenly, in the mid-western and south-western states of the United States of America, an outbreak of paralysis characterized by bilateral foot- and wrist-drop. During March and April of that year almost 4,000 cases were reported in the Press throughout the United States of America. During the whole year 16,000 people were affected, and of these ten died. A connexion was immediately recognized between this paralysis and the ingestion of adulterated samples of a popular alcoholic drink known as *Jamaica ginger* or *jake*. The quantity of ginger fluid consumed was not the determining factor in the severity of the symptoms which follow; a single drink is known to have produced the same result as that following the use of the beverage for many days.

Illness Develops by Three Stages

The clinical picture develops by three stages. In some cases there are early transient gastro-intestinal symptoms including nausea, vomiting, diarrhœa and abdominal pain. These clear up and a symptom-free interval follows lasting from five to twenty-one days, the average being ten days. This interval is followed by soreness of the muscles below the knees, and numbness of the toes and fingers lasting several days and followed by weakness of the toes and bilateral foot-drop. After another interval of about ten days, weakness of the fingers and wrist-drop follow. This paralysis is not usually as severe as that in the feet and legs. In the upper extremities paralysis does not extend above the elbows. The thigh muscles may be involved in advanced cases. Loss of sphincter control is unusual.

Toxic Effects on Animals

By July 1930 Smith and Elvove proved that the adulterated beverage contained about 2 per cent of TOCP and that this caused the paralysis. The reason for including this substance as one of the ingredients is not known. It may have been used deliberately on account of its physical properties, or it may have been an accidental contaminant. By subcutaneous injection of samples of the adulterated drink, as well as of pure synthetic TOCP, Smith and Elvove succeeded in producing a paralysis comparable to that seen in human beings in a variety of laboratory animals including hens, rabbits, calves, dogs and monkeys. Later, in 1930, Smith and Elvove showed that the specific attack of TOCP on the motor nerves is not shared by the *meta-* or *para*-cresyl esters nor by the phenyl ester. The minimal lethal dose of TOCP was approximately thirty times less than that of triphenyl phosphate.

Follow-up of 316 Cases

Zeligs (1938) had the opportunity to follow up 316 cases of *jake* paralysis during six years. His description of the clinical picture in 1930 and later in 1936 shows that the poison may attack the anterior horn cells and the pyramidal tracts in addition to the peripheral motor nerves. In 1930 all the patients had typical foot-drop, the degree of paralysis varying from slight muscular weakness to complete flaccid paralysis of all the muscles of the feet and legs. In about three-fourths of the cases the upper extremities became similarly involved, wrist-drop being common. The ankle-jerks were absent, the knee-jerks present and in many cases over-active. There were no abnormal plantar responses and no ankle clonus. Sensory changes were absent. During the next six years many of the patients recovered completely, and others improved sufficiently to be able to use their hands and feet adequately.

Patients permanently Crippled

Out of 316 patients admitted to the Cincinnati General Hospital in 1930, a group of sixty men were found still in institutions in 1936. They hobbled about with the aid of sticks. Physical examination showed spastic paralysis with adductor spasm, paralytic talipes, exaggerated tendon reflexes and extensor plantar responses. In the upper extremities there was marked atrophy of the extensors of the wrists and of the interossei, with bilateral claw hands. In severely poisoned cases in addition to the peripheral motor nerves, the anterior horn cells, the pyramidal tracts and the spino-cerebellar tracts may be involved. Extreme muscular wasting tends to mask the involvement of the upper motor neurone. When muscular activity is partially restored the spastic signs of the previously hidden upper motor neurone lesion become clinically apparent. In such cases the end-result resembles amyotrophic lateral sclerosis.

Adulteration of Apiol in 1931

In 1931 ter Braak reported in Holland an outbreak of some forty cases of paralysis from the use of apiol (*Petroselinum sativum*) as an abortifacient. During 1931 and 1932 fifty more cases were published from Germany, France, Switzerland and Jugoslavia. Samples of apiol were found to be adulterated with TOCP to the extent of 28–50 per cent (Germon, 1932). Nobody knows why this substance was chosen as an adulterant. Neither in colour, taste nor odour do the two oils resemble each other. In the women affected there was a lower motor neurone paralysis of the distal muscles of the extremities, without sensory loss.

Adulteration of Soya-bean Oil in 1937

In 1937 there occurred an outbreak affecting sixty-eight people who had partaken of soya-bean oil used for salads and for cooking. Forty-one of these people lived in Natal and the other twenty-seven travelled to London in a steamship, the *Jean L.D.*, which had been provisioned in Durban (Sampson, 1938, 1942). This oil was found to contain 0·4 per cent of TOCP. The victims first had gastro-intestinal symptoms, and seven to fourteen days later developed cramps in the calves of their legs. Ultimately lower motor neurone paralysis of the feet and hands supervened, but sensation was unimpaired.

Tragic Accident in the Swiss Army in 1940

In 1940 a tragedy occurred involving eighty officers and men of a company of machine gunners in the Swiss army. Twelve litres of TOCP issued for anti-rust treatment of the bands of the machine guns were added in error to the cooking oil used to make cheese fritters. Within a few hours of eating the meal the victims were prostrated with gastro-enteritis, and after a week they had pain and severe stiffness in muscles followed by flaccid paralysis of the feet and legs and occasionally of the hands and arms too. The existence of a primary lesion of skeletal muscle was proved by biopsy investigations. Histological examination revealed waxy degeneration followed by regeneration of muscle fibrils. In thirty-eight cases the syndrome of muscular pseudospasticity persisted after five years, at which time fourteen only of the cases were completely well and fifteen were still totally incapacitated (Walthard, 1946).

Shortage of Fats in Germany in 1942

Owing to shortage of fats in Germany in the Second World War, cases of TOCP poisoning occurred in Munster. The patients were factory workers who had obtained a fat substitute from their place of work. They had taken it home and, because of the shortage of natural animal and vegetable fats, had used it to fry potato pancakes. They developed nausea, vomiting, abdominal cramps and diarrhœa, followed in ten days by rapidly increasing weakness of the feet, legs and then arms. There was progressive atrophy of the muscles. As a result of this outbreak, a warning was issued to factory medical officers in Germany, who were instructed to prevent recurrences by education and propaganda (Humpe, 1942).

Adulteration of Cotton-seed Oil in 1946

In 1946 an outbreak occurred of twenty-one cases in North Wales and nineteen cases on Merseyside of bilateral foot-drop with weakness of the hands and wrists, but without sensory changes. Most of the patients gave a history of gastric symptoms about ten days before the onset of the weakness in the limbs. The TOCP was traced to cotton-seed oil used in frying, and it was presumed but not proved that the poison reached the oil from second-hand containers previously used for industrial purposes (Holston, 1946).

Mass Poisoning in Morocco in 1959

In the autumn of 1959 more than 10,000 cases of tri-*ortho*-cresyl phosphate poisoning occurred in seven different towns in Morocco. The clinical picture was one of acute peripheral neuritis in which the distribution of the weakness was distal. In addition there were less striking signs of an upper-motor-neurone lesion. Smith and Spalding (1959) were convinced on a visit to Meknes, where the standard of living was low, that the distribution of cases did not correspond to the spread of an infection. The doctor in charge of the dispensaries there told that he had recently seen samples of cooking oil which were as dark as old motor oil and that some patients believed that this oil was responsible for the illness. Samples of oil bought at the grocer's shop in Meknes were analysed and found to contain phosphates and cresols. The lubricating oil was man-made and tri-*ortho*-cresyl phosphate had been added to it to stand the very high temperatures pertaining to turbo-jet aircraft engines. The fraudulent adulteration was traced to Moroccan dealers who had purchased military surplus stocks at a US air base.

Cases of Poisoning in the Chemical Industry in 1942

In the early part of the Second World War black-out regulations in Great Britain imposed as a precaution against air attack led to the occurrence of polyneuritis in three workmen employed in a manufacturing plant (Hunter, Perry and Evans, 1944). All three of these men worked in a room about 25 feet long, 12 feet wide and 12 feet high, which owing to black-out regulations was totally enclosed during the hours of darkness although it was provided with a roof vent. During daylight, doors and windows were open. The men worked at wash-tanks which were roughly cubic vessels about 5 feet in width with a partially open top. The closed-in portion of the top supported the various fittings, one of these being a 6-inch vent-pipe extending through the roof to the open air.

Exposure Hazards

Crude tricresyl phosphate entered these tanks at a temperature of approximately 60° C. At this stage it contained hydrochloric acid which gave it an unpleasant, irritating odour. However, it was immediately cooled by treatment with an equal volume of cold water, this operation being carried out by opening a valve and shutting it at the appropriate moment. The washing was automatic, but it was nevertheless possible for the men to inhale vapour from the tanks. The cold tricresyl phosphate is of low volatility, having a very small vapour pressure at ordinary temperatures. The *ortho*-isomer content of the finished product was about 60 per cent. The three affected men also handled triphenyl phosphate.

Atmosphere Concentration of Tricresyl Phosphate

It was not possible at the time the men were poisoned to determine the concentration of tricresyl phosphate which was present in the atmosphere. This, however, was estimated at a later date when conditions were arranged to reproduce those in operation at the time. The injectors, fans and air-conditioning plant were shut off, the covers of the washing vats left open and the water drained from the cooler. The determinations were carried out during daytime, and also during simulated and actual black-out conditions. The highest concentration of tricresyl phosphate was found in the room containing the washing vats after the hot liquid had been blown over from the reaction vessels into the washing vats. It amounted to no more than 0·6 parts per million by volume.

Symptoms and Signs

Our three patients had been at work for two and a half years, eight months, and six months respectively. The toxic condition started with cramp-like pains in the hands and feet, difficulty in walking and attacks of diarrhœa sometimes accompanied by abdominal pain. The typical physical signs of polyneurit is developed with weakness of muscles in all four limbs slight wasting, hypotonus and a high-stepping gait. Sometimes fibrillary tremors were seen in muscles, especially in the thighs. The plantar responses were always flexor. In the acute stage the tendo-achillis and calves were tender on pressure, but there was no loss of sensation to pin-prick or cotton-wool touch, and the appreciation of posture and vibration of a tuning fork were unimpaired. The cerebrospinal fluid was normal. After rest in bed and treatment by massage, foot-drop was corrected by fitting uplifting toe springs to the boots. All three patients recovered completely in periods of twelve months, four years, and ten months respectively.

Toxic Effects in Domestic Fowls

Flinn (1943) was able to produce paralysis in twenty-eight days in domestic fowls fed with cellophane, containing 11 per cent of TOCP, in amounts of one gram per kilo of body weight. Hunter, Perry and Evans (1944) attempted to confirm these experimental observations. Twelve twelve-week-old hens were fed with gelatin-coated capsules containing 0·5 gram of triphenyl phosphate or of one of the pure isomers of tricresyl phosphate. Four hens were used as controls, and two each were fed with tri-*meta*, tri-*para*, and tri-*ortho*-cresyl phosphate and triphenyl phosphate. Unfortunately two of the controls developed fowl paralysis after the others had had two grams of the substance under test. It was noticed, however, that the two hens which received the TOCP became completely paralysed in the wings and legs. The fowl paralysis in the controls rendered this experiment unsatisfactory, and it was therefore repeated with twelve twelve-week-old cockerels. After receiving 3 grams of TOCP two cockerels became paralysed (fig. 145) and died four days after receiving

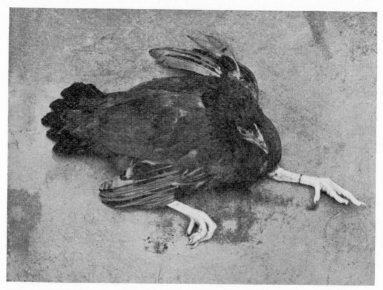

Fig. 145.—Cockerel paralysed by Polyneuritis 14 days after a dose of 2 grams of Tri-*ortho*-cresyl Phosphate

3·5 grams. After 12·5 grams the two cockerels fed with tri-*meta*-cresyl phosphate showed considerable weakness of the legs, and after 15·5 grams they developed respiratory paralysis. Being grossly emaciated they were then killed. The cockerels which were fed with tri-*para*-cresyl phosphate and triphenyl phosphate showed no evidence of ill health after they had received 25 grams.

Experiments on Skin Absorption

Hodge and Sterner (1943) estimated the amount of TOCP that can be absorbed through unbroken skin, and how rapidly the absorption occurs. TOCP containing radioactive phosphorus was used and the absorption measured in two human subjects and one dog. The human subjects applied 0·22 gram and 0·11 gram of the TOCP with radioactivity of 395,000 counts per min. per 0·1 gram. The first had 13 micrograms of TOCP per 100 ml. of blood at the end of one hour, and he excreted 7 micrograms in the urine in the first hour, and continued at 35 micrograms an hour for the next twenty-four hours. He excreted 797 micrograms or 0·36 per cent of the amount applied. The second had 4 micrograms per 100 ml. of blood at the end of one hour, and excreted 143 micrograms or 0·13 per cent of the amount applied.

Distribution of TOCP in the Tissues

2·094 grams of TOCP was applied to the abdomen of a bitch, and the blood level quickly established itself at 8 micrograms per 100 ml., and maintained this for twenty-four hours. The urinary excretion began equally promptly, being 44 micrograms in the first hour, rising after seven hours to a maximum of 1,312 micrograms. The radioactive phosphate was distributed in the various tissues of the dog twenty-four hours after its application to the abdominal surface. Retention was in the following order: visceral organs, muscles, brain and bone.

Hazard of Absorption through the Skin

These authors consider that the magnitude of absorption of TOCP through human skin is such that a real hazard exists in industrial operations permitting a considerable or repeated exposure to this compound. A safe industrial hygiene control requires that measures be taken to prevent such skin contact, and that all workmen exposed to the compound be instructed as to the hazard, and the necessity for preventing skin contamination.

Hazard of Absorption by Inhalation

Because of the low volatility of TOCP and the low vapour pressure at ordinary temperatures, it has been argued that poisoning cannot occur from inhalation. However, the fact that in our cases the symptoms were precipitated by the introduction of black-out conditions suggested that the poisoning may arise in this way. Further, in order to try to prevent recurrence, the firm employing the men fitted the wash-tank room with ventilators and a fan. The tanks were closed in and the vents fitted with ejectors, so that the vapours might be quickly transferred to the open air. Since these precautions have been taken no further cases of poisoning have occurred, and it is therefore possible that the lungs were the portal of entry of the poison in our cases. However, the black-out conditions in the plant raised the temperature, and the introduction of a more elaborate ventilating system substantially lowered this temperature. In view of the low atmosphere concentrations found, a more probable explanation is that increased sweating caused greater absorption through the skin.

Preventive Measures

Since there is experimental evidence that TOCP can be absorbed through the skin, it is important, as a measure of prevention, that workers with this compound and its isomers should wear elbow-length gloves to protect their hands and arms, and should change into special clothing during their working hours. Both smoking and eating while at work must be forbidden. Bathing facilities for use at the end of the work period are desirable. Education of the workmen, propaganda and routine medical examination are essential. Since the respiratory tract may also be a portal of entry, all rooms where the substances are used should be provided with exhaust ventilation. Tanks should be enclosed and the vents fitted with ejectors so that the vapours may be quickly transferred to the open air. The mixing of lacquers containing TOCP as a plasticizer should be carried out under an exhaust draught, particularly if the ingredients are heated (Hamilton, 1934).

Case 12. Chemical works' technician—exposure to tri-ortho-cresyl phosphate for six months—multiple neuritis.

(Hunter, Perry and Evans, 1944.) E. R., a man aged 41. He had been employed for six months in a chemical factory making tri-*ortho*-cresyl phosphate and triphenyl phosphate. He had handled cresol, phenol, phosphorus oxychloride, caustic soda and sulphuric acid. He took on the work in 1940 at a time when the process was speeded up because of the war and the plant production rose by 30 per cent. In addition to six days a week he worked every Sunday, instead of one Sunday in four. *Two weeks* before admission he had suffered for two days from lower abdominal pain accompanied by diarrhœa, in which he passed three pale, watery stools a day. *Five days* afterwards he found quite suddenly that he could not walk properly and was unable to lift up his toes and, consequently, his feet dragged along the ground. This disability progressed until eventually he was unable to stand without the help of a stick. *Five days* after the feet were affected he found that he had weakness of the fingers of both hands so that he was unable to do up buttons. There was occasionally a tingling sensation and a numb feeling in the calves of both legs.

On examination: robust man. Weakness of hand-grips and of

dorsiflexion of both wrists; slight symmetrical wasting of thenar, hypothenar and first dorsal interosseus muscles; reflexes in upper limbs normal; great weakness of dorsiflexors and plantar flexors of ankles; slight symmetrical wasting of calves; flail ankle joints; knee-jerks brisk and equal; ankle-jerks absent; plantar responses flexor: slow, high-stepping, rather stamping gait; two-point discrimination normal; appreciation of pin-prick, cotton-wool touch, vibration and posture normal.

Blood count: normal; blood Wassermann reaction: negative; cerebrospinal fluid: normal; urine: no albumin nor sugar, no tricresyl phosphate detected.

Progress: for six months he was treated with rest in bed and massage. He then learned to walk with a stick and his shoes were fitted with uplifting toe-springs. Complete recovery occurred twelve months after the onset of symptoms. In order to try to prevent further harm, the firm employing the man fitted the wash-tank room with ventilators and a fan. The tanks were closed in and the vents fitted with injectors, so that the vapours might be quickly transferred to the open air.

(*d*) Organic Phosphorus Insecticides

Modern methods for the control of insect pests include the use of insecticides in which the active substances are organic compounds of phosphorus (fig. 146). The first work on these compounds was carried out in Germany in 1939. Since 1945 there have been major advances in the

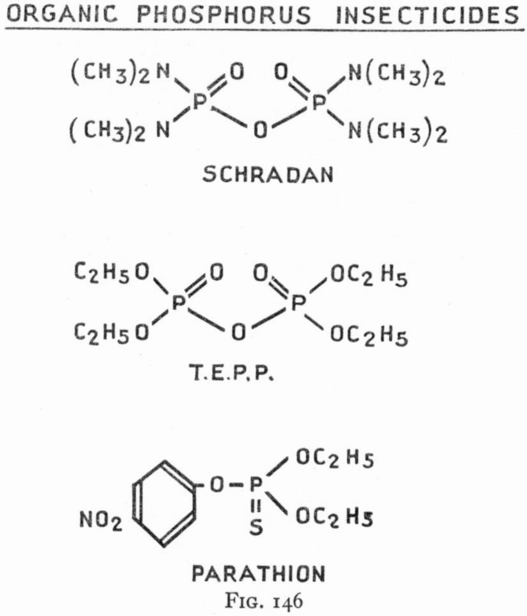

ORGANIC PHOSPHORUS INSECTICIDES

SCHRADAN

T.E.P.P.

PARATHION

FIG. 146

United Kingdom, Germany, U.S.A. and elsewhere but nearly all of this stemmed from the work of Schrader in Germany.

Powerful Cholinesterase Inhibitors

Preparations in common use contain tetra-ethyl-pyrophosphate (TEPP), hexa-ethyl-tetraphosphate (HETP) and diethyl-*para*-nitrophenylthiophosphate (*parathion*, E 605 f., DPTF, or *bladan*) which act as contract insecticides. Octamethyl pyrophosphoramide (*schradan* or OMPA), *bis*-(mono-*iso*propylamino)-fluorophosphine oxide (*mipafox*), *bis*-(dimethylamino)-fluorophosphine oxide (*dimefox*) and diethyl thiophosphate of ethylmercaptoethanol (*demeton*) act as systemic insecticides. They are related in chemical structure and physiological action to di-*iso*propylfluorophosphonate (DFP) which is a powerful cholinesterase inhibitor used in the treatment of myasthenia gravis, paralytic ileus and glaucoma. The insecticidal properties of TEPP, HETP and *parathion* are similar to those of nicotine. The effects of HETP are almost certainly due to contamination of the manufactured product by TEPP.

Systemic Insecticides

Schradan, mipafox, dimefox and *demeton* are systemic insecticides which do not inhibit cholinesterase *in vitro*. After they are absorbed by the leaves, seeds, roots, stems or branches of the plant they are transported by the sap stream and they render the whole plant toxic to sapsucking insects and mites. They differ in their readiness to enter the plant by one or other of these routes. Most of them are specific for certain groups of sapsucking insects, but some show also marked contact insecticidal action for a wider range of insects. When the systemic action of the insecticide is employed, selective action is observable as between the pest and the parasitic and predacious insects, the so-called beneficial insects; this has enabled a more complete and prolonged control to be achieved than would otherwise be the case. Predators which we are not sapsucking, for example ladybirds, remain unharmed because of course the surface of the plant is free from insecticide. Absorption of the systemic insecticide into the plant also means that new growth is continuously protected as long as the insecticide persists; this has resulted in improved control of virus diseases of many plants, for example strawberries and sugar beet, by the better control of the aphid vectors.

Uses

Early in 1945 when there was a world shortage of nicotine, a pilot plant for the production of organic phosphorus insecticides was built in Leverkusen. Soon after the end of the Second World War the manufacture of these insecticides was started in the United States of America and in Great Britain. Since 1948 parathion has been used in the United Kingdom on a commercial scale for the control of *Pentatrichopus fragariæ* on strawberries, *Brevicoryne brassicæ* on brussels sprouts, *Phorodon humuli* on hops, *Myzus persicæ* on broccoli to prevent the spread of broccoli mosaic and *Aphis fabæ* on sugar beet to prevent the spread of sugar beet virus (fig. 147). In California parathion is used to control innumerable aphides, lice, mites, spiders, moths, flies, thrips, leafhoppers, beetles, maggots, worms and caterpillars, many of them specific to a particular plant or tree. The crops sprayed include apple, pear, plum, peach, apricot, cherry,

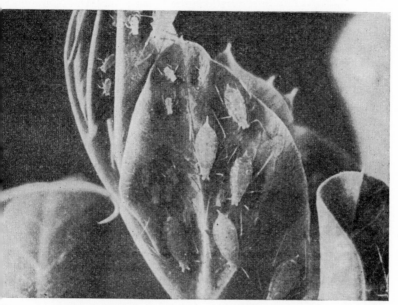

FIG. 147.—Different Aphides specific to various Plants not only suck the Juices of the Plants but also act as Carriers, especially of Virus Diseases

orange, grape, fig, mango, strawberry, raspberry, blackberry, blueberry, dewberry, gooseberry, cranberry, pineapple, carrot, cabbage, broccoli, cauliflower, lettuce, kale, spinach, turnip, celery, cucumber, squash, melon, pea, onion, potato, beetroot, tomato, paprika, sweet corn, peanut, walnut, pecan, artichoke, eggplant (aubergine), alfalfa, tobacco, soya bean, sugar beet and cotton. In the West Indies sugar cane is sprayed to kill the froghopper (*Æneolamia varia saccharina*). In Japan rice plants are sprayed to combat rice-stem borer.

Exposure Hazards

Exposure to as little as 0·3 grams daily has been estimated as dangerous to man. The lethal dose by mouth for man is approximately 100 milligrams of TEPP or *parathion*, and symptoms follow the administration of more than 10 milligrams (DuBois, 1951). HETP and TEPP hydrolyse rapidly in the presence of water or alkaline solutions. Danger of poisoning from these two substances is most likely to occur when the concentrated materials are handled in manufacture or in mixing with suitable wetting agents. *Parathion* is more stable and 168 cases of poisoning, seven of them fatal, were reported from the United States of America in 1950 (Committee on Pesticides Report).

Worldwide Misuse of Parathion

The use and misuse of parathion has become worldwide. Care must be taken when mechanics are employed to service machinery which has been used to spray fields or orchards with parathion. Two men in California using a steam gun in a tank belonging to such machinery were both poisoned for want of protective clothing. In another part of California after aerial dusting of a cotton crop the pilot of the aeroplane employed was ill from inhalation of the dust he was using. In Florida a worker applying a parathion spray rolled his own cigarettes all day and died the next day. Fruit pickers have been poisoned by parathion. *Apple-thinners' disease* has occurred among orchard workers who were thinning green apples that had been sprayed with parathion. Spraying was introduced in Japan in 1952 to combat the rice-stem borer. In the initial year 1800 sprayers were poisoned but by scrupulous control the figure was reduced by 1966 to 300 (Ueda, 1966). However, not all the cases occur in field operations. Young children have died after playing with tins of parathion or with sacks of the wettable powder. This constitutes gross carelessness on the part of the parents who as farmers were in a position to know better than to leave such highly poisonous materials within the reach of youngsters. In Finland there were eighty-eight suicides from parathion in 1956 and in Denmark there were thirteen in the same year. In Germany, Switzerland, Japan and Australia many cases of suicide and of accidental poisoning have occurred. Contaminated food is often responsible for poisoning. In Italy a woman was ill after eating paprika gathered near an orchard which had been sprayed with parathion. In South Africa a woman ate a dish of green beans previously sprayed with parathion and she died. In Greece where 400,000 olive trees were sprayed in 1954 a man noticed that the fleas were killed on one of his arms after it had become soaked with parathion. Spreading the good news he caused many deaths among fellow sprayers and members of their families by urging them to use parathion to kill fleas, bed bugs and head lice in their homes. An outbreak of parathion poisoning from food in Kerala in India in the spring of 1958 created a panic. There were 828 cases with 106 deaths. The first incident occurred in a village where ten people died four hours after eating bread and biscuits. From six of fifty-five polythene carboys the insecticide had leaked over large consignments of flour and sugar in the hold of a ship (Karunakaran, 1958). It is therefore clear that in all countries a stricter control of the sale of organic phosphorus insecticides is urgently to be sought.

Public Concern about Dangerous Pesticides

There is increasing public concern about the death of wood pigeons and other wild birds and in turn their predators (foxes, badgers, cats and dogs) following their eating spring-sown grain treated with insecticides and fungicides. It is difficult to see in true perspective the effects of the ecology of plant and animal life of the widespread use of such pesticides. As an example how does the use of di-nitro-*ortho*-cresol on fields seeded with spring corn alter the course of nature? The DNOC effectively wipes out charlock, the flowers of which normally feed the bullfinch. This bird therefore eats the flower buds of certain fruit trees in the following order— Cox's orange pippin, Worcester pearmain, greengage and Victoria plum. The improper use of pesticides should be brought under control. Much harm is done by failing to read the maker's instructions on bottles and cartons and by inexpert spraying. Clearly those farmers who can afford to do so should pay pest control experts to undertake spraying for them.

International Control of their Sale and Transport

But in addition to damage to wild life there is a considerable hazard to human life including an unnecessary and increasing number of deaths (Hunter, 1962). The increased manufacture and widespread use of fungicides, herbicides, insecticides, larvicides, miticides, molluscicides, ovicides, parasiticides, pesticides, acaricides, defoliants, tickicides, vermin poisons and week-killers cannot but be regarded with anxiety. Public concern would be less if the worst of these substances were to be manufactured only under licence. Conditions for the granting of a licence must include adequate protection for the worker in factory and field, the distributor, and the consumer of sprayed food. In distribution those responsible for transport must be able to produce the licence on demand. It is an utter disgrace that a ship's captain can be unaware that he is carrying dangerous poisons; the containers may leak and contaminate food in the hold of the ship with disastrous results (see p. 398). But the mishandling of these poisons is a greater danger in the home than anywhere else. For instance the mortality from parathion by suicide, homicide and accident is excessive. Modern communities should protect themselves against this tragedy by insistence on the use of clear warning labels.—WARNING: POISON: *Keep this container away from children. When not in use lock it up in a cupboard.* All people young and old alike should refrain from putting poisonous fluids in Coca Cola bottles or poisonous solids in food tins.

Mode of Absorption

Insecticides containing organic compounds of phosphorus are poisonous to man and animals. In a single dose they are less toxic than nicotine, but the effects of absorbing small amounts of these anticholinesterase substances are prolonged and result in increased susceptibility to absorption of further amounts of any cholinesterase inhibitor. All types of preparation penetrate rapidly through the skin, producing only slight local irritation. Absorption may also occur from inhalation and ingestion.

Symptoms and Signs

The early symptoms of poisoning are mild and non-specific, and may include headache, nausea, anorexia and unusual fatigue. These may be accompanied by pin-point constriction of the pupils. The symptoms are aggravated by smoking or taking food. From two to eight hours later nausea, abdominal cramps, vomiting, diarrhœa, muscular twitching, coma, convulsions and signs of pulmonary œdema may develop. Incontinence of urine and fæces is common. Death may result in as short a time as one hour after the onset of symptoms.

Extensive Paralysis following Acute Poisoning

The statement that there are no sequelæ to poisoning by organic phosphorus compounds used as insecticides has proved to be erroneous. In Great Britain three people developed acute poisoning while engaged on a pilot plant in the manufacture of a new substance in this group, *bis*-(mono-*iso*propylamino) fluorophosphine oxide (*mipafox*) (Bidstrup, Bonnell and Beckett, 1953). Recovery from the acute phase of the illness followed the administration of atropine in large doses, but in the third week after the onset of symptoms two of the patients developed paralysis of the limbs similar to that which follows poisoning by tri-*ortho*-cresyl phosphate. Petry (1951) has described this type of paralysis following repeated exposure to *parathion* in the fumigation of greenhouses in Germany. People who have had acute poisoning by organic phosphorus compounds should be kept under close observation until the cholinesterase activity of the blood has returned to normal.

Antidotal Treatment

Atropine is an antidote to the muscarinic and central nervous system effects of this form of poisoning and even minor cases should immediately be treated with it. It should be given in doses of 1–2 milligrams ($\frac{1}{60}-\frac{1}{30}$ gr.) at hourly intervals until the pupils are dilated; in severe cases this may require $\frac{1}{3}$ gr. (20 milligrams) or more. Oxygen, under slight pressure to overcome bronchial spasm, should be administered at the first sign of pulmonary œdema. The fibrillary twitching of muscles appears to affect particularly the diaphragm, and artificial respiration may be necessary. This effect upon striated muscle is due to the nicotine-like action of these compounds. No antidote to this effect is known, and death may occur from neuro-muscular paralysis even though the muscarine-like effects and the signs of involvement of the central nervous system have been controlled by atropine.

Use of Cholinesterase Reactivators

In severe cases it is essential that a cholinesterase reactivator should be given intramuscularly or intravenously as early as possible and preferably at the same time as the atropine. Two such agents are available—namely, P2S and P2AM (PAM). The recommended initial dose of P2S is 1 g. dissolved in 5 ml. of water for injection *B.P.*, which can be used intramuscularly and intravenously. Further 1 g. doses of P2S and P2AM (PAM) may be necessary at intervals of 3–4 hours. Once the clinical condition permits, decontamination should be quick and thorough. The clothing should be removed, wearing rubber gloves, and the skin bathed with soap and water, to which washing soda or baking soda may be added. When the poison has been swallowed the stomach should be emptied, preferably by lavage with sodium bicarbonate solution.

Protective Clothing and Exhaust Ventilation

Strict precautions are necessary to protect workers engaged in handling these insecticides. Protection is more easily arranged and applied in factories than in field operations (fig. 148). In factories where an organic

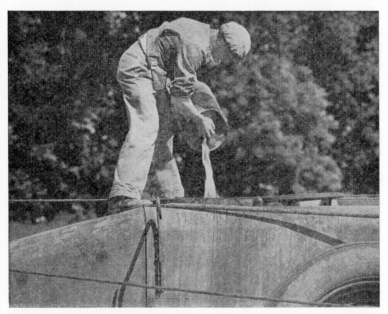

FIG. 148.—To handle Parathion carelessly is to court disaster. The man pouring the Concentrated Substance into the Spraying Tank shows lack of skill. He is splashing the Liquid over his Clothes. He is untidy, wrongly clothed and smoking. He should be wearing Protective Clothing, Rubber Gloves, Rubber Boots and a Mask. The man is untrained and is quite unsuited to handle toxic Chemical Substances

phosphorus insecticide is made, mixed with wetting agents or incorporated in dusts or wettable powders, exhaust ventilation should secure that this substance is absent from the atmosphere. Protective clothing must include overalls, gloves, boots, cap and underwear, which are laundered each day and changed immediately if accidentally splashed. Ordinary clothing must be protected from possible contamination. Respirators should be available in factories for use in emergency; in field operations they must be worn during dusting operations and the diluting of wettable powders (fig. 149). It is

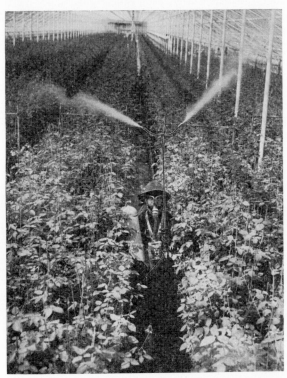

FIG. 149.—Correct Use of Protective Clothing by workman spraying a Hothouse with Parathion. Note Helmet, Rubber Gloves, Rubber Boots and Canister Mask

necessary that the workers should wash thoroughly before eating or smoking, and a bath should be taken at the end of a day's work. These instructions, together with an account of the symptoms of poisoning, must appear on the labels of containers (fig. 150). The attention of all workers exposed to risk should be directed repeatedly to the toxic properties of these compounds (fig. 151).

Protection of the Worker by Law

The Ministry of Agriculture, Fisheries and Food has issued regulations under the *Agriculture (Poisonous Substances) Act, 1952*, and *The Agriculture (Poisonous Substances) Regulations, 1956*, as amended in 1966, which prohibit the use of organic phosphorus compounds unless the men working with them are wearing protective clothing. The number of hours during

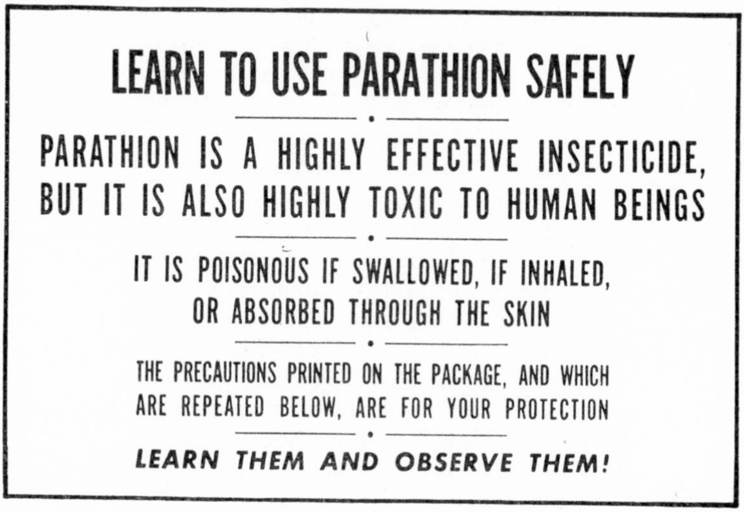

LEARN TO USE PARATHION SAFELY

•

PARATHION IS A HIGHLY EFFECTIVE INSECTICIDE, BUT IT IS ALSO HIGHLY TOXIC TO HUMAN BEINGS

•

IT IS POISONOUS IF SWALLOWED, IF INHALED, OR ABSORBED THROUGH THE SKIN

•

THE PRECAUTIONS PRINTED ON THE PACKAGE, AND WHICH ARE REPEATED BELOW, ARE FOR YOUR PROTECTION

•

LEARN THEM AND OBSERVE THEM!

FIG. 150.—Main Headings of a Warning Notice issued to users of Parathion by the Cyanamide Co. of New York

which workers can be employed is restricted to ten in any one day and sixty during seven days. The employment of any worker under the age of eighteen is prohibited. The regulations also contain requirements about

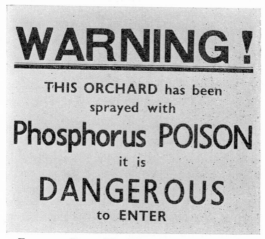

FIG. 151.—Poster Warning against the Danger of Parathion

the provision and maintenance of protective clothing, the provision of washing facilities for workers, the notification of sickness and absence, the training and supervision of workers and the keeping of registers. The regulations do not make adequate provision for the medical supervision of workers. Since the early symptoms and signs of poisoning are vague and indefinite and do not occur until potentially dangerous quantities of the poisons have been absorbed, routine blood tests on the workers would serve to detect absorption of significant amounts before the onset of symptoms, which are often irreversible.

Routine Cholinesterase Estimations in Blood

Absorption of TEPP, *parathion* and *schradan* results in depression of the cholinesterase activity of both red blood cells and serum before symptoms or signs of poisoning occur. People at risk should have the blood cholinesterase activity estimated at frequent intervals. The normal range of cholinesterase activity for the general population has been determined (Callaway, Davies and Rutland, 1951), and the finding of a lowered cholinesterase in a workman who has been handling organic phosphorus insecticides in the factory or in the field is an indication for removing him immediately from further exposure. He should not be allowed to return to work with these substances until the cholinesterase activity has been shown to be within the normal range.

Case 13. Research chemist—exposure to organic phosphorus insecticides—multiple neuritis—inhibition of cholinesterase activity.

(Bidstrup, Bonnell and Beckett, 1953.) M. W., a lady of 28, L.H· Reg. No. 35865/1951, a research chemist, had been employed on the development of organic phosphorus compounds for twenty-one months and lately had been caught up in the race to be the first to produce a systemic insecticide. During this time she had handled a number of substances in this group, and although her exposure to them was mainly in the laboratory, she was concerned occasionally in the manufacture of small amounts of new compounds in pilot plants. She had experienced symptoms of mild organic phosphorus poisoning on at least three occasions during this time, and she was away from contact with organic phosphorus compounds for two or three weeks in June 1951, following one of these attacks.

At about 8 p.m. on 15th August 1951, when she had been working long hours on the pilot-scale production of *bis*-(mono-*iso*propylamino)-fluorophosphine oxide (*mipafox*) for three days, she began to feel sick and tired. She attributed these symptoms to fatigue, and continued at work although the symptoms became gradually worse. She left the factory at 12 midnight and returned to lodgings where she was quite alone. At about 2 a.m. on 16th August 1951 she began to suffer from vomiting and involuntary defæcation, and this continued at intervals of a few minutes until 3.30 p.m., when she was given $\frac{1}{60}$ gr. atropine by intramuscular injection and admitted to Addenbrooke's Hospital under the care of Dr. A. P. Dick. The vomiting and involuntary defæcation were accompanied by cramps in the muscles of the legs, and by 5 a.m. generalized muscular weakness was so marked that she was unable to get out of bed to seek assistance.

The administration of atropine relieved the vomiting and diarrhœa within half an hour, but nausea and muscular twitchings persisted.

On admission to hospital on 15.8.51, significant findings were suffusion of the conjunctivæ, pin-point pupils, twitching of the facial and sternomastoid muscles, and diminished tendon reflexes. On 17th August 1951 hypotonia of all muscles was still a striking feature.

17.8.51	*Cholinesterase activity*		*Normal*
	—red blood cells (true cholinesterase 9 units		75–142
	—plasma	(pseudo cholinesterase 1 unit)	51–128

The gastro-intestinal symptoms were controlled by atropine administered at frequent intervals, but this did not affect the muscular twitchings. The total amount of atropine administered was 0·9 gr. given in the following doses:

$$16.8.51 \quad \tfrac{1}{50} \text{ gr.} \times 7$$
$$17.8.51 \quad \tfrac{1}{50} \text{ gr.} \times 9$$
$$\tfrac{1}{100} \text{ gr.} \times 4$$
$$18.8.51 \quad \tfrac{1}{75} \text{ gr.} \times 1$$
$$\tfrac{1}{30} \text{ gr.} \times 1$$
$$\tfrac{1}{50} \text{ gr.} \times 20$$
$$19.8.51 \quad \tfrac{1}{50} \text{ gr.} \times 4$$

On 19th August 1951 the patient developed delusions and hallucinations, which were attributed to overdosage with atropine. When the atropine was discontinued, her mental state returned to normal. She was symptom-free after four days and was discharged from hospital on 31st August 1951, the sixteenth day after her illness began. For several days she had been out of bed and had walked about the ward, apparently well.

As she walked downstairs to leave hospital she noticed for the first time weakness and unsteadiness of her legs. During the next three or four days there was little change in her condition, which then began to deteriorate. The weakness in the legs increased and she noticed weakness of the hands and arms. These symptoms became gradually worse and she was readmitted to hospital on 10th September 1951.

On examination she was found to have a flaccid paralysis of both legs, and weakness of the muscles of the thighs. The knee-jerks were diminished and the ankle-jerks absent. There was no plantar response. Although the legs and feet were cold and the muscles tender to palpation, there was no change in cutaneous sensation to pin-prick or light touch. Weakness of the muscles of the right hand was present.

The paralysis progressed and the patient was transferred to the London Hospital on 15th September 1951. At this time there was complete flaccid paralysis of the lower limbs. The knee-jerks and ankle-jerks were absent and the plantar reflexes could not be elicited. Tone and power in the arms, forearms and hands were greatly reduced. The biceps-jerk was just present but neither the supinator nor the triceps-jerk could be elicited. The trunk muscles were also weaker than normal. Cranial nerves were normal, there were no signs of involvement of the central nervous system and no disturbance of cutaneous sensation could be demonstrated. All muscles, particularly those of the calf, were tender to palpation, and muscle twitchings were observed in the deltoids, facial muscles and muscles of the legs.

19.9.51 *Lumbar puncture*—normal.

20.9.51 *Pyruvate tolerance test*—normal

10.10.51 *Electrocardiogram*—physiological tracing.

19.9.51 The electromyogram showed a reduced interference pattern, but the individual motor units were normal. There was no activity at rest. Muscle stimulation showed complete reaction of degeneration in the lower limbs and partial reaction of degeneration in the thenar eminence.

21.9.51 Further examination showed the electrical responses to be equivocal and not definitely sluggish. Some polyphasic motor unit potentials were found in the forearm extensors, but no fibrillation potentials were found. This is against a lesion producing lower motor neurone degeneration.

Progress: power returned gradually to the muscles of the thighs, arms and forearms. By 20th October 1951 power and tone were normal in the arm muscles, and the tendon reflexes were present and brisk. There was weakness of the long extensors of the fingers, and the lumbricals and interossei were wasted and completely paralysed. In the lower limbs power and tone had returned to some extent in the thigh muscles and flexors of the hip, but the muscles of the leg below the knee were still flaccid and completely paralysed. There was marked wasting of the small muscles of the feet. Although there was no spasticity, the knee-jerks were exaggerated and patella clonus could be elicited without difficulty. The ankle-jerks were absent. Fasciculation was still present in the deltoids, facial muscles and muscles of the legs, and the patient complained of cramp-like pains affecting particularly the muscles of the lower limbs. Alternating vasodilation and vasoconstriction resulted in subjective symptoms of burning and coldness in the hands and feet, and these were accompanied by flushing or pallor and cyanosis.

In the first week in November the clinical picture was complicated by subjective evidence of sensory changes of glove and stocking distribution. On repeated examination the distribution of these changes was not constant, and at times the pattern was bizarre. It is possible that these symptoms were functional in origin and they disappeared completely within a few weeks. Plasma cholinesterase activity was normal for the first time.

Between November 1951 and February 1952 slow improvement continued in the groups of muscles which had already begun to regain their normal function, but the muscles of the legs and feet remained completely paralysed. The wasting of the small muscles of the hands became increasingly obvious (fig. 152) and it seemed likely at this time that no recovery could be expected in these muscles or in the muscles of the legs and feet.

7.12.51   The electromyogram showed no response to 1 millisecond nerve stimulation. Response to 100 millisecond stimulation weakening on repetitive contraction. Spontaneous muscle fibre activity. Motor unit potentials were of short duration and all polyphasic. These findings are comparable with those found on the administration of a depolarizing drug such as decamethonium iodide and suggest a state of neuro-muscular block due depolarization of the end-plate increasing on muscle contraction.

From the first week in April 1952, however, the small muscles of the hands began to recover. Power returned slowly to the lumbricals, interossei and opponens pollicis, and by July 1952 the wasting was much less marked (fig. 153). In May 1952 the ankle-jerks were first elicited, and this was followed within a few days by the return of slight movements of the toes.

21.5.52   The electromyogram showed no decrease of muscle contraction on repetitive stimulation now demonstrable. Muscle fibrillation potentials present, definite evidence of lower motor neurone lesion. Picture of peripheral neuritis. Probably some fibrosis of muscle, particularly in the gastrocnemius.

June 1953: The upper limbs are normal. Power in the muscles of the thighs is almost normal but is greater in the flexors than in the extensors. Although patella clonus can still be elicited, it is much more difficult to demonstrate. Exaggerated ankle-jerks and ankle clonus are readily elicited and the plantar response is extensor on both sides. Movements of the toes are gradually increasing, and inversion and eversion at the ankle joints are present but weak. Plantar flexion is strong, but there is little evidence of the return of power of dorsiflexion.

July 1953: She left hospital but continued to receive physiotherapy as an out-patient. The clinical picture is essentially that of a paraplegia with persistence of weakness and wasting of the extensor and peroneal muscles. April 1954: The patient is able to go out in a wheel-chair, and to stand with support. With superb courage she has learned to drive a car with hand controls and has undertaken a research post in biochemistry.

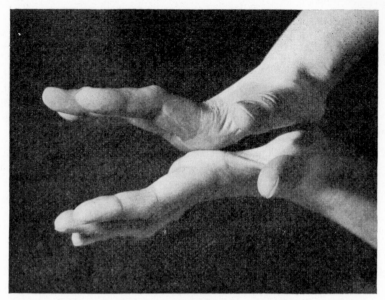

FIG. 152.—Case 13. Wasting of Small Muscles of Hands six months after *Mipafox* poisoning

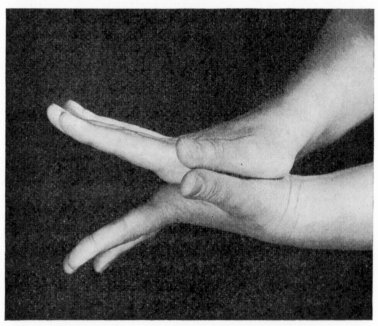

FIG. 153.—Case 13. Recovery in Hands five months later

March 1956: The gait is still spastic and walking is possible only with the aid of a stick and toe-springs. The patient continues to pursue her researches in biochemistry. Throughout the illness the right side has been more severely affected than the left in both upper and lower limbs and is recovering more slowly. There has been a striking absence of trophic changes in the skin over the paralysed muscles. The cranial nerves have been unaffected at all stages of the illness and there has been no tremor nor ataxia present at any stage.

March 1957: Her university has appointed her Junior Lecturer in Biochemistry and she has completed the Ph.D. degree in this subject.

April 1959: Still improving she has now discarded the right uplifting-toe-spring.

August 1959: Left toe-spring discarded.

April 1960: Much improved she has given up the hand controls for driving her car. Her university has promoted her to Senior Lecturer in Biochemistry.

November 1961: Walking is still unstable without the aid of a stick. The power of dorsiflexion of both feet is still improving. Eversion of each foot is now possible but is weak on both sides, the left being worse than the right. Physiotherapy is being continued twice a week.

SILVER

Ornaments of silver, Ag, were found in the royal tombs of Chaldæa built in the fourth millennium B.C. It is the most lustrous of the metals and ranks highest in thermal and electrical conductivity. Silver is only slightly less malleable and ductile than gold. In spite of these valuable properties it is largely wasted as bullion stored in underground vaults. It forms a natural primary alloy with gold in the mineral electrum. Much of the world's silver is recovered during the treatment of gold ores. It is an essential constituent of gold telluride, calaverite, $(AuAg)Te_2$. Silver is also obtained as a by-product from argentiferous lead, zinc and copper ores, in which it occurs as silver sulphide, argentite, Ag_2S.

Uses

Pure silver is too soft for coinage, ornaments, spoons and forks, plate and jewellery, and for all these purposes the metal is alloyed with copper to harden it. It is extremely resistant to acetic acid, and therefore silver vats are used in the acetic acid, vinegar, cider and brewing industries. It is used in busbars and windings of electrical plants, in silver solders, brazing alloys, dental amalgams, military insignia, engine bearings, Christmas-cracker making, the silvering of glass beads and the manufacture of lunar caustic pencils. Silver is almost universally employed in the manufacture of formaldehyde, acetaldehyde and higher aldehydes by the catalytic dehydrogenation of the corresponding primary alcohols. In many installations the catalyst consists of a shallow bed of crystalline silver of extremely high purity. An important use of silver is in photography, especially since the rapid expansion of the motion-picture industry, in which many millions of feet of film are used annually. It is the unique and instantaneous reaction of the halides of silver on exposure to light that makes the metal virtually indispensable for films, plates and photographic printing paper.

ARGYRIA

Silver produces no constitutional symptoms, but it can lead to lifelong disfigurement. The dust of the metal or its salts once absorbed becomes precipitated in the tissues in the metallic state, and in this form it cannot be eliminated. Reduction to the metallic state takes place either by the action of light on the exposed parts of the skin and visible mucous membranes, or by means of sulphuretted hydrogen in other tissues.

Occupations involving the risk of argyria can be divided into two groups: (a) including workmen who handle a compound of silver, either the nitrate, fulminate or cyanide, which, broadly speaking, give rise to generalized argyria from inhalation and ingestion of the silver salt concerned; (b) including workmen who handle metallic silver, small particles of which accidentally penetrate the exposed skin, giving rise to local argyria by a process equivalent to tattooing.

(a) Generalized Argyria

Occupations giving rise to generalized argyria include the manufacture of silver nitrate, the wrapping of lunar caustic pencils, Christmas-cracker making, the silvering of glass beads, mirror plating, electroplating and photography.

(i) *Silvering of Glass Beads.* Schubert, in 1895, reported two cases of generalized argyria occurring in glass-bead silverers in Bohemia. Their occupation consisted in stringing the beads together, dipping them into a reducing solution such as lactose and then sucking a silver compound into them. A small glass tube, 3–4 cm. long, was used for sucking up the silver compound, which consisted of a solution of silver nitrate, ammonia and potassium hydroxide. Unless they were very careful, the workers sucked up some of the solution, and although they used to wash out their mouths with a saline solution a bitter taste remained. In consequence of the constant contact of the solution with the mouth, fissures appeared round the lips and in the mouth generally, and the teeth were stated to become black within eight days, gradually to soften, to break to pieces and to come out painlessly within a few years. The tongue showed the earliest sign of pigmentation. The first discoloration of the skin began after three or four years and appeared round the eyelids as a blue-black corona, gradually increasing both in extent and intensity.

The first case described by Schubert was that of a man who had been silvering beads for twenty-three years before he became pigmented. The skin of the whole body showed a diffuse blue-black colour, the surface of the skin being shiny like graphite. The scalp, neck, nose and ears were the parts most affected. In the upper extremities the colour was most marked on the hands and decreased towards the shoulders. The axillæ, scrotum and nipples were no more affected than other places. Both palpebral and ocular conjunctiva showed a blue-black discoloration, shared by the plica semilunaris. The mucosæ of the lips, gums, tongue, palate, pharynx and epiglottis were blue-black. The second case was similar to the first. The pigmentation appeared eight years after the man began the work, and slowly increased for four years until he left it. Schubert states that forty or fifty other men were known to be affected before the employers forbade the use of the method. He points out the resemblance between these cases and those occurring in medicinal argyria. Now that glass beads made are and silvered by machinery, argyria has disappeared from Bohemia (Teleky, 1914).

(ii) *Christmas-cracker Making.* The use of silver fulminate in the manufacture of Christmas crackers involves the risk of conjunctivitis, accompanied by pain and lachrymation, and also of permanent pigmentation of the conjunctiva (Bridge, 1920). A patient doing this work was admitted to the London Hospital in 1901 showing generalized argyria (Harker and Hunter, 1935). She was a girl of eighteen, and had been employed for ten years in making by hand the detonators of the crackers. Two narrow strips of thin card were supplied to her already sanded and stuck together. She applied powdered silver fulminate to the sanded part and wrapped a strip of tissue paper round it to afford protection. Her fingers seem to have been abnormally dry, and in order to facilitate the wrapping of the tissue paper she moistened them on her lips. None of her fellow workers found it necessary to lick the fingers, and none of them developed discoloration of the skin. The occupation followed by these girls is no longer carried out manually.

(iii) *Manufacture of Silver Nitrate.* Lewin (1886) mentions one case of generalized argyria occurring in a silver-nitrate worker in Berlin who for twenty-five years handled crystals with bare hands. In Great Britain the condition has been recorded in a man who had been employed for many years in the manufacture of silver nitrate (Adamson, 1924).

In 1935 Harker and Hunter described six cases, five of whom had been occupied in the old process of producing silver nitrate, while the sixth worked in the silver-nitrate packing-room. For technical reasons the old process was abolished in 1926, and replaced by a method which is not only less wasteful, but is also less harmful to the workmen.

The old process: Finely divided silver was dissolved in nitric acid in open dishes of porcelain or platinum, standing over gas-burners. Each dish held fifty ounces of silver, and there were as many as thirty of them in one room. The dishes were covered by sloping glass hoods connected with pipes which led to a shaft. No mechanical exhaust system existed. When the acid was poured on to the silver, the room was filled with dense fumes. The burners were lit under the dishes, and when the mixture had evaporated to a certain specific gravity it was poured into other porcelain pans and left overnight. This pouring process caused a lot of splashing, against which neither leather nor rubber gloves afforded complete protection. Next day the mother liquors were poured off, leaving the crystals of silver nitrate to dry. The crystals were then broken up, washed with distilled water and placed in drying ovens. The door of the oven was opened from time to time and the crystals broken up. This process sometimes caused silver nitrate to spatter over the faces of the workmen. The crystals were then sifted through a fine sieve, with the result that fine particles of silver nitrate were present in the atmosphere over long periods.

The new process: On the top floor of the works, silver and concentrated nitric acid are mixed in a closed apparatus. The solution of silver nitrate is passed by pipes to the floor below, where it is concentrated in an apparatus known as the *climbing film evaporator*. This consists of a series of tubes, made of stainless steel jacketed with steam, and forming a closed system. Its use has entirely replaced the method of evaporation in open dishes, which was so frequently a cause of occupational argyria in the past.

Silver-nitrate packing: This process has not altered since about 1890, but owing to the increase in the photographic industry the work done by the packers has been doubled since 1910. In the weighing and packing-room, crystalline silver nitrate is done up into packets which may contain from 50 to 600 ounces. When the workman shoots the material into bags from a folded piece of paper, like a grocer weighing sugar, he creates a dust which loads the atmosphere continuously with finely divided particles of silver nitrate.

Clinical Manifestations

Workers affected by generalized argyria are called by their fellow-workers *blue men*. The face, forehead, neck, hands and forearms are of a dark slaty-grey colour, uniform in distribution and varying in depth according to the degree of exposure. Pale scars up to about 6 mm. across may be found on the face, hands and forearms, due to the caustic effects of silver nitrate (fig. 154). The finger-nails are a deep chocolate-brown colour. The buccal mucosa is slaty-grey or bluish in colour. Very slight pigmentation may be detected in the covered parts of the skin. The toe-nails may show a slight bluish discoloration.

Changes in the Eyes

The conjunctivæ vary from a slight grey discoloration to a deep brown colour, the lower palpebral portion being particularly affected—*argyrosis conjunctivæ* (fig. 155). The posterior border of the lower lid, the caruncle and the plica semilunaris are deeply pigmented and may be almost black. Examination by means of the slit-lamp reveals a delicate network of faint grey pigmentation in the posterior elastic lamina (Descemet's membrane) of the cornea—*argyrosis corneæ* (fig. 156). In cases of long duration Larsen (1927) also found *argyrolentis*. In one such case he described a sunflower

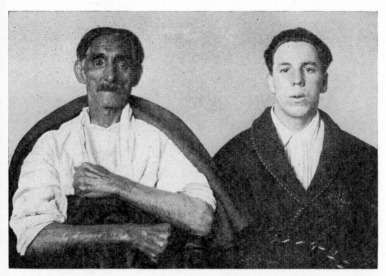

FIG. 154.—Case 14. Generalized Argyria in a maker of Silver Nitrate. The Face, Forehead and Forearms are of a dark slaty-grey colour, uniform in distribution except for Small Scattered Scars of Caustic Burns. The man on the right is a normal person for comparison

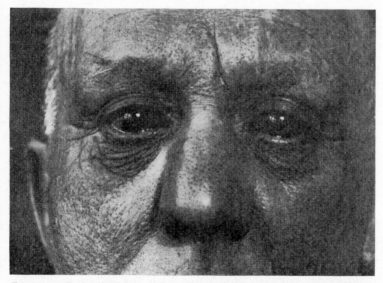

FIG. 155.—Generalized Argyria in a man of 68 who had packed Silver Nitrate Crystals for 42 years. The deep brown Pigmentation of the Conjunctivae contrasts with the slight involvement found in cases of Argyria from taking Silver Salts by mouth

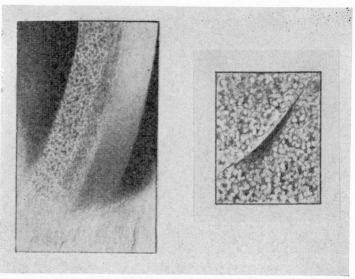

FIG. 156.—Generalized Argyria in a man of 52 who had made Silver Nitrate for 25 years. Note the delicate Network of faint grey Pigmentation in the Posterior Elastic Lamina (Descemet's Membrane) of the Cornea as seen by Slit-lamp Examination

cataract in the anterior capsule of the lens. Slit-lamp examination shows a yellow reflex from the anterior capsule of the lens, a diffuse yellow coloration of the posterior capsule and of the outermost layers of the posterior cortex. In cases with corneal involvement of long duration Larsen also found slight pigmentation of the vitreous, the retina and the optic disc.

Case 14. Silver-nitrate maker—exposure to dust of silver nitrate for twenty-four years—generalized argyria.

(Harker and Hunter, 1935.) S. N., a man aged 63, L.H. Reg. No. 33373/1927. This man was admitted with signs and symptoms of carcinoma of the cæcum. He showed extensive cutaneous pigmentation, and stated that for twenty-four years he had manufactured silver nitrate by the old process, and that for fifteen years he had noticed a grey discoloration of the skin, gradually becoming darker. He stated quite clearly that the whites of his eyes were the first part of the body to be affected.

On examination: The face and forehead were of a dark slaty-grey colour, uniform in distribution except for a few scattered pale areas up to 6 mm. across. These pale areas were the scars of burns from the caustic effect of silver nitrate. The conjunctivæ were a deep brown colour, the lower palpebral portion being particularly affected. The posterior border of the lower lid, the caruncle and the plica semi-lunaris were almost black. The skin of the ears, neck and upper chest was affected to a less degree than that of the face. The hands were more deeply pigmented than the forearms (fig. 154). On admission the finger-nails were a deep brown colour, but during his stay in hospital non-pigmented nail gradually appeared from the base downwards (fig. 157). The forearms showed many scars of caustic burns, and these were non-pigmented. The patient was edentulous;

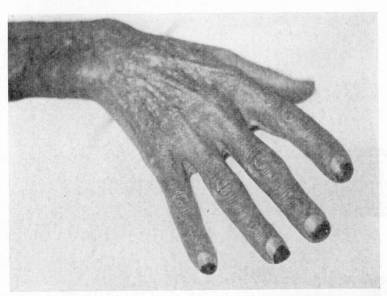

FIG. 157.—Case 14. Generalized Argyria in a maker of Silver Nitrate. The uniformity of the slaty-grey Pigmentation of the Skin is interrupted by innumerable small rounded Scars of Caustic Burns. During his stay in Hospital normal Finger Nail has grown and stands in contrast to the black pigmented Nail of his working life

no pigmentation of the gums, tongue or buccal mucosa was seen. Slight pigmentation could be detected in the skin of the rest of the body, and the toe-nails showed slight bluish discoloration.

Progress: Soon after admission he was operated upon, an ileo-colostomy and an ileostomy being performed because of carcinoma of the cæcum. He died of lobar pneumonia.

Necropsy: (L.H. P.M. 25/1928) Lobar pneumonia, carcinoma of cæcum; operations—ileo-colostomy, ileostomy. Generalized argyria. Marked black pigmentation of nasal mucosa (fig. 158), slight of mucous membrane of maxillary antra, considerable impregnation by silver of patchy grey mucosa of larynx, trachea and bronchi. Very faint grey patches in endocardium of left ventricle. Distinct deposit of silver in pulmonary artery and branches and throughout aorta and large branches. Faint suggestion of pale grey patches in inferior vena cava. Dark blue-

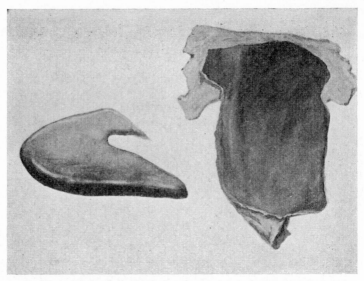

FIG. 158.—Case 14. Generalized Argyria in a maker of Silver Nitrate. Greyish-black Pigmentation of Mucosa of Turbinate Bone and Nasal Septum
(*London Hospital Medical College Museum*)

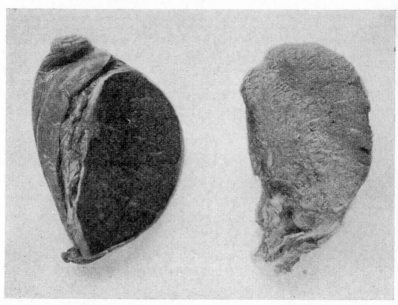

FIG. 159.—Case 14. Generalized Argyria in a maker of Silver Nitrate. Greyish-black Pigmentation of Testis; normal Testis on the right for comparison
(*London Hospital Medical College Museum*)

grey intima of intra-hepatic vena cava. Considerable dusky black deposit in intermediate zone, 0·3 cm. broad, of kidneys, and in a focal area in tip of each medullary pyramid. Faint irregular fine streaked deposit in cortex. Faint grey coloration of bladder and ureters. Conspicuous greyish-black pigmentation of testes and of globi majores of epididymes (fig. 159). Apparently abundant silver in small black

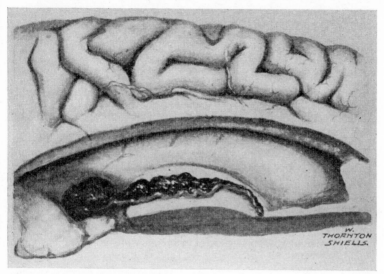

FIG. 160.—Case 14. Generalized Argyria in a maker of Silver Nitrate. Dense black Pigmentation of Choroid Plexus of Lateral Ventricle

glands throughout mesentery. Abundant deposit in black choroid plexuses of lateral and fourth ventricles (fig. 160). Brain substance normal. Moderate deposit in greyish-black anterior lobe of pituitary.

Morbid Anatomy and Histology

At necropsy cases of generalized argyria show grey pigmentation of the skin, buccal and nasal mucosæ, larynx, trachea, bronchi, endocardium, intima of the large elastic arteries and great veins, mesenteric glands, intermediate zone of the kidneys, ureters, bladder, testes, epididymes and of the choroid plexus. The histological picture shows amorphous black granules of silver distributed throughout the internal elastic lamellæ of the arterioles, in the elastic fibres of connective tissues in general, in the basement membranes of the sweat glands of the skin (fig. 161) and between the muscle fibres of the myocardium (fig. 162). The fibro-elastic tissue surrounding the acini of the testes is picked out, as also are the basement membranes of the collecting tubules of the medulla of the kidney and of the ependyma cells of the choroid plexuses.

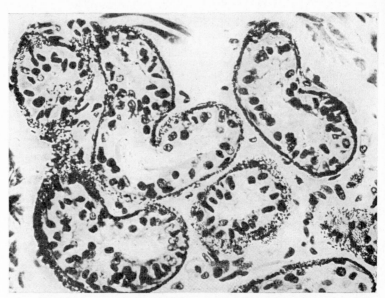

FIG. 161.—Generalized Argyria. Coil Glands of the Corium showing Silver Granules in the Connective Tissues adjoining the Epithelium (Magnified 500 diameters)

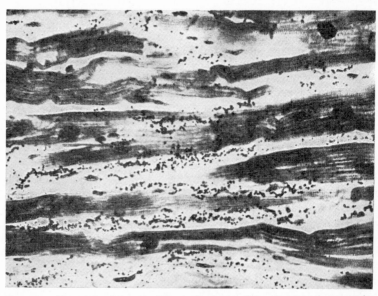

FIG. 162.—Generalized Argyria. Myocardium with Silver Granules between the Muscle Fibres (Magnified 500 diameters)

(b) Localized Argyria

A local form of argyria was noted by Koelsch (1934) amongst workers ngaged in the preparation of silver-leaf. The buccal mucosa was stained lark brown and the teeth greyish-brown in colour. Where a man works vith metallic silver, small particles may accidentally penetrate the exposed kin surface, giving rise to small pigmented lesions by a process equivalent

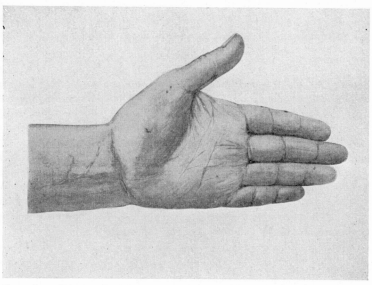

FIG. 163.—Case 15. Dark blue Silver Tattoo Marks on the hand of a man employed for 20 years as a Repairing Silversmith

o tattooing. The occupations responsible are the filing, drilling, hammer-ng, turning, engraving, polishing, forging, soldering and smelting of ilver.

The left hand of the silversmith is more affected than the right, and the ·igmentation occurs at the site of injuries from instruments (Lewin, 1886). Many of these, such as engraving tools, files, chisels and drills, are sharp nd pointed and are liable to produce skin wounds. The piercing saw, an nstrument resembling a fret saw, may break and run into the worker's and. If the file slips, the worker may injure his hand on the silver article n which he is working; this is especially the case with the prongs of forks. man drawing silver wire through a hole in a silver draw-plate gets splin-ers of silver in his fingers. The pigmented points vary from tiny specks to reas 2 mm. in diameter or more. They may be linear or rounded and in arying shades of grey or blue. The tattoo marks remain for life and cannot e removed. The use of gloves is usually impracticable.

Case 15. Repairing silversmith—exposure to dust of silver for twenty years—silver tattoo marks on hands.

(Harker and Hunter, 1935.) G. B., a man aged 35. He had bee. employed as a repairing silversmith for twenty years. He used a pierc ing saw, which sometimes broke and penetrated the skin, especiall that of the left hand.

On examination: Left hand: dark blue spots resembling tatto marks, largest 3 mm. in diameter, on thumb, first two fingers an palm (fig. 163). Right hand: one blue spot on ball of thumb. Eyes an gums normal. Slit-lamp examination negative.

ZINC

Zinc, Zn, is a hard, brittle metal which takes on a white, metallic lustr upon polishing, but the surface quickly tarnishes to the familiar blue-gre tinge. At bright red heat the liquid metal boils, and therefore in the camp fires of primitive man it became a vapour and rapidly oxidized to a cloud c white fume which mixed with the smoke and was not identified. For thi reason zinc was not isolated for many hundreds of years after the discover of brass. It is quite likely that from very early times brass was made acci dentally owing to the admixture of zinc ores with those of copper, but wa not recognized as distinct from bronze. The Romans made coins of bras and it had become an important article of commerce in the Low Countrie by about A.D. 300. By contrast, zinc was first made in China probably i the sixteenth century and reached England about 1740. The chief source c zinc is the mineral, sphalerite, or zinc blende, ZnS, which occurs i association with lead minerals especially galena, PbS.

Uses

Zinc is used for roofing, kitchen fittings, food safes, organ pipes, dr batteries and collapsible tubes. It is made into pressure die castings fc motor cars and is used extensively for galvanizing iron and steel. The ob jects proofed against rust include iron sheets, iron wire, wire netting, wir fencing, tubes, chains, bolts, nuts, screws and nails. Iron articles ma also be coated with zinc by heating them and spraying them with zinc dus This is known as *sherardizing*. The alloys of zinc include brass, gunmeta delta-metal, white metal, german silver and manganese bronze. Zinc dus is used as a reducing substance in the chemical industry, and zinc oxid zinc sulphide and lithopone are used in the paint, rubber and linoleur industries. Zinc sulphate is used as a mordant in dyeing, zinc chloride as wood preservative and other zinc salts as pharmaceutical preparations.

Exposure Hazards

No long-term poisoning occurs in industry from handling zinc com pounds. Metal-fume fever is usually due to inhalation of zinc oxide fum but its effects are temporary and never serious. However, exposure to th fume of certain other zinc compounds may be dangerous and this is true of the chloride.

(a) Metal-fume Fever

Metal-fume fever is an acute disability of short duration which occurs when fume is inhaled from a metal heated to a temperature above its melting-point. The condition was first recognized by Potissier in 1822 and has been called *brassfounders' ague, braziers' disease, spelter shakes, brass chills, zinc chills, zinc oxide chills, galvanizers' poisoning, welders' ague, copper fever, Monday fever, foundry fever* and *the smothers*. It is now known that many metals can cause the syndrome. Zinc, copper and magnesium

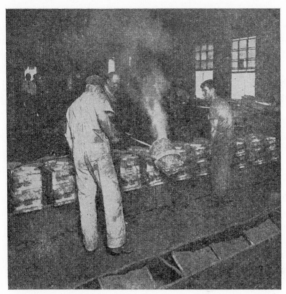

FIG. 164.—Workman pouring molten Brass in a Brass Foundry. Note the White Fume of Zinc Oxide

are the commonest of these, but aluminium, antimony, cadmium, iron, manganese, nickel, selenium, silver and tin may produce it too.

Exposure Hazards

Typical metal-fume fever has occurred in men employed in shipbreaking. They were using the oxy-acetylene flame to cut armour plating when the plates had been galvanized (Bridge, 1921). In 1931 cases were discovered in manganese bronze welders, the zinc content of the bronze being approximately 39 per cent. Typical ague has been observed in men rolling red-hot copper ingots (Koelsch, 1923) and melting copper in an electric furnace (Hanson, 1916). Metal-fume fever can be produced with freshly sublimed magnesium oxide (Drinker, Thompson and Flinn, 1927). Schiøtz (1947) described it in men engaged on electric welding during which they were exposed to iron fume, and in men working in a paint and lacquer factory where pure cuprous oxide was pulverized. Zinc smelting, galvanizing, the welding of zinc or galvanized iron and working up dross from galvanizing tubs are other processes where the hazard exists from exposure to zinc fume.

Brassfounders' Ague

Brassfounders are particularly liable to develop metal-fume fever because zinc melts at a much lower temperature than copper (fig. 164). In making brass, which is an alloy of copper and zinc, fume from the zinc is produced long before the copper begins to melt (Hamilton, 1945). In his famous *Essay on the Effects of the Principal Arts, Trades and Professions on Health and Longevity* (1831), Thackrah, who will always be considered as a pioneer of industrial medicine in England, tells of an ague or intermittent fever attacking the brassfounder once a month or once or twice a year. He did not know the cause of this condition, and it was left to Blandet in 1845 to attribute this form of industrial poisoning to the zinc in brass.

Symptoms and Signs

In 1862 Greenhow made an exhaustive study in the brass industry in Sheffield, Wolverhampton, Leeds and Birmingham. He found that brassfounders are exposed to the risk of shivering attacks with irregular fever accompanied by profuse sweating. The onset is with nausea, thirst, headache, pains in the limbs and a feeling of exhaustion. The attack is of short duration, complete recovery occurring usually before twenty-four hours and always before forty-eight hours. The frequency and severity of the attacks are affected by the regularity of exposure, for those who work continuously in the trade seem to acquire a tolerance which, however, is only transient since it may be lost during a week-end away from work. In such cases the relapse of symptoms after working on a Monday gives rise to the name *Monday fever*. The attacks depend on the density of the zinc fume in the air. Brassfounders suffer most, and the higher the proportion of zinc the worse the symptoms.

Experimental Metal-fume Fever

Drinker (1922) worked experimentally on the question of metal-fume fever. He believes that an important element in the production of zinc oxide poisoning is the breathing of the fumes as they are evolved. That there is a definite difference in the effects produced by inhaling the fume of freshly burned zinc oxide and those produced by inhaling the dust of ordinary zinc oxide powder is shown by the numerous reports of investigators who have administered the latter in doses many times greater than the amount absorbed by brassfounders, without producing anything like the same results. Drinker believes the difference is largely physical, a question of the size of the particles.

Effect of Particle Size

Ordinary zinc oxide consists of particles which have become flocculated and are large and heavy, tending to settle along the walls of a tube and stick there, while the particles formed by the oxidation of vaporized zinc are not only dry and finely dispersed, but also possess enhanced surface activity. On passing through glass tubes they have little tendency to adhere to the sides of the tubes even if there are many sharp bends. This freshly-produced zinc oxide is therefore in the optimum condition to pass through the nose or mouth into the trachea and down into the lungs without clinging to the walls of the trachea. Drinker was able to produce the symptoms practically at will among persons who had not been affected with them for five days previously. The most prominent symptoms were fever as high as 102·5° F., with leucocytosis up to 18,000 cells per c.mm. The shivering and fever are similar in many respects to the phenomena observed following intravenous injections of typhoid vaccine or a foreign serum.

Preventive Measures

Beginning in 1902, exhaust ventilation was installed in the workshops of Birmingham. This resulted immediately in a reduction in the incidence of brassfounders' ague and an improvement in the general health of the workers. Modern methods of prevention include thermostatic control for the zinc pots in brass foundries to reduce the fume which results from overheating of the zinc. Sometimes ammonium chloride is used. It forms a thick layer over the zinc, making a foam which prevents the escape of fume. On foggy or rainy days, workers should wear respirators or air-line masks as an added precaution.

(b) Zinc Chloride

In the open, zinc chloride smoke is held to be innocuous though it is known to be dangerous in confined spaces.

Exposure Hazards

In Malta in 1943 a few people developed minor symptoms on exposure in the open to the concentration of zinc chloride used in screening the harbour. The symptoms, which lasted a few hours, consisted of slight respiratory distress with a feeling of constriction in the chest, dryness of the throat and perhaps a slight cough. On one occasion ten deaths and twenty-five cases of non-fatal injury occurred among seventy persons exposed in a tunnel to zinc chloride fume resulting from the burning of seventy-nine smoke generators stored eighty yards from the entrance. The astringent nature of the zinc chloride was the most potent noxious factor, but the harmful effect of the smoke was enhanced by the heat of the particles, as these were given off in such high concentration and in so confined a space.

Symptoms and Signs

The symptoms were dyspnœa, a feeling of constriction in the chest, retrosternal and epigastric pain, hoarse voice, stridor, lachrymation, cough, expectoration and sometimes hæmoptysis. There was pale grey cyanosis and reddening of the conjunctivæ, nasopharynx and larynx, together with aphonia. The patients were agitated and restless and all had a pulse rate over 100. The pale cyanosis persisted and the temperature rose as broncho-pneumonia developed. About the fourth day moist adventitious sounds appeared in the lungs. At the end of the first week purulent sloughs of mucous membrane appeared in the sputum. Most of the patients began to recover on the tenth day and were up and about six weeks after the incident.

Acute Fatalities and Morbid Anatomy

The deaths occurring immediately after the accident or within a few hours were apparently the result of shock, together with a profuse outpouring of secretion which waterlogged the lungs. In two necropsies the mucous membrane lining the larynx, trachea and bronchi was red and œdematous and in places necrotic. The bronchi were filled with yellow pus, and the lungs showed broncho-pneumonia and œdema. Evans (1945) felt that the particulate nature of the irritant was responsible for the fact that the air passages were far more damaged than the lung itself.

BIBLIOGRAPHY

Arsenic

(a) Arsenic

AGRICOLA, G. (1556), *De Re Metallica*, Basel.

BALTHAZARD, V. (1930), *Occupation and Health*, I.L.O., Geneva, **1**, 159.

HAERTING, F. H., and HESSE, W. (1879) *Vjschr. gerichtl. Med.*, **30**, 296; **31**, 102.

HENRY, S. A. (1934), *Industrial Maladies*, T. M. Legge, London, p. 83.

HILL, A. B., and FANING, E. L. (1948), *Brit. J. indust. Med.*, **5**, 2.

HOLMQUIST, I. (1951), *Acta Dermato-Venereologica*, **31**, Suppl. 26, Stockholm.

HUTCHINSON, J. (1888), *Trans. path. Soc. London*, **39**, 352.

LEGGE, T. M. (1903), *Annual Report of the Chief Inspector of Factories and Workshops for 1902*, London, p. 262.

MORRIS, M. (1902), in OLIVER, T., *Dangerous Trades*, Murray, London, p. 378.

NEUBAUER, O. (1947), *Brit. J. Cancer*, **1**, 192.

O'DONOVAN, W. J. (1928), *Report of the International Conference on Cancer*, London, p. 293.

PARIS, J. A. (1820), *Pharmacologia*, London, p. 282.

PINTO, S. S., and McGILL, C. M. (1953), *Indust. med. and surg.*, **22**, 281.

PYE-SMITH, R. J. (1913), *Proc. R. Soc. Med.*, **6**, Clin. Sect., p. 229.

(b) Arseniuretted Hydrogen

BALTHAZARD, V. (1930), *Occupation and Health*, I.L.O., Geneva, **1**, 159.
BOMFORD, R. R., and HUNTER, D. (1932), *Lancet*, **2**, 1446.
BRIDGE, J. C. (1932), *Annual Report of the Chief Inspector of Factories and Workshops for 1931*, London, p. 81.
DUDLEY, S. F. (1919), *Journ. Industr. Hyg.*, **1**, 215.
GLAISTER, J. (1908), *Poisoning by Arseniuretted Hydrogen or Hydrogen Arsenide*, Edinburgh.
JONES, N. W. (1907), *J. Amer. med. Ass.*, **48**, 1099.
KOELSCH, F. (1920), *Zbl. GewHyg.*, **8**, 121.
LEGGE, T. M. (1923), *Annual Report of the Chief Inspector of Factories and Workshops for 1922*, London, p. 64.
LEVVY, G. A. (1947), *Quart. J. exp. Physiol.*, **34**, 47.
LONING, F. (1931), *Zbl. inn. Med.*, **52**, 833.
LUNDSGAARD, C., and SCHIERBECK, K. (1923), Amer. J. Physiol, **64**, 210.

(c) Organic Arsenic Compounds

BIGINELLI, P. (1901), *Gazz. chim. ital.*, **31**, 58.
CHALLENGER, F. (1935), *J. Soc. chem. Ind.*, **54** (*Chem. and Ind.*, vol. 13), 657.
EHRLICH, P. (1909), *Uber den jetzigen Stand der Chemotherapie, Ber.*, **42**, 17.
GOLDBLATT, M. W. (1945), *Brit. J. industr. Med.*, **2**, 183.
LONGCOPE, W. T., LUETSCHER, J. A., WINTROBE, M. M., and JAGER, V. (1946), *J. clin. Invest.*, **25**, 528.
PETERS, R. A., STOCKEN, L. A., and THOMPSON, R. H. S. (1945), *Nature*, **156**, 616.
SARTORI, M. (1940), *The War Gases*, London.

Calcium

CAROZZI, L. (1930), *Occupation and Health*, I.L.O., Geneva, **1**, 332.
DREESSEN, W. C. (1934), *Publ. Hlth. Rept.*, Wash., **49**, 724.
GARDNER, L. U., DURKAN, T. M., BRUNFIEL, D. M., and SAMPSON, H. L. (1939), *J. industr. Hyg.*, **21**, 279.
HENNELL, T. (1946), *British Craftsmen*, Collins, London, p. 12.
HEPPLESTON, A. G. (1946), *Brit. J. industr. Med.*, **3**, 253.
KOELSCH, F. (1930), *Occupation and Health*, I.L.O., Geneva, **1**, 334.
MARCHAND, M. (1945), *Arch. Mal. prof.*, **6**, 132.
MINTON, J. (1949), *Occupational Eye Diseases and Injuries*, Heinemann, London, p. 44.
OPPENHEIM, M. (1935), *Wien. klin. Wschr.*, **48**, 207.
PIERACCINI, G. (1906), *Patologia del lavoro e terapia sociale*, Milan, p. 137.
TURANO, L. (1930), *Silicosis Studies and Repts.*, Series F., *Industr. hyg.*, No. 13, p. 509.

Phosphorus

(a) Phosphorus

BARON, R. (1944), *Brit. dent. J.*, **76**, 331.
COLLIER, R. (1965), *The General next to God*, Collins, London, p. 194.
COLTART, G. (1931), *Lancet*, **2**, 829.
DEARDEN, W. F. (1899), *Brit. med. J.*, **2**, 270.

HAMILTON, A. (1925), *Industrial Poisons in the United States*, Macmillan, New York, p. 315.
HEIMANN, H. (1946), *J. industr. Hyg.*, **28**, 142.
KENNON, R. (1944), *Brit. dent. J.*, **76**, 343.
KENNON, R., and HALLAM, J. W. (1944), *Brit. dent. J.*, **76**, 321.
OLIVER, T. (1902), *Dangerous Trades*, Murray, London.
PICKERILL, H. P. (1923), *Brit. J. Surg.*, **10**, 380.
SÉVÈNE, H., and CAHEN, E. D. (1898), *Rev. Proc. Chim.*, **1**, 210.
WARD, E. F. (1928), *J. industr. Hyg.*, **10**, 314.

(b) Phosphoretted Hydrogen

BELL, A. (1961), Personal communication.
BRUYLANTS, G., and DRUYTS, H. (1909), *Bull. Acad. roy. Méd. Belg.*, **23**, 26.
COPEMAN, S. M. (1909), *Report on Ferro-Silicon, Supplement to 38th Report of the Local Government Board*, London.
GESSNER, O. (1937), *Samml. Vergiftungsf.*, **8**, 13.
HAKE, H. W. (1910), *Lancet*, **2**, 220.
MÜLLER, W. (1940), *Arch. exp. Path. Pharmak.*, **195**, 184.
THIELE (1921), *Zbl. GewHyg.*, **9**, 94.
ZANGGER, H. (1930), *Occupation and Health*, I.L.O., Geneva, **1**, 742.

(c) Tri-*ortho*-cresyl Phosphate

BLOCK, H. (1941), *Helv. med. Acta.*, **8**, Suppl. 7, 17.
TER BRAAK, J. W. G. (1931), *Ned. Tijdschr. Geneesk.*, **75**, 2329.
EARL, C. J., and THOMPSON, R. H. S. (1952), *Brit. J. Pharmacol.*, **7**, 261.
FLINN, F. B. (1943), Personal communication.
GERMON, G. (1932), *Intoxication mortelle par l'Apiol*, Thèse de Paris.
HAMILTON, A. (1934), *Industrial Toxicology*, New York, p. 195.
HODGE, H. C., and STERNER, J. H. (1943), *J. Pharm. exper. Ther.*, **79**, 225.
HOTSTON, R. D. (1946), *Lancet*, **1**, 207.
HOTTINGER, A., and BLOCH, H. (1943), *Helv. chim. Acta*, **26**, 142.
HUMPE, F. (1942), *Munch. med. Wschr.*, **89**, 448.
HUNTER, D., PERRY, K. M. A., and EVANS, R. B. (1944), *Brit. J. indust. Med.*, **1**, 227.
LOROT, C. (1899), *Les combinaisons de la creosote dans le traitement de la tuberculose pulmonaire*, Thèse de Paris.
ROGER, H., and RECORDIER, M. (1934), *Ann. Méd.*, **35**, 44.
SAMPSON, B. F. (1938), *Bull. Off. Int. Hyg. Publ.*, **30**, 2601; (1942), *S. Afr. Med. J.*, **16**, 1.
SMITH, HONOR V., and SPALDING, J. M. K. (1959), *Lancet*, **2**, 1019.
SMITH, M. I., ELVOVE, E., and others (1930), *Publ. Hlth. Rept.*, *Wash.*, **45**, 1703, 2509.
WALTHARD, K. M. (1946), *Arch. suisses de neurologie et de psychiatrie*, **58**, 189.
ZELIGS, M. A. (1938), *J. nerv. ment. Dis.*, **87**, 464.

(d) Organic Phosphorus Insecticides

BIDSTRUP, P. L., BONNELL, J. A., and BECKETT, A. G. (1953), *Brit. med. J.*, **1**, 1068.
CALLAWAY, S., DAVIES, D. R., and RUTLAND, T. P. (1951), *Brit. med. J.*, **2**, 812.

ommittee on Pesticides of the American Medical Association Council on Pharmacy (1950), *J. Amer. Med. Ass.*, **144**, 104.

uBois, K. P. (1951), *Proceedings Ninth Internat. Congr. of Entomology*, Amsterdam.

ARUNAKARAN, C. O. (1958), *J. Indian Med. Assoc.*, **31**, 204.

ETRY, H. (1951), *Zbl. Arbeitsmed. Arbeitsschutz*, **1**, 86.

EDA, K. (1966), Brit. med. J., **2**, 1132.

Silver

DAMSON, H. G. (1923–4), *Proc. R. Soc. Med.* (Sect. Dermatol.), **17**, 8.

RIDGE, J. C. (1920), *Annual Report of the Chief Inspector of Factories and Workshops*, H.M.S.O., London, p. 134.

ARKER, J. M., and HUNTER, D. (1935), *Brit. J. Derm.*, **47**, 441.

OELSCH, F. (1934), *Occupation and Health*, I.L.O., Geneva, **2**, 871.

ARSEN, B. (1927), *v. Graefe's Arch. Ophthal.*, **118**, 145.

EWIN, G. (1886), *Berl. klin. Wschr.*, **23**, 417.

CHUBERT, L. (1895), *Z. Heilk.*, **16**, 341.

ELEKY, L. (1914), *Zbl. GewHyg.*, **2**, 128.

Zinc

LANDET (1845), *Ann. Hyg.*, **34**, 222.

RIDGE, J. C. (1921), *Annual Report of the Chief Inspector of Factories and Workshops for 1920*, Cmd. 1705, p. 70.

RUTON, D.M. (1967), Brit. med. J., **1**, 757.

RINKER, P. (1922), *J. industr. Hyg.*, **4**, 177.

RINKER, P., THOMSON, R. M., and FLINN, J. L. (1927), *J. Industr. Hyg.*, **9**, 98.

VANS, E. H. (1945), *Lancet*, **2**, 368.

REENHOW, E. H. (1862), *Med.-chir. Trans.*, **45**, 177.

AMILTON, A., and JOHNSTONE, R. T. (1945), *Industrial Toxicology*, Oxford Loose Leaf Medicine, New York, p. 614.

ANSON, W. C. (1916), *Diseases of Occupation*, by Kober, G. M., and Hanson, W. C., Philadelphia.

ARRIS, D.K. (1951), Lancet, **2**, 1008.

OELSCH, F. (1923), *J. industr. Hyg.*, **5**, 87.

CHIØTZ, E. H. (1947), *Tidsskrift for den Norske Laegeforening*, Oslo, 67/17 451.

HACKRAH, C. T. (1831), *Essay on the Effects of the Principal Arts, Trades and Professions on Health and Longevity*, London.

CHAPTER VII

THE NEWER METALS

OF the metals newly introduced into industry a good deal is known about the ill-effects of chromium, manganese, nickel, radium and thorium, and the toxicity of many others is at present under study. So far no toxic effect has been discovered in workers handling cæsium, cerium, columbium (niobium), gallium, germanium, hafnium, indium, lanthanum, molybdenum, rhenium, rhodium, rubidium, strontium, tantalum, titanium, wolfram (tungsten) and zirconium. On the contrary, toxic effects are already known in the case of beryllium, cadmium, osmium, platinum, ruthenium, selenium, tellurium, thallium, uranium, vanadium and a large number of radioactive compounds. Browning (1961) has written a comprehensive review of the toxicity of the metals used in industry.

BERYLLIUM

In 1798 the French chemist Vauquelin discovered that the mineral beryl contained an earth similar to alumina, which he called *glucine* or *glucina* because its salts tasted sweet. The element was isolated later and became *glucinum*, a name still used principally in France. In other countries it is called *beryllia*, BeO. The element beryllium, Be, is a hard, shiny metal resembling steel in appearance and lustre. It is remarkably light in weight, having a slightly greater density than magnesium. Its chemical properties are similar to those of aluminium or magnesium.

Sources

Beryllium occurs in nature as beryllium aluminium silicate or beryl $3BeO.Al_2O_3.6SiO_2$. There are three well-known varieties of beryl—namely the precious stone emerald, which is coloured green by chromium oxide, the greenish-blue gem stone aquamarine and the yellow chrysoberyl. The more usual cloudy green, white or yellowish crystals occur in feldspar quarries in the Argentine, Brazil, the United States of America, India and South Africa. At rare intervals very large crystals of the mineral have been found: one in Maine was 18 feet long, 4 feet in diameter, and weighed 19 tons. A few others almost as large have been found in Namaqualand, South Africa. More commonly the amounts of beryl are so small that until about 1935 when beryllium became an important metal, beryl deposits were worked only when other minerals such as feldspar or mica were the chief products.

Uses

It was the appreciation of the properties of the alloys of beryllium which first increased its value. The principal alloy is beryllium-copper, also referred to as beryllium-bronze, but beryllium-nickel and beryllium-aluminium are also in use. When 2 to 3 per cent of beryllium is added to copper, the alloys produced are hard, corrosion-resistant, non-rusting, non-sparking and non-magnetic, and they have good elastic properties. They can be temper-hardened and then they behave like spring steel, having a tensile strength which is six times that of copper. In addition, they are characterized by a high fatigue limit, while their electrical conductivity is but little different from that of copper. Metallic beryllium is employed as a deoxidizer in steel making. In the atomic-energy industry, pure beryllium rods are essential to the efficient working of the graphite pile. Industrial radiography has created a demand for pure beryllium foil for the windows of X-ray tubes, since the metal is seventeen times more transparent to X-rays than aluminium.

Recovering the Metal from the Ore

In recovering the metal from the ore, the beryl is run through a dry crusher and then through a wet ball mill which reduces it to powder. The wet powder is then mixed with soda ash and sodium fluosilicate. Briquettes are made from this mixture, and these are passed through a furnace at high temperature where sodium beryllium fluoride is formed as the only water-soluble constituent of the briquettes. They are then crushed and ground in a wet ball mill, and the sodium beryllium fluoride is extracted with water. The resulting solution is then treated with caustic soda which precipitates beryllium hydroxide. The precipitate is filtered off and heated in a furnace for conversion to beryllium oxide. In the production of beryllium-copper alloys, a mixture of beryllium oxide, copper oxide, copper and carbon is heated in an electric furnace. The temperature is increased to above the melting-point until a homogeneous mixture is formed. The furnace charge is then poured into metal moulds to form pigs of a master alloy containing about 4 per cent of beryllium. In the foundry trade these pigs are remelted with more copper to make castings containing smaller amounts of beryllium up to 0·4 per cent. In all these processes, exposure to fume and dust may occur in crushing the briquettes, handling the furnace dross, and knocking-out, cleaning and grinding the castings (Walworth, 1949).

Exposure Hazards

A considerable hazard exists in preparing and mixing the powders used as phosphors for coating the tubes of fluorescent strip lamps and certain tubes used for electric signs. In this industry the compounds involved are zinc beryllium manganese silicate, zinc beryllium silicate and beryllium oxide. The tubing is coated on the inside by pumping into it a liquid suspension of the phosphor, excess of which is then drained away. Dry mixing of the powder, spillage of the liquid suspension and brushing clean the ends of the tubes may produce considerable amounts of dust (fig. 165). Other occupations involving exposure to beryllium compounds

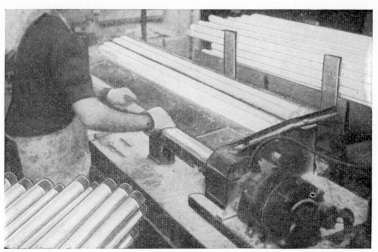

Fig. 165.—Manufacture of Fluorescent Lamp Tubes. The woman is removing from the end of each Tube a white Phosphor containing Beryllium Salts. Exhaust Ventilation has been applied locally to the Brush used
(*By courtesy of General Electric Company, 1949*)

are the extraction of the metal from the ore, the manufacture and cutting of beryllium-copper alloys and the making of beryllium-containing crystals for wireless apparatus. In addition, exposure may occur to beryllium oxide used as a refractory for making crucibles and to beryl in the manufacture of electrical porcelain.

Historical Summary

The first men poisoned by beryllium compounds in industry suffered from an acute respiratory disease—namely, bronchitis and bronchiolitis. They were German workmen employed in extracting beryllium from the ore (Weber and Engelhardt, 1933). Working in Milan in 1935, Fabroni gave animals beryllium carbonate and produced a modified form of pneumoconiosis which he called berylliosis. By 1936 the dust of beryllium fluoride, $5BeF_2.2BeO$, was causing trouble. At this time animal experiments supported the erroneous view that the beryllium ion was non-toxic. Because the dust of beryllium fluoride was toxic to animals, it was too readily assumed that the acid radical was to blame.

The Dust of Beryllium Fluoride

Much of the early experience of handling beryllium compounds in industry came from the preparation of beryllium steel. Here a certain amount of dust is continually given off by the molten salt electrolytic baths. The dust consists of sodium silico-fluoride, barium fluoride, beryllium oxide, and beryllium fluoride. In 1936 Gelman in Moscow described cases of occupational poisoning by beryllium oxyfluoride. He said that it was not easy to separate the action of beryllium and its fluorides from that of other fluorides. He observed a mild irritant action on the skin, mucous membranes and conjunctivæ. There was also bronchiolitis with cough, moist râles in the chest and an X-ray picture resembling that of miliary tuberculosis.

The Dust of Phosphors of Fluorescent Lamps

The first cases of the acute disease which occurred in the United States of America were reported by Van Ordstrand, Hughes and Carmody in 1943. In 1946 Hardy and Tabershaw described cases of a chronic lung disease occurring among the employees of a firm manufacturing fluorescent lamps in Salem, Massachusetts. It was the resemblance between these cases and sarcoidosis which had led to the designation *Salem sarcoid*. In 1949 Machle reported more than 400 cases of lung disease which had occurred in beryllium workers in the United States of America. One hundred and twenty-three of these patients showed the delayed pneumonitis known as chronic berylliosis or pulmonary granulomatosis of beryllium workers.

The Dust of the Metal and the Oxide

In 1949 Aub and Grier reported seven cases of acute pneumonitis in metallurgical workers exposed to the dust and fume of pure beryllium metal and beryllium oxide. The occurrence of such cases supports the view that the beryllium ion is toxic in its own right and that the poisonous effects of soluble beryllium salts are not to be attributed to the acid radicals. It would seem that the more soluble compounds of beryllium, particularly those containing a strongly electro-negative group such as the fluoride or sulphate, are likely to cause acute disease, whereas the less soluble compounds may cause chronic disease (Machle, 1949).

Few Cases in Great Britain

In Great Britain, fortunately, beryllium and its compounds have been handled on what is relatively a small scale and therefore the number of cases of beryllium poisoning has been small and is likely to remain so. Agate (1948) described a case with beryllium granulomatosis of the lungs and liver in a London physicist who has since died. He had worked on the development of fluorescent lamp tubes which were coated on the inside with phosphors containing zinc beryllium manganese silicate and magnesium tungstate.

Acute Beryllium Poisoning

In 1933 Weber and Engelhardt reported cases of dermatitis and of an acute respiratory illness occurring among workers handling beryllium compounds in Germany. A number of clinical syndromes has since been recognized and attributed to exposure to beryllium. These are conjunctivitis, irritation of the upper respiratory tract, dermatitis, subcutaneous granulomata and acute and chronic forms of lung disease (Machle, 1949). Conjunctivitis is frequently associated with dermatitis of the face. It follows exposure to soluble salts of beryllium in plants where the ore is processed or where the halides and acid salts are handled. On removal from contact the lesions readily heal. Exposure to the soluble salts may also give rise to irritation of the nose and throat, with epistaxis, and swelling and redness of the mucous membranes. Tracheitis and bronchitis may develop, together with anorexia, dyspnœa and loss of weight. The symptoms and signs clear up completely within two or three weeks after exposure ceases and no special treatment is required.

Beryllium Dermatitis

Dermatitis may be severe, and sensitization, once established, is permanent. It follows that a person once affected should not work again with beryllium compounds. The lesion is usually an œdematous papulo-vesicular eruption appearing mainly on the exposed surfaces. Healing occurs promptly on removal from contact and is hastened by local treatment of the lesion.

Beryllium Granuloma of the Skin

Subcutaneous granulomata occur when beryllium compounds are introduced beneath the skin (Grier, Nash and Freiman, 1948). Such lesions may occur in persons who have cut themselves on broken fluorescent lamps, After the glass splinters have penetrated the skin, healing may occur at once, and the granulomata appear much later, even as long as four years (Lederer and Savage, 1954). The swellings may measure as much as 2·5 centimetres in diameter (fig. 166). There is no pain nor tenderness; occasionally the lesion ulcerates through the skin. It is necessary to excise the granulomatous mass and to remove completely all beryllium from the lesion for fear that healing may be delayed.

Chemical Pneumonitis

The respiratory symptoms of the acute disease are those of a chemical pneumonitis. They occur during employment. In the early stages cough with blood-stained sputum is accompanied by retro-sternal pain, dyspnœa, cyanosis and loss of weight. Non-productive cough may be present for several days before dyspnœa, on exertion, and later at rest, becomes obvious. Rapid respiration, anorexia and marked prostration follow. Usually there is no fever, but cyanosis and tachycardia are present and râles are heard over both lungs. Death may occur within two weeks.

Morbid Anatomy of the Acute Disease

The morbid anatomy of the lungs is similar to that of acute chemical pneumonitis from other causes except that there is less evidence of necrosis. The alveoli are filled with exudate composed of œdema fluid and fibrin containing macrophages. Collections of lymphocytes and plasma cells occur in the septa. In cases where death has occurred after several weeks, there are large areas of fibroblastic proliferation such as are seen in or-

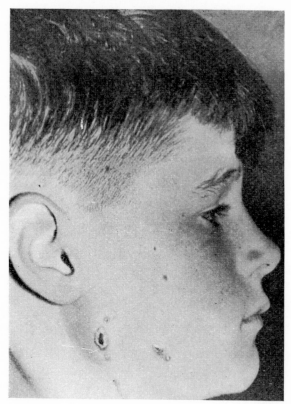

FIG. 166.—Subcutaneous Beryllium Granulomata in a boy aged 12, following a Cut from a broken Fluorescent Lamp Tube

(After Dr. P. H. Nash, 1949)

ganizing pneumonia. More commonly, resolution begins in the third week of the illness and is complete in from five weeks to five months. Serious sequelæ are unusual, but attacks of the acute illness have been followed by the onset of chronic berylliosis after two years (Machle, 1949).

Radiographic Changes

In the acute disease symptoms and signs precede radiological changes in the lungs by several weeks. Increased linear markings and a granular ground-glass appearance suggesting pulmonary congestion appear first. The shadows are diffuse, but may be less marked at the apices and bases owing to compensatory emphysema. Consolidation may follow. As the clinical signs disappear, the lung lesion becomes granular and nodular with conglomerate masses. In from one to four months these disappear, leaving residual fibrosis in some cases.

Chronic Beryllium Poisoning

The first symptoms of the chronic disease are variable and may not appear for as long as six years after the last exposure to beryllium compounds. The majority of cases have occurred in employees in the fluorescent lamp industry, but two laboratory workers and at least ten people living in the neighbourhood of factories using beryllium compounds have been affected. Less than 5 per cent of the persons exposed have developed the disease. This suggests that some people are unduly susceptible to the effects of absorption of small amounts of beryllium. Vague ill health, slight but persistent loss of weight, weakness and lack of energy, or an unusually persistent upper respiratory tract infection may herald the onset of the disease.

Physical Signs and Prognosis

It may be weeks or months before abnormal signs appear in the lungs. Weakness, anorexia and progressive loss of weight, which may be as much as 20 or 30 lb. in a month, become prominent symptoms and persist throughout the illness. Cough, with little sputum, worse in the mornings or on exertion, is constantly present and bears no relationship to the severity of the disease or to the radiographic signs. Dyspnœa is extreme and may be the presenting symptom. Tachycardia, particularly when there is cyanosis, is associated with a normal or low blood-pressure. Clubbing of the fingers develops in the later stages. Cardiac failure occurs, increasing the dyspnœa and later causing orthopnœa and œdema of the extremities. Approximately one-third of the patients die, while one-third are permanently disabled and remain in great respiratory distress. The rest lose their symptoms, the lung changes resolving to some extent.

Radiographic Changes

In the chronic disease the earliest change in radiographs is a diffuse, finely granular appearance homogeneously distributed through both lungs. Both apices and bases are involved. Paratracheal masses and enlarged hilar shadows are seen in many cases. As the disease progresses, fine nodulation appears on a granular background (Pl. I). Confluence of nodules may occur, but it is much less evident than in silicosis. Later, there is lobular emphysema, particularly at the apices and bases. Signs of cor pulmonale may develop, and spontaneous pneumothorax, without pleural effusion, has occurred in a few cases. The X-ray appearances alone are not diagnostic.

Morbid Anatomy of the Chronic Disease

The pathological findings in chronic berylliosis resemble closely those found in sarcoidosis. The lungs are grossly emphysematous, with universally scattered fine, grey, granulomatous, miliary nodules and diffuse interstitial fibrosis. The granulomata are formed within the alveolar spaces by organization of exudate. They have a fibrinoid centre with peripheral fibrosis and varying degrees of mononuclear infiltration, together with numerous giant cells of the Langhans type. Similar lesions have been found in the skin and subcutaneous tissues (fig. 167), in hilar and axillary lymph nodes, and in the liver. Mid-zonal necrosis is also found in the liver.

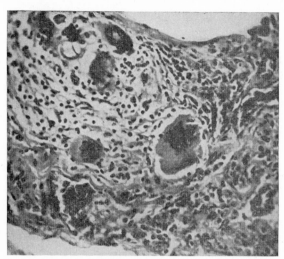

FIG. 167.—Chronic Beryllium Granuloma showing Giant Cells from the case described in Fig. 166. (Magnified 250 diameters)

(*After Dr. P. H. Nash, 1949*)

All these changes serve to prove that beryllium poisoning is a systemic disease and not merely an affection of the lungs.

Diagnostic Criteria

Diagnosis depends upon an occupational history of significant exposure to beryllium compounds, a characteristic onset and course of the disease, X-ray findings and the presence of beryllium in urine and tissues. Spectrographic methods for analysis of beryllium are now sensitive to 0·3 microgram of beryllium per 100 milligrams of tissue, and to 0·1 microgram per litre of urine (Cholak, 1943). Amounts of beryllium excreted in the urine have ranged from 0·1 microgram per litre to 2·0 micrograms per litre. The higher values occur in the acute cases. No method is available by which beryllium can be detected in the tissues or excreta of persons who have not been exposed. Beryllium inhaled into the lung appears to remain there for a considerable time. This may explain the long latent interval before symptoms of the chronic disease begin. In one patient, who died five years after the termination of exposure, the lungs contained 20 micrograms per 100 milligrams of lung tissue although the urinary excretion was less than 0·1 microgram per day.

Differential Diagnosis

Differentiation from sarcoidosis, chronic miliary tuberculosis, fungus infections, primary pulmonary fibrosis, diffuse nodular silicosis, miliary carcinomatosis and mitral stenosis with hæmosiderosis (see Pl. XIV) may be difficult. A diagnosis of chronic berylliosis can be made only by considering the whole picture together with evidence of significant exposure to beryllium compounds.

Hazard in the Neighbourhood of Factories

The United States Atomic Energy Commission has investigated the contamination of the atmosphere in the neighbourhood of a plant producing beryllium oxide, beryllium copper and beryllium metal. During the previous ten years 1,600 workers had been employed. Compared to five known cases of the chronic disease within the factory, ten cases with at least one death occurred in persons living within three-quarters of a mile of the plant, though they had never worked there. The atmosphere concentration of beryllium three-quarters of a mile away from the factory ranged from 0·01 to 0·1 microgram per cubic metre (Eisenbud and others, 1949). The existence of the hazard of non-occupational beryllium poisoning in the neighbourhood of factories handling this substance presents a challenge not only to the guardians of health in industry but also to public health authorities in industrial communities in general. Indirectly, therefore, the splitting of the atom has given us new and grave responsibilities besides those connected with radioactive substances. In Great Britain the Alkali Inspectorate enforces the provision laid down by the Clean Air Act of 1956 that the maximum concentration of beryllium allowed in the outside effluent of a factory is 0·01 microgram per cubic metre of air.

Deaths in Animals dusted with Beryllium Salts

Policard (1950) found that both beryl and beryllium metal proved harmless when inhaled by guinea-pigs and white rats. On the other hand, inhalation of beryllium oxide containing traces of beryllium fluoride caused death within a few hours. Necropsy showed intense pulmonary congestion and œdema, and severe lesions of the bronchial mucosa. The initial lesions may have been due to hydrofluoric acid formed by hydrolysis in the pulmonary epithelium. About twenty days after heavy dusting with pure beryllium oxide of particle size less than one micron, hyperplasia of histiocytes had produced the typical granulomata of chronic berylliosis. In animals which recovered, the lesions resolved completely.

Pulmonary Granulomata in Rats

Lloyd-Davies and Harding (1950) introduced amorphous beryllium oxide into the lungs of twenty-three rats by means of intratracheal injection of 50 milligrams of beryllium oxide of which 75 per cent of particles measured less than one micron in size. These authors believe that the occurrence of granulomata in the lungs of such experimental rats is associated with the rate of solution of the particles and that this is determined by the size of the particle and the solubility of beryllium. Beryllium oxide is relatively insoluble and disappears slowly from the lung. All work on beryllium granulomatosis must therefore include consideration of the particle size and solubility.

Multiple Sarcomata of Bone in Rabbits

In animal experiments after intravenous injection, very little beryllium is excreted. Instead, it collects in the liver and spleen, where it produces minimal tissue response (Barnes, 1949). Beryllium is capable of displacing magnesium in the tissues and of inhibiting the activity of alkaline phosphatase (Grier and others, 1949). Multiple sarcomata of bone have been found in rabbits eight months after intravenous injection of a suspension of beryllium silicate or of zinc beryllium silicate (Gardner and Heslington, 1946). Repeating this work, Barnes (1949) showed that three out of six rabbits developed multiple sarcomata of bone after similar injections. In tracer experiments with small laboratory animals, Wilson (1948) showed that the radioactive isotope of beryllium accumulates in bone. As yet, no case of sarcoma of bone has occurred among human victims of beryllium poisoning (Hardy, 1953).

Safe Substitutes for Phosphors and Beryllium Alloys

Since the poisonous nature of beryllium and its compounds has been known only since 1933, there is much room still for education of those who handle it. At a time when cases of beryllium poisoning in the United States fluorescent-lamp industry were occurring with greatest frequency, the phosphors contained beryllium in percentages ranging from 4 to 12. Later, the figure was reduced to 2 per cent, and now halo-phosphates containing no beryllium are available as safe substitutes for the poisonous phosphors of the past. Calcium halophosphate consists of a mixture of calcium phosphate, chloride and fluoride with a small amount of a manganese salt as activator. Since chronic berylliosis has occurred in smelters of beryllium and copper and in others who machine the finished alloy, it is imperitave to use efficient apparatus for exhaust ventilation of fume in the foundries concerned. Those who machine the metal or the finished beryllium-copper alloy must work with their hands and arms inserted into glove boxes to which are attached effective systems of suction ventilation. In Great Britain in 1949 poisoning by beryllium and its compounds was added to the list of diseases prescribed under the *National Insurance (Industrial Injuries) Act 1946*. In 1967 it was made notifiable under the *Factories Act*.

Preventive Measures

These are set out at length in a review of the subject by Stokinger (1966). In all industries where beryllium and its compounds are used, strict measures for dust suppression must be enforced. There is evidence that cases of disease will occur when exposure to beryllium as oxide exceeds

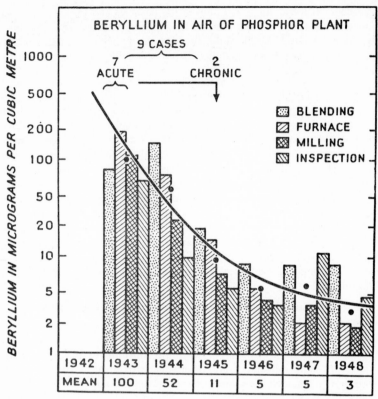

FIG. 168.—Concentration of Beryllium Compounds in the Atmosphere of a factory making a Phosphor for use in Fluorescent Strip-lamps. Note diminishing incidence of cases as Protective Measures are introduced. This correlation fails to take into account cases where the onset of symptoms and signs is long delayed

(*After Machle and others, 1949*)

100 micrograms per cubic metre of air (fig. 168). Every effort must be made by engineering methods to keep the atmosphere concentration in the working environment lower than 2 micrograms per cubic metre of air. Protective clothing and adequate laundry services should be provided. No factory effluent must be allowed to endanger the health of people living in the neighbourhood. Since subcutaneous granulomata have developed in persons who have cut themselves on broken lamps, caution must be exercised in the disposal and salvage of burnt-out fluorescent tubes. It is best to break them under water (fig. 169) and to bury the fragments in the ground.

Routine Medical Examination and Radiography

Workers at risk should be examined at regular intervals by a doctor and questioned about suggestive symptoms. Accurate case records should be kept. All persons exposed must be weighed at monthly intervals and have

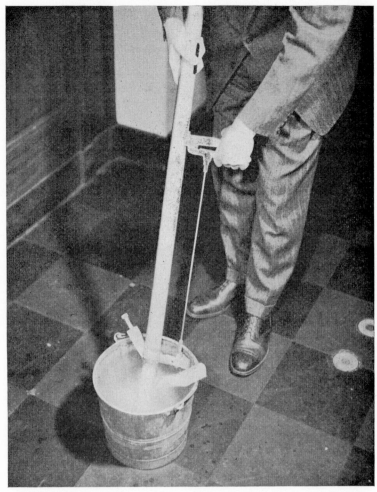

FIG. 169.—Apparatus known as a Bazooka used to destroy burnt-out Fluorescent Lamp Tubes under Water. This aims at the prevention of Beryllium Granuloma of the skin following cuts

(*By courtesy of Dr. L. Greenburg, 1949*)

the chest X-rayed at least once a year. Repeated medical and X-ray examinations must be made of all workers who have unexplained symptoms, particularly when these suggest disease of the respiratory system.

Treatment of the Acute Disease

A patient with acute pneumonitis must be treated for many weeks in bed. Before the serious nature of the disease was appreciated, several patients died from a relapse of pulmonary symptoms and signs which occurred on getting them up too soon. Treatment is symptomatic. The patient should be propped up with a canvas bed-rest and sedatives should be given for the cough. In those severely affected, oxygen is necessary to relieve the dyspnœa. Penicillin-streptomycin aerosol therapy has relieved secondary bacterial infection but has no other beneficial effect. Prolonged convalescence up to four or six months is necessary; it must continue until X-rays of the chest show no abnormality.

Treatment of the Chronic Disease

In the chronic disease, certain patients, although losing weight and suffering from mild dyspnœa, are capable of some type of work, perhaps only part time. Attempts to increase the rate of elimination of beryllium with injections of 2,3-dimercaptopropanol (BAL) have not been successful. The course of the chronic illness may often be influenced favourably by treatment with prednisolone the dosage of which must be reduced as the clinical response allows. In spite of the fact that spontaneous recovery is known to occur in some patients with severe and progressive loss of weight and dyspnœa, treatment by corticosteroids does not cure the disease, although relief of symptoms is undoubted. In the case of granulomata of the skin following cuts from broken fluorescent tubes, the need for total excision of the swellings has already been emphasized (p. 432).

Case 16. Research physicist—exposure to beryllium compounds for four years —latent interval of three years—death after three years' illness from granulomatous fibrosis of the lungs with right heart failure.

(Agate, 1948.) J. P., a man aged 36, was engaged in research on mercury-vapour lamps from his graduation in 1936 until 1941. He was slightly exposed to dust between 1938 and 1941, when he was filling some 200 lamps with powdered sulphides of zinc and cadmium. He noted no ill effects from this. Between December 1941 and December 1942 he worked on the development of tubular fluorescent lamps. He handled about 500 tubes, which had already been coated internally with phosphorescent powders containing zinc beryllium, manganese silicate and magnesium tungstate. He had to clean the last 3 inches of each tube with a duster; from time to time he shook out the duster and a cloud of dust arose. The next state—the sealing-in of electrodes and exhaustion of the tube—was not without risk, because he sometimes had to suck at a side tube and could have inhaled powder. He was working in a small laboratory, but the coating processes were all done in a separate room. During October and November 1942 small quantities of these phosphor powders containing beryllium were prepared, ground and heated in his laboratory, only a few feet from his bench. This increased the risk to which he was exposed. After December 1942 his contact with phosphors was negligible; for the next two years he worked in other rooms and only occasionally walked through the laboratory.

In November 1945, three years after his last significant exposure, he had a feverish cold, and a dry cough developed when he returned to work three days later. After another month the cough became productive, yielding a little yellow-green sputum, and he began to be dyspnœic on exertion; he could neither run for a bus nor climb a hill. At the same time he began to lose weight rapidly, and by February 1946 was already 23 lb. below normal. Radiography of his chest then led to a tentative diagnosis of miliary tuberculosis. He could walk only about 30 yards on the level. He was admitted to hospital, where miliary tuberculosis was excluded and pulmonary sarcoidosis diagnosed. All of many sputum examinations were negative for tubercle bacilli; a Mantoux test at 1 : 1,000 dilution was positive; and a blood count showed 6,000,000 red cells per c.mm. and Hb 130 per cent. He attended various hospitals for a year and a half after his discharge. His weight was still falling, his appetite was poor, and he had to be absent from work repeatedly because of attacks resembling acute bronchitis. His chief symptom, which varied in severity, was dyspnœa on exertion and at rest.

On examination in February 1948, he weighed 7 st. 5 lb. He was dyspnœic at rest and slightly cyanosed. There was no clubbing of the fingers. The cardiovascular system was normal except for an accentuated second heart sound in the pulmonary area. The chest expansion was only 1 inch. The percussion note of the chest was resonant, but multiple rhonchi and coarse crepitations could be heard in all areas. The liver edge was palpable 1½ inches below the costal margin, but the upper limit of hepatic dullness in the chest was displaced downwards. The spleen was not palpable, and only one small lymph-gland was felt in the neck. No glands were discovered elsewhere, and the parotids and uveal tracts were normal.

During a stay in hospital of three weeks there was no fever, but there was considerable dyspnœa at rest, and the respiratory-rate varied between 18 and 38 per minute. On the slightest exertion there was dyspnœa to the point of distress.

Vital capacity: 1,470 ml. A healthy man of this patient's height and weight might have had a vital capacity of 3,800 ml.

Sputum: repeatedly negative for *Myco. tuberculosis.*

Erythrocyte-sedimentation rate: 7–13 mm./1 hour (Wintrobe).

Mantoux test: 1/10,000 negative and 1/1,000 negative.

Blood count: Hb 112 per cent, red cells 6,412,000 per c.mm., white cells 5,300 per c.mm. (polymorphs 44 per cent, eosinophils 1 per cent. lymphocytes 45 per cent, large hyaline cells 10 per cent.).

Electrocardiogram: right ventricular preponderance.

Circulation-time: arm to breath (ether min. 5) = 7–9 sec., arm to face (histamine phosphate 0·1 mg.) = 25–8 sec.

Glucose-tolerance test: within normal limits.

Liver-function tests: van den Bergh, indirect reaction 0·5 mg.

bilirubin per 100 ml. Alkaline phosphatase, 6 units. Thymol turbidity, 6 units. Cephalin cholesterol flocculation, 1. Serum colloidal gold, 0.

Plasma-proteins: total 6·6 g. per 100 ml. (albumin 4·4 g. and globulin 2·2 g. per 100 ml.).

Urine: on admission, no beryllium detected. After a course of 2,3-dimercaptopropanol (BAL), no beryllium detected.

Radiography: X-ray films of the patient's hands and feet in April 1946 and April 1948 showed no abnormality.

Radiography of the chest *four months* after the onset of the illness showed a fine punctate or granular marking scattered throughout both lung fields, the lesions being 0·5–1·0 mm. across. The cardiac outline was normal. *Eight months* after the onset there was a similar uniform fine punctate marking, with some evidence of a reticular pattern. *Seventeen months* after the onset there was more definite appearance of reticulation in all areas with some small scattered nodules, 2 mm. across, at the periphery of the mid zones. The right interlobar septum had been drawn upwards. There was broadening of the upper half of the cardiac shadow, especially in the region of the pulmonary artery: the hilar vessels were prominent. *Twenty-one months* after the onset more definite fine nodulation was apparent in the upper mid-zones, though the other appearances were unchanged. *Thirty months* after the onset there was some clearing of the lower zones, where the appearances suggested emphysema. In the upper and mid zones there was a coarse reticular pattern with much increase of linear striæ, suggesting fibrosis; nodulation was less in evidence. The diaphragm was flattened in the shape of a cone, the mediastinal shadow was broad and the hilar vessels were prominent. There was no enlargement of the left auricle on screening in the oblique positions with opaque emulsion in the œsophagus.

Drill biopsy of the liver showed focal granulomatous areas scattered throughout the tissue. These areas consisted mainly of macrophages and small round cells, with a few fibroblasts and occasional epithelioid cells, but no giant cells. There was no necrosis or fibrosis. The surrounding liver parenchyma was normal.

Ultraviolet microscopy showed aggregates of sharply defined spiculate particles with a bright white fluorescence in the middle of some of the granulomatous lesions. These were seen only in the abnormal tissue. In specimens of normal liver obtained from necropsies and examined by this method, single fluorescent bodies were sometimes seen in the sinusoids and small aggregates in the region of the portal vein, but these bodies were rounded and often had a yellowish tint. Possibly the particles within the lesions in the present case consisted of the original fluorescent powder, but the test cannot yet be considered conclusive.

The patient remained remarkably dyspnœic, and cough and expectoration increased. He could do only light laboratory work and was often absent as a result of minor respiratory infections which drove him to bed. In September 1948 he took two weeks' holiday, but became worse and was readmitted to hospital six months after his last discharge.

On examination in October 1948 he weighed 7 st. 2 lb., having lost 54 lb. in all. There was laboured dyspnœa at rest, and the respiratory rate varied between 28 and 42 per minute. His general condition soon became worse, he was frail and often drowsy. The illness remained afebrile throughout. Two weeks later cyanosis appeared. There was pitting œdema of the legs and back, and the liver became enlarged and tender. From this time he became much worse, and died on the 4th November 1948, after an illness which had lasted three years.

Dr. W. W. Woods made the necropsy, of which the following is a summary.

Necropsy: (L.H. P.M. 378/1948). Small pulmonary emboli. Cardiac thrombosis. Failure of hypertrophied right heart. Granulomatous fibrosis of lungs due to inhalation of a beryllium silicate.

About one-third or one-half of upper lobe of each lung in its posterior part considerably contracted (8 cm. from apex to lower border posteriorly on left, and 11 cm. on right) and showing areas of black carbon-impregnated fine reticular fibrosis, in places confluent, in others more widely separated nodules (0·4 cm. diam.) and trabeculæ, some areas especially in subpleural zones showing a coarse spongework of bronchiolectasis (0·5 cm. diam.); apices less affected and lower posterior parts most. Less numerous black nodules and trabeculæ (0·4 cm. diam.) in upper posterior areas (about 6 cm. from above down) in each lower lobe. Similar lesions, but quite few and scattered, in rest of upper and lower lobes and middle lobe: moderate œdema of lower lobes of lungs. Pronounced emphysema with a few bullæ (up to 2 cm. diam.) in both lower lobes. Moderately tough fibrous pleural adhesions and fibrous thickening of the visceral pleura (0·05 cm. thick) over upper posterior one-third of left upper lobe. Delicate fibrous tags over left lower lobe. Lightly adherent thrombotic embolus riding bifurcation of artery to right upper lobe; another in a small artery in left upper lobe. Small atheromatous buttons (0·6 cm. diam.) and numerous fat flecks in hypertrophied, dilated pulmonary arteries. Thin clear, pale yellow pleural effusions (24 oz. right; 8 oz. left). Viscid clear grey mucus in main bronchi, but none in small bronchi or bronchioles. Considerable enlargement of bronchial, cardinal and lower paratracheal lymph glands (up to 3·5 × 1·2 × 0·7 cm.), but mostly by heart failure œdema, though smooth, grey, rubbery areas in the largest. About the same degree of enlargement of lower posterior mediastinal glands. Foramen ovale closed. Clear yellow pericardial fluid (5 oz.). Considerable hypertrophy and dilation of right ventricle, forming apex of heart, and also of right auricle. Central softening of ante-mortem thrombus filling the innermost area (4 cm. diam.) of right auricular appendage; another (3 cm. diam.) in lower postero-anterior part of right auricle. Left ventricle and auricle of normal size. Valves normal. Milk spot (4 × 2 cm.) on anterior surface of right ventricle and a small one on posterior surface of left. Pulmonary artery 8 cm. circumf. Aorta 6·5 cm. circumf. Moderate atheroma; fat flecks in mitral; few small buttons in ring; area of large confluent fat flecks at start of anterior descending coronary and of large left horizontal, one of them calcified in anterior descending; no atheroma in congenitally small right coronary; few fat flecks at orifices of branches of arch; powder streaks in distal carotids; numerous fat flecks at their bifurcation; white patch of slight fibrosis of intima at bifurcation of left; fat flecks around orifices of descending thoracic aorta, and numerous, with two buttons, in abdominal aorta. Conspicuous, but minute, specks of central congestion, with focal paradoxical lobulation, in liver; three cough furrows (1 cm. deep) on upper part of right lobe; no granulomatous nodules, nor fibrosis, seen in liver. Chronic congestion of very firm spleen and kidneys. Plaque (0·2 cm. diam., 0·05 cm. deep) of ectopic suprarenal cortex under capsule of anterior surface of right kidney just above the middle. Group of three subacute gastric ulcers (2 × 2 cm. and 3 × 1·5 cm. and 1 × 0·5 cm. respectively, and up to 0·3 cm. deep) on lesser curve of stomach 1·5 cm. from duodenum, without peritoneal fibrosis over them; another (0·8 cm. diam., 0·2 cm. deep) about middle of posterior wall of body; subserous cyst (0·7 cm. diam.) on peritoneal surface of the larger ulcers. A few shallow erosions (0·3 cm. diam.) in stomach. Subacute ulcer (2 × 1·4 cm.) with undermined edges and slight fibrosis of serosa on anterior wall of duodenum, immediately beyond stomach. Severe congestion and mucous catarrh of mucosa of stomach. Congestion of small intestine; a few streaked areas of hæmorrhage in mucosa of ileum. Considerable œdema and slight congestion of large intestine. A few marginal hæmorrhoids (0·6 cm. diam.). Two calcareous mesenteric glands (0·6 cm. diam.) in ileo-cæcal angle. Ascites 10 oz. Firm, congested pancreas. Abundant lipoid, dark pigment zone and moderate amount of medulla in suprarenals. Abundant colloid in normal thyroid. Testicles, prostate and urethra normal. Red marrow (floats) in upper one-third of shaft and in neck of femur. Premature senile atrophy of frontal convolutions. Slight dilatation of lateral ventricles, with very slight granulation of ependyma. Meninges normal. Aqueduct of Sylvius normal. Yellow anterior lobe and white posterior lobe in normal pituitary. Middle ears, nose and accessory sinuses normal. Considerable pitting œdema of legs, thighs and lumbar regions. Very wasted man.

CADMIUM

Cadmium, Cd, is a by-product of zinc refining, and the level of production is entirely dependent upon the rate of operation of the world's

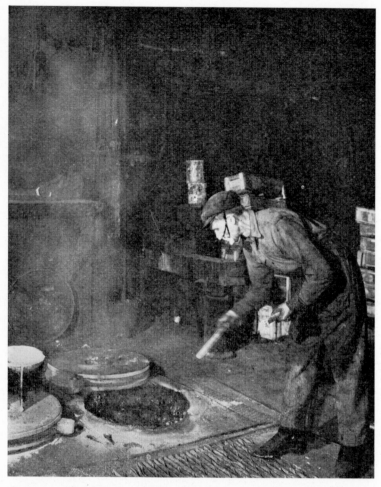

FIG. 170.—Manufacture of Master Alloy of equal parts of Copper and Cadmium. The Crucible in the Pit is heated by an Oil Furnace and contains Molten Copper. The workman is adding slugs of Cadmium and will later stir the Alloy. The yellow Fume of Cadmium Oxide is poisonous
(*By courtesy of British Insulated Callender's Cables, Ltd.*)

zinc smelters. The U.S.A., Canada and Australia are the chief producers of the metal. It was isolated by Stromeyer in 1817, and cadmium sulphide, its most characteristic compound, was first recorded by Guy-Lussac. It is a bluish-white lustrous metal sufficiently soft to be cut with a knife. It is resistant to corrosion and withstands wear. Many zinc ores contain up to 3 per cent of cadmium sulphide, and the cadmium is extracted from them in the course of smelting. Since cadmium is more volatile than zinc, the first portions of dust collecting in the receivers of zinc furnaces in

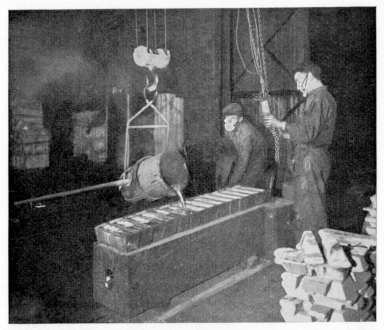

Fig. 171.—Pouring into Moulds a Master Alloy of equal parts of Copper
and Cadmium
(*By courtesy of British Insulated Callender's Cables, Ltd.*)

which ores containing cadmium are reduced will contain most of the
cadmium. Cadmium is also obtained from the rare mineral greenockite,
CdS. This mineral nowadays is little used as a pigment; greenockite,
obtained from deposits in Greece and Bohemia, was, however, used 2,000
years ago by artists and painters.

Uses

It is used in the manufacture of certain bearing alloys for motor-car,
aircraft and marine engines. It is added to silver to prevent staining and
serves as an ingredient in brazing alloys (see p. 163). Together with either
silver or lead and tin, cadmium is used in solders. When added to the
extent of 1 per cent to copper it forms an alloy which improves strength and
wear resistance without seriously reducing the electrical conductivity of
such material as trolley wire. It is employed as an active constituent of the
negative plates of alkaline electric accumulators and in making cadmium
vapour lamps. The rustproofing of iron and steel articles such as tools,
fittings, bearings and hardware by the method of cadmium electroplating
has to some extent replaced that of coating with zinc. Yellow and orange
pigments derived from cadmium sulphide and red pigments from cadmium
sulpho-selenides are used in paints, artists' colours, rubber, plastics,
printing inks, wallpaper, leather, glass and vitreous enamels.

Exposure Hazards

The principal industrial hazards arise in the smelting of ores, the manufacture and welding of alloys, the firing or welding of cadmium-plated
metals (figs. 170 and 171), the manufacture of alkaline accumulators and
of cadmium sulphide and cadmium sulpho-selenide pigments for colouring
plastics and ceramic glazes.

Cadmium Poisoning by Ingestion

The careless use of cadmium-coated vessels as containers for food and
drink may lead to acute poisoning. The symptoms appear suddenly within
fifteen minutes to two hours after ingestion, and everybody who has eaten
the contaminated food is affected. Increased salivation, severe nausea and
vomiting are the first symptoms. In severe cases there is collapse with signs
of shock, and sometimes hæmatemesis. Later, diarrhœa occurs, sometimes
with tenesmus. Recovery usually takes place within seven hours and is invariably complete within twenty-four hours. Beyond fluid replacement no
treatment is required. Anti-rust treatment by cadmium plating of the trays
of domestic refrigerators should be abandoned.

Acute Cadmium Poisoning

In 1924 Legge reported three cases of cadmium poisoning, one of them
fatal, in men in a paint factory where ingots of cadmium were melted
during a period of three hours in a poorly ventilated room. All three men
complained of dryness of the throat, headache and nausea. The urine was
coloured brown. A necropsy on the man who died showed hyperæmia of
the bronchi, gastro-intestinal tract and kidneys. In 1942 Nasatir reported
a fatal case. Death occurred on the fifth day after exposure to cadmium
fume caused by burning off, with an oxy-acetylene flame, deposits of metal
containing a high percentage of cadmium. The symptoms consisted of a
feeling of constriction of the chest, increasing dyspnœa and cough, which
became much worse before death.

Symptoms and Signs

In 1944 Spolyar and others wrote an extensive report on cases of cadmium poisoning resulting from flanging operations on cadmium-plated
pipe. The resulting exposure to cadmium-oxide fume led to five cases,
including one death. On the basis of the fifty-nine cases reported up to that
date the mortality rate of industrial cadmium poisoning appears to be 15
per cent. In 1948 Johnstone reported the case of a young Mexican labourer
who was sent to hospital following the use of an oxy-acetylene torch on the
inside walls of a furnace in which cadmium residues had been recovered
from scrap metal. The patient was extremely ill with severe dyspnœa and
exhaustion, and he gave a history of headache, cough and pain in the chest.
The temperature rose to 104° F., the pulse to 140 and the respiratory rate
to 50. Patchy signs appeared in the chest and bronchopneumonia was re-

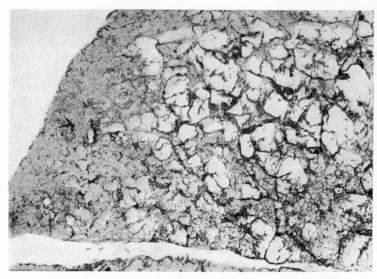

Fig. 172.—Chronic Cadmium Poisoning in the manufacture of Copper, Cadmium Alloy. Section of the Lung, natural size, showing chronic Emphysema in a man of 52 exposed for 14 months to Cadmium Oxide fume. A section of normal lung prepared by the same technique is seen in fig. 370
(By courtesy of Professor R. E. Lane and Professor J. Gough)

vealed by X-rays. Cyanosis and increasing respiratory distress preceded death. At necropsy the lungs showed confluent bronchopneumonia.

Mass Poisoning by Cadmium-oxide Fume

In 1944 Ross described mass poisoning due to cadmium-oxide fume affecting twenty-three workers. Finely divided cadmium dust from a cadmium recovery chamber became ignited owing to red-hot cigarette ash carelessly dropped by one of the workers. In a few minutes the cadmium dust became incandescent and emitted clouds of cadmium-oxide fume. The victims complained of irritation of the eyes, headache, vertigo, dryness of the throat, cough, constriction of the chest and weakness of the legs. Three hours later a set of delayed effects was observed. These included shivering, sweating, nausea, epigastric pain and dyspnœa. No case was fatal.

Renal Necrosis in Acute Cadmium Poisoning

In 1966 Beton and others described five cases of acute cadmium poisoning with one death from bilateral renal necrosis. The men were steel erectors building a bridge. The team of five was employed inside the top of a tower to dismantle a frame of girders. Cadmium-plated nuts, bolts and washers had been used to construct the frame and it was decided to do the job by melting away these steel bolts with an oxyacetylene burner. Dismantling took five hours. The working space was enclosed and had neither natural nor induced ventilation. No masks were worn and nothing in the exposure gave the men reason to suspect the seriousness of what they were doing. The man who died had symptoms on the day of exposure, namely, cough, breathlessness and a feeling of malaise. He went to work the next day, when he found that his mates had the same symptoms, but during the next two days he seemed to be getting worse than they were. On the third day he called his doctor saying that he had been gassed by carbon dioxide at work. The doctor found him in bed breathless and cyanosed with a temperature of 101° F. and a pulse rate of 98 per minute. Finding reduced breath sounds at the bases of the lungs and deciding that the patient looked much worse than the clinical signs suggested he treated him for broncho-pneumonia. He became worse and died on the fifth day of the illness. At necropsy extensive bilateral cortical necrosis of the kidneys was found together with severe pulmonary œdema. Nobody in the whole consortium of bridge builders had any idea of the grave danger of burning cadmium-plated bolts in an enclosed space but the circumstances of the case led the pathologist to the truth. The lungs were found to contain 0·25 g. cadmium oxide per 100 g. wet specimen. The other four men consented to hospital investigation and treatment; they were less seriously affected and they recovered.

Preventive Treatment

When cadmium is heated, dangerous quantities of cadmium oxide are formed and volatilized. Therefore in the smelting of cadmium ores, the welding of alloys and the firing of cadmium-plated metal, precautions should be taken to remove all fume by means of adequate exhaust ventilation. It has been suggested that all cadmium-coated metal should bear a warning label. While this measure is effective for large pieces, it is somewhat difficult to ensure that small objects so coated are labelled (Fairhall, 1946). Rustproofing by cadmium electroplating of steel sheet, pipes, girders, nuts, bolts, washers, rivets and motor-car and motor cycle components had better be abandoned rather than deaths should continue to occur in men who apply blow-pipe flames to such surfaces. Symptomatic treatment is directed specifically against broncho-pneumonia when it occurs.

Chronic Cadmium Poisoning

Chronic cadmium poisoning in workers exposed to the dust of cadmium oxide while making alkaline storage batteries in Sweden (Friberg, 1948) led to loss of weight, cough and dyspnœa, together with gross pulmonary emphysema (fig. 172) and the appearance in the urine of a protein of low molecular weight. The lungs may be so severely affected that they push the liver and spleen down, rendering them easily palpable in the abdomen. There is staining of the teeth in the form of a golden-yellow ring and a raised erythrocyte sedimentation rate. Baader (1951) suggested that the symptom complex of a running nose with soreness and prickling should be called *cadmium rhinitis* since it occurs so frequently. The sense of smell becomes impaired or abolished—*cadmium anosmia*—and in such cases there is usually atrophy of the nasal mucosa. It is the oxide in the form of dust which attacks the nasal mucosa in this way; where fume is inhaled from the molten metal the nose escapes.

An Unusual Proteinuria

In the majority of men suffering from chronic cadmium poisoning an unusual protein is found in the urine. It is quite unlike the protein present in the urine in cardiovascular-renal disease or the Bence Jones protein. When the boiling test is applied to such urine the result is sometimes positive and sometimes negative or inconclusive. The albustix test is positive. Non-specific protein precipitants such as 25 per cent salicyl-sulphonic acid give positive reactions. Friberg (1950) studied the physico-chemical properties of this protein in 15 of 35 men affected and found it had a molecular weight in the range 20–30,000. Kekwick (1955) examined the protein in the urine in four of the cases described by Bonnell. The electro-phoretic pattern showed many ill-defined components with mobility ranges similar to those of serum proteins. Despite this the protein sedimented in the ultracentrifuge as a single component, corresponding to a molecular weight in the range 20–30,000, which is much lower than that of any known serum-protein. The *cadmium proteinuria* has been found to remain static and symptomless for periods up to ten years in men employed in the manufacture of alkaline accumulators (Malcolm, 1966), cadmium-copper alloys (Holden, 1966) and cadmium pigments (Hughes, 1966). It seems that progress of the renal tubular lesion giving rise to renal insufficiency occurs only with prolonged and excessive exposure of the workman. Happily this is now a thing of the past (see p. 453). Clarkson and Kench (1956) showed that workmen exposed to the dust of cadmium oxide also exhibit marked amino-aciduria, the concentrations of the hydroxy-amino-acids threonine and serine being particularly increased. They put forward the view that this state of affairs may arise as a result of blockage by the toxic cadmium ions of the reabsorptive pathways of the amino-acids in the renal tubular cells. In a group of workers exposed to cadmium oxide dust in an alkaline accumulator factory, Ahlmark, Axelsson, Friberg and Piscator (1960) found impaired renal function as shown by low inulin clearance values and a diminished capacity of the kidneys to concentrate urine. These abnormalities were related to length of exposure to cadmium oxide.

Proteinuria and Emphysema

Bonnell (1955) examined men exposed to cadmium oxide fume in two English factories where alloys of copper and cadmium are manufactured (figs. 170 and 171). The health of 100 of these men was compared with that of similar groups who worked in the same factories but had never been exposed to cadmium. No significant abnormalities were found in the control groups. Of those exposed to cadmium 19 showed evidence of poisoning; 9 had emphysema and proteinuria, 3 had emphysema only and 7 had proteinuria only. Four other men, including 2 with proteinuria, who were too ill to work were investigated in hospital. In one man, symptoms had developed 10 years after his last exposure, and his urine still contained cadmium. In a follow-up survey four years later, Bonnell, Kazantzis and King (1959) found twenty-four new cases of chronic cadmium poisoning, making a total of forty-three cases in a group of 100 exposed men. Eighteen of these new cases had proteinuria alone, the remainder had emphysema with proteinuria. A deterioration was found in the condition of those men who had originally been diagnosed as having emphysema despite the fact that no further exposure to cadmium oxide had occurred in the intervening four years. Kazantzis (1961) found five cases of proteinuria in a group of twelve men who had been engaged in the manufacture of cadmium sulphide and cadmium sulpho-selenide pigments. The proteinuria was distinctive and was similar to that found in patients with renal lesions of predominantly tubular type. Three of these men subjected to more detailed study showed impairment of renal tubular function. While they showed no evidence of clinical emphysema, the three men had mild breathlessness on exertion, and respiratory function tests gave abnormal results.

Chronic Emphysema the Main Disability

Like the proteinuria the emphysema developing in men poisoned by cadmium may be delayed in onset until months or years after the last exposure. It differs from the chronic hypertrophic emphysema associated with chronic bronchitis. In *cadmium emphysema* breathlessness develops slowly and insidiously without cough and attacks of bronchitis which so often precede and accompany chronic hypertrophic emphysema. In patients with chronic cadmium poisoning breathlessness may develop suddenly after an isolated acute infection of the upper respiratory tract; and chronic bronchitis may follow, but almost invariably shortness of breath comes first (Bonnell, 1955). There are also differences from the common emphysema in the respiratory function tests (Kazantzis, 1956; Buxton, 1956). At necropsy, in one case, Lane and Campbell (1954) found fundamental pathological differences. No emphysematous bullæ were seen at the periphery of the lungs, but there was a narrow zone of normal lung tissue under the pleura, and chronic bronchitis was neither widespread nor severe (fig. 172). These findings have been confirmed by Smith, Smith and McCall (1960) who reported the necropsy findings on five men who had been intermittently exposed to cadmium fume. On detailed examination of the respiratory organs they found no histological evidence of chronic bronchitis and concluded that emphysema results from the direct effect of cadmium fume on the alveolar wall.

Evidence from Animal Experiments

Friberg (1951) exposed twenty-five rabbits to cadmium oxide dust for from two to three hours daily for a period of from seven to nine months. Proteinuria was found in most of the animals after six months' exposure ; the protein was of the same type as that found in the men employed in the accumulator factory. At necropsy chronic rhinitis was found in 16 cases and tracheitis in 20. Chronic bronchitis and emphysema was present in all the animals and nephrosis was found in the majority. Friberg suggests that cadmium excreted in the urine is in some way linked with protein. Repeated administration of small doses of cadmium chloride by intraperitoneal injection in rats was shown by Bonnell, Ross and King (1960) to lead to renal lesions consisting essentially of tubular atrophy and interstitial fibrosis. Rats in which the administration of cadmium salts had been discontinued after five months of the experiment developed seven months later lesions as severe as those animals which had been dosed for twelve months. The renal lesions were attributed to cadmium even though a severe chemical peritonitis had been produced. Kazantzis (1961) gave cadmium sulphide by intratracheal injection to a group of rats on a single occasion. Discrete nodules of fibrous tissue were found in the lungs, and renal lesions developed over a period of months. These lesions included tubular dilatation and epithelial atrophy, and, at a later stage, hyalinization of glomeruli. The rats excreted in the urine a protein of distinctive electrophoretic pattern quite unlike the physiological proteinuria of the normal rat.

Morbid Anatomy and Histology

In a man aged 39 years who had been exposed to cadmium oxide dust for eight years in an accumulator factory, Baader (1951) found at necropsy severe emphysema, fatty infiltration of the liver and toxic nephrosis. The renal lesion is not described in detail. Friberg and Nystrom described the death of five of their cases in 1952; in two this was due to emphysema. Two others died as the result of coronary atheroma and thrombosis but evidence of advanced renal damage was found at post mortem. The fifth man died of acute pancreatitis but the lungs were found to be emphysematous. Bonnell (1955) described the case of a man of 54 who had been employed for 32 years casting alloys of copper and cadmium. He died of a progressive renal lesion with a blood urea of 454 mgm. per 100 ml. There was no hypertension. The patient was observed for 18 months before death and repeated tests showed cadmium proteinuria but never albuminuria. Histological examination of the kidneys showed changes similar to those of chronic nephritis.

Preventive Treatment

The preventive treatment of acute cadmium poisoning is described on p. 449. All processes involving the escape into the working atmosphere of cadmium oxide dust or fume and of the dusts of cadmium sulphide and

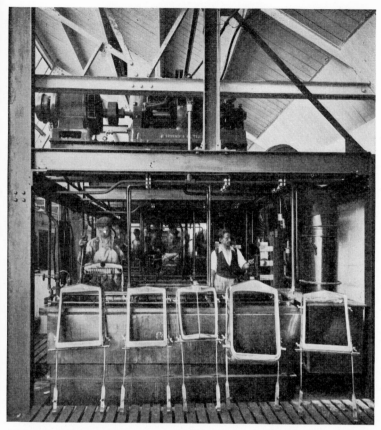

Fig. 173.—Electrolytic Bath for Chromium Plating of Motor-car Radiator Shells. The longitudinal Exhaust Chamber is connected through the Tank on the right to the Ducting which leads to an Exhaust Fan. The whole installation is now obsolete

sulpho-selenide must be strictly controlled by adequate exhaust ventilation. In the manufacture of these compounds men will continue to be affected by chronic cadmium poisoning, unless the whole process of manufacture and of handling and packing is completely enclosed. The insidious onset and the severe disability caused by chronic cadmium poisoning emphasizes the importance of its early recognition. In 1956 it was added to the list of prescribed diseases under the *National Insurance (Industrial Injuries) Act, 1946*. In 1967 it was made notifiable under the *Factories Act*. Periodic medical examination of workers exposed must include questioning as to dyspnœa on exertion, physical examination, X-ray of chest, respiratory efficiency tests and electrophoresis of the urine where proteinuria is found. Alternative work away from all risk must be found for any man in whom emphysema or proteinuria is discovered.

CHROMIUM

Chromium, Cr, derives its name from the Greek χρῶμα, meaning *colour*, because its compounds are nearly all brightly coloured. It is a silver-white, hard, brittle metal. The only workable source of the element is the ore chromite or chrome ironstone, $FeO.Cr_2O_3$, which is mined in Russia, Turkey, Southern Rhodesia and South Africa.

Uses

Approximately 45 per cent of the world's supply is used for alloys, about 40 per cent for refractories and 15 per cent for chemical purposes. Chromium is an essential component of the hard, high-strength steels used in engineering, and also of stainless and rustless steels. Corrosion-resistant alloys, such as stainless chromium-nickel steel, are extensively used in the chemical industry. The alloy steels are manufactured directly from ferro-chrome, a chromium-iron alloy prepared by reducing chromite in an electric furnace in the presence of carbon. Nickel-chromium alloys are used for making resistance wires for electric fires (see p. 166), copper-chromium alloys for electrical switch gear and cobalt-chromium-molybdenum alloys for use in jet-turbine engines and in orthopædic surgery (see p. 166). For refractory purposes the crude ore is embodied in bricks, cements and plasters in the construction of furnaces. The only commercial use of pure chromium metal is in the form of electroplate, the method for which was perfected in 1925 by Finck in the United States of America and introduced the same year into England by Sir Ernest Canning. The chromates of lead, zinc and barium are known as chrome pigments and are extensively used for colouring paints, linoleum, rubber and ceramics. Chromium sulphate is important in tanning, and potassium dichromate in the dyeing of wool, silk and leather. Chromium compounds are used in photography, in making safety matches and as catalysts in the manufacture of aviation petrol and methanol.

Monochromates and Dichromates

Chromium compounds used in chemical industry are obtained from the basic chromates, sodium and potassium dichromate or monochromate. These compounds are prepared from chromite, which is crushed, mixed with dolomite and the carbonate of sodium or potassium, and heated in a rotary furnace for eight hours at a temperature of 1,200° C. The introduction of the rotary furnace to replace the reverberatory furnace has taken place in many factories only since 1938. The oxide is converted to monochromate and the frit from the furnace is carried to washing or leaching tanks arranged in series. The monochromate is dissolved out by repeated washings with water and the concentrated liquor containing monochromate is treated with sulphuric acid. Dichromate is formed by double decomposition and sodium sulphate is a by-product of the process. In some factories in Germany and the United States of America the residue from the leaching tanks is dried, crushed and used over again in the process.

This residue contains up to 1 per cent of monochromate. In Great Britain no attempt is made to extract this small remaining quantity of chromate; the residue is removed from the leaching tanks in a moist state and discarded.

Chromium Plating and Anodizing

The toxicity of chromium compounds is determined by the valency of the metal radicle. The toxic action is confined to the compounds of hexavalent chromium. Trivalent chromium salts such as the phosphate and carbonate are harmless (Akatsuka and Fairhall, 1934). Air contaminated with chromic-acid mist or with the dust from chromates or bichromates is the principal source of exposure in industry. The process of chromium plating consists in wiring the articles to a frame ready for the plating vat, the initial plating, which lasts up to fifteen minutes, and the unwiring, swilling and polishing of the plated articles (fig. 173). The solution in the plating tank contains 50 per cent of chromic acid, and during electrolysis

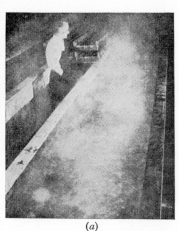
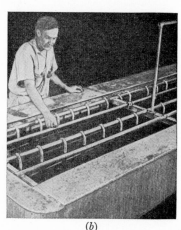

(a)   (b)

FIG. 174.—Chromium Plating and Anodizing. (a) Chromic-acid Mist produced during anodic oxidation of aluminium. (b) Removal of Chromic-acid Mist in Chromium Plating by Exhaust Ventilation locally applied
(*After R. T. Johnstone, 1948*)

reddish-brown fumes which contain 60 per cent of chromic acid are forced up in the form of a mist by the evolution of hydrogen at the cathode. In anodizing, a coating highly resistant to corrosion is formed on aluminium and its alloys through the anodic oxidation of the aluminium. Chromic acid is used as the solution in which the anodizing operations are carried out (fig. 174), and the hydrogen liberated at the cathode carries a significant amount of chromic-acid mist into the atmosphere along with it (Zvaifler, 1944).

Dermatitis and Chrome Ulcers

Lesions of the skin due to chromium salts have been known since 1827, when Cumming described *chrome holes* on the fingers and hands of bichromate workers in Glasgow. Wutzdorff (1897) pointed out that similar lesions were found in 1889 by the German factory inspectors amongst workers in the newly opened chromate works at Griesheim. A good deal of attention was directed to the subject during the manœuvres of the German Army in 1894, when eighty-four men in Anhalt who were called to the colours were found to be unfit for service because of chrome ulcers! The chromates and bichromates of potassium and sodium and chromic acid may cause either dermatitis or localized ulceration, according to whether trauma is present or not. Exposure to these substances occurs in chromium platers, colour workers, French polishers, calico printers, photographers, litho-etchers and chrome tanners. Dermatitis may occur on the hands, arms, face and chest. The onset is sudden, but it is unusual for an attack

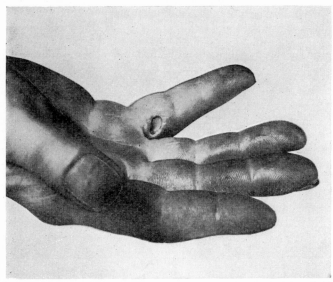

FIG. 175.—Chrome Ulcer in a man aged 46 years who had handled Sodium Bichromate for 7 years as a Colour Worker

to occur until the operator has been at the work for at least six months. In severe cases the face is intensely red and swollen, and the affected parts itch a great deal and may become painful (Trumper, 1931). Fair-haired people are particularly prone to a chrome dermatitis, and their presence at a chromium-plating bath calls for peculiar care (Horner, 1934).

Chrome ulcers begin in abrasions of the skin and are most commonly found at the root of the finger-nail, the knuckle of the hand or the dorsum of the foot. They are circular in shape, clear-cut, usually one centimetre or less in diameter, and looking as if punched out, hence the name *chrome hole* (fig. 175). They have a strong tendency to heal but may penetrate very deeply, even to bone. Although painless, they itch intolerably at night. If neglected, an ulcer may give rise to infection of the adjacent joint, causing

oss of a finger. There is no tendency towards malignant change. The dust
of chromium salts and the mist of chromic acid may produce ulcers on the
eyelids or the edge of the nostrils. Maloof (1955) reported the successful
treatment of chrome ulcers by an ointment containing 10 per cent edath-
amil calcium (calcium EDTA).

Perforation of the Nasal Septum

The mucous membrane of the nose is commonly affected, in which case
perforation of the nasal septum occurs. Usually this causes no inconvenience and is discovered accidentally. Legge (1902) examined 176 men employed in the manufacture of potassium bichromate. In 126 the septum
was perforated, and in 20 it was ulcerated. In none of the 30 men in whom
the septum was found to be normal was the immunity attributable to
shortness of employment, and one-half of them had been employed for
upwards of ten years. Legge was not in doubt that the mucous membrane
covering the septum is attacked more readily in some persons than in
others, and he inclined to the view that an immunity may be acquired if
the first few months pass without ulceration taking place. The condition
usually appears between the sixth and twelfth months after beginning work.
Less commonly it comes on within six weeks to three months of the first
exposure. The site of election for the ulceration is a point about a quarter
of an inch from the lower and anterior margin of the septum, and from this
point it extends upwards and backwards. The limitation of the perforation
to the cartilage of the septum is accounted for by the fact that the mucous
membrane covering it is adherent, forming the perichondrium, and is far
less vascular than the mucous membrane lining the rest of the nasal fossa.
Once the mucous membrane is destroyed, the blood supply to the cartilage
is cut off and necrosis ensues. When the ulceration has progressed upwards
as far as the junction of the septum with the ethmoid and backwards to the
vomer, it becomes arrested. Healing then takes place without the bone
being attacked, and the scar usually becomes covered with a crust of mucus.
Since the anterior or lower border of the septum is never destroyed, the
rigidity of the parts is maintained and deformity does not occur. The onset
of the process is ushered in by sneezing and by the symptoms of nasal
catarrh. The pain accompanying the ulceration appears to be insignificant.
It is never severe enough to necessitate absence from work or to call for
treatment. Once the perforation is established the only inconvenience is the
formation of plugs of mucus in the nasal passages. The general health is
unaffected by the condition. Greenburg and others (1942) carried out a
survey of 106 painters in an aeroplane factory and found five cases of perforation of the nasal septum as a result of spray painting with a paint containing zinc chromate.

Cancer of the Lung

A high incidence of cancer of the lung in the chromate-producing
industry has been reported from Germany, the United States of America

and Great Britain. The possibility that chromates can cause cancer of the respiratory system had been denied for many years, and Legge (1922) supported this opinion. He stated that although constant irritation of the skin and mucous membranes by chromium compounds resulted in chronic ulceration and the active destruction of tissues, epitheliomatous change did not occur in such lesions. In 175 cases of chrome ulceration recorded in the English industry at this time, no single case showed any sign of epithelioma. Newman (1890) had already recorded the occurrence of adenocarcinoma originating in the nares in a man aged forty-seven who had worked for twenty years in the chromate industry in Scotland. He had the perforation of the nasal septum found in many chromate workers. This is the first reported case of cancer of the respiratory system in a chromate worker.

Incidence of Lung Cancer in Chromate Workers

No further cases were noted until 1912, when Pfeil observed two cases of lung cancer in workers in a factory in Germany where basic chromates were made or used in the manufacture of quinones. In 1935 he reported these and five additional cases among workers in the same factory in Ludwigshafen. Ten more cases occurred in chromate workers in Griesheim between 1926 and 1936 (Alwens, Bauke and Jonas, 1936). Gross and Alwens (1939) and Gross and Koelsch (1943) reported a total of forty-seven cases from several factories and estimated that 3·9 per cent of the workers at risk in the industry since 1880 had developed cancer of the lung. The incidence of perforation of the nasal septum appears to bear no relationship to the incidence of cancer of the lung. Machle and Gregorius (1948) found that in workers in the chromate-producing industry in the United States of America, deaths from lung cancer were occurring at sixteen times the normal rate, with incidence rates in individual factories varying from thirteen to thirty-one times the normal. Baetjer (1950) Mancuso and Hueper (1951) and Gafafer (1952) confirmed these findings. In England, Bidstrup and Case (1956) reported a six-year follow-up study of workmen first examined in 1949. They found that the incidence of lung cancer was 3·6 times the normal at that time but stated that with the observed latent interval of twenty-one years this value may not be the final one. Thus there is no doubt that cancer of the lung is an occupational risk in the chromate-producing industry, although the chemical agent or agents have not yet been identified. There is evidence that one or more of the furnace products, such as an intermediate form of chromate or a component of the residue, may be responsible.

Preventive Treatment

The preventive measures necessary in handling chromic acid, chromates and bichromates include the removal of dust and mist, cleanliness, regular medical supervision, and the covering up of cuts and abrasions with suitable dressings. The prevention of danger in chromium plating and anodizing depends on the correct design of the vats to include exhaust ventilation (fig. 174). It may often be necessary to provide rubber gloves, boots and apron for a person working round the chromic-acid tanks, but these are not always of real value. The workers have to reach up to lift out the metal parts and hang them on hooks, and if the gloves are loose at the wrists the solution that drips on to the arms may, when the hands are lowered, run down inside the gloves. The solution may also run down inside the boots if they are loose at the top (Hamilton and Hardy, 1949). The exposed skin should be washed and carefully dried. Application of an ointment made up of equal parts of lanolin and soft paraffin is useful. Soft paraffin should be freely applied through the anterior nares to the nasal septum. Weekly inspection of the nasal passages should be regularly carried out for all workers by the nurse, and less frequent inspection should be made by the works' doctor.

MANGANESE

Manganese, Mn, when pure is a silvery-white metal, but as usually prepared it is reddish-grey, brittle and intensely hard. Its most important ore is the black dioxide, MnO_2, known as pyrolusite. Less important manganese minerals are the oxides braunite, Mn_2O_3, manganite, $Mn_2O_3.H_2O$, and hausmannite, Mn_3O_4. The ores are mined in Russia, India, Morocco, Egypt, Ghana, South Africa, Canada, Brazil, Chile and Cuba. By 1954 the annual world production was of the order of 7,000,000 tons of saleable ore.

Manganese Alloys

It was in 1888 that manganese was first added to steel to toughen it; today about 95 per cent of the world production of manganese is used for metallurgical purposes, particularly the manufacture of manganese alloy steels (p. 161). The metal industry could not dispense with it and uses an average of 14 kilograms of manganese per ton of ordinary steel. Its most important alloys are ferro-manganese, spiegeleisen, silico-manganese, silicospiegel and manganese-bronze. During the process of steel making, ferro-manganese is added to the furnace charge to prevent the formation of iron oxide and sulphide in the finished steel. A small amount of manganese in steel increases its elastic limit and tenacity so that steels containing about 1 per cent of manganese are commonly used in structural work. For rock-crushers, dredger buckets, railway points and crossings, clutches, steel helmets and in certain mining equipment requiring high-tensile strength and resistance to shock and abrasion, high-manganese steel with about 12 per cent of manganese is employed. At the Baker Street junction of the London Underground Railway ordinary steel rails used to need replacement every nine months, but manganese steel lasts twenty-two years. Alloys are also made with aluminium, tin, arsenic, antimony, bismuth and boron.

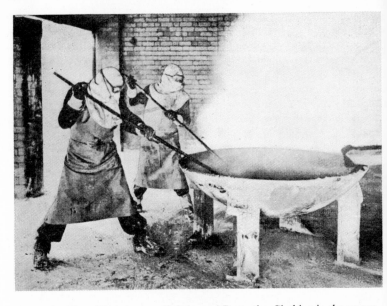

FIG. 176.—Use of Respirators, Goggles and Protective Clothing in the prevention of Manganese Poisoning and Alkali Burns. Workers stirring Manganese
Dioxide, melted Caustic Potash and Lime, in the manufacture of Potassium
Permanganate. In the violent reaction which ensues, volumes of steam and
quantities of dust are emitted

(By courtesy of Boots Pure Drug Co., Ltd.)

Manganese Compounds

The dioxide is the starting-point in the manufacture of all manganese
preparations. It is used in decolorizing glass stained by traces of iron compounds, for the violet colour of manganese silicate masks the complement-
ary green tint of the iron. The pyrolusite used for this purpose is known as
glass makers' soap. It is much used in the manufacture of dry batteries and
in the pottery and soap industries. Manganous chloride, $MnCl_2$, is used in
dyeing; and manganous sulphate, $MnSO_4$, in calico printing. The insoluble
colours formed in the dye vats are referred to variously as *manganese brown*,
manganese bistre and *manganese violet*. Manganates and permanganates,
especially potassium permanganate, $KMnO_4$, are used for preserving wood,
for bleaching textiles and for oxidizing and disinfecting purposes (fig. 176).
Condy's fluid is a mixture of sodium manganate, $Na_2MnO_4.10H_2O$, and
permanganate, $NaMnO_4$. Although manganese dioxide is still used to
oxidize hydrochloric acid to chlorine on a laboratory scale, the Weldon
process is obsolete in industry, the electrolysis of brine having replaced it.
A cyclopentadienyl-manganese derivative is employed as an anti-knock
compound.

Exposure Hazards

Cases of manganese poisoning have been seen from the inhalation of excessive amounts of dust in the mining, grinding, sorting, sieving, packing and loading of manganese ores and in the manufacture of manganese steel in which the manganese is first fused in an electric furnace. In Great Britain no case has been recognized in the manufacture of dry batteries. Of a number of persons exposed, few are susceptible to the disease. Manganese poisoning produces two entirely different effects: the first is an attack on the brain with strict localization to the extrapyramidal motor system, a condition discovered in France in 1837; and the second an increased incidence of pneumonia first noted in Germany in 1921.

Historical Summary

In 1837 Couper described five cases of poisoning in men employed in grinding manganese dioxide in the manufacture of chlorine for bleaching powder in France.

Their skin is constantly covered with a layer of the oxide, and the air which they breathe is impregnated with a multitude of molecules of this oxide which are introduced into their lungs by respiration. In 1821 a young man apparently in good health, being employed at this work, presented symptoms of paraplegia which, becoming worse, forced him at the end of some months to stop work. After having tried without effect the medicines used in paralysis, he absented himself from the neighbourhood for a year, and at the end of this time, having returned, it was evident that he had made little progress toward recovery. In the following year another workman, similarly employed in grinding manganese and apparently enjoying the best of health, fell equally ill. It not being suspected that manganese produced poisonous effects, he was permitted to work for several months, with the exception of short intervals employed in treatment. As the paralysis increased, manganese was finally suspected to be the cause and the workman moved to another region. After this time there was no augmentation of symptoms and at the end of six years the patient was in good health. During the height of the disease the weakness of the contractile muscles was much greater in the legs than in the arms. It was of such nature that the patient reeled in walking and leaned forward when he wished to walk. The arms were somewhat weak and there was difficulty in speech. He was not able to make himself understood by a person at a little distance. Other sensations and intelligence were unaffected. The trunk muscles had the appearance of a paralytic. Saliva ran from the mouth during speech. There was no trembling of any part of the body, no colic, constipation nor derangement of digestion. He was given mercurials, vesication of the head and dorsal spine, and strychnine, but all without effect.

Parkinsonism in Manganese Dioxide Workers

It is a point of great interest that Parkinson's famous *Essay on the Shaking Palsy* which first laid down the clinical characteristics of extra-pyramidal motor disease was published in 1817, four years before Couper first observed a case caused by manganese dioxide. But what he wrote was overlooked, and in 1901 von Jaksch described three cases resembling disseminated sclerosis in men employed in drying manganese dioxide in Austria. In 1919 in Boston, U.S.A., Edsall, Wilbur and Drinker published an article on manganese poisoning resulting from inhalation of manganese dust in a separating mill. The first cases recognized in Great Britain were reported by Charles in 1922. They were three men who had been exposed to the dust of manganese ores from nine months to three years. They had developed spastic paralysis of the lower limbs which had incapacitated them for work from three to five years. Cases of manganese poisoning were still occurring in England in 1934 when four men, exposed for years to the dust of pyrolusite, showing classical Parkinsonism, were seen on Merseyside by Owen. By 1945 Fairhall was able to find in the literature 353 cases of manganese poisoning which had occurred since the first report by Couper in 1837. At least 118 more cases have been published since 1945, so that the disease can no longer be called very rare.

Poisoning in Manganese Miners

The symptoms and signs include languor and sleepiness by day but insomnia by night, muscular pains, including cramps in the calves, unsteady gait, weakness and stiffness of the limbs, and involuntary movements varying in degree from a fine tremor of the hands to gross rhythmical movements of the arms, legs, trunk, jaw and head which may be severe enough to shake the bed. Occasionally uncontrollable laughter or crying occur and there may be impulsive acts such as running, dancing, singing and uncontrolled talking. Sometimes forced movements occur in which the patient falls without being able to make the effort necessary to save himself. Attacks of aggressiveness, unprovoked irritability and euphoria are known. The handwriting is tremulous, the letters and words cramped, and micrographia is common. Speech disturbances include disappearance of the pauses between words, monotonous tone of voice and in severe cases aphonia. Occasionally deglutition is impaired. In Cuban mines drilling and blasting an ore containing 45 per cent of manganese impotence is one of the commonest manifestations of poisoning (Peñalver, 1955). In mines at Gowari Wadhona in India, where the ore is braunite and dry drilling was used fifteen cases of poisoning occurred in men from twenty to twenty-five years of age. The symptoms and signs were tremor, Parkinsonism, shuffling, festinant gait, monotonous speech and uncontrollable spasmodic laughter with dribbling of saliva (Berry and Bidwai, 1959). But in various parts of India there are 619 manganese mines, some of them opencast pits. From these mines Wadir (1961) examined twenty-eight men aged from seventeen to forty-four years who had been exposed to the dusts of dry drilling from six months to fourteen years; all of them had the illness described above.

Poisoning in the Manufacture of Alloys

In 1953 Dogan and Beretić described ten cases of manganese poisoning which occurred in a factory making manganese alloys in Yugoslavia. The men had been exposed for periods between eighteen months and twelve years to the dust of pyrolusite and to fume from furnaces making ferro-manganese, spiegeleisen, silicomanganese and silicospiegel. All cases gave a history of weakness of the legs; sometimes there was weakness of the arms too. Nearly all the patients complained of muscle cramps. They showed a mild form of Parkinsonism; in two cases the signs were uni-lateral. There was a slapping gait with retropulsion and propulsion, and in one case the *cock-walk* of von Jaksch. Rhythmic rotatory tremor of the hands, tremor of the extended tongue and increased muscle tone of the lead-pipe type were present. The tendon reflexes were not increased and the plantar responses were flexor. The patients had mask-like facies and sialorrhœa but no disturbances of ocular movement. Cohen (1934) pointed out that diminution of convergence accommodation response so characteris-tic of post-encephalitic Parkinsonism does not occur in chronic manganese poisoning.

Prognosis

Although men seriously poisoned are lifelong cripples, the condition is not lethal. Charles (1922) agreed with others as to the similarity between this form of poisoning and progressive lenticular degeneration, except that in manganese poisoning the condition remains stationary or improves when exposure ceases. The emotional alterations are usually transient only; the extra-pyramidal symptoms and signs persist. In any group of workmen showing neurological symptoms and signs it is unusual for as many as 10 per cent to recover sufficiently to resume work. In the remainder the weak-ness, spasticity and tremor render impossible any return to the former employment.

Morbid Anatomy and Histology

The pathological changes in the body of a manganese worker who died of cardiovascular-renal disease at the age of sixty-nine, after fourteen years of disability from manganese poisoning, were described by Canavan, Cobb and Drinker (1934). There was atrophy of the frontal lobes of the brain, shrinkage and distortion of the basal ganglia and internal hydrocephalus. Histological studies showed gliosis and degenerative lesions of the nerve-cells, particularly in the optic thalamus, globus pallidus, lenticular nucleus, caudate nucleus and the putamen. In the ten patients exposed to the dust of pyrolusite described by Dogan and Beretić (1953), liver function tests revealed no abnormality. Of five cases subjected to liver biopsy, four showed no histological changes and one showed pigmentation by a substance which gave a negative iron reaction.

Experimental Manganese Poisoning

In 1924 Mella produced manganese poisoning experimentally in four monkeys by administering every day for a period of eighteen months manganous chloride by intraperitoneal injection. The animals developed choreic movements, passed into a state of rigidity and finally developed tremor resembling paralysis agitans. Gross morbid changes were found in three animals in the lenticular nucleus and the liver. These experiments afford an explanation of the symptoms in most of the cases described. The extrapyramidal motor system is picked out by the poison, hence the rigidity, difficult gait, retropulsion, propulsion, mask-like facies, sleepiness, Parkinsonian tremor and uncontrollable laughter.

High Incidence of Pneumonia near a Factory

In 1921 Brezina first drew attention to the unusually high incidence of pneumonia in men handling manganese ores. He reported that five out of ten men working in a pyrolusite mill had died of pneumonia in two years. In 1933 Baader ascribed the high incidence of pneumonia amongst dry battery workers to manganese dioxide, while Heine (1943) pointed out the high incidence of pneumonia in men handling pyrolusite in German factories. The erection, in 1923, of an electrical plant for manganese smelting at Sauda in Norway was followed by a tenfold increase in the mortality rate for pneumonia in that area. A pall of smoke which overhung the town was found to contain particles, less than 5 microns in size, of oxides of manganese (Riddervold and Halvorsen, 1943).

Pneumonia in Men making Potassium Permanganate

Lloyd-Davies (1946) described his observations on men employed in the manufacture of potassium permanganate. The manganese content of the atmospheric dust to which they were exposed, expressed as manganese dioxide, varied from 41 to 66 per cent; practically all the particles were below 1 micron in size, and 80 per cent were below 0·2 micron. During eight years the number of men exposed varied between forty and 124. Besides a high incidence of pharyngitis and bronchitis, they showed an incidence of pneumonia which varied from 1,500 to 6,300 per 100,000 in the period 1938 to 1945, compared with an average of seventy-three for the same period amongst the rest of the male employees. The response to sulphonamides and resolution of the lung were slower than in ordinary lobar pneumonia, but no persisting pulmonary lesions were observed either clinically or radiographically. Exposure of mice to the dust of oxides of manganese led to interstitial infiltration of the lung with mononuclear cells and finally to consolidation with necrosis and hæmorrhage.

Preventive Treatment

In the mining of manganese ores adequate ventilation and wet rock drilling are essential precautions underground. Baths and changing rooms must be provided on the surface. In factories manganese poisoning can be prevented by the application of local exhaust ventilation, both at the furnaces to remove fume and at the packing and sieving apparatus to remove dust. Respirators may be worn which combine active charcoal for absorbing vapours and a cotton-wool filter to trap dust. Personal hygiene is important and the worker must wear protective clothing and gloves, since the occurrence of skin absorption is established. Adequate supervision and routine medical examination are essential. These measures are attended with good results. Applied in one particular factory they removed all risk of poisoning encountered by the workers over a period of six years.

Symptomatic Treatment

No effective method to increase manganese excretion is known. Both 2,3-dimercaptopropanol (British Anti-Lewisite, BAL) and calcium EDTA are without effect. Symptomatic treatment includes simple anodynes for muscular pain and barbiturates for insomnia. For the rigidity, gentle exercise, passive movements and massage are useful. Some relief may be obtained by hyoscine hydrobromide given three times a day as a tablet of gr. $\frac{1}{100}$. This usually renders movements more free and relieves the tremor for a few hours after each dose is taken. Patients often become bedridden and therefore need institutional treatment. It is then necessary to take great care of the skin, since the immobility of the trunk greatly increases the liability to the formation of bed-sores.

NICKEL

Nickel, Ni, was first isolated in 1751. It is a hard, silver-white, corrosion-resistant metal which takes a high polish. It is malleable, ductile and very tenacious. It is sometimes found in meteorites alloyed with iron, but in the earth's crust it does not occur in the metallic state. The name nickel originated in the Harz mountains, when the early copper miners found ores which seemed to be contaminated and could not readily be reduced into workable metallic copper. They attributed this to the power of Old Nick, and one of the contaminated ores was called Kupfer-nickel or devil's copper. It was later found that this evil influence was due to the presence of a compound of arsenic with another element, which was therefore named nickel. More than four-fifths of the world's supply of nickel is mined in the Sudbury district of Ontario, Canada, from ore deposits containing nickel, copper and iron sulphides, especially pentlandite, $(FeNi)S$. The deposits occupy a basin thirty-six miles long and sixteen miles wide, and the ore reserves are estimated to be over 200,000,000 tons (fig. 177). In Canada nickel is refined by electrolysis and the process yields as a by-product the greatest supply of platinum and platinum-group metals in the world.

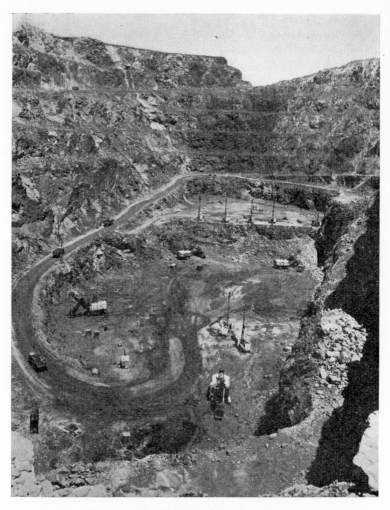

FIG. 177.—Frood-Stobie open pit nickel mine
(*By courtesy of International Nickel Company of Canada, Ltd.*)

Uses

Pure nickel is used principally in electroplating, either as the complete coating as in the case of sewing needles or as an undercoat to a chromium finish as in the case of motor-car bumpers. It forms an unusually large number of alloys of technical importance. Nickel is a metal similar to iron in some of its properties, having rather greater strength and hardness and being magnetic, though to a smaller degree than iron. Ferro-nickel alloys have a wide range of magnetic, electrical and thermal properties, depending on the percentage of nickel used. Thus *invar*, with 36 per cent nickel, has the remarkable property of not expanding or contracting appreciably with ordinary changes of temperature. It gets its name because it is invariable at all air temperatures. It is useful for standards of length, measuring tapes and chronometer parts (see p. 165). *Platinite*, with 46 per cent nickel, has the same coefficient of expansion as glass and can therefore be used as a substitute for platinum for the lead-in wires of electric-light bulbs. Nickel is used in stainless steels, and to add strength and toughness to steel alloys for motor cars, aircraft, gun forgings, armour plate and machine tools, including cemented carbide cutting tools. It is alloyed with copper and other metals to make condenser tubes and coins. Our so-called silver coins are made of an alloy which is copper 75, nickel 25; and so is the United States 5-cent coin known as a *nickel*. Together with zinc and copper it forms *nickel silver*, the basis of silver-plated tableware, hence the letters E.P.N.S., or electroplated nickel silver, seen on spoons and forks. *Monel metal* is an alloy of nickel with copper and small quantities of iron, manganese, silicon and carbon. It is malleable and of high-tensile strength, and is used for kitchen ware, laundry fittings, food-handling plant, pump bodies and turbine blading (see p. 166). Of the alloys acting as permanent magnets, *alcomax* is composed of nickel, iron and aluminium, and *alnico* of nickel, cobalt and aluminium. Alloyed with chromium, it is used to make heating elements for electric fires and surgical and dental instruments. In the Second World War modifications of the binary alloy nickel 80, chromium 20, were developed to withstand the combination of high stresses and high temperatures met with in gas-turbine engines and at the same time to resist corrosion by the products of combustion. They are known as the Nimonic series. In *Nimonic 75*, which is used for flame tubes and nozzle guide vanes, the alloy is stiffened by the precipitation of titanium carbide caused by the presence of about 0·3 per cent of titanium and 0·1 per cent of carbon. Finely powdered nickel is used as a catalyst in a number of chemical reactions, especially in the hydrogenation of oils to form solid fats. Nickel and its salts are used in alkaline storage batteries and in the manufacture of enamels.

Exposure Hazards

Three distinctly different hazards are known:

(*a*) contact with solutions of nickel salts in refining the metal and in electroplating may give rise to dermatitis;

(*b*) inhalation of nickel carbonyl, a gas which is highly poisonous and may cause hæmorrhagic bronchopneumonia, and

(*c*) inhalation of dust in the refining of nickel, giving rise to cancer of the lung and nasal sinuses, especially the ethmoid.

(*a*) Nickel Salts

Nickel sulphate is obtained by dissolving nickel waste in sulphuric acid and then evaporating the filtered solution. In aqueous solution it is used for electroplating copper, brass and iron. In chromium plating the metal has usually been electroplated first with nickel.

Nickel Itch in Miners and Electroplaters

Rambousek (1908) graphically described the *nickel itch* which occurs in nickel-plating establishments. It also affects nickel miners, smelters and refiners. It begins as a pink, papular erythema in the web of the fingers. There is itching, soreness, burning and sometimes swelling of the parts affected. The itching is worse at night and in hot weather. The eruption may spread on to the fingers, wrists and forearms, and at times on to the chest and face. In extreme cases pustulation, ulceration and weeping occur. As a rule recovery takes place after a week, although cases are known where the condition has lasted for three months.

Some Workers develop Sensitivity

Rarely, the patient complains of a bitter metallic taste in the mouth, with loss of energy both physical and mental (Hamilton and Hardy, 1949). There is a heavy preponderance among fair-skinned employees. Some persons are extraordinarily susceptible to nickel salts and others become sensitized only after having worked as electroplaters for years. One man in three seems to be immune. If a man has once been affected, he is almost sure to have another attack in which the lesions are slower in healing than in the first. Such a man may be compelled to abandon the occupation for good.

Dermatitis from wearing Nickel-plated Metal Objects

Nickel dermatitis may occur from wearing nickel-plated and chromium-plated articles, including wrist-watches, metal bracelets, garter buckles (*suspender dermatitis*), shoe buckles, spectacle frames (*spectacle dermatitis*), ear-rings (fig. 178), brooches, hairpins, safety pins and necklaces. The repeated handling of nickel coins and nickel-plated padlocks, pokers, shovels and other implements also may produce nickel dermatitis. The nickel salt concerned is produced by sweating; removal of the offending article leads readily to cure. Nickel dermatitis has been described in the same man from his spectacle frames and from the buckle of his wrist-watch. Patch testing incriminates nickel and not chromium. Susceptible persons are rare, and familial susceptibility has been observed, for example, in two sisters who developed nickel dermatitis on their wrists. Markičević (1960) described the case of a woman chemical engineer, aged thirty-five, working in an electroplating establishment in Zagreb who began to suffer from recurrent nickel dermatitis and conjunctivitis four weeks after entering the factory. She gave a history of primary nickel dermatitis which had occurred years before when the skin of the thighs had come in contact with her suspender buckles. In Denmark Marcussen (1960) found that 14 per cent of the nickel-sensitive occupational cases examined in the Finsen Institute had been previously sensitized in this way in private life.

Preventive Treatment

Women should refuse to buy suspenders fitted with nickel-plated buckles and demand nylon ones. Persons who are sensitive or show pre-

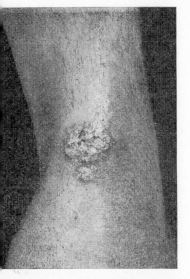
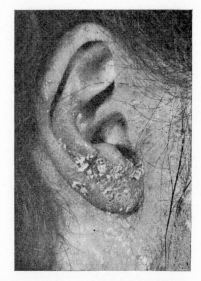

FIG. 178.—Nickel Dermatitis in a woman aged 21 years. A rash appeared at the site of the metal strap of a wrist-watch. Three weeks later a similar rash appeared on the lobes of the ears where she had been wearing metal ear-rings. Patch tests with nickel were positive

(*By courtesy of Dr. Brian Russell*)

vious susceptibility to nickel dermatitis should be excluded from working on electroplating vats. Discipline and regular medical supervision should ensure minute cleanliness on the part of the workmen. Cuts and abrasions should be covered by suitable dressings. The exposed skin should be washed, carefully dried and treated with an ointment of lanolin and soft paraffin. If the workmen wear gloves, boots and aprons, they should understand how to use them properly. Removal of dust and mist from the atmosphere is essential. It depends on the correct design of the vats to incorporate exhaust ventilation.

(*b*) Nickel Carbonyl

The discovery of the metallic carbonyls and their industrial development is an interesting chapter in the history of pure and applied science. In the year 1888, at the Brunner Mond chemical works in Cheshire, an experimental plant was set up for the decomposition by distillation of ammonium chloride. Trouble developed in certain nickel valves which became leaky through the formation of a black crust. Dr. Ludwig Mond took a sample of this black substance with him to the laboratory in his private house in London, where he instructed his assistant, Dr. Carl Langer, to study its properties (Mond and others, 1890). That examination was to lead to the discovery of a novel type of chemical reaction, to the production of an entirely new series of metallic compounds and to the development of an efficient method of obtaining certain metals from their ores in a state of purity previously impossible on a commercial scale.

History

The plant had recently been erected to operate a new process for obtaining chlorine and ammonia from ammonium chloride. The chloride was being produced in quantity in the ammonia-soda process at the works, and Dr. Ludwig Mond wished to utilize the contained chlorine for the manufacture of bleaching powder. Ammonium chloride was passed over magnesia mixed with a little potassium chloride, magnesium chloride and ammonia being formed. By passing heated air over the magnesium chloride this was reconverted into magnesia, and chlorine was liberated.

In developing the process a plant had to be constructed for volatilizing ammonium chloride, and this was a difficult problem, since the vapour of this substance not only acts on oxides and salts but also violently attacks most metals. The difficulty could be overcome in the reaction vessels by lining them with glazed tiles, but valves were required for changing the current of ammonium chloride vapour to hot air and vice versa. The valves had to be very tight to prevent loss of ammonia, and it was found that they could be made of nickel, this metal not being attacked at all by ammonium chloride vapour. On a laboratory scale the valves worked perfectly, but when placed in the large manufacturing plant they very soon became leaky, the surface being covered with the black scale. The laboratory examination revealed that the scale contained carbon, derived from the small percentage of carbon monoxide present in the carbon-dioxide gas used to sweep the ammonia out of the apparatus before admitting the hot air.

Investigation of a Luminous Flame, 1888

The further experiments which led up to the isolation of a new compound of nickel may be told in Dr. Ludwig Mond's own words:

About 1888 I was engaged with my collaborator, Dr. Langer, in trying to find a method for eliminating the carbon monoxide from hydrogenous gases which we wanted for use in our gas battery. We tried to avail ourselves for this purpose of the remarkable property of nickel we had just discovered, and found, to our satisfaction, that by passing gases containing hydrogen, carbon monoxide, and a certain quantity of steam over finely divided nickel at a temperature of 400° C. we could completely convert the carbon monoxide into carbon dioxide, containing its equivalent of hydrogen, which was just what we wanted.

This led to a more elaborate study of the action of carbon monoxide upon nickel, with a view to determining whether a definite compound of nickel and carbon was formed. We found that a small quantity of nickel decomposed a very large quantity of carbon monoxide, so that we could obtain a product containing only 15 per cent of nickel and 85 per cent of carbon, the nickel in which was only partially soluble in acids.

In the course of these experiments finely divided nickel, formed by reducing nickel oxide at 400° C. with hydrogen, was treated with pure carbon monoxide in a glass tube at varying temperatures for a number of days, and was then cooled down in a current of carbon monoxide before it was removed from the tube. In order to keep the poisonous carbon monoxide out of the atmosphere of the laboratory, we simply lit the gas escaping from the apparatus. To our surprise we found that, while the apparatus was cooling down, the flame of the escaping gas became luminous and increased in luminosity as the temperature got below 100° C. On a cold plate of porcelain being put into this luminous flame, metallic spots were deposited similar to the spots of arsenic obtained with a Marsh apparatus; and on heating the tube through which the gas was escaping we obtained a metallic mirror, while the luminosity disappeared.

At the first moment we thought that there must be an unknown element in our nickel giving rise to the production of this effect, but when we examined the mirrors we found them to consist of pure nickel. As it seemed so very improbable that so heavy a metal as nickel should form a readily volatile compound with carbon monoxide, we purified our carbon monoxide as perfectly as possible, but still obtained the same results.

We now endeavoured to isolate this curious and interesting substance by preparing the nickel with great care at the lowest possible temperature, and treating this nickel with carbon monoxide at about 50° C., and thus we gradually increased the amount of the volatile nickel compound in the gases passing through the apparatus. We absorbed the excess of carbon monoxide by cuprous-chloride solution, and thus obtained a residue of several cubic centimetres, containing the volatile nickel compound mixed with a little nitrogen. By passing this gas through a heated tube we separated the nickel, obtaining an increased volume of gas, and found in this a quantity of carbon monoxide corresponding to about four equivalents for one equivalent of nickel (fig. 179).

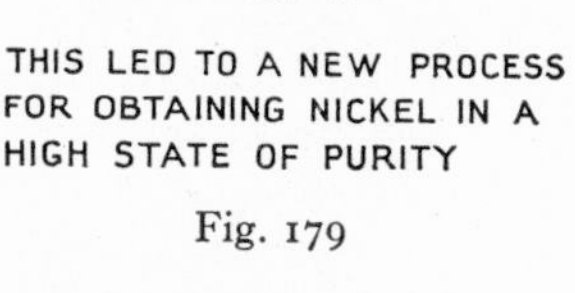

By further improving our method of preparing the finely divided nickel and by passing the resulting gas through a refrigerator, cooled by snow and salt, we at last succeeded in liquefying this compound, and were able to produce it with ease and facility in any quantity we desired (Mond, 1930).

MOND NICKEL PROCESS

IN 1888 LUDWIG MOND
DISCOVERED A GASEOUS
METALLIC COMPOUND
NICKEL CARBONYL

$$Ni + 4CO \underset{180°C}{\overset{80°C}{\rightleftharpoons}} Ni(CO)_4$$

THIS LED TO A NEW PROCESS
FOR OBTAINING NICKEL IN A
HIGH STATE OF PURITY

Fig. 179

Carbonyls of Metals

The compound which was thus isolated in quantity for the first time was given the name nickel carbonyl, and the term carbonyl is now applied to all similar compounds of the metals with carbon monoxide. Mond and Langer tried unsuccessfully to form other gases in a similar way by passing carbon monoxide over metals such as iron and cobalt. The fact, previously unheard of, that a heavy metal could be converted into a gas was an intensely interesting and important discovery. Mond quickly saw that if nickel could easily be turned into nickel-carbonyl gas whilst no other metal was affected by carbon monoxide in the same way, it might be possible by this means to separate nickel from other metals, particularly cobalt, which is invariably found in nickel-containing ores. Then, by heating the nickel carbonyl to 180° C., the nickel could be recovered in an exceptionally pure state, all the other metals and impurities remaining behind.

A Pilot Plant for Nickel Refining, 1892

Mond and Langer set to work on evolving a process for refining nickel in this way. By 1892, satisfied with the results obtained in the laboratory, Mond erected a pilot plant in a nickel works near Birmingham. After many difficulties in the design and control of this plant had been surmounted, Mond was convinced that his process could be made to operate on an industrial scale, but how and by whom was this to be undertaken since he himself was now nearly sixty? In the years since he had arrived, an unknown young scientist in England, he had with John Brunner built up the great chemical company which bore their name. His many industrial and scientific interests kept Mond more than fully occupied and he was disinclined at his age to embark once again upon the hazardous and laborious task of developing an entirely new process. He tried to interest existing concerns in the nickel process but nobody had sufficient faith to support him. Realizing that he must develop the nickel process himself, he threw all his energy into the new venture.

Continuous Process for Nickel Refining, 1900

He and Langer embarked upon the formidable task of designing an entirely new type of refinery. They devised a mechanized continuous process which, with modifications, is still the basis of operations in South Wales and an acknowledged masterpiece of chemical engineering. Since it had to deal with two poisonous gases, carbon monoxide and nickel carbonyl, the whole of the operation had to be carried out in a sealed circuit and entirely automatically. Regular supplies of ore were obtained from mines purchased by Mond in Sudbury, Ontario, where a smelting plant was erected together with houses, railways and other necessary services. A site for the refinery itself was found at Clydach in the Swansea valley, with abundant local supplies of anthracite and with excellent road, rail and water transport to Swansea. This is a convenient port to which to ship the concentrated ore or matte from Canada and from which to export refined nickel overseas. So it was that in 1900 the Mond Nickel Company Limited came into existence eleven years after the investigation of the luminous flame in the private laboratory. The origin of this company provides a classic example of how a small unusual occurrence may, in the hands of highly trained scientists, ultimately lead to the founding of a new industry. The story is remarkable, not only as part of the history of science, but also from the human point of view, for without Ludwig Mond's unswerving confidence, indomitable energy and far-sighted vision, the carbonyl process might well have remained a scientific curiosity, instead of becoming the basis of the nickel industry in Great Britain.

Volatilizers and Decomposers

The concentrated nickel-copper sulphide matte imported from the smelting works at the Sudbury mines is calcined at Clydach. This converts the sulphide into the corresponding oxide. After intimate contact with dilute sulphuric acid, copper is extracted as copper sulphate. The filtered solution passes to driers and the powder is subjected to reduction in sealed towers. The mixture obtained goes to volatilizers where a current of carbon monoxide combines with the nickel and yields nickel carbonyl. The mixture of nickel carbonyl and carbon monoxide coming from the volatilizers is first passed through filters to eliminate any dust particles that may have been carried with it, and is then blown, by means of a fan, into decomposers (fig. 180). It is kept at a suitable temperature above the decomposition temperature of the carbonyl, so that it breaks up, liberating the carbon monoxide, which re-enters the cycle, and nickel, which is deposited on small pellets which seal the towers. These pellets are kept continually moving so that they grow into an approximately spherical shape and do not adhere together. Periodically, the stream of gas is cut off from each decomposer and the pellets it contains are extracted. These are then sorted, those of suitable size being packed for the market, and the others being returned for further nickel to be deposited on them. The pellets are sold when they reach a diameter of 1 cm., and they take from six to eight months to reach that size.

Nickel-carbonyl Poisoning at Clydach and Port Colborne

Nickel carbonyl, $Ni(CO)_4$, is a clear, pale, straw-coloured liquid volatilizing at room temperature and solidifying into crystalline needles at 23° C. When it is heated to 150° C. it gives off a peculiar odour like soot, which is perceptible when the air contains one part in two million. In the Clydach factory in 1902 thirty-seven cases of poisoning due to nickel carbonyl occurred, two of them fatal (Mott, 1907). This incident brought to light hitherto unsuspected physiological effects of nickel carbonyl, attended by a train of symptoms unlike those produced by any known substance. The factory was new and amply provided with ventilation. Arrangements had been made for the processes to be carried on automatically in a closed apparatus. No serious cases of poisoning took place so long as the automatic working was not interrupted. On two occasions, however, owing to the

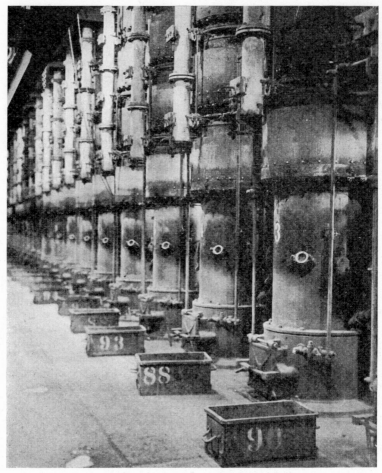

Fig. 180.—View of Decomposers in the Clydach Works showing Inspection
Dead-lights and Draw Boxes for Nickel Pellets

breaking of a chain it became necessary to substitute hand labour for the
automatic arrangements. The break in the continuity of the system allowed
escape of nickel-carbonyl gas. The proportion of carbon monoxide was
believed to be about 10 per cent. For several years little further trouble
was experienced, but between 1922 and 1930 forty-two cases, including
two deaths, were reported, all due to escapes during repairs or to fractures
of pipes and leaks in joints subsequent to general repairs and cleaning of
the plant. The International Nickel Company of Canada at Port Colborne,
Ontario, makes small amounts of pure nickel by the carbonyl process.
In 1950 ten men were exposed to an escape of the gas and three of them
died (Cunningham, 1954).

Animal Experiments

Experimental investigations have shown that the poisonous effects are entirely due to the nickel of the compound and not to the carbon monoxide (Armit, 1907). Rabbits die in sixty-five minutes after breathing air containing 0·018 per cent of nickel carbonyl, dogs and cats in from twelve to fourteen hours. The animals treated by Armit died when their blood contained not more than 0·072 to 0·16 per cent of carbon monoxide, and were not poisoned by iron carbonyl, which contains more carbon monoxide than nickel carbonyl. Its peculiar toxicity is due to the fact that when nickel carbonyl enters the respiratory tract it splits up, depositing nickel as a slightly soluble compound in a very fine state of subdivision over the immense respiratory surface of the lungs. It there sets up irritation, congestion and œdema. Some writers have attributed the toxic action of nickel carbonyl to carbon monoxide, which can easily be detected in the blood of the victim, rather than to any specific action of nickel. Whether this be so or not, the toxicity of nickel carbonyl is at least five times as great as that of carbon monoxide (Amor, 1932).

Symptoms and Signs

The symptoms in man come on immediately after the inhalation of the gas, and consist of giddiness, slight dyspnœa, nausea and vomiting, all of which pass off rapidly in the open air. Then, after twelve to thirty-six hours the dyspnœa returns, with cyanosis, rise in temperature and cough, sometimes accompanied after the second day by blood-stained expectoration. The rise in the pulse-rate is not proportional to the rise in the respiration-rate, which may reach a figure as high as sixty. Abnormal physical signs in the lungs are usually absent. Although at the time exertion causes considerable distress in breathing, there is no permanent disability and most of the men affected are absent from work for a short time only. In fatal cases delirium develops with death on the fourth to the twelfth day. At necropsy extensive hæmorrhages are found, especially in the lungs, the corpus callosum and the spinal cord. The cause of death is usually œdema of the lungs.

Preventive Treatment

The escape of gases must be prevented by carrying on the process in a completely closed system of iron chambers and pipes. Air containing 0·5 per cent of nickel carbonyl is dangerous. Compressed air should be supplied on each floor of the works and suitable joints provided at frequent intervals for fixing a face-piece and tube through which to breathe air whenever repairs become necessary. The air should be delivered into the face-piece at sufficient pressure to keep out any gas. The workmen should be instructed to test for the presence of nickel carbonyl by holding the blue flame of a methylated-spirit lamp against the air suspected (fig. 181). In the event of a large leak the flame turns yellow, and with a small leak a yellow film forms on the surface of the blue flame. This test detects a proportion

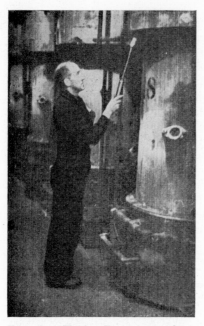

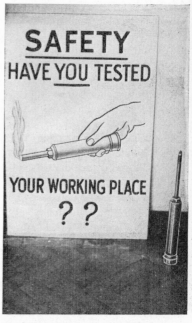

Fig. 181.—Testing Decomposers for a leak of Nickel Carbonyl

Fig. 182.—Poster warning Workmen to test for Nickel Carbonyl

of one part in 400,000 of air. Workmen should be instructed by word of mouth and by posters (fig. 182) about the toxic properties of nickel carbonyl and the great need to take care.

(c) Dust in the Refining of Nickel

A high incidence of cancer of the respiratory system has been recognized in men exposed to dust in the refining of nickel. It is not known which component of the dust is carcinogenic, but arsenic compounds as well as nickel compounds are under suspicion. At the Mond nickel works in Clydach, South Wales, Amor (1939) reported the occurrence of cancer of the lung and ethmoid in men employed in refining nickel from ores containing metallic arsenides. In Great Britain seventy-seven cases of cancer of the lung, and forty-seven cases of cancer of the nasal sinuses, especially the ethmoid, have been recorded since 1921. For a period of twenty-five years, nickel ores from Sudbury, Ontario, had had the copper extracted by the addition of sulphuric acid which had not been freed from arsenic.

Suppression of Arsenical Dusts and Metallic Arsenides

These ores were subsequently ground and calcined in Clydach and much dust escaped from the apparatus employed. It is possible that arsenic was the carcinogenic agent in these cases, and measures to exclude metallic arsenides from the process have been in force since 1925. In addition, strenuous efforts are made to suppress all dust at every stage of the process, since nickel ores and nickel carbonyl cannot be completely ignored as possible causes of cancer of the respiratory system in this industry. Pneumonectomy for carcinoma of the lung has been performed successfully on two of these workers. Both were squamous-celled carcinoma, and the arsenic content of the lungs, the hair and the urine of these men was greater than normal (Perry, 1947).

COBALT

In the sixteenth century the miners of Saxony were puzzled and disappointed when they smelted smaltite, $CoAs_2$, because it gave off poisonous arsenical fumes and yielded no silver in spite of its metallic-white appearance (see p. 333). They thought there was a *kobold* or *goblin* in the ore which accounted for its unreasonable behaviour, and this, of course, is the origin of the word cobalt (Mellor, 1953).

Sources

Practically all the world's cobalt is recovered as a by-product from copper and silver mining. The cobalt is present usually in the form of sulphides, arsenides, and sulpharsenides. The most important cobalt minerals are linnæite, Co_3S_4, smaltite, $CoAs_2$, and cobaltite, CoAsS, which occur as primary minerals. The chief sources of cobalt are the copper deposits of Katanga in the Congo Republic and of Zambia. In these two countries the chief primary cobalt mineral is linnæite. The deposits in Katanga carry from 2 per cent to 4 per cent cobalt, as against an average of about 0·5 per cent in the Zambian ores. The cobalt is recovered during the metallurgical treatment of the copper ores in the form of copper-cobalt-iron alloys containing some 40 per cent cobalt. In 1961 the Congo Republic supplied 58 per cent of the total world production.

Uses

Until recent years the principal use of cobalt and its compounds was in the manufacture of pigments, especially blues, for colouring glass, enamel, pottery glaze, and paints. Cobalt oxides are still used in ceramics but cheaper pigments have been substituted for them in paints other than artists' colours. It is in the metallurgical field that cobalt now finds greatest application, especially in the manufacture of rustless alloys and for cobalt steels (see p. 162). The most important use of the metal is in stellite alloys for high-speed cutting tools, a typical alloy of which contains 60 per cent tungsten or molybdenum. Cobalt alloys are now used under high-temperature conditions, especially for jet-engine parts. A cobalt-chromium-molybdenum alloy known as *vitallium* is used in orthopædic surgery in view of its resistance to corrosion by body fluids (see p. 166).

Cobalt steels possess many of the valuable properties of nickel and tungsten steels (see p. 166). Certain ferrous and non-ferrous cobalt alloys are utilized for making strong and remarkably permanent magnets capable of lifting heavy loads, sixty times the weight of the magnet. So rapid has been the increase in the use of the metal in permanent magnet alloys that this is now its largest single use. Corrosion-resisting steels suitable for safety-razor blades and surgical instruments frequently contain cobalt. The best binder for tungsten carbides and similar very hard cutting materials is stated to be cobalt. As a catalyst, cobalt is now rapidly gaining favour especially as a drier for promoting the oxidation of vegetable oils in paints. The hard and brilliant surface produced by cobalt in electroplating has been known for many years (Jones, 1963).

Hard Metal Disease

Hard metal is manufactured by a process of powder metallurgy from tungsten and carbon with cobalt as a binder. The industry, starting in Germany after the first world war, continues greatly to increase in size (Fair hall, 1957). Experience in a number of hard metal factories has shown that there have been complaints of cough, expectoration, shortness of breath and tightness in the chest. In the majority of workers these symptoms are comparatively mild. A few individuals experience well-marked respiratory distress towards the end of the working day. At an early stage such symptoms may be reversible on withdrawal from exposure. The majority of those developing severe symptoms leave and are thus excluded from the industry. In 1962 Bech, Kipling and Heather made clinical and radiological investigations in six cases, one of whom died. X-ray changes are slight and usually show increase of linear markings with scattered nodular opacities in the lungs. In two of the cases physiological studies indicated mild alveolar diffusion defects. In the man who died necropsy showed mild interstitial fibrosis of the lungs with carcinoma of the bronchus. Histological examination revealed diffuse pulmonary interstitial fibrosis with marked peribronchial and perivascular fibrosis and bronchial epithelial hyperplasia and metaplasia. The agent responsible for hard metal disease is as yet unknown. In animal experiments cobalt has been shown to produce pulmonary lesions, hyperglobulinæmia and erythrocytosis and to be the toxic constituent in hard metal. In man cobalt is known to produce a skin allergy and an erythrocytosis. Post-mortem analysis of the lungs of hard metal workers has shown the presence of tungsten but cobalt has not been found.

OSMIUM

Osmium, Os, occurs among the platinum group of metals (p. 481) as the alloy osmiridium. It was discovered in 1802 by S. Tennant and is named from the Greek ὀσμή, a smell. It is the densest of all known substances, being nearly three times as heavy as iron. Osmiridium is excep-

tionally hard and is therefore used for the tips of the gold nibs of fountain-
pens. It is also used for electrical contacts, as a catalyst in the preparation
of synthetic ammonia and for measuring the rapidity of explosion of guncotton.

Effects of Osmium Tetroxide on Nose and Conjunctiva

Osmium itself is innocuous, but the volatile osmium tetroxide, commonly called osmic acid, is slowly formed on exposure of the spongy metal
to air. Osmium tetroxide has a very irritating odour resembling bromine,
which attacks the nose and eyes. The vapour has a sudden vigorous effect
on the mucosa of the nose, pharynx and bronchi likened by workmen to the
kick of a mule. If fairly high concentrations are inhaled, there is a sense of
momentary constriction of the chest and inability to breathe, the aftermath
of which may persist for twelve hours. Deville and Debray (1859), the first
chemists to make an extensive study of osmium compounds, described
how the vapour of osmic acid attacked their eyes. One of them had conjunctivitis which interfered with vision for some weeks.

Death from Bronchopneumonia

Raymond (1874) reported a fatal case of poisoning which occurred in a
Paris workman. The vapour of osmium tetroxide had given rise to capillary
bronchitis followed by bronchopneumonia. Necropsy revealed purulent
bronchitis and confluent bronchopneumonia. Brunot (1933) exposed himself to the vapour of osmic acid and found that a smarting sensation in the
eyes was followed by lachrymation and the appearance of haloes around
bright lights.

Animal Experiments

He then exposed rabbits until they died of bronchopneumonia.
Necropsy showed dark red consolidation with scattered purple areas in the
lungs. The bronchi were filled with pus. The kidneys showed cloudy
swelling. He also placed one drop of 1 per cent osmium tetroxide in water
into the conjunctival sacs of rabbits. After twenty-hours there was œdema
and swelling of the eyelids, with profuse purulent discharge and a metallic
brown stain on all parts of the conjunctiva. After forty-eight hours there
were superficial ulcers in the conjunctiva and the cornea was milky and
semi-opaque. Ten days after the exposure the acute stage had subsided,
but there was corneal opacity and a pannus began to form which after one
month slowly extended towards the centre of the cornea.

Headache and Haloes round Lights

McLaughlin, Milton and Perry (1946) recorded the effects of osmium
tetroxide in seven men engaged in refining osmiridium. The hazard arose
from the fine mist or spray containing osmic acid which came off from the
reaction vessels when the ore containing the precious metals was dissolved

in aqua regia. The men exposed had smarting of the eyes with lachrymation and sometimes frontal or orbital headache. They saw haloes round
lights, one man saying they were green in the centre and red round the outside. At the height of the symptoms they were unable to read or to see the
images on a cinema screen. The eyes were always normal by the next day.
Only one man complained of cough and expectoration. No chronic or
cumulative effects were noted. Histologists who use osmic acid as a stain
for myelin and fat are familiar with headache, which comes on if the bottle
is left unstoppered on the bench. Because of the blackening of osmium
tetroxide in contact with oil and fat, an aqueous solution of osmic acid was
at one time used for taking finger-prints. The method was given up because
it was soon realized that its use in contact with the skin caused dermatitis.

Preventive Treatment

Preventive treatment of osmic-acid poisoning consists of the proper
ventilation of reaction vessels and other apparatus giving off osmium
tetroxide. Clearly the vapour of this substance must not be allowed to enter
the atmosphere of the workroom.

PLATINUM

Platinum, Pt, is a silver-white metal, tenacious, malleable, ductile and
softer than silver. Its coefficient of linear expansion is similar to that of
glass. It was discovered by the Spaniards about 1735 in Colombia, South
America. The term *platina* is the diminutive form of the Spanish *plata*,
silver, and it was applied in allusion to the silvery colour of the metal.
Platinum is now mined in the Ural Mountains of Russia, in Sudbury,
Ontario, at Potgietersrust and Rustenburg in the Transvaal, in Rhodesia,
Abyssinia, Australia, Indonesia and Japan. It occurs both in metallic
form and as the arsenide *sperrylite*, $PtAs_2$. Sometimes along with it palladium is found as arsenide or selenide. *Platinum concentrates* consist of
rounded grains which show signs of cubic crystallization and flattened
scales containing up to 76 per cent of platinum, and also iridium, rhodium,
palladium, osmiridium, gold, copper and iron.

Uses

Platinum is used in the electrical, chemical, glass, petroleum, dental
and decorative industries. It is manufactured into sheet, wire and foil, and
used for laboratory apparatus such as crucibles and dishes. It may be
prepared in the form of a black powder known as platinum black, and as a
spongy mass known as platinum sponge. It is used as a supportive catalyst
in the manufacture of sulphuric acid in which platinized asbestos or
platinized silica gel effects the oxidation of sulphur dioxide to the trioxide.
Platinum catalysts are used extensively in the petroleum and pharmaceutical industries. Because it has exceptional resistance to corrosion, being
superior even to gold in this respect, it finds application for parts where
the slightest corrosion would be detrimental, as in sparking plugs, magneto

nd other contacts and electronic tubes. Because its lustre is permanent
n air, it is very suitable for jewellery. The properties which distinguish
he platinum metals can be summed up in the word *permanence*. This
ccounts for their use as national and international standards of weight
nd length which are of hard platinum-iridium, and for temperature
measurement.

Salts of Platinum

Platinum salts are handled in industry both dry and as aqueous solu-
ions. The chemical industry uses considerable quantities of hexachloroplatinic acid, H_2PtCl_6, in the manufacture of platinum catalysts. The
electroplating industry deposits platinum from aqueous solutions contain-
ng various platinum salts such as sodium hexahydroxy-platinate,
$Na_2Pt(OH)_6$. In photography, use is made of a paper sensitized with a
mixture of potassium chloroplatinite, K_2PtCl_4, and ferric oxalate. Barium
platinocyanide, $BaPt(CN)_4$, is used in X-ray fluorescent screens.

The Platinum Metals

Platinum is the commonest member of a group of six metals which includes also palladium, osmium (p. 478) iridium, ruthenium and rhodium.
All are usually found in intimate association and, except in rare instances,
platinum, as found in nature, is invariably alloyed with other metals of
the platinum group and with gold and iron. Osmium (1802) and iridium
(1803), so named from the Greek ἴρις, a rainbow, from the varying tint of
its salts, were discovered by S. Tennant. Rhodium (1803), so named from
the rose-red colour of it salts, and palladium (1804) were discovered by
the English physician and chemist William Hyde Wollaston (1766–1828)
in his successful attempts to purify platinum. Ruthenium (1845) was
discovered by K. Claus and is named after *Ruthen*, Russia. Osmium, iridium
and platinum, in that order, are the three heaviest metals known and,
with the exception of palladium, the members of the group are characterized by their insolubility in ordinary acids. In addition, their high melting-
points, their resistance to heat and to oxidation at ordinary temperatures
endow them with valuable properties. All six are highly resistant to corrosive chemicals; they are in fact basically non-reactive, which entitles
them to the designation *noble metals*. In the First World War, when platinum was urgently needed for other purposes, *white golds* were invented as
substitutes for use in jewellery. They are alloys of gold with palladium or
nickel. Owing to its relative cheapness, twice as much palladium as platinum has been used in the electrical industry since 1936. Palladium is
exceedingly malleable and is used in the form of palladium-leaf. It is used
as a catalyst in the hydrogenation of many organic compounds. Rhodium
electroplating is used for searchlight reflectors, watch-cases, trophies,
medals and silver ceremonial tableware. Rhodium is used as an electro-
deposit on silver for sliding contacts handling radio frequency currents.
Rhodium-iridium alloys are used as catalysts in the manufacture of sul-

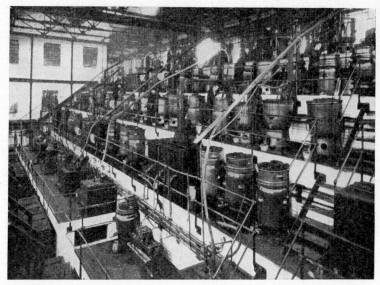

FIG. 183.—The wet-process department in a precious metals refinery

phuric acid. Osmiridium, platinum-iridium, and platinum-ruthenium-tungsten are used for the tips of fountain-pen nibs. Thermocouples made up of platinum-rhodium, iridium-rhodium, platinum-ruthenium and iridium-ruthenium are in common use. Ruthenium is alloyed with platinum or palladium as a hardener for jewellery and electrical contacts. When ruthenium is heated in air a volatile tetroxide is formed. Like osmium tetroxide, but to a much lesser degree, this irritates the conjunctiva and the mucous membrane of the nose (Cooper, 1922).

Exposure Hazards

The hazard arises from the dust, droplets, spray or mist caused by the complex salts of platinum and not of the metal itself. Workmen are exposed in the metallurgical and chemical processes for preparing the metal and its salts (fig. 183). Sometimes the complex salts are handled in dry form and sometimes by a wet process. If they get into the atmosphere in the dry process it is in the form of dust, and if centrifuges are used in the wet process the salts are thrown into the atmosphere in the form of droplets or fine spray. Spongy platinum is prepared by igniting ammonium chloroplatinate, $(NH_4)_2PtCl_6$, or some other complex salt of platinum. After ignition, the subsequent process of sieving the spongy platinum causes a dust of metallic platinum. Chemists and technicians are exposed in handling platinum dioxide, PtO_2, and in making platinum catalysts. Photographers face a hazard when using potassium chloroplatinite in plate toning. Men employed in platinum electroplating are exposed to hexachloroplatinic acid, the *platinum chloride* of commerce, both in the plating baths and as mist arising from them. Jewellers face risks when dissolving platinum in aqua regia, adding ammonium chloride and heating the product to make spongy platinum.

Symptoms and Signs

In 1911 Karasek and Karasek, examining the workers in forty photographic studios in Chicago, found eight cases of poisoning characterized by pronounced irritation of the throat and nasal passages, causing violent sneezing and coughing. There was also bronchial irritation causing respiratory difficulties so great that some individuals were entirely unable to use the paper containing potassium chloroplatinite. Irritation of the skin causing cracking, bleeding and pain was also observed. In 1945 Hunter, Milton and Perry described the same syndrome in men working in four precious-metals refineries in England. They found that fifty-two out of ninety-one workers exposed to the dust or spray of complex salts of platinum suffered from running of the nose (*platinum rhinorrhœa*), sneezing, tightness of the chest, shortness of breath, cyanosis, wheezing and cough (*platinum asthma*). Thirteen of the men complained of a skin eruption. In mild cases this was an erythema or urticaria of the hands and forearms; in the more severe cases the face and neck were involved also (*platinum urticaria*). Collectively these three allergic phenomena occurring in the nasal mucosa, bronchi and skin may be referred to as *platinosis*. None of these symptoms or signs was apparent in the workers exposed to metallic platinum dust only, or to the complex salts of the other precious metals, including palladium. The platinum content of the air samples taken at various stations throughout the works was determined spectrographically and found to vary from 5 to 70 micrograms per cubic metre (Fothergill and others, 1945). *Platinosis* has been observed in Switzerland by Jordi (1951) in three men exposed to the dust of ammonium chloroplatinate and in England by Roberts (1951) in men employed in a refinery process in which they handled sodium chloroplatinate. Sheard (1955) records the case of a woman who developed contact dermatitis from wearing rings made of platinum, iridium and ruthenium and plated with rhodium. In Spain Lide-Dunipe (1957) reported sensitization of the skin to platinum in a solderer. In addition, chemists and their technicians (Marshall, 1952), electroplaters and jewellers have all been found to suffer from platinum dermatitis or asthma or both.

Preventive Treatment

Prevention of this syndrome can be achieved by not allowing the complex salts of platinum to reach the atmosphere of the workshop or laboratory either in the form of dust or spray. Dust is worse than spray; therefore, unless it is necessary for technical reasons, it is advisable that the double salts of platinum should not be dried. In precious-metals refineries an adequate system of exhaust ventilation must be installed. Chemists and their technicians should work with platinum salts only in fume chambers with an adequate draught. Methods involving the use of centrifuges should be abandoned. Masks give some protection, but since they introduce the human factor, they are unsatisfactory. To protect the skin, gloves and barrier creams may help, but they must be used under supervision.

Symptomatic Treatment

The patient must be removed from exposure to the dust or spray. It is advisable to wash away the salts from the nose with water. Fresh air relieves the symptoms more quickly than anything else. Oxygen may help to relieve symptoms; and intramuscular injections of adrenalin may be useful to relieve a severe attack. It is unlikely that a workman, technician, chemist, electroplater or jeweller who has shown sensitivity will ever again be able to do work which exposes him to the hazard of inhalation of the complex salts of platinum.

SELENIUM

Selenium, Se, was discovered in 1817 by Berzelius and named from the Greek σελήνη, the moon, owing to its resemblance to tellurium, which had been discovered a few years before and named after the earth. It is a nonmetal which has certain metallic properties and belongs to the same periodic group as sulphur. Compounds of selenium must not be confused with selenite which is calcium sulphate (p. 371).

Allotropic Forms

Like sulphur, it exists in a number of allotropic forms. Metallic selenium is silver-grey, giving a black powder which is red when very fine. Vitreous selenium is opaque, black and lustrous, giving a red powder. Amorphous selenium is a dark red powder and colloidal selenium is a red solution. Two monoclinic crystalline varieties are known, both of them red. Selenium occurs in nature as selenides of lead, copper, mercury and silver. The principal source of selenium is the anode mud in the electrolytic refining of copper. The biggest supplies come from Noranda in Quebec.

Stench of Organic Selenides

Garlicky breath is a characteristic effect of the absorption of selenium compounds. This fact led to the discovery of selenium by Berzelius in Gripsholm, Sweden (fig. 184). His housekeeper had complained that he was eating too much garlic for lunch, whereas he had been examining a selenium-bearing deposit formed from pyrites in a sulphuric-acid chamber. The volatile compound exhaled in the breath is probably dimethyl selenide, $(CH_3)_2Se$. The amount of selenium which must be absorbed before a garlicky odour appears in the breath is greater than is the case with tellurium (p. 491). The unpleasant odour also occurs in the sweat, the urine and the fæces. Selenium compounds are sometimes added to non-odorous, poisonous commercial gases such as methyl chloride and carbon monoxide, so that their stench will act as a warning. For this reason they are known as *stenching agents*.

A Revolting Odour in Cambridge

In 1909 W. J. Pope and J. Read undertook much spectacular but unprofitable work on the stereochemistry of organic derivatives of sulphur and selenium. Starting with methylethylthetine bromide, $(CH_3.C_2H_5S.CH_2.COOH)Br$, they hoped to prepare its selenium analogue methylethyl-selenetine bromide, $(CH_3.C_2H_5Se.CH_2.COOH)Br$, and thus to determine the effect produced upon the optical rotary power of an asymmetric molecule by changing its central asymmetric atom from sulphur to selenium. Unhappily, although this final product of their search is an inoffensive substance, they were obliged to isolate at an intermediate stage methylethyl selenide, $CH_3.C_2H_5.Se$, which is a volatile liquid with a revolting odour. Transferring their work to the open roof of the University Chemical Laboratory, Cambridge, they were soon the cause of annoyance to business men in Petty Cury, who found it necessary to close their offices and send their staffs hurriedly on holiday, and then unhappily the notorious odour reached the nostrils of the guests at garden parties which were part of the Darwin Centenary celebrations of June 1909. Widespread protests were aroused and it was decided to continue the work in the open country of the fens. In the end the scientific results were judged to be too indefinite to warrant publication and, partly on account of its unpleasant nature, the research was abandoned (Read, 1947).

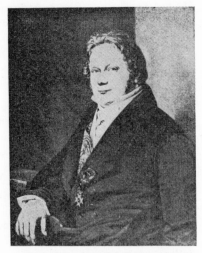

Fig. 184.—Jöns Jakob Berzelius, 1779–1848

Photo-electric Equipment

The electrical conductivity of the grey form of selenium is poor, but is greatly increased on exposure to light. This property makes possible all the fascinating uses to which the selenium cell is put. When an object intercepts a beam of light shining on a selenium cell, a change in electrical resistance occurs and is instantaneously registered. The selenium cell makes it possible to transmit photographs and sketches along a wire to illustrate papers, to make synchronous records of sounds and moving pictures for cinemas, and to construct street lamps, buoys and electric signs which light themselves up at dusk and extinguish themselves at dawn. It is also used for burglar alarms and for opening and closing doors without touching them, to enable the blind to read ordinary type by ear by means of the optophone, and to register precisely the moment at which the runner touches the tape or the racehorse passes the finishing post.

Other Uses

Selenium is one of the substances employed by glassware manufacturers to produce various shades of red as well as to neutralize the greenish tint due to compounds of iron. Selenium compounds find a place in the production of coloured paints, inks and plastics. They are employed to supplement sulphur as vulcanizing agents to produce hard durable rubber. They give improved belt flexing and oil resistance as well as increased tensile abrasion resistance. In the manufacture of stainless steels and of commercial copper these metals are alloyed with selenium to give improved machining properties. Sodium selenate was at one time used in the United States of America as a systemic insecticide to keep down aphides, red spider and thrips. It was used especially by commercial growers of chrysanthemums and carnations. After application to the soil in dilute solution it was absorbed through the roots and conveyed in the sap to every part of the plant. It was argued that these plants are never eaten by man or beast and that, if care is taken in the disposal of the soil, no harm can result. Unhappily, sodium selenate is both a very poisonous and a very stable substance, and adding it to the soil is, in ordinary circumstances, most undesirable.

Selenium Poisoning in Animals

Selenium poisoning in animals was formerly called alkali disease, because farmers associated it with alkali seeps and waters of high salt content. It was first described in 1856 in horses by Madison, an army surgeon stationed at Fort Randall, in what is now South Dakota, U.S.A. It has also been reported from the states of North Dakota, Montana, Wyoming, Kansas, Nebraska, Colorado, New Mexico, and from parts of Canada. It does not occur in Great Britain, but the disease of livestock known in Ireland as *dry murrain* is evidently the same condition. The symptoms in livestock were not definitely ascribed to the consumption of selenium-contaminated grain until the relationship was demonstrated by Franke in 1934. The animals affected are horses, cattle, sheep, pigs and chickens.

Seleniferous Soils and Plants

Soils which have been derived from certain geological formations contain selenium, up to four parts per million. This is absorbed by plants which concentrate it so that they become toxic to animals which consume them. The poisonous vegetation causes considerable livestock losses and is directly and indirectly a hazard to health in certain areas. The selenium in toxic cereals is associated with the proteins of the cereals. It is an integral part of the protein molecule, and consequently there has been much speculation regarding the possibility of selenium replacing sulphur in cystine and methionine. Such substitution for sulphur in the sulphur-containing amino-acids of proteins affords a possible explanation of the

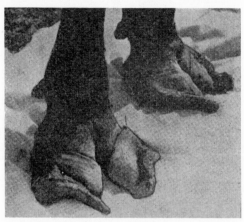

FIG. 185.—Chronic Selenium Poisoning in South Dakota, U.S.A. Bizarre deformity of the Hoofs of a Cow living in a District where the Soil, Grain and Forage contain Selenium Compounds
(*By courtesy of Dr. A. L. Moxon*)

poisoning of animals, for they show focal necroses of the liver in acute forms of the disease, and cirrhosis of the liver in chronic poisoning.

Acute Poisoning in Animals

Acutely poisoned animals are found in parts of Wyoming, where plants may contain several thousand parts per million of selenium. The acute illness is called *blind staggers*. In the early stages the animal may stray from the herd because of impairment of vision and difficulty in judging nearness of the objects in its path. Later, the blindness increases and there is profuse lachrymation with œdema of the eyelids. There is also a depraved appetite with a desire to chew wood, bone and even metal objects. The tendency to wander increases and weakness of the limbs occurs, but there is no involvement of the hoofs. There is evidence of abdominal pain, and death results from failure of respiration.

Chronic Poisoning in Animals

The chronic type, *alkali disease*, is predominant in South Dakota, where the vegetation, grain and forage contain up to 25 parts per million of selenium. Lack of vitality and loss of hair from the mane and tail are the first symptoms. There may be stunting of growth and inability to reproduce. The hoof elongates and assumes shapes so bizarre that animals often have to graze on their knees (fig. 185). It has been suggested that this deformity results from the replacement of sulphur, which is present in high concentration in the hoof, by selenium. Because of erosion of the growing ends of the long bones of the limbs the animals become stiff and lame. Death ensues from anæmia and emaciation. Sometimes sheep grazing over seleniferous areas produce lambs with abnormal eyes and deformed feet. In affected chickens the eggs are either sterile or they produce a high percentage of monstrosities (Moxon and Rhian, 1943).

Few Symptoms in Man

The effects of ingestion of selenium compounds by man have yet to be fully explored. Many of the inhabitants of the highly seleniferous areas of South Dakota and Nebraska show garlicky breath and gastro-intestinal symptoms, believed to be associated with the ingestion of selenium contained in meat, eggs, milk and vegetables. Urinary analyses showed that many persons in the affected areas of these two states excreted from 20 to 198 micrograms of selenium per 100 ml. (Smith and Westfall, 1937).

High Incidence of Dental Caries

In the state of Oregon there are two counties called Clatsop and Klamath. The children of Klamath have the best teeth in the state, but those of Clatsop have the worst. Dentists are no fewer in Clatsop than in Klamath, and there is just as much fluorine in its water. It was difficult to explain the difference, but when the excretion of selenium in twenty-four boys and girls from Clatsop was compared with that in twenty-nine from Klamath, it was found that the children born and bred in Clatsop county had more selenium in their urine. The preliminary survey suggests that the ingestion of selenium compounds in the diet leads to a higher rate of dental caries (Hadjimarkos and others, 1952).

Exposure Hazards

In addition to the element itself some of the commonly used compounds are: selenium dioxide, selenium oxychloride, sodium selenide, hydrogen selenide; selenious acid, H_2SeO_3, and its salts sodium and potassium selenite, and selenic acid, H_2SeO_4, and its salt sodium selenate.

Symptoms and Signs

In industry where workers have been exposed to selenium in copper refineries, a number of symptoms such as metallic taste in the mouth garlicky odour of the breath and perspiration and irritation of the nose and throat have been encountered. Many selenium compounds are acid in reaction and act as vesicants. Dudley (1938) studied selenium oxychloride $SeOCl_2$, and found it to be a vesicant producing in one human experiment a third-degree burn of the skin which was extremely painful and slow to heal. Middleton (1947) described the case of a chemist who was sprayed by accident with a solution of selenium dioxide, SeO_2, sustaining burns of both eyes, the entire face and the back of the neck. In spite of repeated irrigation of the eyes with isotonic solution of sodium chloride and of local næsthetics he suffered severe, persistent, intolerable pain in both eyes, with lachrymation and photophobia lasting twenty-four hours. There were first-degree burns of the eyelids, intense chemosis of the bulbar conjunctiva and clouding of the lower half of each cornea. Complete recovery occurred within ten days.

In workers exposed to selenium dioxide in the manufacture of telephone apparatus, Pringle (1942) reported five cases of burns, dermatitis and paronychia. The molten metal produced lesions of less severity than its salts. He found that the fingers, teeth and hair may become stained red from the precipitation of minute amounts of amorphous selenium in the tissues. He also stated that where workers are exposed to finely divided selenium, the dust of the metal tends to collect in the upper nasal passages where it may cause anosmia, catarrh and epistaxis.

Exposure to Selenium Fume

Clinton (1947) reported an incident in which a group of workers engaged in smelting scrap metal were suddenly and unexpectedly exposed to high concentrations of selenium fume. When the dross from the furnace was stirred up, a cloud of reddish fume arose from the material and billowed up around the hood to the roof, where it spread out and then gradually settled to the ground. The fume was intensely irritating to the eyes, nose and throat, and the works' chemist was notified at once. He immediately ordered the premises to be evacuated until the fume had dispersed. Fortunately, no worker was exposed for more than two minutes. The fume disappeared in about thirty minutes, leaving reddish streaks on the floor about the furnace. In the afternoon of the same day the melt in the furnace was poured into ingots without incident.

Symptoms and Signs

All exposed workers noticed immediate and intense irritation of the eyes, nose and throat, and an unpleasant sour garlic-like odour to the fume. The more heavily exposed workers complained of a severe burning sensation in the nostrils, like a hot poker, a dryness of the throat, followed after about two hours by severe headache, mainly frontal, lasting until the following day. Several men observed immediate sneezing, cough and headache, followed for some hours by nasal congestion, dizziness and redness of the eyes. Most of the men noticed an unpleasant taste in the mouth, and a similar odour of the skin and clothing. All of them recovered within three days, and there were no sequelæ.

Exposure to Hydrogen Selenide

Selenium hydride or hydrogen selenide, H_2Se, is a gas of obnoxious odour, less stable and more poisonous than hydrogen sulphide. It is particularly liable to cause laboratory accidents, though death is rare. Both Berzelius and Professor P. Bruylants of Louvain University were overcome while handling this gas. It causes extraordinary and persistent irritation of the mucous membranes, lasting for about fifteen days. Bruylant almost completely lost his sense of smell during a period of more than four weeks. In 1947 Buchan reported five cases of industrial selenosis due to less than 0·2 parts per million of hydrogen selenide in the atmosphere. The men were handling an etching ink containing selenium, and the penetrating putrid odour of hydrogen selenide was detectable at the etching machine.

Symptoms and Signs

The predominating symptoms were nausea, vomiting, metallic taste in the mouth, garlic odour of the breath, dizziness and extreme lassitude. Selenium compounds were detected in the urine. Clinical recovery occurred when a harmless etching ink was substituted for that containing selenium compounds.

Treatment

Workers exposed to selenium compounds should be given ascorbic acid daily in doses of 10 milligrams per kilogram of body weight. Such treatment aims at removing the garlicky odour from the breath and often succeeds. In workshops where selenium and its compounds are handled, all dust should be properly removed by exhaust ventilation and suitable protective clothing worn as necessary. It is sometimes essential for the workmen to wear a helmet with positive air pressure. Suitable washing facilities should be provided and no food should be consumed in the shop.

Disposal of Residues

The disposal of surplus selenium compounds presents a difficult problem. Burning must not be carried out in a residential area, because the smoke has an obnoxious and persistent smell. If the material is merely dumped and allowed to drain into streams, there is the obvious danger of creating seleniferous areas. Amor and Pringle (1945) point out that in theory it would seem most satisfactory to reclaim the selenium for further use.

TELLURIUM

Tellurium, Te, was discovered in 1782 by Muller von Reichenstein and named by Klaproth in 1798 from the Latin *tellus*, the earth. It belongs to the same periodic group as sulphur and is therefore similar to sulphur in its general chemical behaviour. Sulphides and tellurides often have similar properties. Tellurium is obtained mainly from the anode mud in the electrolytic refining of copper. The biggest supplies come from Butte in Montana and Noranda in Quebec.

Uses

As small a quantity as 0·05 per cent of tellurium added to lead hardens it and improves its resistance to acids. When fully toughened, tellurium-lead has a tensile strength which is twice that of ordinary lead and this enables sheets to be bent double and hammered flat without fracture. Compared with ordinary lead, tellurium-lead pipes have twice the resistance to bursting by frost. Minute amounts of tellurium added to cast iron increase the chill depth hardness. When added either to stainless steel or to copper it imparts improved machining properties. The nozzles of oxy-hydrogen torches are made of tellurium-copper (p. 239, fig. 70). Tellurium compounds are employed in rubber compounding to improve ageing, oil resistance, tensile strength and durability at elevated temperatures.

Stench of Organic Tellurides

Much smaller quantities of tellurium compounds are needed to produce a garlicky odour in the breath than is the case with selenium (p. 484). Gmelin (1824) was the first to observe the presence of a garlic-like odour in the breath of animals after administration of inorganic compounds of tellurium. In 1884 Reisert gave men 0·5 microgram of tellurium dioxide by mouth and showed that they had garlicky odour of the breath in one hour and a quarter; this lasted thirty hours. Ingestion of 15 micrograms produced a garlicky odour still obvious after 237 days.

Workers become Social Outcasts

Chemists and workmen who suffer from the remarkably objectionable tellurium breath state that when travelling in public vehicles passengers who sit next to them get up and choose another seat at a distance. Their wives will not sleep with them nor kiss them. Laboratory technicians handling sodium tellurite as a medium on which to grow diphtheria bacilli may develop the garlicky breath. In 1920 several men were poisoned by fume in silver refining. A garlicky odour was noticed both in the breath and in the urine. There was dry mouth and skin, somnolence, anorexia and vomiting.

Deaths from Sodium Tellurite

In 1946 a tragedy affecting three soldiers, of whom two died, was recorded by Keall, Martin and Tunbridge. In some army supplies certain bottles had lost their labels and had evidently been wrongly relabelled. This led to retrograde pyelograms being done with sodium tellurite instead of sodium iodide. The soldiers had garlicky breath, renal pain, cyanosis, vomiting, stupor and coma, and two of them died within six hours. The amount of sodium tellurite used was approximately 2 grams.

Effect of Ascorbic Acid

In 1947 de Meio studied the appearance of garlicky breath after oral administration of a sodium tellurite solution, in a group of thirteen men and seven women. While in some cases garlicky breath appeared in from twenty to thirty minutes, with an intake of 1 microgram of tellurium, as sodium tellurite, in other individuals it was necessary to increase the dose to 10, 25 and even 50 micrograms to obtain the same effect. This difference in behaviour was not related to body weight or sex. From the beginning of his work with tellurium de Meio became convinced that a much larger dose of elementary tellurium than of tellurite was necessary to produce the garlicky breath in rabbits. He thought that by reducing tellurite to elementary tellurium he could probably eliminate the garlicky breath. He chose ascorbic acid for the purpose because it reduces tellurite to elementary tellurium at room temperature (Levine, 1936). Ascorbic acid probably acts by reducing tellurite, tellurous acid and possibly other tellurium compounds to elementary tellurium, thereby decreasing the formation of di-methyl telluride, $(CH_3)_2Te$, the compound responsible for the garlic-like odour.

De Meio found that in two cases out of three the garlicky breath disappeared, following the administration of ascorbic acid in doses of 10 milligrams per kilogram of body weight. Four workers exposed to tellurium dust and suffering constantly from garlicky breath were given 750 milligrams of ascorbic acid three times daily at three hours' interval, and the garlicky breath was considerably reduced in strength or completely disappeared. The garlicky breath returned after treatment with ascorbic acid ceased.

Treatment

In workers exposed to tellurium compounds a daily dose of 10 milligrams of ascorbic acid per kilogram of body weight usually suffices to abolish the garlicky odour of the breath. Amdur (1947) described the accidental exposure of three metallurgists to tellurium fume for ten minutes while melting and pouring an alloy of 50 per cent tellurium and 50 per cent copper. Garlicky breath and sweat appeared within a few hours of the accident and next day all the men had become social outcasts even in their own homes. They were treated with a course of injections of 2,3-dimercaptopropanol (BAL). In spite of the fact that treatment did not begin until forty-eight hours after the accident, they lost all trace of the garlic-like odour in fourteen, thirteen and eleven days after their common exposure.

THALLIUM

Thallium, Tl, was discovered in 1861 by Crookes and is named after the brilliant green line distinguishing its spectrum (Greek θαλλσς, green shoot). In a pure state it is a silvery white metal but when molten it is black on account of the formation of oxide. It is found in nature as crookerite which is a selenide of thallium, copper and silver. Thallium is recovered as a by-product from the treatment of zinc ores mined in Canada.

Uses

In industry the metal is converted to thallium sulphate, which is used as a rodenticide and for the extermination of ants and other insects. In the optical-glass industry thallium is used for the manufacture of lenses since

ts salts are characterized by their unusually high refracting power.
Together with barium it also has some application in the manufacture of
phosphorescent colours. It is also used in alloys, as a chemical catalyst, in
photo-electric cells, in the manufacture of fireworks and as a fungicide and
depilatory. Fused crystals of sodium iodide containing 5 per cent of thallous
iodide are used as scintillation counters. The radioactive isotope ^{204}Tl is
used as a static eliminator, particularly in cellophane paper manipulation
Hudson, 1956).

Poisoning by Ingestion

Thallium is well recognized as a very poisonous substance and is considered to be more toxic than lead and almost as toxic as arsenic. Its effect
is cumulative. In children the therapeutic use of thallium acetate as a
temporary depilatory in ringworm of the scalp has repeatedly caused
severe poisoning. A number of cases of suicide or murder have been reported, as well as accidental cases, many of which proved fatal. Most of
these cases resulted from ingested rodenticides or insecticides containing
thallium sulphate (Teleky, 1928). In acute fatal cases following ingestion
of a large dose there is swelling of the feet and legs with pain in the joints,
abdominal colic, vomiting, sleeplessness, hyperæsthesia and paræsthesia
of the hands and feet with mental confusion and terminal convulsions.
Smaller doses have a more gradual effect with striking loss of hair from the
head and trunk and polyneuritis. Ocular lesions are common and include
retrobulbar neuritis with scotomata for red and green, primary optic
atrophy and lens opacities (p. 870). In 1964 in Guasave, Sinaloa, Mexico
nine members of three families living on a sugar-cane estate were poisoned
by eating oats baited with thallium sulphate as a rat poison. The incident
occurred in spite of strict instructions forbidding anybody to use the oats
as food. One family fed their dog with it too. The dog lost its hair, and all
the children in varying degree had alopœcia and polyneuritis. The mother
who by preference gave all her food to her children remained normal
Viniegra and Márquez, 1964).

Poisoning by Inhalation

In industry thallium compounds may be absorbed by inhalation of
dust and fume, absorption through the mucous surfaces from contact with
thallium in any of its physical states, and ingestion, as when individuals
indulge in smoking and eating during the handling of these materials. In
1927 Rube and Hendriks reported severe poisoning among men recovering
thallium from the flue-dust of a sulphuric acid works. Six men developed
pain in the joints, loss of appetite, fatigue, albuminuria and loss of hair.
The one who was most severely affected had, in addition, a posterior
adhesion of the iris, with cloudiness of the lens at the point of adhesion and
slowly progressive pallor of the optic discs. He suffered loss of vision in
both eyes, which was unchanged two years later although he had recovered
from the other symptoms. Other effects which have been observed are

tingling and weakness of the hands and feet with physical signs of poly
neuritis, papular erythema of the exposed skin, lymphocytosis an
eosinophilia (Carozzi, 1934).

Poisoning by Skin Absorption

Four patients investigated in Stockholm had been engaged in th
manufacture of rodenticides and came from four different workshops
Thallium sulphate had been employed partly in a dry state, partly i
solution for the impregnation of corn. The patients had been careless i
handling the powder without gloves, and may well have spilt the solutio
on skin and clothes. Sensory changes in the distal parts of the limbs wer
accompanied by only minor and uncertain signs of polyneuritis. In onl
one case was alopecia definitely demonstrable. One of the patients was
woman, aged 48, who had handled thallium for four years. After about
week's continuous exposure to thallium she complained of tingling in he
hands, fingertips in particular, in the soles of her feet and toes. In the ab
sence of signs of polyneuritis her symptoms were at first regarded a
climacteric, and it was not until thallium was found in the urine that th
correct diagnosis was established. It then transpired that the patient'
symptoms had varied from time to time with the degree of exposure t
thallium (Glömme and Sjöström, 1955).

Preventive Treatment

Adequate means such as exhaust ventilation must be used to captur
and remove dust and fume of thallium compounds. All chemical manipu
lations should be carried out in properly draughted fume cupboard
Furnaces used to fuse the halides of thallium must be built into fum
chambers and thermostatically controlled. The men working them mus
wear canister gas-masks. Gloves and other protective clothing must be wor
washing facilities provided and smoking and eating at work forbidde
The men should be informed of the hazard and periodical medical exam
ination instituted (Sessions and Goren, 1947). There is no known specif
treatment for thallium poisoning.

URANIUM

The uranium ore which occurs in black masses like pitch was calle
pitchblende in 1770, the word being an adaptation of the German *pec*
pitch; and *blenden*, to deceive. A new substance isolated from it by M. l
Klaproth in 1789 was called uranium in honour of Herschel's discovery
the planet Uranus in 1781. The substance was in fact uranium oxide an
the metal itself was not obtained from this oxide until 1842. Uranium, l
is a hard, heavy, nickel-white metal. It occurs as pitchblende or uraninit
U_3O_8, as carnotite, $KUO_2(VO_4).3H_2O$, and in several other mineral
Uranium ores are mined at Joachimsthal in Czechoslovakia, in the Cong
Republic, in Colorado, in Canada and in Australia.

Discovery of Radioactivity

In 1896 Henri Becquerel showed that the salts of uranium emitted radiations capable of reducing the silver salts of a photographic plate even when they were separated by black paper or thin sheets of metal. Shortly afterwards Marie Curie found that some uraniferous minerals are more radioactive than the uranium they contain. This was particularly marked in pitchblende from Joachimsthal, and she traced the effect to a new element more than a million times more radioactive than uranium to which she gave the name radium.

Uranium Fission Products

Ordinary uranium is radioactive and isotopes with atomic weights of 234, 235, 238 and 239 are known. The isotope of weight 235 has been utilized in the so-called atomic bomb since, when bombarded with slow neutrons, it is capable of undergoing fission with explosive violence. Before 1940 the expanding use of radium tended to create a surplus of uranium products. Henceforth radium is likely to have a subordinate position because of the availability of a great number of uranium fission products which can furnish a large array of types and intensities of radiation. The non-military uses of uranium include its application for colouring materials in ceramics as well as its use in photographic chemicals and as a catalytic agent.

Exposure Hazards

The high incidence of carcinoma of the lung in the Schneeberg and Joachimsthal miners may be due to the radon in the air they breathe. Chronic exposure to radon levels of the order of 10^{-9} curies per litre may result in damage to the lung. It is probable that the radon daughters attached to dust particles in the air impinge on and are held by the moist surfaces of the air passages in the lungs. Uranium hexafluoride fumes on exposure to air and is highly corrosive to glass and metal. Inhalation of the fume must therefore be strictly avoided (Fairhall, 1946).

Uranium Nephritis in Animals

Uranium and its salts are highly toxic; animal experiments indicate that they attack the arteries, kidneys and liver. Numerous studies of uranium nephritis in animals have been made since Leconte (1854) first showed that absorption of small amounts over long periods of time caused chronic nephritis. In dogs injured with uranium nitrate the renal lesions are associated with acute necrotizing arteritis, a process which is widespread throughout the arterial tree and especially affects the large elastic arteries (Holman, 1941). In dogs poisoned with uranium, hepatic degeneration occurs, and sometimes the animal can repair the hepatic injury (MacNider, 1936). Dogs receiving sodium citrate can survive an otherwise lethal dose of uranyl nitrate, because such treatment facilitates the excretion of uranium in the urine (Gustafson, Koletsky and Free, 1944).

Preventive Measures

Sultzer and Hursh (1954) measured the polonium excreted in the urine of miners working in the uranium mines of the Colorado Plateau. The Po^{210} in the urine is believed to come from the Pb^{210} stored in bone, which in turn is derived about equally from radon daughter products deposited in the lung and radon accumulations in the body fat. These authors suggest that urinary polonium estimations may prove to be a useful method of checking how much radon has been inhaled by uranium miners. All workers handling uranium must be under constant supervision, and frequent blood counts should be taken.

VANADIUM

Vanadium, V, was discovered in 1830 by N. G. Sefström in the iron ore of Taberg, Sweden, and named after Freya Vanadin, a Scandinavian goddess. H. E. Roscoe in 1867 isolated the metal and established its relationship to the nitrogen family of elements. Pure vanadium is difficult to obtain, even on a small scale, on account of the high temperature necessary and the tendency to re-oxidation.

Sources

The ores of vanadium are distributed mainly in Peru, Colorado, Utah, South-west Africa and Zambia. They occur as patronite, vanadium sulphide, VS_4, carnotite, potassium uranyl vanadate, $KUO_2(VO_4).3H_2O$, and vanadinite, a lead vanadium compound, $Pb_5(VO_4)Cl_3$. It occurs also in certain coals, lignites, shales, fireclays, asphalts and crude petroleum oils. It is also present in certain terrestrial plants, in sea water and in marine muds.

Vanadium in Crude Petroleum

Vanadium occurs regularly in the blood of certain *Ascidiacea*, or sea squirts, and *Holothuroidea*, or sea cucumbers, where it forms up to 10 per cent of the blood cell pigment. These creatures live fixed to rocks, and their fossilized remains account for the presence of vanadium in petroleum found in certain parts of the world. The percentage of vanadium in the ash of crude oils varies a good deal. Thus in samples from Venezuela it may be as high as 45 per cent, Oklahoma, 22 per cent, Iran, 14 per cent, and California, 5 per cent (Thomas, 1938). More than 20 tons of vanadium pentoxide are recovered annually from soot which collects in the boilers and smoke stacks of ships burning Venezuelan and Mexican fuel oil.

Uses

Vanadium was first used in the manufacture of special steel alloys in 1907. In that year Henry Ford, seeking to make a light car of great strength, was delayed for want of a steel strong enough for his purpose. By accident he came upon a piece of vanadium steel which was not then made in the U.S.A. With that steel in 1909 he designed his touring (T) model and by

1927 he had produced 15 million cars of this model. By 1936 about 95 per cent of the world's supply of vanadium was being consumed in the manufacture of special alloy steels. In the form of ferro-vanadium it is added to steel to promote fineness of grain, toughness and resistance to torsion and high temperature. The tensile strength of steel is raised from 7·5 to 13 tons per square inch by the addition of 0·5 per cent of vanadium. This property commends itself in the manufacture of forgings for locomotive and motor-vehicle parts, including transmission shafts, gears, axles and springs. Vanadium bronze is used for armaments as well as for aircraft propeller bushings. Vanadium pentoxide is used as a catalyst in the oxidation of naphthalene and is replacing platinized asbestos in the contact process for the manufacture of sulphuric acid.

Exposure Hazards

In 1911 Dutton described vanadium poisoning in a factory where vanadium ore was ground. In 1939 Symanski made a study of nineteen cases which occurred in a metallurgical works in Germany. He claimed that it is only the pentoxide of vanadium which gives rise to a toxic dust. Balestra and Molfino (1942) reported respiratory symptoms in labourers handling petroleum ash containing vanadium pentoxide. Wyers (1946) described ten similar cases among ninety workers making vanadium pentoxide. In 1951 the Department of Industrial Hygiene in Peru studied the health of vanadium miners and others processing the ore at Mina Ragra at an altitude of 15,700 feet in the Andes. Thirty-nine workers exposed to vanadium-bearing ore after roasting, and to the final product, vanadium pentoxide, showed the characteristic symptoms and signs of mild vanadium poisoning (Vintinner and others, 1955). Exposure to vanadium compounds in the cleaning of oil-fired boilers was first pointed out by Williams in 1952. The workmen concerned entered the combustion chambers and dislodged the fine soot from the brick-lined walls and from the heating tubes. Similar exposure in men cleaning the boilers of Esso oil tankers was reported by McTurk and others (1956) in New Jersey. On Tyneside, Browne (1955) described 12 cases in men working inside a gas turbine heat exchanger cutting away with pneumatic chisels metal tubes covered with a deposit containing up to 20 per cent of vanadium pentoxide. However, it is important to note that in addition to vanadium compounds boiler soot may contain high percentages of sulphuric acid, and it could be the acid rather than the vanadium compounds which causes the acute respiratory disorder.

Symptoms and Signs

In 1938 Molfino showed that vanadium anhydride has a strongly irritant action on the respiratory tract of animals. It is absorbed, and excreted in the urine. The clinical picture as Dutton recorded it in man included loss of appetite, anæmia, emaciation, diarrhœa, dimness of vision, melancholia, dry paroxysmal cough, hæmoptysis and albuminuria. Vanadium was found in the urine, fæces and saliva. In the men he examined

Symanski observed severe conjunctivitis, often with suppuration. There was chronic bronchitis with a feeling of constriction in the chest, persistent cough, profuse expectoration and sometimes hæmoptysis. The men described by Wyers had complained of shortness of breath, pain in the chest, palpitation on exertion and paroxysmal cough rarely with hæmoptysis. On examination they showed greenish-black discoloration of the

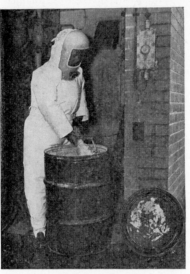

tongue, tremor of the fingers and arms and rhonchi throughout both lungs. Three of them developed pneumonia, of which one died. Sjoberg (1950) described the symptoms in 36 workers in a vanadium pentoxide factory in Sweden. They included cough, shortness of breath, irritation of the conjunctivæ, throat and nose but no gastro-intestinal symptoms. Five of the men had pneumonitis and in one there was a greenish-black discoloration of the tongue.

Preventive Treatment

In order to prevent poisoning by vanadium compounds in industry, mechanization and enclosure of all dusty processes must be strictly enforced. In boiler scaling the operator must stand outside the boiler using a long rabble or compressed-air lance.

FIG. 186.—Workman handling vanadium pentoxide while protected by means of a polyvinyl chloride air-fed pressure suit.
(*By courtesy of Siebe, Gorman & Co., Ltd.*)

The soot must be drawn away from him into the flue by an induced draught fan. In cases where certain parts of a boiler cannot be reached by this method, men entering the boiler must wear protective clothing and suitable dust masks. Men handling vanadium pentoxide in chemical works must be protected by means of a polyvinyl chloride air-fed pressure suit (fig. 186). All men exposed to vanadium compounds must be under medical supervision and must be re-examined periodically. Pre-employment examination should include radiographic examination of the chest and a patch test of the skin with a 2 per cent solution of sodium vanadate.

BIBLIOGRAPHY

The Newer Metals
BROWNING, E. (1961), *Toxicity of Industrial Metals*, Butterworth, London.

Beryllium
AGATE, J. N. (1948), *Lancet*, **2**, 530.
AUB, J. C., and GRIER, R. S. (1949), *J. industr. Hyg.*, **31**, 123.

BARNES, J. M. (1949), *Proc. Ninth Internat. Congr. Industr. Med., London,* Wright, Bristol, p. 630.

CHOLAK, J. C., and HUBBARD, D. M. (1948), *Analytical Chemistry,* **20**, 73.

EISENBUD, M., WANTA, R. C., DUSTAN, C., STEADMAN, L. T., HARRIS, W. B., and WOLF, B. S. (1949), *J. industr. Hyg.,* **31**, 282.

FABRONI, M. S. (1935), *Med. d. Lavoro,* **26**, 297.

GARDNER, L. U., and HESLINGTON, H. F. (1946), *Federation Proceedings,* **5**, 221.

GELMAN, I. (1936), *J. industr. Hyg.,* **18**, 371.

GRIER, R. S., HOOD, M. B., and HOAGLAND, M. B. (1949), *J. Biol. Chem.,* **180**, 289.

GRIER, R. S., NASH, P., and FRIEMAN, D. G. (1948), *J. industr. Hyg.,* **30**, 28.

HARDY, H. L. (1953), *Proc. R. Soc. Med.,* **44**, 257.

HARDY, H. L., and TABERSHAW, I. R. (1946), *J. industr. Hyg.,* **28**, 197.

LEDERER, H., and SAVAGE, J. (1954), *Brit. J. industr. Med.,* **11**, 45.

LLOYD-DAVIES, T. A., and HARDING, H. E. (1950), *Brit. J. industr. Med.,* **7**, 70.

MACHLE, W., BEYER, E. C., and TEBROCK, H. (1949), *Proc. Ninth Internat. Congr. Industr. Med., London,* Wright, Bristol, p. 615.

POLICARD, A. (1950), *Brit. J. industr. Med.,* **7**, 117.

STOKINGER, H. E. (1966), *Beryllium: Its Industrial Hygiene Aspects,* Academic Press, New York.

VAN ORDSTRAND, H. S., HUGHES, R., and CARMODY, M. G. (1943), *Cleveland Clin. Quart.,* **10**, 10.

WALWORTH, H. T. (1949), *Industr. med. and surg.,* **18**, 428.

WEBER, H. H., and ENGELHARDT, W. E. (1933), *Zbl. GewHyg.,* **10**, 41.

WILSON, S. A. (1948), *Occup. Med.,* **5**, 690.

Cadmium

AHLMARK, A., AXELSSON, B., FRIBERG, L., and PISCATOR, M. (1960), *13th Internat. Congr. Occup. Hlth.,* New York.

BAADER, E. W. (1951), *Proc. Tenth Internat. Congr. Industr. Med., Lisbon.*

BETON, D. C., ANDREWS, G. S., DAVIES, H. J., HOWELLS, LEONARD, and SMITH, G. F. (1966), *Brit. J. industr. Med.,* **23**, 292.

BONNELL, J. A. (1955), *Brit. J. industr. Med.,* **12**, 181.

BONNELL, J. A., KAZANTZIS, G., and KING, E. (1959), *Brit. J. industr. Med.,* **16**, 135.

BONNELL, J. A., ROSS, J. H., and KING, E. (1960), *Ibid.,* **17**, 69.

BUXTON, R. ST. J. (1956), *Brit. J. industr. Med.,* **13**, 36.

CLARKSON, T. W. and KENCH, J. E. (1956), *Biochem. J.,* **62**, 361.

FAIRHALL, L. T. (1946), *Brit. J. industr. Med.,* **3**, 207.

FRIBERG, L. (1950), *Acta med. Scand.,* suppl. no. 240.

FRIBERG, L., and NYSTRÖM, A. (1952), *Svenska Läk T.,* **49**, 2629.

FRIBERG, L. (1951), *Proc. Tenth Internat. Congr. Industr. Med., Lisbon.*

HOLDEN, H. (1966), *Personal communication.*

HUGHES, E. G. (1966), *Personal communication.*

JOHNSTONE, R. T. (1948), *Occupational Medicine and Industrial Hygiene,* St. Louis, p. 268.

KAZANTZIS, G. (1956), *Brit. J. industr. Med.,* **13**, 30; (1961), *Personal Communication.*

KEKWICK, R. A. (1955), *Brit. J. industr. Med.,* **12**, 196.

LANE, R. E., and CAMPBELL, A. C. P. (1954), *Brit. J. industr. med.*, **11**, 118.
LEGGE, T. M. (1924), *Annual Report of the Chief Inspector of Factories for 1923*, H.M.S.O., London, p. 74.
MALCOLM, D. (1966), *Personal communication.*
NASATIR, A. V. (1942), *U.S. Publ. Hlth. Rept.*, **57**, 601.
ROSS, P. (1944), *Brit. med. J.*, **1**, 252.
SMITH, S. P., SMITH, J. C., and McCALL, A. J. (1960), *J. Path. Bact.*, **80**, 287.
SPOLYAR, L. W., KEPPLER, J. F., and PORTER, H. G. (1944), *J. industr. Hyg.*, **26**, 232.

Chromium

AKATSUKA, K., and FAIRHALL, L. T. (1934), *J. industr. Hyg.*, **16**, 1.
ALWENS, W., BAUKE, E. E., and JONAS, W. (1936), *Arch. Gewerbepath. Gewerbehyg.*, **7**, 69.
BAETJER, A. M. (1950), *Arch. Industr. Hyg.*, **2**, 487, 505.
BIDSTRUP, P. L., and CASE, R. A. M. (1956), *Brit. J. industr. Med.*, **13**, 260.
CUMMING (1827), *Edinb. med. J.*, **26**, 134.
GAFAFER, W. M. (1952), Publication 192, Federal Security Agency, Washington. U.S. Pub. Hlth. Service.
GROSS, E., and ALWENS, W. (1939). *Report of the Eighth Internat. Congr. for Indust. Accidents and Occup. Diseases, Leipzig*, **2**, 966, 973.
GROSS, E., and KOELSCH, F. (1943) *Arch. Gewerbepath. Gewerbehyg.*, **12**, 164.
GREENBURG, L., MAYERS, M. R., HEIMANN, H., and MOSKOWITZ, S. (1942), *J. Amer. med. Ass.*, **118**, 573.
HAMILTON, A., and HARDY, H. L. (1949), *Industrial Toxicology*, Hoeber, New York, p. 47.
HORNER, S. G. (1934), *Lancet*, **2**, 233.
LEGGE, T. M. (1902), in Oliver, T., *Dangerous Trades*, Murray, London, p. 447; (1922), *Brit. med. J.*, **1**, 1110.
MACHLE, W., and GREGORIUS, F. (1948), *U.S. Publ. Hlth Rept.*, **63**, 1114.
MALOOF, C. C. (1955), *Arch. industr. Hlth.*, **11**, 123.
MANCUSO, T. F. and HUEPER, W. C. (1951), *Industr. Med. Surg.*, **20**, 358.
NEWMAN, D. A. (1890), *Glasgow Med. J.*, **33**, 469.
PFEIL, E. (1935), *Dtsch. med. Wschr.*, **61**, 1197.
TRUMPER, H. B. (1931), *Brit. Med. J.*, **1**, 705.
WUTZDORFF (1897), *Arb. a. d. kaiserl. Gesendheutsamt*, **13**, 328.
ZVAIFLER, N. (1944), *J. industr. Hyg.*, **26**, 124.

Manganese

BAADER, E. W. (1933), *Arch. Gewerbepath. Gewerbehyg.*, **4**, 101.
BERRY, J. N., and BIDWAI, P. S. (1959), *Neurology, India*, **7**, 34.
BREZINA, A. (1921), *Internationale Übersicht über Gewerbekrankheiten nach den Berichten den Gewerbeinspektionen der Külturlander über das Jahr 1913*, Berlin, p. 40.
CANAVAN, M. M., COBB, S., and DRINKER, C. K. (1934), *Arch. Neurol. and Psychiat.*, **32**, 500.
CHARLES, J. R. (1922), *J. Neurol. Psychopath.*, **3**, 262.
COHEN, H. (1934), *Lancet*, **2**, 990.
COUPER, J. (1837), *J. chim. méd.*, Paris, **3**, 233; (1837), *Brit. Ann. Med. Pharm.*, **1**, 41.

DOGAN, S., and BERITIĆ, T. (1953), *Arhiv za Higijenu Rada*, **4**, 139.
EDSALL, D. L., WILBUR, F. P., and DRINKER, C. K. (1919), *J. industr. Hyg.*, **1**, 183.
FAIRHALL, L. T. (1945), *Physiol. Rev.*, **25**, 182.
HEINE, W. (1943), *Z. Hyg. InfektKr.*, **125**, 76.
VON JAKSCH, R. (1901), *Wien. klin. Rdsch.*, **15**, 729.
LLOYD-DAVIES, T. A. (1946), *Brit. J. industr. Med.*, **3**, 111.
MELLA, H. (1924), *Arch. neurol. and psychiat.*, Chicago, **11**, 405.
OWEN, D. (1934), *Lancet*, **2**, 989.
PARKINSON, J. (1817), *An Essay on the Shaking Palsy*, Sherwood, Neely and Jones, London.
PEÑALVER, R. (1955), *Industr. med. and surg.*, **24**, 1.
RIDDERVOLD, J., and HALVORSEN, K. (1943), *Acta path. microbiol. scand.*, **20**, 272.
WADIR, N. (1961), *Proc. VII Internat. Congr. Neurol.*, Rome.

Nickel

AMOR, A. J. (1932), *J. industr. Hyg.*, **14**, 216; (1939), *Report of the Eighth Internat. Congr. for Indust. Accidents and Occup. Diseases, Leipzig*, **2**, 248.
ARMIT, H. W. (1907), *J. Hyg.*, *Camb.*, **7**, 525; (1908), *ibid.*, **8**, 565.
CUNNINGHAM, J. G. (1954), *Personal Communication*.
HAMILTON, A., and HARDY, H. L. (1949), *Industrial Toxicology*, Hoeber, New York, p. 205.
MARCUSSEN, P. V. (1960), *Brit. J. industr. Med.*, **17**, 65.
MARKIČEVIĆ, A. (1960), *Arh. Hig. Rada*, **11**, 147.
MOND, L., LANGER, C., and QUINCKE, F. (1890), *J. chem. Soc.*, **57**, 749.
MOND, R. L. (1930), *J. Soc. chem. Ind., Lond.*, **49**, 271.
MOTT, F. W. (1907), *Arch. Neurol., Lond.*, **3**, 246.
PERRY, K. M. A. (1947), *Thorax*, **2**, 91.
RAMBOUSEK, J. (1908), *Zbl. GewHyg.*, Nr. 8, S. 185.

Cobalt

BECH, A. O., KIPLING, M. D. and HEATHER, J. C. (1962), *Brit. J. industr. Med.*, **19**, 239.
FAIRHALL, L. T. (1957), *Industrial Toxicology*, 2nd ed., Williams and Wilkins, Baltimore.
JONES, W. R. (1963), *Minerals in Industry*, 4th ed., Penguin Books Ltd., Harmondsworth, Middlesex.
MELLOR, J. W. (1953), *A Comprehensive Treatise on Inorganic and Theoretical Chemistry*, **14**, 419.

Osmium

BRUNOT, F. R. (1933), *J. industr. Hyg.*, **15**, 136.
DEVILLE and DEBRAY (1859), *Ann. Chem.*, **56**, 385.
MCLAUGHLIN, A. I. G., MILTON, R., and PERRY, K. M. A. (1946), *Brit. J. industr. Med.*, **3**, 183.
RAYMOND, F. (1874), *Progr. méd.*, **2**, 373.

Platinum

COOPER, R. A. (1922), *J. Chem. Met. Soc. S. Africa*, **22**, 152.
FOTHERGILL, S. J. R., WITHERS, D. F., and CLEMENTS, F. S. (1945), *Brit. J. industr. Med.*, **2**, 99.
HUNTER, D., MILTON, R., and PERRY, K. M. A. (1945), *Brit. J. industr. Med.*, **2**, 92.
JORDI, A. W. (1951), *Schweiz. Med. Wschr.*, **81**, 1117.
KARASEK, S. R., and KARASEK, M. (1911), *Rep. Ill. State Commiss. Occ. Dis.*, p. 97.
LIDO-DUNIPE, E. (1957), *Act. dermo-sifliogr.* (Madrid), **48**, 583.
MARSHALL, J. (1952), *S. Afr. Med. J.*, **26**, 8.
ROBERTS, A. E. (1951), *Arch. industr. hyg.*, **4**, 549.
SHEARD, C. (1955). *Arch. dermat. Syph.*, **71**, 357.

Selenium

AMOR, A. J., and PRINGLE, P. (1945), *Bull. Hyg.*, **20**, 239.
BUCHAN, R. R. (1947), *Occup. Med.*, **3**, 439.
CLINTON, M. (1947), *J. industr. Hyg.*, **29**, 225.
DUDLEY, H. C. (1938), *U.S. Publ. Hlth. Rept.*, **53**, 281.
FRANKE, K. W. (1934), *J. Nutr.*, **8**, 597.
HADJIMARKOS, D. M., STORVICK, C. A., and REMMERT, L. F. (1952), *J. Pediat.*, **40**, 451.
MIDDLETON, J. M. (1947), *Arch. Ophthal.*, **38**, 806.
MOXON, A. L., and RHIAN, M. (1943), *Physiol. Rev.*, **23**, 305.
PRINGLE, P. (1942), *Brit. J. Derm.*, **54**, 54.
READ, J. (1947), *Humour and Humanism in Chemistry*, Bell, London, p. 288.
SMITH, M. I., and WESTFALL, B. B. (1937), *U.S. Publ. Hlth Rept.*, **52**, 1375.

Tellurium

AMDUR, M. L. (1947), *Occup. Med.*, **3**, 386.
GMELIN, C. (1824), *Versuche über die Wirkungen des Baryts, Strontians, u. s. w. auf den thierischen Organismus*, Tübingen, p. 43.
KEALL, J. H. H., MARTIN, N. H., and TUNBRIDGE, R. E. (1946), *Brit. J. industr. Med.*, **3**, 175.
LEVINE, V. E. (1936), *Proc. Soc. exp. Biol.*, **35**, 231.
DE MEIO, R. H. (1947), *J. industr. Hyg.*, **29**, 393.
REISERT, W. (1884), *Amer. J. Pharm.*, **56**, 177.

Thallium

CAROZZI, L. (1934), *Occupation and Health, I. L. O.*, Geneva, **2**, 1038.
GLÖMME, J., and SJÖSTRÖM, B. (1955), *Svenska Läkartidningen*, no. 22, 1436.
HUDSON, H. E. (1956), *J. roy. inst. chem.*, **80**, 187.
RUBE and HENDRIKS (1927), *Med. Welt*, **1**, 20.
SESSIONS, H. K., and GOREN, S. (1947), *U.S. Naval Med. Bull.*, **47**, 545.
TELEKY, L. (1928), *Wein. med. Wchnschr.*, **78**, 506.
VINIEGRA, G., and MARQUEZ, R. E. (1964), *Intoxicacion par sulfato de talio*, Secretaria de Salubridad y Asistencia, Dirección de Higiene Industrial, México, D.F.

Uranium

FAIRHALL, L. T. (1946), *Brit. J. industr. Med.*, **3**, 207.
GUSTAFSON, G. E., KOLETSKY, S., and FREE, A. H. (1944), *Arch. intern. Med.*, **74**, 416.
HOLMAN, R. L. (1941), *Amer. J. Path.*, **17**, 359.
LECONTE, C. (1854), *Gaz. des hôp.*, Paris, **27**, 157.
MACNIDER, W. de B. (1936), *J. Pharmacol.*, **56**, 359.
SULTZER, M., and HURSH, J. B. (1954), *Arch. Industr. Hyg.*, **17**, 359.

Vanadium

BALESTRA, G., and MOLFINO, F. (1942), *Rass. Med. Lav. Industr.*, **13**, 5.
BROWNE, R. C. (1955), *Brit. J. industr. Med.*, **12**, 57.
DUTTON, W. F. (1911), *J. Amer. med. Ass.*, **56**, 1648.
MCTURK, L. C., HIRS, C. H. W., and ECKARDT, R. E. (1956), *Industr. Med. and Surg.*, **25**, 29.
MOLFINO, F. (1938), *Rass. Med. Lav. Industr.*, **9**, 362.
SJOBERG, S. G. (1950), *Acta med. Scand.*, **138**, *suppl. no.* 238.
SYMANSKI, H. (1939), *Arch. Gewerbepath. Gewerbehyg.*, **9**, 295.
THOMAS, W. H. (1938), in Dunstan, A. E., and others, *The Science of Petroleum*, vol. 2, p. 1053, Oxford Univ. Press, London.
VINTINNER, F. J., VALLENAS, R., CARLIN, C. E., WEISS, R., MACHER, C. and OCHOA, R. (1955), *A.M.A. Archives of Industrial Health*, **12**, 635.
WILLIAMS, N. (1952), *Brit. J. industr. Med.*, **9**, 50.
WYERS, H. (1946), *Brit. J. industr. Med.*, **3**, 177.

CHAPTER VIII

THE AROMATIC CARBON COMPOUNDS

WE have seen (p. 88) how the close of the Industrial Revolution coincided with the birth of organic chemistry, and (p. 150) how the manufacture of coal gas laid the foundations of the coal-tar chemical industry which was destined to have far-reaching results on account of its by-products. In Great Britain the development of gas lighting is associated with the name of William Murdoch (1754–1839) and its commercialization with the names of Boulton and Watt. The first public display of gas lighting with the use of flaming open burners took place in London in 1802.

Rapid Advance of Coal Tar Chemistry

By 1812 Great Britain already had a gas industry. In 1825 Michael Faraday discovered benzene in gas prepared from whale oil by the Portable Gas Company. It was Hofmann (p. 150) who first proved conclusively that coal-tar contains benzene and he made this fact public in 1845. We have seen (p. 152) how Mansfield, one of Hofmann's pupils, undertook a systematic study of coal-tar (1849) and devised a still for fractionating tar oils by the reflux principle. Work in the rich field of coal-tar chemistry reached an exhilarating pitch with the preparation from coal-tar aniline (p. 151) of the dyes mauveine in 1856, alizarin in 1868, and di-brom indigo in 1890 (p. 152). Parallel progress was made in the preparation of explosives, perfumes, flavouring essences (p. 153) and pharmaceutical compounds. Since 1890 the coal-tar derivatives have become so numerous and complex that it has been difficult for the toxicologist to keep pace with the chemists who produced them (fig. 188). The following compounds will be discussed—benzene, hexachlorobenzene, nitrobenzene, dinitrobenzene, trinitrotoluene, dinitrophenol, hexachlorocyclohexane, phenol, quinone, hydroquinone, *para*methylaminophenol sulphate, dinitro-*ortho*-cresol, aniline, trinitrophenylmethylnitramine and phenylenediamine.

Relationship of Chemical Structure to Toxicological Effect

It is sometimes possible to predict from the chemical composition of the simpler members of this group what their toxicological action is likely to be. Addition of a *nitro-* or *nitroso*-group usually produces a more toxic compound, but it does not follow that toxicity will continue to increase as more *nitro*-groups are added. Thus 2,4-dinitrophenol is toxic, whereas trinitrophenol is practically harmless. The position of the substituent groups in the benzene ring may have an effect on the toxic action. Thus the toxic properties of 2,4-dinitrophenol are not shared by any of the other isomers. When a *nitro*-compound is reduced to an amine, as when nitro-benzene is reduced to aniline or nitrotoluene to a toluidine, the toxic character remains much the same, but the intensity of the action is lessened. Sulphonation renders a compound non-toxic; as soon as aniline is sulphonated, it ceases to give trouble (Hamilton, 1925).

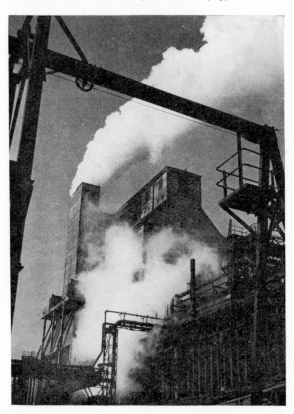

FIG. 187.—Coke Ovens of a Gas Works
(*Crown Copyright: Central Office of Information*)

No Inflexible Rules as to Toxicity

But there is no inflexible rule for judging the toxicity of isomers. Where the substituent group is in the *para*-position, the compound is likely to be more toxic than the corresponding *ortho*- or *meta*-isomer (Fraenkel, 1912). This is true of *para*- phenylenediamine, but in the case of tricresyl phosphate the *ortho*-isomer is the toxic one, and *meta*-nitraniline is more poisonous than *para*-nitraniline. Toxic activity depends not only on chemical constitution, but also on physical properties. It may be that toluene is harmless compared to benzene, merely because of its higher boiling-point and lower vapour pressure.

BENZENE

The story of the discovery of benzene and its isolation from coal-tar is told on p. 504. It is a hydrocarbon of the aromatic series, a colourless, highly refractile liquid with a distinctive odour; its formula is C_6H_6. The arrangement (p. 150) of six carbon atoms as the closed ring of the benzene nucleus was determined by Kekulé in 1866. It was named *benzin* or *benzine* by Mitscherlich, *benzol* by von Liebig and *benzene* by Hofmann.

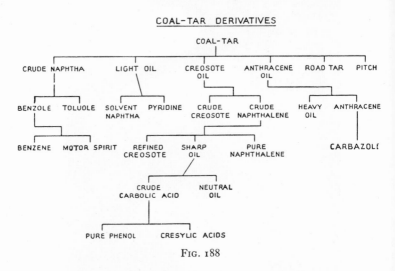

COAL-TAR DERIVATIVES

Fig. 188

English chemists follow Hofmann and use the term *benzene*, though *benzol* is favoured in Germany and the U.S.A., and *benzole* in France. In English usage *benzole* means the crude fraction in which the hydrocarbon benzene is the chief constituent. Commercial benzoles contain toluene and xylene, and traces of phenol and carbon disulphide. *Coal-tar benzene* must be carefully distinguished from *benzine*, a term used for the light distillate of petroleum better known as *petroleum-benzine* and containing chiefly hexane and heptane (fig. 189).

Uses

Benzene is handled in industry in two distinctly different ways. In the first, it is used in large quantities in closed mechanical systems, and the industries involved include the distillation of coal and coal-tar, the blending of motor fuels, and the chemical industries. In the second, it is used as a solvent or diluent, and the industries involved include the rubber industry, the boot and shoe industry, artificial leather manufacture, photogravure colour-printing, the manufacture of paints and varnishes, the aeroplane, linoleum and celluloid industries, the manufacture of artificial manure and glue, and the extraction of certain alkaloids (p. 1156).

Outstanding Toxicity of Benzene and Not of Toluene or Xylene

Of all the hydrocarbons, benzene is outstanding because of its serious toxic effect on the bone-marrow. Any doubt that this effect is due to impurities in crude benzoles has now been settled. The response of dogs and guinea-pigs exposed to crude and commercial benzoles is characteristic of benzene poisoning, and the toxicological effect is due primarily to the benzene content of the solvent used and not to impurities (Schrenk, Yant, Pearce and Sayers, 1940). Toluene, xylene and petroleum distillates containing no benzene have no such action. Commercial toluol may contain up to about 15 per cent of benzene, and this may explain serious toxic effects in industrial workers which have been attributed to the inhalation of toluene. Many of the distillates both of coal-tar and petroleum exert dangerous acute narcotic effects, and the outcome may be fatal if they are inhaled in sufficient concentration.

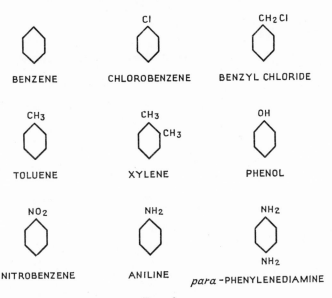

FIG. 189

Great Volatility aids Quick Drying

Under industrial conditions, however, only benzene and mixtures containing benzene produce aplastic anæmia. The risk of poisoning from this group of industrial solvents depends, therefore, on their benzene content. The greater volatility of benzene as compared with its higher homologues has obvious commercial advantages in aiding quick drying of paints, coloured printing inks, lacquers and rubber cements. This is an obstacle to the substitution of the higher homologues for benzene. Much, however, has been achieved in this direction in Great Britain, particularly in the rubber industry and in the manufacture of cellulose lacquers, so much so that it is rare for more than one or two cases to be notified annually.

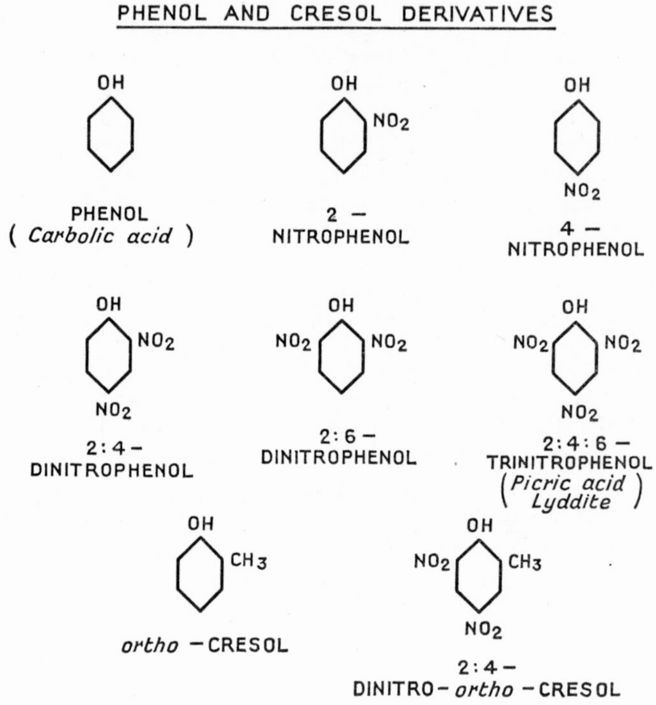
PHENOL AND CRESOL DERIVATIVES
OH
PHENOL
(Carbolic acid)
OH
NO2
2 –
NITROPHENOL
OH
NO2
4 –
NITROPHENOL
OH
NO2
NO2
2:4 –
DINITROPHENOL
OH
NO2
NO2
2:6 –
DINITROPHENOL
OH
NO2
NO2
NO2
2:4:6 –
TRINITROPHENOL
(Picric acid
Lyddite)
OH
CH3
ortho – CRESOL
OH
NO2
CH3
NO2
2:4 –
DINITRO – ortho – CRESOL

FIG. 190

Acute Benzene Poisoning

Except for a few cases of accidental or suicidal ingestion, poisoning in industry is due to inhalation of the vapour of benzene. Acute poisoning results from cleaning vats, painting tanks or the breakage of distilling apparatus. The symptoms are excitement, incoherent speech, flushed face, headache, giddiness, nervousness, insomnia, nausea, paraesthesiæ in the hands and feet, and fatigue, which may persist for more than two weeks. If the exposure is continued, narcosis and ultimately death will follow. Muscular exertion, emotion and fear are believed to increase the severity of the intoxication. Treatment consists in rest, warmth, artificial respiration, administration of oxygen by means of an oro-nasal mask, and injection of nikethamide as a respiratory stimulant. After recovery, the patient should not return to work for some days for fear of relapse. Preventive treatment is very important. It is considered under the headings which refer to gassing accidents (pp. 643–5), namely hazards from working in confined spaces, freeing tanks of noxious gases and vapours, rescue methods and artificial respiration.

Chronic Benzene Poisoning

Chronic benzene poisoning arises from the constant day-to-day inhalation of benzene vapour which has escaped into the working environment.

The Beginning of Chronic Benzene Poisoning in Industry, 1897

In the last years of the nineteenth century the use of benzene as a rubber solvent in more than one industrial country led to small outbreaks of purpura hæmorrhagica with a number of deaths from aplastic anæmia. The invention of the pneumatic tyre in 1888 immediately made the safety bicycle popular. Within nine years of the tyre first being manufactured the benzene-rubber cement used to seal its edges had caused four fatal cases of benzene poisoning among nine women engaged in a tyre factory in Stockholm. This was announced to the world in 1897 by the Swedish toxicologist Santesson who read a paper, which has since become a classic, before the Twelfth International Congress of Medicine in Moscow. In 1910 Selling reported three similar cases in a American cannery among girls employed using a solution of rubber in benzene for sealing tins. Selling was the first to point out that the important characteristic of benzene poisoning is not the purpura hæmorrhagica but the leucopænia with extreme reduction of the granular leucocytes caused by aplasia of the bone marrow.

The End of Benzene Therapy in Chronic Leukæmia, 1913

The demonstration by Selling of the leucotoxic action of benzene led to its adoption in the treatment of leukæmia. Korányi of Budapest was the first to undertake this, and in 1913 he read a paper stating his results before the Seventeenth International Congress of Medicine in London. This paper and the discussion which followed it called a permanent and world-wide halt to this drastic treatment. Eighty cases had been treated but good results admittedly were rare. The benzene was given by mouth in gelatin capsules starting with 3 grams a day and increasing to 5 grams if necessary. The ideal result was a gain in weight, shrinkage of the spleen and great reduction of the white cell count. However, after some months' treatment, most patients developed multiple hæmorrhages especially from the fauces and gums, and in the case of women there was troublesome menorrhagia. Often there was severe purpura and an uninterrupted fall of both white cells and red cells in the blood. With advancing anæmia, fever and bleeding these patients died of chronic benzene poisoning, their fate being much worse than it would have been with x-irradiation therapy and simple symptomatic treatment. However, Korányi established another important effect of benzene treatment, namely that repeated small doses of

0·25 gram daily excited erythropoiesis. Happily his suggestion that this method could be used in the treatment of certain anæmias was ignored by the International Congress! He also pointed out the danger of the continuance of the effects of benzene after the dose has been stopped.

Xylene used as a Safe Substitute for Benzene, 1918

In 1911 the Factory Inspectorate of the government of Austria reported two fatal cases of purpura hæmorrhagica due to the use of benzene in a rubber works. The first cases of chronic benzene poisoning to be discovered in Great Britain were reported by Dr. Veitch of Edinburgh to Dr. T. M. Legge of the Factory Department of the Home Office, London, in January 1918. Three men were involved, all had bleeding from the nose, gums, intestines and under the skin, the white cells dropped to 2,000 per c.mm., the red cells to figures below 3 millions per c.mm., and the hæmoglobin to 35 per cent. Necropsy showed the changes of aplastic anæmia in all three. The ages of the first two men were thirty and twenty-nine years and both were apparently healthy. They had been employed in a rubber works spreading balloon fabric, the rubber for this being dissolved in benzene (crystallizable benzol). In each case three months had elapsed between the first exposure to benzene and the onset of acute symptoms. The third man was thirty-three years of age and he died with the same symptoms and signs as the other two. He had been employed for six months in a poorly ventilated establishment coating metal rims with a solution of rubber in benzene in the manufacture of pneumatic tyres. The ventilation of these factories was improved and medical supervision of the workers instituted. On the advice of Dr. H. H. Dale (afterwards Sir Henry Dale) xylene was substituted for benzene and it proved to be quite safe.

The Growing Menace of Benzene Poisoning, 1922

After the First World War in most industrial countries the use of benzene as a solvent increased. In 1922 Alice Hamilton pointed out the growing menace of benzene poisoning in American industry. The chief industries responsible were rubber tyre building, the manufacture of spread rubber goods, the use of rubber cements for fastening rubber heels and soles on boots and shoes, artificial leather manufacture, the dry cleaning industry, the sealing of food cans with a benzene-rubber cement and, in the painting trade, the use of benzene as a solvent and thinner for paints, varnishes and stains and also as a paint remover. In all these industries many workers, both men and women, fell sick with benzene poisoning and nearly half of them died a terrible death from aplastic anæmia. The tragedy was on a much smaller scale in Great Britain where, for example, we had but a small industry putting fruit and vegetables into tins compared to the vast mechanized canning industry of the U.S.A.

Report of U.S. National Safety Council, 1926

We have just seen how Dr. T. M. Legge (afterwards Sir Thomas Legge) in 1918, acting to prevent benzene poisoning in Great Britain, ordered the improvement of the ventilation of rubber factories, instituted medical supervision of the workers, and used xylene as a safe substitute for benzene. Dr. Alice Hamilton secured the same benefits for U.S. citizens. She gives the credit for this to the work of a committee set up in 1922 of the Chemical and Rubber Sections of the U.S. National Safety Council, an association of industrialists and insurance companies. Within six years of her complaint of a growing menace of benzene poisoning she was able to write that this menace to the U.S. workman was lessening (Hamilton, 1928). At the beginning of her campaign one works chemist had told her that the concentration of benzene vapour in his factory was *only five per cent and how could that be poisonous!* A determined effort was made to persuade U.S. industry by means of good exhaust ventilation to keep the concentration of benzene in the atmosphere of workshops *below 100 parts per million.*

U.S.A. adopts Safe Substitutes for Benzene, 1928

The attitude of most U.S. industrialists changed and safe substitutes for benzene were used even where they cost more. Toluene was substituted for benzene in dry cleaning and in the thinners used for quick-drying paints. Cellulose lacquers sprayed on to motor-car bodies were now dissolved in toluene instead of benzene. Many rubber factories returned to the use of petroleum naphtha as a solvent for spread rubber goods and rubber cements. But the greatest triumph of all was the substitution of rubber latex for benzene—rubber cements in the canning and the boot and shoe industries. Latex is the milky fluid which is drawn off from the rubber tree after slitting the bark (p. 633). Originally the practice in rubber plantations was to coagulate it at once and make it into sheets for export. Instead ammonia is added to inhibit the growth of coagulating bacteria and the latex is exported as a liquid rubber.

Hazard to Photogravure Printers, 1933

There is some evidence that the Chinese and Japanese were practising methods of colour-block printing before the inception of printing from movable types. Of the modern colour printing processes machine photogravure was invented in Vienna by Karl Klietsch, a Czech, who used the method for calico printing in Lancaster in 1895. It is a photo-mechanical intaglio process in which prints are obtained from a plate or cylinder upon which the design is etched below the surface. The etched cylinder turns in a trough of printing ink, and as it rotates a fine steel knife, known as the *doctor*, scrapes the surplus ink from the surface leaving it clean. The cells or cavities, however, representing the tones of the design, retain the ink, which is transferred to the paper as it passes through the machine. At first the cylinders were used in flat-bed printing and the ink pigments were dissolved in turpentine, but about 1933 benzene was introduced when quicker drying of the inks was made necessary by the invention of rotary presses which were much faster and turned out copies of magazines in batches of hundreds of thousands.

Careless Use of Vast Quantities of Benzene, 1939

In France the process is called *héliogravure* (Glibert, 1935) and in the U.S.A. *rotogravure*. In 1939 Greenburg, Mayers, Goldwater and Smith found that three such plants in New York City employed 350 men and used in the pressrooms approximately 50,000 gallons of benzene per month. The benzene content of the ink solvents varied from 10 to 75 per cent by volume. Benzene concentrations in the workroom atmosphere ranged from 11 to 1,060 parts per million. Exposure to benzene occurred from evaporation from open troughs on the machines and from the paper web itself. Careless filling of the troughs by means of open pails and funnels led to spilling of the inks in pools on the floor. It was common practice for the printers to use benzene to clean the cylinders and the troughs as well as their own hands. A total of 332 workers was examined in the three plants. Of these 130 showed varying degrees of benzene poisoning. The use of benzene was discontinued because the concentration of the vapour could not be kept within safe limits in the case of such fast moving presses. Safe solvents were substituted and removal of the solvent vapours was ensured by proper ventilation.

Protection of Aircraft Spray Operators, 1944

In Great Britain the outbreak of the Second World War, with the increased demand for aircraft and diversion of toluene to the manufacture of explosives, necessitated a slight relaxation of the high standard of protection against benzene. As a result of this, anxiety was felt that in cellulose spraying some of the *dope girls* might show signs of intoxication. An extensive investigation was therefore carried out involving nearly 1,200 workers in sixteen factories (Hunter and others, 1944). The workers, most of whom were women, were exposed to concentrations of benzene vapour varying between 5 and 15 per cent (fig. 191). It was found impossible to detect any significant changes in the blood or any change in the inorganic total sulphate ratio in the urine of the groups of workers examined. Much work in the past has attributed leucopenia in such groups of workers to benzene poisoning, but this investigation shows that there is no justification for doing so, unless it is proved that the workers were in fact exposed to a toxic concentration of benzene in the atmosphere.

Low Concentrations of Benzene in Dope Shops

In the dope shops examined it was found that the concentration in the general shop rarely rose above 10 parts per million; and even on such specialized jobs as spraying the insides of cockpits, the concentration did not rise above 45 parts per million, and then only for short periods of time.

The toxic level for benzene in the atmosphere is usually stated to be 100 parts per million, but when the possibility of idiosyncrasy is considered, the only level which can be regarded as safe is zero. The situation with regard to benzene in Great Britain during the Second World War may therefore be looked upon with satisfaction and pride. It is most unlikely that any *dope girl* was poisoned with this substance and, indeed, it was difficult to find anybody who was exposed to toxic levels. The staff of the Factory Department of the Ministry of Labour are to be congratulated on the way in which they protected the worker from this hazard.

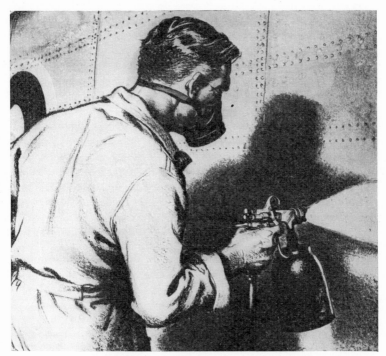

FIG. 191.—Use of the Spray-gun for coating Aircraft with Cellulose Lacquer. The Solvent used contains from 5 to 15 per cent of Benzene
(*By courtesy of the De Havilland Aircraft Co.*)

The Pathogenesis Over-simplified

The early work on chronic benzene poisoning (Santesson, 1897; Selling, 1910, 1916) established the concept of a simple constant picture. This was an over-simplification based on insufficient human material. The attack on the bone-marrow was destructive, affecting first the platelets, then the granular leucocytes and finally the red cells. The settled belief grew up that a diagnosis of benzene poisoning is not justified unless the blood picture shows an aplastic anæmia associated with a thrombocytopænia, and a granulocytopænia; that a leucopænia is more important in diagnosis than a low red-cell count; that cases of benzene poisoning invariably show purpuric manifestations associated with menorrhagia, bleeding gums, epistaxis and retinal hæmorrhages; that the spleen is never enlarged in these cases; that at necropsy the bone-marrow is always in a state of aplasia; that young women are more susceptible than men to the vapour of benzene; and that a concentration of 100 parts per million or less in the air may be considered safe.

Aplastic Anæmia in Advanced Cases

It is true that some advanced cases do show many of these features. On the other hand we have seen how Korányi (1913) established the fact that bezene taken by mouth can in certain circumstances excite erythropoiesis. In 1934, when only thirty cases of industrial benzene poisoning had come to necropsy, Dr. Alice Hamilton prophesied that when the blood pictures in this disease had been studied as intensively as those produced by radium or X-rays they would show the same infinite variety. In 1939 a series of detailed studies appeared, which not only fulfilled her prophecy but swept away many long-cherished beliefs about benzene poisoning.

Hyperplasia of Red Marrow in Certain Cases

These studies were all undertaken upon workmen exposed to benzene and were published by Hunter, who investigated eighty-nine cases, by Erf and Rhoads, who investigated nine cases, and by Mallory, Gall and Brickley, who examined histological sections from nineteen cases, fourteen of these being necropsies and five biopsies. The authors last mentioned found the picture in the bone-marrow to vary from severe hypoplasia to the most extreme hyperplasia, and they even recorded extramedullary hæmopoiesis. In spite of the old view, hyperplasia proved the more common of the two reactions. It was found only in patients with prolonged exposure, whereas hypoplasia followed either short or long contact. Sex appeared to play a part, for hyperplastic reactions were distinctly more common in the male, and hypoplastic ones in the female subject. Although splenomegaly was rarely apparent clinically, the spleen was often enlarged at necropsy. Lymph nodes were frequently prominent and dusky-pink on cut section, but occasionally they were grossly enlarged. Purpura of the skin, mucous membranes and serous surfaces was often noticed. Gangrenous stomatitis was present in some of the worst cases.

Indications of Hæmolysis of Red Cells

There are many indications that circulating red cells may be destroyed at an abnormally rapid rate in patients poisoned with benzene. Many authors have recorded increased numbers of circulating reticulocytes, a finding which was assumed to indicate abnormally active hæmopoiesis. The plasma-bilirubin is raised and an increased excretion of urobilinogen in the urine has been reported. Hæmosiderosis of the liver, spleen, kidneys and bone-marrow is a frequent pathological alteration, both in human beings and in experimental animals dead of benzene poisoning. In the cases reported by Erf and Rhoads the hæmatological findings were very variable. Thus, in nine patients the hæmoglobin values ranged between 47 per cent and 81 per cent, the red-cell count from 1,850,000 to 4,130,000 per c.mm., the white-cell count between 1,750 and 6,500 per c.mm., the platelet count from 18,000 to 150,000 per c.mm., and the reticulocytes from 3·8 to 14 per cent. Free hydrochloric acid was found in the gastric juice of all the patients, though two were achlorhydric until histamine was injected.

Leucopænia Inconstant as an Early Sign

From experience of photogravure colour-printing in which benzene was used as an ink solvent, Greenburg, Mayers, Goldwater and Smith (1939) deprecated reliance on the leucocyte count as a rapid means of detecting cases of poisoning; leucopænia, they said, is more often found in severe than in early cases. They regarded a reduction in the number and an increase in the size of the red cells as earlier and more sensitive signs of poisoning, and they looked with suspicion on a macrocytosis in a benzene worker even in the absence of other abnormalities. Eosinophilia, erythrocytosis and leucocytosis occasionally accompany the condition, but rarely stand as isolated phenomena. Of ninety-eight cases they examined, twenty-four had an eosinophil count over 3 per cent, seven had a red-cell count over 5,200,000 per c.mm. and twenty-eight had a white-cell count over 9,900 per c.mm.

Does Chronic Exposure to Benzene cause Leukæmia?

The evidence that chronic exposure to benzene produces leukæmia in human beings is still incomplete, but it is accumulating rapidly and to a volume which commands serious consideration. Penati and Vigliani (1938) were able to collect ten cases of leukæmia in patients exposed to benzene. All varieties of the leukæmic state have been recorded—chronic myeloid, chronic lymphatic and acute myeloblastic. Four more cases may now be added to this list—namely, two published by Hunter, one by Mallory, Gall and Brickley, and one by Erf and Rhoads, all in 1939. One of Hunter's patients showed a typical acute leukæmia; he had been heavily exposed to benzene for four years, lightly for a further six years, and not at all for the twenty months before his illness. Mallory tells of leukæmia in a boy of twelve years who repainted his toys after taking off the old paint with a solvent found to contain benzene. Fourteen cases of leukæmia developing among the many thousands of people exposed to this solvent do not seem impressive, but they gain in significance when we bear in mind that Lignac (1932) produced leukæmia in mice poisoned with benzene. Salter (1940) suggested that the leukæmia may be due to a tumour of the bone-marrow in which benzene plays the rôle of a carcinogen.

Rapid Onset in Susceptible Persons

Victims of benzene poisoning often constitute a small minority of the workers. A single susceptible individual may develop fatal poisoning in an environment which does not give rise even to mild poisoning in others (Ronchetti, 1922). The factors responsible for the great variations in susceptibility are unknown, but the original idea that women are more susceptible than men has been disproved (Hunter, 1939). Changes in the blood may begin from two days to one month after the first exposure, and may progress or develop after exposure has ceased. Death may occur within three weeks of the onset of symptoms. The death-rate is as high as 10 per cent. Occasionally a severe case ends in recovery. Hayhurst and Neiswander (1931) recorded a case in a rubber worker in whom the red cells were 900,000 per c.mm., hæmoglobin 10 per cent, white cells 850 per c.mm., bleeding time more than 25 minutes, and platelets 100,000 per c.mm. Treatment by blood transfusion and iron was followed by recovery, and three and a half years later the blood count was normal except for slight granulocytopænia.

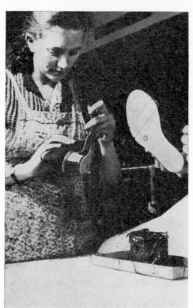

FIG. 192.—Worker using Shoe-cement made up with Benzene as Solvent at the Bata Works, Zlin, Czechoslovakia, 1947

(*By courtesy of Dr. J. Roubal*)

Preventive Measures

The prolonged inhalation of any concentration of benzene is dangerous (fig. 192). Where workers are exposed to benzene vapour, monthly medical examination must be a routine and must include a full blood count. It would be better to prevent poisoning by abandoning its use as a solvent, and from medical investigators all over the world comes the plea to use one of the many harmless substitutes. As rubber solvents, petroleum, toluene, xylene, cyclohexane or trichlorethylene often can be substituted for benzene. Toluene can replace benzene satisfactorily in lacquers, and xylene can be used in coloured printing inks, cyclohexane or methylene chloride in paint removers, and petroleum naphtha in rubber cements and in lacquer diluents. Rubber latex is a perfect substitute for benzene-rubber cements. Where no substitute can be found, benzene should be used only under the best conditions of ventilation, and its characteristic odour in a workshop should be regarded as a danger signal. In other words the safe concentration of benzene vapour in a factory or workshop is ZERO parts per million.

Treatment

Patients with chronic poisoning should be treated by a rapid series of blood transfusions, since the toxic influence may persist even after removal from exposure. Unhappily nothing can be done for the thrombocytopænia. Infection must be dealt with by the use of penicillin. No patient who has suffered from poisoning should ever return to work involving exposure to benzene.

Case 17. Cellulose sprayer—exposure to benzene for five months—death from aplastic anæmia.

C. I., a man aged 19. For five months he had worked about fifty hours a week spraying leather hides with a pneumatic spray gun in a large workshop. The solution used was a nitro-cellulose lacquer containing 25 per cent benzene. Any evaporating solvent was carried away by means of fans blowing conditioned air into the room from behind the workmen and exhausting it at the base of the opposite wall. By this means the air was changed forty times per hour (fig. 193). After three months at the work he began to have repeated nose-bleeding and was weak and shaky. After four months' exposure he was admitted to hospital with a high temperature and very ill.

On examination: the skin and mucous membranes were pale. There were purpuric spots and ecchymoses in the skin over the trunk and limbs. The nose and gums were bleeding and there was hæmorrhagic stomatitis. Blood count: red cells 2,000,000 per c.mm., hæmoglobin 48 per cent, colour index 1·2, white cells 2,400 per c.mm., polymorphs 6 per cent, platelets 14,000 per c.mm. In spite of three blood transfusions the hæmoglobin dropped to 28 per cent and the white-cell count to 100 white cells per c.mm. He died two weeks after admission to hospital.

Necropsy: aplastic anæmia. Petechial hæmorrhages in skin, trachea and under pericardium; altered blood in stomach; fatty degeneration of myocardium; yellow marrow throughout shaft of femur. No other bones were examined, neither were histological investigations made.

Case 18. Leather doper—exposure to benzene for sixteen years—death from acute myeloid leukæmia.

J. G., a man aged 40. He had been employed by a firm of curriers for sixteen years. For the first thirteen years he worked as a varnisher, and exposure to benzene was slight only. October 1933: he began leather doping with a brush or swab. In this process he applied to hides spread flat on a table a nitro-cellulose lacquer containing 7 per cent of benzene. Any evaporating solvent was carried away by means

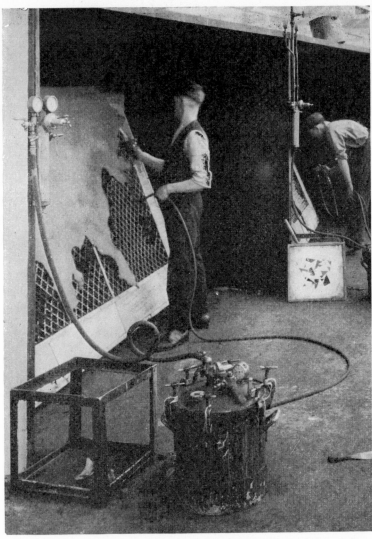

FIG. 193.—Case 17. Cellulose Colour-spraying of Leather for the Upholstery of Motor Cars. The Hides are spread on Steel Horses. The men are seen at work with Compressed-air Pistols. The use of Benzene as a Solvent should be avoided

(*By courtesy of Connolly Bros. (Curriers) Ltd.*)

of fans blowing conditioned air into the room near one end of the table and exhausting it at the base of the opposite wall. By this means the air was changed forty-three times per hour. July 1934: routine blood examination showed hæmoglobin 87 per cent. 8th November 1935: nose began to bleed, hæmoglobin 55 per cent. 19th December

1935: admitted to hospital because of bleeding gums, pallor and vomiting.

On examination: great pallor of skin and mucous membranes, petechial hæmorrhages in skin of arms and legs, hæmorrhagic stomatitis with areas of necrosis of buccal mucosa. Great swelling of right superior maxilla, and smaller swelling in left mandible, without discoloration of skin. Fundi pale; gross retinal hæmorrhages. Spleen and liver not felt. No œdema of legs. Blood count: red cells 3,610,000 per c.mm., hæmoglobin 58 per cent, colour index 0·81, white cells 6,900 per c.mm, polymorphs 30 per cent, myeloblasts 41 per cent, normoblasts 21 per cent. He became progressively weaker, the temperature rose to 101°, and he died three weeks after admission to hospital.

Necropsy: Dr. J. R. Gilmour made the necropsy (L.H. P.M. Appendix 524/1935), of which the following is a summary, and later wrote short notes upon the histology which Professor H. M. Turnbull has amplified at his request.

Bronchopneumonia. Anæmia and considerable purpura.
Myeloid leukæmia.

Very slightly enlarged myeloid spleen (5 oz.); pulp tinged with grey and rather cellular looking. Greatly enlarged myeloid upper cervical glands (up to 5 by 3 by 1·5 cm.); cut surface white and cellular. No enlargement of pinkish grey cœliac, lumbar and, slightly myeloid, axillary glands (up to 0·6 by 0·4 by 0·2 cm.). Cellular-looking, pinkish-grey marrow in lumbar vertebræ. Patches of red, partly hæmorrhagic, marrow (sinks in water) in surgical and anatomical necks, and under corticalis throughout shaft of femur. Œdema, albuminous degeneration, central lipoidaffin pigmentation and slightly fatty degeneration in somewhat brown liver; slight myeloid infiltration of a few portal systems. Œdema, anæmia and a few petechiæ in kidneys; severe albuminous and dropsical degeneration of first convoluted tubules and ascending limbs of Henle; very slight fatty degeneration of the latter and the second convoluted tubules. Large discoloured foul slough over absent teeth of right superior maxilla, surrounded by slight inflammatory induration; great myeloid infiltration beneath slough. Upper incisors loose; their gums retracted. Small tonsils. Slight granular laryngitis over vocal cords. Mucous bronchitis. Œdema, acid digestion and purulent bronchitis on lower and posterior part of lower lobe of left lung. Area (4 cm. diam.), in lower posterior angle of right upper lobe, of bronchopneumonia, characterized by fibrinous plugs in alveoli and fibrin or leucocytes in respiratory bronchioles only; myeloid infiltration of wall of a bronchiole. Clear pleural effusion (2 oz.) on left. Petechiæ in pleura over right upper lobe. Numerous petechiæ in visceral pericardium. Pericardial effusion (1 oz.) containing flakes of fibrin. Œdema of myocardium. Slight atheroma of aorta, and carotid and right coronary arteries. Pituitary, thyroid, parathyroid and suprarenal glands normal in size and appearance. Œdema of pancreas. Great involution of thymus. Distension of bladder by clear urine; numerous petechiæ in mucosa. Scar in urethra 5 cm. from external meatus. A few petechiæ in stomach and colon. Grey (from medicinal iron) semifluid fæces. Scar in scalp continuous through a trephine opening in skull (1·5 cm. diam. and 4 cm. above and to right of nasion) with œdematous scar tissue filling a defect (2 cm. diam.) in the subjacent brain. Scattered hæmorrhages (to 1 cm. diam.) in leptomeninges of sulci over convexities of brain; diffuse hæmorrhages over upper surface of left lobe of cerebellum. Middle ears, sphenoidal and ethmoidal sinuses clean. Smear of mucopus over somewhat swollen, discoloured, mucous membrane of right nasal cavity and maxillary antrum. A few petechiæ on trunk and limbs. General pallor. Moderately wasted man.

Microscopical examination: Marrow. In the upper end of the shaft of the *femur* adipose cells are relatively very sparse. Myelocytes preponderate over hæmocytoblasts. The latter are seldom present in compact groups, but as many as twelve or even twenty are occasionally in close proximity and in general they are numerous. Neutrophil myelocytes are much more numerous than eosinophil. There are a few metamyelocytes and leucocytes. There are no dark islands of erythropoiesis; but normoblasts and occasional primary erythroblasts lie singly or, occasionally, three to five in close proximity. Megakaryocytes are sparse. In the marrow, therefore, leucopoiesis predominates greatly over hæmopoiesis, and granular cells are more numerous than non-granular.

In the lower third of the femur, four rounded areas of hæmopoietic marrow free from adipose cells lie in a considerably larger area of adipose tissue containing areas of slight diffuse hæmopioesis. The marrow resembles that in the upper end of the shaft.

In a *lumbar vertebra* there are no adipose cells. The marrow has the characteristics of that in the femur. Myelocytes are perhaps relatively more numerous. Only fourteen megakaryocytes were enumerated in 45 square millimetres of the section.

Spleen. The Malpighian bodies are sparse and very small, having been encroached on or obliterated by a myeloid reaction. The pulp strands are packed with neutrophil and much less numerous eosinophil myelocytes, relatively few hæmocytoblasts, a few metamyelocytes, many leucocytes and a relatively small number of scattered erythroblasts, for the most part orthochromic normoblasts. Similar cells lie beneath the endothelium of veins in trabeculæ, and are numerous with or without erythrocytes in the sinuses, and with erythrocytes in the veins. Megakaryocytes are very sparse; only two were found in 3·2 square centimetres of the section. There is much hæmosiderosis of the pulp.

Upper cervical gland. The portion cut is 3 by 1·7 cm. The capsule is very thick and fibrotic, and is greatly infiltrated with myeloid cells. The septa and hilar tissue are almost obliterated by such infiltration. A very few small rounded areas are occupied by small lymphocytes. Myelocytes are numerous but the proportion of cells with non-granular basophil cytoplasm is greater than in the spleen and marrow. Among these basophil cells micromyeloblasts are more numerous than hæmocytoblasts. There are a few scattered normoblasts. Only one megakaryocyte was observed.

The axillary glands are small and atrophied. Lymphadenoid tissue is scanty so that much of the reticular tissue contains few or no lymphocytes and appears fibrotic. Myelocytes and more numerous meta-myelocytes and leucocytes are present in small numbers in the sinuses where lymphadenoid tissue is present, and are abundant in the more fibrotic tissue free from lymphocytes, making this tissue conspicuously myeloid.

Liver. The smaller portal systems are slightly infiltrated with lymphocytes; in the larger systems the infiltration is greater and a few myelocytes are present.

Kidney. There is no myeloid infiltration.

Superior maxilla. A deep zone of the soft tissue is completely necrosed or hæmorrhagic or densely infiltrated with neutrophil leucocytes. The tissue beneath this consists of voluntary muscle, adipose tissue and a mucous gland. In it there is a great myeloid infiltration in which the cells resemble in type and relative number those in the cervical gland.

Upper lobe of right lung. There is extensive fibrinous, partly hæmorrhagic, bronchopneumonia. Myeloid infiltration occupies the submucosa and adventitia of a large bronchiole which lies in partially collapsed lung between two bronchopneumonic areas.

The *blood* in the renal capillaries contains numerous myelocytes and leucocytes, many micromyeloblasts, a few hæmocytoblasts, large and small lymphocytes and metamyelocytes, and a very few monocytes and normoblasts; one primary erythroblast was seen. The blood in the hepatic sinusoids is very similar but contains many normoblasts.

Other microscopical changes in the liver, kidney and lung are incorporated in the summary of necropsy.

HEXACHLOROBENZENE

Hexachlorobenzene, C_6Cl_6, also called perchlorbenzene, is a white crystalline solid applied dry as a fungicidal dressing to seed grain, notably wheat. Its use is limited to moist seed grain, for in the presence of water alternative fungicides, especially organic mercury compounds, are phyto-toxic. Care must be taken not to confuse hexachlorobenzene with hexachlorocyclohexane, $C_6H_6Cl_6$, also called benzene hexachloride, which is

widely used as an insecticide (p. 524). In Britain the use of hexachlorobenzene has decreased in recent years until very little is now used. Although in the spring of 1961 reports of damage to wild life following the
eating of seed grain by birds incriminated hexachlorobenzene in addition
to the more toxic insecticides and fungicides, consideration of the amounts
involved and its relatively low toxicity suggests that this accusation is false.
Increasing public concern about the death of wood pigeons and other wild
birds and in turn their predators (foxes, badgers, cats and dogs) following
their eating spring-grown grain led to a Ministry of Agriculture rule
restricting the use of aldrin, dieldrin and heptachlor to autumn-or winter-
sown wheat and then only when there is a demonstrable risk from wheat
bulb fly.

Epidemic Cutaneous Porphyria in Turkey

Although hexachlorobenzene has done no harm to men manufacturing
it nor to those using it in the field we must nevertheless notice a local
outbreak of chronic poisoning affecting thousands of people. This has
given rise to two new clinical conditions known as kara yara (blackwound)
and pembe yara (rosewound) which were first observed in 1955 as an
epidemic outbreak widely distributed in villages and towns in south-east
Turkey (Çam, 1959). Kara yara occurs in adults and children more than
three years old. The syndrome consists of blistering and epidermolysis of
the skin, involving the exposed parts of the body and particularly the face
and hands. The skin is unusually sensitive both to light and to minor
mechanical trauma. The cutaneous lesions heal poorly and become easily
infected. If healing does take place during the winter season, pigmented
scars are formed, and contractures are frequently observed in areas where
tissue loss has occurred. Moreover, infected lesions may give rise to a sup-
purative arthritis and osteomyelitis, affecting particularly the digits.
Invariably, the patients exhibit hyperpigmentation, which is most
noticeable on the face and hands but also involves other parts of the body.
In addition, there is usually marked hypertrichosis, which is not limited
to the exposed parts of the skin but covers the trunk and extremities with
a fine layer of dark hair. Loss of weight and hepatomegaly are frequently
present, but abdominal pain and neurological complications are conspicuously absent. The urine in all cases contains coproporphyrin. The
disease may last for several years and is rarely fatal (Schmid, 1960). Pembe
yara occurs only in breast-fed children. The characteristic skin lesions
are patches of rose-pink papules on the hands and legs. Porphyrinuria
seldom occurs, and when it does there is less coproporphyrin than in kara
yara. There is frequently diarrhœa and bronchitis and the disease may last
for several years. The fatality rate is about 10 per cent (Kantemir, Çam
and Kayaalp, 1960).

Toxic Origin of Kara Yara and Pembe Yara

The probable ætiology of this peculiar syndrome was first suggested by Dr. Cihad Çam, the director of the Skin Clinic in Diyarbakir. In taking dietary histories of many hundreds of his patients he discovered that virtually all of them had consumed wheat treated with the fungicide hexachlorobenzene. High-quality seed wheat mixed with fungicidal and insecticidal agents is distributed annually to the farmers. Since 1955 the wheat supplied in the districts of Urfa, Diyarbakir and Mardin contained 0·2 per cent *Chloroble* or *Sürmesan A*, in addition to mercurous and mercuric chloride, which had been used in previous years. These two commercial preparations contain about 10 per cent hexachlorobenzene, a fungicidal agent used against *Tilletia tritici*. In the winter of 1956 some of the treated wheat was used for human consumption instead of being reserved for planting purposes. At first this occurred only in the rural areas outside the townships, but local observers believe that some of the wheat containing hexachlorobenzene gradually reached the local markets where it was distributed among a much larger segment of the population. Dr. Çam examined over 600 patients with porphyria, all living in his district. He estimates that in the three districts involved, the number of cases may have been as high as 5,000.

Acquired Porphyria in Experimental Animals

Investigators in Ankara gave 10 per cent hexachlorobenzene as Sürmesan alone or mixed 2:1000 with wheat to rats. They died after being fed for one to two months with 20 gm. per day of the wheat mixture, all showing marked porphyrinuria. Rabbits fed daily with Sürmesan showed coproporphyrinuria after six days, which increased, leading in some cases to death with convulsions in about two weeks. At necropsy liver damage was observed (Kantemir, Gener, Kayaalp and Timlioglu, 1960). Similar experiments in rats carried out by Harvard workers showed that daily ingestion of hexachlorobenzene resulted in a profound disturbance of porphyrin metabolism, characterized by increased amounts of porphyrins and porphyrin precursors in the liver and excreta, with histological evidence of hepatocellular degeneration. These findings support the suggestion, derived from epidemiological data, that hexachlorobenzene ingestion is the cause of the outbreak of porphyria in Turkey. This experimental result is of particular interest in that, hitherto, human porphyria was assumed to be genetically determined, because conclusive evidence for the existence of a purely acquired form of this disease has been lacking. The widespread appearance of porphyria among three genetically distinct populations in south-eastern Turkey—domestic Turks, Kurds and Turks repatriated after several centuries of residence in the Balkans—makes its dependence on an inherited abnormality extremely unlikely (Ockner and Schmid, 1961).

Hexachlorocyclohexane

Benzene hexachloride, hexachlorocyclohexane, $C_6H_6Cl_6$, also known as hexachlorane, BHC, 666, and lindane exists in five isomeric forms of which only the gamma isomer has a powerful insecticidal effect, hence the additional names gamma hexachlorocyclohexane and gammexane. The substance here described should not be confused with hexachlorobenzene, C_6Cl_6, which is used as a fungicide for seed grain (p. 521).

Uses

Gammexane was a British discovery of the Second World War. It is a powerful insecticide which kills lice, fleas, flies, mosquitoes, cockroaches and other insects. It acts in very low concentrations being about nine times as toxic to houseflies as DDT and about eighteen times as toxic as the pyrethrins. However, it does not possess the long-lasting toxicity of DDT and to overcome this lack of residual effect it may be combined with DDT in insect powders. It is particularly effective against the cotton boll weevil, the cotton flea hopper and cotton aphides. It is one of the few compounds that will kill both cattle lice and eggs at the same time. It is a valuable soil insecticide but should not be used for potatoes for it may impart to them a disagreeable taste.

Effects of Crude BHC on the Skin

As is the case with DDT the record for BHC is one of widespread use without evidence of occupational poisoning. Improperly used it has produced toxic effects in man but instances of this have been rare. The handling, particularly in the summer months, of a mixed insecticide known as *cotton dust* caused toxic and allergic skin injuries in factory workers (Behrbohm and Brandt, 1959). The powder consisted of crude benzene hexachloride, DDT, sulphur and a filler. It is not known which component was responsible, but, on the basis of patch tests, it is assumed that impurities in the BHC were to blame. The lesions were localized especially in folds of the skin, such as the elbows, where sweating was most marked. Allergic eczema was related to the severity and duration of the first attack. It sometimes recurred after an interval away from work when clothes which smelt of crude BHC were worn again.

Acute Poisoning by BHC

Accidental poisoning has occurred in a variety of circumstances including the use of BHC as a vermifuge. After a dose of 45 mg. one man felt ill and another had a fit. On the other hand a man who took 40 mg. daily for ten days suffered nothing worse than a mild burning feeling in the tongue. Schmiedeberg and Wasserburger (1953) recorded fits and loss of consciousness in a man who took 1000 mg. In these and other episodes of acute poisoning recovery was rapid. Much is to be learned from the misuse of BHC which led to acute poisoning in a farmer's wife (Heiberg

PLATE I

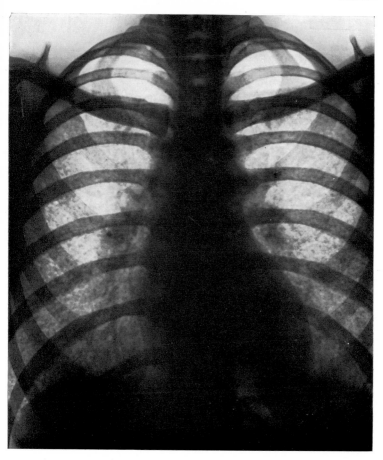

Chronic Beryllium poisoning in a woman aged 25, who had been exposed in a Laboratory three years previously to the Dust of Zinc Beryllium Silicate for three weeks only. She became desperately ill with intense Dyspnœa, Apathy, Loss of Appetite and Loss of Weight. Five years after cessation of exposure she was recovering rapidly and had gained forty pounds in weight

(By courtesy of Dr. W. N. Rogers)

PLATE II

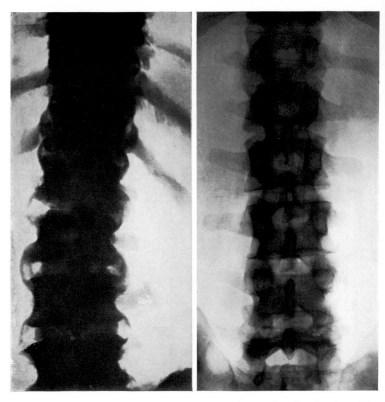

Fluorosis of Bones and Ligaments in a Copenhagen Cryolite Crusher. The osseous pattern of the Vertebræ is completely effaced and replaced by dense opaque shadows. There is evidence of Calcification of Ligaments, and around the Inter-vertebral and Costo-vertebral Articulations are calcified shadows resembling Osteophytes. The picture on the right is a normal Spine for comparison

(*By courtesy of Dr. Sk. V. Gudjonsson*)

PLATE III

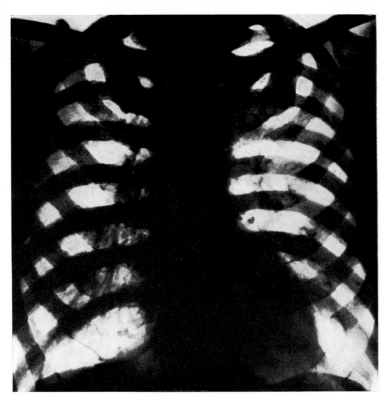

Fluorosis of the Ribs in a Copenhagen Cryolite Crusher. There is uniform increase of density, the structure of the Bone having been altered in such a way that the outline of Cortex and Spongiosa has completely disappeared. There is pronounced Calcification of the Costal Cartilages. The Ribs show excrescences due to Calcification of the attachments of the Intercostal Muscles

(By courtesy of Dr. Sk. V. Gudjonsson)

PLATE IV

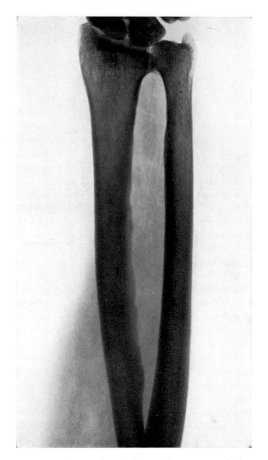

Case 23. Fluorosis of Bones in a man of 63,
exposed to Cryolite Dust for 43 years as Furnaceman in the manufacture of Aluminium. The
Radius and Ulna show extensive amorphous and
granular shadows with loss of Trabecular Pattern.
The adjacent borders of the Bones show gross
irregularity of Subperiosteal Bone

PLATE V

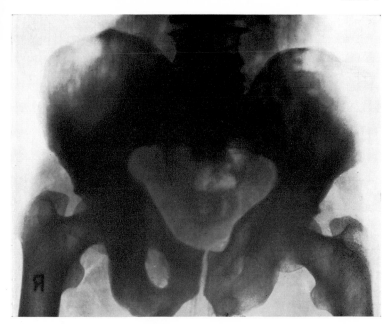

Case 24. Fluorosis of the Skeleton in a man of 37. For five and a half years, as Furnaceman in a Magnesium Foundry, he had been exposed to molten Fluoride Fluxes used in open Crucibles of Magnesium

(Bowler, R. G., and others (1947), Brit. J. industr. Med., 4, 216)

PLATE VI

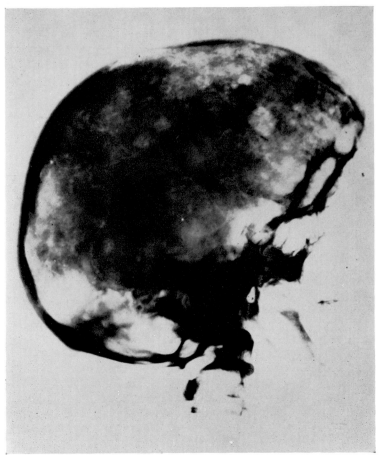

Radiation osteitis in a woman aged 74 who had worked as a dial
painter for 3 years (1919-1922) when she was 31 to 34 years of
age. She had never put the brush in her mouth. In 1962 she
complained of mild pain in the left hip. The calvaria shows a
number of large and small rounded areas of bone resorption

(By courtesy of Dr. R. J. Hasterlik and the editor of
The Medical Clinics of North America)

PLATE VII

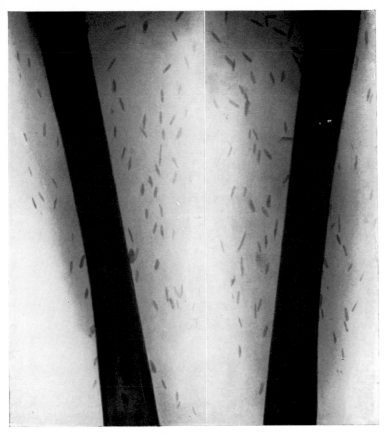

Cysticercus Epilepsy in a man aged 64, who had served in the Army in India.
The elliptical shadows, roughly uniform in size and density, are tough fibrous
Cysticerci, sometimes partially calcified

PLATE VIII

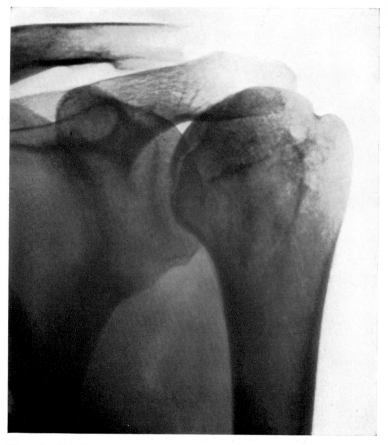

Necrosis of the Head of the left Humerus in a soft-ground Miner, aged 40, who had worked in Caissons for 18 years. While working on the Dartford-Purfleet Tunnel he had constant pain in the left Shoulder unrelieved by Recompression and slow Decompression. Note the faint linear translucency below the Articular Surface of the Head of the Humerus. When the Joint was opened the Articular Cartilage was necrotic and had separated with a thin layer of Bone. This portion was excised

PLATE IX

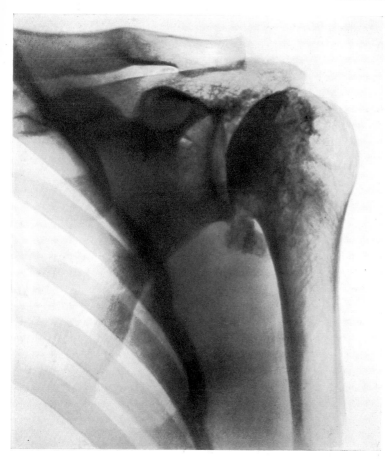

Condition of left Shoulder in the same man three years after Operation. Note distortion of the Head of the Humerus, the shadow of a Foreign Body in the Joint, and the lipping of Osteo-arthritis

PLATE X

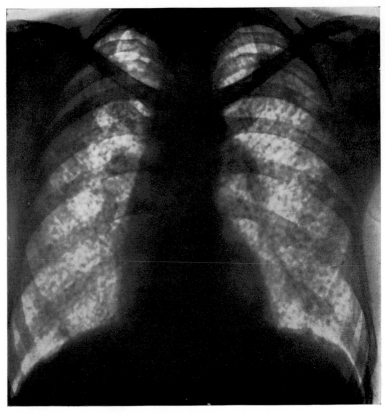

Silicosis in a Knife Grinder, a man of 46, who had worked for 25 years, often with dry Sandstone Wheels. The whole of both Lung Fields are occupied by nodular shadows and occasionally these have coalesced to form larger, more dense opacities

PLATE XI

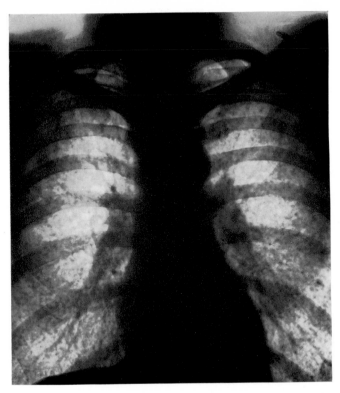

Silicosis in a Cornish Tin Miner, a man of 54, who had worked at the rock face for 28 years. Besides universal nodular shadows, in part obscured by Emphysema, there are increased hilar shadows and linear markings

PLATE XII

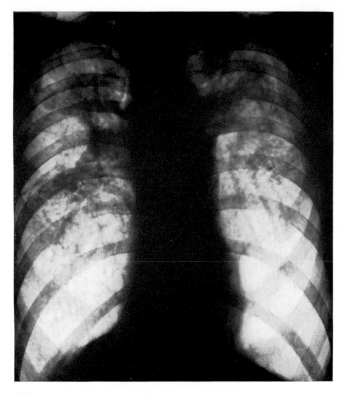

Silicosis complicated by Chronic Pulmonary Tuberculosis in a Cornish Tin Miner, aged 48, who had worked for 20 years hewing and shot-firing. Besides Nodulation and Emphysema there are dense, irregular shadows of Tuberculosis at both Apices

PLATE XIII

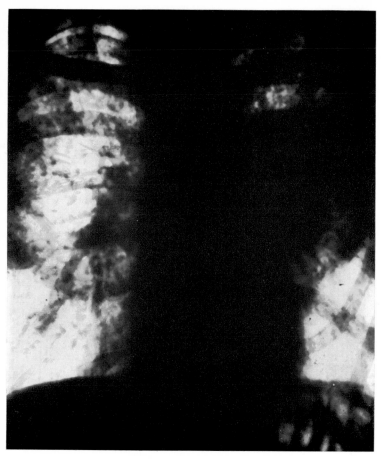

Silicosis and Carcinoma of the Lung in a man who had worked for 15 years in the Schneeberg Mines. Nodulation is universal and coexists with the large, dense shadow of Carcinoma occupying the Mediastinum, Hilum and upper part of the left Lung

(By courtesy of Professor D. Saupe)

PLATE XIV

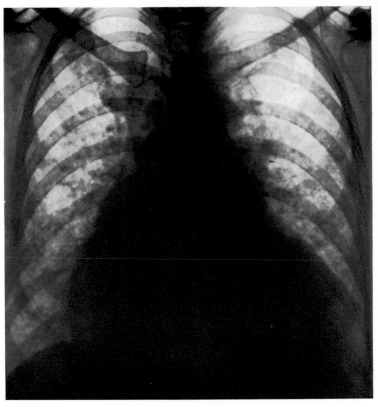

Hæmosiderosis in a woman of 68 with Chronic Heart Failure, Rheumatic Carditis, Mitral Stenosis and Tricuspid Incompetence. Note scattered irregular shadows of Hæmosiderin leaving Apices free. The great enlargement of the Heart shadow is due to the effects of Rheumatic Heart Disease, including Aneurysmal Dilatation of the left Auricle

PLATE XV

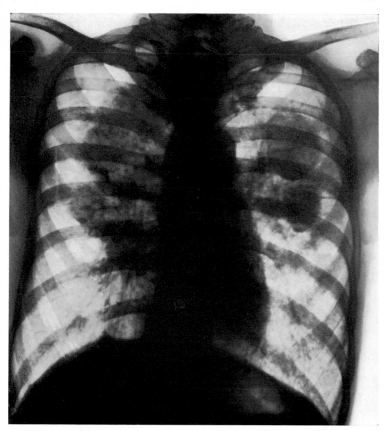

Progressive massive Fibrosis of the Lungs of a Welsh Coal Miner, a man of 58, who had worked for 40 years at the coal face hewing Steam Coal. The large, well-defined, homogeneous, smooth, rounded shadows in the Upper Zones are characteristic. Finer shadows are in part obscured by Emphysema

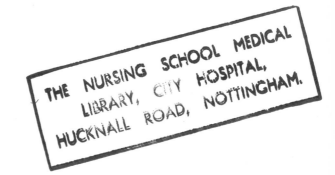

PLATE XVI

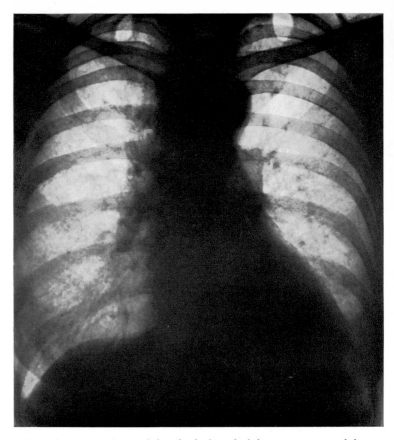

Asbestosis in a woman aged 60 who had worked for 5 years as an Asbestos
Spinner 33 years before. She had been short of breath on exertion for 14 years.
At both Bases and to a less extent throughout the Lungs there are shadows of a
close network as fine as a cobweb. It has made part of the outline of the Heart
appear slightly shaggy

and Wright, 1955). Two days before she was ill this woman had helped her husband treat calves for two hours using a solution of BHC dispensed by a veterinarian in unmarked bottles with verbal instructions only for its use. She soaked rags in the BHC and washed the calves with her hands and arms bare to the elbows. Her skin and part of her clothing were soaked. About twelve hours after the washing two of the calves had convulsions and died, and a third became blind. The following afternoon the patient helped her husband spray cattle in an unventilated barn. Her hands were wet with the spray, some of which she inhaled. The same evening she complained of a burning sensation in the throat and chest, and these symptoms were followed by a convulsion which lasted two minutes. On the third day the urine was found to contain 4·95 mg. BHC per 100 ml. For fear of further fits she was treated with phenobarbitone, and she made a rapid and complete recovery.

Chronic Poisoning by BHC

In Greece in the summer of 1951 mass poisoning occurred from the improper use of BHC as an insecticide. Seventy-nine persons became affected, 61 slightly and 18 seriously. There were 6 deaths. The powder contained 60 per cent of magnesium silicate and 40 per cent of the alpha, gamma, and delta isomers of BHC. Those affected had used either the powder itself or concentrated solutions in petroleum. The idea was to control house pests by sprinkling the floors and walls of their houses as well as their bedcovers, clothes and in some cases even their own bodies. The initial symptoms were lassitude, headache, vertigo, pain in the limbs, stomatitis, intestinal colic and diarrhœa. Then followed symptoms and signs in the nervous system including cerebellar ataxia, adiadochokinesia, asynergia and tremor. One patient had a temporary paraplegia and another became totally blind. Probably the most significant lesion was aplasia of the bone marrow with diminished production of normoblasts, reticulocytes and red cells. The platelets were said to be normal. Unhappily the authors of the paper describing this outbreak (Danopoulos, Melissinos and Katsas, 1953) give no particulars of the necropsies carried out, nor in the physical examination of patients do they record those essential physical signs which would indicate whether the origin of the blindness was cortical or peripheral. In one case they state that the condition was optic atrophy but no description is given of the changes seen in the ocular fundi nor in patients partially sighted were the fields of vision charted.

Prevention and Treatment of Poisoning by BHC

Adequate exhaust ventilation, avoidance of working at all in very hot weather, strict cleanliness in the working conditions, provision and frequent changing of overalls, adequate washing facilities, and above all daily supervision of what is happening should remove the hazard of dermatitis. Every effort must be made to educate people to read warnings on the labels attached to cartons and bottles and to abide by the instructions laid down. The dispensing of insecticides in unlabelled containers must be forbidden. It is unsafe to impregnate clothing with BHC because the concentration needed to kill insects also could cause absorption through the skin of the wearer. Conditions of ordinary application to food-stuffs will leave but negligible and therefore harmless quantities to be ingested. The essential treatment of a patient with convulsions is the repeated use of phenobarbitone, if necessary by subcutaneous injection (Nicholls, 1958).

TOLUYLENE DI-*ISO*CYANATE

Organic di-*iso*cyanate compounds are used in the making of adhesives, of synthetic rubbers, of polyurethane paints and lacquers and in the manufacture of printers' rollers. Their most important application, however, is in the plastics industry in the making of flexible and rigid urethane foams. These are used for a variety of products ranging from toys to the insulation of ships' holds. The di-*iso*cyanates owe their useful properties to the presence of the two highly reactive *iso*cyanate (NCO) groups in the molecule, which allow them to react with a large number of different organic compounds. In the making of plastic foams di-*iso*cyanates are allowed to react with a resin containing free carboxyl and hydroxyl groups, producing a high polymer. The carbon dioxide evolved during the reaction is trapped in the form of bubbles in the mass and produces the foamed plastic. A large number of di-*iso*cyanates can be made, but relatively few have found industrial applications. The first of these compounds to be introduced into industry was hexamethylene di-*iso*cyanate (H.D.I.). This aliphatic di-*iso*cyanate was highly volatile, and soon caused considerable respiratory symptoms as a result of which it has now been withdrawn from sale in Great Britain. The next compound to be introduced was toluylene di-*iso*cyanate (T.D.I.), generally in mixtures of varying proportions of the 2:4 and 2:6 isomers. This compound is also highly volatile, but it was some time before it was realized that very small atmospheric concentrations could cause respiratory symptoms. In spite of this, however, methods of handling have been evolved which enable T.D.I. to be used with relative safety, and this material is used in most systems for the manufacture of flexible urethane foams. A later introduction is 4:4'-di-*iso*cyanato-diphenyl methane (M.D.I.), which being much less volatile than the earlier di-*iso*cyanates, is virtually without vapour hazard, and does not require the special handling precautions necessary with T.D.I. The major use of M.D.I. is in the manufacture of rigid urethane foams, though it is also used in various surface coatings (Williamson, 1964).

Clinical Effects of Di-*iso*cyanates

Of the di-*iso*cyanates used in industry both H.D.I. and T.D.I. act as direct irritants and also as allergens. The irritant effects include rhinitis, pharyngitis, bronchitis and in cases of excessive exposure bronchiolitis obliterans. Breathlessness and cough, often severe, with fatigue and night sweats are accompanied by rhonchi and râles in the chest (Hama, 1957). Cyanosis may occur especially if there is pulmonary œdema or broncho-pneumonia. In 1956 Baader described 100 cases with 4 deaths. Less commonly the onset is with an attack of asthma, usually beginning with a feeling of tightness in the chest. In practically all reported cases chest symptoms and signs have cleared rapidly after the patient has been removed from contact with H.D.I. or T.D.I. But in many of those who have recovered, the symptoms have recurred, often in a violent form, after further contact with even very low concentrations of H.D.I. or T.D.I. Permanent disability seems to be rare, but a few cases have been reported (Munn, 1965), and some of these followed repeated exposure to T.D.I. after recovery from an earlier attack. The clinical evidence, especially bronchospasm and the recurrence of symptoms on renewed contact, suggests an allergic mechanism, so does the occasional occurrence of purpura and of appreciable eosinophilia. The asthma usually responds to *iso*prenalin inhalations.

Protective Measures

The maximum allowable concentration (M.A.C.) for T.D.I. was originally 0·1 p.p.m., but experience soon showed the need for an even lower value, and the present M.A.C. of 0·02 p.p.m. must be regarded as realistic. Work situations where this value is exceeded, except for short periods, are unsatisfactory. The prevalence of respiratory symptoms due to T.D.I. cannot be estimated at present, because the condition is not a notifiable industrial disease, and the connection between a man's work and his symptoms may not be recognized. Estimates of prevalence in factories have ranged from 100 per cent of the work force when working conditions were bad to 4 per cent of the exposed population in eighteen months in good conditions (Williamson, 1965). Most of the handling of di-*iso*cyanates is in industrial processes, but paints and lacquers containing these materials have wider applications, including domestic use. T.D.I. and H.D.I. were formerly used in paints; but, because of their high volatility, conjugates of these compounds are now used instead, and the better preparations are now free from hazard (Piper, 1965). In a proportion of cases of di-*iso*-cyanate poisoning the cause of the illness is unrecognized. If a man has respiratory symptoms which can reasonably be ascribed to working with di-*iso*cyanates, he must be advised to avoid all further contact with these materials to prevent the possibility of permanent disability. It is clear that the di-*iso*cyanates, especially the more volatile T.D.I. and H.D.I., are toxic substances, but they can be handled safely; to do so requires great care in the planning of equipment and methods of work and constant vigilance to eliminate unsatisfactory working practices.

PHENOL

Phenol, C_6H_5OH, also known as hydroxybenzene or carbolic acid *carbo*, coal; *oleum*, oil) is a colourless, deliquescent, crystalline solid often reddish from impurities. It has a peculiar odour and a sweetish, pungent taste. It is soluble in water but much more so in ethyl alcohol. *Liquid carbolic* consists of 100 parts of phenol with water to produce 115 parts.

History

The antiseptic and disinfectant properties of coal-tar were recognized in France in 1815. Phenol was discovered in 1834 by Runge in coal-tar. In 1840 creosote was used to preserve railway sleepers and ship timbers. In 1851 in England phenol was successfully used for the preservation of dead bodies. The effective use of carbolic acid as a deodorant and disinfectant for sewage in Carlisle led Lister in Glasgow in 1866 to adopt it in the treatment of compound fractures. The success which followed this venture is one of the epic stories of medicine (Godlee, 1924). Carbolized gauze and lint were devised as surgical dressings and carbolic lotion (1 in 20) was used in operating theatres as a cold sterilizing fluid for surgical instruments. The surgeon rinsed his gloved hands in this fluid and used it in diluted form to irrigate wounds. In the practice of surgery phenol lotions remained in universal use for seventy-five years. The carbolic spray (1 in 40) had a much shorter life. Lister first publicly recommended it in 1871 and its use spread all over the world, until in 1887 he abandoned it. In 1872 Bayer showed that phenol reacted with formaldehyde to yield a hard resinous substance. About 1905 Dr. L. H. Baekeland took up this discovery and in doing so gave a *new look* to organic chemistry. By 1916 the first heat mouldable powder was made and its use heralded the advent of the new plastics industry. Since then the production of phenolic and related products has expanded enormously and the word *Bakelite* as applied to thermohardening plastics has become a household word. Today the plastics industry uses phenol on such a large scale that industrial countries have increased their production to ten times the 1935 figure; and indeed a proportion of the phenol used now comes not from the fractional distillation of coal-tar but from a synthetic process starting with monochlorobenzene.

Uses

Sixty-five per cent of the phenol used in industry goes to the production of bakelite and other phenol-formaldehyde plastics. Insecticides and disinfectants absorb about 10 per cent and the extraction of lubricating oils and the manufacture of dyes and dye intermediates each absorbs about 5 per cent. Among other uses are the manufacture of explosives, perfumes, paints, lampblack and pharmaceutical substances (Fairhall, 1957). It is used also by brewers, calico printers, etchers, coal-gas purifiers, reclaimers of rubber and as a paint remover and wood preserver.

Effects on the Skin

Phenol exerts a strong corrosive action on the skin and serious caustic burns may result from skin contact unless it is removed promptly and thoroughly either by sponging with ethyl alcohol or by copious prolonged irrigation with warm water. The first skin reaction is tingling and local anæsthesia with a feeling of numbness which lasts some hours. Because of this the patient may feel nothing until serious damage has been done. The affected area becomes opaque white and if the application is prolonged a whitish-grey slough results from the coagulating action of phenol on the proteins of the skin. There is no vesication. In severe cases where there has been prolonged exposure gangrene of the deeper tissues may occur. Even if a dilute solution of phenol is applied to the skin for several hours gangrene may occur; it is the result of constriction of the smaller vessels supplying the part. Chronic dermatitis may result from repeated or prolonged contact with low concentrations of phenol. This causes about 20 per cent of the cases of dermatitis in the industry making phenol-formaldehyde plastics. Dermatitis also is prevalent among creosoters of wood (Schwartz, Tulipan and Birmingham, 1957).

Pigmentation of the Urine, the Cartilages and Fibrous Tissues

Phenol is readily absorbed by ingestion, inhalation and through the skin. Following absorption it is partly oxidized to hydroquinone and pyrocatechin which are excreted in the urine and tend to be oxidized to coloured substances which cause the urine on standing to become a dusky green colour, changing to brown or even black like black coffee, a condition referred to as *carboluria*. Cartilages and tendons also may be pigmented, a condition known as *ochronosis*, identical with that of alkaptonuria which is an inborn error of metabolism (Garrod, 1909). The clinical, biochemical and morbid anatomical identity of these two conditions is evident. In both, the blackened cartilages of the ears show dark blue through the normal skin. *Ocular ochronosis* occurs as a raven-black pigmentation of the sclera in small roughly triangular patches of which the base is near the cornea. In severe cases a blue-grey batswing area is seen over the nose and malar eminences, and similar pigmentation occurs on the knuckles of the hands, the extensor tendons of the fingers, the thenar and hypothenar eminences and the nail-beds. Their biochemical identity is seen in the fact that the homogentisic acid found in the urine of patients with alkaptonuria is known by the alternative name hydroquinone acetic acid, and this is the substance found in the urine of patients showing chronic poisoning by phenol, hydroquinone (p. 532) and metol (p. 558). Lastly in both conditions necropsy reveals blue-grey pigmentation of cartilages including the ears, trachea, bronchi, articular cartilages, intervertebral discs and costo-chondral junctions. Fibrous tissues such as the tendons, the sclerotics and the nail-beds also may be pigmented (Pope, 1906).

Chronic Phenol Poisoning

During the sixteen years or so when Lister's carbolic spray was in use it affected the health of surgeons and their theatre assistants all over the world. *Carboluria* was common among them, some had dermatitis and those who used hand-operated sprays suffered repeatedly from cold, numb fingers (Godlee, 1924). According to Zangger (1934) *phenic marasmus* or *carbolmarasmus* was described for the first time by Czerny in 1882. It was a condition affecting doctors and their assistants who used the carbolic spray regularly, and it occasionally occurred also among workmen who manufactured carbolic dressings. The patient suffered from anorexia with progressive loss of weight. Carboluria occurred and often there was a progressive dermatitis due to phenol. Other symptoms were headache, vertigo, salivation, nausea, vomiting and diarrhœa. Sometimes the condition was fatal especially where albumin, red cells and casts were found in the urine. Czerny and others considered that more doctors died from this cause than was generally recognized. Unfortunately *chronic carbolism* persisted after the use of the carbolic spray had ceased. Thus Beddard (1909) described the case of a woman who developed varicose ulcers of the legs in 1891. Between 1900 and 1909 she used, on an average, more than seven pints of carbolic oil per week soaked in lint and applied to the ulcers. On admission to hospital she had the classical signs of *ochronosis* namely dark urine, together with blackening of the cartilages of the ears and of the sclerotics. The case of a woman who for thirty-five years continuously used 5 per cent phenol dressings for two very large varicose ulcers near the ankles was recorded by Berry and Peat (1931). She had carboluria, severe ochronosis and pain in the back and knees suggesting the presence of *osteo-arthritis ochronotica*.

Lethal Effect of Absorption of Liquid Carbolic through the Skin

The mishandling of phenol can easily result in serious consequences; the hazard of rapid absorption especially through the skin must never be underestimated. If the skin be splashed with phenol solutions, especially liquid carbolic, acute toxic symptoms rapidly supervene. They are profound muscular weakness, headache, dizziness, dimness of vision, ringing noises in the ears, irregular and rapid respiration and a weak pulse. A state of collapse with subnormal temperature may be followed by convulsions. The urine may be as dark as black coffee and oliguria may develop. Approximately half the reported cases of acute phenol poisoning have ended fatally. Severe acute intoxication occurred in a three-year-old child whose scalp was treated accidentally with pure phenol instead of a dilute solution. The mistake was discovered four minutes after application, when the child became unconscious (Brown, 1895). A nurse, whose thumb and index finger were contaminated with pure phenol, accidentally touched the groin of a seven-day-old infant, leaving two patches, one 3 cm. and the other 1 cm. diameter. Severe convulsions were observed within five minutes, ending fatally ten hours later (Abrahams, 1900). A thirteen-year-old girl accidentally poured pure phenol over the scalp and cheek; she died within two hours (Gibson, 1905). A man accidentally broke a bottle of dilute phenol in his pocket. The contents ran down his thighs, and he showed signs of systemic intoxication within five minutes. The toxæmia was characterized by severe cyanosis, stertorous breathing, vomiting, coma, the abolition of reflexes, pin-point pupils and lowering of body temperature (Turtle and Dolan, 1922).

Acute Phenol Poisoning in Industry

Alice Hamilton (1925) describes the case of a young chemist who stepped into a pool of phenol waste in which his leg became soaked. Soon he began to complain of ringing in the ears, dizziness and dyspnœa. Then he became dazed and excited and was allowed to leave the building. Evidently he soon lost consciousness, for the next morning he was found dead on the road his leg being discoloured greenish—black up to the knee. In 1945 a case was reported from a U.S. oil refinery. A pipefitter was removing a gasket from a flange when some phenol splashed on his face, neck, shoulders and arms. Within a few minutes he lost consciousness and was taken at once to the plant hospital where he was washed first with water and then for half an hour with ethyl alcohol. This probably saved his life for he was so severely poisoned that he showed muscular twitching and cyanosis. He was comatose for three hours but the pulse was good and the breathing normal. During the week which followed there were red cells, white cells and casts in the urine. Unfortunately a burn in the left eye led to permanent partial loss of vision (Hamilton and Hardy, 1949). Evans (1952) reported from a chemical works in Yorkshire the case of a general worker, a man of twenty-two, who suffered from acute phenol poisoning as a result of spraying weeds with the effluent from a chemical plant the phenol content of which was 43·5 per cent. A faulty coupling caused the operative to be sprayed with the fluid. He was wearing goggles, gloves, waterproof coat and gum-boots, but had omitted to put on his protective trousers. Areas of skin exposed to this fluid included most of both thighs and the scrotum. The patient developed symptoms of shock within half an hour. The temperature fell to 97·2° F., the pupils were contracted and for a period of half an hour there were convulsive movements of the left leg. Prompt rescue and medical treatment saved his life. The superficial burns on the skin rapidly healed.

Treatment of Phenol Poisoning

Wherever phenol is handled all concerned must know exactly what to do if splashing occurs from a broken carboy or as the result of some apparatus having exploded. In treating such a case speed is of paramount importance. Contaminated clothing must be quickly removed and the affected areas of the skin flooded with warm water. Since phenol is only slightly soluble in water swabbing with ethyl alcohol or methylated spirits should at once follow to remove all phenol and the surface coagulum containing it. The patient must be put to bed and kept warm with hot water bottles and hot fluids to drink. The smell of phenol on the skin may persist for two hours or more, but the alcohol treatment must go on until such odour is no longer detectable. Only then should oil dressings be applied. Skin burns or gangrene must be treated in the same fashion as thermal burns.

PENTACHLORPHENOL

This is a crystalline solid of poor solubility. It is frequently used as the sodium salt, which is freely soluble in water. It is used as a preservative for timber, as an insecticide to control termites and snails, as a herbicide and cotton defoliant, and as a mildewcide in emulsion and tropical paints (Piper, 1965). Its action resembles that of the dinitrophenols (p. 555) and consists of an increase in the metabolic rate leading to a marked increase in body temperature, collapse and death. In 19 cases the time from the first symptoms to death ranged from 3 to 30 hours, the average being 14 hours. It is claimed that one man drank a glassful of a 2 per cent solution of the sodium salt with no effect except a hangover. One man died after working 6 days as a mixer preparing a 2·1 per cent cotton defoliant from a 40 per cent concentrate. Nine men died after dipping timber by hand and without any protection, in a 2 per cent solution for periods varying from 3–30 days; this is typical of several other situations in which accidents have occurred. Necropsy shows parenchymatous degeneration in the liver and kidneys and venous congestion of the lungs. In one case of fatal occupational poisoning, pentachlorphenol was found in concentrations of 97 p.p.m. in the liver and 84 p.p.m. in the kidney. Campbell (1952) described seven cases in Bristol all from the use of a domestic wood preservative. They showed peripheral neuritis and retrobulber neuritis and all recovered within six months. Non-fatal cases have shown up to 10 p.p.m. of pentachlorophenol in the urine and sometimes traces of albumin (Hayes, 1963). The use of this substance as a herbicide is controlled by the Ministry of Agriculture, Fisheries and Food. They specify the wearing of gloves and face-shield when the concentrate is used, immediate removal of contaminated clothing, avoidance of all contact by mouth and no working in the spray mist. The washing of hands and exposed skin before eating, drinking and smoking and after work are emphasized.

QUINONE AND HYDROQUINONE

Quinone, *para*-benzoquinone, is a yellow crystalline solid with a characteristic irritating odour suggesting chlorine. It is an intermediate in the manufacture of hydroquinone and dyes and is used in tanning (quinone leather). Hydroquinone, quinol, 1,4-dihydroxybenzene is a white crystalline solid extensively used as a photographic developer and as a dye intermediate, and is the base for a number of chemical syntheses. It is an antioxidant and stabilizing agent for preventing deterioration of fats, oils and resin monomers (Fairhall, 1957).

Corneal and Conjunctival Injury

The vapour of quinone and the dusts of hydroquinone and metol (p. 558) can cause injury to the cornea and conjunctiva of men who manufacture these substances. In 1931 Velhagen gave an accurate description of the eye lesions found in six men employed on a plant making hydroquinone in Germany. In 1947 Sterner, Oglesby and Anderson described eye injuries in fifty men making hydroquinone in a factory in Kingsport, Tennessee. Then in 1954 Miller described the same thing in sixteen men employed on this work in London. The conjunctival lesion consists of pigmentation in the interpalpebral fissure varying from a slight yellow tinge to a deep brown. The cornea develops a brown sepia-like stain across the area exposed to light. The stain, though most marked in the corneal epithelium, traverses the whole thickness of its substance extending to Descemet's membrane. A further change is a superficial milky-white precipitate leaving permanent opacities in the cornea. Its whole structure may be deformed with appreciable loss of visual acuity. Occasionally the cornea breaks down in frank ulceration with all its acute symptoms. Miller (1954) showed that in advanced cases there is staining of the sclera as well as of the conjunctiva. This gives rise to discrete black patches on either side of the cornea separated from it by a clear area, a condition identical with *ocular ochronosis*. However, there is no record of systemic symptoms in these patients, neither do they pass black urine nor are their cartilages involved; the abnormality is purely local. Patients who have swallowed hydroquinone may pass black urine for many days.

Prognosis of the Eye Lesions

The conjunctival and scleral pigmentation disappears gradually over a period of years and leaves no ill effect. The prognosis as to vision is in dispute. Sometimes a man who has only slight corneal lesions will suffer no loss of visual acuity if he is removed from exposure. Banks Anderson (1947) and Miller (1954) do not believe this often happens; they hold a less hopeful view as to prognosis, and indeed some of their patients had been put on other types of work for three years without improvement in visual acuity. One characteristic of the corneal change which is particularly damaging to accurate vision is the appearance of vertical folds in Descemet's membrane. This may be associated with progressive astigmatism. In some cases the fitting of a contact lens is helpful; in others corneal grafting should be undertaken.

Prevention of Ocular Staining

In 1961 this eye condition was scheduled as a prescribed disease under the *National Insurance (Industrial Injuries) Act*. The main factor in the prevention of ocular staining is the introduction of entirely enclosed machinery. Fundamentally, the manufacturing process is a two-step operation. In the first step, aniline is oxidized to quinone in the presence of an excess of manganese dioxide and sulphuric acid. In the second step, quinone is steam distilled from the reaction liquor and immediately brought into contact with a water suspension of iron dust that reduces the quinone to hydroquinone. Emphasis must be placed on prevention of

leaks of quinone vapour and on the removal at source of dusts by ventilation. Daily changes of working clothes and washing facilities are necessary.
The constant use of goggles would, of course, prevent the appearance of
this syndrome altogether, but goggles are easily steamed up by escaping
vapours and have to be removed from time to time.

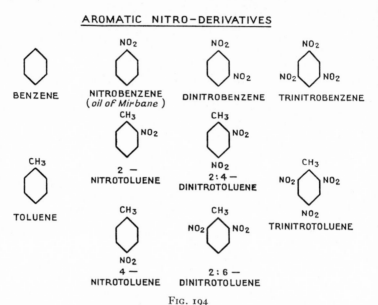

FIG. 194

AROMATIC NITRO- AND AMINO-DERIVATIVES

Most of the aromatic nitro- and amino-derivatives, and especially nitrobenzene, dinitrobenzene, and aniline, act on the blood converting hæmoglobin into methæmoglobin (fig. 194). Methæmoglobinæmia has been
observed in poisoning by a great variety of compounds, including tetra-
nitro-methane, di-nitro-ethylene glycol, nitrobenzenes, nitrotoluenes,
aniline, dimethylaniline, tetra-nitro-methyl aniline, *para*-nitraniline,
ethanolaniline, *para*-phenylenediamine, phenylhydrazine, acetyl phenylhydrazine, toluidines, nitrophenols, *para*-aminophenol, *para*methylaminophenol (p. 558), pyrogallic acid, antipyrine, acetanilide, phenacetin,
sulphanilamide, sulphapyridine, sulphathiazole, sulphonal, trional, potassium chlorate, nitrites, methylene blue and plasmoquine (fig. 195).

Anilism in Chemical Factory Workers

The convenient terms *anilism* or *anilinism* are sometimes used to cover
all cases in which methæmoglobinæmia has occurred from exposure to any
one of this group of substances. Workers in English chemical factories
affected in this way sometimes refer to themselves as being *blued up.*

Methæmoglobin is an isomer of oxyhæmoglobin; the two substances have the same chemical composition but their structures are different (Henderson and Haggard, 1943). Methæmoglobin holds oxygen much more firmly than does hæmoglobin; it is not dissociated even by a vacuum. This

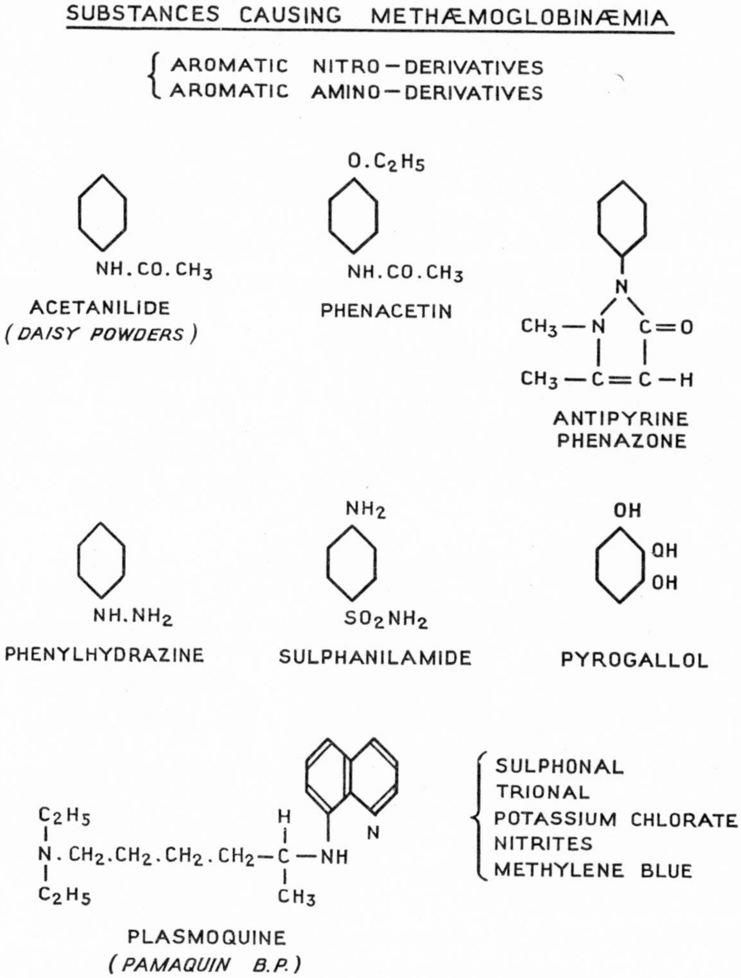

SUBSTANCES CAUSING   METHÆMOGLOBINÆMIA

$\begin{cases} \text{AROMATIC} & \text{NITRO}-\text{DERIVATIVES} \\ \text{AROMATIC} & \text{AMINO}-\text{DERIVATIVES} \end{cases}$

NH.CO.CH$_3$

ACETANILIDE
(*DAISY POWDERS*)

O.C$_2$H$_5$

NH.CO.CH$_3$

PHENACETIN

$CH_3 - N \quad C = O$
$CH_3 - C = C - H$

ANTIPYRINE
PHENAZONE

NH.NH$_2$

PHENYLHYDRAZINE

NH$_2$

SO$_2$NH$_2$

SULPHANILAMIDE

OH
OH
OH

PYROGALLOL

C_2H_5
$N.CH_2.CH_2.CH_2.CH_2-C-NH$
C_2H_5 CH_3

PLASMOQUINE
(*PAMAQUIN B.P.*)

$\begin{cases} \text{SULPHONAL} \\ \text{TRIONAL} \\ \text{POTASSIUM CHLORATE} \\ \text{NITRITES} \\ \text{METHYLENE BLUE} \end{cases}$

FIG. 195

stability of methæmoglobin prevents it from performing the normal function of hæmoglobin, that of transporting oxygen in the body. For this reason the formation of large amounts of methæmoglobin causes asphyxia of the tissues. The minimum amount of methæmoglobin in the blood causing cyanosis is 5 grams per 100 millilitres. When large amounts occur in the blood, its colour is altered to chocolate brown. The skin then shows cyanosis of a distinctive tint, most noticeable on the cheeks, ears, tip of the nose and finger-nails. It is a bluish-grey colour varying in intensity from lilac to a deep leaden hue, and quite different from the blue colour of cyanosis due to lack of oxygen.

Formation of Methæmoglobin promoted by Para-aminophenol

After the substance producing methæmoglobin has been eliminated from the body, the methæmoglobin may be converted back to oxyhæmoglobin. The serious consequences of poisoning by substances causing methæmoglobin formation probably occur from a specific toxic effect of such substances upon the tissues. Methæmoglobin, however, serves to some extent as an index of the severity of the intoxication. If the destruction of red cells is severe there is, of course, anæmia. Such destruction may result also in injuries to the kidney and liver. The formation of methæmoglobin may be due, not to the intact nitro-compound, but to the product into which it is broken down by the liver. Thus aniline, which may cause marked formation of methæmoglobin in the body, does not do so when added to blood in a test-tube. The intermediate products believed to be primarily responsible for the formation of methæmoglobin are amino-compounds such as *para*-aminophenol. This substance promotes the formation of methæmoglobin *in vitro*. It is probable also that these intermediate products are in some measure responsible for the other toxic effects induced by aniline and similar substances.

Contradictory Ideas about Methæmoglobin in Relation to Cyanosis

Much of the work done on methæmoglobinæmia has produced contradictory results. This arose through difficulties in the accurate identification and quantitative determination of methæmoglobin in the blood. Price-Jones and Boycott (1909) thought that methæmoglobin disappeared by the time cyanosis was fully developed, but Schmidt (1930) stated that the bands of methæmoglobin appear only when 40 per cent of the oxyhæmoglobin is transformed into methæmoglobin, and that death occurs when 75 per cent of the oxyhæmoglobin is transformed. Then, in 1932, Peters and Van Slyke in work upon acute nitro-benzene poisoning suggested that the pigment formed is some other hæmoglobin derivative, possibly a direct combination with nitrobenzene.

Spectrophotometric Measurements of Methæmoglobinæmia

In 1938 Hamblin and Mangelsdorff published an accurate method for measuring the percentage of methæmoglobin in venous blood. Using a recording spectrophotometer, they demonstrated methæmoglobinæmia in concentrations varying from 1 to 100 per cent. These authors made a large number of methæmoglobin measurements on the blood of patients who had been exposed to nitrobenzene, dinitrobenzene, aniline, dimethylaniline, *para*nitraniline and mixed toluidines. In every case the severity of the clinical picture increased in direct proportion to a rising concentration of methæmoglobin and decreased with a falling concentration.

Studies of Sulphæmoglobinæmia

The study of sulphæmoglobinæmia has been hampered for want of reliable methods. In order to distinguish between cyanoses produced by methæmoglobin and sulphæmoglobin, careful measurements must be made on a good spectroscope—for instance, a Hartridge reversion spectroscope. The mechanism of sulphæmoglobin formation *in vivo* is not understood, though it probably involves an oxidation, and Michel (1938) has shown that at any rate *in vitro* the presence of soluble sulphides is necessary. The factors which favour sulphæmoglobin rather than methæmoglobin formation following ingestion of a large variety of amino- or nitro-benzene derivatives are quite unknown. Sulphæmoglobin is most commonly observed clinically and in animals after ingestion of acetanilide or phenacetin. With TNT or sulphonamides the number of cases in which sulphæmoglobin is found in the blood is about 2 per cent of those in which methæmoglobin is observed.

Slow Elimination of Sulphæmoglobin

If cyanosis is due to methæmoglobin, as much as 35 per cent of the total blood pigment may be in a non-oxygen carrying form, but recovery after removal of the causative agent is effected rapidly by the reducing enzyme systems within the red cells. In slight cases this may be complete in twenty-four hours, and in more severe cases in four or five days. In cyanoses due to sulphæmoglobin, not more than 7 per cent of the blood pigment is immobilized. Jope (1946) showed that, although the amount of sulphæmoglobin encountered is slight, it is over three months before it is entirely eliminated from the body. The disappearance of sulphæmoglobin from the blood of seven TNT workers studied was found to be related to the fixed life-span of the red cell—namely 116 days. This figure is to be contrasted with that of two to five days occupied in the removal of methæmoglobin from the circulating blood of the same men.

Significance of Heinz Bodies in the Blood

Three types of change in the red cells usually accompany methæmoglobinæmia—namely, punctate basophilia, polychromatophilia (polychromasia) and the appearance of Heinz bodies (fig. 196). It was shown by Malden as early as 1907 that punctate basophilia of the red cells is as valuable an early sign of poisoning by dinitrobenzene and aniline as it is of lead poisoning. In 1942 Gross, Bock and Hellrung suggested that to search for Heinz bodies was more useful in diagnosis than to look for methæmoglobin in the blood. In 1890 Heinz described for the first time protein inclusion bodies seen in the erythrocytes of rabbits during phenylhydrazine poisoning. Twenty-four hours after the injection of 0·1 gram of phenylhydrazine a large number of red cells of the blood showed small rounded highly refractile inclusions in their cytoplasm. The inclusions were generally situated eccentrically near the periphery of the cell, but some were

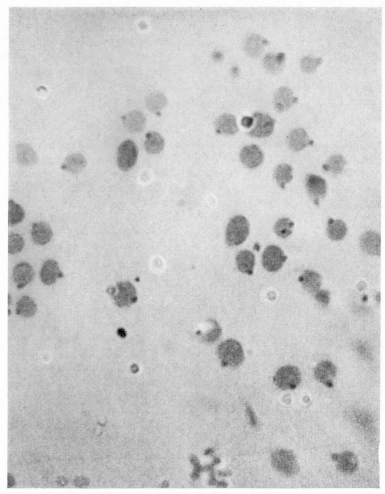

Fig. 196.—Heinz Bodies stained with Brilliant Cresyl Blue in the Blood of a
man exposed to DNB in Bomb Disposal
(*By courtesy of Professor J. Teisinger, Prague, 1947*)

found floating free in the plasma. The nature and origin of the protein
which makes up the inclusion is not known, but it is probably denatured
globulin. The subject has been reviewed by Webster (1949), Buckell and
Richardson (1950) and Fertman and Fertman (1955).

Chemical Substances giving rise to Heinz Bodies

The method of dark-ground illumination shows them to be distinct
from the substance of the reticulum of the reticulocyte. They have been
found in malaria and blackwater fever. The following chemical substances

give rise to Heinz bodies: hydroxylamine, nitrobenzene, dinitrobenzene, dinitrochlorbenzene, dinitrotoluene, trinitrotoluene, aniline, chloraniline, ethyl aniline, anisidine, toluylenediamine, phenylenediamine, ethylamino-benzoate, phenylhydrazine, acetyl phenylhydrazine, phenetidine, acetanilide (antifebrin), sulphanilamide, sulphapyridine, ethyl nitrite, glycol-mononitrate, glycol-dinitrate, nitroglycerine, sodium nitrite, sodium nitrate, diethylene glycol dinitrate (DEGN). The last substance named is a new propellant explosive more stable than nitroglycerine and used by the Germans in the Second World War.

Importance of Skin Absorption

In addition to their action upon the blood the nitro-substitution products act, to some extent, upon the central nervous system, causing stimulation and then paralysis. With the amino-compounds this action is much less pronounced. Unlike most other industrial poisons, the aromatic nitro- and amino-derivatives are absorbed not only through the respiratory tract, but also through the skin. The importance of the skin as a channel of absorption was shown for dinitrobenzene in 1901 by Prosser White and John Hay, and for trinitrotoluene in 1918 by Benjamin Moore. These investigators rubbed their own skins with the substance to be tested. It has often been observed clinically that the poisonous effect of the aromatic nitro- and amino-derivatives is increased by the simultaneous intake of alcohol, even in relatively small amounts. The work of Rejsek (1947) explains this. He found that small doses of alcohol caused nitro-bodies to appear in the blood, both of rabbits and of men previously exposed to DNB (p. 545).

(a) Nitrobenzene

Nitrobenzene or mononitrobenzene is referred to in commerce as mirbane, oil of mirbane, essence of mirbane, or artificial oil of bitter almonds. It is an oily liquid almost colourless or faintly yellow, with an odour of bitter almonds which is still present in great dilution.

Uses

It is used in the manufacture of aniline dyes and explosives, as a constituent of shoe polish and floor polish, and, on account of its odour, as a perfume in cheap soaps and other toilet articles. It is even used as a substitute for the natural essence of bitter almonds in confectionery and liqueurs.

Acute Lethal Effect of Skin Absorption

Nitrobenzene is regarded by experienced men as more dangerous than aniline. The most important portal of entry is through the skin, but the respiratory and digestive tracts may be responsible. In acute occupational poisoning, skin absorption occurs from the wearing of clothes badly soiled by splashing, or from lack of cleanliness on the part of the workman who does not change his working clothes sufficiently often. Hamilton (1919) recorded the case of an elderly man who was at work in a soap factory in

Boston, carrying a five-gallon can of oil of mirbane. He spilt some of the fluid on his trousers, became shaky and suddenly collapsed, spilling more of the fluid on himself. His mirbane-soaked clothing was not removed before he was sent to hospital, and it is not surprising that his condition was serious when he arrived there. He was unconscious, with slow irregular breathing but a good pulse. The pupils were small, irregular and fixed. The skin was a pale, grey-blue colour. Some blood withdrawn from a vein was as brown as chocolate. Respiration failed but the pulse was good until just before death, which occurred one hour after admission.

Involvement of the Nervous System

Nitrobenzene is more poisonous to the nervous system than is dinitrobenzene. The symptoms include fatigue, vertigo, headache, vomiting, general weakness, buzzing in the ears and numbness in the limbs. In serious cases there is loss of consciousness followed by deep coma in which the pupils are contracted at first and react sluggishly to light, but later dilate and react no more. The pulse is rapid and weak, and the skin damp and cold. Respiration is quickened at first, but it slows as the patient becomes unconscious. Death may supervene during profound coma. In patients who recover, consciousness returns generally in the first twenty-four hours. The pulse and respiration improve, but the nervous symptoms may persist for a week or more.

Changes in the Blood

The blood changes include conversion of hæmoglobin into methæmoglobin, and this gives rise to the characteristic lilac cyanosis. In grave poisoning the number of red cells may drop in six days to 2,000,000 per c.mm., with a diminution in the content of hæmoglobin to as little as 30 per cent. Polychromatophilia, punctate basophilia, anisocytosis and poikilocytosis are found, and where the anæmia is severe normoblasts may appear. The colour index may be high for a time. The worst stage of the anæmia is usually passed by the end of the first or second week, and thereafter the blood count returns rapidly to normal.

Cases with Jaundice and Splenomegaly

About the third day there may be jaundice and the spleen may be slightly enlarged. At the end of the second week the jaundice persists only in the conjunctivæ and gives place to the pallor of anæmia. The enlargement of the spleen disappears after several weeks as the blood count returns to normal. Sometimes, after the poisoning has been overcome, there is a reactive erythrocytosis with a red-cell count as high as 7,000,000 per c.mm. In serious cases the urine may have a pronounced odour of nitrobenzene. It may show a dark-brown tint from the presence of methæmoglobin, and this colour may deepen still more on the surface on exposure to air. Albumin and casts may be found, and in the jaundiced cases bilirubin is present.

Subacute and Chronic Poisoning by Nitrobenzene

Subacute and chronic forms of poisoning may follow upon repeated absorption of small doses of nitrobenzene. Anæmia is the leading feature of the clinical picture, and pallor is a more prominent sign than in aniline workers. If cyanosis is present, it disappears rapidly after cessation of work. Fatigue, headache and loss of appetite are commonly seen. Redness and swelling of the exposed skin and even a pustular eruption have been recorded. Complete recovery from the anæmia and the nervous symptoms may require several weeks (Engel, 1934).

Preventive Measures

For reasons of health it is necessary in the manufacture of nitrobenzene to use closed apparatus. Transport, as well as the emptying of receptacles. should be effected either by the use of compressed air or by aspiration, Good natural ventilation should be provided and, in hot weather, this must be artificially reinforced. Floors should be impermeable and not made of asphalt or tar, because these materials absorb the nitrobenzene. The workman should be provided with suitable clothing, and this should be changed so often that it does not become unduly impregnated with nitrobenzene. Gloves are necessary and should be frequently changed and cleaned. Cloakrooms, washing-rooms and baths are essential. Workmen should be instructed as to the care of any victim of an accident in which the clothing becomes suddenly soaked with the liquid. It is imperative that such a workman should have his clothes removed and be given a bath at once. All workers should be informed of the danger which may follow indulgence in alcohol. Regular medical inspection of workmen is desirable, and medical assistance should at all times be within easy reach.

Case 19. *Shoe-polish maker—exposure to nitrobenzene for three weeks— methæmoglobinæmia and anæmia with punctate basophilia.*

D. S., a married woman aged 33, L.H. Reg. No. 40274/1942. She had worked eight hours a day for three weeks in a workshop 30 by 12 by 8 feet, inadequately ventilated by small windows and doors. The concentration of the vapour of nitrobenzene to which she was exposed was such that its odour could be detected not only in the workshop but also for ten yards down the street. At one end of the workshop various waxes were placed in a 15-gallon pot, dissolved in a fluid containing 15 per cent nitrobenzene and kept warm over a gas burner. No exhaust ventilation was provided. The patient's duties included filling small steel moulds from a kettle containing the wax, and she found it necessary repeatedly to blow down the spout of the kettle when the wax solidified and blocked it. A good deal of her time was occupied in removing the shoe polish from the moulds and packing it in cartons. In both these operations she used her bare hands. *After ten days' exposure* she had throbbing frontal headache, giddiness, palpitation, shortness of breath and occasional vomiting. In the third week she noticed that her face was pale and her lips mauve. She had four children, and her menstrual and obstetric histories were normal.

On examination: skin pale, lilac cyanosis of lips, tongue, fauces and finger-nails. No jaundice of skin or conjunctivæ. Hands stained yellowish-brown with the dye of brown boot polish. Blood-pressure 140/95. Spleen not felt. No œdema. Blood count: red cells 3,060,000 per c.mm., hæmoglobin 60 per cent, colour index 1·0, white cells 9,040, per c.mm., differential count normal; two normoblasts seen in counting 200 white cells; considerable punctate basophilia, polychromatophilia and anisocytosis, moderate poikilocytosis; reticulocytes 3·4 per cent, platelets 149,000 per c.mm., bleeding time and coagulation time normal. Indirect van den Bergh 0·5 mg. per 100 c.c. Urine: a trace of albumin, a few leucocytes; hæmoglobin, bilirubin and lead absent. Fæces: lead absent. The patient was treated with iron and ammonium citrate. The cyanosis disappeared completely in three days. Within seven days the red-cell count rose to 3,550,000 per c.mm., and the hæmoglobin to 78 per cent. Seen *five months later,* the patient was well and a blood count showed: red cells 4,700,000 per c.mm., hæmoglobin 90 per cent, colour index 0·95, white cells 8,320 per c.mm., differential count normal.

Of five other workers examined clinically, all showed slight lilac cyanosis of the lips and cheeks. Two of these who had worked for two years in an atmosphere charged with the vapour of nitrobenzene agreed to have blood counts made. The first, a chemist aged 45 years, who habitually siphoned nitrobenzene from a drum by sucking it through a rubber tube until it touched his lips and who repeatedly got the fluid on to his hands, showed: red cells 4,530,000 per c.mm., hæmoglobin 84 per cent, colour index 0·93, white cells 13,080 per c.mm., differential count normal; no punctate basophilia nor polychromatophilia. The second, a woman worker aged 30, who did the same work as the patient described above, showed: red cells 3,860,000 per c.mm., hæmoglobin 80 cent, colour index 1·04, white cells 7,800 per c.mm., polymorphs 44·5 per cent; one normoblast seen in counting 200 white cells; moderate punctate basophilia and polychromatophilia; slight anisocytosis and poikilocytosis. Notification was followed by considerable improvement in the ventilation of this workshop.

(b) Dinitrobenzene

Of the three isomers of DNB, it is only *meta*-dinitrobenzene which is used commercially. It is a solid at ordinary temperature and, in the pure state, it forms inodorous, colourless flakes. The commercial product is slightly yellow.

Uses

It is used extensively in the manufacture of dyes and explosives. Owing to its deficiency in oxygen, its explosive properties are not marked and detonation is difficult to bring about. Mixed with potassium chlorate, DNB forms *cheddite*, with ammonium nitrate, *roburite*, and, with guncotton, a smokeless powder called *indurite*. A mixture of potassium chlorate and DNB is known in the United States of America by the expressive name of *rack-a-rock*.

Effect of Skin Absorption of DNB

Since DNB is a solid, cases of poisoning develop less rapidly and are less severe than in the case of nitrobenzene. Poisoning occurs among men who either shovel or melt DNB. An attack usually develops some hours after a man has left the plant and rarely during work. Skin absorption was proved by White and Hay as early as 1901. Hay gives the following account of the experiment performed upon himself:

On 8th October, before dressing, I anointed my groins with a small portion of the 25 per cent DNB ointment, weight 400 milligrams, containing 0·1 gram of DNB. I repeated this in the evening before going to bed. On the 9th I noticed very marked blueness about the lips and the finger-nails; the tongue was also markedly blue. There were no subjective sensations. Before dressing I anointed my groins again with a similar quantity, but at 12 noon, owing to the cyanosis increasing in intensity, I carefully washed off all the ointment. At 1 p.m. the lips were a livid blue and the nails and skin generally of a deadly hue. The pulse was 100 to 120; it was regular in time and force and with its tension apparently raised and fuller. There was a feeling of fullness in the head and some throbbing headache, increased by movement. There was no obvious alteration in the urine. On cutting the thumb the blood appeared of a distinctly brown and darker colour than is normal. At 6 p.m. the pulse was still full and bounding, from 96 to 98, regular in time and force. There were a rather metallic taste in the mouth and frontal and orbital headache, accompanied by a feeling of fullness, increased by movement, especially when running up and down stairs. Oxygen was inhaled for five minutes without any relief or alteration in the appearance of the lips and skin. The veins of the hands and the ears were full and engorged. A distinct tremor of the hands was present. On the 10th there was still some cyanosis of the lips, but not so marked as on the 9th. The headache had almost disappeared and there was no tremor. The pulse was still somewhat frequent. On the 11th my health was practically normal, with the exception of a slight tendency to headache.

Changes in the Blood and Urine

The main effect of DNB is the conversion of oxyhæmoglobin into methæmoglobin. This may progress to the extent of making the blood a chocolate colour. Spectrophotometric measurements show that the severity of the clinical picture increases in direct proportion to the rising concentration of methæmoglobin in the blood. Malden (1907) described the blood counts in twenty-one men engaged in the manufacture of DNB. The red cells were reduced in numbers and showed marked punctate basophilia. The hæmoglobin was proportionately decreased, the colour index being normal. The total white cells were increased, but with a relative decrease in the polymorphonuclear cells. DNB undergoes in the body a change into *meta*-nitraniline, and is eliminated in this form by the urine (Lupschütz, 1920). In addition, methæmoglobin, hæmoglobin, porphyrins and sometimes albumin have been found in the urine. A workman may notice that he passed smoky urine soon after his first contact with DNB.

Acute Poisoning by DNB

In acute poisoning there is rapid onset of headache, vertigo and vomiting. Depression is followed by exhaustion, numbness of the legs, a staggering gait, somnolence and then loss of consciousness. Profound bluish-grey cyanosis develops and the skin is moist and cold. Respiration becomes fast and deep, the pulse is weak and rapid, and the blood-pressure drops. If consciousness is lost, the pupils become dilated, the temperature falls and death may occur within twenty-four hours from central respiratory paralysis. If acute poisoning terminates in recovery, the symptoms remain much longer than in poisoning by aniline. There is more exhaustion, and cyanosis and vertigo may persist for days or weeks, whereas in aniline poisoning a man recovers in forty-eight hours.

Deaths in the First World War

In Bavaria from 1915 to 1918 there were fully 1,000 cases of DNB poisoning. Many of the victims had from two to five attacks, and there were 113 deaths. In Great Britain before 1914 there were only two or three factories making *nitro*-derivatives of benzene. The factory where the manufacture was on the largest scale gave rise to more anxiety than any other, since there was not sufficient other employment to allow alternation of work. One factory had to close during a hot summer because there were not enough healthy men left to carry on the work. In another factory, hot weather, inadequate ventilation and overtime led to twenty-eight cases of illness, with two deaths in the course of a few weeks. With reduction of contact to four hours a day, no further cases occurred (Legge, 1917).

Chronic Poisoning by DNB

In subacute and chronic poisoning the symptoms are weakness, weariness, headache, dyspnœa, nausea, vomiting and slight fever in the evening. The skin and mucous membranes are pale as well as cyanosed, and the patient shows a low-colour-index anæmia. In many cases there is increased sensitivity to the poison as exposure continues. The patient shows cyanosis after working one week with dinitrobenzene, on the second exposure he is blue after four days and on the third exposure he is affected on the first day. Acute exacerbation of his symptoms occurs on exposure to the heat of the sun and after taking alcohol, even a glass of weak beer.

DNB mobilized by Alcoholic Drinks

Rejsek (1947) described Czech workers who filled German bombs with DNB in the Second World War. The explosive was run through a tap from a container in which it had been melted. The melt frequently ran over so that DNB adhered to the walls and was left on the floor. The workshops were cleaned twice a day and this involved scrubbing the walls. The workers had DNB on their clothing, in their hair, and also under their finger-nails and toe-nails. One of them had a relapse of cyanosis after lying in the sun for half a day, and another collapsed while riding a bicycle in full sunlight. Rejsek was able by the polarographic method to detect nitro-compounds in the blood of these men both after giving them alcoholic drinks and after exposing them to the sun. In rabbits he confirmed these observations and also showed that the DNB was stored in fat and mobilized by benzene, chloroform, alcohol and diathermy.

Acute Necrosis of the Liver due to DNB

Jaundice is unusual. When it appears, it produces a peculiar appearance owing to the coexistence of cyanosis. In deeply jaundiced patients, enlargement of the liver may be detected. Death from acute necrosis of the liver, previously thought to be rare (Engel, 1930), was encountered frequently in Germany and Czechoslovakia in the Second World War (Rejsek, 1947).

Preventive Measures

In building a factory which is to be perfect from both technical and hygienic points of view, it is important that doors, windows, walls, partitions and platforms should be so arranged as to allow of free natural ventilation. Nitration tanks should be provided with airtight lids for charging and with adequate exhaust ventilation. Special attention must be paid to the removal of steam containing the toxic substance. All flooring should be even and made of an impermeable material. These arrangements may fail in summer and on windless days, when the heat is oppressive. On such days it is not uncommon to see the whole personnel of a DNB factory affected with slight cyanosis.

Protective Clothing and Personal Cleanliness

There must be a constant campaign against careless and dirty habits. Working garments, gloves and boots must be changed and cleaned regularly as soon as soiled by the poisonous product. Cloakrooms and baths must be provided, and stress laid upon the urgent necessity for changing at once and taking a bath whenever the garments have been soiled more than usual. Workmen who do not change their working clothes on returning home may sit before the fire and absorb DNB from the evaporation of crystals or from the material in solution on their clothing. Absorption from the alimentary canal is more rapid if the stomach is empty, and it is therefore desirable that men should have a meal before they begin work. Clear warning should be given as to the danger of taking alcohol even in ordinary amounts. Workers should be made aware of the risks of hot baths or exposure to the heat of the sun. On account of the frequency of subacute and chronic poisoning, strict medical supervision is of great importance.

(c) Trinitrotoluene

2,4,6-trinitrotoluene or *alpha*-TNT is a pale yellow crystalline solid. Commercial TNT is handled in blocks from which an objectionable oily exudation arises as a result of impurities, including small amounts of other trinitrotoluenes and traces of dinitrotoluene.

Use as an Explosive

The wide adoption of TNT as an explosive is indicated by its many synonyms, which include such names as *trilit, trinol, tritolo, triton, trolite, trotyl* and *Füllpulver*-02. Its main use is as a bursting charge in shells, bombs and mines. Owing to its very marked deficiency in oxygen it is more often used mixed with substances rich in oxygen; *amatol* and *ammonal* contain ammonium nitrate, and *baratol* contains barium nitrate.

Importance of Skin Absorption of TNT

The main route of absorption of TNT is through the skin, but, of course, ingestion of the substance and absorption through the respiratory tract of dust and fume cannot be ignored. Absorption is greater in hot weather, not only because the worker exposes his arms and neck to a greater extent, but also because sweat helps to dissolve the TNT dust on the skin, so hastening its absorption. Because TNT is absorbed through the skin, amatol is more productive of poisoning than TNT alone. Ammonium nitrate is hygroscopic and keeps the skin of the hands and forearms moist, thus dissolving TNT (Hamilton and Johnstone, 1945).

Nitro-derivatives excreted in the Urine

The fate of TNT in the body has been studied, but with little result. In 1916 Webster devised a test for a derivative of TNT—namely, 2,6-dinitro, 4-hydroxylamino-toluene—which is excreted in the urine. Webster and others have since improved the test, making it sensitive to 1 part in 10,000 (Ingham, 1941). The urine of practically all workers in TNT contains the substance identified by Webster, but in some there is only a minute trace, in others an intense reaction, and there may be a considerable reaction where there is no sign of TNT illness, or illness with only a moderate degree of reaction.

Effects of rubbing Amatol into the Human Skin

In 1917 Legge satisfied himself by studies of the precise occupation of workers with toxic jaundice that the skin had been the route of absorption.

Benjamin Moore (1918) investigated the problem of skin absorption of TNT by experiments upon himself. After showing that the Webster test of his urine was negative, he went into an orchard attached to a factory and rubbed into the palms of his hands intermittently for about six hours an *amatol* pellet containing 20 per cent TNT. He was careful to refrain from going near any part of the factory where there was TNT dust or fume. After two hours a specimen of urine was passed and this showed a positive Webster test. This reaction went on increasing until next day when its intensity was about the same as that given by the urine of the shop-worker. The TNT reaction remained and gradually increased in intensity for a period of ten days, although he neither rubbed TNT in again nor went near any source of dust or fume. The first morning after rubbing in the *amatol* he woke with all the symptoms of a minor attack of TNT illness. He had marked frontal headache, with a feeling of nausea and intermittent abdominal pain. This abated shortly, but a feeling of malaise and drowsiness persisted for about two days. After a fortnight, and when his urine had become free from TNT reaction, he repeated the experiment, with the same result as before.

Symptoms and Signs

The clinical manifestations of TNT poisoning include dermatitis, cyanosis, gastritis, toxic jaundice and anæmia. The hands and sometimes the face and hair are stained orange with TNT, causing an appearance easily distinguishable from jaundice. Dermatitis arises on the parts exposed—namely, the hands, forearms, legs, wrists and ankles. It begins between the fingers and on the thenar eminence as a pink papular eruption on an erythematous background. As it spreads over the wrists and forearms, the papules become confluent. Desquamation is the rule, and if it is severe it may lead to exfoliation. The irritation is so intense that removal from contact is essential.

Methæmoglobinæmia and Sulphæmoglobinæmia

A great number of workers show minor degrees of cyanosis, with little or no pallor. Very often the condition is symptomless. Occasionally a worker who looks quite purple declares that he has never felt better in his life. The more serious cases present the TNT facies, a condition brought about by the combined effects of methæmoglobinæmia and vasomotor changes. It has been described by Moore (1918) and Roberts (1941). There is slight pallor, but the striking change is a lilac cyanosis of the lips, tongue, lobes of the ears and curve of the helix. The appearance is so difficult to detect in artificial light that inspection of night-shifts is valueless. It is lessened by excitement or by mild exercise, and for this reason it is best detected by the medical officer when in the department during work rather than on a medical parade. Some of these cases develop symptoms such as breathlessness on exertion, lassitude and a tightness behind the sternum. In studies of the blood of TNT workers, Jope (1946) encountered about one case showing sulphæmoglobin to forty showing methæmoglobin. The magnitude of this sulphæmoglobinæmia is so slight as to rob it of clinical significance (see p. 537).

Toxic Gastritis due to TNT

Toxic gastritis is a definite syndrome. The patient is weary and miserable and has a heavy ache in the epigastrium together with loss of appetite. He is constipated, has nausea and vomiting which may be unrelated to food, looks ill, worried and wretched, and may show the TNT facies. In the cases falling into this group Lane (1942) found the liver enlarged and tender. Investigations disclosed little. The lævulose tolerance test was usually normal, barium and fractional test meals showed no abnormality, and blood examination was normal. The urinary coproporphyrin, however, was raised in over half the cases.

Treatment of TNT Poisoning

The patient must be removed to hospital. A thorough bath is followed by scrubbing of hands, fingers, feet and toes with ether until no pink reaction is obtained with alkaline alcohol. The nails should be closely cut. The bowels should be moved as soon as possible and kept open. A bland diet is allowed as soon as it can be tolerated. Fluids are given in large quantities with as much fresh fruit and vegetables as can be obtained. These cases usually clear up so far as the major symptoms are concerned after a few days' rest in bed. In a few of the worst cases it has taken two or three weeks before the patients have been sufficiently free from symptoms to get up. In nearly all cases, however, the fatigue has persisted and it is almost always the last symptom to disappear. Cases of this sort should never be allowed to return to contact with TNT.

Toxic Jaundice due to TNT

Toxic jaundice is a rare complication, but it has a mortality of 30 per cent and so it must be treated seriously. If cyanosis occurs in one in ten of the workers, jaundice attacks one in 500. The greatest incidence of jaundice is in the third month of employment. Sometimes a latent interval occurs between removal from exposure and the onset of jaundice; thus, a woman who left work owing to an injury developed jaundice five weeks later (Panton, 1917). Premonitory symptoms such as drowsiness, giddiness, depression and dark urine are sometimes present, or the attack may be heralded by cyanosis or toxic gastritis. But it may arise without warning, and some patients even maintain that they feel perfectly well. The intensity of the jaundice varies; the stools are light-coloured and the urine dark. The liver is palpable at some stage of the illness in most of the cases. Sometimes it is soft and tender in the early stages, but it usually becomes firm and non-tender at the end of the illness. The serum bilirubin figure may rise as high as 15 milligrams per 100 millilitres. The lævulose tolerance test is of little help, and the lack of a simple yet comprehensive test of liver function is a great disadvantage.

Fatal Cases and Morbid Anatomy

The one investigation which shows a definite abnormality is the urinary coproporphyrin (Rimington and Goldblatt, 1940). In two fatal cases described by Lane in 1942, the figure was some fifty times greater than normal. The estimation was carried out some weeks before death and is therefore a striking finding. The prognosis is always uncertain, but grave symptoms of hepatic insufficiency sometimes appear rapidly. The morbid appearances are those of yellow and red necrosis of the liver, with great reduction in its size and weight. The necrosis of the liver cells may be associated with infiltration and subsequent fibrosis resembling ordinary portal cirrhosis. There is little attempt at regeneration (Turnbull, 1917). However, typical multiple nodular hyperplasia of the liver has been described in a TNT worker who died of aplastic anæmia four months after her attack of toxic jaundice (Davie, 1942).

Incidence of Aplastic Anæmia

Aplastic anæmia sometimes occurs among TNT workers, but its incidence is very small. In 1917 Panton investigated thirty-four cases of sickness arising among workers in TNT. Of these, twenty-eight had toxic jaundice, six had aplastic anæmia and four had gastritis. Toxic jaundice and anæmia appeared to be separate pathological states. Anæmia might occur without jaundice, and only about 17 per cent of the jaundiced patients became anæmic. The latency of the blood changes was even longer than the latency of the jaundice, for it was found that anæmia could develop as long as nine months after exposure to TNT had ceased. The anæmia was always fatal. Lane (1942) described three cases of aplastic anæmia, all in men. Each case presented a profound normocytic anæmia associated with agranulocytosis and a low platelet count, all the blood-forming elements being affected.

Treatment of Aplastic Anæmia due to TNT

Liver and nucleotide therapy was attempted without improvement, the only measure which met with any success being repeated blood transfusions. In this way, one of the patients was kept alive for some months until his marrow began to regenerate. When examined nine months after the beginning of his illness, and four months after his last transfusion, this man had retained his red-cell count at the same level and his hæmoglobin had increased by 20 per cent. His white-cell count remained in the neighbourhood of 6,000 per c.mm., with a normal differential count, and his platelets also had returned to normal. He still had an enlarged liver and his spleen had become palpable.

Aplasia and Hyperplasia of the Marrow at Necropsy

In two cases of TNT aplastic anæmia, Turnbull (1917) found at necropsy fatty marrow throughout all the bones. In each case the liver was rusty-brown from an excess of iron pigment, and multiple petechial hæmorrhages were present in the tissues. There seems to be some evidence as in the case of benzene, that an early effect of TNT may be to stimulate the bone-marrow. Thus Davie (1942) described a necropsy on a woman TNT worker who showed acute toxic purpura and died at home without any hæmatological examination prior to death. At necropsy she presented the features of purpura hæmorrhagica. No anæmia was apparent, but the liver showed very early acute necrosis. Her marrow was markedly hyperplastic, the femur containing red marrow throughout the upper three-quarters of its length, and microscopically all the elements of the marrow were represented.

Evidence of Hæmolysis of Red Blood Cells

Stewart (1943) examined a number of students who had volunteered to fill shells with TNT during their vacation. Their chief subjective complaints were nausea, with variable loss of appetite, diffuse abdominal pain, vomiting and diarrhœa, fatigue, and nasal and throat irritation. The symptoms came on after an initial period when there was an increased sense of wellbeing accompanied by a voracious appetite. There was evidence of

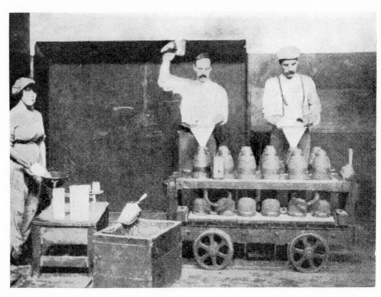

Fig. 197.—Stemming Shells with TNT in 1915. The Workers handled the Powder without Protection and spilt it over both the Apparatus and the Floor

hæmolysis in over 85 per cent of the students, with a fall in hæmoglobin, red-cell and hæmatocrit readings. There was also an increase in reticulocytes, bilirubinæmia with urobilinuria, and a marked erythroblastic response in the marrow. The reticulocyte response was not maximal until a few days after exposure had ceased. This suggests that TNT, in addition

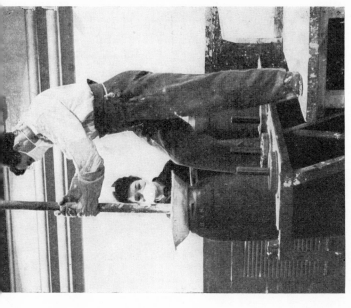

Fig. 199.—Stemming Bombs with TNT in 1945. Note the Gloves and other Protective Clothing

(By courtesy of the Director of Filling Factories)

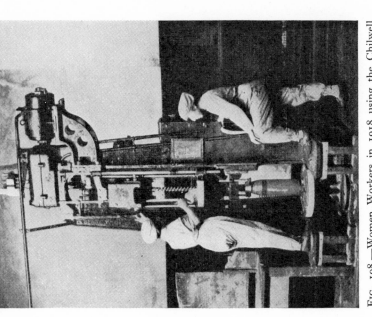

Fig. 198.—Women Workers in 1918 using the Chilwell Stemming Machine for filling Shells. Note the Protective Clothing and the absence of Contamination of the Machine or the Floor with TNT

to a destructive action on the circulating red cells, also affects the bone marrow.

Preventive Measures developed in the First World War

Experience in industry goes to show that when a poison is absorbed through the skin the application of effective measures of prevention is most difficult (fig. 197). In 1917 Legge minimized the risk of TNT poisoning not by any single precaution, but by the combination of several, of which alternation of employment, periodical medical examination, ventilation and clean working conditions were the chief. Success was not achieved until mechanical means were substituted for the hand carriage of shells

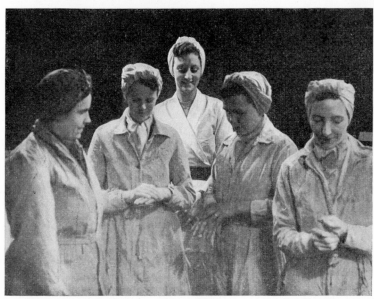

FIG. 200.—The Beauty Parlour of a Shell-filling Factory in 1944. Operatives applying Barrier Cream to the Skin under Supervision of a Woman Foreman. Note the Protective Clothing
(By courtesy of Dr. A. J. Amor, Ministry of Supply)

combined with measures of cleanliness which were so precise as to prevent the contamination of the outside of the shells by TNT (fig. 198).

Methods of the Second World War

Unfortunately, in 1939, hand contact again became widespread. In filling factories TNT is used either molten, powdered or in pellets known as biscuit. In the preparation of *amatol* and *baratol*, in filling shells, bombs and mines, and in the breaking of biscuit, both contact with the skin and the production of dust are inevitable. In these processes further dangers are involved because solid TNT is spilled on the benches and it adheres to stemming rods, pouring cans and funnels (fig. 199). Also, the cleaning of these tools and the shops themselves, unless done properly and under supervision, very often entails worse contact than the filling itself (Swanston, 1942). Fume hazard occurs where TNT is melted and where shells and anti-tank mines are filled. In ill-ventilated shops with dust and fume constantly present in the air, a certain amount of TNT must be inhaled and ingested. In 1942 Himsworth and Glynn made experimental observations which suggest that a high fat diet renders rats more susceptible to TNT poisoning. It seems advisable, therefore, to arrange for TNT workers a diet of high protein and carbohydrate content with low fat.

Summary of the Principles of Prevention

In Great Britain between 1916 and the end of 1941, 475 cases of TNT poisoning were notified. Of these, 125, or 26·3 per cent, ended fatally. In many factories the conditions still need to be improved by better ventilation, especially local dust extraction, and by the provision of better tools and the introduction of machine filling. Washing facilities must be extended and the supply of protective clothing improved. There should be a stricter supervision of the workers by people who are sufficiently intelligent and interested to appreciate the dangers of the work and the methods by which they can be avoided. Workers and supervisors must be trained to the job and penalized if rules are not obeyed (fig. 200). Bridge (1942) summarized the principles for the prevention of TNT illness as cleanliness of the air breathed, secured by effective ventilation or, if that is impossible, filtration through an effective respirator; cleanliness of the implements used and cleanliness of the person, secured by protective clothing and by personal attention to the skin.

Case 20. Munitions worker—exposure to TNT for five weeks—death from necrosis of the liver.

(Turnbull, 1916.) E. S., a boy aged 14, was employed in Woolwich Arsenal filling bags with trotyl, a powder of crude TNT. No protective clothing was provided nor was special ventilation installed. After five weeks' exposure he complained of nausea and was found to be jaundiced. He was transferred to other work, but a week later the jaundice was more marked and he was admitted to hospital. Two months after the onset of symptoms he died of hepatic insufficiency.

Necropsy: Professor H. M. Turnbull made the necropsy of the liver (L.H. P.M. 724/1915), of which the following is a summary.

Trinitrotoluene poisoning. The liver (fig. 201) weighs 1 lb. 4½ oz. —that is, less than one-third the normal. The gall-bladder contains a few drops of dark-brown bile. The mucosa is dark green and honeycombed. The hepatic portion of the inferior vena cava has a smooth lining, the orifices therein of the hepatic veins are patent. The whole of the left lobe and lower third of the right lobe are greatly shrunken; the surface is greatly wrinkled; the capsule is opaque and no lobular pattern is visible through it. The upper two-thirds of the right lobe

form a mass which is 14 cm. broad, 9 cm. from above down, and projects 5·5 cm. above the level of the shrunken portions. The greater
part of the surface of this mass has a thin capsule through which a
large lobular pattern, of a pale yellow colour, is visible. Portions, however, of the surface of the mass are slightly shrunken, and show a
small lobular pattern, in which the centres of the lobules are dark
reddish brown and the peripheries are pale yellow. These sunken areas
on the surface of the mass are irregularly distributed; in places they

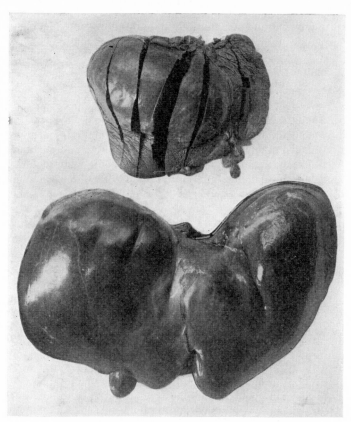

Fig. 201.—Case 20. Acute Necrosis of the Liver due to TNT. The Liver
below is a normal control. The Patient was a boy of 14 who in 1915
filled Bags with TNT for 5 weeks. He became Jaundiced and died of
Hepatic Insufficiency two months after the onset of symptoms
(*London Hospital Medical College Museum*)

surround and isolate small nodules of the large lobular pattern. Vertical sections through the liver show that the raised mass in the right
lobe corresponds to an area of soft swollen tissue, in which there are
large lobules of canary-yellow colour with darker, redder centres. The

shrunken lower third of the right lobe, and the shrunken left lobe have a flat, firm surface, on which small grey portal systems lie close together in a red ground. Beneath the sunken areas which were seen on the surface of the large mass are areas of similar tissue. The posterior quarter of the right lobe, behind the large mass, is similar. The atrophied hepatic tissue therefore occupies the left lobe and considerably more than a third of the right lobe.

Microscopic: the sunken areas with small obular pattern are found, to be areas in which the hepatic parenchyma has undergone necrosis following a degeneration which is largely fatty. The parenchyma has been destroyed completely with the exception of pseudo-bile canaliculi which pass from portal bile ducts and end blindly in expansions lined by small hepatic cells. The destruction is associated with an active inflammatory reaction, demonstrated by a fibrosis which is densest in the portal zone.

The raised areas with large lobular pattern differ. Destruction is less extensive and the inflammation has generally reached a later stage, and regenerative hypertrophy of the surviving parenchyma has taken place; the infiltration of the portal systems by neutrophilic leucocytes is absent.

Case 21. Munitions worker—exposure to TNT for seven months—death from aplastic anæmia.

(Panton, 1917.) I. E., a girl aged 21, L.H. Reg. No. 41104/1917. admitted to the London Hospital under the care of Dr. Robert Hutchison. She had been working on the manufacture of trinitrotoluene for seven months, and until a fortnight previously when the works closed down. It was stated that she had been overcome on several occasions by the fumes developed in the nitrating process. She had been sufficiently in contact with trinitrotoluene to have absorbed a poisonous dose through the skin. A girl who worked with her was said to have recently developed toxic jaundice. Ten days before admission she began to bleed from the vagina, and subsequently from the rectum and mouth. *On admission* she was extremely ill, was bleeding profusely and had a purpuric rash over the limbs and trunk. Blood count: red cells 1,200,000 per c.mm., hæmoglobin 8 per cent, colour index 0·3, white cells 480 per c.mm. Of the white cells 75 per cent were lymphocytes, and only 10 per cent polynuclears. The blood picture in stained films was that of aplastic anæmia. The patient died two days later, and at necropsy no liver necrosis was present. The vertebral marrow was grey, and there was less than the normal amount of red marrow in the humerus and femur.

(d) Dinitrophenol

Of all the dinitrophenols it is only the 2,4- or alpha isomer which has toxic properties. It is a pale yellow crystalline powder used as an explosive, in the dye industry and for the preservation of timber. Mixed with picric acid it forms the French explosive *mélinite*. In France it was handled extensively in shell-filling factories during 1915 and 1916, and many cases of poisoning occurred, including twenty-seven deaths.

Absorption and Excretion of DNP

Absorption may take place through the respiratory tract, the alimentary canal and the skin. Heat aids absorption and therefore more cases of poisoning occur in the warm days of summer. Alcohol influences the development of toxic phenomena in man; cases of poisoning are more numerous the day after a holiday and among alcoholics. 2,4-dinitrophenol does not produce methæmoglobinæmia, though many mononitro- and dinitrophenols do so. Very little is known of the fate of DNP in the body. It is excreted, apparently in conjugation with sulphate or glycuronate, mostly unchanged, but partly after reduction of one or both nitro groups. Derrien's test, which was widely used by the French as an indicator of excessive DNP intake by munition workers, depends on the presence in the urine of 2-amino-4-nitrophenol. The specificity of the test has been called in question.

Symptoms and Signs

Workers show yellow staining of the face, legs and forearms, and especially the palms and soles. French experience of the manufacture of DNP suggests that staining of those parts of the body not in direct contact with the powder indicates a dangerous accumulation of the compound in the body. In a small proportion of workers a rash appears on the exposed skin. It is a pink papular or maculo-papular eruption. Mild poisoning is characterized by lassitude, slight headache, night sweats and fatigue on the least exertion. Workmen may lose weight from the time they first take up the work. Acute intoxication comes on suddenly with a sensation of extreme weariness in the limbs and painful constriction in the chest, a burning thirst, abundant sweats, and an agitation and anxiety which is characteristic. Other signs are pallor, dyspnœa and scanty urine, which may be a deep orange colour owing to the presence of 2-amino-4-nitrophenol.

Acute Fatalities and Morbid Anatomy

In more severe cases death may take place in a few hours after a rise of temperature to 104° F. or over. The victim has severe sweating, intense thirst and sometimes colic and diarrhœa. The state of anxious terror and restlessness is typical, and is followed by coma, convulsions and death. Temperatures as high as 109·4° F. have been recorded, and in some cases there was a rise of several degrees after death (Perkins, 1919). Necropsy reveals no characteristic lesions. When the dose is not fatal, the symptoms rapidly improve and many workers develop a tolerance to the poison (Martin, 1930).

Effects in Experimental Animals

The mode of action of the dinitrophenols has been investigated by animal experiment. It was discovered in 1885 that certain nitrophenols possess marked influence on metabolism (Cazeneuve and Lépine). In 1929 this work was amplified by Heymans and Bouckaert, who showed that nitrophenols not only cause a great increase in oxygen consumption, but if the administration be pushed there is also a rise in temperature terminating in a fatal hyperpyrexia.

Toxic Effects in the Treatment of Obesity

In 1933 Cutting, Mehrtens and Tainter used 2,4-dinitrophenol in the treatment of obesity. The compound, administered to patients in doses of 3 milligrams per kilogram of body weight, caused a rise in basal metabolic rate and loss of weight, unattended by tachycardia. The treatment became very popular and, within a year, some 100,000 persons in the United States of America had used this substance for obesity. Proprietary preparations appeared under various names, such as *aldinol, dekrysils, dinitrenal, dinitrolac, dinitrole, dinitrose, dinitroso, nitraphen, nitrobese, nitromet, redusols, slendite* and *slim*. Toxic symptoms were soon reported, including urticaria, exfoliative dermatitis (Hitch and Schwartz, 1936), jaundice (Sidel, 1934), neutropenia (Davidson and Shapiro, 1934), fatal agranulocytosis (Silver, 1934), peripheral neuritis (Nadler, 1935) and loss of the power to discriminate between sweet and salt tastes (Tainter, Stockton and Cutting, 1933). The literature was reviewed by Hardgrove and Stern (1938). Albuminuria, cloudy swelling of the renal tubules, fall in blood-pressure, electrocardiographic changes, fullness in the ears, deafness and decrease of sugar tolerance have also been described.

Total Blindness from Cataract

After DNP had been in use for four years, cataract was found to be a late complication of the use of the drug. The shortest time reported before its appearance was three months, and the longest eighteen months. The smallest total amount of DNP taken in these cases was 9 grams and the largest 123·5 grams. The change is bilateral and the lens fibres alter so quickly that the cataract swiftly progresses to total blindness (Horner, Jones and Boardman, 1935). No case has shown spontaneous resolution and most have progressed to complete opacity within about three months in spite of withdrawal of the drug. Altogether not less than 100 cases of cataract occurred in the United States of America and some writers have reckoned the incidence as between 0·1 and 1 per cent of those treated with DNP. This final disastrous effect of DNP, together with the fact that it could be obtained only by a physician's prescription in most countries, brought to a close the unfortunate popularity of this drug. Deaths have been rare and where they have occurred the dose of DNP has been excessive—for example, 10 milligrams per kilogram of body-weight. repeated for four or five days (Poole and Haining, 1934).

Preventive Measures

In 1918, when it became necessary in Great Britain to use DNP, the manufacturers profited by the experience in France and took extensive precautions. The men employed were provided with underclothes and overalls into which they changed from their ordinary clothes, a separate cubicle being provided for each man. The washing and bathroom facilities were all that could be desired. Exhaust ventilation was applied locally to remove the fume in melting the compound and also in filling the shells. Dust which collected round the margin of the shell was removed by a vacuum cleaner. As a result of these measures, combined with daily examination of the urine, little or no trouble has occurred from handling DNP in Great Britain (Legge, 1934).

Symptomatic Treatment

No antidote to DNP is known. There is no point in using thiouracil, for it has no effect on the raised metabolism. The state of anxiety must be allayed by repeated doses of phenobarbitone. The patient must be kept cool by tepid sponging; fluids and electrolytes which have been lost by profuse sweating must be replaced.

(e) *Para*methylaminophenol Sulphate (Metol)

The aminophenols are used as photographic developers, in the manufacture of azo-dyestuffs and of phenacetin. Metol alone, or in combination with hydroquinone, has been one of the most popular of all photographic developers since its introduction by Hauff in 1891. It occurs as a white crystalline powder which darkens on exposure to air.

Photographers' Dermatitis due to an Impurity

Fig. 286 on p. 796 shows how metol stains the nails and fingers dark brown. Although Wyers (1952) observed men working on a metol plant for eleven years he saw dermatitis from sensitization once only. He and many other authors agree that the dermatitis of photographers from contact with metol is due to the presence of n,n-dimethyl-p-phenylenediamine as an impurity; dermatitis never occurs with pure metol. The backs of the fingers are affected first, followed by the back of the hand and the interdigital spaces. The eruption is papulo-vesicular; the lesions sometimes ulcerate and then become encrusted. Once sensitization has occurred relief is secured only by completely avoiding contact with the substance concerned.

Systemic Poisoning in a Chemical Factory Worker

Wyers (1952) describes the case of a man manufacturing metol who became poisoned by inhalation of dust. He was thickly clad and wore gloves. His mask proved to be ineffective against the passage of fine dust, particularly when working in a high concentration and with physical exertion requiring rapid breathing. He voided black urine, sometimes towards the end of the shift and at other times on the morning after he had been mixing batches of powder. The staining by airborne dust of the skin of the hands, the fingernails and the interpalpebral conjunctiva were the same as in men exposed to the dust of hydroquinone (p. 532). The lips, tongue and cheeks were cyanosed, the colour being the bluish-grey tint of methæmoglobinæmia as in other cases of poisoning by aromatic amino-compounds (p. 534). On removal from exposure he recovered rapidly in a few days.

Accidental Poisoning of Patients in an X-ray Department

In Zagreb a mistake in a department of X-ray diagnosis led to systemic poisoning by metol of two patients given an opaque meal, and of two others given an opaque enema (Palmović and Frketić, 1955). Of the second group of patients one died. To the barium sulphate contrast medium, by mistake, about 1 per cent of metol, stored on one of the shelves of the department, was added. Each patient given an opaque meal received 2 to 3 grams of metol. Within ten minutes each suffered nausea, vomiting, abdominal discomfort, weakness and drowsiness. Cyanosis of the lips and fingers occurred after one hour, and within six hours the urine was as dark as black coffee, signs which began to clear up after twenty-four hours. Both patients were normal by the next day. The patients given a barium enema each received 10 to 12 grams of metol. The first one had immediate abdominal discomfort, diarrhœa, nausea, weakness and cyanosis. The urine became dark the same day. After six days there was no further diarrhœa and she slowly recovered. The patient who died collapsed at once, becoming weak, dizzy and cyanosed. There was diarrhœa with abdominal discomfort, subnormal temperature and collapse of the circulation. Apathy, restlessness and delirium were followed by unconsciousness and she died after twelve hours. Necropsy showed a peritoneal exudate of 600 ml. of translucent brown fluid which revealed methæmoglobin by spectroscopy. The rectal mucosa was greyish-violet and swollen. The colon showed old ulceration and fresh surface necrosis. In lesser degree the inflammatory changes affected the terminal two metres of the ileum. The brain showed œdema especially in the region of the basal ganglia.

(f) Dinitro-*ortho*-cresol

This compound is called 3,5-dinitro-*ortho*-cresol by the Chemical Society of London. It is referred to also as 2,4- or 4,6-dinitro-*ortho*-cresol. The confusion arises from alternative methods of numbering (fig. 202). It is yellow crystalline solid.

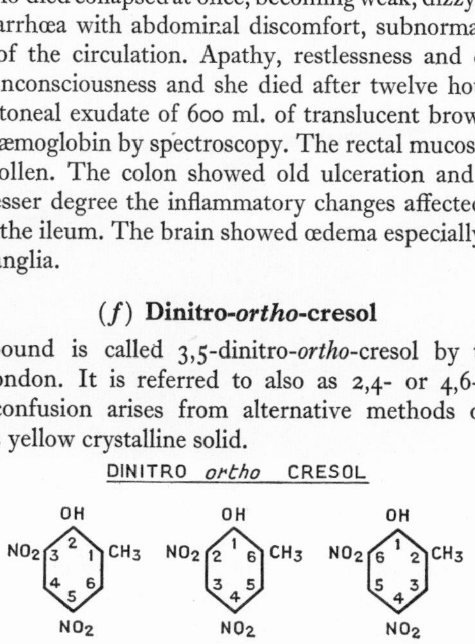

FIG. 202

Uses

It was introduced in 1892 as the active constituent of a preparation *antinonnin* for use against the nun moth. The work which led to its commercial development was done in 1925 by Tattersfield, Gimingham and Morris. It was first used as a synthetic selective herbicide in Great Britain in 1940 (Ripper, 1960). It is applied in agriculture in the spring as an aqueous solution of the sodium salt especially to destroy the field poppy (*Papaver rhœas*), yellow charlock (*Sinapis arvensis*), white charlock (*Raphanus Raphanistrum* and cornflower (*Centaurea cyanus*). As an insecticide, ovicide and fungicide, it is used in orchards as a dilute winter wash. Applied as a spray, this kills such pests as aphides, especially the woolly aphis (*Eriosoma lanigerum*), the apple capsid bug (*Plesiocoris rugicollis*), the winter moth (*Operophtera brumata*), the red spider mite (*Oligonychus ulmi*) and the ova of the apple sucker (*Psylla mali*). For locust control it is used as a dust or as a solution in oil (fig. 203). The wide adoption of DNOC is indicated by its many trade names, including *amdinoc, capsine, cresosin, cudinoc, denoc, denocate, denocol, dinocide, dytrol, elgetine, elgetol, hibernoc, ovamort, sinox* and *sodinoc*. In 1933 Dodds and Pope recom-

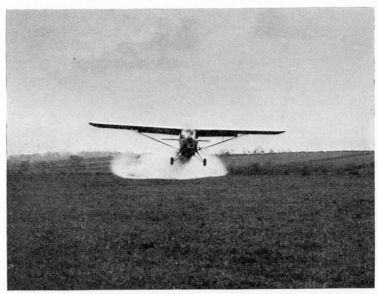

FIG. 203.—Where DNOC is sprayed from Aeroplanes as a Dust in Locust Control, great care must be taken to protect the Pilot and other Operatives

mended DNOC for the treatment of obesity as being more effective and less toxic than dinitrophenol, but by 1937 the dangers from its ingestion were widely recognized and it passed into disrepute.

Exposure Hazards

Overdosage of DNOC, taken for obesity, has caused at least three deaths in Great Britain, and its industrial and agricultural use at least nine more. Deaths and cases of severe intoxication in industrial and agricultural workers have been reported from Germany, Hungary, France, the United States of America, India and Africa. Non-fatal cases of poisoning with DNOC have occurred from medicinal and from industrial exposure. Merewether recorded fourteen cases of DNOC poisoning which occurred in a factory in Great Britain in 1943 during the height of the summer. For two years it had been manufactured in paste form with no harmful effects to the worker, but on this occasion a dust was being prepared for use against locusts. After the introduction of locally applied exhaust ventilation and periodic medical examination of workers in the factory concerned, only one further case of mild severity was reported.

Hazards in the Spraying of Cereal Crops

Spraying orchard trees against aphides, red spider and caterpillar with dilute winter washes of DNOC in cold weather involves but little risk. It is the spraying of cereal crops on a large scale, especially in hot weather, which constitutes a serious hazard. The nozzles of the booms of the spraying machines emit droplets widely differing in size. The microscopic droplets form a mist or drift. The spray from a machine working on the atomizer principle emitted 10 feet from the ground into a ten-mile-an-hour wind will drift coarse droplets 25 feet, fine droplets 150 feet, and fog and mist over a mile. A certain proportion of the droplets settle as fine dust which readily flies in the atmosphere. This drift is an important factor in poisoning the spray operators as well as wild animals and birds; it may also kill neighbouring crops and stain the washing hanging out to dry in the villages. Crop spraying by helicopter was introduced in 1949, and aerial spraying by unmanned robot machines was first used in 1957. Crop protection by helicopter has the advantage that liquid sprays are more effective than dry dusts (Ripper, 1960).

Effect on the Rate of Metabolism

The actions of DNOC and DNP are qualitatively similar in all respects. The acute lethal effect of each substance is due to excessive stimulation of the general metabolism. DNOC may be considered about twice as active pharmacologically and about twice as toxic as DNP. When an animal is given a moderate dose of DNOC—say, 1 milligram per kilogram of body weight—the basal rate of metabolism is raised by about 40 per cent. The only abnormalities observed are moderate flushing of the skin and increased pulmonary ventilation. The effect comes on within a few minutes of injection or within fifteen minutes when the DNOC is ingested, and reaches its peak within an hour; its duration appears to vary with the size of the animal, being about two hours in the rat and from one to four days in man.

Effects of Large Doses of DNOC in Animals

With larger doses, all the mechanisms of the body which control heat loss are brought into action. If these are inadequate, the temperature rises and remains high until the metabolic rate begins to decline. The increase in metabolism is always much greater than can be ascribed to the fever itself. There is usually hyperglycæmia associated with a fall in liver and muscle glycogen. When a lethal dose is given, the metabolism and the respiratory minute volume may increase to ten or more times the normal, and the temperature may rise to 105° F. or more. The increase in breathing and in cardiac output become inadequate to supply the needs of the tissues for oxygen and to carry off the excess of heat and metabolites. Finally, death occurs from heat stroke or cerebral œdema, respiration and the heart failing almost simultaneously. Rigor mortis sets in at once. At the moment of death the temperature may exceed 110° F.

Cumulative Effect of DNOC in Man

It is possible to correlate physiological effects with the concentration of DNOC in the blood (Harvey, Bidstrup and Bonnell, 1951), and routine estimation of the blood DNOC level in persons at risk should be included among the measures adopted for the prevention of DNOC poisoning. DNOC can be estimated accurately in 0·1 millilitres of blood obtained by finger-tip or ear-lobe puncture using the method described by Parker (1949) adapted by Harvey (1952). Studies of the comparative rates of elimination of DNOC by the rat, the rabbit and man confirm the clinical observation that this substance is a cumulative poison in man and is eliminated slowly. The figures show the need for caution in the interpretation

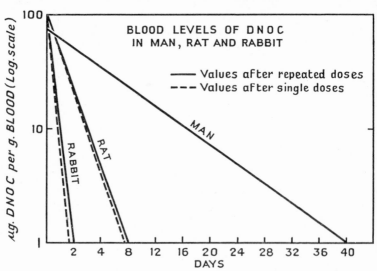

FIG. 204

of animal experiments. When DNOC intoxication is present in the three species (fig. 204) and is represented by initial blood levels of from 60 to 80 micrograms per gram, the concentration will approach zero in two days in the rabbit, eight days in the rat and forty days in man (King and Harvey, 1953).

Symptoms and Signs

The earliest symptom of DNOC poisoning is an exaggerated feeling of well-being, but this is difficult to assess. It is likely to be present when the concentration of DNOC in the blood is of the order of 20 micrograms per gram of blood. Later manifestations are loss of weight, unusual thirst, excessive sweating and fatigue, symptoms which are frequently attributed to other causes such as hot weather and long hours of work. The temperature rises with the rise in metabolism, and both reach a peak between the first and fourth day of the illness. The height of the basal rate of metabolism varies between 120 and 400 per cent of normal, and the figure is always higher than can be ascribed to the fever itself. Dyspnœa occurs and may be present at rest, with a corresponding rise in the rate of respiration. The skin is flushed and dyed yellow where exposure has recurred, especially on the hands, face, feet and knees. There is anxiety tachycardia, profuse sweating, but no tremor nor exophthalmos.

Occasional Clinical Findings

A papular dermatitis is common in workers handling DNOC, and burns of the skin of the hands have been reported (Gate and Chenial, 1936). Nasal irritation was noted by an entomologist applying DNOC treatment in locust-control experiments (Gahan, 1942), and both cough and dyspnœa have been complained of by industrial workers after inhaling DNOC dust. Although some of the cases reported as jaundice following exposure to DNOC have been merely the yellow dyeing of the skin due to the compound itself, there seems no doubt that severe liver damage can occur. Agranulocytosis seems not to have been reported as an effect of DNOC poisoning. The fact that cataract has been recorded only once may be merely a reflection of the less extensive or more cautious use of DNOC for slimming as compared with DNP (Horner, 1941). In Kenya polyneuritis has been recorded in the case of two men who had been employed cleaning the spraying apparatus of aircraft which used a 20 per cent solution of DNOC in oil for locust control. The skin exposure to the hands was heavy and in both cases they were affected more severely than the feet. Systematic symptoms were minimal. Stott (1956) therefore put forward the view that the polyneuritis was due to local absorption of DNOC.

Acute Fatalities and Morbid Anatomy

In fatal cases the symptoms, signs and necropsy findings have been similar in all cases. Typically the worker felt ill late in the day, began to sweat profusely and to be very thirsty, went home and lay down, but grew rapidly worse, with high fever, weakness, anxiety and great hyperpnœa. From two to eight hours after stopping work the fatal heat stroke observed in animals came on, death being preceded by a brief period of coma. Rigor mortis set in immediately. At necropsy the changes noted were yellow pigmentation of all the tissues, dehydration, petechial hæmorrhages in the brain and lungs, and parenchymatous degeneration of the liver and kidneys (Bidstrup and Payne, 1951).

Examples of Clinical Cases

Parsons (1948) saw three cases of severe DNOC intoxication from the group described by Merewether (1943). One was a man aged thirty-seven who had been employed for seventeen days pouring DNOC powder from kegs into a grinding mill. He wore an ill-fitting mask. In one day his hands were stained yellow, and in three days his feet, ankles and knees were yellow too. He was well until two days before admission to hospital. The first symptom was sweating at night; next day he felt suffocated, became dyspnœic and weak, and complained of a dry mouth. On examination there was profuse sweating, the temperature was 100° F., the pulse rate 130, and the respiratory rate 38 per minute, but there was no tremor or exophthalmos. The basal metabolic rate, determined twenty-four hours later, was 180 per cent. He recovered completely within forty-eight hours. McDonald (1943) reported the case of a Negro factory worker whose palms and soles were yellow and who had recently lost 20 lb. in weight. He had a temperature of 102° F., a phenomenal basal rate of metabolism of 400 per cent, rapid pulse, rapid respiration, profuse sweating, shortness of breath and cough. An examination of his place of work showed that he had been exposed to 4·7 milligrams of DNOC dust per cubic metre of workroom air per day. The man recovered. Pollard and Filbes (1951) recorded an acute case with recovery in a spray operator who had been applying DNOC to cereal crops. He recovered, but even seven days after he was free from symptoms the basal metabolic rate was still 180 per cent.

Preventive Measures

Since DNOC is so extremely toxic, the search for safe substitutes is an important matter; it is to be hoped that substances as harmless to man as the hormone weed-killers will soon be found to destroy poppy and charlock in our wheat fields and locusts in Africa and elsewhere. Measures adopted to reduce the incidence of DNOC poisoning include education and periodic medical examination of the workers. In carrying this out, a record should be kept of the weight of each man; since many spray operators lose weight during the cereal-crop spraying season, this record may be unreliable as a warning of DNOC poisoning. Arrangements should be made with the local hospital to estimate at intervals the level of DNOC in the blood of all men exposed.

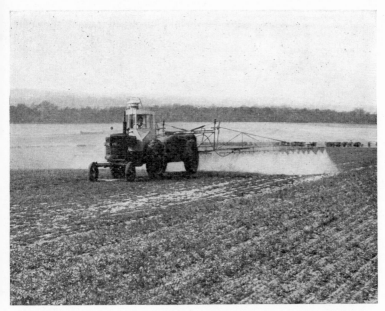

FIG. 205.—Driver in a Gas-proof, Air-conditioned Tractor Cab spraying a
Wheat Field with DNOC

Protection against Dust and Spray Mist of DNOC

Locally applied exhaust ventilation should be installed in factories.
Spray operators must be provided with protective clothing, and the tractors
they use should be made with enclosed cabins. The ideal tractor cabin is
gas-proof, air-conditioned and water-cooled, and is designed in such a way
that it will not operate with the door open (fig. 205). Although DNOC is
absorbed through the skin, relatively small amounts gain entrance to the
body by this route, and in the cases of poisoning recorded, inhalation of
spray mist or DNOC dust has been the most likely method of absorption
of DNOC. Some form of respirator should therefore be worn by all persons
at risk of absorbing DNOC through the respiratory tract, and is an essential
part of protective equipment for men spraying cereal crops and for supervisors and all other persons who come into the vicinity of spraying operations.

Deadly Habits of DNOC Spray Operators

Individual workers have different methods of handling DNOC, both
in mixing the spray and in correcting faults such as blockage of nozzles on
the spray boom. Mixing and spraying should be done across wind so that
spray and dust are carried away from the operator. Often there is no agita-
tor in the spray tank to keep the DNOC in suspension, so that the nozzles
of the spray boom frequently become clogged. A spray operator on such a

machine was observed during most of one day to correct this fault by jumping from the moving machine, running into the spray and hitting blocked nozzles with a spanner while the machine and spraying continued. This was specifically forbidden by his employers, but adequate supervision of individual workmen in this type of work is difficult to arrange. In one fatal case it was discovered that the man had quenched his thirst with water contaminated with DNOC.

The Agriculture (Poisonous Substances) Act, 1952

The workmen are warned that they are handling a dangerous substance, and spray crews are instructed in spraying methods and in the early symtoms and signs of DNOC poisoning. In spite of these precautions, cases of DNOC poisoning continued to occur (Steer, 1951) and a new law was enacted to protect the workmen. The *Agriculture (Poisonous Substances) Act, 1952*, and the *Agriculture (Poisonous Substances) Regulations, 1956*, place upon the employer responsibility for providing adequate means of protection from absorption of dangerous amounts of DNOC and other toxic chemical substances used in agriculture, and for ensuring that these precautions are carried out by all members of spraying teams. Unhappily, the Act failed to provide for the measurement and control of the level of DNOC in the blood of the worker.

Estimation of DNOC in the Blood

As a result of experimental work on volunteers (Harvey, Bidstrup and Bonnell, 1951) and the estimation of DNOC in single samples of blood collected from men engaged in the manufacture of DNOC or in its use as a late-winter wash on fruit trees or as a selective weed-killer in cereal crops (Bidstrup, Bonnell and Harvey, 1952), it is possible to state that when the concentration of DNOC in the blood is about 20 micrograms per gram of blood or more, the man should be removed from further contact with DNOC for at least six weeks. To avoid false high or peak values, the blood should be collected not less than eight hours after the last exposure to DNOC. Since the workman will have no symptoms he may continue to work, provided he agrees not to handle any substance known to be toxic.

Safe Level of DNOC in the Blood

When the blood DNOC level is between 10 and 20 micrograms the man may continue to work, but close supervision is necessary to ensure that he obeys strictly all the precautions recommended for the safe handling of DNOC. The blood DNOC estimation should be repeated in forty-eight hours, and if there is any increase the man should be removed from further contact. The exaggerated feeling of well-being is likely to be present when the blood DNOC level is above 15 micrograms, but unless the workman is well-known to the observer, this change is difficult to assess. If the blood DNOC concentration is less than 10 micrograms, the man may continue at work and no extra precautions need be advised.

Symptomatic Treatment

No antidote to DNOC is known. Early diagnosis is essential, and treatment on general lines will often result in recovery, even in serious cases. The patient must be kept cool by tepid sponging; fluids and electrolytes which are lost in the profuse sweating which characterizes the illness in its acute stages must be replaced; barbiturates should be administered in

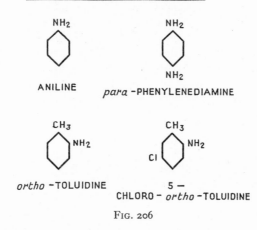

AROMATIC AMINO-DERIVATIVES

ANILINE

para -PHENYLENEDIAMINE

ortho -TOLUIDINE

5 — CHLORO - *ortho* -TOLUIDINE

Fig. 206

doses adequate to allay the anxiety. Treatment with thiouracil has no effect because the raised metabolism is a direct effect upon the cell and has nothing to do with hyperthyroidism.

(g) Aniline

Aniline is a colourless oily liquid, with a distinctive aromatic odour. It turns brown on exposure to air and light (fig. 206). It is handled in the manufacture of dyes, explosives, perfumes, pharmaceutical products and photographic chemicals. It is used in dyeing, calico printing, painting, varnishing and rubber processing.

Ready Absorption of Aniline through the Skin

The high lipoid solvent power of aniline leads to its ready absorption through the intact skin. Experience has shown that in factories most of the serious cases of acute poisoning occur when the workers have had their clothing or skin soiled by aniline. Its absorption by the respiratory tract also occurs, especially after the breaking of vessels containing aniline, or where a workman enters a chamber filled with the vapour. Danger from aniline vapour is much greater during hot weather. At these times, when the work is over, numerous cases of headache and slight cyanosis are observed. Many homologues of aniline, especially the *nitro*-anilines, are absorbed through the skin, and those which are sufficiently volatile are dangerous if inhaled. *Para*-nitraniline seems to be considerably more poisonous than aniline. In the absence of efficient locally applied exhaust ventilation, this substance must not be packed in powder form for fear it should produce systemic symptoms, dermatitis or conjunctivitis. The aniline sulphonic acids are harmless.

Symptoms and Signs of Aniline Poisoning

In a mild case of aniline poisoning the face flushes, the man experiences a sense of fullness and throbbing in the head, burning in the throat, tightness in the chest, and then violent headache with dizziness and noises in the ears. The flushed face becomes bluish-grey, and the nose, ears, lips, tongue and nails turn lilac. There is a sensation of weakness in the knees, and a staggering gait. If the man is promptly removed from all contact with aniline, recovery is rapid and the cyanosis disappears within twenty-four hours. This disappearance is more rapid than in poisoning by *nitro*-derivatives of the aromatic series, probably because aniline becomes changed more quickly into hydroxylated products capable of being eliminated in the urine (Engel, 1930).

Curve of Methæmoglobin in the Venous Blood

The recording spectrophotometer gives an exact picture of what happens to the methæmoglobin in the blood in these circumstances. Hamblin and Mangelsdorff (1938) recorded the case of a man who disregarded instructions and wore leather shoes which became contaminated with aniline oil while he was cleaning up the liquid spilled from a tank. He worked at this job for about four hours and then reported sick, complaining of severe headache, dizziness, weakness and aching all over. He showed deep, bluish-grey cyanosis, his pulse was 112, and his respiration 22. A curve of his venous blood plotted on the recording spectrophotometer showed 61 per cent of methæmoglobin. This curve, repeated two hours later, showed a drop to 59 per cent. After resting quietly for four hours, the patient still had severe headache and was deeply cyanosed. However, his pulse had dropped to 80 and he was less lethargic. A blood curve at this time showed 34 per cent of methæmoglobin. The following morning he felt well, had no headache and his colour was normal. The blood curve then showed 5 per cent of methæmoglobin. The following day the patient remained well, and the curve showed 3 per cent of methæmoglobin.

Punctate Basophilia a Delicate Sign of Poisoning

Punctate basophilia is a valuable early sign of aniline poisoning. In 1907 Malden investigated the cases of thirteen men employed in aniline black dyeing. There was so much aniline vapour in the atmosphere in which they worked that all unpainted deal woodwork was stained bright yellow. Of the thirteen men, none had been employed for less than one year and all had suffered at some time or other from symptoms of aniline poisoning. The blood in six of the thirteen men showed punctate basophilia. The number of cells affected varied from two or three in the whole film in the slight cases to ten or twelve in every field of the microscope in the more pronounced cases. These observations have often been confirmed. Thus, Agasse-Lafont, Feil and de Balsac (1926) found fine basophilic granules in the red cells of one-third of a series of men exposed to aniline.

Symptoms and Signs of Severe Poisoning

In more severe cases, the colour of the face is a deep bluish-grey, and the lips and tongue are livid or almost black. The victim trembles and staggers, and complains of weakness in the knees. These symptoms may be followed by nausea, vomiting and cramps in the abdomen. Extreme weakness comes on, and sometimes a few hours after the onset of the attack consciousness is lost. The respiration is shallow and quick, the pulse small, rapid and irregular, the skin is cold and the blood-pressure drops. If coma persists, the respiration and pulse grow progressively slower. There is involuntary defæcation and micturition, and convulsions usually come on just before death. It is a characteristic feature that the attack seldom takes place while the man is at work, but almost always while he is on his way home or even some hours later (Hamilton, 1925). In serious poisoning the blood turns brown and may even be the colour of chocolate. The urine is either dark brown or the colour of port wine because it contains hæmoglobin and methæmoglobin. Often in the first days of the poisoning, strangury occurs and the urine then contains red blood cells.

Symptoms and Signs of Chronic Poisoning

Prolonged absorption of small quantities of aniline leads to chronic poisoning. In such cases cyanosis does not persist after the patient leaves his daily work, but he shows the weakness, fatigue and slight giddiness and dyspnœa of anæmia. The blood shows a mild, low colour-index anæmia, sometimes with polychromatophilia and punctate basophilia.

Preventive Measures

The manufacture of nitrobenzene and the reduction of nitrobenzene and nitrotoluene to aniline and toluidine must take place in closed vessels. The escape of small quantities of aniline into the atmosphere is very difficult to prevent and so ample ventilation must be provided. In addition to the technical regulations, there must be insistence on cleanliness of the workrooms, personal cleanliness on the part of the workers and provision of baths and changes of clothing. Contact with aniline, especially on the skin, must be carefully avoided, and the spilling and splashing of the liquid forbidden. All workers must be instructed as to the symptoms of aniline poisoning and the steps to take should it occur. Regular medical inspection of workmen is desirable.

Instruction in First-aid Methods

Workers, especially those newly employed, must be under supervision in order that help may be given on the first sign of poisoning. Medical assistance should be within easy reach. Systematic instruction should be given in first-aid methods and the use of apparatus for oxygen and carbon-dioxide inhalation. The possibility of skin absorption must always be borne in mind. A victim whose skin or clothing has been splashed with aniline may turn blue in the face and begin to stagger. Someone may take him out to the fresh air or administer oxygen, when what he most needs is to have his clothes removed and be given a bath. Workers entering stills and similar chambers should always be equipped with breathing apparatus and a supply of oxygen. Other aids, such as safety belts which are held by helpers, involve certain risks, especially as the rescuer is easily induced to spring to the assistance of his unfortunate mate without the necessary breathing equipment. The frequency of such accidents calls urgently for the provision of breathing apparatus.

(h) Trinitrophenylmethylnitramine

Trinitrophenylmethylnitramine, N-nitro-N-methyl-2,4,6,trinitraniline or tetranitromethylaniline, is the explosive *tetryl* or *tetralite*. It is known in the fighting services as *composition exploding* or *CE*. It is a pale yellow crystalline powder, very stable when pure, but it undergoes detonation readily and is frequently used as a primer in detonators.

Symptoms and Signs of Tetryl Poisoning

Tetryl causes yellow staining of the hands of workers in from one to three days and of the face, neck, scalp and hair in from one to three weeks. The colour deepens to orange on exposure to sunlight. New workers sometimes complain of a sharp tingling sensation in the nose. This causes sneezing and, rarely, epistaxis. These symptoms are due to the irritating effect of the crystals on the nasal mucous membrane. The commonest complaint from *tetryl* workers is dermatitis. This starts as an erythema, followed by a pink papular eruption accompanied by some exfoliation. It generally affects the face first, especially at the sides of the nose and around the eyes and the corners of the mouth. Later the condition spreads to the chin, neck and back of the head, causing severe irritation. In some cases there is conjunctivitis and even gross œdema of the eyelids which may prevent the patient from opening the eyes for two or three days. Mild cases clear up in a few days, but in severe cases the rash often persists for two or three weeks. Suspension from work is seldom necessary. *Tetryl* rarely gives rise to any constitutional symptoms. A certain number of new workers complain of epigastric pain with nausea or vomiting. These symptoms bear no relation to food and are seldom severe enough to keep the patient away from work (Hilton and Swanston, 1941).

Preventive Measures

Protective clothing should be provided, and it is necessary to insist upon frequent changes of underclothes. Workrooms must be well ventilated and the atmosphere dry. Great care should be taken to avoid raising dust.

The hands should be washed thoroughly in running water before the face is washed. The addition of 5 per cent sodium sulphite will assist removal of *tetryl* by converting it into a soluble substance (Silver, 1938). Workers should be warned against the use of proprietary ointments. A water-soluble skin varnish can be used on the face and arms before beginning work. Calamine lotion should be applied. Oils and ointments aggravate the condition and must be avoided except after the acute inflammation has subsided, when the affected parts may be cleansed with olive oil. Workers who recover from an acute attack in less than a fortnight may be allowed to resume contact work after a further week. If a second or third attack occurs, it is an indication that the patient is susceptible and should be removed permanently from handling *tetryl*. A worker who develops œdema of the face and peri-orbital tissues is a bad risk, and must be removed permanently from contact at the first outbreak of the eruption.

(i) Phenylenediamine

Of the three isomers of phenylenediamine, the *ortho*-compound is of little importance. The dye *ursol* as used in the fur industry is a mixture of the *meta-* and *para*-isomers. *Para*-phenylenediamine is a colourless crystalline solid which rapidly oxidizes in the air, darkening in colour (fig. 206). At various times it has been used in dilute aqueous solution as a constituent of hair dyes, including proprietary preparations such as *inecto*, *koorpa* and *primal*.

Dermatitis and Asthma

It is well known that this dye may cause dermatitis and sometimes asthma. In 1929 Mayer and Forster examined 181 persons employed in the fur trade in which *para*-phenylenediamine was used as a dye, and found that 111 had suffered from dermatitis or asthma. It seems that the asthma is due to direct stimulation of the bronchi rather than to allergy, since Hanzlik (1923) was able to demonstrate constriction of the intact bronchi of dogs and guinea-pigs.

Skin Eruption due to Sensitization

The skin eruption is an eczematous dermatitis appearing as minute pink papules on the face, neck and forearms. Moist points, such as the lips, corners of the mouth, angles of the eyelids and orifices of the nose, especially suffer (White, 1924). In discussions of the ætiology of fur dermatitis many authors dismiss personal idiosyncrasy as irrelevant. However, Ingram (1932) demonstrated delayed reactions to patch tests and claimed that the dermatitis must therefore be a sensitization phenomenon. The tests were made with pieces of lint saturated with 1 per cent aqueous solution of *para*-phenylenediamine. Approximately 4 per cent of 1,000 normal subjects showed dermatitis, which appeared from twenty-four hours to twenty-four days after the test was applied.

Systemic Effects of *Para*-phenylenediamine

The systemic effects of *para*-phenylenediamine are less common and have received little attention. Nott (1924) described a case of systemic poisoning without dermatitis in the proprietor of a hairdressing saloon. This patient had suffered for three years from attacks of weakness and vomiting, sometimes followed by unconsciousness. After a night's rest the effects disappeared. He was seen in a severe attack, when his face was cyanotic and swollen. The lips were violet, the tongue swollen and the gums purple. After three months' avoidance of exposure to the dye, he had no further symptoms.

Subacute Necrosis of the Liver

Israëls and Susman (1934) recorded the death of a girl aged twenty-one years who for five years had worked in a hairdressing department as a dyer. She used *para*-phenylenediamine and was provided with rubber gloves, but after she had applied the dye she had to shampoo the hair, and for this the gloves were removed. At no time had she experienced any skin reaction directly traceable to the dye. She developed toxic jaundice and died of hepatic insufficiency after an illness lasting seven months. At necropsy the liver was small and showed the changes of subacute atrophy with regeneration nodules. The patient was evidently unusually susceptible to the poison.

Refractory Anæmia caused by *Para*-phenylenediamine

Baldridge showed in 1935 that anæmia may follow the use of *para*-phenylenediamine as a hair dye. At least four cases have been described, and in all of them the anæmia was of the macrocytic, high colour-index type, and refractory to treatment with iron or liver. One of these women repeatedly showed a red-cell count below 1,000,000 per c.mm., and though she improved temporarily after eight blood transfusions, her condition remained unchanged four years after the onset of symptoms (Bomford and Rhoads, 1951).

Dermatitis from Colour Developers

Workers who handle photographic colour developers consisting of substituted *para*-phenylenediamines are liable to two morphologically differentiated skin diseases. In some patients, the eruption is eczematous and in others it is lichenoid. Fry (1965) described these rashes as appearing on hands or forearms, suggesting direct contact as the cause. In a few patients the eruption may appear at other sites. Oral lesions were not observed. Out of 20 patients 13 had eczematous and 7 lichenoid eruptions with atypical lichen planus histology. Patch tests were positive in 17.

Preventive Measures

The use of *para*-phenylenediamine for cosmetic purposes and as a dye for furs, stockings and blouses might with advantage be forbidden. Short of this, care must be taken to remove surplus *para*-phenylenediamine from dyed fabrics by thorough washing. The workers who dry or cut fur must be protected from dust containing the dye, and where those exposed to risk are men they should be clean-shaven. Patch testing of the skin should be carried out on all applicants for the job of ladies' hairdresser; perhaps one in a hundred will show a positive result and must therefore be rejected. Hairdressers handling the dye must wear rubber gloves. So also must photographers whenever they handle developers.

BIBLIOGRAPHY

The Aromatic Carbon Compounds

FRAENKEL, S. (1912), *Die Arzneimittel Synthese auf Grundlage der Beziehungen zwischen chemischem Aufbau und Wirkung*, Berlin.

HAMILTON, A. (1925), *Industrial Poisons in the United States*, Macmillan, New York, p. 490.

Benzene

ERF, L. A., and RHOADS, C. P. (1939), *J. industr. Hyg.*, **21**, 421.

GLIBERT, D. (1935), *Brux.-méd.*, **16**, 194.

GREENBURG, L., MAYERS, M. R., GOLDWATER, L., and SMITH, A. R. (1939), *Ibid.*, **21**, 395.

HAMILTON, A. (1928), *J. industr. Hyg.*, **10**, 227; (1934), *Industrial Toxicology*, New York, pp. 162, 195.

HAYHURST, E. R., and NEISWANDER, B. E. (1931), *J. Amer. med. Ass.*, **96**, 269.

HUNTER, D., MILTON, R., PERRY, K. M. A., BARRIE, H. J., LOUTIT, J. F., and MARSHALL, T. S. (1944), *Brit. J. industr. Med.*, **1**, 238.

HUNTER, F. T. (1939), *J. Amer. med. Ass.*, **21**, 331.

K. K. *Gewerbe-Inspectoren* (1911), p. 490.

KORÁNYI, Baron Alex. von (1914), *Seventeenth Internat. Congr. Med.*, Lond., 1913, Med., Part 2, Sect. 6, Oxf. Univ. Press.

LEGGE, T. M. (1919), *Annual Report of the Chief Inspector of Factories and Workshops for the year 1918*, H.M.S.O., London, Cmd. 340, p. 78.

LIGNAC, G. O. E. (1932), *Krankheitsforsch*, **9**, 403.

MALLORY, T. B., GALL, E. A., and BRICKLEY, W. J. (1939), *J. industr. Hyg.*, **21**, 355.

PENATI, F., and VIGLIANI, E. C. (1938), *Rass. med. Industr.*, **9**, 345.

RONCHETTI, V. (1922), *Atti. Soc. lombarda Sci. med. biol.*, **11**, 322.

SALTER, W. T. (1940), *New Engl. J. Med.*, **222**, 146.

SANTESSON, C. G. (1897), *Arch. Hyg.*, **31**, 336.

SCHRENK, H. H., YANT, W. P., PEARCE, S. J., and SAYERS, R. R. (1940), *J. industr. Hyg.*, **22**, 53.

SELLING, L. (1910), *Bull. Johns Hopk. Hosp.*, **21**, 33; (1916), *Johns Hopk. Hosp. Rep.*, **17**, 83.

Hexachlorobenzene

ÇAM, C. (1959), *Dirim*, Istanbul, **34**, 11.

KANTEMIR, I., ÇAM, C., and KAYAALP, O. (1960), *Türk Ijiyen ve Tecrübi Biyoloji Dergisi*, Ankara, **20**, 79.

KANTEMIR, I., GENER, S., KAYAALP, O., and TIMLIOGLU, Ö. (1960), *ibid.*, **20**, 31.
OCKNER, R. J., and SCHMID, R. (1961), *Nature*, **189**, 499.
SCHMID, R. (1960), *New Engl. J. med.*, **263**, 397.

Hexachlorocyclohexane

BEHRBOHM, P., and BRANDT, B. (1959), *Arch. f. Gewerebepath. u. Gewerbehyg.*, **17**, 365.
DANOPOULOS, E., MELISSINOS, K. and KATSAS, G. (1953), *Arch. Industr. Hyg. and Occup. Med.*, **8**, 582.
HEIBERG, O. M. and WRIGHT, H. N. (1955), *Arch. Industr. Health*, Chicago, **11**, 457.
NICHOLLS, R. W. (1958), *Med. J. Austral.*, **45**, 42.
SCHMIEDEBERG, J. and WASSERBURGER, H. J. (1953), *Anz. Schädlingsk.*, **26**, 129.

Toluylene Di-*iso*cyanate

BAADER, E. W. (1956), *Med. Sachverst.*, **70**, 128.
HAMA, G. M. (1957), *A.M.A. Archiv. industr. Hyg.*, **16**, 232.
MUNN, A. (1965), *Ann. occup. Hyg.*, **8**, 163.
PIPER, R. (1965), *Brit. J. industr. Med.*, **22**, 247.
WILLIAMSON, K. S. (1964), *Trans. Ass. industr. med. Offrs.*, **14**, 81; (1965), *ibid.*, **15**, 29.

Phenol

ABRAHAMS, R. (1900), *Pediatrics*, **9**, 241.
BEDDARD, A. P. (1909), *Quart. Journ. Med.*, **3**, 329.
BROWN, W. H. (1895), *Lancet*, **1**, 543.
CZERNY (1882) quoted by Zangger, H. (1934), *Occupation and Health*, I. L. O., Geneva.
EVANS, S. J. (1952), *Brit. J. industr. Med.*, **9**, 227.
FAIRHALL, L. T. (1957), *Industrial Toxicology*, 2nd ed., Williams and Wilkins, Baltimore.
GARROD, A. E. (1909), *Inborn Errors of Metabolism*, 2nd ed., Hodder and Stoughton, London.
GIBSON, W. (1905), *Queen's med. Quart.*, **10**, 133.
GODLEE, Sir Rickman J. (1924), *Lord Lister*, Clarendon Press, Oxford.
HAMILTON, A. (1925), *Industrial Poisons in the United States*, Macmillan, New York.
HAMILTON, A., and HARDY, H. L. (1949), *Industrial Toxicology*, Hoeber, New York.
POPE, F. M. (1906), *Lancet*, **1**, 24.
SCWARTZ, L., TULIPAN, L., and BIRMINGHAM, D. J. (1957), *Occupational Diseases of the Skin*, 3rd ed., Kimpton, London.
TURTLE, W. R. M., and DOLAN, T. (1922), *Lancet*, **2**, 1273.
ZANGGER, H. (1934), *Occupation and Health*, I.L.O., Geneva.

Pentachlorphenol

CAMPBELL, A. M. G. (1952), *Brit. med. J.*, **2**, 415.
HAYES, W. J., Jr. (1963), *Clinical Handbook on Economic Poisons*, U.S. Dept. of Health, Education and Welfare, Atlanta, Georgia.
PIPER, R. (1965), *Brit. J. industr. Med.*, **22**, 247.

Quinone and Hydroquinone

FAIRHALL, L. T. (1957), *Industrial Toxicology*, 2nd ed., Williams and Wilkins, Baltimore.

MILLER, S. J. H. (1954), *Trans. Ophthal. Soc.*, **74**, 349.

OGLESBY, F. L., STERNER, J. H., and ANDERSON, B. (1947), *J. Industr. hyg. and tox.*, **29**, 74.

STERNER, J. H., OGLESBY, F. L., and ANDERSON, B. (1947), *Ibid.*, **29**, 60.

VELHAGEN, K. (1931), *Klinische Monatsblatter f. Augenheilkunde*, **86**, 729.

WYERS, H. (1952), *Trans. assoc. industr. med. off.*, **11**, 109.

Aromatic Nitro- and Amino-derivatives

BUCKELL, M., and RICHARDSON, D. (1950), *Brit. J. industr. Med.*, **7**, 131.

FERTMAN, M. H., and FERTMAN, M. B., (1955), *Medicine, Baltimore*, **34**, 131.

GROSS, E., BOCK, M., and HELLRUNG, F. (1942), *Arch. exp. Path. Pharmak.*, **200**, 271.

HAMBLIN, D. O., and MANGELSDORFF, A. F. (1938), *J. industr. Hyg.*, **20**, 523.

HEINZ, R. (1890), *Virchows Arch.*, **122**, 112.

HENDERSON, Y., and HAGGARD, H. W. (1943), *Noxious Gases*, Reinhold, New York.

JOPE, E. M. (1946), *Brit. J. industr. Med.*, **3**, 136.

MALDEN, W. (1907), *J. Hyg.*, **7**, 672.

MICHEL, H. O. (1938), *Journ. biol. Chem.*, **126**, 323.

MOORE, B. (1918), *Spec. Rep. Ser. med. Res. Com., Lond.*, No. 11.

PETERS, J. P., and VAN SLYKE, D. D. (1932), *Quantitative Clinical Chemistry, Interpretations*, Baltimore, **2**, 623.

PRICE-JONES, C., and BOYCOTT, A. E. (1909), *Guy's Hosp. Rept.*, **63**, 309.

REJSEK, K. (1947), *Acta med. scand.*, **127**, 179.

SCHMIDT, P. (1930), *Occupation and Health*, I.L.O., Geneva, **1**, 252.

WEBSTER, S. H. (1949), *Blood*, **4**, 479.

WHITE, R. P., and HAY, J. (1901), *Lancet*, **2**, 582.

(a) Nitrobenzene

ENGEL, H. (1934), *Occupation and Health*, I.L.O., Geneva, **2**, 334.

HAMILTON, A. (1919–20), *J. industr. Hyg.*, **1**, 200.

(b) Dinitrobenzene

ENGEL, H. (1930), *Occupation and Health*, I.L.O., Geneva, **1**, 567.

LEGGE, T. M. (1917), *Proc. R. Soc. Med.*, **10**, i, Gen. Repts., Spec. Discussion, **1**.

LIPSCHÜTZ, W. (1920), *Z. f. physiol. Chem.*, **109**, 189.

MALDEN, W. (1907), *J. Hyg.*, **7**, 672.

REJSEK, K. (1947), *Acta med, scand.*, **127**, 179.

WHITE, R. P., and HAY, J. (1901), *Lancet*, **2**, 582.

(c) Trinitrotoluene

BRIDGE, J. C. (1942), *Proc. R. Soc. Med.*, **35**, 553.

DAVIE, T. B. (1942), *Ibid.*, **35**, 558.

HAMILTON, A., and JOHNSTONE, R. T. (1945), *Industrial Toxicology*, Oxford Loose-Leaf Medicine, New York, p. 661.

HIMSWORTH, H. P., and GLYNN, L. E. (1942), *Clin. Sci.*, **4**, 421.
INGHAM, J. (1941), *Lancet*, **2**, 554.
JOPE, E. M. (1946), *Brit. J. industr. Med.*, **3**, 136.
LANE, R. E. (1942), *Proc. R. Soc. Med.*, **35**, 556.
LEGGE, T. M. (1917), *Ibid.*, **10**, i, Gen. Rept., Spec. Discussion, 1.
MOORE, B. (1918), *Spec. Rep. Ser. med. Res. Com., Lond.*, No. 11.
PANTON, P. N. (1917), *Lancet*, **2**, 77.
RIMINGTON, C., and GOLDBLATT, M. W. (1940), *Ibid.*, **1**, 73.
ROBERTS, H. M. (1941), *Brit. med. J.*, **2**, 647.
STEWART, A. (1943), Personal communication.
SWANSTON, C. (1942), *Proc. R. Soc. Med.*, **35**, 553.
TURNBULL, H. M. (1917), *Ibid.*, **10**, i, Gen. Rept., Spec. Discussion, 47.
WEBSTER, T. A. (1916), *Lancet*, **2**, 1029.

(d) Dinitrophenol

CAZENEUVE, P., and LÉPINE, R. (1885), *C.R. Acad. Sci. Paris*, **101**, 1167.
CUTTING, W. C., MEHRTENS, H. G., and TAINTER, M. L. (1933), *J. Amer. med. Ass.*, **101**, 193.
DAVIDSON, E. N., and SHAPIRO, M. (1934), *Ibid.*, **103**, 480.
HARDGROVE, M., and STERN, N. (1938), *Industr. med.*, **7**, 9.
HEYMANS, C., and BOUCKAERT, J. J. (1929), *Arch. intern. Pharm. et de Therap.*, **35**, 63.
HITCH, J. M., and SCHWARTZ, W. F. (1936), *J. Amer. med. Ass.*, **106**, 2130.
HORNER, W. D., JONES, R. B., and BOARDMAN, W. W. (1935), *Ibid.*, **105**, 108.
LEGGE, Sir T. (1934), *Industrial Maladies*, Oxford University Press, London.
MARTIN, E. (1930), *Occupation and Health*, I.L.O., Geneva, **1**, 576.
NADLER, J. E. (1935), *J. Amer. med. Ass.*, **105**, 12.
PERKINS, R. G. (1919), *Publ. Hlth. Rept., Wash.*, **34**, 2335.
POOLE, F. E., and HAINING, R. B. (1934), *J. Amer. med. Ass.*, **102**, 1141.
SIDEL, N. (1934), *Ibid.*, **103**, 254.
SILVER, S. (1934), *Ibid.*, **103**, 1058.
TAINTER, M. L., STOCKTON, A. B., and CUTTING, W. C. (1933), *Ibid.*, **101**, 1472.

(e) *Para*methylaminophenol Sulphate (Metol)

BUSATTO, S. (1939), *Deutsche Stschr. f.d. ges. gerichtl. Med.*, **31**, 285.
PALMOVIĆ, V., and FRKETIĆ, J. (1955), *Arkiv Hig. Rada*, **6**, 135.
WYERS, H. (1952), *Trans. assoc. industr. med. off.*, **11**, 109.
ZEIDMAN, I., and DEUTL, R. (1945), *Amer. J. med. sci.*, **210**, 328.

(f) Dinitro-*ortho*-cresol

BIDSTRUP, P. L., BONNELL, J. A. L., and HARVEY, D. G. (1952), *Lancet*, **1**, 795.
BIDSTRUP, P. L., and PAYNE, D. J. H. (1951), *Brit. med. J.*, **2**, 16.
DODDS, E. C., and POPE, W. J. (1933), *Lancet*, **2**, 152.
GAHAN, J. B. (1942), *Journ. econ. Ent.*, **55**, 669.
GATE, J., and CHANIAL, G. (1936), *Bull. soc. franc. Derm. Syph.*, **41**, 1305.
HARVEY, D. G. (1952), *Lancet*, **1**, 796.

HARVEY, D. G., BIDSTRUP, P. L., and BONNELL, J. A. L. (1951), *Brit. med. J.*, **2**, 13.
HORNER, W. D. (1941), *Trans. Amer. ophth. Soc.*, **77**, 405.
KING, E., and HARVEY, D. G. (1953), *Biochem. J.*, **53**, 196.
MCDONALD, J. M. (1943), *Baltimore Health News*, **20**, 9.
MEREWETHER, E. R. A. (1943), *Annual Report of the Chief Inspector of Factories*, H.M.S.O., London, Cmd. 6563, p. 51.
PARKER, V. H. (1949), *Analyst*, **74**, 646.
PARSONS, F. B. (1948), *Personal communication*.
POLLARD, A. B., and FILBEE, J. F. (1951), *Lancet*, **2**, 618.
RIPPER, W. E. (1960), *Personal communication*.
STEER, C. (1951), *Ibid.*, **1**, 1419.
STOTT, H. (1956), *Brit. med. J.*, **1**, 900.
TATTERSFIELD, F., GIMINGHAM, C. T., and MORRIS, H. M. (1925), *Ann. appl. Biol.*, **12**, 218.

(g) Aniline

AGASSE-LAFONT, E., FEIL, A., and DE BALSAC, F. H. (1926), *Pr. méd.*, **34**, 1169.
ENGEL, H. (1930), *Occupation and Health*, I.L.O., Geneva, **1**, 567.
HAMBLIN, D. O., and MANGELSDORFF, A. F. (1938), *J. industr. Hyg.*, **20**, 523.
HAMILTON, A. (1925), *Industrial Poisons in the United States*, New York, p. 493.
MALDEN, W. (1907), *J. Hyg.*, **7**, 672.

(h) Trinitrophenylmethylnitramine

HILTON, J., and SWANSTON, C. N. (1941), *Brit. med. J.*, **2**, 509.
SILVER, A. L. L. (1938), *Journ. R. Army med. Cps.*, **71**, 87.

(j) Phenylenediamine

BALDRIDGE, C. W. (1935), *Amer. J. med. Sci.*, **189**, 759.
BOMFORD, R. R., and RHOADS, C. P. (1941), *Quart. J. Med.*, **10**, 175.
FRY, L. (1965), *Brit. J. Derm.*, **77**, 456.
HANZLIK, P. J. (1922–3), *J. industr. Hyg.*, **4**, 386, 448
INGRAM, J. T. (1932), *Brit. J. Derm.*, **44**, 422.
ISRAËLS, M. C. G., and SUSMAN, W. (1934), *Lancet*, **1**, 508.
MAYER, R. L., and FÖRSTER, M. (1929), *Zbl. GewHyg.*, **6**, 171.
NOTT, H. W. (1924), *Brit. med. J.*, **1**, 421.
WHITE, R. P. (1924), *Journ. State Med.*, **32**, 16.

CHAPTER IX

THE ALIPHATIC CARBON COMPOUNDS

In the history of chemical industry we have seen (p. 154) how the use of petroleum (fig. 207) as a raw material has come to rival that of coal. Crude petroleum contains a high proportion of aliphatic compounds, that is to say, open-chain hydrocarbons (fig. 208). This group of substances, of which methane is the simplest representative, includes many natural gases, light petroleum derivatives and higher paraffins (fig. 209). The number of

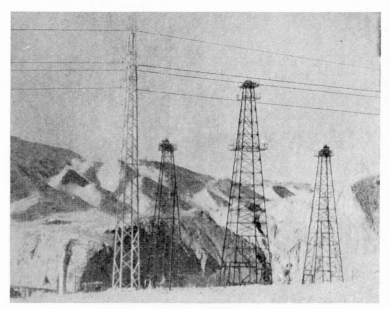

Fig. 207.—Derricks of Petroleum Wells at the Abadan Oilfield
(*By courtesy of J. Arthur Rank Organisation, Ltd.*)

aliphatic hydrocarbons and more particularly of their derivatives is, of course, very large. The following compounds will be discussed—methyl alcohol, nitroglycerine, nitrocellulose, the halogenated hydrocarbons, ethylene chlorhydrin, diethylene dioxide, carbon disulphide and acrylonitrile.

Methyl Alcohol

Methyl alcohol or methanol, CH_3OH, is a clear, colourless, volatile, inflammable liquid with a burning taste and an odour somewhat resembling that of ethyl alcohol. It is also known as wood alcohol, wood spirit, wood naphtha, carbinol, acetone alcohol, colonial spirit, methylated spirit, pyroxylic spirit, Columbian spirit, Eagle spirit, Hastings spirit, Lion d'Or or Manhattan spirit.

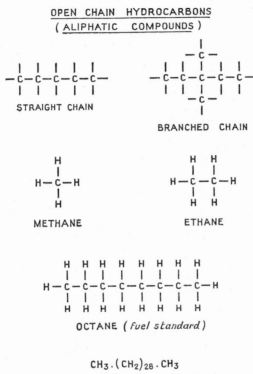

FIG. 208

Uses

In timber-producing countries, natural methanol to the extent of 25,000 tons annually is still produced by the destructive distillation of wood in retorts. Synthetic methanol is made to the extent of 300,000 tons annually by a process first developed by I.G. Farbenindustrie in 1924 and now worked throughout the world. It involves passing a mixture of carbon monoxide and hydrogen at high pressure and temperature over a catalyst such as zinc oxide or copper. It is used in antifreeze for motor-car radiators, as fuel for racing cars, as a denaturant of ethyl alcohol, as a solvent for paints, varnishes, shellacs and paint removers, and in dry cleaning. By far the largest amount is used in the manufacture of formaldehyde; smaller amounts are used to make synthetic indigo, explosives, felt hats, shoes and linoleum.

PETROLEUM

METHANE
ETHANE
PROPANE
BUTANE
} NATURAL GAS

PETROL (gasoline, motor fuel)
PETROLEUM BENZINE
PETROLEUM NAPHTHA (solvent naphtha)
PARAFFIN OIL (kerosene, lamp oil)
} LIGHT PETROLEUM

FUEL OILS (diesel oil)
LUBRICATING OILS
LIQUID PARAFFIN
SOFT PARAFFIN (petroleum jelly, vaseline)
PARAFFIN WAXES
} HIGHER PARAFFINS

FIG. 209

History of Poisoning

Although a case of poisoning was reported in 1855, the toxicity of methanol was not really appreciated until well into the present century. One of the principal reasons for this is the extreme variation in the individual response to a dose taken by mouth. Thus it has been known since 1911 that one man may be blinded by drinking 4 millilitres of 40 per cent methanol and another who drinks 4 litres may suffer from mild transient gastro-intestinal symptoms only. As late as 1910 methyl alcohol was freely substituted for the more expensive ethyl alcohol, and in many wines, brandies and whiskeys sold on New York's East Side the proportion ranged from 24 to 43 per cent. Occasional instances of poisoning after ingestion of methanol were attributed to contaminants such as acetaldehyde, allyl alcohol, acetone or fusel oils. So little did doctors think of wood alcohol as toxic that Ehrlich once used it as a solvent for salvarsan. And although it was demonstrated in 1923 that a group of dock workers in Hamburg had been poisoned by chemically pure methanol, doubts as to its toxicity were still voiced as late as 1936.

A Poison which was peculiarly American

In industry, methanol has been peculiarly an American poison. Up to 1904 in the United States of America the use of ethyl alcohol in industry was illegal. Since denatured ethyl alcohol, so commonly used in Europe, was unknown in American industry, methyl alcohol became the customary solvent. The law providing for the use of tax-free ethyl alcohol came about as a result of cases of death and of blindness from inhalation of the vapour of methyl alcohol by men employed in varnishing the interior of beer vats (Patillo, 1899; Hale, 1901). But denatured grain alcohol was very slow in displacing wood alcohol in industry, so much so that in 1915 no fewer than 2,500,000 workers in the United States of America came in contact with wood alcohol in the course of their work. Poisoning caused either by inhalation or by absorption through the skin was common. It was not until the days of prohibition when cases of death and blindness from drinking bootleg liquor occurred again and again that the danger of methyl alcohol loomed large in the public mind and many manufacturers hastened to give up its use (Hamilton and Hardy, 1949). Meanwhile there were many instances where the employer wrongly asserted that the poisoned men had drunk the solvent.

Toxicology of the Alcohols

The alcohols used in industry are methyl, ethyl, isopropyl, normal butyl and amyl. Of this series methyl alcohol, the member with the lowest molecular weight, is the only one to be feared. In spite of misleading animal experiments dating back as far as 1869 and suggesting the contrary, it is perfectly clear to the clinical worker that the toxicity of this alkyl series diminishes with increasing molecular weight. Thus a man who drinks or inhales methyl alcohol, CH_3OH, is readily blinded or killed, whereas ethyl alcohol, $CH_2.CH_3OH$, only makes him drunk and *iso*propyl alcohol, $CH_2.CH_2.CH_3OH$, won't even make him happy. In industry, great importance attaches to the fact that these alcohols are volatile in inverse proportion to their molecular weight. The fact that methyl alcohol is so volatile enhances the hazard of its use as a solvent for paints and varnishes, especially when they are used in spray guns.

Symptomatology

When methyl alcohol is ingested there follows a latent period usually of about twenty-four hours before the onset of symptoms. In industrial cases a few days' exposure is often enough to cause irritation of the skin and conjunctiva, dizziness, staggering gait, headache, anorexia, nausea, vomiting, severe colicky upper abdominal pain and blurring of vision. The trouble with the eyes begins usually with pain in the eyeballs and tenderness on pressure, slight photophobia, and then indistinct vision with dancing spots, snowstorm effects or flashes before the eyes. If loss of vision progresses, there is concentric constriction of the fields both for form and for colour. When the concentration of methyl alcohol inhaled is very high, the worker may suffer a degree of poisoning equal to that when it is taken by mouth. Severe headache is rapidly followed by blindness, delirium, stupor, acute mania with retrograde amnesia, coma convulsions and death in respiratory failure (Bennett and others, 1953).

Physical Signs

The patient is apprehensive and uncomfortable. The condition is afebrile, the skin cool, with profuse perspiration and a rubeose cyanosis. Although in all severe cases acidosis is an outstanding feature, the incidence of overbreathing is low and dyspnœa never a major complaint. The pupils are dilated and react sluggishly. Both deep-seated pain on rotation of the eyeballs and paralysis of extra-ocular muscles with diplopia and ptosis are rare. Colour scotomata and concentric constriction of the fields of vision are seen and, of course, total loss of light perception may occur. Opththal-moscopic examination shows hyperæmia of the discs without swelling and with peripapillary radial grey streaks of retinal œdema extending sometimes to the macula. These changes often subside in two weeks. The blind who survive ultimately show the white discs and attenuated vessels of primary optic atrophy.

Diagnosis

The severity of the changes in the fundi is a better index of the degree of acidosis than any other clinical finding. Patients with confusion, stupor or coma often have, in addition, headache, vomiting and neck rigidity so that their condition resembles meningitis. Severe abdominal pain is often accompanied by striking rigidity and tenderness of the abdominal muscles resembling the acute abdomen. Bradycardia indicates the onset of a fatal termination, but often the blood-pressure remains normal and the heart-beat may continue after respiration has ceased (Bennett and others, 1953).

Effects of Ethyl Alcohol on the Metabolism of Methyl Alcohol

Much of our modern knowledge of the treatment of methanol poisoning originates in the careful clinical observations of a Norwegian ophthalmolo-gist Røe, who in 1943 obtained detailed histories as to the exact types and quantities of alcoholic drink consumed by three Oslo friends. He concluded that the great individual variation in the duration of the latent period and in the response to methyl alcohol depended on the simultaneous or subse-quent ingestion of ethyl alcohol which, he believed, delayed or prevented the oxidation of methyl alcohol, and thus the onset of acidosis. A large amount of experimental work, mostly in animals, confirms and amplifies the clinical observations of Røe. Zatman (1946) studied the effect of ethanol on the metabolism of its methyl homologue, demonstrating that alcohol dehydrogenase was able to oxidize methanol at only one-ninth of the rate for ethanol, and that ethanol in equimolar concentration completely in-hibited the oxidation of methanol.

Mechanism of Methyl-alcohol Poisoning

The following tentative hypothesis of the mechanism of methyl-alcohol intoxication may be advanced. In the body methyl alcohol is partly oxidized to the much more toxic products, formaldehyde and formic acid. The latent period between ingestion of methyl alcohol and onset of symptoms repre-sents the time during which these toxic oxidation products are accumulat-ing. The oxidation products of methyl alcohol then poison certain oxida-tive processes in the cells, possibly by combining with iron in the respiratory oxidase. This results in failure of formation of carbon dioxide, together with the accumulation of organic acids, which accounts for the extreme acidosis. If, however, even a little ethyl alcohol is present in the blood-stream, it competes successfully with the methyl alcohol for the available alcohol dehydrogenase in the liver (Bartlett, 1950). In this way the oxidation of methyl alcohol is delayed until all the ethyl alcohol has been meta-bolized, and this explains the prolongation of the latent period when ethyl alcohol is consumed together with or after methyl alcohol. All the symp-toms of methyl-alcohol poisoning, except amblyopia, are directly due to acidosis. The degree of amblyopia is parallel to the degree of acidosis. The retinal changes are due primarily to hypoxia, which develops early in the retina because this tissue contains less iron in relation to its oxygen re-quirement than any other part of the body (Røe, 1946).

Treatment

This hypothesis is by no means proved, but it at least allows us to formulate a policy for treating acute methyl-alcohol poisoning. Immedi-ately the patient is admitted to hospital the alkali reserve should be esti-mated, and in severe cases intravenous infusion of sodium bicarbonate should be started without waiting for the result. The amount administered should be controlled by serial estimations of alkali reserve, or, if this is impossible, by testing the pH of the urine. The required amount should be given quickly; in severe cases 60–70 grams is necessary in the first instance. A watch should be kept both for recurrence of acidosis and for such overdose effects as tetany, hypokalaemia and sodium retention. It is unprofitable to give sodium bicarbonate by mouth to nauseated patients, and this route should be used only in the mildest cases. For parenteral treatment, sixth-molar sodium lactate seems quite effective. There seems to be good theoretical justification for giving small quantities of ethyl alcohol four-hourly; but massive alkalinization is the outstanding life-saving and sight-saving measure against acute methyl-alcohol poisoning in man.

Preventive Treatment

As a solvent, except where it can be used in closed systems, methy alcohol should be replaced by safe substitutes. The application of wood-alcohol shellac or any other comparable varnish or paint by means of brushes or spray guns should be forbidden except where adequate exhaust ventilation is installed. Because methanol is a cumulative poison forming in the body formic acid and formaldehyde, continued exposure to re-peated small doses may be more harmful than a single large dose. It is for this reason that men who use varnish with this solvent in small airless spaces are exposed to a deadly risk. Workers must be warned that if they spill methyl alcohol on their clothing they must at once remove that clothing, for men who have neglected this precaution have been blinded.

NITROGLYCERINE

Nitroglycerine is an ester of glycerine and nitric acid, glyceryl trinitrate. It is a pale yellow oil, has a sweet burning taste and is poisonous. The Swedish chemist, Scheele (1742–86), whose early life was spent as a struggling apothecary, discovered glycerine in 1779. The Italian chemist, Ascanio Sobrero of Turin, was the first to make nitroglycerine in 1847. Inhalation of its vapour produces violent headache, and the same effect is often caused by handling dynamite. Although a nitrate, its pharmacological actions resemble those of nitrites such as amyl nitrite, but it has the advantage of acting more slowly.

Alfred Bernhard Nobel, 1833–96

Alfred Bernhard Nobel, the outstanding figure in the history of explosives, was born in 1833 in Stockholm, and died in 1896 at San Remo, Italy. He was therefore a contemporary of William Henry Perkin (1838–1907). His father was an architect and inventor. Four years after his third son, Alfred, was born, he went to St. Petersburg where he invented land mines filled with gunpowder for the Russian army. Thus Alfred went to Russia when he was nine years old, having attended a formal school for two terms only when he was a boy of eight. For the following eight years he had two private tutors—a Swede first, then a Russian; he never attended a university. At sixteen he stood head and shoulders above other boys of his age, as to both knowledge and intellectual maturity. Though trained as a chemist, he always called himself a civil engineer. He was a remarkable linguist, speaking English, French, Swedish, Russian, German and Italian. He was a sickly, dreamy and introspective youth who preferred to be alone.

Dynamite Factories in Many Countries

He created great business enterprises which developed the manufacture of nitroglycerine, dynamite, smokeless powder and other high explosives; between 1871 and 1873 he put up ten dynamite factories in different European countries, and in Great Britain alone he took out 122 patents. He and his brothers were financially interested in the Baku oil fields and in many other industries. He worked hard at his inventions, never leaving a particular idea until he had modified it in such a way as to make it succeed. Nobel had to a marked degree the gifts of a poet, deep feeling and considerable powers of imagination. He was at heart a pronounced optimist, and he believed not only in a happier and healthier humanity in the future but also that the conquests of natural science would create happiness for coming generations. He was an idealist and a cynic, a brilliant conversationalist and a shy recluse, a man of almost feminine sensitivity who at times sacrificed lives without flinching. He knew well that it was useless to expect an explosive substance to come into general use without waste of life.

Foundation of the Nobel Prizes

The creator of dynamite was no dynamic personality, he would never have been noticed in a crowd. He was a little man, repressed, inhibited, self-effacing and colourless (Pauli, 1947). Although he lived for many years in Paris, he was the loneliest millionaire on earth, spending a great deal of time in hotels and trains. He never married and he ended his days surrounded only by his French servants. No relative or close friend was with him when he died. The contradiction in his life was that he was a great inventor of war material who was interested in peace. This conflict he partly solved when he left the bulk of his fortune in trust for the foundation of the Nobel prizes in physics, chemistry, medicine, literature and peace. His estate amounted to more than 33,000,000 crowns, of which nearly 10 per cent was taken in taxes. The first Nobel prizes were awarded in 1901.

Modern Blasting Explosives

Nobel began to apply nitroglycerine as a blasting explosive in 1863. During the next few years so many accidents attended the manufacture, transport and use of *Nobel's blasting oil* that in some countries, including Great Britain, it was prohibited. It was dangerous also because it tended to creep into fissures in the rock and remain unexploded. Nothing daunted, Nobel tried solid absorbents, of which kieselguhr was the most satisfactory. Dried kieselguhr is able to absorb three or four times its weight of nitroglycerine. *Kieselguhr dynamite* was first made in 1866. Nobel admitted that in 1875 he applied collodion, which is nitrocellulose dissolved in ether and alcohol, to a cut on his finger and that this gave him the idea to make *blasting gelatine*. The usual blend is nitroglycerine 93 and collodion cotton 7. Blasting gelatine is a light-yellow solid, translucent and elastic, an explosive unrivalled for blasting hard rock. Then followed *gelignite*, which is nitroglycerine 60, collodion cotton 5, potassium nitrate 27 and wood meal 8.

Slow-burning Propellents

In 1888, by uniting the two lines of research which had started from glycerine and from cotton, Nobel showed that the explosive properties of nitrated cotton could be tamed for propellent purposes by gelatinizing the fibrous material with nitroglycerine; the result was *ballistite*, one of the earliest of the nitroglycerine smokeless powders. This discovery, that the two most powerful explosives then known could be blended to furnish a slow-burning propellent, represented the apex of Nobel's genius. Ballistite was a precursor of *cordite*, produced in 1889 by Sir Frederick Abel and Sir James Dewar; it is nitroglycerine 58, guncotton 37 and soft paraffin 5 (Read, 1942).

A Model Dynamite Factory at Ardeer

In 1873 the British government allowed Nobel to build a works in which to make nitroglycerine at Ardeer, Ayrshire. It was on a peninsula fronting on the Firth of Clyde. Alarik Liedbeck came from Sweden to lay out the plant, and he created a model for all future high-explosives factories. The principle adopted was dispersal; wide stretches of land isolated all danger zones. All manufacturing processes were carefully separated and distributed over a number of small scattered buildings connected by a private railway. On each house and hut a notice was posted stating the maximum quantity of explosives and the maximum number of workers allowed inside at one time. Ardeer became the only one of the world's

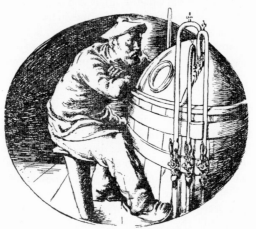

Fig. 210.—At one time the worker who controlled the manufacture of nitroglycerine sat on a one-legged stool. If he became sleepy he fell off and woke up.

(*By courtesy of Imperial Chemical Industries, Ltd.*)

great dynamite factories that never had an accident of catastrophic proportions (fig. 210).

Precautions taken in the Process of Nitration

Not only is nitroglycerine made in segregated buildings but also the apparatus used is fitted with elaborate safety devices. One of the most efficient methods of manufacture utilizes a nitrator-separator, which is a cylindrical leaden vessel with a sloping bottom and a conical roof provided with observation windows and carrying a thermometer which acts as a guide to the operator (fig. 211). The glycerine, owing to its viscosity, is thinned by being warmed to about 30° C. before being admitted gradually into the nitrating acid. The liquid is kept in constant agitation by the introduction of compressed air through a coil provided with several holes and lying at the bottom of the vessel. The water-cooling coils are also kept in operation, and the glycerine is added at such a rate that the temperature is kept between 22° C. and 25° C. Nitric-acid fumes arising from the mixture are drawn away and recovered in a condensing tower. If the temperature gets out of control and exceeds 30° C., local decomposition is indi-

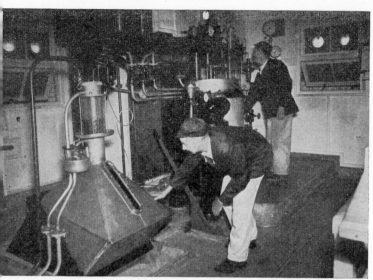

FIG. 211.—Underground Nitrating House for the manufacture of Nitroglycerine. For an hour at a time one of two men on duty watches a Dial indicating the Temperature of the Charge. If this gets out of control he pulls a Safety Lever causing the Charge to be drowned in excess of Cold Water

(*Crown Copyright*)

ated, and the charge is immediately drowned in a large excess of cold ater contained in a tank below the apparatus. Some modern types of itrator permit of continuous working and can nitrate as much as 1,100 . of glycerine within an hour (Read, 1942).

egulations for handling High Explosives

The *Explosives Act, 1875*, followed. Among its provisions was one uthorizing port authorities in the United Kingdom to adopt rules and egulations for the handling of high explosives in harbours. The port of eith adopted a code requiring dynamite carts to be drawn by horses earing flannel shoes and driven by men clad in suits without pockets, aetal buttons or buckles, certified to be of sober habits and able to stand xamination in the by-laws. The pier had to be laid with a carpet and overed with an awning before any dynamite was brought on it, and all angerous material was doused with water before and after loading. Dis-ersal among small scattered buildings and protection by means of mounds f earth and blast walls are principles which have been adopted in planning ll high-explosives factories subsequent to this Act.

Titroglycerine Headache

Apart from ingestion by mouth, nitroglycerine is absorbed both by ihalation and through the skin (Rabinowitch, 1944). Its vapour has a powerful pharmacological effect even when much diluted with air. When he discovered it, Sobrero placed a small quantity of it on his tongue and at once it gave him a violent pulsating headache. From his laboratory work and occasional visits to quarries, Nobel suffered from *dynamite headache* over a period of many years. In the manufacture of nitroglycerine, work in the washing-house and mixing-rooms is particularly prone to produce headache. Men handling sticks of dynamite and charges of cordite, which are essentially nitroglycerine and nitrocellulose, also suffer from it, especially in hot weather. Beginning as a severe, throbbing, frontal headache, it spreads to the vertex and is associated with flushing of the face, palpitation a fall in blood-pressure and the passing of copious pale urine. Nausea frequently occurs, but vomiting and abdominal pain are less usual.

Susceptibility and Immunity

There is a wide variation in susceptibility to nitroglycerine. Thus, of eight sailors who handled aged cordite in a small, hot, airtight compartment, one was quite unaffected throughout prolonged trials (Weiner and Thomson, 1947). This immunity is said to be lessened by hot weather and by indulgence in alcohol. The headache affects the new-comer only, for in all but 2 or 3 per cent of workers an immunity is acquired in three or four days (Ebright, 1914). Nevertheless, this freedom from headache is lost by a few days' absence from nitroglycerine, so that on resumption of work the operator will again suffer severe headache.

In *A Blind Hog's Acorns*, Carey P. McCord tells the following story of cases of dynamite headache:

> In industry, wherever occupational disease exposures prevail, one or more engineers are likely to be included in those exposed. Let one engineer tell his own medical history, much as he told it to me.
>
> "I'm one of the engineers building the hydro-electric dam down on the Setan River. I am sick, Doctor, and my wife and children are sick. We're all pretty badly shaken. It must be something communicable. I got it first, and then quickly one child after another, and then my wife. We have frightful headaches, just as though something was on the inside of our heads boring out. At times I have been willing to dash my head against a stone wall, believing that there would be less pain from the outside than came from the inside. This has been pretty hard on the children. At the same time, our hearts beat very fast. I am not a doctor, but I can count pulse, and our heartbeats are so fast at times that I can't count them. They must run at times 140 or 150. I took our temperatures with the thermometer, but everyone of us was perfectly normal. What is this all about? I think maybe we all have meningitis or infantile paralysis."
>
> Since other members of the household were involved, for the moment I was off guard and did not expect an occupational disease but as part of the routine questions I inquired,

"What is your particular work at the dam?"

Back came the illuminating reply, "I'm the firing boss. I supervise all of the drilling for explosion shots; I'm in charge of the dynamite dump, I supervise the loading of all firing holes and the placing of fuse wires."

Then came my inquiry, "Have you been at this work long?"

"No," the engineer replied, "only for a few months. The old boss retired just before this new contract started. I had been in the cost estimating department for years and was in line for a promotion. This new job is a real advance for me."

By this time I believed I knew the answer, but it would have been foolish to have jumped to a conclusion. There were many more questions, examinations, visits with the engineer's wife and children. Then came the diagnosis.

"You have a 'dynamite head.' Your headaches come from the explosives at your work. Every explosive worker is apt to have this experience. You are fairly new, not yet enough experienced."

The incredulous engineer said, "That's foolish, Doctor, my wife and children aren't engineers. They don't come around the dam more than once a month."

"No, it isn't foolish. On your clothing you carry enough powder dust to your home two or three times a week to bowl them over with the same disease. With you it is a disease of the trade. For them that is not so—it is just a disease that father brings home."

"Maybe you're right, Doctor, but what can we do about it?"

"Well, sir, there is a strange thing about dynamite. When it is around you all the time, you don't have the disease. Seemingly, intermittent exposure is necessary. I'm telling you what to do. Slip two or three grains of powder under your hat-band and forget about them. Take a few more grains and safely hide them about the house. The chances are there won't be any more headaches."

And so it all worked out, but several days later back came the engineer. "Doctor, my family and I are all right now. We're cured, but everybody that calls on us at my house gets a hell of a headache. What are we going to do about that?"

And now I was at the end of my row.

"Possibly," I proposed, "you ought to go back to being the cost accounting engineer."

Treatment

All men working with nitroglycerine, dynamite and cordite should wear impermeable rubber gloves and aprons. Where possible they should work only where a system of exhaust ventilation has been installed. To avoid *Monday headache*, workers sometimes rub nitroglycerine into their hatbands. Sometimes the wife of an operator in the nitrator room will suffer from severe headache unless her husband washes his hair on arriving home each night (Critchley, 1949). Tablets of amphetamine sulphate, mg 15, or of ephedrine hydrochloride, gr. ½, have been adopted as prophylactics for nitroglycerine headache, but both are useless once a headache has started. Strong coffee helps to relieve the pain, and tablets of aspirin and caffeine should be given too. Alcohol must not be given with the idea of relieving the pain, for it may then cause great agitation with a state of confusion and even delirium, the so-called *dynamite encephalosis*.

NITROCELLULOSE

In 1838 Pelouze obtained a highly inflammable material by treating cotton with strong nitric acid, thereby opening the way to the study of materials which became known as nitrocelluloses. They are not true nitro compounds and, strictly speaking, they should be referred to as cellulose nitrates—for example, cellulose trinitrate and cellulose dinitrate. The nitro celluloses of commerce are mixtures and their properties vary through a fairly wide range according to the degree to which they have been nitrated.

Historical Summary

The second half of the nineteenth century witnessed developments which brought nitrocellulose products into use all over the world. In 1845 Schönbein of Basel improved the process of nitration by using a mixture of nitric and sulphuric acids which produced *guncotton*. The practical difficulties in making and using this substance as an explosive were overcome by Sir Frederick Abel by the year 1865. About the same time Alexander Parkes of Birmingham rather surprisingly used nitrocellulose as an ingredient of the first synthetic plastic. He obtained a solid product which he called *xylonite*, by mixing nitrocellulose, camphor and castor-oil. It fell to the American Hyatt to make the first commercially useful product, which was named *celluloid* in 1872. This opened the way for *cellulose lacquers*, which were soon to become of such value in the motor-car industry. In 1884 the Chardonnet process made *artificial silk* a reality, and in 1892 the viscose process was developed.

Guncotton and Cordite

As a raw material in industry, cellulose is used chiefly in the form of cotton waste from the spinning mills. The short fibres of the ripe cotton seed capsule separated in the process of ginning and known as *cotton linter* also are used. Cotton cellulose has the great advantage of uniformity of composition and texture. Guncotton is a mixture of nitrated celluloses and contains about 13 per cent of nitrogen, whereas collodion cotton contains about 12 per cent. *Cordite* and *smokeless powders* in general are made from guncotton and collodion cotton by gelatinization with nitroglycerine (see p. 585). Some types of collodion cotton dissolve completely in a mixture of three volumes of ether and one volume of alcohol, forming viscid solutions of *pyroxylin* or *surgical collodion*. Such specimens also dissolve completely in nitroglycerine, as in the manufacture of *blasting gelatine* (see

p. 585). Nitrocellulose, containing about 11 per cent of nitrogen, is used to make the celluloid plastics, including photographic film.

Cellulose Lacquers

Dissolved in amyl acetate, carbitol, ethyl acetate, ethylene glycol, methyl acetate, nitroethane or triethanol, nitrocellulose forms a series of cellulose lacquers which are used for spray-painting. When the solvent evaporates from the solution it leaves the nitrocellulose as a hard, glossy film on the metal or leather surface to which the lacquer has been applied. Artificial leather or *leathercloth* is made by spraying a cellulose lacquer on to cloth.

Comte Hilaire de Chardonnet (1839–1924)

The age of artificial silk really began with Comte Hilaire de Chardonnet (1839–1924), who was a student of Pasteur at the time of his investigations into silk-worm disease. This was the source of the inspiration which started Chardonnet on his life work. After thirty years of effort he took out his first patent for nitrocellulose, collodion or Chardonnet silk in 1884. As raw material he used cotton linters. His method was to nitrate the cotton, and squirt the nitrocellulose dissolved in alcohol and ether through spinnerettes into a setting bath of water which coagulated the jets to threads. Since nitrocellulose is both inflammable and explosive, he removed the nitro-groups from the spun threads by immersion in a bath of sodium sulphide. Happily, the process exposed the workmen to no toxic hazard. His factory at Besançon was in operation by 1901, and by 1907 he was making a ton a day. Chardonnet silk has since been displaced by other kinds of cellulose silks such as viscose silk (see p. 626) and acetate silk.

The Manufacture of Guncotton and Collodion Cotton

In the manufacture of guncotton and collodion cotton, scrolls of paper or cotton waste are dipped in mixtures of sulphuric acid and nitric acid. The precise method of nitration that will provide a collodion cotton having the requisite properties has to be found by experiment, but in general the cotton is nitrated with a weaker and warmer acid, and for a shorter time, than in the production of guncotton (Read, 1942). The dipping is done in an earthenware bath fitted with an aluminium hood open at one side to allow the work to be carried out. The dipper stands here, pushes cotton waste through the opening and dips it under the surface of the acid with a stainless-steel fork. A man or woman usually does this for four hours at a time and then pushes trucks loaded with wet washed nitrated cotton to the boiling vats.

Hazard of Nitrogen Dioxide Fumes

There is a tendency for the incompletely nitrated material to decompose spontaneously; it then smoulders and evolves fumes of nitrogen dioxide. If such a fire occurs, the dipper must immediately extinguish it. Unfortunately, it is not easy for the dippers in the neighbourhood to move away, because unattended and incompletely dipped cotton waste will readily decompose (Lynch and Bell, 1947). All operatives must therefore be protected against this danger.

Hazards of Dental Erosion

Erosion of the teeth of workers in acid fumes, a process quite distinct from caries, has been known in chemical industry over many years. The occupations involved are the manufacture of nitric, sulphuric and hydrochloric acids, the forming of electric accumulators, the carroting of rabbit skins in the hatters'-furriers' trade and the nitrating of explosives (see p. 802). In 1947 Lynch and Bell found the condition in forty-five out of 126 workers employed in the dipping-rooms of a factory manufacturing guncotton. Similar erosion among acid dippers in explosives factories has been reported by Simpson (1919) in Canada and by Muzi (1927) in Italy.

Symptoms and Signs

The degree of erosion increases with the length of the period of employment. Its site suggests the direct action of the acid fume on those teeth exposed by talking or mouth-breathing. The teeth affected are the upper and lower incisors and sometimes the canines. The erosion begins on the incisal edges of the teeth and extends on to the labial surface. The eroded surface is smooth and polished and never pitted. When the enamel has been destroyed, the dentine is attacked and there is brown or black discoloration of the affected teeth, but they retain their polished appearance. While the erosion is taking place, the pulp chamber shrinks and the condition is painless except in rare cases where the erosion is so rapid that bacterial invasion of the pulp cavity occurs with abscess formation (Lynch and Bell, 1947).

Preventive Measures

The aim of prevention is so to design the plant that there is no escape of fume; usually this ideal is not achieved. Mouth-breathers should be excluded from the work. Excessive talking and singing should be discouraged, the reason for this being explained to the workers. It would be difficult to continue to do the work in a mask or respirator, but a transparent plastic face shield could be worn with benefit. Alkaline tablets may be tried, both to increase salivary flow by the mechanical process of sucking and as neutralizing agents. All workers should be encouraged to clean their teeth before and after shifts and also at meal breaks. Suitable breathing apparatus must be provided to protect the workers against the hazard of inhaling nitrogen dioxide. Both canister gas-masks kept close at hand or gas-masks connected through a hose to a fixed supply of compressed air are suitable. In the case of photographic film it should be noted that cellulose acetate which is non-inflammable is now used as a safe substitute for cellulose nitrate. All old collections of cellulose nitrate X-ray film should be suitably destroyed to avoid a fire in which nitrogen dioxide is evolved, as happened in the shocking accident at the Cleveland Clinic in 1929.

DIMETHYLNITROSAMINE

Dimethylnitrosamine is used in industry as a solvent. In man and animals it produces severe liver injury in the form of centrilobular necrosis. In animals it is carcinogenic producing tumours in liver, kidney, lung and urinary bladder.

Effects on the Liver in Man and Animals

Alice Hamilton (Hamilton and Hardy, 1949) observed that it had poisoned two men who were employed in an automobile factory in the U.S.A. It produced jaundice with ascites. One of the men was violently ill but recovered. The other was less severely affected and was recovering when he developed an infection from the paracentesis and died. At necropsy there was cirrhosis of the liver with regeneration nodules. Because of this finding the physician in charge tested DMN on dogs. Acute symptoms came on immediately, death occurred in hypoglycæmia, and necropsy showed severe liver destruction. In 1954 Barnes and Magee recorded poisoning in two out of three men working in a research laboratory where for 10 months they had handled DMN One of the men had died of bronchopneumonia, and cirrhosis of the liver was an incidental finding at necropsy. The second man with a long-standing history of dyspepsia had a laparotomy after five months' exposure to DMN. At that time no note of any abnormality of the liver was made. Six months later he was examined for an incisional hernia that had developed in the operation scar. It was then recorded that the liver felt hard and was suspected of being cirrhotic. Liver function tests carried out at this time showed evidence of damage. When repeated three months later after all further exposure to DMN had ceased these tests indicated an improved liver function. The third man had remained in good health but had had no liver function tests carried out on him. Animal tests showed hæmorrhagic liver necrosis following administration by any route other than skin application. In dogs, rats and guinea pigs a striking feature is hæmorrhage into the gut and peritoneal cavity. The toxic action of the nitrosamines is due to the release of powerful alkylating agents in the liver. They also inhibit protein synthesis and alkylate liver protein and ribonucleic acid. In all cases the effective agent appears to be a metabolite.

Carcinogenic Effects in Animals

So far as is known no case of malignant disease in man has yet resulted from the handling of the dialkylnitrosamines. In the laboratory carcinogenic effects have been demonstrated in animals mainly rats. The various dialkylnitrosamines are remarkably consistent in their action and it is easy to cause tumours with them in most of a group of animals tested (Heath and Magee, 1962). The organs affected depend upon both the dose rates and the strain of rat. Liver tumours are mainly liver cell carcinoma and kidney tumours adenocarcinomas. Œsophageal, bladder and stomach tumours are all squamous carcinomas. Malignant tumours have been found in the trachea and lungs of golden hamsters fed DMN. Diethylnitrosamine produces liver and kidney carcinomas in rats. Tumours do not develop only in those organs in which either acute or chronic necrotic damage is most marked. For example, dimethylnitrosamine causes little acute damage to lungs or kidneys, but causes tumours there as readily as in the liver; and diethylnitrosamine caused hæmorrhages in lungs, thymus, para-aortic lymph nodes, and gastric mucosa when given over long periods by mouth, but only caused liver tumours. DMN has been shown to cause kidney tumours and dibutylnitrosamine to cause bladder tumours after a single dose (Druckrey and others, 1962). This *one-shot* carcinogenic effect is a particular hazard of the nitrosamines. If man is like the rat in his response not only long-term exposure but also a single serious incident may give rise to unpleasant sequelæ years later. In this case the evidence from animal experiments is so definite as to call for a total ban to be placed on the manufacture or use of the dialkylnitrosamines. It surely must be possible to find safe substitutes.

THE HALOGENATED HYDROCARBONS

The rapid growth of the moulded-plastics and cellulose-lacquer industries has led to the extensive use of many new solvents, most of which were little more than chemical curiosities before about 1925. Amongst these are the chlorinated hydrocarbons which have flooded the market largely because the alkali industry requires an outlet for its by-product chlorine. The various halogenated hydrocarbons are useful as refrigerants, as degreasers of metals, fire-extinguishers, cleansers of textiles, solvents for rubber and thinners of cellulose lacquers. Because they are non-inflammable, non-combustible and non-explosive, they are often labelled *safe* but although they are safe from causing fire they are far from harmless in their effects on the human body.

Historical Summary

The action of carbon tetrachloride has been extensively studied because of its use in the treatment of hookworm disease. Tetrachlorethane dramatically attracted attention in the aircraft industry in England in 1914. Methyl bromide caused fatalities in the Swiss chemical industry in 1920. A mass poisoning from leaking refrigerators in Chicago in 1929 led to an increase in knowledge of the action of methyl chloride. Trichlorethylene has been studied because of its extensive use in dry cleaning. It led to trouble in German industry in 1931. Chlorinated naphthalenes caused no serious harm until 1937.

Chlorination increases Toxicity

The entrance of chlorine into an aliphatic hydrocarbon increases its toxicity, whereas the reverse is the case with an aromatic hydrocarbon.

Thus, chlorobenzene is less toxic than benzene and causes no trouble in industry. The toxic effects of the chlorinated hydrocarbons increase with their molecular weight, though this is compensated to some extent by a decrease in volatility. The effects of the *chloro*-compounds may be related to the activity of the halogen contained in them. Chlorine is certainly more active in the aliphatic than in the aromatic compounds. For instance, the *chloro*-derivatives of the paraffins are hydrolysed by boiling with aqueous alkali, whereas chlorobenzene is scarcely affected by this process. The *chloro*-derivatives of naphthalene hold an intermediate position between the aliphatic *chloro*-compounds and chlorobenzene, both as to stability and toxicity.

Phosgene a Decomposition Product

It is well known that at high temperatures and in an excess of air the halogenated hydrocarbons are decomposed. The decomposition products may contain free halogen, hydrogen halide and carbonyl halide. As these gases are all highly toxic, there is some risk to health where gas burners are present or welding processes are carried out in proximity to sources of the vapour of chlorinated hydrocarbons. As to smoking, it has often been asserted that phosgene is formed when trichlorethylene passes through burning tobacco.

No Risk from Smoking

The work of Elkins and Levine (1939) throws doubt upon the danger of smoking in the presence of these vapours. They found that the extent of decomposition into the corresponding halide of trichlorethylene, dichloro-benzene, carbon tetrachloride, ethylene bromide and ethyl bromide, occur-ring as a result of smoking cigars or cigarettes in the presence of their vapours, is of a low order and does not constitute a risk to health. It is essential that all illnesses occurring among workers exposed to the chlor-inated hydrocarbons should be carefully recorded. Accurate case records are necessary in order to establish clear clinical pictures which can be readily recognized in the future. Only in this way can diagnosis be im-proved and workers' lives saved.

Some Halogenated Organic Compounds attack the Liver

A large number of halogenated organic compounds are either definitely known to be liver poisons or are under suspicion. They include bromethol (avertin), carbon tetrachloride, chlorbutol (chloretone), chlorinated di-phenyl, chlorinated naphthalene, chloroform, dichloromethane, ethyl chloride, ethylene dichloride, iodoform, methyl chloride, monoiodoethane, tetrachlorethane and trichlorethylene. It is not suggested that all these sub-stances are industrial poisons, but some of them are used in therapeutics as sedatives and anæsthetics and must be avoided in patients whose work exposes them to the chlorinated hydrocarbons.

Exposure to Other Potential Liver Poisons

Workers with a past history of jaundice, even mild infective hepatitis, or of any other liver disease should not handle these substances, nor should workers with a past history of typhoid fever, malaria, gall-stones or other diseases known to attack the liver. Workers receiving arsphenamine treatment for syphilis, or those who are taking drugs believed to be injurious to the liver, should not be further exposed in their work to potential liver poisons. Neither should pregnant women be exposed to the chlorinated hydrocarbons because the liver in pregnancy is peculiarly susceptible to injury. Sedatives such as chloral hydrate and chlorbutol should be avoided, as also should the anæsthetics chloroform, trichlorethylene, bromethol (avertin) and ethyl chloride. No worker who has received such an anæsthetic should go back to his former occupation until after a long interval.

Treatment with *dl*-methionine

Where poisoning has actually occurred from exposure to a chlorinated hydrocarbon, treatment with *dl*-methionine should begin at once. Four grams a day should be given by mouth for three days, followed by 2 grams a day for six days. In desperate cases 15 grams should be given intravenously (Beattie, Herbert, Wechtel and Steele, 1944). Alkaline glucose drinks, together with large doses of calcium lactate up to 15 grams a day, should be given. Calcium gluconate may be given by intramuscular injection.

Treatment with Calcium Gluconate

The use of sugar and calcium salts is based upon the accidental discovery of Minot and Cutler (1929) that, though carbon tetrachloride causes a severe intoxication in dogs on a meat diet, the addition of calcium salts to such a diet produces a high degree of tolerance to the drug. The symptoms of poisoning are gastro-intestinal irritation and hyperexcitability followed by depression. There is retention of guanidine in the blood and hypoglycæmia. The relief and protection given by calcium salts seem to depend upon their antagonistic effect to the retained guanidine. These authors found that when calcium salts were administered to poisoned animals, the nervous symptoms were relieved and the blood-sugar was restored to normal. However, if the blood-sugar was raised by the administration of glucose, the hyperexcitability persisted until calcium salts were given in addition.

(*a*) Methyl Chloride

Methyl chloride, or monochloromethane, CH_3Cl, is a colourless gas with a faint ethereal odour. It is used in the dye industry and in the preparation of chloroform. As a refrigerant it is superior to ammonia and sulphur dioxide. Its advantages for this purpose are its stability and low boiling-point, and that it is non-corrosive to metals, relatively non-inflammable, non-explosive and non-injurious to food, furs or textiles.

Early Cases in Chemical Industry

The first cases of its poisonous action in industry were reported by Gerbis in 1914. The patients were two men working in a chemical plant, who suffered from nausea, vomiting and extreme somnolence. The first patient slept for twenty-four hours with three interruptions for meals. The second patient was restless and ran excitedly about the factory doing everthing the wrong way. He had dimness of vision which did not clear up for fourteen days after leaving work. Subsequently, forty-one cases were reported in Switzerland, Germany and the United States of America, all of them being persons employed upon making, installing or repairing refrigerators.

Cases in Refrigerator Workers

It is to Kegel, McNally and Pope (1929) of Chicago that we owe the fullest clinical description. Their paper is based upon twenty-nine cases, many of them severe, with ten deaths. In 1927 Baker described twenty-one milder cases amongst the employees of an American firm of refrigerator manufacturers and in 1930 a further seventy-five non-fatal cases. In Great Britain ten cases were described between 1930 and 1935. A clinical account of seven further cases was written by Jones in 1942. These occurred amongst a small number of travelling refrigerator repairers; six of the cases were of moderate severity and the seventh was the first severe case to be reported in this country.   ·

Symptoms and Signs

In mild cases, exposure to the gas is followed by staggering gait, dizziness and headache. Anorexia, nausea and vomiting occur next day. The patient is rarely prevented from working. In a case of moderate severity the patient is ill for several weeks. The staggering and dizziness are accompanied by drowsiness, malaise and weakness. Ocular symptoms occur in about half of the cases, but their appearance is usually delayed for twenty-four hours. They include misty vision, diplopia and difficulty in accommodation. Vomiting sometimes occurs for a week or more, and diarrhœa has been described. Depression, diplopia and misty vision have been known to persist for two months. In more severe cases epileptiform convulsions occur and may lead to death. Ptosis, strabismus and diplopia are common, but optic atrophy does not occur. Slurred speech, amnesia, drowsiness by day and delirium by night are occasionally seen.

Persistence of Certain Signs

There is a rise of temperature, pulse and respiratory rate. In the worst cases there is oliguria, occasionally with suppression lasting up to forty-eight hours. Fifty per cent of cases have albumin and red cells in the urine. The detection of formic acid in the urine is not of diagnostic value as was at one time thought. No case showed jaundice, though in necropsies fatty degeneration of the liver was seen. Anæmia occurs in some of the men affected, the red cells dropping as low as 3,100,000 per c.mm. and the hæmoglobin as low as 50 per cent. Sometimes there is leucocytosis with a normal differential count. Sequelæ such as ataxia, diplopia, misty vision, headache, drowsiness and amnesia sometimes persist for as long as eight months.

Use of a Stenching Agent

Poisoning in refrigerator factories can be eliminated by exhaust ventilation. Unfortunately it is difficult to convince the refrigerator repairer that an almost inodorous non-irritating gas can be poisonous. He must be forbidden to stay in a room after he has heated liquid methyl chloride in the blocked evaporator of a refrigerator. The suggestion has been made that a small percentage of some pungent detector substance such as acrolein or methyl selenide should be added to the methyl chloride. The use of such a stenching agent would draw attention to the dangerous nature of the gas, facilitate the education of those who handle it and warn the householder of a leak from his refrigerator. Unfortunately, it would afford no protection to infants, the infirm or refrigerator repairers.

Dichlorodifluoromethane a Safe Refrigerant

The discovery of safe refrigerants has progressed systematically. Chemists set out deliberately to discover a non-toxic, non-corrosive, non-inflammable, non-irritant refrigerant which would be safe to put in domestic refrigerators. It was found in dichlorodifluoromethane, known also by the trade name *freon*. Sayers, Yant, Chornyak and Shoaf (1930) showed that prolonged exposure of dogs, monkeys and guinea-pigs to air containing 20 per cent by volume of dichlorofluoromethane vapour does not lead to any ill effects. It is therefore probable that the use of this refrigerant involves little risk to the health of the worker.

(b) Methyl Bromide

Methyl bromide, CH_3Br, is a colourless, non-inflammable gas at normal temperature and pressure. It has but little odour, successive exposures dull the olfactory sense to its presence, and therefore no warning of danger may be apparent to workers handling it. It comes on the market compressed into containers, in which it assumes the liquid condition. When released it readily vaporizes and in this form is some 3·3 times heavier than air, a point of importance with reference to industrial exposure.

Uses

Unhappily methyl bromide is used as a fire extinguisher, refrigerant, fumigant and insecticide. The chemical industry sometimes uses it as a methylating agent, but the iodide is preferred owing to its higher boiling-point. In fire-fighting its density enables it to act as a blanket around burning objects, in this way excluding oxygen and putting out the fire. Bulk for bulk, less is required for the purpose than of any other known substance. It has, further, the advantage of being self-trajectory. A mixture with carbon tetrachloride is frequently used; methyl bromide is recommended for fires involving celluloid or volatile hydrocarbons. It is capable of protecting against insects a wide variety of substances including food, grain, plants and textiles. Entomologists favour its use in pest control because it is highly toxic to insects in all stages of their development. It is particularly effective in the extermination of lice, bed-bugs and weevils. By its use to destroy rats and ground squirrels, together with their parasites, the hygienist can control plague. It is useful in the fumigation of warehouses, flour mills, railway food vans, greenhouses and even of the soil itself. Its swiftly penetrating powers enable it to attack pests in sacks of grain, the pulp of fruit or the depths of a cheese in effective concentrations, and thereafter to dissipate quickly, leaving no smell or taste behind it. As there is no fire hazard, its value to the warehouseman is considerable.

Historical Summary

In spite of three cases of methyl-bromide poisoning which occurred in 1893 and were recorded by Jacquet in 1901, the condition remained a medical curiosity until about 1920 when cases appeared in the Swiss and German chemical industries. In Danbury, Connecticut, in 1926, two people died in an apartment house owing to the escape of the vapour of methyl bromide from a refrigerator. From 1925 onwards, cases have occurred in chemical works and in men charging and repairing refrigerators and filling and using fire extinguishers. In the Second World War thirty-three cases were reported in the Royal Navy with six fatalities, and others in the Royal Air Force. The skin lesions were first described in 1940 in a French soldier.

Exposure Hazards

Methyl bromide can be emitted from fire extinguishers either as liquid before volatilization or as vapour. The former can contaminate floors, furniture, hands and clothing, and both can be inhaled. It is extensively used in fire extinguishers in aeroplanes and ships. Its density and lack of smell make it extremely dangerous should a leak occur in the fire-fighting apparatus of a ship or launch where the cabins are small and below water-level. Aircraft mechanics are exposed to a special hazard owing to the fact that methyl bromide is played automatically on to the carburettors of aircraft engines to lower the flash-point of the petrol. Any process, whether of manufacture or filling, which is carried out inside a building is potentially dangerous. The process of filling containers from distributor cylinders must never be carried out in a confined space nor even in the open air on hot days. Cylinders of methyl bromide should not be stored in a workroom. In factories, such faults as ill-fitting joints, fractures in delivery pipes and the displacement of vapour-laden air from collecting vessels are among the commonest defects. The great volatility of methyl bromide permits large quantities of gas to escape through a small leak. A workman with insufficient training and experience in chemical process work may be careless in spilling the liquid or in allowing accidental overflow from a still (Wyers, 1945).

Systemic Action Delayed

Systemic effects are produced by inhalation of the vapour; they involve the nervous system, lungs and kidneys. Skin lesions arise through contact with the liquid or vapour. Cases of poisoning are commoner in hot weather than in cold. It is important to realize that methyl bromide is a deadly and insidious poison with a delayed action like phosgene and nitrogen dioxide. The latent interval varies from four to forty-eight hours. Many cases are recorded where men who have worked with methyl bromide have suffered only minor symptoms and then later have been seized with convulsions and died. Prain and Smith (1952) described six deaths among eight boys who broke bounds from an approved school in Dundee. The police discovered six of these boys huddled together in varying degrees of unconsciousness in a small cabin aboard a disused Royal Air Force launch. A recently discharged methyl-bromide fire extinguisher was found on the spot. One of the boys walked $3\frac{1}{2}$ miles home without feeling more than vaguely ill and yet died of poisoning within fifteen hours.

Symptoms and Signs

In contrast to the chlorinated hydrocarbons, methyl bromide has very little narcotic action. After the latent interval the patient is seized abruptly with nausea, vomiting, headache, vertigo, dimness of vision, diplopia, euphoria and delirium. In severe cases pulmonary œdema, oliguria, suppression of urine, convulsions and even acute mania may occur. The skin is pale, the temperature normal, sweating is profuse, trismus and even opisthotonus may be seen. The pupils are dilated; optic atrophy has never been recorded. The blood bromide is usually raised. In prognosis much will depend on the concentration of the vapour inhaled and on the length of the exposure. Mild cases usually recover, but where there is œdema of the lungs, convulsions, anuria or severe burns, the outcome is often fatal. Among the sequelæ recorded are apathy, depression, sleeplessness, amnesia, hallucinations, tremor of the hands and tongue and polyneuritis.

Causes of Skin Lesions

Early in the Second World War a French soldier who extinguished a fire with methyl bromide in an armoured car developed a pink papular erythema on his arms and abdominal wall, together with extensive burns on his feet, which took over four weeks to heal. In a study of ninety workers engaged in the filling and sealing rooms of a factory manufacturing methyl bromide, Watrous (1942) found twenty-two cases showing skin lesions. Four of these had vesicles which healed without dermatitis; eleven had both vesicles and dermatitis, and seven had dermatitis only. In 1945 Butler and others described how two soldiers driving an armoured car carrying ammunition used a methyl-bromide fire extinguisher to deal with a small fire under the dashboard. In doing this one driver contaminated his feet and also the well of the car where his companion put his feet. They took little notice of this and drove on for five hours to their destination. They then noticed their feet were sore, and on removal of their anklets, socks and boots found them red, tender and covered with blisters up to 4 inches in diameter.

Dermatitis, Vesication and Burns

In the incidence of skin lesions idiosyncrasy plays a part, for many workmen repeatedly use methyl bromide to remove grease from their hands without ill effect. The incubation period in the formation of blisters varies from four to ten hours. The vesicles are at first tiny and grouped together but they become confluent and may then measure from 1 to 4 inches across; they contain clear straw-coloured fluid. Premonitary pruritus is characteristic and may be intense. Methyl-bromide burns are superficial, rarely extending deeply enough to destroy the whole dermis. They are characterized by excessive vesication with reddening and swelling of the surrounding skin. Healing readily occurs and in most cases there is considerable desquamation. In mild cases an itching, pink, papular erythema is all that occurs; it usually heals within seven days. Any influence retarding evaporation, such as soaked clothing, will favour absorption by prolonging the time of contact. Methyl bromide will penetrate ordinary fabrics and even leather boots. Happily, no case has so far been recorded in which constitutional symptoms have occurred from skin absorption. Methyl bromide readily dissolves in rubber and adhesive tape. Watrous (1942) refers to workers who acquired burns by resting their elbows on sponge rubber pads which could only have been contaminated by occasional drops of methyl bromide. Surgical dressings applied to the skin, especially adhesive tape, also take it up and vesication then occurs beneath the dressing.

Animal Experiments

Animal experiments show methyl bromide to be by far the most toxic of the four organic halides, methyl bromide, methyl chloride, ethyl bromide and ethyl chloride. Sayers and others (1929) found that the signs of poisoning in guinea-pigs were excitement, loss of equilibrium, weakness, rapid pulse and respiration, râles and, in some cases, a bloody exudate from the nostrils. The pathological findings were congestion of the lungs with hæmorrhages and œdema, parenchymatous degeneration of the myocardium and liver, and congestion of other viscera such as pancreas, kidneys, intestines, meninges and brain. Irish and others (1940) investigated the action of methyl bromide on animals of different species including rats, rabbits, guinea-pigs and monkeys. Rabbits were more sensitive than the other animals and death occurred with pulmonary œdema.

Morbid Anatomy and Histology

Prain and Smith (1952) carried out necropsies on five victims who died within eighteen hours of exposure. They found cyanosis, petechial hæmorrhages in the respiratory organs, small bilateral blood-stained pleural effusions and intense œdema of the lungs with discrete hæmorrhages in the lung substance. The liver, kidneys and meninges showed congestion; there were small subdural, subarachnoid and cerebral hæmorrhages. Histologically, the œdema of the lungs was accompanied by general distension of alveolar capillaries as in phosgene poisoning. The kidneys showed coagulative necrosis in the epithelium of the first convoluted tubules, in rather fewer of the second convoluted tubules and in the loops of Henle, particular the ascending limb. The tubulo-venous communications seen in the kidney of carbon-tetrachloride poisoning were not found in these cases, but this change may depend upon a much longer time of survival.

Symptomatic Treatment

If there is cyanosis, little can be done except to administer oxygen. Lumbar puncture should be carried out in order to examine the bromine content in the cerebrospinal fluid. In cases showing mild systemic symptoms, fresh air and two days' rest in bed with three weeks' convalescence will usually be adequate as treatment. The burns have been treated with 2 per cent tannic acid in triple-dye solution with propamidine isethionate cream and with calcium penicillin. All these methods are satisfactory, but the propamidine cream is painless, whereas calcium penicillin causes tingling (Butler and others, 1945).

Preventive Measures in Factories

Methyl bromide is so extremely toxic and its action so insidious that the search for safe substitutes is imperative. Hygiene of the place of work and especially the prevention of leaks is vital. The siting of plant in the open air, preferably in a passage between two buildings, is of the greatest importance. Where possible, pipe-work should be of copper as this metal does not flake and block delivery tubes. Heavy rubber or neoprene tubing may be used. Methyl bromide has a solvent action on grease, and soap should therefore be used for the lubrication of threaded pipe-work. It has been suggested that volatile colouring agents or substances with penetrating odours or lachrymatory effects might be added to methyl bromide as safety measures. Technical difficulties here are very great. The colouring substance would require to be at least as volatile as the substance it was intended to betray, whilst an odour should be of such character that it did not escape too readily and yet would give sufficient warning of danger (Wyers, 1945). Periodic medical examination should be instituted. Instruction of chemists and workmen as to the dangerous properties of the substance is of first importance. The incidence of poisoning among inexperienced workmen is strikingly higher than among old hands. It should be the responsibility of one man to issue, examine periodically and repair gas-masks.

Protection of the Skin

Bathing the hands in a weak solution of sodium carbonate may help to prevent skin lesions by promoting the decomposition of methyl bromide. In the manufacture of the substance, prevention has been largely achieved by education and supervision of the workmen. No attempt should be made to protect the hands of workers with gloves, particularly rubber gloves, and no one should be allowed to handle methyl bromide with surgical dressings on his hands. Owing to its use in fire-fighting, firemen and members of H.M. Services must be made aware of its dangers. Notices must be placed on all fire extinguishers containing methyl bromide warning the user of the danger of the liquid getting on the hands, in the eyes and on the clothing. If the latter is contaminated, it must at once be removed and not used for two days. Warning notices should be posted when fumigation is in progress, and the men carrying it out should work in pairs and not singly. When it is used as a fumigant the trucks, ships, store-houses, barns or other buildings must be thoroughly ventilated on the completion of the process.

(c) Trichlorethylene

Trichlorethylene, $CHCl.CCl_2$, is a colourless liquid with a faint aromatic odour. It is used for degreasing metals, in the extraction of oils and fats, in painting, enamelling, dyeing and dry-cleaning, in the boot and shoe industry, in textile manufacture and the printing industry, as an insecticide, a disinfecting agent, an impregnation material, in cleaning films, photographic plates and optical lenses, in the chemical industry, in gas purification and as a rubber solvent.

Many Trade Names

In all these processes trichlorethylene may be used pure or as an addition to other solutions under various proprietary names, such as *benzinol, blanco-solv, chlorylene, cinco-solv, cocolene, crawshawpol, dukeron, flock-flip, gemalgene, lanadin-lap, lith lithurin, Lithuin E, pern-a-chlor, tetraline, trethylene, trielin, triklone, trilene, triol, tripur, vestrol* and *westrosol*.

No Significant Lesions in Experimental Animals

The outstanding result of animal experiments with trichlorethylene is the absence of any severe lesion of the liver and kidneys, such as is found with other halogenated hydrocarbons like tetrachlorethane. Only Castellino (1932) appears to have produced a slight fatty degeneration of the liver and granular degeneration of the kidneys in inhalation experiments. Nevertheless, the case of an adult man who died of acute necrosis of the liver eleven days after prolonged trichlorethylene anæsthesia has been recorded (Herdman, 1945).

Action as a Powerful Narcotic

There can be no doubt that the chief danger of trichlorethylene in industry is that of acute narcosis following prolonged exposure to high concentrations. Since 1935 it has been used as an inhalation anæsthetic and for this purpose resembles chloroform, but is less potent and less toxic (Hewer and Hadfield, 1941). Stüber (1931) recorded no fewer than 284 cases of poisoning from trichlorethylene, including twenty-six deaths, in German industry. She described the powerful narcotic effect of trichlorethylene, loss of consciousness having occurred in 117 cases. Twelve of the deaths occurred in men who failed to recover consciousness after prolonged exposure to a large dose. Sometimes residual symptoms such as headache, giddiness and loss of appetite occur, but it is difficult to decide whether these are not functional manifestations.

Cranial Nerve Palsies

There is little evidence of the cumulative action of trichlorethylene, though it is possible that it has a special affinity for nervous tissue. Lesions of the second, fifth and twelfth cranial nerves have been described, but there is some suspicion that they may have been due to an associated poison and not to trichlorethylene itself. Of Stüber's 284 cases, ten showed fifth-nerve paralysis and nine optic disturbances. These included blindness from optic atrophy in two cases, and retrobulbar neuritis with disturbances of the colour fields in the others.

Corneal Anæsthesia and Ulceration

German factory inspectors have described corneal ulcer resulting from a foreign body in the eye, the workman not having been aware of its presence because of anæsthesia of the cornea. The use of capsules of trichlorethylene for trigeminal neuralgia is inadvisable. After its introduction about 1925 this mode of therapy remained popular for some time, but eventually proved disappointing. More recently it has been used to try to relieve anginal pain, but with a similar disappointing result.

A Case of Polyneuritis

Isenschmid and Kunz (1934) described the case of a man aged fifty-six years who had been exposed for a year to the vapour of trichlorethylene in the process of cleaning steel cylinders. He developed retrobulbar neuritis, accompanied by left-sided paralysis of the tongue and polyneuritis of all four limbs.

Danger of Closed-circuit Anæsthesia

Seventeen cases have been reported in which cranial-nerve palsies, sometimes with herpes, developed after general anæsthesia (Humphrey and McClelland, 1944; Carden, 1944). In all of these a closed-circuit apparatus was used, and, despite the fact that thirteen out of fifteen of the cases of Humphrey and McClelland did not have trichlorethylene as the anæsthetic, the notorious reputation of this substance led to its being suspected as the noxious agent. When trichlorethylene is passed over soda-lime, dichloracetylene is formed. This substance is highly toxic to rabbits (Humphrey and McClelland, 1944) and also to rats (Milton, Graham, Perry and Hunter, 1944).

Dichloracetylene in the Soda-lime Canister

Trichlorethylene must never be used in a closed-circuit anæsthetic apparatus. Not only is dichloracetylene a highly toxic substance and dangerous to the person being anæsthetized, but it is stored in the soda-lime canister and may be volatilized by a later anæsthetic, particularly if ether is used. It may thus have toxic or even fatal results, even though no trichlorethylene be used in the subsequent anæsthetic. It seems probable that the trigeminal anæsthesia in German industry which seemed at one time such a mystery must be due to dichloracetylene either present as an impurity or formed by the close proximity of alkali.

Trichlorethylene unlikely to attack the Liver

Trichlorethylene is less likely to attack the liver than tetrachlorethane, carbon tetrachloride or chloroform. In many cases in which toxic jaundice is recorded, the evidence for attributing it to trichlorethylene is not definite. Stüber went so far as to state that the liver is never affected. Roholm (1933) stated that acute hepatitis may occur as late as sixty hours after the initial exposure and may produce acute necrosis of the liver like that due to delayed chloroform poisoning. Bridge (1933) reported the case of a boy who developed jaundice after six months' exposure to trichlorethylene in a degreasing process. There was a smooth enlargement of the liver, especially of the left lobe. Inquiry of the firm supplying the fluid precluded the possiblity of tetrachlorethane having been substituted by mistake for trichlorethylene.

Jaundice of Uncertain Origin

Willcox (1934) described a case of toxic jaundice in a boy aged sixteen years who had been employed dipping safety-razor blades into a tub containing trichlorethylene. Before admission to hospital he had been jaun-

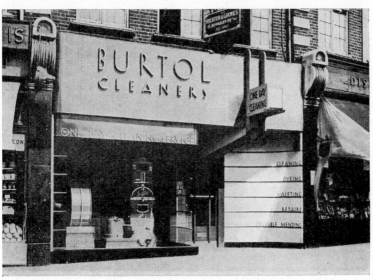

Fig. 212.—Dry-cleaning Shop using Trichlorethylene. Ventilation of the Establishment and of Individual Machines must be adequate
(*By courtesy of Burtol Cleaners, Ltd.*)

diced for a month and had frequently vomited. The temperature was normal and the liver enlarged. There was albumin in the urine. Gradually the jaundice cleared up and the liver became normal in size. The history and physical signs in these cases do not justify the conclusion that trichlorethylene was the causative agent to the exclusion of some other cause of jaundice.

Dermatitis due to Degreasing Effect

Dermatitis was found by Stüber in eighteen of her 284 cases, but she stated that in fact it was more frequent than this. It presented no special features, but like all dermatitis due to such substances was caused by the solvent action of trichlorethylene upon the fat in the skin.

Addiction to Trichlorethylene

Continued exposure to low concentrations of trichlorethylene causes a pleasant feeling of mild intoxication without nausea and may lead to a craving for further exposure. Such addiction was described by Baader in 1927 and has been frequently observed since.

Preventive Treatment

Premises in which trichlorethylene is employed for dry-cleaning must be amply ventilated and the individual machines provided with exhaust ventilation (fig. 212). Degreasing vats must be constructed in such a way as

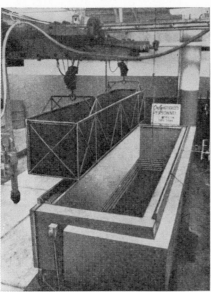

to prevent the escape of vapour into the general atmosphere; horizontal pipes through which cold water circulates serve to condense the vapour so that it returns to the vat as drops of fluid (fig 213). Accidents with trichlorethylene occur under abnormal circumstances, such as cleaning out a sump without the fan running, or entering a tank or cleaning apparatus without protection. When solutions containing trichlorethylene are applied to the interior of closed vats, the men should work in pairs, relieving each other frequently. The man in the enclosed space should be provided with a lifebelt, and also with an apparatus such as a hose-mask, through which he can breathe air from outside.

FIG. 213.—Trichlorethylene Vat for degreasing Metals. The Wire Cage is filled with Metal Objects and lowered into the Vat. Note Horizontal Water Pipes to condense the Vapour

(*Johnstone, R. T., 1948, Occupational Medicine and Industrial Hygiene, The C. V. Mosby Company*).

Case 22. *Owner of dry-cleaning business—exposure to trichlorethylene for three years—recurrent attacks of narcosis—contact dermatitis of hands and forearms.*

E. G., a man aged 44 years, seen in consultation with Dr. J. P. Reid in June 1954 (L.H. 20675/54). During three years day by day he entered the cleaning cabinets in his shop and frequently dipped his hands and forearms into an open tank of tricholorethylene. Although often drowsy towards the evening he never suffered from giddiness, headache, nausea or abdominal pain. On two occasions, six weeks and eight days previously, he had lost consciousness at work but had promptly recovered without further ill-effect. For five weeks he had had an itching eruption on both hands and forearms. The lesions were scattered red, slightly scaly discs up to two inches in diameter, and the skin was excoriated by scratching. Dr. Brian Russell considered that they had the appearance of a discoid eczema and that they had been initiated by the degreasing effect of trichlorethylene. There were no other abnormal physical signs. The Wassermann test of the blood and X-ray examination of the chest were both negative. The itching was arrested by fractional X-ray exposures and the lesions healed in 6 weeks.

(*d*) Carbon Tetrachloride

Carbon tetrachloride, or tetrachloromethane, CCl_4, is a colourless liquid with an odour somewhat resembling that of chloroform. Its vapour is 5·3 times heavier than air.

Uses

Commercial dry-cleaning accounts for 8 per cent of the annual output of carbon tetrachloride, 56 per cent is used in the manufacture of *freon* for refrigerators, 12 per cent for fire extinguishers and 4 per cent for grain fumigation. It is used as a solvent in the rubber, leather, chemical, pharmaceutical and paint industries, as a cleansing agent in the dry-cleaning industry and as a constituent of fire extinguishers (*pyrene*). Its value as a fire extinguisher, especially about electrical equipment, is increased by its high resistance to the passage of an electric current, thus preventing a short circuit through the extinguishing medium. This prevents shocks and burns to the operator of the fire extinguisher. The further fact that it dissolves petrol, benzene and coal-tar naphtha, thus lowering their flash-point, makes it especially valuable as an extinguisher of fires in motor cars, ships and aeroplanes. It has a low surface tension with a high specific gravity, and these properties give it high qualities of penetration for fibrous material such as textiles, leather and seeds. It is easily recovered and completely separated from extracted material or from insoluble residue. It is non-irritating and without corrosive action on metal parts. It is used in machine shops and printing plants for the removal of grease, as a solvent in the extraction of oils from seeds and fats from bones, as a parasiticide for certain cereals while in storage, as a dry shampoo for the hair, as a household

cleaning fluid under such trade names as *beaucaire, carbona, CTC, dabito*
and *thawpit,* and internally as an anthelmintic.

Exposure Hazards

One of the earliest reported cases of carbon-tetrachloride intoxicatio
was that of a man who entered a reservoir, and later showed excitement an
delirium followed by mild narcosis, with recovery in eight days (Lehmann
1903). Boveri (1930) reported from Milan five cases in men preparing a
insecticide which contained carbon tetrachloride. Two were poisone
severely, enlargement of the liver, albuminuria and urinary casts bein
noted. Subsequently, profound diuresis occurred and both patients re
covered. Henggeler (1931) reported six cases of poisoning in one family i
Switzerland. For three days they worked long hours cleaning and waxin
the floors of a school. The wax, which contained carbon tetrachloride, wa
heated by the man and then applied hot by the entire family. All th
patients suffered by the end of the third day from nausea, headache an
malaise. The man, who had undoubtedly breathed more of the vapou
than the others, became dangerously ill and showed mental confusio
headache, hiccup, nausea, vomiting, diarrhœa and scanty urine loade
with albumin. At the end of three weeks he was exhausted and emaciated
having lost 29 lb. in weight, but he gradually recovered after three months

Dry-cleaning in Confined Spaces

In 1932 McGuire reported from Boston seven cases of poisoning amon
workers passing felt through a warm mixture containing 33·3 per cent o
carbon tetrachloride to remove spots of grease. The symptoms were smart
ing around the eyes and mouth, headache, nausea, vomiting and diarrhœa
with acute nephritis in one case and jaundice with liver enlargement in two
All the patients recovered, the two with subacute necrosis of the live
remaining jaundiced for two months. A mass poisoning of eighty-eigh
soldiers who used carbon tetrachloride to clean their rifles in closed barrack
rooms was described by Perry in 1942. Five men were severely affected an
two of them died. In warships it is common for sailors to use *pyrene* ob
tained from fire extinguishers in order to remove grease spots from thei
clothes in the confined space of small cabins. Many such cases, includin
occasional deaths, occurred in the Royal Navy (Woods, 1946), and other
in the United States Navy (McGill, 1946), in the Second World War.

Extinguishing Fires in Confined Spaces

Dudley (1935) described two exposures to the vapour of carbon tetra
chloride sprayed from *pyrene* fire extinguishers in confined spaces i
British warships, and one exposure in a large, well-ventilated workroon
(fig. 214). Four men were poisoned in the first two exposures and were kep
under observation in hospital. They all showed impairment of renal func
tion, but they all recovered. One suffered from oliguria and jaundice, and
ten days after exposure developed convulsions. The blood-urea rose to 30

milligrams per 100 millilitres and the patient was practically moribund when, on the thirteenth day, polyuria developed, followed by recovery. Another man had almost complete anuria for ten days, but no other symptoms of renal insufficiency and no jaundice. None of the fourteen men who were exposed in the large workroom developed any untoward symptom or showed any impairment of renal function. The use of a *pyrene* fire extinguisher for about half an hour in the interior of a motor car had similar effects (Hagen and others, 1940).

Symptoms and Signs

Although carbon tetrachloride is not the most harmful of the chlorinated hydrocarbons it is nevertheless a dangerous poison. In a series of cases exposed to risk, personal idiosyncrasy is striking. There may be little or no relation between the amount of exposure and the severity of symptoms. In animal experiments it has been shown to cause necrosis of the liver (Lamson, Robbins and Ward, 1929). In man it may attack both liver and kidneys, but in most clinical histories the symptoms of renal injury overshadow those of hepatic injury. The early stages of the illness are characterized by persistent headache, nausea, vomiting, diarrhœa and tenderness over the liver, but such symptoms are often followed by oliguria, suppression of urine and uræmia. The blood urea rises, but a figure as high as 746 milligrams per 100 millilitres is compatible with recovery.

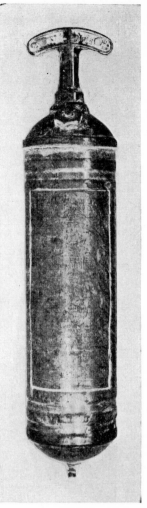

FIG. 214.—Veteran Pyrene Fire Extinguisher

Albumin, casts and red blood cells are sometimes found in the urine. Dermatitis is mentioned by Davis (1934) and is regarded by him as being due to the solvent action of carbon tetrachloride upon the fat in the skin. Although the majority of workmen dislike its odour, mild addiction to the vapour of carbon tetrachloride as a narcotic has been found to occur in men exposed to concentrations of from 100 to 160 parts per million (Hamilton and Hardy, 1949). Deaths in industry from the narcotic effects of carbon tetrachloride are seldom encountered, though they have occurred from the use of this substance as a dry shampoo for the hair.

Œdema of the Lungs

In some of the fatal cases following the use of fire extinguishers, œdema of the lungs has been found. It has been suggested that this is caused by the decomposition product phosgene, but it should be noted that œdema of the lungs has been found where there had been no contact of the carbon tetra-chloride with any agents likely to bring about decomposition. Nevertheless, carbon tetrachloride does decompose at 250° C., forming phosgene, and therefore its use as a fire extinguisher must be held in certain circumstances to involve the risk of phosgene poisoning.

Simulation of the Acute Abdomen

Simulation of an acute abdominal emergency has been recorded (Graham, 1938). The patient had been working with a dry-cleaning appa-ratus which was leaking. Epigastric pain and vomiting were accompanied by oliguria and tenderness in the left loin. The pulse rose to 130 and the patient showed the Hippocratic facies with abdominal distension and tenderness. It was only the increasing tenderness in the loins and the blood-cells in a scanty urine which tipped the balance in favour of medical treatment rather than laparotomy. Witts, Stewart and Kemp (1943), investigating a group of workmen exposed to carbon tetrachloride, showed by means of X-rays using opaque meals that there was hypermotility of the intestines associated with spasm.

Retrobulbar Neuritis

Toxic amblyopia has been described by Wirtschafter (1933). All his patients already showed gastro-intestinal disturbances, and three out of five complained of blurring of vision and spots before the eyes. Examination by perimetry showed bilateral constriction of the colour fields. Wirt-schafter suggested the routine of perimetric examination of the visual fields of workers to detect intoxication at an early stage. Out of ninety-three men whose visual fields were examined, Smyth, Smyth and Carpenter (1936) found ten with extensive and sixteen with slight constriction, which was not closely correlated with the degree of exposure.

Post-neuritic Optic Atrophy

Retrobulbar neuritis with post-neuritic optic atrophy following in-halation of the vapour of carbon tetrachloride was described by Smith (1950) in three workers in New York City. One of these patients had dipped electric razors into a mixture of gasoline and carbon tetrachloride for four months, the second was an electrician who for five months had cleaned silver busbars with rags dipped in carbon tetrachloride, and the third was a dressmaker who had removed spots from dress materials with a solvent consisting of 20 per cent carbon tetrachloride and 80 per cent petroleum naphtha. In one of the cases constitutional symptoms preceded the failure of vision; in the two others there were no such symptoms. All three showed great diminution of visual acuity, constriction of the visual fields, scoto-mata and blurring of the edges of the optic discs. The dressmaker recovered normal acuity of vision, but the two other patients developed optic atrophy and remained almost blind.

Morbid Anatomy and Histology

The necropsy findings, of course, differ according to whether death has occurred from hepatic or from renal insufficiency. With severe liver injury there is both extensive necrosis of cells and fatty degeneration with hæmorrhages. In the three cases described by Woods (1946), necrosis was confined to the centres of the liver lobules with evidence of regeneration about the central foci. The liver therefore appeared to have entered a stage of repair. The blood urea had risen before death to 266, 374 and 365 milligrams per 100 millilitres respectively in the three cases. Clearly the renal lesions had been responsible for death. The kidneys showed severe degeneration, with loss of cells and evidence of early regeneration in the second convoluted tubules and ascending limbs of Henle, and abundant casts seemingly derived from fragmented red corpuscles together with orange-brown or café-au-lait pigmented casts. These characteristics are found also in the crush syndrome, and Woods pointed out that the analogy was completed by the tubulo-venous communications which he found in two of his three cases.

Preventive Measures

The problem of prevention concerns the correct design of plant, the use of exhaust ventilation at appropriate points and good general ventilation everywhere. Stewart and Witts (1944) suggest that alternation of work with successive weeks in and out of exposure to carbon tetrachloride may increase efficiency. As a precaution against poisoning routine medical examination should be carried out on all workers exposed to the vapour. Household cleaning fluids, paint and shellac removers, and solutions for cleaning floors should not be sold under misleading trade names without labels to give warning of their poisonous nature. Firemen and first-aid workers must be taught as part of fire rescue to seek promptly the householder or other victim who may lie anæsthetized at the point where he attempted to extinguish the fire. An occasional accident occurring in a confined space cannot be used as an argument against the employment of carbon tetrachloride as a fire extinguisher. The prompt use of this liquid has saved countless people from death by burning or asphyxia from the poisonous gases normally present in the smoke from fires; while, on the other hand, the victims of poisoning from the vapour of carbon tetrachloride, even those who are very ill, usually recover.

Symptomatic Treatment

In the treatment of cases narcotized by exposure to the vapour it is important that the patient should not be placed upon the floor of the room where the accident occurred, for the vapour, being heavier than air, accumulates on the floor. Hepatic insufficiency has been treated by daily intravenous injections of glucose, calcium gluconate, protein hydrolysates and vitamin supplements. Methionine therapy is of doubtful value. For renal insufficiency, hot packs have been applied to the flanks, and dried blood plasma, equivalent to 500 millilitres of whole blood dissolved in 300 millilitres of sterile water, has been given intravenously.

(e) Ethylene Dichloride

Ethylene dichloride, or *sym*.-dichlorethane, $CH_2Cl.CH_2Cl$, is a colourless liquid with an odour like chloroform.

Uses

It is used in industry as a solvent for oils, fats, waxes, turpentine, rubber, some resins, benzyl cellulose, benzyl abietate, soft copals, sandarac and mastic, as an insecticide and fumigant especially for furs, in fire extinguishers and in household cleaning fluids.

Toxic Effects in Animals

Its toxicity after inhalation is not very high, ranking above trichlorethylene and slightly below carbon tetrachloride. It is a powerful narcotic and was used as an anæsthetic by Simpson in 1848. In animal experiments Müller (1925) claimed to have produced fatty degeneration of the liver and kidneys, but no changes in the liver other than congestion and cloudy swelling have been recorded by other workers. In their extensive studies in animals, Heppel and others (1946) found that guinea-pigs, mice, rats and rabbits were more susceptible than dogs. They remained uncertain as to the real cause of death in animals exposed to heavy concentrations of the vapour. Often there was no severe change in any organs, and the hepatic lesions characteristic of poisoning by carbon tetrachloride and chloroform were never seen. They called attention to the fact noted by a number of previous investigators that exposure of dogs to the vapour of ethylene dichloride causes bilateral turbidity of the cornea. Repeated exposures, separated by rest periods, produced tolerance to the vapour so that eventually no cloudiness developed.

Morbid Anatomy

Hueper and Smith (1935) described a case in which death followed twenty-two hours after drinking 2 oz. of ethylene dichloride. The patient showed dizziness, increasing stupor, cyanosis, a rapid pulse and heart failure. The urine contained albumin and sugar. At necropsy the kidneys showed extensive tubular necrosis with calcification resembling that seen in mercury-perchloride poisoning. These authors suggested that this finding indicated excretion by the kidney of the substance itself or of a decomposition product, presumably oxalic acid. The liver showed fatty degeneration and, in addition, there was extensive hæmorrhagic colitis. The necropsy described by Bloch (1946) in the case of a man who drank a fatal dose of ethylene dichloride also showed fatty degeneration of the liver. Ethylene dichloride is therefore capable of producing liver damage after ngestion, but for man its hepatotoxic action is less than that of tetra-chlorethane or carbon tetrachloride.

Symptoms and Signs

Bridge (1933) recorded the case of a patient who suffered from acute symptoms after exposure to the vapour of ethylene dichloride. The man was fitting a coil in a glycol plant when he complained of vomiting, diarrhœa, giddiness, drowsiness and slight breathlessness. In 1939 Wirt-schafter and Schwartz reported three cases of ethylene dichloride poisoning which were due to exposure to an open vat of this substance when cleaning yarn in a knitting factory. After four hours the men complained of dizziness, nausea, vomiting, epigastric pain, weakness and trembling. They were removed to hospital one hour later. In one case the liver was enlarged and tender but there was no jaundice; liver damage was suggested by very low blood-sugar levels. Leucocytosis was present in all cases. All three patients showed a severe dermatitis of the hands which presented a raw scalded appearance. It was thought to be due to the solvent action of ethylene dichloride upon the fat in the skin. There was no evidence of kidney involvement.

Treatment

On admission to hospital the patients were given injections of 10 per cent calcium gluconate, with immediate relief of the epigastric pain and vomiting. All the patients recovered after one week and were discharged with instructions to take a high-calcium, high-carbohydrate diet.

(f) Tetrachlorethane

Tetrachlorethane, or acetylene tetrachloride, $CHCl_2.CHCl_2$, is a colourless liquid with an odour resembling that of chloroform. Its vapour is 5·8 times as heavy as air. It attacks iron, copper, lead and nickel slightly and aluminuim vigorously. At various times it has been sold under proprietary names such as *alanol, cellon, emaillet, novania, quittnerlack, tetraline* and *westron.*

Uses

It is a good solvent for cellulose acetate and nitrate films and lacquers, for bitumen, waxes, resins, pitch, tar, sulphur, rubber and oils. It is used as a fire extinguisher and to make artificial silk, safety glass, leather and artificial pearls. It is also used as a dry-cleaning agent usually mixed with benzene, sometimes under the name *benzinoform,* and as a parasiticide, especially in hair-washes for dogs. It is used in the rubber industry, in the manufacture of gas-masks, shoe cements and floor waxes, and for the impregnation of furs and skins.

Historical Summary

In 1914 Jungfer reported the first cases of industrial poisoning from tetrachlorethane. They occurred in Germany in an aeroplane plant where eight men were employed in spraying a solution of cellulose acetate over the linen which covered the wings in order that they should be waterproof. Four of the men became jaundiced, and one died. This incident saved the Germans from serious trouble in aeroplane manufacture, for before the outbreak of war in 1914 they prohibited the use of this solvent in aeroplane doping. In England the first cases came to light in November 1914, when nineteen workers developed jaundice in an aeroplane works at Hendon. One man died after working for eleven weeks as a doper, and it was proved that his death was due to tetrachlorethane (Willcox, 1915). The large number affected at the same time was due to the fact that a plenum system of ventilation was installed in the works and blew the heavy vapour into every corner of the large shed where the work was being done. Aeroplane works were springing up all over the country, overtime was being worked to the utmost and all the dope used contained the noxious ingredient. Periodic medical examination at fortnightly intervals in the fifty or sixty factories was organized. Exhaust ventilation by fans which changed the air in the doping-rooms twenty-five to thirty times an hour was insisted on, and alternation of employment was recommended. Conditions were ameliorated to such an extent that no outbreak affecting so large a number of workers in any factory occurred subsequently, but there were many isolated cases and deaths, and many workers continued to be suspended at the medical examinations. By 1917 seventy cases, with twelve deaths, had been reported (Legge, 1917).

Prohibition in many Countries

Attempts to solve the problem by reducing the quantity of tetrachlorethane in the dope failed, for even as little as 10 per cent proved to be dangerous. Pressure was brought to bear to find a substitute for tetrachlorethane, and in July 1917 the War Office and Admiralty were able to announce that no aeroplane dope containing tetrachlorethane was being made or used. Similar cases occurred in France and Holland, and the use of tetrachlorethane in dope was forbidden in those countries too. In the artificial-pearl industry the use of tetrachlorethane collodion, known in France as *essence d'orient*, to impart lustre comparable to that of the natural pearl, has also been forbidden in many countries.

Morbid Anatomy

In 1911 Lehmann proved that tetrachlorethane is the most dangerous of all the chlorinated hydrocarbons, being about four times as toxic as chloroform and nine times as toxic as carbon tetrachloride. In three cases of poisoning after its ingestion, the patients all became unconscious and died within twelve hours from central respiratory paralysis (Forbes, 1943). Complete narcosis can also occur when tetrachlorethane is absorbed through the skin (Schwander, 1936). In industry the normal route of absorption is through the respiratory tract. In 1915 the investigations of Willcox, Spilsbury and Legge established the clinical picture as that of toxic jaundice resulting from hepatic insufficiency; necropsy showed the underlying lesion to be acute necrosis of the liver. The necrosis is found in the form of acute red and yellow atrophy. The liver is much reduced in size and may weigh 26 oz., or even only 19 oz. The kidneys may be pale, swollen and fatty. Hæmorrhages into serous membranes and the heart muscle may be present.

Symptoms and Signs

Two groups of cases of tetrachlorethane poisoning may be recognized in which the predominating symptoms are gastro-intestinal and nervous. Patients in whom nervous symptoms predominate, usually, though not invariably, show no liver disturbance. The course of the gastro-intestinal or hepatic form of the disease may be divided into four stages. In the first stage there is loss of appetite, fatigue, headache, vomiting and abdominal pain, occasionally so prominent as to suggest lead colic. In the second stage there is jaundice, with clay-coloured stools and constipation. Most of the workers have to cease work at this stage through increasing fatigue. There may be a slight rise in temperature, vomiting, albuminuria and even œdema of the legs. In the third stage the jaundice increases, the liver becomes enlarged and tender, and toxic symptoms appear. These include somnolence, delirium, convulsions and coma, leading usually to death. The fourth stage is that of ascites, but death often occurs before this is reached.

Toxic Polyneuritis

The nervous lesion is toxic polyneuritis. The illness begins with numbness and tingling of the fingers and toes. There is weakness of the interossei, and of the flexors and extensors of the fingers. Hypoæsthesia of the hands and feet is present, and sometimes tremor (Zollinger, 1931). Polyneuritis has occurred especially in the artificial-pearl industry, where the workers are exposed to tetrachlorethane, not only by inhaling the vapour, but also in manipulating the liquid with their hands. Léri and Breitel (1922) suggested that the lesion in the peripheral nerves may be a direct result of cutaneous absorption, since, in their series of cases, many who were exposed to the vapour suffered only from giddiness, while the two who showed polyneuritis developed it a month after first handling the liquid. Minot and Smith (1921) found that the blood changes in mild poisoning consist of an increase of large mononuclear cells up to 40 per cent, with a slight elevation of the white-cell count.

Preventive Measures

Amyl acetate can often be used as a solvent in place of tetrachlorethane. Closed apparatus should be used for cleaning purposes and adequate ventilation installed. The workers must be warned as to the dangers of the substance they are using and against eating food in rooms where cleaning processes are carried out (fig. 215). A canister gas-mask containing activated charcoal provides excellent protection against the concentrations usually

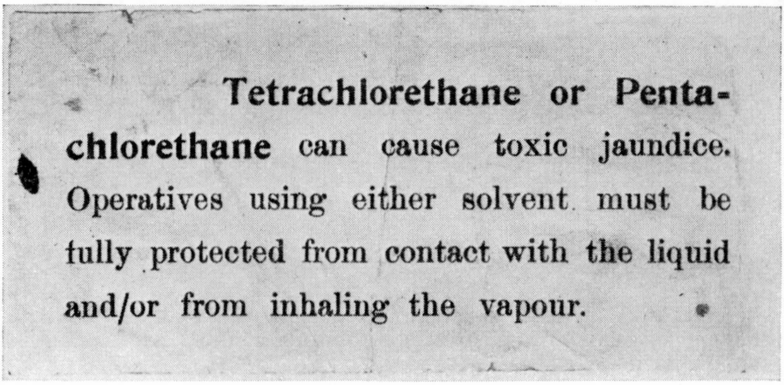

Tetrachlorethane or Penta-chlorethane can cause toxic jaundice. Operatives using either solvent must be fully protected from contact with the liquid and/or from inhaling the vapour.

FIG. 215.—Warning Notice issued by a Manufacturer of Chlorinated Hydrocarbons

found in factories where tetrachlorethane is used. Special precautions in the artificial-pearl industry have been suggested in the form of glass cases with openings for the arms of the worker manipulating the pearls. Such a worker must wear rubber gloves. Prophylactic measures include routine medical examination, with removal of workers from exposure on the earliest appearance of anorexia, malaise, headache, constipation, drowsiness or vomiting. Parmenter (1921) made routine blood counts in order to detect early poisoning among the workers in an artificial-silk factory.

(g) Chlorinated Naphthalenes

In the chlorination of naphthalene, as more hydrogen atoms are replaced by chlorine, so mono-, di-, tri-, tetra-, penta- and hexa-chloro-naphthalenes are produced. According to the amount of chlorine introduced, the chlorinated products vary in physical state from a freely mobile liquid to a crystalline or amorphous wax. In industry chlorinated diphenyls are used in conjunction with chlorinated naphthalenes. When diphenyl is chlorinated, one or more of the hydrogen atoms is replaced by chlorine forming mono-chlorodiphenyl, di-chlorodiphenyl, up to deca-chlorodi-phenyl. The greater the amount of chlorine introduced, the higher the melting-point and the more the substance becomes resinous or waxy in nature.

Uses

Such waxes have wide application in industry owing to their special insulating and water-resistant properties, their chemical stability and their flame resistance. They are used as dielectrics on condensers, as an insulating coat on wires and cables, or on metal bars to circumscribe the action of plating processes—for example, in chromium plating. They are sold under such trade names as *arochlor*, *halowax* and *seekay*. Certain insoluble cutting oils are treated with sulphur and solid chloronaphthalenes when they are required for use in heavy cutting or gear-grinding operations.

Exposure Hazards

The chlorodiphenyls are used in conjunction with the chloronaph-thalenes as insulators for electric wires and on condensers. The wax is usually melted in a bath and the articles may be dipped in the bath directly or the wax applied to them by means of a brush. When highly chlorinated cutting oils are used in engineering, a mist of oil is seen around the machines and it falls on the workers, soaking their clothing.

Chlor-acne an Unsuitable Name

The term *chlor-acne* was first used by Herxheimer in 1899 to describe an eruption composed of comedones and small sebaceous pustules which occurred on the arms and faces of workers manufacturing chlorine gas electrolytically, using carbon electrodes. It was natural to assume that the chlorine was the causative agent. Later, some authors suspected various chlorobenzene derivatives such as hexa-chlorobenzene, hexa-chlorethy-lene, *para*nitrobenzene, perchloronaphthalene (*perna*) and probably others. Chlorinated naphthalenes were first indicted by Wauer in 1918 as a cause of acneiform eruptions of the skin, the condition being called *Pernakrank-heit*. Workers engaged in the manufacture of these substances are exposed to fume of the molten mass and also to the sublimated dust. The majority of writers on the subject, particularly White (1934), have felt that chlorine as such has little to do with the formation of the comedones and cysts, and they have repeatedly referred to tar and products of the distillation of tar as the prime causative factors. White rebuked authors for using the term *chlor-acne* at all, and expressed the belief that the process is one of the manifold cutaneous reactions produced by tar and its derivatives.

Chloronaphthalene Acne

Jones (1941) emphasized that the acne is due to the chloronaphthalenes themselves. In the absence of cleanliness, these substances irritate the sebaceous glands, causing an excess of cell growth and secretion, fol-lowed by plugging of the glands and possible secondary infection. Cleanli-ness is therefore a most important factor. In men who manufacture the chloronaphthalenes the typical skin condition starts on the face, around the angles of the jaws or over the malar prominences, and from there spreads on to the sides of the face and on to the sides and back of the neck. The skin lesions in a typical case are comedones, papules, pustules and, in severe cases, small cysts (fig. 216). Sometimes the eruption spreads on to the shoulders and forearms. It differs from ordinary acne because it itches, and the men call it *blackhead itch*. Schwartz (1943) reported an outbreak of *halowax acne* or *cable rash* among electricians installing and stripping heat- and flame-proof cables in ships. Engineering workers exposed to the mist of highly chlorinated cutting oils develop acne on the face, neck, anterior surface of the trunk, the arms, the penis, scrotum and other places where the oil-soaked clothing touches the skin (Schwartz, Tulipan and Peck, 1947).

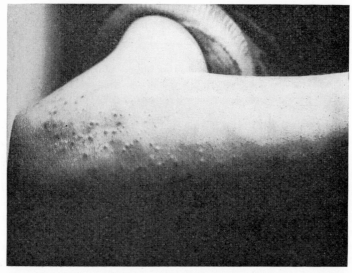

FIG. 216.—Chloronaphthalene Acne in a man aged 35, after 3 months'
Exposure
(*By courtesy of Dr. A. Thelwall Jones*)

Toxic Effects in Animals

Systemic effects from chlorinated naphthalenes were first pointed out
by Lehmann in 1919. He found that animals which were fed on these substances, or inhaled them, lost appetite and at death showed liver lesions.
Drinker, Warren and Bennett (1937) administered chlorinated hydrocarbons by inhalation, subcutaneously and by mouth to white rats. Tri-,
tetra-, penta- and hexa-chloronaphthalenes and chlorinated diphenyls
were used. These experiments showed that tri- and tetra-chloronaph-
thalenes produced relatively unimportant pathological changes in the liver
until extremely high concentrations were used. Animals exposed for six
weeks to the more highly chlorinated compounds in relatively low concentrations regularly showed minor degrees of liver damage, even though,
as a group, they gave no clinical evidence of such toxicity while alive.
Exposed to still higher concentrations, the rats lost weight and appetite,
and began dying after eight days of exposure, many with severe jaundice.
Examination of the liver at necropsy revealed marked fatty degeneration
with necrosis of cells, at the centres of the lobules.

Systemic Effects in Man

For twenty years acne remained the only industrial injury from the use
of these waxes, but about 1935 there was a change in the type of product
used from the lower to the higher chlorinated members. And then in 1936
three fatal cases of jaundice in workers handling chlorinated naphthalenes
were recognized in the United States of America (Flinn and Jarvik, 1936;
Drinker, Warren and Bennett, 1937). All three of the men were young, and

n none could any predisposing cause other than the industrial exposure be ound to account for the illness. Two of the men who had worked side by ide died within two months of each other. Both had been exposed to mixtures of penta- and hexa-chloronaphthalene, and one had been exposed o a mixture of tetra- and penta-chloronaphthalene with 10 per cent hlorinated diphenyl. In both, the diagnosis of acute yellow atrophy of the iver was made at necropsy. In the third case no necropsy was reported, but leath occurred after an acute illness characterized by jaundice. In one case cne had preceded the jaundice. In addition to these fatal cases, Drinker, Warren and Bennett also mentioned four cases of non-fatal jaundice mong subjects with similar exposure. No details were given.

atal Cases and Morbid Anatomy

Greenburg, Mayers and Smith (1939) recorded three fatal cases in oung people working with chlorinated naphthalenes and diphenyl. Two f the patients apparently had suffered from at least one previous attack of epatitis, followed by a certain degree of improvement, before the fatal ttack. McLetchie and Robertson (1942) and Collier (1943) recorded a atal case of toxic jaundice in a woman of forty-one years who worked in an ngineering establishment in Scotland and had been exposed to the fume nd dust of chlorinated naphthalenes for six months. Some of her fellow vorkers had the usual acne, but there was no other case of jaundice. The llness came on slowly, jaundice appeared and increased, the patient passed nto coma and died in the fifth week. Necropsy showed acute red and ellow necrosis of the liver, which weighed 650 grams, the normal being ,500 grams.

reventive Measures

By attention to ventilation and medical supervision of workers, the hlorinated naphthalenes and diphenyls can be handled in industry with afety. Education of the workers as to the cause of the acne must be undertaken and the necessity for personal cleanliness emphasized. Lightcoloured, highly starched, closely woven overalls with full-length sleeves hould be provided. These must be changed and laundered at least once a veek. Adequate washing accommodation and locker space must be provided. The work-people must be taught not to touch the skin with the hands and not to use rags for wiping the nose and the face. They must vash before meals and take food only in special rooms set aside for the ourpose.

Medical Supervision

Medical selection of workers must aim at avoiding adolescents and all persons with oily skins, established acne or seborrhœa. Medical examination must be carried out at least once a week. All early cases of acne or aundice must be removed from contact with the toxic substance. Prevention of systemic effects turns upon exhaust ventilation to remove fume nd dust, and avoidance of over-heating of the wax.

Protection of Machine Operators

Machine operators using chlorinated cutting oils must be provided daily with clean clothes made so that the anterior surfaces of the trunk and arms are protected by aprons and sleeves of impermeable material. Prevention of acne depends upon cleanliness of the person, of the clothes, of the machines and of the oil. Adequate locker space, washing facilities, towels, hot and cold running water, and shower baths should be provided, and the men compelled to use them under supervision (Schwartz, Tulipan and Peck, 1947).

THE GLYCOL GROUP

About 1925 a great new aliphatic chemical industry grew up and rapidly became bigger than the coal-tar or aromatic industry (fig. 217). One result of this was the introduction of a host of new solvents, including ethylene chlorhydrin, dioxan, cellosolve, cellosolve acetate, methyl cellosolve, butyl cellosolve, carbitol and butyl carbitol (Browning, 1953). The first two of these substances will be described since they have caused poisoning in man. The others of the group may be toxic too. Acute poisoning by ethylene chlorhydrin first attracted attention in a paper factory in Germany in 1927. Five deaths occurred in 1934 from exposure to diethylene dioxide in the manufacture of cellulose acetate silk yarn in the Midlands.

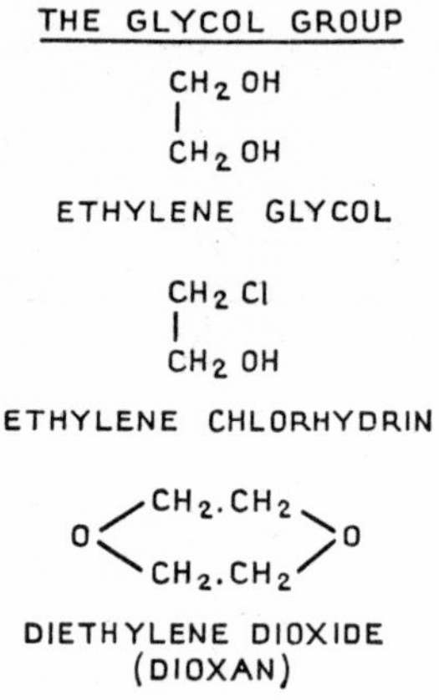

THE GLYCOL GROUP

CH_2OH
|
CH_2OH

ETHYLENE GLYCOL

CH_2Cl
|
CH_2OH

ETHYLENE CHLORHYDRIN

$O \diagdown \genfrac{}{}{0pt}{}{CH_2 \cdot CH_2}{CH_2 \cdot CH_2} \diagup O$

DIETHYLENE DIOXIDE
(DIOXAN)

Fig. 217

(a) Ethylene Chlorhydrin

Ethylene chlorhydrin, 2-chloro-ethyl alcohol, $CH_2Cl.CH_2OH$, also known as glycol chlorhydrin, is a clear, glycerine-like fluid with an odour resembling that of a mixture of ethyl alcohol and ether. Its vapour has a specific gravity 2·8 times that of air. It is intensely poisonous, the maximum allowable concentration in the working environment being 2 p.p.m. of air.

Uses

The greater part of the ethylene chlorhydrin produced is used as an intermediate for the production of such substances as ethylene glycol, amines, carbitols, indigo, malonic acid, novocaine and, in general, for the introduction of the hydroxyethyl group in organic syntheses. Owing to its solvent action for cellulose acetate, resin and wax, it is used in the lacquer industry especially as an addition to plasticizers for paint and varnish; also in the dyeing and cleaning industry, and in the linoleum, paper and pharmaceutical industries. It is used for treating potatoes, especially sweet potatoes, before planting in order to activate sprouting.

Toxic Effects in Animals

Rats, mice, guinea-pigs, rabbits and cats are all readily poisoned by ethylene chlorhydrin after ingestion, application to the skin, intraperitoneal injection or inhalation. After oral administration, death is delayed in onset and no true narcosis occurs. There is general prostration and spasmodic movements occur. Depression and convulsions are followed by respiratory paralysis. In chronic poisoning the cells of the convoluted tubules of the kidney are attacked but the glomeruli escape. Goldblatt (1944) suggests that the effect of ethylene chlorhydrin on the kidneys is that of a vascular poison. The liver shows congestion and fatty degeneration.

Fatal Cases following Ingestion

In a fatal case recorded by Ballotta and others (1953), ingestion of a small amount caused death. The victim merely aspirated a mouthful of ethylene chlorhydrin through a rubber tube, spat it out at once and rinsed his mouth thoroughly with water. Half an hour later he had nausea and headache, followed in three hours by excitement and mania, ending in coma in which he died seven hours after the accident. Necropsy showed hyperæmia of the brain, liver and kidneys. Güthert (1943) described two cases where ingestion was fatal; in the one where death was longer delayed the kidneys showed severe nephrosis.

Non-fatal Acute Cases

Numerous cases of acute poisoning by ethylene chlorhydrin have been reported in which recovery occurred. Chronic intoxication has not been observed. Poisoning occurs either from inhalation or from absorption through the skin. Koelsch (1927) described seven non-fatal cases which occurred from inhalation of the vapour. In most of these, nausea, vomiting, drowsiness and weakness were followed by recovery after some days. In those least affected there was no symptom other than slight irritation of the eyes. Goldblatt and Chiesman (1944) described nine non-fatal cases which occurred during the actual manufacture of ethylene chlorhydrin. The symptoms and signs were nausea, epigastric pain, repeated vomiting, cough, headache, giddiness and confusion. In severe cases there was erythema on the skin of the arms and trunk, and also transient albuminuria. The vapour absorbed was a mixture of ethylene chlorhydrin and ethylene dichloride, but the very minor narcotic effects suggest that the latter was not the principal cause of the symptoms.

Acute Fatal Cases and Morbid Anatomy

Two fatal cases, one in a paper factory and the other in a linoleum factory, were reported from Germany by Koelsch (1927). In the first case the workers cleaned the cylinder of a paper machine with cloths dipped in ethylene chlorhydrin. The symptoms began with nausea, vomiting and drowsiness. Some hours later severe headache and slight stupor developed, with vomiting. There was no fever, but râles were present in the lungs, and death occurred in syncope. At necropsy there was engorgement of the lungs and liver. The kidneys were unaffected. The case of the linoleum worker showed a latent period in the development of symptoms. The patient had slight vomiting and drowsiness in the morning and was then examined by a doctor, who found nothing abnormal. In the afternoon dyspnœa developed and he died the same evening. At necropsy there was œdema of the lungs and brain, and acute gastro-intestinal catarrh.

Renal Involvement in a Case of Subacute Poisoning

Of the two fatal cases described by Goldblatt and Chiesman (1944), one occurred in a foreman who repaired a fault in a concentration tower for ethylene chlorhydrin, thus exposing himself, strictly against instructions, to a high concentration of hot vapour for an hour and a half. He collapsed and died within fourteen hours. Necropsy showed marked œdema of the cerebral hemispheres, but the kidneys and liver were normal. The other case was that of a process worker exposed for two months to the vapour of ethylene chlorhydrin. The illness was subacute, with headache, confusion and ultimately hæmaturia. An incomplete necropsy showed renal changes, especially necrosis of the convoluted tubules with much debris in the lumen of the tubules.

Absorption through the Skin

In one of the fatal cases described by Koelsch (1927) there must have been considerable contact with the skin, for the man cleaned a machine for two and a half hours with a rag soaked in ethylene chlorhydrin. Middleton (1930) recorded a fatal case where the toxic effects appear to have been due not only to inhalation of the vapour, but also to absorption through the skin, the patient having entered a still in a dye works to mop up water containing ethylene chlorhydrin in solution. The initial symptoms were vomiting and drowsiness. Death took place about twelve hours after removal from exposure. Necropsy showed œdema of the lungs and bronchopneumonia. In the fatality reported by Dierker and Brown (1944) the patient was exposed to a concentration of vapour of 305 p.p.m., but skin absorption also occurred. Necropsy showed kidneys described as deeply congested.

Preventive Measures

Since ethylene chlorhydrin is intensely poisonous, the correct design of plant for its manufacture is of major importance. Leaks, overflows and escape of vapour should be avoided. There must be good general ventilation, and local exhaust ventilation at specially hazardous points. The necessity for periodic sampling from reaction vessels requires arrangements which do not involve the opening of points where escape of vapour is inevitable. Routine estimation of the concentration of the vapour at working-places is necessary. Goldblatt and Chiesman (1944) take the view that no concentration which is capable of chemical determination should be regarded as satisfactory. Routine medical examination, report by workers of untoward symptoms and detection of susceptible subjects are all essential as measures of protection for the worker.

(b) Diethylene Dioxide

Diethylene dioxide, or *dioxan*, $O{<}^{CH_2.CH_2}_{CH_2.CH_2}{>}O$, is a colourless liquid with a faintly pungent odour. It is used as a degreaser, especially for wool, as a solvent in the textile, lacquer and celluloid industries, and in the manufacture of polishes, pastes, cements, glues, shoe-creams and cosmetics. In addition, it is a paint remover, preservative, fumigant and deodorant.

Toxic Effects in Animals

In experiments carried out on guinea-pigs, Yant, Schrenk, Waite and Patty (1930) were unable to demonstrate lesions of the kidneys or liver. Acute poisoning from the vapour caused irritation of eyes, nose, throat and bronchi, and even narcosis. Their report suggests that owing to its low toxicity in small concentrations and its irritant effect, health hazards from breathing the vapour under ordinary conditions are slight. In 1934 Fairley, Linton and Ford-Moore exposed rats, mice, guinea-pigs and rabbits over long periods to mixtures of *dioxan* and water in the approximate ratio of four to one. The animals inhaled the vapour in the form of a spray. Lesions were observed, sometimes of great severity, in the kidneys and liver. They were present even in animals exposed to a non-lethal concentration of 1 in 1,000 of the mixture.

Exposure Hazards

Barber (1934) recorded the death of five men which occurred within a fortnight from exposure to *dioxan* in the manufacture of cellulose-acetate silk yarn in a works near Derby. The process on which they were employed had been in use for nearly sixteen months, but for five weeks before they became ill, exposure to the vapour was intensified by the speeding-up of the machine on which they worked. Diethylene dioxide is not highly volatile under ordinary conditions, but here the men found it necessary to put their heads into the vat containing the noxious substance. There was a possibility of exposure in eighty other men, and detailed inquiries showed that some of these had suffered from anorexia, nausea and vomiting. No jaundice had been present in either the fatal cases or in exposed workers examined, but in one of the latter the liver was palpable and a trace of albumin and a few red-blood cells were found in the urine. There was also a trace of albuminuria in 65 per cent of those much exposed and in 50 per cent of the others.

Fatal Cases and Morbid Anatomy

In the five fatal cases the premonitory symptoms were nausea, vomiting and abdominal pain. In two cases an acute abdominal emergency was simulated. In no case was there jaundice to indicate necrosis of the liver. From about the third day of the illness the urine was scanty, and in one case it was found to contain blood and albumin. The symptoms of uræmia with suppression of urine were predominant after the first few days, and death occurred in about a week. In one case the blood-urea reached 346 milligrams per 100 millilitres. The blood counts in three cases showed no anæmia or change in the red cells, but the white-cell counts varied between 21,400 and 38,000 per c.mm., with a high percentage of polymorphs. In the four cases submitted to necropsy the kidneys showed hæmorrhagic nephritis with necrosis of the outer part of the cortex. The destruction was vascular in distribution and dependent on hyaline thrombosis of the vessels in the renal cortex. There were areas of necrosis of the liver without bile staining or fatty change. Histologically, there was complete necrosis of the inner half of each lobule. The absence of fatty degeneration was in striking contrast to that found with liver poisons such as chloroform. Absorption evidently occurred by inhalation, and the severity of the changes in the kidneys suggests that death was due to the great increase of the dose which occurred when the process was intensified.

Symptoms and Signs

Henry (1934) divided intoxication into three stages. The earliest effects include irritation of the nasopharynx with cough, of the nose with coryza and of the conjunctivæ with misty vision. Even if the inhalation is continued, this irritation may subside and thus give rise to a false sense of security. Drowsiness, vertigo, headache, loss of appetite, nausea and vomiting follow. If at this stage a rest of twenty-four hours is taken, the ill effects tend to pass off quickly. In the second stage the gastric symptoms become more severe. There is pain and tenderness in the abdomen and lumbar region, and enlargement of the liver. After removal from exposure for a week or so, these effects pass off gradually. In the third stage there is acute hæmorrhagic nephritis, which may lead to suppression of urine, uræmia, coma and death.

Preventive Measures

Where the use of *dioxan* cannot be confined to enclosed apparatus, adequate exhaust ventilation must be provided and large evaporation surfaces forbidden. Since animal experiments show that diethylene dioxide is absorbed through the skin, plant design must ensure that the skin of the worker is not contaminated. The use of gloves gives partial protection.

CARBON DISULPHIDE

Carbon disulphide, CS_2, was discovered in 1796 by W. A. Lampadius of Freiberg while studying the action of pyrites on carbon. Pure carbon disulphide is a colourless, mobile, refractive liquid with a boiling-point of 46° C. It has an aromatic smell, not displeasing and somewhat like that of chloroform. The crude technical product is a yellowish liquid with a disagreeable odour which has been likened to that of decaying radishes. It evaporates at room temperature, giving a vapour which is 2·62 times as heavy as air and therefore collects near the ground. It is very dangerous, highly inflammable and must be handled with great care.

Danger of Fire and Explosion

The flash-point of carbon disulphide is below −20° C. and it has an extremely low ignition temperature. Contact with a warm steam-pipe or electric-light bulb, or even a heavy blow, may be sufficient to cause ignition of the vapour. The minimum explosive mixture in air is nineteen volumes in 1,000. Precautions against fire include the exclusion of naked lights, hot pipes and other hot plant from places where carbon disulphide is stored. Ordinary safety lamps are *not* safe in an atmosphere containing carbon disulphide. To reduce the risk of explosion, non-sparking tools—for example, those made of beryllium-copper—must be used (fig. 218). All

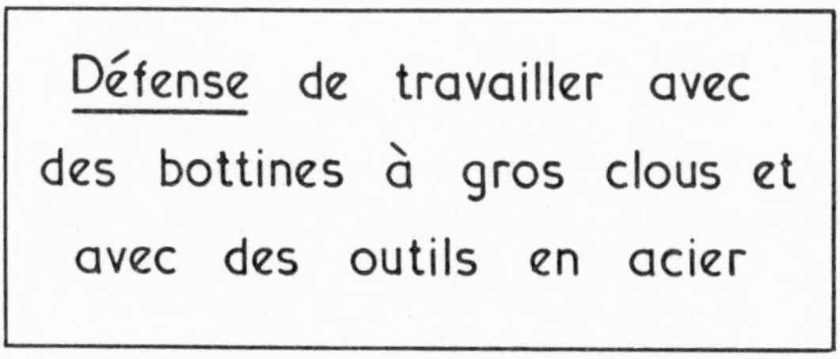

Défense de travailler avec des bottines à gros clous et avec des outils en acier

Fig. 218.—Notice in use in the churn room of a viscose silk factory in Belgium
(*By courtesy of S. A. Fabelta, Tubize, Belgium*)

electrical apparatus should be outside the room or area where carbon disulphide is present. Electric lights should be outside windows or sealed behind plate-glass in order to prevent the passage of carbon disulphide vapour to the fittings. Static electricity may accumulate during the flow and agitation of carbon disulphide in pipes, and under certain conditions may cause sparking. Metal pipes and tanks should therefore be efficiently bonded at all joints and earthed. Static charges are dissipated if the relative humidity is not allowed to fall below 60 per cent (Factory Department Memorandum, 1943). Fire extinguishers of the foam type must always be available. If carbon disulphide catches fire in an enclosed space, such as in a room where people are present, extinguishers containing carbon tetrachloride or methyl bromide must not be used.

Storage and Conveyance

Storage and conveyance of carbon disulphide should be under water, in which it is only slightly soluble. In the Martini and Hüneke system an inert gas is used to replace air in the outer of two pipes, the inner one of which carries liquid carbon disulphide. The liquid is forced through the inner pipe by pressure applied through the outer pipe to the surface of the

liquid in the storage tank. The escape of large quantities of carbon disulphide cannot occur, since a leak in the inner pipe results in escape of the
liquid to the outer pipe and its return to the storage tank. If the leak is in
the outer pipe, the pressure drops and liquid is no longer forced into the
inner pipe.

Uses

In the first half-century after its discovery carbon disulphide was used
in medicine in the treatment of a variety of diseases, and was tried as an
anæsthetic agent before chloroform was discovered. It mixes in all proportions with alcohol, ether, benzene and essential oils. It is also a good
solvent for sulphur, phosphorus, iodine, bromine, camphor, gums, resins,
waxes, fats and rubber; and it is largely employed in the industries on
account of its solvent properties. It is also used as an insecticide. Its two
most important uses are in the cold curing of rubber and in the manufacture of artificial silk by the viscose process.

Cold Curing of Rubber

When rubber is vulcanized by heating it for some time with flowers of
sulphur, carbon disulphide is not employed. However, in the cold-curing
process used in making surgical appliances, thin strips of rubber are dipped
into a solution of sulphur monochloride in carbon disulphide. The carbon
disulphide does not take part in the reaction but has the advantage over
other solvents of causing considerable swelling of the rubber, thus allowing
greater impregnation of the interstices with sulphur. Since it is volatile it
is easily recoverable and can therefore be used again.

The Viscose Process

After 1890, owing to the immense expansion of newspaper production,
wood-pulp, a comparatively pure form of cellulose, became available in
abundance at little cost. In 1892 the viscose process for the manufacture of
artificial silk was developed. It employs the cheap cellulose of wood-pulp
instead of the more expensive pure cotton cellulose used in the Chardonnet
process (see p. 591). The wood-pulp is treated with alkali and the product
is dissolved in carbon disulphide. Courtaulds began the industrial operation of the viscose process in 1906, and by 1954 viscose rayon made in
many different countries was providing three-quarters of the world's
artificial silk. The immense industrial importance of rayon may be measured
by the fact that world production is approximately a million tons a year.
About half of this is made in the United States of America; the next
largest producer is Great Britain.

Xanthation of Cellulose Crumbs

In the viscose process the wood-pulp is mercerized with caustic-soda
solution, shredded to form alkali cellulose crumbs and, after an interval of
ageing, subjected to a process termed xanthation. This process takes place

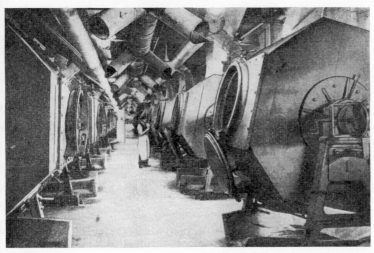

FIG. 219.—Churns for making Cellulose Xanthate—a stage in the production
of Rayon Fibres by the Viscose Process
(*By courtesy of Courtaulds, Ltd.*)

n revolving drums called churns, where the crumbs enter into a chemical
reaction with carbon disulphide to form cellulose xanthate. The reaction
generates heat, and the rise of temperature causes a rise of pressure within
the churn. Leakage of carbon disulphide vapour may occur because of the
solvent action of the carbon disulphide on the rubber gaskets round the
doors of the churn (fig. 219).

Cleaning the Xanthate Churns

At the next stage the cellulose xanthate is taken from the churn to the
mixer. For a variable time before the churn is opened, air is drawn through
it to remove the carbon disulphide vapour. The xanthate may be dry and
crumbly, or so moist and sticky that it has to be shovelled out of the churn.
Moreover, the churns must be cleaned after each xanthation and this is
recognized as dangerous work, during which the workmen should be protected by constant air suction. The risk varies according to the character
of the xanthate and the type of churn. It may be necessary for the man to
climb inside the churn to clean it. Xanthate crumbs spilled on the floor of
the churn room are a further source of carbon-disulphide vapour. There
may be leaks from the churn or from the pipe supplying carbon disulphide
to it. The supply pipe should be straight and free from traps or U-bends
where carbon disulphide will collect and continue to vaporize after the
churn is opened.

Hazards in the Spinning Rooms

The xanthate is dissolved in a dilute solution of caustic soda, and carbon
disulphide is liberated. The resulting product is viscose, a syrupy fluid

which is filtered and ripened in a series of tanks before being spun. In the spinning-room the viscose is forced through spinnerets into a bath containing sulphuric acid, sulphate and other substances. The viscose coagulates and decomposes, releasing pure cellulose which is drawn out as a thread and wound on bobbins. Carbon disulphide and sulphuretted hydrogen are formed and, unless the spinning machines are enclosed, high concentrations of these two gases occur in the air over the spinning baths. The danger of absorption is increased by the heat and high humidity which commonly exist in the spinning-rooms (Hamilton, 1940). Further processes include drying, reeling, washing, desulphuring, bleaching and staple- or fibre-cutting. There may be a hazard from carbon-disulphide vapour at any of these stages, but the main risks are in the churn and spinning-rooms.

Charcot's Sulphide of Carbon Neurosis

In 1851 Payen directed attention to the danger to workers using carbon disulphide in the cold-curing of rubber in factories in France. In 1856 Delpech gave an accurate description of the symptoms and signs of carbon disulphide poisoning. In 1889 Charcot demonstrated cases of what he called sulphide of carbon neurosis, saying that while some of the symptoms described by Delpech were probably due to carbon disulphide, most of them were undoubtedly due to hysteria. The first case of industrial origin was reported from Germany in 1866 by Harmson. In 1885 Frost published the results of an earlier investigation in rubber factories in England in which he described thirty-three cases of nervous and mental disturbance. Twenty-four of these patients showed evidence of damage to the optic nerve.

Cases in Poland, Italy and France

Many cases of carbon-disulphide poisoning have been reported from European countries. In 1947 Paluch described two outbreaks of carbon-disulphide poisoning in Poland, one occurring during the German occupation and the other shortly after the end of the Second World War. In the first of these, 148 known cases occurred and there were probably more which were not published. It is alleged that more than one case of acute psychosis occurred each month in a factory established by the Germans in Lodz in 1940. These cases were sent direct to psychiatric hospitals and no traces remain of them, since all mental patients were killed by German police before the end of the war and the case records destroyed. In France there were sixty-two fatal cases in 1945, compared with 252 in 1942, a steady decline in both serious and fatal cases occurring between these two dates (Auffert, 1946). Serious cases do still occur, however, in France and other European countries, and Vigliani reports 100 cases in Italy in 1946 six of whom had psychosis. In England, carbon-disulphide poisoning has been compulsorily notifiable since 1924, and only twenty-five cases had been reported up to 1951.

Ieadache, Somnolence and Acute Mania

Oliver (1902) described the poisoning as occurring in two forms:

In one the symptoms which are slowly developed are dizziness, headache, vomiting, lassitude, and not infrequently paralysis of the arms or legs. Many female workers complain of tasting the nauseous bisulphide in their food. The appetite thus becomes impaired. In the other form of poisoning, which may be spoken of as acute, the individual is really intoxicated. Girls have told me that on leaving the factory at night they have simply staggered home, fallen as if drunk, or at the end of a day's work they have had a splitting headache, and on reaching home have sat down, tired out, and fallen asleep before touching their evening meal. This sleep is heavy and non-refreshing. In the morning they drag themselves to the factory. Sad as this state of things is, it is nothing to the extremely violent maniacal condition into which some of the workers, both male and female, are known to have been thrown. Some of them have become the victims of acute insanity, and in their frenzy have precipitated themselves from the top rooms of the factory to the ground. In consequence of bisulphide of carbon being extremely explosive, vulcanization by means of it has generally to be carried on in rooms, one side of which is perfectly open. This open front is usually protected by iron bars.

3ymmetrical Polyneuritis

Polyneuritis is the commonest manifestation of carbon-disulphide poisoning, both motor and sensory nerves being involved. The limbs are nore often affected than other parts of the body. Increasing fatigue and veakness, particularly of the legs, are associated with numbness and coldness in the feet, and wasting of the muscles. Aching or cramp-like pain in he distribution of the affected nerves may be intolerable and may cause nsomnia. The signs are those of a symmetrical polyneuritis in which all our limbs may be involved. In 1948 Paluch described the case of a worker n a Polish factory, making viscose rayon since 1945. He was employed in his factory since 1922 and had been engaged in the rayon staple-fibre plant ince 1941. He last worked for several weeks at the desulphuring baths. When visited at home on 27th February 1946 he said that he had been ill 'or three weeks. Since the middle of December 1945 he had felt increasing veakness in his legs, and had had to stop and sit down when walking to the actory and back. Finally, he could not walk at all. The physician of the 3ocial Insurance Scheme called at his home, advised him to go to hospital ind gave him a letter stating that he was suffering from paresis of the ower extremities of unknown cause. The patient did not like to follow this idvice and called a private practitioner who treated him at home. He was ible to sit up in bed but could not stand or walk unless strongly supported. There was tenderness on pressure over the muscles and nerve trunks of the ower extremities. The knee-jerks and ankle-jerks were absent on both

sides. There was loss of sensation of touch, pain and temperature in th
region of both peroneal nerves. There were no other changes either nervou
or psychic. The course of the disease is slow, much slower than in alcoholi
polyneuritis. There may be no improvement in years, and sometimes th
condition progresses. These variations do not appear to be related eithe
to the initial severity of the symptoms or to the age of the patient.

Visual and Auditory Changes

Eye changes have been recognized since the report by Frost in 1886
They include diminished reaction of the pupils to light, central scotom
and concentric narrowing of the visual fields. Very rarely there is blurrin
of vision with no change in the appearance of the fundus oculi. Auditor
symptoms include dizziness, tinnitus and deafness. There is, however
little objective evidence of damage to the ear and the symptoms may b
due to lack of concentration. Audiometric tests reveal no significant im
pairment for tones in the speech-range of frequencies (300–3,000 cycle
per second). Audiograms show impairment of perception in the C_5 are
(4,096 cycles per second). There is some evidence of involvement of th
vestibular apparatus.

Headache, Insomnia and Melancholia

The early symptoms of carbon disulphide psychosis may pass unnotice
by the patient and an attack of acute mania occur, apparently withou
warning. In all such cases careful inquiry from relatives and workmate
will reveal the presence of early symptoms such as irritability, uncontrol
lable anger and changes of temperament. Among men supposedly norma
and continuing at work, Braceland (1942) reports, in addition to irritability
marked defect of memory, severe insomnia and depression of sexual func
tion in individuals far below the normal age for loss of libido. The insomni
is due either to jerking movements, which may be severe enough to throw
the patient out of bed, or to frequent bad dreams so terrifying that sleep i
dreaded in spite of intense fatigue. Frontal headache, transient excitemen
and slight delirium may occur, and progress through depression, apath
and melancholy to acute mania or melancholia with delusions of persecu
tion. Recovery may occur, or an incurable dementia result.

Parkinsonism and Epigastric Pain

In 1929 Trossarelli reported a case of psychosis from the insane asylum
in Turin of a woman aged thirty-one, who had worked for ten months in a
viscose rayon factory. She complained first of headache, vertigo and insomnia, and then that her neighbours sent ghosts into her bedroom to
electrify her. She was admitted restless, exhausted and suffering from
auditory hallucinations, but after eight months she was convalescent and
she subsequently recovered completely. In some cases the basal ganglia are
affected and the Parkinsonian syndrome develops. Gastro-intestinal disturbances are usually overshadowed by the nervous symptoms and signs,

but some authors describe epigastric pain resembling that of duodenal ulcer and occurring in a high percentage of workers exposed.

Vesicant Action on the Skin

Carbon disulphide is a vesicant and may cause blisters on the hands, especially at the tips of the fingers. They occur in men working in the spinning- or reeling-rooms in viscose-rayon plants and resemble second- or even third-degree burns. Unusual forms of poisoning may occur, particularly following fresh exposure of a patient who already has the chronic form of the disease. Thus Baader (1932) described a case with severe headache, confusion, nausea, vomiting, slow pulse, blurred vision and papilloedema.

Albuminuria and Renal Insufficiency

During 1940–1 in the viscose rayon factories of Piedmont, 100 cases of carbon disulphide poisoning were observed amongst workers exposed to concentrations ranging from 0·2 to 1·5 mg./litre. The commonest manifestation observed was polyneuritis (88 per cent of the cases), followed by gastric disturbances (28 per cent), headache and vertigo (18 per cent), sexual weakness and tremors (16 per cent); in 15 per cent myopathic changes in the calf muscles were noted; in 6 per cent of the cases mental deterioration, and in 3 per cent extrapyramidal symptoms were observed. Many cases of chronic vascular encephalopathy developed in workers exposed from 10 to 30 years to atmospheres containing CS_2 vapour in concentrations which during the years of the Second World War had been beyond the maximum allowable. During the period 1946–53 in four factories in Lombardy forty-three such cases were seen. Patients with chronic encephalopathy showed symptoms and signs either of pseudobulbar paralysis with mental deterioration or of extrapyramidal involvement, or of focal cerebral thrombosis. Sixteen cases were associated with hypertension and five had albuminuria with renal insufficiency. Clinical features, electroencephalograms, and cerebral arteriograms in several cases and necropsy in three others revealed that the encephalopathy was vascular in nature and due to a sclerosis of the small arteries and capillaries of the brain and spinal cord (Vigliani, 1954).

Differential Diagnosis

The diagnosis of psychosis due to carbon disulphide may be difficult because so many of the symptoms are subjective. The hazard is so great that nervous symptoms in a worker exposed to carbon disulphide should be regarded as occupational in origin, the assumption being that carbon disulphide has either caused the psychosis or accelerated the change in an individual already predisposed to mental disorder. The objective findings which will assist in diagnosis are visual-field defects, alteration of tendon reflexes, sensory changes and tremor, which is increased by muscular effort but disappears in sleep. Carbon disulphide may be estimated in the urine, using the xanthate reaction. Neurosyphilis must be considered in the differential diagnosis. The Argyll-Robertson pupil, loss of vibration sense and a positive Wassermann reaction will help in distinguishing between the two conditions, but the possibility of their occurring together must be borne in mind.

Treatment of Symptoms

Acute cases, with collapse, coma and cessation of respiration, are rarely seen. Obviously the patient must be removed at once from the room in which the accident has occurred, since the greatest concentration of the vapour is near the ground. Artificial respiration and inhalation of oxygen may be necessary. Cases of psychosis require appropriate mental rehabilitation and those of polyneuritis treatment along the usual lines. The risk of early and severe relapse on re-exposure is so great that a different occupation should be sought after recovery.

Preventive Treatment

In industries where carbon disulphide is used, precautions must be taken against the risks of fire and explosion, as well as against the toxic hazard. The most important measures in the prevention of poisoning are the establishment of efficient exhaust ventilation to remove the vapour as it is formed, regular alternation of employment so that exposure to the hazard is not continuous over a long period, and routine medical examination of workers at intervals of not more than one month.

Exhaust Ventilation through Hoods

In rubber works, arrangements must be made for the supply of fresh air to the workrooms. Benches for the cold curing of rubber must be provided with hoods connected to an efficient system of exhaust ventilation. The mixing of the carbon disulphide with sulphur monochloride must be done either on these benches or in the open air. The exhaust fans must be so placed that discharged vapour cannot re-enter any room.

Restricted Hours of Work

Auffert (1946) advises that workers selected for employment where carbon-disulphide exposure may occur should be robust and properly fed. There is evidence that young and very old persons are particularly susceptible. In England no person under eighteen years of age may be employed in a process where carbon disulphide is used or its vapour given off. The hours of employment are limited to five in one day, and to not more than two and a half at one time (Factory Department Memorandum, 1943).

Exhaust Fans at Floor Level

Respirators should be worn in the recognized dangerous jobs such as churn cleaning. Efficient exhaustion of carbon-disulphide vapour from the churn should be accomplished before the churn is opened for discharge, and the vapour-air mixture exhausted in contact with water to lessen the risk of explosion. Churn rooms should be ventilated by exhaust fans at floor level on one side of the room, with inlet openings at a higher level on the opposite side to maintain a cross-current of air.

Rules for entering Tanks

Routine examinations to determine the concentration of carbon disulphide in the air in various parts of the factory should be made, especially near the carbon-disulphide supply pipe, at the churn outlet and in the spinning-room in viscose rayon factories. The highest permissible concentration is twenty parts per million. Workers should not be allowed to enter any tank which has contained carbon disulphide without wearing a respirator and a rescue belt, unless it has been ascertained that the tank is free from vapour. Similarly, breathing apparatus and lifeline should always be worn by a person entering a tank in which sludge is present.

ACRYLONITRILE

Acrylonitrile, vinyl cyanide, $CH_2 = CHCN$ is a stable colourless liquid; the commercial product has a smell somewhat resembling phosphorus. It is a poisonous substance comparable in its toxicity to a molecular equivalent of hydrocyanic acid. It is used in the manufacture of special synthetic rubbers known as Buna N and Butakon (I.C.I.). Also it is polymerized to form *acrylic fibres* such as Acrilan (Chemstrand) and Courtelle (Courtaulds).

Early History of Raw Rubber

It was during his second visit to South America that Columbus was astonished to see the native Indians amusing themselves by bouncing a black ball made from a vegetable gum. About 1730 French explorers of the Amazon Valley reported that the material came from the *latex* (the Spanish word for *milk*) of the wild *hevea tree*. Some of this material found its way to Europe and Joseph Priestley, about 1780, showed that it would rub out pencil marks. Therefore he gave it the name rubber or indiarubber, and it was for use as a pencil eraser that it was first marketed. The rubber industry began to give promise of importance about 1820 when Charles Macintosh, a Scottish chemical manufacturer, by showing that rubber was soluble in benzene was able to cement it together in sheets between two layers of cotton fabric for the purpose of making waterproof cloth. But his *macintoshes* were soft and sticky in the hot weather and hard to the point of cracking in the cold weather.

Vulcanized Rubber and the Pneumatic Tyre

It remained for Charles Goodyear, a Connecticut hardware merchant, in 1839, to discover that rubber melted with sulphur resulted in a dough-like product unaffected by hot and cold weather. Goodyear called his process *vulcanizing* from the Roman god of fire (p. 8) and to the product he gave the name *gum elastic*, a name still applied to certain catheters, as also to *gum boots*. Meanwhile a niece of Macintosh who had married a Frenchman in Clermont-Ferrand gave her children a rubber ball obtained from her uncle. This so aroused the interest of her husband's partner in business that he set up a small factory which his grandchildren, Édouard and André Michelin, in 1886 succeeded in making prosperous, so much so that their home town is now *la cité du pneu*. The first rubber tyres belonged to racing bicycles and they were solid. In 1888 J. B. Dunlop, a Belfast veterinary surgeon, patented a pneumatic bicycle tyre (p. 509) and this gave cycling a widespread popularity. Then with the beginning of the twentieth century came the motor car, demanding a phenomenal increase in world rubber production, stimulating the production of plantation rubber and ultimately of synthetic rubber.

Successful Production of Plantation Rubber

As early as 1850 it became clear that the wild *Hevea brasiliensis* of the Para district of the Amazon Valley would not long provide enough rubber for world demands. Rubber-producing trees were known to grow all round the world in a belt about ten degrees on either side of the equator, but the quantity and quality of their latex could not measure up to that of the hevea tree of the Amazon Valley. About 1876 H. A. Wickham (afterwards Sir Henry Wickham), evading the vigilance of the Brazilian government, displayed much enterprise and care in bringing successfully to Kew Gardens a consignment of 70,000 seeds of *Hevea brasiliensis*. Hot houses were summarily emptied and within two weeks there were over 2,000 young plants ready for despatch to Ceylon, where they have since grown to useful trees. *Plantation rubber* was such a success that in Ceylon, Malaya and the Dutch East Indies 600,000,000 hevea trees were under cultivation by the year 1935.

Synthetic Rubber competes with Plantation Rubber

Synthetic rubber was being made before the Second World War in Germany, the U.S.A. and Russia, but as recently as 1941 production amounted only to about 100,000 tons. When Japan entered the war nearly all the supply of natural rubber was cut off from the Allies, and it became necessary to turn to synthetic rubbers for nearly all our requirements. In 1944 the U.S.A. and Canada made 900,000 tons, equivalent to the production of nearly five million acres of plantations. Today rubber trees planted at the rate of about 100 to the acre cover some 9,000,000 acres of south-east Asia, mainly in Malaya, Indonesia and Ceylon, and an average yield of about 500 pounds of dry rubber is obtained per acre. On the other hand, four synthetic rubber factories each producing 50,000 tons a year yield as much as a million acres of plantations (Gibbs, 1961).

Chemical Structure of Buna S Rubber

It had been known for many years that natural rubber yields on distillation the diolefin, isoprene which is closely related to the petroleum hydrocarbon, butadiene. Chlorobutadiene polymerizes to neoprene, a substance much like a vulcanized soft rubber and later used in paints, adhesive cements and as crêpe soles for shoes. Still more useful rubbers were obtained by making polymers from two different substances, the one a diolefin and the other a substituted ethylene. Such compounds are called co-polymers. One of the first of these was made from butadiene and styrene. This rubber was made in Germany under the name Buna S, with sodium (Na) as catalyst. Buna S was thus an abbreviation for butadiene-Na-styrene. The proportions of the two components can be varied considerably to give products varying from rubbers to resins and plastics. The high-styrene polymer is much used as a material for soling shoes and the normal polymer as a general-purpose rubber for car-tyres, rubber-proofing fabrics and for rubber-based paints. But instead of styrene, other substances, for example acrylonitrile (vinyl cyanide), can be used to make butadiene co-polymers referred to by such names as Buna N and Butakon (I.C.I.).

Special Properties of Buna N Rubber

This is more expensive to produce than Buna S but its properties are such that it has become a synthetic rubber of considerable importance. This is chiefly due to its remarkably good resistance to oil and petroleum. It can be used as hoses to carry these materials and for tank linings, gaskets and other goods that must not deteriorate in contact with oil. During the war it was particularly useful for self-sealing petrol tanks in aeroplanes. Until the end of 1959 the United Kingdom had to import acrylonitrile, but a plant now operated by Imperial Chemical Industries at Billingham supplies the Company's Plastics Division, which uses it for making Butakon rubbers. The consumption of synthetic rubber in Great Britain was almost negligible before the war but it has increased greatly in the last few years. Until 1958 it was mainly imported as the home manufacture has had to wait for the extension of refinery facilities and is only now beginning on a large scale. Much new plant came into production during 1958 and 1959 and it is expected that by 1963 enough will be made to meet all requirements.

Poisoning by Acrylonitrile

In the manufacture of synthetic rubber acrylonitrile presents definite hazards of vapour toxicity and of toxic absorption. The studies of Dudley (1942) in guinea pigs, rabbits, cats, dogs and monkeys show clearly that it is a poison in the same sense as is hydrocyanic acid. Repeated exposures of these animals to 153 p.p.m. of acrylonitrile in air led to a significant increase in serum and urinary thiocyanate and were lethal. Wilson (1944) found that in spite of all precautions to protect workmen some became exposed. They suffered from nausea, vomiting, weakness, fatigue and diarrhœa. Mallette (1943) described a manufacturing process for Buna N in which exposure to acrylonitrile vapour occurred from the heat of driers. Brieger and his associates (1952) were able to demonstrate in the blood of their patients both cyanide and cyanmethæmoglobin, proving that the toxic action of acrylonitrile is based on the formation of cyanide in the body. Dudley recommended a maximum allowable concentration of 20 parts per million in air. Although no fatal cases have occurred in industry it is felt that sufficient exposure either to the vapour or through skin absorption would cause the death of an operative. (Fairhall, 1957).

Prevention and Treatment of Poisoning by Acrylonitrile

Transport of acrylonitrile in bulk is carried out by road tankers; smaller quantities are handled in drums. Men discharging the liquid from road tankers into stock tanks and all those who handle it in factories must wear either air-fed pressure suits (fig. 186) or some other form of protective clothing in conjunction with compressed-air masks. All such clothing must be made of some impermeable material such as polyvinyl chloride. In every case there must be on the same job a second man similarly equipped even if he has nothing to do but watch. In cases where the interior of a tank or autoclave must be inspected also there must be two men, but in such cases in addition to protective clothing with compressed-air masks both must be equipped with safety harness and life line. First-aid cabinets and clear notices as to the procedure to be followed must be provided, as in the case of men handling other cyanides. If a man is overcome, amyl nitrite inhalations must be given without delay. If necessary an intravenous injection of sodium nitrite followed by sodium thiosulphate must follow promptly (p. 666).

Other Toxic Hazards of the Rubber Industry

We have seen (p. 273) how the invention of litharge rubber removed the risk of lead poisoning from rubber compounding. Some antioxidants (p. 769) and acrylonitrile (Schwartz, 1945) may cause dermatitis. Benoquin, an antioxidant used in processing white rubber gloves, can act as a de-pigmenting agent, causing patches of occupational leucodermia on the hands of negro workmen (p. 788). Malignant tumours of the bladder in men exposed to *beta*-naphthylamine have occurred in the manufacture of rubber tyres and electric cables (p. 828). The manufacture of xenylamine for use as an antioxidant has been condemned because it is carcinogenic both in animals and man. It has already caused sixteen cases of bladder tumour among seventy-one workers (p. 829). Indirectly rubber has been responsible for many cases of chronic benzene poisoning but safe substitutes for this solvent are now in use (p. 516). Rubber is soluble in tetrachlorethane but this solvent is so dangerous to life (p. 615) that it must never be used for such a purpose.

ACRYLAMIDE

Acrylamide $CH_2 = CHCONH_2$, a white crystalline powder, is a vinyl monomer which exhibits the usual reactions of the amide group and readily undergoes polymerization. The monomer is a powerful neuro-toxin; the polymer is non-toxic. These substances are handled in the manufacture of flocculators. A flocculator aids the separation of suspended solids from aqueous systems, which may be useful in mining, soil stabili-zation, the disposal of industrial wastes, and on any filtration or centrifugal process. There is a use for smaller quantities of acrylamide in the dyeing, photographic, plastic, paper, textile, ceramic and paint industries.

The first mention of acrylamide poisoning in man was by Stokinger (1956). He speaks very briefly of a man who suffered from disturbed gait, postural tremors, visual and auditory hallucinations, and muscular atrophy. Kuperman (1958) who worked solely with cats indicates that these pharmacological studies were undertaken as a result of cases of accidental poisoning in workers in the U.S.A. but details evidently had never been published. The cats developed ataxia, postural and ataxic tremors, signs of polyneuritis and what he took to be chronic intoxication in the mesencephalic tegmentum. A report on further extensive toxi-cological studies on rats, rabbits, guinea-pigs, cats, and monkeys was published by McCollister and others in 1964. They found that acrylamide was toxic whether absorbed cutaneously, orally, or parenterally. All species showed involvement of the nervous system. Most of his animals developed weakness of the hindquarters so that they could not grip the mesh floor or climb the sides of their cages. Recovery often began 100 days later. Some of them were well after 123 days. Fullerton and Barnes (1966) published a paper which throws considerable light on the peripheral neuropathy that occurs in chronic acrylamide poisoning in rats, but they make no reference to the possibility of a central disturbance.

There are two published reports on human cases in Japan. One describes intoxication in 10 out of 18 workers in a factory making acryl-amide from acrylonitrile, but the description is incomplete in a number of respects (Fujita and others, 1960). There is a further very brief report of a single case in a Japanese factory making flocculators. The author infers that there were other cases in the factory but gives no details. A Canadian report (Auld and Bedwell, 1967) describes peripheral neuropathy in one man using acrylamide in a grouting process, stressing the excessive sweating of the extremities. Garland and Patterson (1967) describe six cases of poisoning in workers handling the monomer acrylamide. All occurred during the process of polymerization of the monomer in the manufacture of flocculators. Absorption was evidently through the skin of the hands. The clinical picture was that of polyneuritis and a midbrain disturbance. The main signs and symptoms were loss of weight, numbness and paræsthesiæ in the limbs, sometimes with generalized tremors, slurring of speech and bladder disturbance; weakness, most marked in the lower limbs; increased sweating of the hands, with erythema and peeling of the palms; and unsteadiness and lethargy without obvious personality change. Removal from exposure was followed by complete recovery in the less severely poisoned, but this took from 2 to 12 months.

BIBLIOGRAPHY

Methyl Alcohol

BARTLETT, G. R. (1950), *Amer. J. Physiol.*, **163**, 619.

BENNETT, I. L., CARY, F. H., MITCHELL, G. L., and COOPER, M. N. (1953), *Medicine*, Baltimore, **32**, 431.

HALE, A. B. (1901), *J. Amer. med. Ass.*, **37**, 1450.

HAMILTON, A., and HARDY, H. L. (1949), *Industrial Toxicology*, Hoeber, New York.

PATILLO, R. S. (1899), *Ophthal. Rec.*, **8**, 599.

RØE, O. (1943), *Acta med. scand.*, **113**, 558; (1946), *Ibid.*, suppl., 182.

ZATMAN, L. J. (1946), *Biochem. J.*, **40**, 67.

Nitroglycerine

CRITCHLEY, A. M. (1949), Personal communication.

EBRIGHT, G. E. (1914), *J. Amer. med. Ass.*, **62**, 201.

MCCORD, C. P. (1945), *A Blind Hog's Acorns*, Cloud Inc., Chicago.

PAULI, H. E. (1947), *Alfred Nobel*, Nicholson and Watson, London.

RABINOWITCH, I. M. (1944), *Canad. med. Ass. J.*, **50**, 199.

READ, J. (1942), *Explosives*, Penguin Books, London.

WEINER, J. S., and THOMPSON, M. L. (1947), *Brit. J. industr. Med.*, **4**, 205.

Nitrocellulose

LYNCH, J. B., and BELL, J. (1947), *Brit. J. industr. Med.*, **4**, 84.

MUZI, E. (1927), *Stomatologia*, **25**, 107.

READ, J. (1942), *Explosives*, Penguin Books, London.

SIMPSON, R. S. (1919), *Dominion Dental Journ.*, **31**, 94.

WILLIAMS, T. I. (1953), *The Chemical Industry*, Penguin Books, London.

Dimethylnitrosamine

BARNES, J. M. and MAGEE, P. N. (1954), *Brit. J. industr. Med.*, **11**, 167.

DRUCKREY, H., PREUSSMANN, R., SCHMÄHL, D. and MÜLLER, M. (1962), *Naturwissenschaften*, **49**, 19.

HAMILTON, A. and HARDY, H. L. (1949), *Industrial Toxicology*, 2nd ed., Paul B. Hoeber, New York.

HEATH, D. F. and MAGEE, P. N. (1962), *Brit. J. industr. Med.*, **19**, 276.

The Halogenated Hydrocarbons

BEATTIE, J., HERBERT, P. H., WECHTEL, C., and STEELE, C. W. (1944), *Brit. med. J.*, **1**, 209.

ELKINS, H. B., and LEVINE, L. (1939), *J. industr. Hyg.*, **21**, 221.

MINOT, A. S., and CUTLER, J. T. (1929), *J. clin. Invest.*, **6**, 369.

(a) Methyl Chloride

BAKER, H. M. (1927), *J. Amer. med. Ass.*, **88**, 1137; (1930), *J. publ. Hlth.*, **20**, 291.

GERBIS, H. (1914), *Münch. med. Wschr.*, **61**, 879.

JONES, A. M. (1942), *Quart. J. Med.*, *N.S.*, **11**, 29.

KEGEL, A. H., McNALLY, W. D., and POPE, A. S. (1929), *J. Amer. med. Ass.*, **93**, 353.

SAYERS, R. R., YANT, W. P., CHORNYAK, J., and SHOAF, H. W. (1930), *Toxicity of Dichloro-difluoro-methane; a New Refrigerant*, United States Bureau of Mines Report, No. 3013.

(b) Methyl Bromide

BUTLER, E. C. B., PERRY, K. M. A., and WILLIAMS, J. R. F. (1945), *Brit. J. industr. Med.*, **2**, 30.

IRISH, D. D., ADAMS, E. M., SPENCER, H. C., and ROWE, V. K. (1940), *J. industr. Hyg.*, **22**, 218.

JAQUET, A. (1901), *Dtsch. Arch. klin. Med.*, **71**, 370.

PRAIN, J. H., and SMITH, G. H. (1952), *Brit. J. industr. Med.*, **9**, 44.

SAYERS, R. R., YANT, W. P., THOMAS, B. G. H., and BERGER, L. B. (1929), *Publ. Hlth Bull.*, *Wash.*, **42**, 185.

WATROUS, R. M. (1942), *Industr. med.*, **11**, 575.

WYERS, H. (1945), *Brit. J. industr. Med.*, **2**, 24.

(c) Trichlorethylene

BAADER, E. W. (1927), *Zbl. GewHyg.*, **4**, 385.

BRIDGE, J. C., (1933), *Annual Report of the Chief Inspector of Factories and Workshops for 1932*, H.M.S.O., London, p. 107.

CARDEN, S. (1944), *Brit. med. J.*, **1**, 319.

CASTELLINO, P. (1932), *Folia med.*, **18**, 415.

HERDMAN, K. N. (1945), *Brit. med. J.*, **2**, 689.

HEWER, C. L., and HADFIELD, C. F. (1941), *Ibid.*, **1**, 924.

HUMPHREY, J. H., and McCLELLAND, M. (1944), *Ibid.*, **1**, 315.

ISENSCHMID, R., and KUNZ, Z. (1934), *Schweiz. med. Wschr.*, **65**, 530, 612.

MILTON, R., GRAHAM, J., PERRY, K. M. A., and HUNTER, D. (1944), *Brit. med. J.*, **1**, 341.

ROHOLM, K. (1933), *Ugeskr. Laeg.*, **95**, 1183.

STÜBER, K. (1931), *Arch. Gewerbepath. Gewerbehyg.*, **2**, 398.

WILLCOX, Sir W. H. (1933–4), *Proc. R. Soc. Med.*, **27**, 455.

(d) Carbon Tetrachloride

BOVERI, M. P. (1930), *Le Méd. du Travail*, **2**, 280.

DAVIS, P. A. (1934), *J. Amer. med. Ass.*, **103**, 962.

DUDLEY, S. F. (1935), *J. industr. Hyg.*, **17**, 93.

GRAHAM, W. H. (1938), *Lancet*, **1**, 1159.

HAGEN, W. S., ALEXANDER, H. A., and PEPPARD, T. A. (1940), *Minn. Med.*, **23**, 715.

HAMILTON, A., and HARDY, H. L. (1949), *Industrial Toxicology*, Hoeber, New York.

HENGGELER, A. (1931), *Schweiz. med. Wschr.*, **61**, 223.

LAMSON, P. D., ROBBINS, B. H., and WARD, C.B. (1929), *Amer. J. Hyg.*, **9**, 430.

McGILL, C. M. (1946), *Northwest Med.*, **45**, 169.

McGUIRE, L. W. (1932), *J. Amer. med. Ass.*, **99**, 988.

PERRY, W. J. (1942), *Army Med. Bull.*, No. 64, p. 71.

SMITH, A. R. (1950), *Arch. Industr. Hyg.*, **1**, 348.
SMYTH, H. F., SMYTH, H. F., JR., and CARPENTER, C. P. (1936), *J. industr. Hyg.*, **18**, 277.
STEWART, A., and WITTS, L. J. (1944), *Brit. J. industr. Med.*, **1**, 11.
WIRTSCHAFTER, Z. T. (1933), *Amer. J. publ. Hlth.*, **23**, 1035.
WITTS, L. J., STEWART, A., and KEMP, F. H. (1943), *Quart. J. Med. N.S.*, **12**, 261.
WOODS, W. W. (1946), *J. Path. Bact.*, **58**, 767.

(e) Ethylene Dichloride

BLOCH, W. (1946), *Schweiz. med. Wschr.*, **76**, 1078.
BRIDGE, J. C. (1933), *Annual Report of the Chief Inspector of Factories and Workshops for 1932*, H.M.S.O., London, p. 104.
HEPPEL, L. C., NEAL, P. A., PERRIN, T. L., ENDICOTT, K. M., and PORTERFIELD, U. S. (1946), *J. industr. Hyg.*, **28**, 113.
HUEPER, W. C., and SMITH, C. (1935), *Amer. J. med. Sci.*, **189**, 778.
MÜLLER, J. (1925), *Arch. exp. Path. Pharmak.*, **109**, 276.
WIRTSCHAFTER, Z. T., and SCHWARTZ, E. D. (1939), *J. industr. Hyg.*, **21**, 126.

(f) Tetrachlorethane

FORBES, G. (1943), *Brit. med. J.*, **1**, 348.
JUNGFER (1914), *Zbl. GewHyg.*, **2**, 222.
LEGGE, T. M. (1917), *Proc. R. Soc. Med.*, **10**, i, Gen. Repts., Spec. Discussion, 1.
LEHMANN, K. B. (1911), *Arch. Hyg.*, **74**, 1.
LERI, A. T., and BREITEL (1922), *Bull. et mém. Soc. méd. Hôp. Paris*, **46**, 1406.
MINOT, G. R., and SMITH, L. W. (1921), *Arch. intern. Med.*, **28**, 687.
PARMENTER, D. C. (1920–1), *J. industr. Hyg.*, **2**, 456.
SCHWANDER, P. (1936), *Arch. Gewerbepath. Gewerbehyg.*, **7**, 109.
WILLCOX, W. H. (1915), *Lancet*, **1**, 544.
WILLCOX, W. H., SPILSBURY, B. H., and LEGGE, T. M. (1915), *Trans. med. Soc. of London*, **38**, 129.
ZOLLINGER, F. (1931), *Arch. Gewerbepath. Gewerbehyg.*, **2**, 298.

(g) Chlorinated Naphthalenes

COLLIER, E. (1943), *Lancet*, **1**, 72.
DRINKER, C. K., WARREN, M. F., and BENNETT, G. A. (1937), *J. industr. Hyg.*, **19**, 283.
FLINN, F. B., and JARVIK, N. E. (1936–7), *Proc. Soc. exp. Biol. N.Y.*, **35**, 118.
GREENBURG, L., MAYERS, M. R., and SMITH, A. R. (1939), *J. industr. Hyg.*, **21**, 29.
HERXHEIMER, K. (1899), *Munch. med. Wschr.*, **46**, 278.
JONES, A. T. (1941), *J. industr. Hyg.*, **23**, 290.
LEHMANN, K. B. (1919), *Kurzes Lehrbuch der Arbeits und Gewerbehyg.*, Leipzig, p. 215.
MCLETCHIE, N. G. B., and ROBERTSON, D. (1942), *Brit. med. J.*, **1**, 691.
SCHWARTZ, L. (1943), *J. Amer. med. Ass.*, **122**, 158.
SCHWARTZ, L., TULIPAN, L., and BIRMINGHAM, D. J. (1957), *Occupational Diseases of the Skin*, 3rd ed., Kimpton, London.

Wauer (1918), *Zbl. GewHyg.*, **6**, 100.
White, R. P. (1934), *The Dermatergoses or Occupational Affections of the Skin*, 4th ed., Lewis, London.

The Glycol Group

Browning, E. (1953), *Toxicity of Industrial Organic Solvents*, Industrial Health Research Board, M.R.C. Report No. 80, H.M.S.O., London.

(a) Ethylene Chlorhydrin

Ballotta, F., Bertagni, P., and Troisi, F. M. (1953), *Brit. J. industr. Med.*, **10**, 161.
Dierker, H., and Brown, P. G. (1944), *J. industr. Hyg.*, **26**, 277.
Goldblatt, M. W., and Chiesman, W. E. (1944), *Brit. J. industr. Med.*, **1**, 207.
Güthert, H. (1943), *Arch. Gewerbepath. Gewerbehyg.*, **12**, 362.
Koelsch, F. (1927), *Zbl. GewHyg.*, **4**, 312.
Middleton, E. L. (1930), *J. industr. Hyg.*, **12**, 265.

(b) Diethylene Dioxide

Barber, H. (1934), *Guy's Hosp. Rept.*, **84**, 267.
Fairley, A., Linton, E. C., and Ford-Moore, A. H. (1934), *J. Hyg.*, **34**, 486.
Henry, S. A. (1934), *Annual Report of the Chief Inspector of Factories and Workshops for 1933*, H.M.S.O., London, p. 67.
Yant, W. P., Schrenk, H. H., Waite, C. P., and Patty, F. A. (1930), *Publ. Hlth. Rep. Wash.*, **45**, 2023.

Carbon Disulphide

Auffert, J. (1946), *Arch. Mal. prof.*, **7**, 181.
Baader, E. W. (1932), *Medizinische Klinik*, **28**, 1740.
Braceland, F. J. (1942), *Ann. intern. Med.*, **16**, 246.
Charcot, H. C. (1889), *Leçons du Mardi*, Paris.
Delpech, A. (1856), *Gazette hébdomadaire de médecine et chirurgie*, **3**, 41.
Factory Department, Ministry of Labour and National Service (1943), London, Form 836.
Frost, W. A., Gunn, R. M., and Nettleship, E. (1885), *Trans. Ophthal. Soc. U.K.*, **5**, 157.
Hamilton, A. (1940), *Occupational poisoning in the Viscose Rayon Industry*, U.S. Dept. of Labor Bull., No. 34.
Oliver, T. (1902), *Dangerous Trades*, Murray, London.
Paluch, E. (1948), *J. industr. Hyg.*, **30**, 37.
Payen, A. (1851), *Précis de chimie industr.*, Paris.
Trossarelli, A. (1929), *Leipziger Monatschrift für Textil-Industrie*, **44**, 5.
Vigliani, E. C. (1954), *Brit. J. industr. Med.*, **11**, 235.

Acrylonitrile

Brieger, H., Rieders, F., and Hodes, W. A. (1952), *Arch. industr. hyg. and Occup. Med.*, **6**, 128.
Dudley, H. C., and Neal, P. A. (1942), *J. industr. hyg. and tox.*, **24**, 27.

FAIRHALL, L. T. (1957), *Industrial Toxicology*, 2nd ed., Williams and Wilkins, Baltimore.
GIBBS, F. W. (1961), *Organic Chemistry Today*, Penguin Books, London.
MALLETTE, F. S. (1943), *Industr. Med.*, **12**, 495.
SCHWARTZ, L. (1945), *J. Amer. med. Assoc.*, **127**, 389.
WILSON, R. H. (1944), *Ibid.*, **124**, 701.

Acrylamide

AULD, R. B. and BEDWELL, S. F. (1967), *Canad. med. Ass. J.*, **96**, 652.
FUJITA, A., et al. (1960), *Japan Medical Report*, Feb. 20, p. 37.
FULLERTON, P. M., and BARNES, J. M. (1966), *Brit. J. industr. Med.*, **23**, 210.
GARLAND, T. O. and PATTERSON, M. W. H. (1967), *Brit. med. J.*, **4**, 134.
KUPERMAN, A. S. (1958), *J. Pharmacol. exp. Ther.*, **123**, 180.
McCOLLISTER, D. D., OYEN, F., and ROWE, V. K. (1964), *Toxicol. appl. Pharmacol.*, **6**, 172.
STOKINGER, H. E. (1956), *A.M.A. Arch. Industr. Hyg.*, **14**, 206.

CHAPTER X

NOXIOUS GASES

FROM the point of view of industrial hygiene a gas may be considered to be any aeroform or completely elastic fluid which does not become liquid or solid at ordinary temperatures. The distinction between gas and vapour is somewhat vague; a vapour is a completely elastic fluid near its temperature of liquefaction. Otherwise expressed, a gas is an elastic fluid at a temperature above its critical temperature, and a vapour is an elastic fluid below its critical temperature but not in a liquid state. Thus, for example, at room temperature a flask partially filled with ethyl ether may contain both liquid ether and ether vapour, while, on the contrary, hydrogen or nitrogen are encountered under these conditions only as gases.

Classification of Noxious Gases

The effects of noxious gases and vapours are best classified on a physiological basis. They include simple asphyxiants, chemical asphyxiants, irritant gases, organo-metallic gases and anæsthetic vapours. The effects of nickel carbonyl (p. 469), arsine (p. 344), dimethylarsine (p. 349) and phosphine (p. 383), and the anæsthesia produced by carbon tetrachloride (p. 607), trichlorethylene (p. 603) and benzene (p. 506) have been discussed elsewhere in these pages. Gases of the irritant group are potent poisons and, since they are irrespirable, workmen exposed to them fly for their lives, so that fatalities are rare. Unfortunately, with gases such as carbon monoxide and arseniuretted hydrogen we are dealing with non-irritant, tasteless, odourless compounds. Here the victims may be overcome without even suspecting danger. It is important to bear in mind that, though one gaseous poison may be more toxic than another, a greater rate of volatility may make the less poisonous one the more dangerous.

Principles of Treatment

In preventive treatment the vapour density of the substance concerned must be taken into account. There are four important toxic gases of less density than air, namely, ammonia, hydrogen fluoride, carbon monoxide and hydrogen cyanide. Equally there are five simple asphyxiants of less density than air, namely nitrogen, helium, hydrogen, methane and ethylene. The toxic gases heavier than air are nitrogen dioxide, chlorine, phosgene, sulphur dioxide, sulphuretted hydrogen and carbon dioxide. Carbon tetrachloride, trichlorethylene and benzene are all denser than air and all act by producing acute narcosis. Since the effects of the four main classes of noxious gases are widely different, the curative treatment will differ too. The general aim will be the rapid elimination of the poison through the same channel as that by which it entered—namely, the lungs. For this purpose augmented breathing is induced by inhalation of oxygen. Both warmth and complete bodily rest are necessary. Such treatment enables the body to obtain and conserve oxygen and, if successful, to escape death by suffocation.

Hazards from Working in Confined Spaces

Work within tanks or other confined spaces requires much more care than is required for work in open areas. Saving a life is worth the extra care. Such confined spaces include tanks, pits, vats, boilers, stills, silos, silage pits, wells, sewers, caves, cellars, vaults, tunnels, caissons, ships' holds and box-cars. All can contribute to accidents from contamination of the atmosphere by toxic gases or vapours. Tanks are often constructed with openings for workmen to enter. Some have a whole side, usually the top, completely open. Even if the entire top be open, air movement within the tank and exchange of air between it and the outside environment is usually very poor. Gases and vapours which are denser than air will remain in confined spaces, especially where the opening is on top. Because gases do not diffuse rapidly there will be little tendency for dilution to occur unless a positive means for ventilation is provided.

Freeing Tanks of Noxious Gases and Vapours

No enclosed space should be entered until it is certain that all the noxious gas or vapour within it has been removed. The tank should be emptied, washed and then steamed or aerated repeatedly until free of atmospheric contaminants or materials which might produce them. It should not be assumed that because a tank has been emptied, steamed and aerated, that it is free of volatile substances. It is possible that the coating material on the inside of a tank will absorb such substances and release them gradually. There may also be less obvious sources for recontamination of the atmosphere within a tank or pit. It is necessary, therefore, to test the atmosphere rather than assume that it is safe. Air in tanks can be tested for oxygen content by means of a flame safety lamp. In the absence of methane, the flame of the lamp will be extinguished at an oxygen content below 16 per cent. There are numerous instruments available for the rapid estimation of inflammable gases and vapours such as carbon monoxide, hydrogen sulphide, sulphur dioxide and chlorinated hydrocarbons. Clean, fresh air should be supplied to the tank after it has been rendered free of contaminants. This is necessary to insure an adequate supply of air for the worker who is to enter.

Workmen trained in Rescue Methods

If it is impossible to remove all atmospheric contaminants from an enclosed space the worker must be provided with respirable air. No person should be allowed to work single-handed in such a place. The man in danger must wear a safety belt or harness with a rope attached. His mate holds the far end of the rope and in no circumstances does he abandon his post. A third worker must be within hailing distance so that the two can lift and remove to safety the man at work, should he show signs of distress. Under certain conditions the worker must wear an apparatus consisting of an oro-nasal mask connected to a hose led out to uncontaminated air. A reviving apparatus must be provided, consisting of a cylinder containing oxygen with the necessary valves, tubing, flexible bag and mask. This apparatus should be in charge of no fewer than three persons, adequately instructed in its use. At least once a month the equipment, and especially the rubber parts, should be examined by them, and this inspection should never be omitted. Unnecessary loss of life can occur because of the thoughtless act of a workman who, when in need of a piece of rubber tubing, has gone to the gas-mask cabinet and cut away part of the rescue equipment. All such cabinets should be kept locked and made with glazed doors so that they can be broken open in emergency. The workmen should be practised in rescue drill, including artificial respiration and the use of the appliances provided.

Courage alone is Not Enough

All responsible persons should be taught that no canister gas mask affords protection against deficiency of oxygen. Where box respirators are provided, a foolproof system of coloured markings must be used whereby the rescue team will promptly and automatically use the correct respirator for the noxious gas concerned. It cannot be too strongly insisted upon that respirators designed to protect the wearer against inhalation of dust are of no avail as a protection against toxic gases. Equally, it is important to realize that reliance on a folded handkerchief has cost many a rescuer his life. Brave rescues are frequently made by workmen, miners, foremen and managers, but courage is not enough unless combined with skill and linked up to training and practice. All workers responsible for rescue work must understand that in resuscitation of persons who have ceased to breathe it is vitally important to apply artificial respiration *promptly*. The physician must be taught to realize that the application of artificial respiration to an average-sized man is hard work. Rescue men generally work in teams of three, each man working for twenty minutes and the team continuing for as long as four hours, or until rigor mortis has obviously begun. A person in any but the best physical condition will find this ordeal extremely tiring.

Methods of Artificial Respiration

The prone pressure method of artificial respiration described by Schafer in 1903 remained in general use for more than thirty years. One distinct advantage that it has over many others is that the massage action used aids venous return and helps support the circulation. However, since 1932, the arm-lift, back-pressure method of Holger Nielsen has been used in Scandinavia with success. Work done in many countries since 1950 has shown that the Schafer method gives inadequate ventilation in many subjects. It is now agreed that the Holger Nielsen method gives a higher uptake of oxygen than does the Schafer method and is easy to teach, accurate in performance and can be readily carried out over long periods. It has therefore been adopted by the International Red Cross and by all three of the Armed Services of Great Britain.

Back-pressure, Arm-lift Method of Artificial Respiration (Holger Nielsen)

In the Holger Nielsen method of artificial respiration the chest is compressed against the ground by pressure applied to the back (expiration), and expanded by taking the weight off the chest and raising the arms (inspiration).

Place the patient face downwards with head turned to one side, arms bent and forehead resting on his hands, so as to keep mouth and nose free from obstruction.

Give one or two firm thumps with the flat of the hand between the shoulders to bring the tongue forward and clear the throat.

Kneel at his head, placing one knee near the head and the other foot alongside the elbow. The operator's mid-line should be in line with that of the patient. From time to time this position can be altered by changing the kneeling knee.

Place your hands on his shoulder-blades with thumbs touching on the mid-line and fingers pointing towards the patient's feet, your arms being kept straight and the heels of your hands over the spines of the shoulder-blades.

Bend forward with arms straight, and apply light pressure by the weight of the upper part of your body while steadily counting "One, Two and Three." Time, $2\frac{1}{2}$ seconds. This forces the air out of the lungs.

Release the pressure gradually and slide your hands to just above the elbows of the casualty, counting "Four." Time, 1 second.

Draw his arms and shoulders towards you by bending backward with your arms straight till you feel resistance and tension, without lifting the chest off the ground, counting "Five, Six and Seven." Time, $2\frac{1}{2}$ seconds. This draws air into the lungs.

Lay his arms down and replace your hands on the shoulder-blades counting "Eight." Time, 1 second.

Repeat the movements with rhythmic rocking at the rate of approximately nine times to the minute, counting as follows:

"One, Two and Three": with hands on shoulder-blades, bend forward and apply pressure ($2\frac{1}{2}$ seconds);

"Four": slide hands to elbows (1 second);

"Five, Six and Seven": bend backward, raising arms and shoulders ($2\frac{1}{2}$ seconds);

"Eight": lay arms down and place your hands on shoulder-blades (1 second).

When breathing is re-established, omit the back pressure and continue the arm raising and lowering alone at the rate of twelve times to the minute, counting as follows:

"One, Two and Three": arm raising (inspiration, $2\frac{1}{2}$ seconds);

"Four, Five and Six": arm lowering (expiration, $2\frac{1}{2}$ seconds).

If there are chest injuries, do the arm raising and lowering procedure only, at the rate of twelve times a minute.

If arms and chest are both injured, do arm raising and lowering, but grasp the arms under the armpits.

Degrees of pressure on the shoulder-blades depend on the sex and age of the patient, ranging from 24 to 30 lb. on an adult to from 12 to 14 lb. for half-grown children and slender women. For infants the pressure should be not more than from 2 to 4 lb.

Prone Pressure Method of Artificial Respiration (Schafer)

Place the patient face down, with one arm extended directly overhead and the other arm bent at the elbow, and with the face turned outward and resting on the hand or forearm so that the nose and mouth are free for breathing. If, as frequently happens, the victim vomits or if fluid comes up into the mouth from the lungs, it runs out freely and no chance is given to hinder the entrance of air.

Place the palms of the hands on the small of the back with fingers resting on the ribs, the little finger just touching the lowest rib, with the thumb and fingers in a natural position and the tips of the fingers just out of sight. The position of your hands is important. You apply pressure to the lowest ribs, which are free to move and are therefore not in danger of breaking when the pressure is given properly. If your hands are too high you operate upon the more thoroughly supported upper ribs, and at times these may be broken even by moderate pressure.

With arms held straight, swing forward slowly so that the weight of your body is gradually brought to bear upon the patient. The shoulder should be directly over the wrist at the forward swing. Do not bend your elbows. This operation should take about two seconds.

When you make the motion in this direction you compress the chest and push the diaphragm upwards. Air is driven out of the lungs. Your active movement causes expulsion of air. In natural breathing the active part of the process enlarges the chest and lets air into the lungs, and, in its turn, breathing out is passive. The prone method of artificial respiration reverses the procedure, air being expelled by pressure and entering the lungs as a result of the passive expansion which follows release of pressure.

Now immediately swing backward so as to remove the pressure completely. When you stop pressing you obviously allow those parts you have compressed to spring back to their normal position, and this in its turn results in enlargement of the chest and an inrush of air. After two seconds swing forward again. You thus repeat deliberately from twelve to fifteen times a minute the double movement of compression and release, a complete respiration in four or five seconds (Clark and Drinker, 1935).

Inhalation of Oxygen

No mistake will be made if the victim be removed immediately from the source of poisoning and be kept quiet and warm. The first and immediate consideration is the restoration of breathing. The delay incident to the removal to a hospital may be fatal, and is justifiable only when there is no one at hand to give artificial respiration. If complications exist or arise which require hospital treatment, artificial respiration should be maintained in transit and after the arrival at the hospital until spontaneous respiration begins. It is often advisable to use oxygen for resuscitation if this is available, irrespective of the method of artificial respiration employed. For resuscitation of subjects exposed to carbon monoxide a mixture of 95 per cent oxygen and 5 per cent carbon dioxide is particularly valuable. This treatment is based on the observation by Henderson and Haggard (1922) that the activity of the respiratory centre may be stimulated by adding 5 per cent of carbon dioxide to the respired air.

Importance of Rest and Warmth

Those responsible for rescue work must be especially warned of the danger of exposing gassed persons to cold, and of walking them up and down. They must realize that rest and warmth are essential in treatment, that the patient must be wrapped in dry blankets and provided with hot water bottles, and that such stupidity as dashing a bucket of cold water over the face may lead to a fatality. It is particularly important to keep the victim quiet if the offending gas is one of the irritant group like nitrous fumes, chlorine or phosgene until it is certain that pneumonia is not going to follow the exposure. In such cases respiration must not be stimulated by the use of carbon dioxide.

The Drinker Respirator

When long-continued artificial respiration is required, the manual method may be replaced advantageously by one of the special instruments known as pulmotors, lungmotors or resuscitators. Of course, they offer the difficulty that some training is required to operate them properly, and they are not as a rule available for instant use. The Drinker respirator makes use of a subatmospheric pressure applied to the outside of the chest to obtain an expansion of the lungs. The body, with the exception of the head, is placed in a chamber in which the pressure is reduced rhythmically by a pump. The thorax and the lungs are expanded by the pressure differential created between the lungs and the exterior of the chest, and in this way

spiration may be kept up indefinitely with no danger of injury to the
ings (Drinker and McKhann, 1929).

SIMPLE ASPHYXIANTS

Gases like nitrogen, methane, helium and hydrogen may cause death
·om simple asphyxia through deprivation of oxygen. They are inert and
xert their action in the lungs merely by keeping oxygen from reaching the
lood. Their effect is proportional to the extent to which their presence
iminishes the partial pressure of oxygen in the expired air. They must be
resent in considerable amounts before they exert any appreciable effect.

(a) Nitrogen

Nitrogen, N_2, is an inert, odourless, tasteless, colourless gas which
onstitutes four-fifths of the total volume of atmospheric air. It has a
pecific gravity 0·97 times that of air. It is the main constituent of the
lackdamp or *chokedamp* of mines. It is used on a very large scale for the
ianufacture of synthetic ammonia. Smaller quantities are used for gas-
lled electric lamps. Nitrogen is also used to provide an inert atmosphere in
ertain industrial processes—for example, in metallurgy to prevent oxida-
on or decarburization.

The Activities of Subterranean Demons

Sudden exposure to an atmosphere almost entirely devoid of oxygen
iay occur in mines, caves, wells, subterranean passages, long-sealed cellars
uilt in rock, the holds of ships and agricultural silos and silage pits. In the
liddle Ages the subject of the effects of noxious gases in mines was
hrouded in superstition of the most primitive character (Rosen, 1943).
Vhen miners were asphyxiated it was thought that subterranean demons
ad destroyed them by the blast of their breath (see p. 28). In the middle
f the seventeenth century superstition gradually gave way to reasoned
eduction from observed facts. Ultimately, the gases encountered in various
ircumstances were identified.

Beating out the Gas

From the thirteenth to the end of the sixteenth century coal mines were
hallow and the means of ventilation imperfect. The only ventilating prac-
ce which can be said to have been general was that known as beating out
ie gas, an operation which consisted in swinging a miner's jacket to and
·o to induce a current of air. The miners were chiefly hampered by the
resence of what they call stythe, chokedamp or blackdamp, which put
ut their lamps, caused panting respiration and sometimes suffocated them.
line gases came to be called *damps* from the German word *dampf*, meaning
fog or vapour.

Composition of Blackdamp

Until the very end of the nineteenth century blackdamp or chokedamp
f mines was thought to be carbon dioxide. In 1899 Haldane and Atkinson

investigated the blackdamp in various coal mines, metalliferous mines an
wells, and found it to consist of nitrogen mixed with small amounts o
carbon dioxide varying from 5 to 15 per cent. These gases are formed b
the oxidation of iron pyrites, FeS_2, and calcite, $CaCO_3$, contained in coa
according to the equation:

$$4FeS_2 + 15O_2 + 8CaCO_3 = 8CO_2 + 8CaSO_4 + 2Fe_2O_3.$$

This yields blackdamp consisting of 87·7 per cent nitrogen and 12·3 pe
cent carbon dioxide, which is approximately the composition of the gase
usually found. The oxygen of air left in contact with coal gradually dis
appears. Hence old workings or spaces of any kind left unventilated soo
become filled with blackdamp.

Blackdamp in Wells

In wells blackdamp is formed in the interstices of the lining materi
and issues up the well whenever a fall of barometric pressure occurs. Thus
the well may be fairly clear of blackdamp at one time, and shortly after
wards full of it. Accidents to well-sinkers commonly occur through ig
norance of this fact. The air is perhaps tested in the morning with a cand
and found clear. In the afternoon a further test is neglected, and if th
barometer has meanwhile fallen, the well-sinkers may descend into black
damp and be asphyxiated or fatally injured, or drowned by falling fror
the ladder.

Extinction of a Flame

Blackdamp is ordinarily recognized by its action in extinguishing
flame. Haldane and Atkinson (1899) showed that a candle held verticall
will not continue to burn if more than 15·8 per cent of blackdamp i
present. This corresponds to an oxygen percentage of 17·6. Blackdamp i
a concentration of 17·7 per cent extinguishes a miner's safety-lamp. C
course, the presence of blackdamp affects the light given by a flame lon
before the point of extinction is reached.

Symptoms and Signs

The effects of blackdamp on men are due mainly to the diminishe
oxygen percentage accompanying the admixture of blackdamp with the ai
There is no noticeable effect until the percentage of oxygen falls to abou
12 per cent, when the breathing begins to be just perceptibly deeper. At 1
per cent, respiration is distinctly deeper and the lips are slightly blue. At
per cent, the lips and face are leaden blue and usually the breathing i
deeper and more frequent. At 5 per cent, there is clouding of consciousnes
and loss of power over the limbs.

The Danger increased by Muscular Effort

The symptoms described are those of a patient at rest. The dange
point is reached much sooner when any muscular effort is made. Even a

5 per cent oxygen there is often shortness of breath and dizziness on exertion, and when the oxygen percentage falls much further fainting is apt to occur. When the oxygen percentage falls below 8 or 10, death may occur in consequence of muscular exertion. Sudden exposure to air containing less than 4 per cent of oxygen causes in men loss of consciousness within about 40 seconds. This is followed by convulsions, and the respirations soon cease. The heart, however, continues to beat for some time longer, and during this period artificial respiration will still restore life.

The Coal Miner protected by Ventilation

Air vitiated simply by diminished partial pressure of oxygen is exceedingly dangerous because the victim suffers hardly any warning symptoms before life is imperilled. Were it not that a flame safety-lamp is usually carried in such air, and that its extinction gives ample warning since it occurs at about 17 per cent of oxygen, accidents would be much more frequent. So far as coal mines are concerned the accumulation of blackdamp is largely prevented by ventilation with powerful centrifugal fans. Haldane (1926) pointed out that it was the need created for better ventilation against firedamp as deeper seams of coal were mined which was the salvation of coal miners from the dangers of blackdamp.

(b) Methane

Methane, CH_4, is a colourless, odourless gas with a specific gravity 0·55 times that of air. It forms mixtures with air which explode on ignition. It is formed by the bacterial decay of vegetation at the bottom of marshy pools, and marsh gas, which is liberated in bubbles when the mud is disturbed with a stick, consists mainly of methane and carbon dioxide. Since the middle of the sixteenth century a pale phosphorescent light seen at night hovering or flitting over marshy ground has been called "an *ignis fatuus* that bewitches and leads men into pools and ditches." Popularly known as *will-o'-the-wisp* or *jack-o'-lantern*, this arises from the spontaneous combustion of methane sometimes mixed with phosphoretted hydrogen. Methane and carbon dioxide are evolved from the fermentation or digestion of sewage solids in sewage tanks and sewers. Methane, also known as *surfet* or *firedamp*, began to create a problem in coal mining in the early part of the seventeenth century when pits were sunk much deeper into coal seams. The gas occurs occluded in the coal and escapes when the pressure is relieved. It often issues in large quantities from *blowers* in the coal, which contain from 80 to 98 per cent of methane with some carbon dioxide and nitrogen. The amount of firedamp varies in different coal mines and in different workings of the same mine.

Dangerous Dilution of the Oxygen of Mine Air

Methane has no physiological action of its own. A mixture of 79 per cent of methane and 21 per cent of oxygen is just as respirable as air. In addition to the risk of explosion, methane presents a further hazard to life in that it may dilute the oxygen of air to a dangerous extent. But since methane is lighter than air, a man affected will, on losing consciousness, usually fall into better air. Were it not for this, fatal accidents from asphyxia would be much more common. In coal mines it often enough happens that a man is temporarily overcome by putting his head upwards into a cavity filled with firedamp. If this contains little or no air, loss of consciousness occurs suddenly and without previous warning. Fatal accidents sometimes occur through a man incautiously advancing without a lamp up a road during attempts to restore ventilation in a district of a mine which has become filled with firedamp. So long as a safety-lamp burns in air containing firedamp, not the slightest harm results from breathing such air (Haldane, 1926).

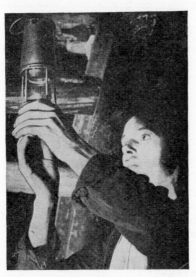

FIG. 220.—Miner places Flame Safety-lamp as near as possible to the Roof of the Mine Working to test the Atmosphere for Methane

Percentage of Firedamp in Mine Workings

Relative safety from methane explosions came in 1816 when the Davy lamp was introduced into coal mines (see p. 1135). Because the density of methane is only half that of air, in detecting its presence in mine workings the flame safety-lamp, which is the modern equivalent of the Davy lamp, is held as near as possible to the roof (fig. 220). The wick of the lamp is lowered until the luminous portion almost disappears; then, upon raising the lamp into a mixture of firedamp and air, a pale blue cap will be seen burning above the luminous flame of the lamp. The height of this cap enables one,

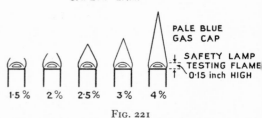

PERCENTAGE OF METHANE IN ATMOSPHERE AS ESTIMATED BY USE OF MINER'S FLAME SAFETY LAMP

PALE BLUE GAS CAP

SAFETY LAMP TESTING FLAME 0·15 inch HIGH

1·5%   2%   2·5%   3%   4%

FIG. 221

with practice, to estimate within 0·25 per cent any concentration of firedamp between 1·5 and 4·5 per cent. In accordance with the Coal Mines Act of 1911 a miner must leave his working-place in the pit if the concentration of inflammable gas, determined by this method, is above 2·5 per cent. Fig. 221, drawn to scale, gives the percentage of firedamp present for caps of different heights, shown on a miner's flame safety-lamp, with a wick half an inch wide, burning a mixture of colza oil and paraffin.

Flame Safety-lamps and Electric Safety-lamps

The safety-lamps at present used in the coal mines of Great Britain are divisible into two classes—namely, flame safety-lamps and electric safety-lamps. Each must be provided with an efficient locking device. In the case of electric lamps, as with all other electrical equipment in coal mines, the switch and other electrical contacts must be contained in flame-tight enclosures. Naturally, all persons entering pits of which the return airway contains inflammable gas must remove from their pockets and give up at the pithead matches, lighters, pipes, tobacco and cigarettes. In coal pits where the return airway never contains inflammable gas, naked lights are allowed.

Effects of Powerful Mechanical Ventilation

In a gassy mine the ventilating system may carry out enormous quantities of methane amounting to four or five million cubic feet a day. Such a powerful system of ventilation removes not only the hazard of firedamp explosions but also that of asphyxia from blackdamp (see p. 649). But neither safety-lamps nor powerful mechanical ventilation alone sufficed to prevent serious colliery explosions. There was no great fall in the number of these disasters until after 1844 when Michael Faraday discovered that firedamp explosions can be greatly aggravated and extended for long distances underground by the ignition of mixtures of coal dust and air. Today such explosions are prevented by the method of stone dusting (see p. 1140).

(c) Carbon Dioxide

Carbon dioxide or carbonic-acid gas, CO_2, is a colourless, inodorous gas with a sharp taste which is present in small quantities in outside air and in very large quantities in certain gaseous emanations from volcanoes and in grottoes. It has a specific gravity 1·53 times that of air. At atmospheric temperature, water dissolves about its own volume of carbon dioxide forming carbonic acid, H_2CO_3. It is produced in industry by decomposing the natural carbonates by means of acids, by calcining limestone to lime, by burning coke, charcoal or heavy hydrocarbons, and in the fermentation of sugar.

Uses

Carbon dioxide is used in the manufacture of alkaline salts, beer, effervescing drinks, sugar, white lead and chemical manures; for sterilizing organic liquors; to produce cold industrially; to preserve perishable products, such as milk, eggs, butter and raisins; to make freezing mixtures in histological and medical work and in the chemical and rubber industries. Carbon dioxide is readily liquefied and is then sold in cylinders for use in the beverage industry, as a fire-extinguishing agent and as blasting material in the soft-explosion method of coal mining. By rapid evaporation of the liquid, solidified carbon dioxide is readily obtained. This is sold in the form of white snowy masses as *dry ice*, *cardice* or *drikold*. Solid carbon dioxide is used as a refrigerating agent, for shrink-fitting metal parts in industry and in the treatment of certain skin lesions.

Exposure Hazards

Danger of exposure to carbon dioxide occurs in mines, tunnels and caissons, in fermenting vats, in breweries, in mineral-water factories, cellars, vaults, wells, tanks, cisterns, ships' holds, blast furnaces, coke ovens, boilers, tannery pits, agricultural silos (fig. 222) and silage pits, and at lime kilns. It is often found mixed with more poisonous gases—for

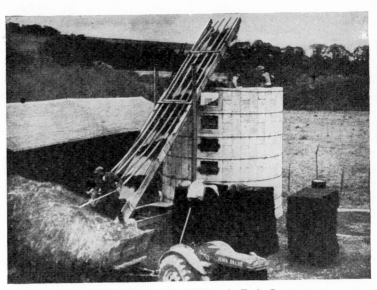

Fig. 222.—Preparation of Silage in Early Summer

example, in illuminating gases, sewer gas, acetylene gas and in the product of combustion and of the firing of explosives. Here it may be carbon monoxide or sulphuretted hydrogen, rather than carbon dioxide, which constitutes the main danger. Where solid carbon dioxide evaporates, the surrounding atmosphere will contain an excessive amount of carbon dioxide which constitutes a hazard when it is confined in an enclosed space such as a store room, box car or motor van.

Symptoms and Signs

Carbon dioxide is a natural excretory product of the body and is not a toxic substance in the usual sense. When it is inhaled even in high concentrations, irritation of the respiratory passages is negligible. Its outstanding effect is the increase in ventilation produced by stimulation of the respiratory centre. The maximum allowable concentration of carbon dioxide in domestic premises is 5,000 parts per million of air. A proportion above 1 per cent in the air is considered as directly harmful, though 2 per cent, which was common long ago in the fermenting vats in breweries, produced no symptoms in the workmen employed there. A proportion of 3 per cent suffices to induce dyspnœa with slight headache; if the proportion is from 5 to 6 per cent, the dyspnœa is pronounced and accompanied by headache and sweating; a proportion of 10 per cent breathed only for a minute sets up headache, visual disturbances, tinnitus, tremor and loss of consciousness. The victim of carbon-dioxide poisoning rapidly becomes unable to stand and passes into coma. Death is not preceded by convulsions.

Treatment

It is important that the patient should not be placed on the floor or on any other equivalent place low down, for the gas, being heavier than air, will accumulate at the lowest point. If breathing has ceased, artificial respiration must be carried out promptly. He must be kept warm and treated by administration of oxygen. The burns caused by solid carbon dioxide are slow to heal. Treatment is the same as for thermal burns.

Preventive Measures

Generally, the mere lowering of a lighted candle into coke ovens, fermenting vats or agricultural silos would suffice as a precaution, extinction of the light indicating an irrespirable atmosphere. Work in such places could be rendered safe by wearing a safety-belt and a breathing apparatus consisting of an oro-nasal mask with tube connexion to the outside atmosphere. The workman must never be alone. His mate must be constantly on the alert and ready at once to rescue him. A third man must be within hailing distance so that should the workman collapse the two can haul him to safety using the rope attached to his safety belt. People handling solid carbon dioxide should wear suitable gloves, otherwise superficial necrosis of the skin rapidly occurs.

Chemical Asphyxiants

Carbon monoxide, sulphuretted hydrogen and hydrogen cyanide each exerts a specific chemical action either on the blood or on the tissues. They do not cause asphyxia by excluding oxygen from the lungs. Their action is prompt even when they are present in minute amounts in the air. They interfere with tissue respiration which is essentially the auto-oxidation of cytochrome oxidase. This is an iron-containing enzyme, the respiratory ferment of Warburg, which makes possible the re-oxidation of reduced cytochrome. Cytochrome also acts catalytically by facilitating a reversible valency change between ferrous and ferric iron. These three noxious gases combine with iron in the cell thereby inhibiting cell respiration.

(a) Carbon Monoxide

Carbon monoxide, CO, is likely to be present wherever man uses fire.

It originates from the incomplete combustion of carbonaceous material. Carbon monoxide is a colourless, tasteless, odourless gas with a specific gravity 0·97 times that of air. The maximal allowable concentration has been placed at 100 parts per million of air for exposures not exceeding a total of eight hours daily.

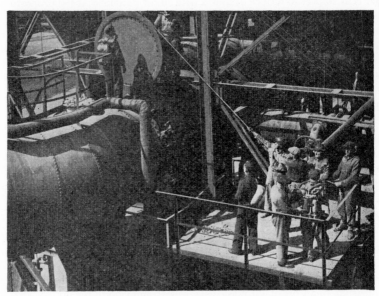

FIG. 223.—*Turning the Goggles* to control the flow of Producer Gas to Blast Furnaces in Ostrava, Czechoslovakia
(*By courtesy of Dr. P. Pachner*)

Exposure Hazards

Coal gas contains about 5 per cent, producer gas about 25 per cent, blast-furnace gas about 30 per cent and water gas (power gas) about 40 per cent of carbon monoxide. These gases are manufactured and widely used for driving gas engines, heating furnaces and boilers, and welding and soldering. Accidents occur amongst workmen on blast furnaces (fig. 223) and amongst persons charging, cleaning and repairing generating plants. The charcoal burner is to some extent exposed (fig. 224). Countless other occupations involve a risk, and even persons working in the offices of iron and steel works may be poisoned by unsuspected escapes from underground flues. Flue gas from boilers, coke furnaces, charcoal braziers and bathroom geysers may cause poisoning through a leak or back draught in the heating apparatus.

Exhaust Gases of Petrol and Diesel Engines

The exhaust gas from internal-combustion engines contains carbon monoxide ranging up to 7 per cent or higher, according to the adjustment of the mixture of petrol and air. A rough estimate of the volume of carbon

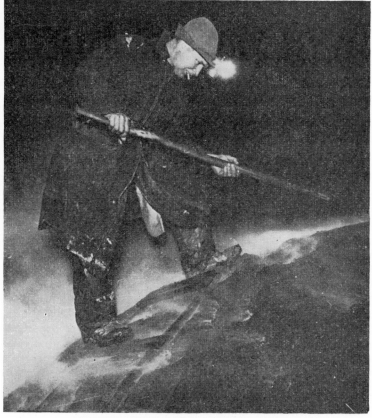

FIG. 224.—Charcoal Burner working at Night
(*Photograph by "Camera Talks"*)

monoxide that a motor car may produce is 1 cubic foot per minute per horse power. This is sufficient to render the atmosphere of a domestic garage deadly within five minutes if the engine is run with the garage doors shut. A man breathing such an atmosphere often falls helpless before he realizes that he is affected; hence many fatalities occur. Diesel engines are widely used in motor buses, lorries and tractors. The exhaust gases from such engines contain carbon monoxide, nitrogen dioxide, nitrogen peroxide and aldehydes. The disagreeable odour is due to aldehydes, which are not very poisonous. When a diesel engine is run on a high fuel-air ratio, carbon monoxide is produced in amounts comparable to those from a petrol engine burning a rich mixture.

Dangers of Fires and of Afterdamp

The smoke of burning buildings, particularly if the fire smoulders in the basement, contains a high percentage of carbon monoxide and may cause poisoning. Where underground fires occur in coal mines, the poisonous constituent of the gas given off is carbon monoxide. The dangerous properties of *afterdamp* produced by explosions of methane and of coal dust are due to carbon monoxide.

$$CH_4 + O_2 = CO + H_2 + H_2O.$$

Examination of the bodies of men killed in three great colliery explosions in 1896 showed that in 95 per cent of the cases death had been due to carbon-monoxide poisoning, though a certain proportion of the men had in addition received burns or other injuries sufficient ultimately to cause death (Haldane, 1926).

Canaries kept at all Coal Mines

As carbon monoxide is odourless, it is important to have some test which will warn miners and others of danger from this gas. The fact that his safety-lamp continues to burn is no proof to the miner of the safety of air in which afterdamp may be present. Haldane introduced the plan of using a small warm-blooded animal such as a mouse or, still better, a small bird to indicate the presence of dangerous proportions of carbon monoxide. The oxidation processes in the small animal or bird are enormously more rapid than in man, consequently it breathes and absorbs carbon monoxide much more rapidly. It therefore shows symptoms of poisoning in a fraction of the time necessary in the case of a man. Hence by watching the bird timely warning may be obtained of the presence of enough carbon monoxide to endanger the life of the miner and his rescuer. It is a legal enactment that canaries must be kept at all coal mines. The cage in which the bird is carried is supplied with a small oxygen cylinder for the purpose of the resuscitation of the bird.

Continuous Carbon-monoxide Recorders

The most convenient method for determining the concentration of carbon monoxide in the air is a portable direct-reading instrument sensitive to 10 p.p.m. of the gas. This employs a catalyst to promote oxidation of the gas, and the corresponding rise of temperature is indicated on a sensitive thermocouple (Elkins, 1950). Carbon-monoxide recorders which operate continuously are installed in up-to-date vehicular tunnels.

Symptoms and Signs

The initial symptoms include giddiness, a sense of oppression in the chest, and loss of power in the lower limbs, the patient falling to the ground unconscious. A simple test can be employed to prove the presence of carbon monoxide in the blood. A greatly diluted solution of the suspected sample is compared with that of normal blood similarly diluted. The latter is yellow, whereas blood containing even very small traces of carboxyhæmoglobin is pink. When the proportion of carbon monoxide in the blood is more than 40 per cent of saturation, spectroscopic examination affords a confirmatory test.

Preventive Measures

Preventive measures must be strictly applied and the structure of buildings regulated in such a way as to obviate unnecessary risk. A competent person should be made responsible for inspecting the plant concerned at stated short intervals. He should see that there is no leakage and must keep a signed and dated record of such inspection. No person should be allowed to work single-handed in a place where exposure is to be anticipated, and a safe form of breathing apparatus must be worn (fig. 225).

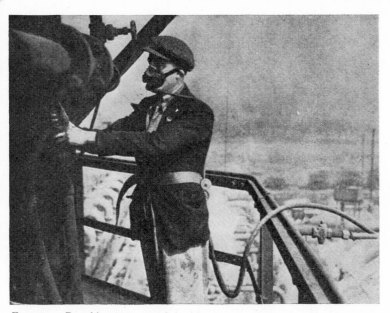

FIG. 225.—Breathing apparatus fed with compressed air—the air main can be seen on handrail of platform fencing. The workman is protected from carbon monoxide while he repairs pipes conveying producer gas

(Factory Department Memorandum on CO Poisoning, H.M.S.O., 1951, by permission of the Controller of H.M. Stationery Office)

Activated charcoal does not effectively protect against carbon monoxide. Respirators must contain a mixture of 50 per cent manganese dioxide, 30 per cent copper oxide, 15 per cent cobaltic oxide and 5 per cent silver oxide, known by the name *hopcalite*. This catalyses the oxidation of the carbon monoxide by the oxygen of the air.

Rescue Squads in Iron and Steel Works

Iron and steel works must have first-aid men constantly on duty, trained to work as rescue squads and taught how to keep all apparatus in good order. Warmth is essential in treatment. The patient should be wrapped in dry blankets and provided with hot-water bottles. Rest is absolutely necessary. The first and immediate consideration is the restoration of breathing, and the second the promotion of warmth and circulation. The use of a mixture of 95 per cent oxygen and 5 per cent carbon dioxide is of great value. It has been shown that the blood of men gassed with carbon monoxide up to 35 per cent and to a 50 per cent hæmoglobin saturation can be brought down to 15 per cent saturation in thirty minutes when the oxygen-carbon-dioxide mixture is inhaled. The same men, gassed to comparable saturations, are relieved very slowly when oxygen alone is inhaled (Henderson and Haggard, 1943).

Sequelæ of Severe Asphyxia

After-effects are headache, cough, depression, and prostration. After severe asphyxia followed by prolonged coma the victim usually dies within thirty-six hours without regaining consciousness. Otherwise he usually recovers completely in a few days. Occasionally prolonged asphyxia permanently damages the brain and the patient survives with paralysis, sensory loss, Parkinsonism or loss of memory. Such sequelæ are due, not to retention of carbon monoxide but to degeneration of nerve cells. The determining factor in their production is the length of time that the tissues have been subjected to oxygen lack. Old people or patients suffering from cardiovascular disease do not stand asphyxia as well as do robust persons.

Acclimatization to Carbon Monoxide

Repeated daily exposure to small amounts of carbon monoxide occurs sometimes in garage mechanics, blast-furnace workers and cooks. They suffer no impairment of health, and they may develop true acclimatization as indicated by compensatory polycythæmia—that is to say, an increase in the red-cell count and hæmoglobin figure. Carbon monoxide is not a cumulative poison. In pure air, and with a sufficient volume of breathing, small amounts of this gas are readily ventilated out of the blood. There is therefore no such condition as chronic carbon-monoxide poisoning.

Validity of Legal Claims

A large number of legal claims of impaired health from exposure to carbon monoxide are unjustified. Such a claim must not be accepted as valid unless three conditions can be established. These are the presence of at least a 50 per cent saturation of the blood or a concentration of carbon monoxide in the air sufficient to induce this; an exposure of at least three hours; and continuous complete unconsciousness lasting for at least six hours after return to fresh air. Short of conditions of such severity, recovery is nearly always complete.

(b) Sulphuretted Hydrogen

Sulphuretted hydrogen, hydrogen sulphide, H_2S, is a colourless gas with a powerful nauseating smell. In mine workings it is called *stinkdamp*. It has a specific gravity 1·19 times that of air and it therefore tends, under stagnant conditions, to accumulate in deep cavities such as tunnels, caissons, vats and cellars. A concentration of 200 parts per million is sufficient to cause symptoms in man, but there is a great variation in individual susceptibility and some men develop symptoms after exposure for some hours to an atmosphere containing less than 100 parts per million (Gerbis, 1927). Exposure to 1,000 parts per million is rapidly fatal. The maximum allowable concentration is 20 parts per million of air.

Occurrence

Wherever sulphur and its compounds are deposited in the crust of the earth, pockets of hydrogen sulphide may be encountered—for example, near volcanoes or in mining lead, gypsum and sulphur. In coal mines it is produced by the decomposition of iron pyrites; it may be liberated by blasting or it may collect in pools of water and rise when the water is disturbed. It is present in natural gas from some oilfields and it is met with in the production, transport and refining of petroleum oil containing sulphur, especially in Mexico and Texas. Measurements of the percentage of hydrogen sulphide in ten adjoining wells in western Texas showed that it ranged from 4 to 14 per cent. All natural life has vanished from these oilfields, and once a sudden shift of wind drove the gas into a corral and killed all the mules. Men have been found lying unconscious in the open to the leeward of a well or in a ravine or near the pumps or tanks (Aves, 1929).

Exposure Hazards

In industrial hygiene the importance of hydrogen sulphide lies in its nuisance value rather than its usefulness. In the coal-gas industry it is encountered in cleaning out tar stills and also the iron-oxide beds used for purification of the gas. The decay of organic matter gives rise to hydrogen sulphide in sewers and waste waters from industrial plants where animal products are handled. The putrefaction of animal and vegetable material may be dangerous as in the storage of green hides, sheep skins and the retting of flax. There has been accidental gassing in tanneries, glue factories, fur-dressing and felt-making plants, abattoirs, beet-sugar factories and breweries. The danger from tanning waste is increased by the presence of sodium and calcium sulphides which are used to remove hair from hides. Hydrogen sulphide is met with in certain industrial processes, such as the production of carbon disulphide and of phosphorus sesquisulphide; in the manufacture of artificial silk by the viscose process; in the action of acids on sulphides; in purifying sulphuric acid; in the manufacture of sulphur dyes; in the vulcanizing of rubber and in repairing and cleaning machinery in chemical and rayon works. The accidental poisoning described by Nau and others (1944) resulted from hosing with water a hot dross which contained arsenic, antimony and sulphur. The gases evolved were arsine, stibine and hydrogen sulphide.

Toxic Action

Death in acute poisoning is as rapid as from poisoning by cyanides; a man inhaling a high concentration drops dead. Its action upon the nervous system, with resulting respiratory paralysis, is exerted only during the

D.O.—22*

time the free hydrogen sulphide is in the blood. Sulphur compounds of hæmoglobin are not important in poisoning by the gas because it does not combine with oxyhæmoglobin but with methæmoglobin, a substance normally present in the blood only in small amounts. On the other hand, sulphmethæmoglobin appears in the blood of cadavers and gives a bluish-green colour to the vessels about the intestines. Hydrogen sulphide, even in low concentrations, exerts a marked irritant action upon the cornea. This is due to the caustic action of sodium sulphide formed in combination with the alkali of the cells in the presence of moisture (Henderson and Haggard, 1943).

Symptoms and Signs

A chemical worker or sewer man inhaling a large dose of the gas falls as if struck by a blow and dies almost instantaneously. Low concentrations of the gas cause irritation of the conjunctiva, nasal mucosa and pharynx, with photophobia, spasm of the eyelids, sneezing, dryness and soreness of the mouth and throat, and increased secretion of tears, saliva and mucus. Headache, giddiness, depression and loss of energy may follow. Hydrogen sulphide is not a cumulative poison, and if a man who has stopped breathing can be revived by artificial respiration there are no systemic sequelæ. Œdema of the lungs and broncho-pneumonia occasionally occur; abdominal colic, vomiting and diarrhœa are rare.

Conjunctivitis and Keratitis

The reaction of the conjunctiva may be extreme, with lachrymation, intense photophobia, pain, chemosis and eversion of the lids. Punctate keratitis produces blurred vision and haziness of the cornea, often accompanied by the formation of bullæ which rupture and are very painful at night. Often there is a warning of the onset of keratitis, in the appearance of increased sensitivity to all kinds of light together with a coloured ring around lights. The eye signs usually recover rapidly within a few days of removal from exposure. Even severe degrees of keratitis usually heal, leaving no injury to the cornea. Corneal ulcers and consequent scarring are rare.

Preventive Measures

To prevent conjunctivitis in the spinning-rooms where viscose-silk yarn is made, it is essential to keep the concentration of hydrogen sulphide down to 20 p.p.m. Moist lead-acetate paper may be used to detect the presence of the gas in the air. At concentrations between 34 and 340 p.p.m. it will darken at once, at 3·4 p.p.m. it will take two seconds to do so. Strict requirements should be laid down in the case of men entering apparatus, such as a tar still, or a settling tank in a tannery, where there is reason to fear the presence of the gas. A hose mask or other suitable breathing apparatus should be used, and a responsible person should see that workmen and, if need be, the rescuers wear a life-belt with the free end of the rope in charge of two men outside, whose sole duty it is to keep watch and to draw out the wearer if he appears to be affected by the gas. In special circumstances the workmen themselves should wear self-contained breathing apparatus—for example, in certain sewers, mine workings, tunnels and wells.

Treatment

In all places where the hazard exists, men must be trained to perform artificial respiration promptly, for although respiratory failure occurs suddenly, the heart continues to beat for several minutes longer and during this period the victim may be saved by prompt measures to restore breathing. He must be kept warm. It may be necessary to combine artificial respiration with administration of oxygen.

(c) Hydrogen Cyanide

Hydrogen cyanide, or hydrocyanic acid, HCN, was discovered by Scheele in 1782. He made it by heating sulphuric acid with Prussian blue, hence the old name *prussic acid*. The term cyanide comes from the Greek word χυάνεος, meaning dark blue. The property referred to is the intense blue colour of the compounds formed with iron.

Properties

It occurs in nature as the glucoside *amygdalin*, which is found in bitter almonds and other plants. Hydrogen cyanide is a colourless, very volatile gas or liquid having an odour of bitter almonds. It is one of the most rapidly acting poisons known, and since many people are unable to recognize its presence by odour they are unaware of danger. The gas has a specific gravity 0·93 times that of air, and it therefore rises and diffuses rapidly. At temperatures below 26·5° C. it is a clear, colourless liquid. The maximum allowable concentration for prolonged exposure is 10 parts per million.

Simple and Complex Cyanides

The cyanide ion is responsible for the toxic action, and this effect is therefore shared by all the soluble inorganic cyanide salts. Potassium cyanide, KCN, sodium cyanide, NaCN, cyanogen, NCCN, cyanogen chloride, CNCl, cyanogen bromide, CNBr, cyanogen iodide, CNI, acetonitrile, CH_3CN, and sodium nitroprusside, $Na_2Fe(CN)_5(NO).2H_2O$, are all intensely poisonous, but they have caused few deaths except by suicide. In addition to the simple cyanides there are a number of complex cyanides, most of which are stable and non-poisonous. Potassium ferrocyanide, $K_4Fe(CN)_6$, potassium ferricyanide, $K_3Fe(CN)_6$, potassium sulphocyanide (thiocyanate), KCNS, ammonium sulphocyanide (thiocyanate), NH_4CNS, and potassium cyanate, KCNO, are among them.

Exposure Hazards

The salts of hydrocyanic acid, chiefly those of potassium and sodium, are extensively used in photography, electro-plating, the case hardening of metals and in the extraction of gold from mineral ores. In processing gold telluride at the Kalgoorlie mines in Western Australia there have been cases of sudden death in men falling into tanks of cyanide slime. Hydrocyanic acid is obtained from the cyanogen compounds found i illuminating gas. Where it is manufactured and handled, precautions shoul be taken against its escape. This applies also to chemical laboratorie Some danger occurs in the following procedures: incomplete combustio of organic nitrogen compounds, exposure of cyanides to the air, decom position of metallic cyanides, gilding and silvering of lace work, stampin of fabrics by means of Prussian blue, manufacture of sulphocyanide an fulminate of mercury, preparation of oxalic acid by treating wood ash with nitric acid, extraction of phosphoric acid from bones and the manu facture of soda by the Leblanc process.

Ulceration of the Skin from Cyanides

During the elutriation of gold by the cyanide method a dilute solutio of potassium cyanide is made to filter through the finely crushed fragmen of ore. The fluid then passes on to boxes filled with shavings of pure zin on which the gold is deposited in the form of slime. The shavings ar scrubbed by hand to extract the gold particles. If a man doing this wor has the slightest abrasion of the epidermis, ulceration which heals only ver slowly may occur. Similar lesions have been found in electro-plating an metal-pickling works. It is possible that this obstinate ulceration of the ski may be due to alkali, for samples of commercial potassium cyanide ofte contain potassium carbonate (White, 1934).

Accidental Deaths from Hydrogen Cyanide

It is only since hydrocyanic acid has come into wide use as a fumigar that accidental deaths from inhalation of the gas have become common. is used for executing criminals and as a fumigating agent to rid close quarters of insect or animal pests (fig. 226). Thus, the holds of ships can b rid of rats and plague-infested fleas, houses of cockroaches or bed bug barns of rats, mice and moles, and greenhouses of insect pests. Even in lo concentrations it kills all forms of animal life and not merely red-bloode creatures as carbon monoxide does. It also kills insects, but is not bactericide.

Fumigation of Houses and Ships

The most convenient means of using the fumigant is as liquid hydro cyanic acid in steel cylinders from which it is forced by air pressure as fine spray which volatilizes immediately. When one of a row of houses being fumigated, the gas may leak through faults in the brickwork, wit fatal results. The fumigation of rooms in dwellings must be conducte with scrupulous care that the gas cannot penetrate to occupied rooms b means of flues, serving hatches, laundry chutes or service lifts. Clearly it use should be entrusted only to those experienced in handling it.

Precautions Necessary in Fumigation

In the practice of fumigation the operators must take the utmost car not to get caught in the building or the hold of the ship after liberation o

he gas has begun, or to return until all spaces have been thoroughly aired.
gas mask with a canister of activated carbon affords effective protection
gainst inhalation. Since the molecular weight of hydrogen cyanide is only
7, less even than the average of the gases in the air, it has a remarkably

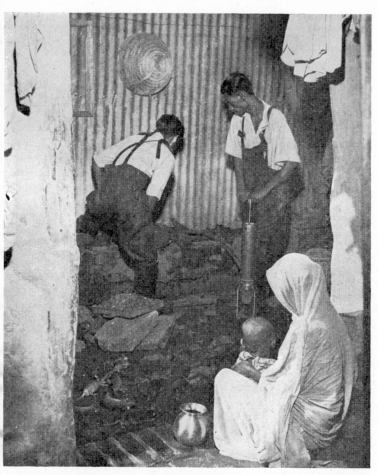

FIG. 226.—Workmen in India exterminating Rats by pumping Hydrogen Cyanide
into a Slum Dwelling
(*By courtesy of United Nations Organisation, Geneva*)

igh capacity to penetrate bedding and other household articles as well as
rerchandise and grain in the holds of ships. Unless fully aired, such material
ray give off enough of the gas to render the air in a confined space danger-
us. Foodstuffs should be aired for at least twenty-four hours, when they
rill be free from injurious effect.

Action of Cyanides

Cyanide poisoning is a form of asphyxia caused by the arrest of internal respiration. The cyanide ion acts on the respiratory ferments of tissue cells incapacitating them in such a way as to prevent their taking up oxygen. It produces an asphyxial death which is unique in that, although the blood is saturated with oxygen, the tissues are rendered incapable of using it. The venous blood is bright red in colour, because oxygen is not abstracted from it in the tissues and it therefore returns in the veins in the arterial condition.

Symptoms and Signs

The symptoms and signs of cyanide poisoning appear within a few seconds or minutes after ingesting compounds or breathing vapours containing the ion. They consist of a sense of constriction in the chest, giddiness, confusion, headache, hyperpnœa, palpitation, unconsciousness, convulsions, feeble rapid respiration and a pulse so weak as to be impalpable. Although large doses are fatal within a few minutes, cases have been reported in which death has been delayed for three hours. In such cases, so long as the heart continues to beat, prompt treatment may save life.

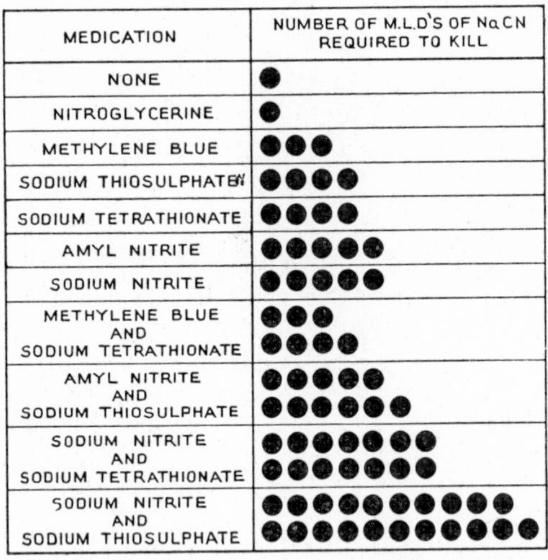

Specific Treatment by Nitrites

Treatment for cyanide poisoning is specific and must be given rapidly if it is to prove effective (fig. 227). It is therefore fortunate that the oil of bitter almonds odour of the breath associated with asphyxia is diagnostic. The objective in treatment is to produce a methæmoglobinæmia. Methæmoglobin combines with the cyanide ion to form cyanmethæmoglobin. In such a combination the cyanide is non-ionized and harmless. Once cyanmethæmoglobin is formed, sodium thiosulphate is given in order to convert to thiocyanate the cyanide which is subsequently released by the dissociation of cyanmethæmoglobin. The best agent to use for the formation of methæmoglobin is sodium nitrite. This is seven times as effective as methylene blue (Chen, Rose and Clowes, 1934).

MEDICATION	NUMBER OF M.L.D'S OF NaCN REQUIRED TO KILL
NONE	●
NITROGLYCERINE	●
METHYLENE BLUE	●●●
SODIUM THIOSULPHATE	●●●●
SODIUM TETRATHIONATE	●●●●
AMYL NITRITE	●●●●●
SODIUM NITRITE	●●●●●
METHYLENE BLUE AND SODIUM TETRATHIONATE	●●● ●●●
AMYL NITRITE AND SODIUM THIOSULPHATE	●●●●● ●●●●●●
SODIUM NITRITE AND SODIUM TETRATHIONATE	●●●●●● ●●●●●●
SODIUM NITRITE AND SODIUM THIOSULPHATE	●●●●●●●● ●●●●●●●●

FIG. 227.—Effects of Treatment on Dogs poisoned with Sodium Cyanide. Note that Sodium Nitrite followed by Sodium Thiosulphate is seven times as effective as Methylene Blue

(Chen, K. K., Rose, C. L., and Clowes, G. H. (1934), Amer. J. med. sci., 188, 767)

Sodium Nitrite given Intravenously

A dose of 0·5 gram of sodium nitrite dissolved in 15 ml. of water is given intravenously over a ten-minute period. If symptoms reappear after having once been controlled, the treatment must be repeated, using half the doses stated. In the event of a prolonged fall in blood pressure, from 3 to 10 minims of 1 in 1,000 adrenalin must be injected subcutaneously. It is unlikely that methæmoglobinæmia will be profound enough to produce severe anoxæmia, but should this occur, inhalation of oxygen or even transfusion of blood may be necessary.

Inhalation of Amyl Nitrite

In the majority of cases the effects of the poison are so rapid that, even if he reaches the scene before death, the practitioner has no time to do anything for his patient. In cases of poisoning by inhalation, subcutaneous or even intravenous treatment is too slow to be effective. The patient should receive an immediate inhalation of amyl nitrite. Glass capsules of this substance should be on hand and their contents liberated by breaking one or more into a handkerchief, which is then held over the patient's face while manual artificial respiration is applied (Henderson and Haggard, 1943).

Following, but not together with, the sodium nitrite, sodium thiosulphate should be given by slow intravenous injection. The dose is 25 grams in a total volume of 50 ml. administered over a ten-minute period.

Recovery of Consciousness after Three Days

The successful use of sodium nitrite followed by sodium thiosulphate in the treatment of poisoning by hydrocyanic acid has been reported by Ingegno and Franco (1937). The patient was a labourer who was removing small trucks loaded with cotton from a large fumigating tank which had recently been filled with hydrogen cyanide. He recovered consciousness five hours after treatment began. A similar case is recorded by Williams (1938). The patient was overcome while spraying liquid hydrocyanic acid into a building. When rescued he was apparently dead. He began to breathe after artificial respiration had been maintained for an hour and a half, and recovered consciousness three days after intravenous injection of sodium nitrite followed by sodium thiosulphate.

IRRITANT GASES

Sulphur dioxide, ammonia, nitrogen dioxide (nitrous fumes), chlorine, phosgene, fluorine and hydrofluoric acid all belong to this group. They are irrespirable in any but very low concentrations and many of them cause immediate irritation resulting in coughing and sneezing. Some of them, such as ammonia, are very soluble in water and in the body fluids, whereas others, such as chlorine, are less soluble. Any gaseous irritant which is highly soluble in water is absorbed from the inspired air by contact with the first moist tissue which it reaches in the respiratory passages. As a consequence, the upper respiratory tract bears the brunt of the action; the lungs are relatively little affected, since the concentration of the irritant which reaches them is greatly reduced by absorption in the upper passages.

Action varies with Solubility

With those gases which have a low solubility, the upper respiratory passages suffer little, for little is absorbed and the main damage is deep in the lungs. A gas of moderate solubility exerts its action more or less uniformly throughout the entire respiratory tract. Thus, as a general rule, the irritant gases are dangerous inversely as their solubility; the less soluble any one of them the more insidious is its action. At the opposite end of the scale we have the soluble gas ammonia, which causes an immediate œdema in the upper respiratory passages, whereas phosgene and nitrogen dioxide have slight immediate effects but subsequent results which are virulent and deadly (Henderson and Haggard, 1943).

(a) Sulphur Dioxide

Sulphur dioxide, SO_2, is a colourless gas possessing a characteristic pungent and irritating odour. It has a specific gravity 2·26 times that of air. It arises from the combustion of sulphur.

Occurrence

It is encountered in the pyrites mines of Tuscany. In adits and galleries where the ventilation is poor the concentration of sulphur dioxide after shot firing can reach more than ten parts per million (Barsotti and Parmeggiani, 1955). The threshold limit in the atmosphere of work rooms is five parts per million. It occurs in the gases issuing from volcanoes and is constantly discharged into the air of towns by the burning of coal and of fuel oil containing compounds of sulphur. Sulphur dioxide is a notable constituent of town fogs. Smog disasters do not occur unless *both the SO_2 and the smoke* content of the atmosphere are greatly increased (fig. 228). Since the introduction of natural gas as fuel in place of coal and fuel oil Pittsburgh has lost her fogs because neither sulphur dioxide nor smoke are produced in its combusion. Sulphur dioxide emitted from smelters as well as that from other chimneys may be injurious to vegetation, particularly to coniferous trees. The effects of atmospheric pollution on limestone and dolomite buildings and the benefits arising from implementing the *Clean Air Act, 1956* have already been discussed (see p. 360).

Uses

Large quantities of sulphur dioxide are produced in the smelting of sulphide ores. Anhydrous sulphur dioxide liquefied under moderate pressure is handled in steel cylinders and in containers holding up to 15 tons. It has been widely used in the liquefied state as a refrigerant, and in the manufacture of sulphuric acid. It is employed for bleaching wool, straw and wood pulp for paper making, in fruit preserving and sugar refining, as a reagent in a number of organic syntheses and also in the refining of

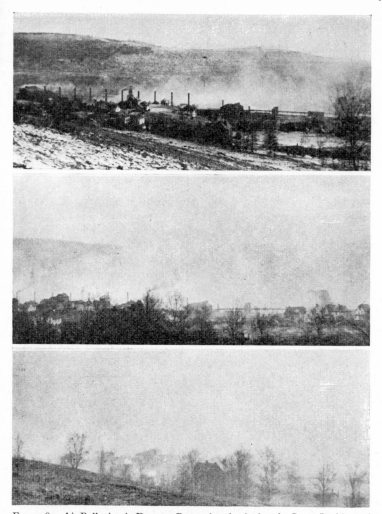

FIG. 228.—Air Pollution in Donora, Pennsylvania, during the Smog Incident of October 1948. Photographs taken at the same time of day to give a comparison of Atmospheric Pollution on different days
(*Photographs by U.S. Public Health Service*)

petroleum. It is used as a fungicide and for fumigation, especially to kill rats as an anti-plague measure. When ships are fumigated, sulphur may be burned either in iron pots in many small lots, or in a specially constructed furnace from which the sulphur dioxide is blown through pipes into the ship.

Symptoms and Signs

Sulphur dioxide is almost irrespirable to those unaccustomed to it, but men who have worked in an atmosphere fairly heavily contaminated acquire a degree of tolerance. Beyond this, irritation of the pharynx may produce cough, and higher concentrations irritate the conjunctiva and bronchi and interfere with taste and smell. Severe acute gassing accidents are rare mainly because sulphur dioxide is so intensely irritating that men run for their lives to escape from its effects. In the case of an overwhelming dose arising from the sudden escape of a large amount of gas from a broken container or a leak in a refrigeration apparatus the victim is asphyxiated, may lose consciousness and, if not removed from the contaminated atmosphere, may die. If he be promptly rescued, he may escape without lung involvement, although œdema of the larynx has been reported. At the worst he may have acute bronchitis, œdema of the lungs or bronchopneumonia, and recover completely within three weeks.

Injuries to the Eyes

Injury to the eyes with sulphur dioxide will vary according to whether the gaseous or the liquid substance is involved. When only the gas is employed, as in magnesium foundries, ocular reactions are mild. This is no doubt due to the warning characteristics of the gas, which enable the worker to avoid excessive exposure. Even in acute exposures severe enough almost to kill the patient, the severe conjunctivitis which occurs recovers completely, leaving no ocular damage. On the other hand, accidental spraying of liquefied sulphur dioxide into the eyes of men working on refrigeration machines may cause permanent reduction of visual acuity from its effect on the cornea. At first there is only minor discomfort even with serious injury, and this is followed by considerable swelling of the eyelids with opacity of the corneal epithelium. After several days this epithelium is shed, revealing infiltration of the stroma together with interstitial vascularization. The complications are corneal scarring, conjunctival overgrowth of the cornea and symblepharon (fig. 229). It has been shown experimentally in rabbits that sulphur dioxide readily penetrates the corneal epithelium and acts, principally as sulphurous acid, by denaturing corneal proteins and inactivating corneal catalase (Grant, 1947).

Effects of Prolonged Exposure

Kehoe and others (1932) studied the effect of prolonged exposure on 100 workmen exposed to this gas in the course of their employment. In forty-seven there had been from four to twelve years' exposure to concentrations up to 70 parts per million by volume. They found an incidence of slight chronic nasopharyngitis significantly higher than was normal, and many of these workmen had partly lost their sense of taste and smell. Although the susceptibility to ordinary colds was no higher than normal, their average duration was two or three times longer than the average for the control group. Other significant differences between the two groups were dyspnœa on exertion and increased fatigue from work.

Symptomatic Treatment

The patient should be kept warm and given artificial respiration if necessary. He should be put to bed and treated by inhalation of oxygen if

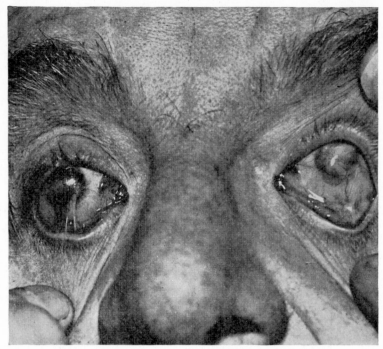

Fig. 229.—Blindness caused by liquid Sulphur Dioxide which splashed into the Eyes when a Refrigerator exploded. Condition ten years later shows Leukomata of both Corneæ with pronounced Symblepharon of both Eyes
(Grant, W. M. (1947), Arch. Ophthal., 38, 755, 762)

the dyspnœa demands this. Tracheotomy is necessary in rare cases. Castor oil or liquid paraffin instilled into the conjunctival sacs will relieve the pain of conjunctivitis. If the liquid substance has been splashed into the eye, prompt and prolonged irrigation with water must be carried out.

(b) Ammonia

Ammonia, NH_3, is a colourless gas with a pungent odour and a vapour density of 0·597. It is easily liquefied and is extremely soluble in water, with which it forms ammonium hydroxide, NH_4OH. The threshold limit for ammonia in air for an eight-hour working exposure is 100 parts per million. It is one of the by-products formed in the destructive distillation of coal for the production of coal-gas, coke and tar. It is made synthetically when nitrogen and hydrogen are mixed and brought in contact with a catalyst, such as specially prepared iron granules at high temperature and pressure.

Uses

It is transported in liquid form in steel cylinders or in tank cars, or in drums or carboys dissolved in water as the hydroxide. It is used as a refrigerant in cold-storage plants and for the manufacture of ice. To some extent it is being replaced in these uses by other refrigerants (see p. 598). If a pipe or joint breaks or leaks, ammonia gas escapes into the air and quickly becomes intolerable to everyone in the vicinity who is not wearing a gas-mask. Contamination of the air may occur also from the bursting or leaking of a cylinder of the liquid in filling, storage or transit. It is used also in petroleum refining, in the treatment of steel, the purification of water, the fertilizer industry, the manufacture of sulphuric and nitric acids, drugs and chemicals, and in bottling plants for household ammonia.

Exposure Hazards

As long ago as 1887 Fairbrother described an accident in a brewery where four men were installing an ice machine and a large vat of ammonia broke, letting the fluid run over the floor and filling the room with the gas. It was about three minutes before the men could be released, and then one of them was found comatose with a barely perceptible heart-beat and he died in fifteen minutes. The second was wildly delirious and unable to stand; he lived for only two hours. The third was conscious and could walk, but developed marked dyspnœa and died in five hours. The one man who survived had suffered a compound fracture which necessitated amputation. Even three months after the accident he was still suffering from chronic bronchitis with hæmoptysis.

Ammonia Burns of the Skin

Burns, which may be severe and even fatal, may follow the splashing of strong ammonia on to the skin. In 1938 Slot described the cases of six women who had been exposed to a pipe-burst in the refrigerator system of an ice-cream factory. All suffered from shock, one from delirium, and three from burns on the skin. In two the burns were not extensive and they healed within a few days. One of these women was left with anxiety symptoms, insomnia and a painful scar. The third woman was extensively burned over the face, neck, chest, left arm and right leg. At first she vomited blood and mucus. There was severe shock, the face was ashen grey and the pulse was often imperceptible. There was laboured breathing, relieved somewhat when she was treated in an oxygen tent, but she remained unable to swallow. Bronchopneumonia developed, and albumin and blood appeared in the urine. She remained very ill and died five weeks after the accident.

Injuries to the Eyes

Ammonia gas has an immediate effect on the conjunctiva, causing smarting pain. If strong aqueous solutions of ammonia splash into the eye, conjunctivitis and keratitis usually occur. Ulceration of the conjunctiva and cornea, scarring of the tissues and corneal and lenticular opacities may interfere with vision or even lead to blindness (Teraskelli, 1927). It can be shown experimentally that ammonia appears in the anterior chamber of the eye within a few seconds of its introduction into the conjunctival sac. Therefore, apparatus to irrigate the eye with water must be installed wherever the hazard of splashing with ammonia exists. Irrigation must be promptly applied and it may be necessary to carry it out continuously for an hour.

Symptoms and Signs

In 1941 Caplin described the mass poisoning of seventy-five people in the cellars of a London brewery which were used as an air-raid shelter. A fragment of flying metal pierced the connecting pipe of an ammonia condenser, causing sudden escape of the gas, which continued for about ten minutes before it was shut off. Those farthest from the leak were mildly affected. They complained of a smarting sensation in the eyes and mouth, and pain on swallowing. All were hoarse and could hardly raise their voices above a whisper. Cough was not a prominent feature. There was a strong smell of ammonia in the breath. The lips, mouth and tongue were reddened and raw, the conjunctivæ reddened and swollen, and the eyelids and fauces œdematous. The group with moderate exposure showed in addition a feeling of tightness in the chest, dysphagia, cough and sometimes blood-stained sputum. There was restlessness, with a slight increase in respiratory rate and a rise in temperature of one or two degrees. There was lachrymation, with more œdema of the eyelids, lips, mouth, tongue and fauces than in the mild cases. Ulceration of the buccal mucosa with the formation of sloughs was a common finding. A few of the patients developed corneal ulcer. Moist sounds were present in the lungs. Some developed œdema of the lungs within six hours, and others bronchopneumonia about the third day. The fatality rate for this group was 22 per cent. The survivors rapidly recovered normal health, although hoarseness tended to clear up only slowly over many weeks.

Fatal Cases and Morbid Anatomy

The most severely affected of Caplin's cases showed symptoms and signs in the eyes, mouth and fauces as in the moderately affected cases, but the signs of shock, restlessness and distress were worse. There was slight cyanosis, intense dyspnœa and persistent cough with much frothy sputum. The pulse was rapid and of poor volume, and the temperature normal. Generalized râles and rhonchi were audible in the chest. Many of these patients became worse and died in two days. The fatality rate for this group was 63 per cent. The necropsy findings included redness and œdematous swelling, with shallow ulcers of the tongue, lips and buccal mucosa, purulent inflammation of the fauces, pharynx, larynx and trachea, with membrane formation affecting both trachea and epiglottis; purulent bronchitis and bronchopneumonia with œdema of the lungs.

Preventive Measures

To prevent accidents at an ammonia refrigerating plant, the following rules must be laid down:

(1) All employees must be instructed as to the dangers from ammonia and trained to avoid them.

(2) Nobody should be allowed to sleep in rooms adjoining the plant.

(3) The refrigerating equipment, including valves and piping, should be regularly inspected at short intervals and necessary repairs made immediately.

(4) The room or rooms in which the machinery is installed should have doors swinging outward and opening directly to the outside air. The relation of this room to other parts of the building should be such that escaping fumes cannot invade the other parts or cut off the escape of persons in them. Regulations should be prominently posted and strictly enforced, requiring that the exits shall never, even for a few minutes, be obstructed by temporary scaffolding, wheelbarrows or other impediments to egress.

(5) Gas-masks with canisters affording protection against ammonia should be provided; they should be stored in some locality readily accessible to, but outside the room in which there is a possibility of the escape of ammonia.

(6) Every workmen engaged in repair work on refrigerating apparatus should be required to carry at all times a gas-mask strapped to his body or hung around his neck in anticipation of the possible escape of ammonia.

(7) A valve arranged to shut off the ammonia at the storage cylinders and to discharge it into the sewers with a large volume of water should be placed where it can be manipulated from the outside of the building (Henderson and Haggard, 1943).

Symptomatic Treatment

In cases of mild exposure the patient recovers promptly on being removed to fresh air. In severe cases the first aim is to relieve restlessness and dyspnœa and to combat shock; the second to neutralize ammonia in the buccal mucosa; and the third to relieve conjunctival and buccal pain. An electric cradle should be used to combat shock, and fluids and morphine given. Where cyanosis and dyspnœa are present, the dose of morphine must be restricted to gr. $\frac{1}{6}$. Oxygen should be administered and, where pronounced moist sounds are present in the lungs, injections of atropine gr. $\frac{1}{100}$ given and repeated two-hourly. The ammonia in the mouth and fauces should be neutralized by a mouth wash and gargle of table vinegar diluted one part in four with warm water. Where there is great pain a cocaine and adrenaline spray is used, otherwise the mouth and nose are treated with liquid paraffin applied on a swab. The eyes should be irrigated with water and a few drops of castor oil instilled into the conjunctival sacs (Caplin, 1941). Where strong ammonia has burned the skin, the treatment of shock may need special care. Local treatment by tannic-acid jelly has proved efficient (Slot, 1938).

(c) Nitrogen Dioxide

The oxides of nitrogen are nitrous oxide, N_2O, nitric oxide, NO, and two forms of nitrogen dioxide, NO_2 and N_2O_4. Nitrous oxide has no irritating action and is used extensively as an anæsthetic. When inhaled without oxygen it acts as a simple asphyxiant. Nitric oxide is a colourless gas, slightly heavier than air and sparingly soluble in water. It does not exist in atmospheric air, for in the presence of moisture and oxygen it is converted into the dioxide. At body temperature the dioxide exists as a reddish-brown vapour consisting of approximately 70 per cent of N_2O_4 and 30 per cent of NO_2. These *nitrous fumes* are given off from fuming nitric acid and are formed when the acid is spilt during handling or storage.

Exposure Hazards

Most cases of industrial poisoning occur in the manufacture of nitric and sulphuric acids and of explosives and other nitro-compounds and various nitrates, in the dipping of brass and copper articles in nitric acid, and from the breaking or upsetting of carboys of nitric acid. Great volumes of nitrous fumes are also liberated by the slow burning or incomplete detonation of nitro-explosives such as cordite, and in the combustion of other nitrated compounds—for example, celluloid. In such circumstances a large number of people may be affected at one time, as happened in Cleveland, Ohio, U.S.A., in 1929, when over a hundred fatalities occurred after the burning of a hospital store containing a large quantity of radiographic films. At the temperature of the electric arc, which is about 3,000° C., atmospheric oxygen and nitrogen combine to form nitrogen dioxide. When electric-arc welding is carried out in confined spaces, fatal poisoning has resulted. Similarly, in the manufacture of bone meal the use of impure sulphuric acid containing a proportion of nitric acid may have the same effect. In *silo-fillers' disease*, as described by Delaney and others (1956), men working in maize silos at certain stages of the fermentation process may be poisoned by nitrogen dioxide, sometimes fatally. The evolution of the gas is enough to produce visible yellow clouds, to stain the forage and unpainted woodwork yellow and to kill animals.

Hazards in Mining

The effects of nitrogen dioxide may be encountered in mining and tunnelling, especially when the ventilation is bad. The risk is only slight in coal mines where the ventilation is likely to be good, but in metalliferous mines cases of poisoning have occurred. When dynamite or gun-cotton burn quietly instead of detonating, nearly the whole of the nitrogen is given off as nitric oxide instead of as free nitrogen. The nitric oxide is at once converted into nitrogen dioxide. In the gold mines of India and the Transvaal accidents involving the loss of as many as twenty men at a time have sometimes occurred from dynamite catching fire underground. Serious results may follow the imperfect detonation of nitro-explosives in any situation where the ventilation is bad. Thus in 1879 two deaths occurred from nitrogen-dioxide poisoning during the construction of the Severn Tunnel (Haldane, 1902). Cases also occur in confined spaces such as gun pits, armoured cars and tanks, and in the burning of cordite in ships set on fire.

Treacherous and Insidious Effects

Since nitrous fumes can be breathed with only slight inconvenience in concentrations which will cause a fatal œdema of the lungs after an ex posure of half to one hour, and since the least concentration of the ga which will provoke coughing is very little less, the margin of safety between appreciation of the risk and exposure to real danger is very small. More over, the initial irritation soon passes off and the worker feels well and is in no apprehension that he may be in a critical condition in a few hours. The gas therefore has most treacherous and insidious qualities, and but for the distinctive colour of the fumes and education of the worker more fatalities would occur.

Mode of Action

Nitrogen dioxide has a direct action upon the alveolar epithelium of the lung, and some hours after its inhalation acute suffocative pulmonary œdema develops. The condition is not only insidious in onset but is pain less and usually severe out of all proportion to the irritation of the upper respiratory tract. A man may, without serious discomfort, breathe an atmosphere containing a concentration of nitrous fumes sufficient to caus death some hours later. After the spilling of nitric acid on a wooden floor or the incomplete explosion of dynamite in a tunnel or some similar slight mishap, a workman inhales some of the fumes for a time but is little in convenienced. He goes home and eats his supper, suffering no ill effects During the night œdema of the lungs overtakes him and before morn ing he may be dead, drowned in the volume of fluid poured out in his lungs.

Initial Symptoms

The initial symptoms—namely, irritation of the eyes and throat, cough tightness of the chest and nausea—are slight and may pass unnoticed especially if the concentration of the gas is low. Although a low con centration will probably be perceived on coming from outside, that appreci ation is soon dulled and symptoms may not be evident until after some hours in the dangerous atmosphere. Usually, however, the presence of the gas has been noted, though little attention may have been paid to it at the time. This is an important diagnostic point for the practitioner called in later to an unconscious man, for the patient may have mentioned the fac to a relative earlier, not because he was feeling really ill but rather because of weariness and a disinclination for any exertion, using it merely as an excuse for resting at home.

Latent Interval

The initial symptoms generally disappear on cessation of exposure and a latent period ensues, during which the patient may even return to work He is then in a highly dangerous situation in which sudden death may follow some quite ordinary exertion. This latent period varies from two to wenty hours; not uncommonly a man finishes his day's work and is at ome for some time before signs of acute illness become manifest.

Physical Signs

At the end of the latent period signs appear. Their onset may be sudden nd precipitated by exertion. Cough, a feeling of constriction in the chest nd difficulty in breathing occur. As the œdema progresses, so do the ymptoms; the cyanosis becomes intense, the air hunger is most distressing nd much blood-stained fluid is coughed up. Unconsciousness usually upervenes, although it may be long in appearing, and then the outlook eems hopeless. So long, however, as there are no signs of failure of the irculation with a thin, soft irregular pulse and the cyanosis taking on a eaden hue, these patients tend to recover, for the œdema begins to recede n the second day and thereafter is absorbed rapidly. Some victims become lelirious; the temperature may be raised two or three degrees. In some he picture when first seen may be that of pallor with a rapid feeble pulse nd a tendency to collapse but without cyanosis or breathlessness. Some of he milder cases may exhibit a picture of acute bronchitis with severe yanosis, and others nausea, abdominal pain and vomiting.

Differential Diagnosis

The earlier a diagnosis is made and appropriate treatment started, the etter the chances of recovery and, since absolute rest is essential, a protracted examination must be avoided. The clinical picture may simulate ther diseases such as pneumonia, acute bronchitis or cerebral hæmorrhage, ut if a history can be obtained it is often so characteristic that a diagnosis an be made on that alone. Usually there has been some reference to gas or umes about the workroom which did not trouble the patient much, then he latent period of some hours, followed by the onset and progressive levelopment of the illness.

Preventive Treatment

Measures must be taken to prevent the escape of fumes and to remove hem as nearly as possible at the point of origin by localized exhaust ventilation. Danger must be reduced to a minimum by special efforts to emove fumes before repairs to dangerous plant are attempted. Approved ypes of breathing apparatus must be provided and maintained for use vhen fumes are noted or apprehended. When any reddish fumes can be een, smelt or appreciated by the conjunctiva or pharynx, there is serious nd imminent danger. All workers, except those properly protected, should e removed from the dangerous area immediately.

Dealing with Spilt Nitric Acid

When spilt, nitric acid may attack wooden floors, refuse or any organic naterial with which it comes in contact, with evolution of the reddish-brown umes. Sawdust, wood shavings or other organic material should not be scattered over spilt nitric acid as they increase the evolution of fumes and ake fire. It should be hosed away with large quantities of water by men wearing efficient breathing apparatus. One must guard against reduction in the ventilation by closing doors and windows, or overcrowding a workroom with additional plant which may so raise the concentration of fumes as to extinguish a small safety margin. Thus, an electrolytic metal-stripping process using weak nitric acid was worked for eight or nine years without accident; during the last two years the number of vats in the room had been increased from six to twelve. The addition of a thirteenth vat resulted in three cases of gassing during the first morning's work.

Treatment of Air in Mines

In rock mining, especially where the rock is exceptionally hard as in the Witwatersrand, the number of shots fired at the rock face, in sinking shaft and in tunnelling, may be phenomenal. Ventilation must therefore deal adequately with the nitrogen dioxide inevitably produced from the ammon dynamite which is used. Happily, at depths as great as 7,000 feet the risk of heat exhaustion is so great that 5 tons of air must be blown into the mine for every ton of rock removed (McIntyre, 1953). Nevertheless, oxides of nitrogen must be removed from the air by forcing it through beds of vermiculite containing adsorbed potassium permanganate and soda ash.

Symptomatic Treatment

In patients seen soon after exposure it may be difficult to decide how much risk has been run. In such cases the patients, in spite of protestations that they are now better and able to carry on, should be kept under observation and at rest for twenty-four hours. Other persons, with or without symptoms, known to have been seriously exposed should be removed to hospital lying flat. Absolute rest is essential; oxygen should be administered as early as possible and continuously, except for the last five minutes in each half-hour, when it may be stopped to observe whether or not the improvement is maintained. If not, the administration should be restarted at once and the routine continued until no adverse effect is noted on temporary cessation. Administration should be by means of a Haldane mask, by nasal catheter or by other means which will ensure maximal efficiency. The rate of flow should be from 3 to 10 litres per minute, the necessary amount being judged by the effect produced. Venesection of patients with purple cyanosis and a full pulse may give much relief to an overloaded right heart but is contraindicated in patients with pallor or grey leaden cyanosis, thin pulse and pulse-rate over 100. Rest, oxygen early and continuously, and venesection when indicated are the three essentials.

(d) Chlorine

Chlorine, Cl_2, is a greenish-yellow gas with a pungent, irritating odour. It has a specific gravity 2·48 times that of air. The maximum concentration allowable for prolonged exposure is one part per million of air.

Uses

It is used in the manufacture of alkali and bleaching powders, in the bleaching of flour, in dye works and paper mills, and in the disinfection of water and sewage. It was the first gas used in chemical warfare. For industrial use it is liquefied under pressure and handled in steel cylinders or special tanks. Poisoning may arise when leakage occurs from stores, particularly during fires when it escapes from the cylinders and is rapidly volatilized. Chlorine cylinders are tested to 3,000 lb. pressure, but are equipped with safety plugs which release the gas slowly before the pressure has reached this point, and thus prevent the bursting of the cylinders. During fires the pressure developed in the cylinders leads to the rapid escape of the gas. Fortunately, fatalities are rare, because the fact that the gas is irrespirable is so well known that at a big escape workers fly for their lives.

Toxic Action

It was at one time supposed that chlorine reacts with the moisture on the tissues to form hydrochloric acid and that its detrimental effects arose from the action of this acid. The similarity between the action of chlorine and hydrochloric acid was pointed out in support of this view. The similarity, however, is more apparent than real. Chlorine is nearly twenty times as toxic as hydrochloric acid, and because of its relatively low solubility, its action is carried over to a much wider area of the respiratory tract than is that of hydrochloric acid.

Symptoms and Signs

Immediate symptoms are a choking, suffocating sensation associated with acute anxiety. There is retrosternal burning pain and a sense of constriction of the chest aggravated by bouts of coughing. The eyes smart and there is burning of the nose and mouth with increased salivation. Headache is intense and epigastric pain is common. Nausea and vomiting follow and syncope may occur. The patient has the appearances of being acutely ill. There is respiratory distress and cyanosis associated with a full bounding pulse and engorgement of the veins of the neck. In most cases cough and respiratory distress persist for about two weeks and patchy infiltration in both lungs is demonstrated by X-rays. Even in severe cases pulmonary œdema or pneumonia occur only rarely. It is probable that in the First World War œdema of the lungs and pneumonia ascribed to chlorine were due to mixtures of chlorine and phosgene. High concentrations of chlorine cause irritation of the skin, but this can occur only if exposure to such concentrations is made possible by the use of a gas-mask.

Treatment

When a man is gassed, complete rest from the moment of exposure is essential. Continuous administration of oxygen should be started as soon as possible and continued as long as signs of anoxia are present. Codeine phosphate by mouth or intramuscular injection (0·03 to 0·12 gram) reduces the cough, and ephedrine gr. $\frac{1}{4}$ relieves bronchial spasm (Chasis and others, 1947). If cyanosis with venous engorgement and right heart failure occur, venesection should be performed. A pint of blood may be safely withdrawn at the first bleeding, but if it is necessary to repeat the venesection, not more than 200 millilitres should be taken on the second occasion. Absolute rest with barbiturates to ensure sleep at night should be continued until the temperature has been normal for forty-eight hours.

Absence of Sequelæ

During the years 1932–48 Jones (1952) observed 820 cases of gassing by chlorine in workers on chemical processes. Of these, 728 were classified as mild and reported to the works' medical department with a painful cough and increased respiration, 81 had considerable respiratory embarrassment, with distended cervical veins and some cyanosis, and 11 were sent home after treatment. The pulse and respiratory rates were raised and the physical signs were those of bronchitis, medium rhonchi and râles being present on auscultation of the chest. Nine cases were severe and required admission to hospital, but even in these cases neither pulmonary œdema nor pneumonia ensued. A follow-up of severe cases from the series revealed no clinical or radiological evidence of permanent damage to the respiratory tract.

Preventive Measures

Men must specially be warned against the breaking-up of cylinders supposed to be empty. Where chlorine is used in industry, effective ventilation is required and the men in charge of the plant should be trained in the use of respirators. The safest system is to provide a compressed-air line with fittings at intervals for the attachment of air-line masks. The fitter who is required to mend a leak can then be instantly and adequately protected by breathing air from this system.

(e) Phosgene

Phosgene, carbonyl chloride, $COCl_2$, is a colourless gas having a characteristic odour resembling that of green corn. It is many times more poisonous than chlorine. It has a specific gravity 3·4 times that of air. The maximum allowable concentration for day-to-day exposure is one part per million of air.

Uses

Its toxic effects have been specially studied in connexion with chemical warfare. More than 80 per cent of the gas fatalities in the First World War were caused by phosgene. It is used in chemical industry as an agent for direct chlorination (fig. 62). As it reacts with organic acids, it is used to make acid chlorides and anhydrides. It is used for preparing numerous other products such as arsenic trichloride, benzoic acid, salol and aniline dyes derived from diphenylmethane. Cases of poisoning occasionally occur in chemical works as a result of accidental leakage. From two factories in which it was manufactured, twenty-seven cases of poisoning were reported in 1917 and sixty-nine in 1918, mainly in workers engaged in repair work.

Toxic Action

In low concentrations it causes little irritation of the upper respiratory tract, so that dangerous amounts may be inhaled before its presence is recognized. Being relatively insoluble, it reaches the lungs before it begins to act. An interval of some hours without symptoms may end with the sudden onset of acute pulmonary œdema accompanied by profound circulatory collapse. The injurious effects of phosgene are materially increased by physical exertion.

Symptoms and Signs

The effect of phosgene is not immediately irritating, and if the victim fails to detect its odour he has no warning of the fact that he is breathing a deadly gas. After exposure for a few minutes he has a feeling of tightness in the chest, and cough, nausea and vomiting occur. As exposure continues, there is irritation of the eyes, nose and pharynx, the patient is restless and very ill, respiration becomes more and more rapid and moist râles are found in the lungs. If pulmonary œdema develops, both coughing and vomiting may result in the removal of œdema fluid from the lungs. Circulatory collapse may occur; it is marked by cyanosis and a rapid pulse which is difficult to feel.

Treatment

Any person who has inhaled phosgene should be carried on a stretcher, put into a warm bed and kept under observation and at absolute rest for twenty-four hours. If no symptoms have developed after forty-eight hours they are unlikely to arise subsequently. Since circulatory collapse commonly occurs in phosgene poisoning, complete rest is essential from the moment of exposure. The patient must lie flat on his back; his clothing should be loosened to allow freedom of breathing. Warmth must be ensured to combat shock and to prevent the muscular exertion of shivering. The oxygen requirement is further reduced by giving by mouth only bland drinks sweetened with glucose.

Continuous Administration of Oxygen

If pulmonary œdema develops, treatment of the anoxia which results is the most urgent need. As long as any degree of anoxia exists, continuous administration of oxygen by an efficient method must be maintained. Such treatment should begin at the earliest sign of cyanosis. Oxygen with carbon dioxide must not be used since the lungs as well as the whole body are in need of rest. Circulatory collapse often occurs simultaneously. It is marked by cyanosis and a rapid, thready pulse. Venesection is indicated in this type of circulatory failure. Nikethamide (coramine) is a useful stimulant, but efficient oxygen therapy is more important. Vomiting always occurs, and much of the fluid from the lungs may be removed in this way.

Measures Ineffective or Harmful

Atropine is not effective, expectorants should not be given and postural drainage is unsafe. If the exudate is so copious that the patient is in danger of drowning, the foot of the bed should be raised on a chair so that the fluid will drain towards the mouth. Cough which is non-productive and exhausting should be controlled by hot drinks and a linctus containing heroin or codeine, so that coughing occurs only periodically and deliberately as a means of removing as much of the œdema fluid from the lungs as possible. Morphine is dangerous since it may abolish the cough reflex and depress the cardio-respiratory centres. Restlessness is better controlled by the administration of oxygen.

Complications and Sequelæ

A rise of temperature after the symptoms of pulmonary œdema have subsided suggests the onset of secondary infection, resulting in bronchitis or bronchopneumonia. Treatment with antibiotics or with full doses of sulphonamides should then immediately begin. Convalescence is slow, and effort syndrome commonly follows an incident of gassing. Patients with persisting tachycardia should not be allowed up too soon. Rehabilitation under medical supervision helps to prevent neurosis as a sequel to phosgene poisoning. Jones (1952) reported the complete recovery of five patients followed up for sixteen years. There was no permanent damage to the lungs as shown by sickness records, clinical and radiological examination.

Preventive Measures

In industrial establishments where it is prepared or handled, measures must be taken to prevent the escape of phosgene from closed apparatus and from piping. Exhaust plant must be installed for the withdrawal of the gas at its point of origin, and adequate ventilation is essential. For emergency use, gas-masks connected through a hose to a supply of compressed air should be installed. Such a hose must be flexible, impervious to oil and petrol, long enough to reach all points of potential danger and strong enough to be used as a life-line if necessary. Frequent change of working clothes is indispensable, since phosgene readily becomes fixed in materials. The skin should be frequently washed and the mouth rinsed with an alkaline mouth-wash in order to prevent traces of phosgene dissolved in the saliva from causing irritation of the stomach.

(f) Fluorine and its Compounds

Fluorine, F_2, is one of the most active elements known; consequently, it does not occur in the free state in nature. The principal fluorine-bearing minerals which are used in large-scale industrial processes are: fluorspar, CaF_2, cryolite, $AlF_3.3NaF$, apatite, $3Ca_3(PO_4)_2.CaF_2$, and sedimentary phosphate rock. Fluorine and some of its compounds are amongst the most reactive substances known and have a highly corrosive action on animal tissues as well as on metals and other familiar materials.

ses

Fluorine and its compounds hydrofluoric acid, HF, hydrofluosilicic cid, H_2SiF_6, silicon fluoride, SiF_4, aluminium fluoride, Al_2F_6, cobalt tri-uoride, CoF_3, sulphur hexafluoride, SF_6, uranium hexafluoride, UF_6, odium fluoracetate, FCH_2COONa, and dichlorodifluoromethane, CCl_2F_2, re all encountered in industry. Hydrofluoric acid is used for clouding lectric-light bulbs, etching glass and pickling metals, especially wire. Jranium hexafluoride is used for the separation of uranium isotopes. Sulhur hexafluoride has remarkable dielectric properties and is used as an nsulator for electric currents of high voltage. Cobalt trifluoride, which eadily gives up one atom of fluorine, is used in the fluorination of hydroarbons. Cryolite, sodium fluoride and barium fluosilicate have found pplication as insecticides. Fluorarsenates of zinc, copper, aluminium and nagnesium have all been recommended as insecticides. Fluosilicates are mployed in the disinfection of hides and as poisons for rats, mice and ockroaches. Of the organic fluorine compounds, sodium fluoracetate is ised as a rodenticide, dichlorodifluoromethane in refrigeration, in air con-litioning and in aerosol bombs, and polytetrafluorethylene as a plastic esistant to attack by chemical substances.

(i) Fluorine and Hydrofluoric Acid

The toxicology of fluorine cannot be considered separately from that of hydrofluoric acid. As a hazard to health, fluorine rarely plays a direct part because atmospheric moisture converts it into hydrofluoric acid. In a similar way, fluorine in contact with a moist mucous membrane immedi-ately forms hydrofluoric acid.

Hazards to Pioneer Chemists

In the middle of the nineteenth century many chemists attempted to isolate fluorine from hydrofluoric acid, and more than one paid with his life for handling too frequently one of the most dangerous of known chemi-cal substances. The danger arose from the volatility of the anhydrous acid and the extremely corrosive nature of its vapour. It is said that G. Knox during his early experiments on the electrolysis of hydrofluoric acid lost permanently the use of his voice, and that T. Knox nearly died of its effects Louyet, 1846).

The Death of Louyet and Nicklès, 1869

The Belgian chemist. P. Louyet, who continued the researches of the Knox brothers, described how his own health deteriorated from using the acid and how it caused him to suffer from cough and hæmoptysis. Accord-ing to Debray (1886) the death of Louyet at the age of thirty-two was a result of his work, but no medical details are available. In 1869 J. Nicklès died from the effects of accidentally inhaling the vapour of concentrated hydrofluoric acid (Gore, 1869). Other courageous pioneers such as L. J. Gay-Lussac and J. L. Thénard also suffered from the ill-effects of inhaling the vapour of hydrofluoric acid. Sir Humphry Davy wrote that he had suffered much from the dangerous effects of hydrofluoric acid, and it is said that he was forced to abandon his attempts to isolate fluorine because of the risk involved.

Isolation of Fluorine, 1886

In spite of these deaths, the search for the fourth halogen went forward. In 1886, after three years' hard work, the brilliant French chemist, Henri Moissan (fig. 230), isolated the element fluorine. The method he used was the electrolysis of a solution of potassium fluoride in anhydrous hydrofluoric acid in an apparatus made wholly of platinum. Even at the low temperature at which the process was operated ($-23°$ C.), 6 grams of platinum were corroded for every gram of fluorine produced.

Large-scale Production of Fluorine, 1941

Following these classical researches, the production of fluorine remained for fifty-five years a small-scale operation that was difficult to manage; the element was still a laboratory curiosity and was not available commercially; and then in 1941 the sudden demand for uranium hexafluoride called for the production of fluorine on a large scale and the electrolytic method was successfully adapted to the manufacture of this element by the ton. It was produced by electrolysis

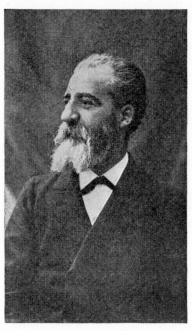

FIG. 230.—Henri Moissan, 1852–1907

of a fused salt bath such as potassium fluoride and hydrogen fluoride at 100° C. with carbon anodes. The discovery, already foreshadowed by Moissan, that with absolutely dry hydrofluoric acid platinum could be replaced by other metals or alloys, was developed by chemical engineers. Electrolytic cells of steel or nickel containing massive carbon electrodes were designed and successfully operated.

Safe Methods of Handling Fluorine

Although dry fluorine can be safely pumped through copper and other metal tubes, absolute cleanliness of all pipes and connexions is essential, since a speck of dirt or grease can initiate combustion and may lead to severe explosions. Safe methods for filling nickel cylinders holding 5 lb. or fluorine at a pressure of 400 lb. per square inch were developed. Specially designed valves which required no greasing were employed, for fluorine under pressure quickly reacts with lubricants, giving rise locally to a heated area at which further attack continues on the metal of the cylinder.

Dangers from Handling Fluorine

Fluorine is a greenish-yellow gas with a characteristic pungent smell. The odour can be detected in concentrations of only a few parts per million. In man, absorption of fractions of a gram can give rise to nausea and vomiting, abdominal pain, salivation, pruritus and diarrhœa. With more than 1 gram these symptoms increase in severity and death supervenes from respiratory paralysis. Owing to their corrosive properties, fluorine and its compounds, hydrofluoric acid, hydrofluosilicic acid and uranium hexa-fluoride, must be handled with every precaution.

Uses of Hydrofluoric Acid

Anhydrous hydrofluoric acid is used extensively by the petroleum industry in the synthesis by alkylation of high octane petrol for use in aircraft piston engines. It is also used in the manufacture of aluminium fluoride which is of importance in the commercial production of metallic aluminium. The manufacture of artificial cryolite, of certain refrigerants, insecticides, the electrolytic refining of metals, the pickling of metals, electroplating operations and the etching of glassware all require the use of hydrofluoric acid.

Dangers from handling Hydrofluoric Acid

The most characteristic property of hydrofluoric acid is that of dis-solving and attacking glass by acting energetically on silica, with which it forms silicon fluoride. Hydrofluoric acid is conveyed in barrels, tarred inside, or else in metal receptacles with a leaden bung. Bottles of polythene or lead are used for small quantities. In industries using processes which give off fluorine the atmosphere contains fluorine, hydrofluoric acid and silicon fluoride. Hydrofluoric acid together with hydrofluosilicic acid is evolved in the superphosphate industry, during the manufacture of phosphorus by treating bones with sulphuric acid and in the production of hydrogen peroxide.

Corrosive Vapour of the Anhydrous Acid

Anhydrous hydrofluoric acid is a liquid which gives off a colourless irritating vapour. Great danger arises from the volatility of the anhydrous acid and the extremely corrosive nature of this vapour. Even when highly diluted with air it causes an intolerable prickling and burning sensation in the nose, mouth and eyes. The local caustic action of fluorine is different on the dry skin and on the moist mucosæ, because in the presence of water, fluorine immediately forms hydrofluoric acid.

Both Attack the Skin, Mouth and Larynx

Both substances if inhaled attack the larynx and the trachea, giving ris
to burning pain behind the sternum, cough, expectoration and even hæmop
tysis; the ultimate result is slow ulceration of the gums, nasal mucos
larynx, bronchi and conjunctivæ. When hydrofluoric acid burns the ski
there is intense pain which is sometimes delayed for several hours. A toug
coagulated area of skin is formed and destruction of the tissue beneath th
may progress for several days (Jones, 1939). There may be ulcers whic
become indurated and take a very long time to heal. Unless handled wit
extreme care the acid may get under the finger-nails, causing great pai
and if a drop comes in contact with this part of the skin, prolonged an
painful ulceration is produced.

Storage in the Tissues

The fate of hydrogen fluoride in the body has been studied in anima
by Machle and Scott (1935). They exposed rabbits to sub-lethal concentr
tions of hydrogen fluoride and showed that fluorine was stored in th
tissues, especially in the bones, the quantities found amounting to as muc
as ten times the normal.

Protection of the Worker

In factories, locally applied exhaust ventilation should be used to re
move the vapour of hydrofluoric acid as near as possible to its point o
origin. Mechanical methods should be substituted for hand labour whereve
practicable. Otherwise, contact with the dangerous substances should, a
far as possible, be avoided by the use of tools, by wearing gloves and b
the application to the skin of lanolin. Baths of hydrofluoric acid for glas
etching should be hooded and arrangements made for efficient ventilation
In the superphosphate industry, precautions must be taken for the with
drawal of gases and fumes from vats, and special care must be taken whe
these have to be entered.

Protective Clothing

Rules dealing with the wearing of goggles, respirators, gloves, overal
and protective footwear must be enforced. Workers must be instructe
about the dangerous properties of the gases to which they are liable to b
exposed and about the precautions to be taken to prevent their escape int
the workshop. Pamphlets giving a brief account of the toxic propertie
of the gases should be distributed and posters displayed.

Treatment of Burns

Any person injured by contact with hydrofluoric acid should be treate
instantly by first-aid. Immediate treatment is of the first importance. Th
burnt area must be thoroughly washed with or immersed in a warm satu
ated solution of sodium carbonate. A paste of magnesium oxide and glyce
ine should be massaged into the burnt area. About 2 millilitres of a steri
10 per cent solution of calcium gluconate must be injected into and und

the coagulum formed by the burn. This precipitates the hydrofluoric acid as inert calcium fluoride and immediately relieves the pain. If the eye is injured it must be thoroughly irrigated for at least an hour with normal saline solution. This treatment is followed by instillation of magnesium-oxide ointment (Jones, 1939).

(ii) Fluorspar

Fluorspar or fluorite is calcium fluoride. It was first described by Agricola in 1556. It is so called because it readily melts at red heat (Latin, *fluo*, I flow). Some varieties of the rock in transmitted light show a delicate violet sheen and this is the origin of the word *fluorescence*. The famous dark-blue variety of fluorspar, *Blue john* or *Derbyshire spar*, formerly used for ornamental purposes, was mined at Castleton. Since 1905 it has been assumed that the multicoloured fluorspars owe their colour to radioactive effects. Przibram (1953) succeeded in tracing the blue fluorescence of fluorspar to the presence of traces of bivalent europium and a red fluorescence band to bivalent samarium. Soon after the introduction of the open-hearth process of making steel (1863) it was discovered that fluorspar was superior to limestone as a flux, and today 70 per cent of the total annual production is used in steel manufacture. It is also used in ceramics and for making hydrofluoric acid.

A Case of Fluorosis of the Skeleton

In Great Britain the bones of those workers in fluorspar, enamel and glass whose chests have been examined radiographically for evidence of silicosis have been found free from fluorosis. The first case of fluorosis of the skeleton discovered in England was reported by Bridge in 1941, in a man who had been engaged for three years in the manufacture of aluminium fluoride. The man had had hæmoptysis and a radiograph of the chest showed abnormal density of the vertebræ. Examination of other bones revealed osteosclerotic changes in the dorsal and lumbar spine and in the pelvis. The bones of the lower limbs showed calcified excrescences resembling osteophytes. Similar changes in the bones were demonstrated in other workers in the same factory.

(iii) Fluorapatite

Millions of tons of superphosphate (see p. 376) are manufactured each year as fertilizer. It is made by treating pulverized rock phosphate with sulphuric acid. Unhappily, this often contains about 4 per cent of fluorine as fluorapatite. It therefore happens that hydrofluoric acid and sometimes hydrofluosilicic acid is evolved, with the corresponding hazard to the workmen. Bauer and others (1937) of Philadelphia were able to estimate the amount of fluorine in the bones of a man of forty-eight who had worked for eighteen years in a fertilizer factory handling finely ground rock phosphate which contained about 4 per cent fluorine. At necropsy the bones of this man showed typical fluorosis—that is, osteosclerosis with osteophytes and roughening and chalky white patches on the cortex. Vertebra, rib, skull and femur contained from 0·29 to 0·70 per cent fluorine, whereas normal bones contain from 0·01 to 0·03 per cent only.

(iv) Cryolite

Cryolite, sodium aluminium fluoride, is a rare mineral found in workable quantities only in Greenland. The word cryolite is derived from the Greek χρύος, *frost*, and means *frost-stone*. It was chosen because of the

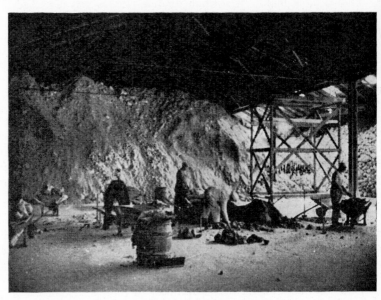

Fig. 231.—Workmen in Copenhagen shovelling Crushed Cryolite
(*By courtesy of Professor K. Roholm*)

resemblance of the mineral to ice. It melts easily, even in a candle flame, hence its value as a flux in metallurgy. It is a natural double fluoride of sodium and aluminium and contains as much as 54 per cent of fluorine. In the crude state it is mixed with a considerable amount of quartz.

Cryolite crushing in Copenhagen

In the vicinity of Copenhagen cryolite is crushed and refined for use in the manufacture of aluminium. After the various accompanying minerals are removed, the cryolite itself is ground down to a suitable fineness. Rough crushing is done by means of hammers, finer crushing under rollers. Conveyance between departments is carried out partly by mechanical devices such as worm-conveyers, bucket elevators and chain transporters. Cryolite is a relatively soft material and, since it is handled dry, every mechanical operation readily produces dust (fig. 231). Crushing, grinding, grading, drying and all handling of fine-grained material produce dust. The conveyance of dry material throughout the factory buildings results in the dust

azard being communicated more or less to all workrooms and thereby to
ll workers in the factory (Roholm, 1937).

Health Survey of Cryolite Crushers

Gudjonsson (1933) was the first to discover fluorosis of the bones and
ligaments in cryolite workers. Assisting Professor P. Flemming Møller in
the Occupational Hygiene Bureau of the Labour Inspectorate in Copenhagen, he was seeking signs of silicosis in radiographs of the lungs of these
workers and found in addition gross changes in the bones of the thorax.
Møller and Gudjonsson (1932) examined seventy-eight employees, all of
whom had been working in a cryolite factory for more than two years.
Symptoms and signs of four distinct lesions were found—namely, silicosis,
fluorosis of the bones and ligaments, anæmia and gastritis. Silicosis due to
the quartz-laden dust in the factory was present in various stages in half
the subjects examined. There was shortness of breath and sometimes
cough. Radiographs of the chest showed silicotic nodules.

Fluorosis of the Bones and Ligaments

Fluorosis occurred in bones and ligaments, giving rise in all severe cases
to pain in the back, stiffness and limitation of spinal movements. There
was no unusual tendency to fracture of bones. In thirty of the seventy-eight
patients, changes of varying extent were found in radiographs of the
skeleton. The osseous pattern of the vertebræ was effaced and replaced by
dense opaque shadows. The transverse processes were covered by calcified
ligamentous excrescences. Around the intervertebral and costovertebral
articulations were calcified shadows resembling osteophytes (plate II).
The ligaments on the lateral aspects of the vertebral bodies were calcified
and showed actual bridges between the vertebræ. The posterior ends of
the ribs were covered by blunt excrescences due to calcification of the
attachments of the intercostal muscles. The shadows of the ribs showed
uniform increase of density, the structure of the corticalis and spongiosa
having been obliterated (plate III). There was pronounced calcification of
the costal cartilages, but the articular cartilages were unaffected. In the
bones of the pelvis the pattern of the spongiosa was obliterated by dense
opaque shadows resembling those seen in the osteoplastic type of secondary
carcinomatosis. Along the periphery of the pelvic bones were blunt
excrescences corresponding to calcified muscular attachments; the ischio-
sacral ligaments and the attachments of the adductor muscles were calcified.
Such changes in the bones, ligaments and muscular attachments are
probably due to the deposition of calcium fluoride, or of a complex salt
such as apatite.

Anæmia in some of the Workers

Complete blood counts were made on all those workers in whom
changes in the bones had been found. In fourteen of the fifty subjects
examined there was a fall in the number of red cells, the average figures

being: red blood cells 3,700,000 per c.mm., hæmoglobin 77 per cen
colour index 1·02. Neither primitive red cells nor basophil punctatio
was discovered. The white-cell count was normal. The general health c
the workers was apparently unaffected by the anæmia.

Nausea and Vomiting

Nausea, loss of appetite and vomiting occurred in forty-two of th
workers examined. These symptoms were supposedly due to the effect o
the mucous membrane of the stomach of hydrofluoric acid liberated from
the swallowed dust of cryolite. They came on acutely soon after beginnin
the dusty work. Thus, one of the managers of the industry, who visite
the factory only occasionally, stated that if he stayed more than te
minutes in a place where the dust was particularly thick, he was obliged t

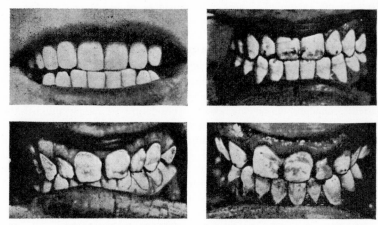

Fig. 232.—Mottled Teeth of Children of female Cryolite workers. The picture, top-left, is a Normal Control. The others show a girl of 15, a boy of 12,
and a man of 24 who, as babies, were suckled for periods varying from one to
two years. The Dental Enamel shows chalky-white and brown Discoloration
and Pitting

(*By courtesy of Professor K. Roholm*)

get out into the open air in order not to be seized with vomiting. Al
symptoms disappeared as soon as the patient reached the open air, an
after working hours no feeling of discomfort remained.

Dental Fluorosis in the Offspring of the Worker

It is to be noted that mottling of the dental enamel can occur only whe
the teeth are subjected to fluorine compounds during their development
In the case of the permanent teeth, exposure must occur before the age o
nine years. It follows that adults absorbing fluorine compounds durin
their work in a factory cannot develop alterations in their dental enamel
However, the irony that female cryolite workers in Copenhagen gave birtl

to children who subsequently showed mottling of the teeth has been pointed out by Roholm (1937). He gave an account of the teeth of five children born of women who either worked at a cryolite factory before or during pregnancy or started to work there soon after childbirth. In three of these children, all of whom were breast-fed for more than a year, the deciduous teeth were normal, but mottling of the enamel was found in the permanent teeth (fig. 232).

Fluorine Compounds excreted in the Mother's Milk

These cases show that fluorine compounds are excreted in the milk of the female after both short and long exposure to cryolite dust. In one of the cases, the mother began to work at the factory only about six weeks after the child was born. The normal enamel of the deciduous teeth may be taken as a sign that fluorine compounds did not pass the placenta, at any rate in the case of the quantities involved here. This seems so far to be the only authentic example of the transmission of an occupational disease to the offspring of a factory worker.

Protection of the Worker

Wherever possible, manual labour with shovel and wheelbarrow should be replaced by mechanical conveyance through closed pipes and chutes. The grinding processes must be carried out in enclosed apparatus under exhaust ventilation; drying stoves and grading plants must be fitted with dust filters or suction ventilators. Dust masks should be supplied to the workers and regular shifts introduced in all the dusty processes. The packing of cryolite into bags by means of shovels should be forbidden and the work done instead by automatic packing machines which make no dust. Separate dust-free dining-rooms and dressing-rooms should be built and proper facilities for washing provided.

Effluents of Iron and Steel Works and Brick and Pottery Kilns

The recognition of fluorosis in farm animals in Lincolnshire, where open calcining of iron ore containing 1,200 p.p.m. of fluorine with coal containing 100 p.p.m. was carried out, led Murray and Wilson (1946) to support the possibility of a human hazard. The human population in the affected area consisted of the occupants of one farmhouse, the window glass of which was etched by the fumes from the burning ore. Cryolite is added as a flux in the manufacture of steel, and the occurrence of outbreaks of animal fluorosis is of increasing frequency and in several areas has been associated with the etching of window glass. Fluorosis of cattle has been found also in the neighbourhood of pottery kilns and brick kilns. This means that the human population is also exposed to a hazard, the magnitude of which is difficult to assess because man is less vulnerable than grazing animals. Neighbourhood fluorosis should receive serious consideration in view of the recent extension of the iron and steel industry.

Neighbourhood Fluorosis affecting Town Populations

In towns or in their outskirts, where there is a concentration of factories, power-stations and gasworks, all or some of which may be emitting fluorine-containing gases, smokes or dusts, the absence of grazing animals may deprive us of what has hitherto been the only means of recognizing the existence of a source of danger. Several cases of marked dental fluorosis have been seen in persons born or bred in the East End of London, where there is a great concentration of industrial undertakings. We have already

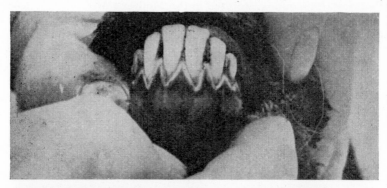

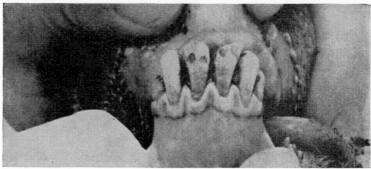

Fig. 233 —Changes resulting from Ingestion of Fluorine Compounds on the Grass at Nevis Bridge Croft, half a mile from the Fort William Factory. Incisor Teeth of Sheep showing Mottling of the Enamel, Distortion and Deformity. The upper picture is a Normal Control
(*By courtesy of Professor G. F. Boddie*)

seen (p. 690) why dental fluorosis cannot be regarded as a sign of industrial fluorosis within a factory. For similar reasons it should be regarded only with reservation as a sign of neighbourhood fluorosis.

Effluents of Aluminium and Superphosphate Factories

Chronic fluorine poisoning has been observed in the form of a disease of the skeleton and teeth of livestock which have grazed in the vicinity of aluminium and superphosphate factories in Denmark, Norway, Germany, France, Switzerland and Italy. Animal fluorosis in the vicinity of factories discharging fluorine-containing gases, fumes or smokes (p. 691) is due to the consumption of herbage on which fluorine compounds have been deposited. Weather conditions, such as the persistence of the prevailing wind and the amount of rainfull, are important.

Investigations at Fort William and Kinlochleven

The occurrence of fluorosis in livestock grazing on land in the vicinity of factories manufacturing aluminium in Inverness-shire led to an investigation by the Medical Research Council (1949) into the risks of exposure to fluorine compounds among workers in these factories and persons living in the neighbourhood. Attention was drawn to the escape of dust and fumes from the aluminium factory at Fort William when a crofter complained that an unknown disease was attacking his sheep. We

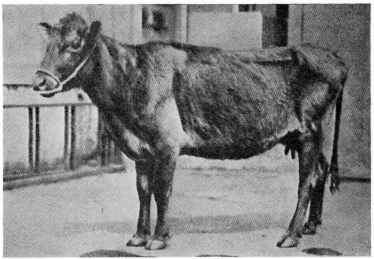

Fig. 234.—Dun Cross Cow from Nevis Bridge Croft, half a mile from the Fort William Aluminium Factory

found that the sheep, and also two cows, all of which grazed in the path of the smoke-cloud, were suffering from fluorosis. Later on the condition was found to exist on other neighbouring farms where animals grazed within two miles of the factory.

Chronic Fluorine Poisoning in Cattle and Sheep

Dental lesions were seen in all the affected animals bred on these farms (fig. 233). Affected cattle and sheep also exhibited wasting, harsh staring coats, reduced milk-yield and bone disorders (fig. 234). Post-mortem bone examination showed that the elasticity, measured by finding the breaking-strength, was much below normal. The radius and ulna of one sheep were found to contain 10,300 p.p.m. fluorine. The radius and ulna of a control sheep contained 279 p.p.m. fluorine.

D.O.—23*

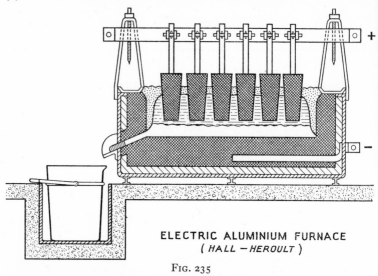

ELECTRIC ALUMINIUM FURNACE
(HALL — HEROULT)

FIG. 235

The Rainfall and Prevailing Winds

At Fort William, aluminium is manufactured by the electrolytic reduction of alumina (bauxite) in molten cryolite (fig. 235). In this process, volatile fluorine compounds and cryolite-contaminated dust are emitted. Factories built for the manufacture of aluminium by this method are generally situated near to a source of water-power. The factory at Fort William in the Western Highlands of Scotland is situated at the junction of four valleys, the largest of which is Glenmore. The smaller factory at Kinlochleven, nine miles to the south, is surrounded on three sides by hills and has Loch Leven on the fourth side. The prevailing wind is south-south-west. At the time of the investigation, the fumes were not scrubbed or treated in any way, and a dense white cloud drifted over the countryside (fig. 236). Fort William has one of the highest rainfalls in Great Britain. Rain, while reducing the persistence of a smoke cloud, would assist leaching of soluble fluorides deposited on the surface of the soil.

The Furnace Rooms

We classified the workmen into three groups, according to degree of exposure of fluorine compounds. The operators in the furnace rooms were considered to be the most exposed (Group I). Into the second category came factory employees not engaged in the furnace rooms (Group II). Lastly, there were villagers not employed by the aluminium company and living at least a quarter of a mile from the works. We subdivided the first group because the three furnace rooms differed from one another in several respects. Furnace room A, the oldest one, lacked artificial ventilation and was hot and dusty. Furnace room C, the newest, had an adequate draught system exhausting the fumes from the furnaces directly and was free from dust. Furnace room B was intermediate in type between A and C.

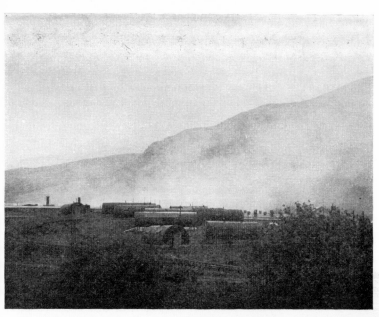

FIG. 236.—View of the Aluminium Factory at Fort William, showing the Smoke Cloud

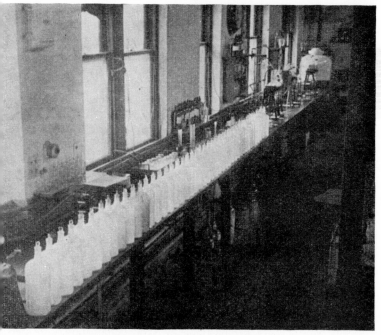

FIG. 237.—Waxed Winchester Quart Bottles for Samples of Urine of Workers in Aluminium Factory, Fort William

Clinical Findings at Fort William

At the time of the clinical investigation, the employees comprised 66 men and 114 women. Minor dyspeptic symptoms were reported by 14·7 per cent of the persons in Group I, by 10·1 per cent of Group II and by 5· per cent of Group III. There was little evidence of abnormal physical sign and none of limitation of movement of the spine. Certain of the X-ra films revealed abnormalities in some of the older furnace men who ha been exposed to fumes for many years (plate IV). Abnormal radiograph were seen in 25·4 per cent of Group I, in 8·3 per cent of Group II and in per cent of Group III. All the schoolchildren examined appeared to b normal. In affected persons the abnormality tended to be in the tibia an fibula. Small irregularities were present at the medial border of the tibi; with sharp upper and lower margins and sometimes bearing small spicules In a dental examination of 373 children, twenty-one were found to hav

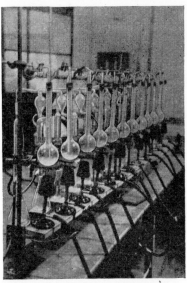

mottled teeth. In no case was th mottling severe and usually it wa very slight. Nevertheless, the num ber of cases affected was slightl greater than that observed in tw other country districts of Scotlan

Estimation of Fluorides in Bloo and Urine

Blood fluoride analysis gav varying results that did not coincid with the positions of the subjects i Groups I, II and III. Hæmoglobi estimations and blood counts, take collectively, showed no abnormalit in any of the groups. Fluorine de terminations carried out on urin samples (fig. 237) showed that mal subjects in Group I excreted abou 8 milligrams of fluoride per twenty four hours, those in Group II ex creted about 1·5 milligrams an those in Group III about 0·8 mill

FIG. 238.—Battery of twelve Steam Distillation Units used for the estimation of Fluorides

gram. The corresponding figure for the schoolchildren was 0·4 milligram per twenty-four hours (fig. 238).

Conclusions

The conclusions drawn were that in the factory the workers in the ol furnace room inhaled considerable quantities of fluorine compounds an judged from the urinary excretion, also absorbed considerable quantitie Although bone changes, demonstrable by X-ray examination, were seen i a proportion of these workers, none of them suffered clinical disabilit attributable to these changes. We felt that some of the workers were exposed to a definite risk and that the conditions within the older type of furnace room were such as to call for determined efforts to reduce the degree of exposure to fluorine compounds. There was less certainty about the risk to human health outside the factory. Clinical examination of a small number of residents in the neighbourhood showed no signs of injury to health, but it would be prudent to site new developments in such a way that, so far as possible, residents are kept out of the zone known to be most liable to contamination. The investigation has drawn attention to the possibility of fluorosis arising in human beings in the neighbourhood of industrial undertakings emitting fluorine-containing fumes and dusts.

Prevention

The danger from fluorine compounds has been recognized by the extension of the manufacturing processes controlled under the *Alkali Works Regulation Act, 1906*, to include volatile organic sulphur compounds and fluorine compounds on the list of noxious or offensive gases, the discharge of which into the atmosphere is controlled; but, until this control becomes really effective and the number of likely sources of fluorine compounds is known, we have no evidence of the extent of the occurrence of neighbourhood fluorosis. A practical point to bear in mind is that an increase of dietary calcium decreases the toxicity of ingested soluble fluorine compounds, presumably by decreasing fluorine absorption, calcium fluoride being relatively insoluble, and therefore milk consumption should be encouraged in all persons exposed to a fluorine hazard.

Manufacture of Magnesium Alloys

There is a risk of fluorosis in men employed in magnesium foundries where castings are made of magnesium-aluminium-zinc, magnesium-aluminium-manganese and magnesium-aluminium-manganese-silver alloys. When these alloys are melted they rapidly oxidize and ignite unless air is excluded from the surface of the molten metal. This is usually done by means of a flux containing about 15 per cent of fluoride (fig. 239). In magnesium foundries the possible sources of danger from fluoride occur in adding the flux to the open crucibles, in applying a fluoride-containing dusting powder to the molten metal, in adding aluminium fluoride to the extent of 2 per cent to the moulding sand, in casting and in knocking out the castings.

Fluorosis of the Skeleton in a Furnaceman

In 1947 Bowler and others investigated the working conditions in a magnesium foundry. Out of 124 workers examined, only forty-seven had been exposed to risk for as long as six years. All who had worked in the foundry for two to six years showed an increase of fluorine compounds in spot samples of urine, the amount increasing with the years of exposure. None had symptoms or physical signs of skeletal disease, and radiological examination showed fluorosis of the skeleton in one case only. This was a

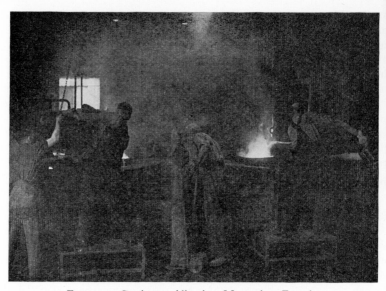

Fig. 239.—Casting an Alloy in a Magnesium Foundry
(By courtesy of High Duty Alloys, Ltd.)

furnaceman who had worked five and a half years on the open crucible furnaces (case 24). Radiological changes in the bones rarely occur until the worker has been exposed to fluorine compounds for more than seven years. Since magnesium alloys have been produced on a large scale only since 1940, the number of men exposed for a sufficient length of time to show such changes must necessarily be few.

Case 23. Furnaceman in aluminium factory—exposure to cryolite dust for forty-three years—fluorosis of skeleton without symptoms.

M. M., a man aged 63, had been a crofter for the first five years of his working life, and went to the South African War for one year. Ever since then he has been in the furnace rooms of the British Aluminium Company Limited. He started at Foyers, was there for eight years as a furnaceman, moved to Kinlochleven thirty-five years ago and has worked there ever since. For the last twenty-four years he has been a foreman. His health has always been excellent, apart from one attack of acute retention of urine. There were no abnormal signs when he was examined, except that his chest was barrel-shaped. He had only six teeth missing and was able to touch his toes with his knees straight. Radiographs of the skeleton showed extensive amorphous and granular shadows with loss of trabecular pattern, especially throughout the pelvis and spine. Similar shadows of lesser density were found in the long bones. The lumbar and lower dorsal spine showed lipping with beak-like exostoses and osseous ridges. The adjacent borders of the radius and ulna showed gross irregularity of subperiosteal bone (plate IV). The urinary fluoride was 14·9 milligrams per twenty-four hours, and the blood fluoride 3·5 parts per million. Forty-three years' exposure had led to extensive changes in the bones without physical disability.

Case 24. Furnaceman in magnesium foundry—exposure to open crucibles for five and a half years—fluorosis of skeleton without symptoms.

(Bowler and others, 1947.) A. B., a man aged 37, had seen service in the army and four years in agricultural work before coming to the magnesium foundry to work as a furnaceman on the open-crucible furnaces, which he had done for the past five and a half years. He had no symptoms and no abnormal physical signs. He had had three teeth extracted; two were carious and six were filled. His blood count showed 5,500,000 red cells and 11,000 white cells, of which 61 per cent were polymorphs, 34 per cent lymphocytes, 2 per cent monocytes, 2 per cent eosinophils and 1 per cent basophils. The hæmoglobin was 112 per cent. His blood contained 4·6 p.p.m. fluorine. The urine was not examined. The radiographs showed a uniform increase of density of the bones, ossification of the ligamentous attachments and increased density of the tips of the spinal processes (plate V).

The Discovery of Mottled Teeth

In many parts of the world a small intake of fluorine compounds in drinking-water is practically unavoidable since igneous rocks contain from traces to 3 or 4 per cent of fluorine. The development of abnormal teeth is a delicate criterion of chronic poisoning by fluorine compounds. In 1916 Black and McKay first called attention to an abnormality of the teeth occurring in various communities in the State of Colorado. They gave to this condition the name *mottled teeth*. It is due to a hypoplasia of the dental enamel and has been called mottled teeth in English-speaking countries, *darmous* in Morocco and *gaddur* in Iceland.

Appearances of the Teeth

The condition consists of greyish and chalky-white blotches and streaks varying in size, scattered over the entire tooth surface and involving all teeth. The surfaces of some teeth are dotted with minute irregular shallow pits in the enamel. Sometimes there is incomplete calcification of the cusp tips. In about 40 per cent of cases this general condition is accentuated by discoloration of the enamel defect ranging from light brown to almost black. It is the permanent teeth which are affected, although occasionally mottled deciduous teeth have been reported. The damage occurs during the process of calcification of the teeth. In man, this process, with the exception of the third molars, occurs during the first nine years of life. The essential malformation is in the cementing substance between the enamel rods on the outermost part of the surface of the enamel. Evidently fluorine compounds exert a direct local action on enamel-forming cells.

World-wide Occurrence of Endemic Fluorosis

The condition was first described as being endemic among the inhabitants of several districts in Colorado, but it has since been observed in many other parts of the United States of America, in Argentina, Morocco, Algeria, the Sudan, the Transvaal, Tunisia, Spain, Italy, Holland, Tibet, China, Mongolia and Japan (Smith and Smith, 1932). In 1931 Churchill reported the results of his work on the spectrographic detection of fluorine in water supplies in various parts of the United States of America, in-

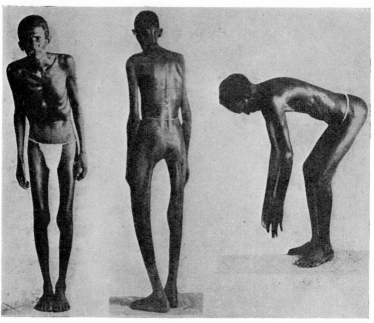

Fig. 240.—Endemic Fluorosis in Madras Presidency. The Cachexia and the Posture are characteristic. The Patient has a Rigid Back and a Permanent Stoop and is unable to bend forward to touch his Toes
(*After Dr. H. E. Shortt and others, 1937*)

cluding areas where mottled teeth occurred. He therefore made the suggestion that fluorine in the drinking-water might be the ætiological factor in the production of mottled teeth. The quantity of fluorine combined as fluorides varied from 2 to 13 parts per million, the degree of mottling tending to vary with the percentage of fluorine, while in the water of immune districts, fluorine, if present at all, in no case exceeded 1 part per million. Ainsworth (1933) made a detailed investigation of cases occurring in Maldon, Essex, where the water supply was shown to contain 4·5 to 5·5 parts per million of fluorine; mottling was also found to occur in other districts of Essex, Suffolk and Somerset.

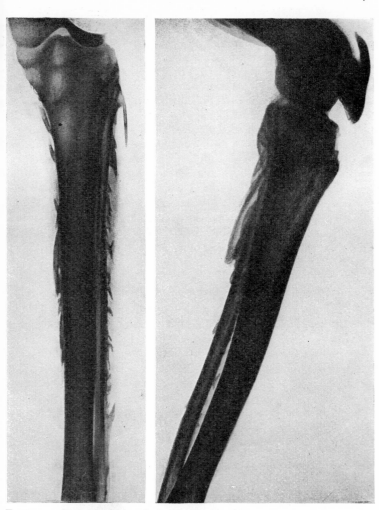

FIG. 241.—Endemic Fluorosis in Madras Presidency. Radiographs showing involvement of the Tibia, Fibula and Patellar Ligament in Calcified Shadows with the characteristic resemblance to Rose Thorns
(*After Dr. H. E. Shortt and others, 1937*)

Endemic Fluorosis of the Spine

In parts of India, China, Africa and Argentina, where the contamination of the water supply is very heavy, the bones and ligaments, as well as the teeth, are affected by fluorosis. Shortt and others (1937) made detailed clinical, radiological and biochemical investigations of ten chronic cases from such an area in India. The people affected had consumed the high fluoride water for from thirty to forty-five years before symptoms of bone changes occurred. Besides mottling of the dental enamel they showed extensive spondylitis with great limitation of flexion and rotation of the spine (fig. 240). Radiographs revealed sclerosis of bones including vertebræ pelvis and some of the long bones, with numerous osteophytes and with well-marked calcification of ligaments. fasciæ and the tendinous insertion of muscles (fig. 241). Ockerse (1941) found a similar state of affairs in an area of the Transvaal. Severe skeletal fluorosis with compression paraplegia has been reported from a small area of the Punjab in India (Singh, Jolly and Bansal, 1961). In a field survey 90 per cent of the population had mottled teeth. Of 46 patients with severe involvement of the skeleton, 2 had paraplegia. Ages ranged from 35 to 75; 43 were men and 3 women. The onset was insidious with stiffness of the back and legs. The thoracic cage showed almost complete immobility; there was kyphosis in 20 cases flexion deformity of the hip-joints in 4 and flexion deformity of the knee in 6. Bony exostoses from 0·5 to 3 cm. diam. were found along the palpable borders of bones in 6 cases. The paraplegia was like any compression paraplegia and was shown at necropsy to be due to deposition of fluorides in the spine leading to narrowing of the spinal canal and compression of the cord.

Experimental Fluorosis of Skeleton and Teeth

A condition in the incisors of rats closely resembling the mottled teeth of human beings has been reproduced experimentally both by the use of water from an endemic district and by the addition of minute amounts of sodium fluoride to the diet. In regions of Morocco, where mottled teeth occur in man, studies of fluorosis (*darmous*) in sheep and other herbivora have shown the bones as well as the teeth to be affected. The teeth of such animals are mottled, the long bones are subject to painful exostoses, and the vertebral column to curvatures (Gaud, Charnot and Langlais, 1934). After volcanic eruptions in Iceland, outbreaks sometimes occur among herbivora of *gaddur*, a dental and osseous disease identical with that found in parts of North Africa.

Changing the Common Water Supply

Treatment of the disfigurement caused by mottling of the enamel is essentially preventive. All that is necessary is to change the common water supply from one containing excessive fluorine compounds to one containing less than 1 p.p.m. By this method, mottling of the dental enamel has been halted in Capua, near Naples, in Oakley, Idaho, in Bauxite, Arkansas, and in Andover, South Dakota.

Fluoridation of Public Water Supplies

There is good evidence that the incidence of dental caries can be reduced by the ingestion from birth of water containing less than 1 p.p.m. of fluorides. In some countries the departments of public health for certain towns have deliberately added fluorides to public supplies of drinking water with the object of improving the teeth in the community. It is obvious that strict precautions must be taken against accidents whereby the consumer could receive more than 1 p.p.m. of fluorine compounds in the water supply.

(v) Organic Fluorine Compounds

Organic fluorine compounds are manufactured for use as rodenticides, refrigerants and plastics. Since 1934 chemists have done a great deal of work on the problem of introducing fluorine into organic compounds, and it was soon recognized that many of the substances produced were highly poisonous.

The Fluoralcohols and Fluoracetic Acid

Replacement of chlorine by fluorine in the comparatively harmless chloracetic acid, $ClCH_2COOH$, yields the very toxic fluoracetic acid, FCH_2COOH. Since 1945 the salts of fluoracetic acid and the urethanes of fluoralcohols have been used for the destruction of rodents. Sodium fluoracetate is the rodenticide in common use. It is known as Compound Number 1080, or simply as *ten eighty*. In animal experiments compounds of the fluoracetate series, after a delayed action, give rise to violent convulsions and death. The work of Peters (1952) has shown by what biochemical mechanism poisoning occurs. Within the mitochondria of certain cells fluorocitrates inhibit the enzyme aconitase, thus interfering with normal intermediary metabolism. In man the first indications of poisoning by sodium fluoracetate are nausea and apprehension, followed within two hours by epileptiform convulsions. In severe cases the patient becomes unconscious and may die from ventricular fibrillation (Chenoweth, 1949).

The Chlorine-containing Fluorocarbons

About 1930 the search for safe refrigerants stimulated investigations into the toxicity of the fluorocarbons including fluorochloromethanes, fluorochlorethanes and fluorochlorethylenes. Dichlorodifluoromethane (*Arcton 6*; *Freon 12*), trichlorofluoromethane (*Freon 11*) and dichloro-tetrafluorethane (*Freon 114*) are in common use as refrigerants. Dichloro-difluoromethane is used as the propellant in aerosol insecticide bombs. The use of dichlorodifluoromethane in domestic and commercial refrigerating appliances and in air-conditioning equipment for public buildings has the advantage of reducing the risk of explosion, but it introduces the possibility that workmen will be exposed to the vapour of an organic fluorine compound. Sayers and others (1930) showed that prolonged exposure of dogs, monkeys and guinea-pigs to air containing 20 per cent by volume of dichlorodifluoromethane vapour leads to no ill effects. It is therefore probable that the use of this substance involves little risk to the health of the workmen.

The Polymeric Fluorocarbons

Polytetrafluorethylene was the first of the polymeric fluorine carbon derivatives to be developed in the plastics industry. It is related to polythene, the hydrogen atoms of which are replaced by fluorine. It is sold under the trade names *fluon* and *teflon* in solid or sheet form, or as a powder which may be sintered under pressure to give complex shapes. Within its working temperature of $-100°$ C. to $250°$ C, it has no solvents and is attacked by only fluorine and molten alkali metals. Its coefficient of friction is so low that bearing surfaces made of it are virtually self-lubricating, while its electrical properties are as good as those of polythene with the additional advantage that arcing or tracking does not leave a carbon path. Above $400°$ C. it depolymerizes to give the monomer and other fluorine compounds.

BIBLIOGRAPHY

Noxious Gases

AVES, C. M. (1929), *Texas State J. Med.*, **24**, 761.

BARSOTTI, M., and PARMEGGIANI, L. (1955), *Med. d. Lavoro*, **46**, 677.

CAPLIN, M. (1941), *Lancet*, **2**, 95.

CHASIS, H., ZAPP, J. A., BANNON, J. H., WHITTENBERGER, J. L., HELM, J., DOHENY, J. J., and MacLEOD, C. M. (1947), *Occup. Med.*, **4**, 152.

CHEN, K. K., ROSE, C. L., and CLOWES, G. H. (1934), *Amer. J. med. sci.*, **188**, 767.

CLARK, W. I., and DRINKER, P. (1935), *Industrial Medicine*, National Medical Book Company Inc., New York.

DELANEY, L. T., SCHMIDT, H. W., and STROEBEL, C. F. (1956), *Proc. Staff Meetings Mayo Clinic*, **31**, 189.

DRINKER, P., and McKHANN, C. F. (1929), *J. Amer. med. Ass.*, **92**, 1658.

ELKINS, H. B. (1950), *The Chemistry of Industrial Toxicology*, New York.

FAIRBROTHER, H. C. (1887), *St. Louis med. and surg. J.*, **52**, 272.

GERBIS, H. (1927), *Zbl. GewHyg.*, **4**, 330.

GRANT, W. M. (1947), *Arch. Ophthal.*, **38**, 755, 762.

HALDANE, J. S. (1902), *Dangerous Trades*, edited by Thomas Oliver, Murray, London; (1926), *Historical Review of Coal Mining*, Fleetway Press, London.

HALDANE, J. S., and ATKINSON, W. N. (1899), *Trans. Inst. Mining Engineers*, **2**, 265.

HENDERSON, Y., and HAGGARD, H. W. (1922), *J. Amer. med. Ass.*, **79**, 1137; (1943), *Noxious Gases*, Reinhold, New York.

INGEGNO, A. P., and FRANCO, S. (1937), *Industr. Med.*, **6**, 573.

JONES, A. T. (1952), *Proc. R. Soc. Med.*, **45**, 609.

KEHOE, R. A., MACHLE, W. F., KITZMILLER, K., and LE BLANC, T. J. (1932), *J. industr. Hyg.*, **14**, 159.

McINTYRE, J. T. (1953), Personal communication.

NAU, C. A., ANDERSON, W., and CONE, R. E. (1944), *Industr. Med.*, **13**, 308, 361.

ROSEN, G. (1943), *The History of Miners' Diseases*, Schuman's, New York.

SCHAFER, E. A. (1903), *Med.-chir. Trans.*, London, **87**, 609.

SLOT, G. M. J. (1938), *Lancet*, **2**, 1356.

TERASKELLI, H. (1927), *Acta Ophthal.*, **4**, 274.

WHITE, R. P. (1934), *The Dermatergoses or Occupational Affections of the Skin*, 4th Ed., Lewis, London.

WILLIAMS, C. L. (1938), *Publ. Hlth. Rept.*, *Wash.*, **53**, 2094.

Fluorine and its Compounds

AGRICOLA, G. (1556), *De Re Metallica*, Basel.

AINSWORTH, N. J. (1933), *Brit. Dental J.*, **55**, 233.

BAUER, J. T., BISHOP, P. A., *and* WOLFF, W. A. (1937), *Bull. Ayer Clin. Lab. Penn. Hosp.*, **3**, 67.

BLACK, G. V., and MCKAY, F. S. (1916), *Dental Cosmos*, **58**, 132.

BOWLER, R. G., BUCKELL, M., GARRAD, J., HILL, A. B., HUNTER, D., PERRY, K. M. A., and SCHILLING, R. S. F. (1947), *Brit. J. industr. Med.*, **4**, 216.

BRIDGE, J. C. (1941), *Annual Report of the Chief Inspector of Factories for 1939*, H.M.S.O., Cmd. 6251, p. 28.

CHENOWETH, M. B. (1949), *J. Pharmacol. and Exper. Ther.*, **97**, 383.

CHURCHILL, H. V. (1931), *J. industr. engng. Chem.*, **23**, 996.

DEBRAY (1886), *Compt. rend. Acad. d. Sc.*, **103**, 850.

GAUD, M., CHARNOT, A., and LANGLAIS, M. (1934), *Bull. de l'Inst. d'Hyg. au Maroc*, No. 1.

GORE, G. (1869), *Phil. Trans.*, **159**, 173.

GUDJONSSON, Sk. V. (1933), *Arch. Gewerbepath. Gewerbehyg.*, **4**, 748.

JONES, A. T. (1939), *J. industr. Hyg.*, **21**, 205.

LOUYET, P. (1846), *Compt. rend. Acad. d. Sc.*, **23**, 960.

MACHLE, W., and SCOTT, E. W. (1935), *J. industr. Hyg.*, **17**, 230.

MEDICAL RESEARCH COUNCIL MEMORANDUM (1949) No. 22, *Industrial Fluorosis*, H.M.S.O., London.

MOISSON, H. (1886), *Compt. ren. Acad. d. Sc.*, **103**, 256.

MØLLER, P. F., and GUDJONSSON, Sk. V. (1932), *Acta Radiologica*, **13**, 269.

MURRAY, M. M., and WILSON, D. C. (1946), *Lancet*, **2**, 821.

OCKERSE, T. (1941), *S. Afr. med. J.*, **15**, 261.

PETERS, R. A. (1952), *Brit. med. J.*, **2**, 1165.

PRZIBRAM, K. (1953), *Verfärbung und Lumineszenz*, Springer, Vienna.

ROHOLM, K. (1937), *Fluorine Intoxication, a Clinical Hygienic Study with a Review of the Literature and some Experimental Investigations*, Copenhagen, p. 121.

SAYERS, R. R., YANT, W. P., CHORNYAK, J., and SHOAF, H. W. (1930), *Toxicity of Dichlorodifluoromethane; a New Refrigerant*, United States Bureau of Mines Report, No. 3013.

SHORTT, H. E., MCROBERT, G. R., BARNARD, T. W., and NAYAR, A. S. M. (1937), *Indian J. med. Res.*, **25**, 553.

SINGH, A., JOLLY, S. S., and BANSAL, B. C. (1961), *Lancet*, **1**, 197.

SMITH, H. V., and SMITH, M. C. (1932), *Univ. of Arizona Coll. Agric. Tech. Bull.*, No. 43.

WOOD, J. R. (1950), *J. Amer. med. Ass.*, **144**, 606.

CHAPTER XI

OCCUPATIONAL DISEASES DUE TO INFECTIONS

EPIDEMIC disease may spread through a factory as easily as through a school. Colds, influenza, scarlet fever, diphtheria and smallpox are liable to spread wherever people are congregated together. Apart from this, there may be special conditions associated with an occupation rendering the worker liable to a given disease. Such is the case with ankylostomiasis and Weil's disease, occurring, for example, in certain mines, and with onchocerciasis in sugar-cane fields in Uganda. In certain occupations direct or indirect human contact is responsible for the transmission of disease. Substitution of machinery for hand labour has rid the glass industry of those occasional cases of syphilis which were at one time contracted by common use of the same blowpipe. The lesion resulting was extra-genital chancre of the lip. In certain occupations the risk of infection from contact with animals is considerable.

Pulmonary Tuberculosis

Conditions peculiar to certain trades may cause disease which predisposes to infections. Thus, silicosis leads to an excessive mortality from pulmonary tuberculosis. There is likewise a heavy mortality from tuberculosis in publicans, cellarmen, barmen, wine waiters, brewers' draymen and others who have ready access to alcohol. The effects of dissipation, however, are marked in only a few occupations, and other factors, such as overcrowding, bad ventilation and lighting, cramped and sedentary occupations, over-fatigue and excessive hours of labour, play their part in spreading tuberculosis.

Carriers of Tuberculosis in Industry

The work of Stewart and Hughes (1949, 1951) shows that local epidemics of pulmonary tuberculosis can result from dissemination of the tubercle bacillus in the working environment. Since 1892, in the Northampton boot and shoe industry, a high pulmonary tuberculosis rate has been known to exist in the absence of any dust hazard. Analysis of the figures of a mass miniature radiography survey revealed, among other factors, that the over-all incidence of tuberculosis was three times higher in factories with over 600 workers than it was in small factories with fewer than 100 operatives. Moreover, a further sub-division of the figures revealed that there was a close correlation between the number of employees *per room* and the incidence of tuberculosis. The findings suggest that under conditions which prevail in the boot and shoe industry, operatives often become infected during working hours and that, in factories with large workshops, *carriers* have actually caused local epidemics of tuberculosis.

Lobar Pneumonia and Chemical Pneumonitis

Workers exposed to great heat such as occurs in the steel and glass industries show a greater liability to pneumonia than other workers. Persons exposed to organic dusts also seem to have a susceptibility to pneumonia. The dusts of bagasse, bone, cotton, derris, feathers, flax, flour, fur, grain, gum arabic, hair, hay, hemp, horn, ivory, jute, leather, linseed, malt, nuts, paprika, seeds, silk, sisal, straw, tea, tobacco, wood and wool may attack the bronchi and thus give rise to an increased incidence of respiratory diseases among the men who work in them (p. 1059). Silicosis is productive of death from pneumonia to a degree only secondary to its influence in predisposing to phthisis. But pneumonia may be particularly fatal to underground workers who are not exposed to silica dust, as is the case with the miners of Broken Hill, New South Wales. Pneumonitis may be determined by the inhalation of chemical substances, especially compounds of beryllium, cadmium, manganese, osmium and vanadium.

Infections of the Fingers

If they prick or cut themselves during operations on infected tissues surgeons are liable to infections of the fingers. This lesion, the so-called *dissection wound*, is usually streptococcal. If the infection remains localized recovery with such deformities as ankylosis of one or more of the joints of the fingers usually occurs. However, before the days of antibiotics the result of the infection was often a fatal bacteriæmia. Innumerable tragedies of this sort are hidden in the history of medicine. For example Jacobus Kolletschka, Professor of Forensic Pathology in Vienna, died in this way in 1847, Ignaz Philipp Semmelweis, Professor of Obstetrics in the University of Budapest in 1865, and Henry Philbrick Nelson, surgeon to the London Hospital in 1936. Such tragedies were the more shocking when, as in Nelson's case, the victim was only 35 years of age. The same hazards of infection face nurses, morbid anatomists and post-mortem attendants. Workers in post-mortem rooms should always use adequate protective clothing in the form of elbow length thick rubber gloves, covered by short, thin cotton gloves. In certain occupations workmen are exposed to the risk of infected wounds. The immediate aseptic or antiseptic treatment of all cuts and abrasions will go far to prevent these infections, and such measures are of great value in reducing disablement in industries where minor injuries are of frequent occurrence, such as the making of barbed wire. A chronic cutaneous form of tuberculosis known as verruca necrogenica or lupus necrogenica sometimes attacks the hands of prosectors (*prosectors' wart*), post-mortem attendants, pathologists, laundry workers and butchers (*butchers' tubercle*). It principally affects the knuckles, and the fingers at the edges of the nails.

Ophthalmia Militaris of Egypt in 1798

A striking feature of the Napoleonic wars in Egypt was an occupational eye disease of French and British soldiers. Napoleon's ill-advised campaign to conquer Egypt was part of a larger plan to capture the sub continent of India. Advancing on Cairo he found drawn up across his path 10,000 horsemen of the Mameluke army superbly drilled and disciplined. In the clash which followed the *yataghan* was no match for the French bayonet; the battle was a bloody rout, and on 25 July 1798 Napoleon entered Cairo. But unfortunately for the invading army Nelson located the French fleet two weeks later and destroyed it at Abukir, thus placing Napoleon in a trap. After fighting on for nearly a year with his troops facing defeat at the hands of the British and the Turks he quietly left Egypt in a frigate. The soldiers he deserted were dogged by misery hunger and disease. Many hundreds of them were blinded by an epidemic eye disease which was probably trachoma secondarily infected by the gonococcus. The malady became such a prominent feature of the expedition that it was called *ophthalmia militaris* (Ceram, 1949). A very high proportion of British troops landed in Egypt in 1799 were attacked by this dread disease, the destructive nature of which can be assessed from the report that of 636 cases in one regiment alone 50 men lost both eyes and another 40 one eye.

The Birth of Moorfields Eye Hospital in 1805

When the troops returned to Britain not only did this infection spread around military quarters but also it spread in the civil population of their home towns. Eye doctors as we know them today did not then exist, but the plight of the returned soldiers and the menace they presented to the community fired some young medical men to start in 1805 a special infirmary in the City of London which in time became the Royal London Ophthalmic Hospital, and is now known all over the world as *Moorfields*. In 1811 teaching started there and the methods of the Moorfields School were copied in similar institutions in Great Britain, and also in New York Boston, Madras, Bombay and Calcutta. Thus did an unforeseen tragedy of the Napoleonic wars play an important part in initiating ophthalmology in its modern form (Davenport, 1961). At present in factories in Great Britain trachoma presents no problem. However, at one time immigrants from the Middle East introduced trachoma which spread in a factory in the United States of America by transmission from one workman to another by the use of the same towel. In factories where the hazard exists sharing of towels must be forbidden.

Epidemic Keratoconjunctivitis in Shipyards in 1941

In 1941 another virus disease of the eye, epidemic keratoconjunctivitis occurred as an outbreak of great economic importance in the shipyard workers of the west coast of the United States—*shipyard conjunctivitis* The causal organism has not yet been identified with certainty. Working

ith corneal epithelial scrapings from one of these patients Sanders (1942)
aimed to have isolated a virus by intracerebral passage in mice. After
vo or three years the major epidemic wave died down and only sporadic
atbreaks were reported. Working with cases which occurred in Cali-
rnia, Jawetz (1955) isolated a new virus called the Trim or type-8 virus.
is important to note that the causal organisms of epidemic keratocon-
nctivitis, whatever they turn out to be, show considerable resistance to
atiseptics so that doctors and nurses must make special efforts to prevent
reading them by their hands and the ophthalmic instruments they use.

ontact Infections in Doctors, Nurses and Veterinary Surgeons

Doctors, bacteriologists, morbid anatomists, nurses, veterinary sur-
ons and laboratory technicians may develop pulmonary tuberculosis in
e course of their work. No person found to react negatively to the
antoux test should be employed in these occupations. Benefit under the
ational Insurance (Industrial Injuries) Act, 1946 is payable to those who
come infected. In addition to tuberculosis doctors and nurses are liable
accidental infection from patients suffering from typhoid, diphtheria,
norrhœal ophthalmia and streptococcal sore throat, as also to bacteriæmia
om puncture wounds and to primary chancre of the finger. In certain
rcumstances they may become infected by poliomyelitis, anthrax,
phus, cholera or plague. In the course of their work veterinary surgeons

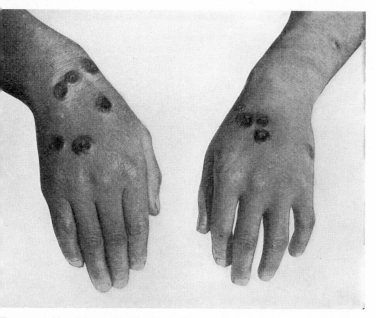

FIG. 242.—Vaccinia on the Hands of a Nursemaid who had charge of an Infant
during Vaccination against Smallpox. She was unvaccinated and became
inoculated with the Virus of Vaccinia from the Arm of the Infant

face the risk of infection by ectothrix ringworms, erysipeloid of Rosenbac
glanders, psittacosis, swine erysipelas, tetanus, tuberculosis, tularæm
and undulant fever. Sometimes a veterinarian gets rabies from doing
post-mortem examination on a rabid dog. The cowman and unvaccinat
nursemaid occasionally suffer from vaccinia, the former infected from t
udders of a cow and the latter from direct contact with a vaccinated ba
(fig. 242).

INFECTIONS FROM CONTACT WITH ANIMALS

Animal infections may be transmitted to man in the course of his wor
Anthrax may occur in men handling carcases, skins, hides or hair
animals that have been infected. Glanders is occasionally derived fro
contact with sick horses. Jute has been the means of conveying tetan
owing to the large number of spores in the soil and dirt with which jute
always mixed. Of ringworms it is the ectothrix trichophyta which a
derived from animals (horses, cattle, deer, pigs, cats and dogs) and bir
They are communicable to man and are seen in cowmen, grooms, ostle
pet-shop salesmen (fig. 243), stockmen and breeders of dogs and ca
They cause lesions in the form of agminated folliculitis on the smooth sk
of the body, the beard and nails, and occasionally on the scalp. T
common varieties of the ectothrices are *Trichophyton mentagrophytes* (sy
T. gypseum), *T. verrucosum* (syn. *T. discoides*), *T. interdigitale* (a variety
T. mentagrophytes) and *T. rubrum* (syn. *T. purpureum*).

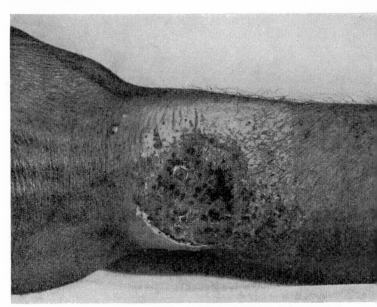

FIG. 243.—Animal Ringworm in a Pet-shop Salesman

Brucellosis

Undulant fever (brucellosis) may occur in men attending cattle and pigs, or handling beef and pork in abattoirs. The common pathogen in cattle is *Brucella abortus* and in pigs *Br. suis*. Operatives in meat-packing plants in the United States of America sometimes eat partially cooked pork during processing and become infected with *Br. suis*. In west Somerset 23 out of 38 patients with undulant fever had had habitual contact with cows. Seventeen were farmers or farm labourers. Five were veterinary surgeons (Boycott, 1964). Veterinarians become infected from the cow and the calf by inhalation from dried secretion on the cow's rump during manual removal of placental remnants and by direct skin contact with foetal parts, amniotic fluid and membranes and placenta. Conjunctival inoculation can occur during these manipulations and accidental inoculation through the skin or the eye during the injection of S19 vaccine. There is also danger from direct contact with contaminated walls and floors of byres and implements (Milliken, 1967). The domestic animal population forms a reservoir of infection for human infection with Brucella organisms. Many countries have eradicated the disease in their animals. Northern Ireland is the first part of the U.K. to make a determined effort to eradicate this infection. The repeated use of S19 vaccine is useless for it prevents abortion without eradicating the disease. The Northern Ireland eradication scheme is based on serological tests of blood, milk and vaginal mucus. The tests used are the agglutination, the complement fixation and the milk ring test. Under a variety of conditions false results are obtained, therefore the interpretation of results is of paramount importance. Reacting animals are bought and slaughtered. Starting from a nucleus of 147 herds selling non-pasteurized milk in 1959 the scheme has progressed to its present stage with four-fifths of the 45,000 herds either classified as Brucella-free or in the process of eradication.

Tularæmia

This is a general infection of small rodents hitherto confined to Norway, the U.S.A., Japan and Siberia. In 1911 during plague work on ground squirrels in California a specific organism was isolated from the blood of infected rodents. The first human case of infection by *Francisella tularensis* occurred in California in 1910 and bacteriological proof was provided by Francis. The infection is conveyed from one animal to another by various blood sucking parasites. In certain parts of north America cooks, market men and hunters may become infected with tularæmia from skinning rabbits. Here *F. tularensis* is transmitted not by the bite of an infected tick but through the skin of the hands or through the conjunctival sac by contamination with the internal organs of the infected rodents. Collett (1895) who published the first account of lemming migrations in Norway, recorded that in many of the affected areas the local people suffered from what they called *lemming fever*. In 1926 three human cases of tularæmia with symptoms like lemming fever were described in

Norway. An epidemic of human tularæmia in Swedish Lapland in 1931 was studied by Olin (1938) who showed that lemmings and mosquitoes carried the disease. In outbreaks which occurred in 1966 Swedish farmers were infected from voles invading their barns in search of hay for food. A 77 per cent incidence of *F. tularensis* was found in the spleens of 20 out of 26 live-trapped voles. A human case of tularæmia almost certainly contracted from lemming occurred in 1966 when the Professor of Zoology in Oslo was bitten by a lemming during field studies in southern Norway. He developed a protracted illness with fever, general malaise and lymphadenopathy (Pearson and Barwell, 1967). In 1931 Thiøtta was able to show, by serological tests, that over fifty people in Norway had had tularæmia, many cases being of men who had handled large numbers of the hares used as food for foxes on fur ranches. Laboratory workers handling the causative organism (p. 1160) are very likely to become infected.

Q Fever

Q fever was first recognized by Derrick (1937) after an outbreak of febrile illness among Brisbane abattoir workers. It was named Q (for Query) fever and the causative organism was identified by (Sir Macfarlane Burnet. It was subsequently named *Coxiella burnetii*. In 1938 *C. burnetii* was recognized in patients with Q fever in Nine Mile Creek, Montana U.S.A. In 1944 Balkan Grippe affected hundreds of allied and axis troops in the Eastern Mediterranean area. In 1949 Q fever was recognized in England. It is primarily an occupational disease of farmers, abattoir workers and veterinary surgeons. *C. burnetii* can be isolated from cows and sheep. In an investigation of occupational infections in the Edinburgh abattoir Schonell and seven others (1966) examined for antibodies the blood of 96 men. Twenty-seven specimens of serum (28·1 per cent) taken from slaughtermen, hide brokers, gut cleaners and clerks contained antibodies to phase 2 antigen of *C. burnetii*. None of these workers was able to recall symptoms which could be attributed to a previous attack of Q fever. In Northern Ireland a nurse had been on holiday at lambing time at a farm where she grew up. The dog brought in bits of sheep placenta to eat in the house, she washed the dog and subsequently developed a severe respiratory infection. At least 64 per cent of patients with Q fever have been in close contact with cattle or sheep (Connolly, 1967). Pigs are an infrequent source of infection and this may explain the absence of antibodies to *C. burnetii* in pig slaughtermen (Schonell, 1966).

Rift Valley Fever and Swineherd's Disease

During epizoötics of Rift Valley fever among the sheep of Kenya, this disease has been contracted by shepherds (Daubney and others, 1931). It is a febrile illness characterized by a short incubation period, acute onset fever of several days' duration, prostration, pain in the extremities and joints, abdominal discomfort and leukopenia. It is of such a mild character that in over 200 cases known to have occurred no untoward sequelæ were observed. The disease does not occur outside the Rift Valley in East

Africa, except in laboratory workers (see p. 1160). Swineherd's disease is a virus disease of young pigs, sometimes attacking young adult farmhands. The illness begins with fever, headache, generalized pain and gastro-enteritis, followed later by meningism, a maculo-papular rash and conjunctivitis. Recovery is complete before the end of the second week Durand and others, 1936).

Distribution of Louping-ill in Britain

Louping-ill (ovine encephalomyelitis, thwarter-ill, trembling ill) is a natural disease of sheep which has been known in Scotland and the North of England since 1807. Because the disease was enzootic in Scotland and because affected sheep developed cerebellar ataxia characterized by a leaping motion it was given the Scottish name louping-ill (*ou* pronounced as in *loud*). The causal virus was discovered in 1930 at the Moredun Institute in Scotland. In 1943 a close serological relationship was demonstrated between the virus of louping-ill and that of Russian spring-summer encephalitis. In 1934 the first infections of human beings were reported; they were laboratory workers investigating the active agent. In 1944 louping-ill was identified in Russia not only in sheep but also in man. The first case of occupational origin in Britain was discovered by Brewis, Neubauer and Hurst in 1949 in a shepherd working on the Cheviot Hills near Otterburn in Northumberland. Since that date further cases in sheep and in man have been found on hill farms in the Lowlands and S.W. Highlands of Scotland including Argyllshire; and in Northern Ireland in the Sperrin Mountains of Co. Tyrone, in the Antrim glens and also in Co. Londonderry and Co. Fermanagh.

Infection of Shepherds and of Workers in Abattoirs

Louping-ill has been found to occur in shepherds, in farmers, in veterinary officers concerned with sheep-dipping, in men employed in killing and skinning sheep in abattoirs and in laboratory workers (p. 1160). The tick *Ixodes riduvius* (Linn.), syn. *Ixodes ricinus* is the vector responsible for the disease in sheep. With the exception of laboratory workers all those named above have been infected through tick bites. It is perhaps surprising that in Great Britain and Northern Ireland natural infection of man with louping-ill has been reported only in nine cases (Ross, 1961). In five of these the clinical illness was a meningoencephalitis and in four an illness closely resembling acute paralytic poliomyelitis (Likar and Dane, 1958). In only five of these nine cases was the illness traceable to the man's occupation, although by contrast there have been eighteen reported examples of the disease in laboratory workers.

Clinical Features of Louping-ill

As in the sheep so in man the disease produces a diphasic fever. During the first phase viræmia occurs; in the second the virus settles in the nervous system. In the preliminary episode, lasting about a week, the patient has

fever, headache, malaise and prostration followed by clinical improveme
which may last a week. Usually he knows that the sheep he handled we
full of tick and that he himself was troubled by them. Often sheep tic
are found on the patient's trunk, particularly in the axillæ and round tl
genitals. Symptoms recur with fever, lethargy, severe headache, phot
phobia, diplopia and vomiting. Physical examination shows mental co
fusion, post-cervical rigidity, ataxia, nystagmus and sometimes intern
strabismus from weakness of the external rectus oculi. The cerebrospin
fluid is under increased tension and shows an increase of lymphocytes ar
of protein. The illness lasts about four weeks and usually terminates
complete recovery.

Prevention of Louping-ill

Clearly as far as possible ticks should be eliminated in flocks of shee
Where they exist shepherds, farmers and veterinary officers can scarce
escape infestation. In the abattoir, where it can be assumed that a propo
tion of sheep admitted for slaughter are tick-infested, infection is probab
conveyed by the bite of an infected tick, although the possibility of tl
virus gaining entrance to the body by infected material contaminating tl
skin is perhaps worth considering. As might be expected, many of tl
employees suffer numerous abrasions and cuts: they should wear clothir
designed to protect them against such lesions. In the laboratory the air
infected by droplets especially where techniques used in the study
viruses include the mechanical fragmentation of infected animal tissue
Such work should be carried out in specially ventilated boxes (p. 1164
The possibility of successful vaccination of susceptible personnel

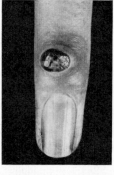

laboratories with repeated doses of formolise
mouse-brain vaccine is being studied.

Outbreaks of Orf in Abattoirs and Shee Stations

Contagious pustular dermatitis is a worlc
wide infectious disease of sheep causing a vesiculc
pustular eruption usually confined to the lips an
adjacent tissues. The virus causing it was isolate
in 1928. It is transmissible to man as a mil
exanthematous malady called orf which affec
farm workers, shepherds, sheep shearer
butchers, abattoir workers and housewives pr
paring sheeps' heads for the table. The earlie
lesion is a dark-red papule on the hand, forear
or face, which enlarges until it reaches 1 t
4 centimetres in diameter (fig. 244). Later
becomes umbilicated and the centre soften
containing at first clear fluid and later pus. Ther
may be local tenderness, headache and mal
aise. Complete recovery occurs within thre

FIG. 244.—The le-
sion of orf (1·0 by
0·8 cm.) in the site
of an abrasion on the
dorsum of the left
ring finger of a girl
of 18, who 6 weeks
before had helped to
skin sheep killed on
a farm in Devonshire

*By courtesy of Dr. Brian
Russell)*

weeks. In 1935 Teleky described forty-seven cases which occurred amongst 300 slaughter-house workers in Odessa. These men had been occupied in removing the skin from sheeps' feet. In 1946 Carne and others described three cases in Australian station-hands who were in close contact with infected lambs. From the lesions in the skin of their hands the virus was recovered and identified. The exudate from the human lesions gave the typical ovine disease in the scarified skin of lambs.

Psittacosis from Parrots and Parakeets

At the time of the French epidemic of 1892 the cause of psittacosis was unknown. During the pandemic which occurred in North and South America, England, France and Germany in 1930, Sir Samuel Bedson in the London Hospital isolated the virus and later photographed it (Bedson and Bland, 1932). Parrots, parakeets, love-birds and budgerigars suffering from psittacosis or merely harbouring the virus may convey infection to those whose work involves handling them. The budgerigar is the Australian grass parakeet *Melopsittacus undulatus*. All parakeets are of course parrots in miniature. More than one type of parakeet is called by dealers a love-bird, but the name is given especially to the West African love-bird, *Agapornis pullarius*, remarkable for the affection it shows for its mate. Pet shop salesmen, gardeners, housewives, veterinary surgeons and research workers may be infected by sick birds.

Clinical Features of Psittacosis

The illness usually sets in rather suddenly after an incubation period of seven to fourteen, and sometimes as long as thirty, days. The rise of temperature is commonly abrupt, and headache is pronounced. Epistaxis sometimes occurs. The patient is generally dull and apathetic, and passes into a condition suggesting a typhoid infection. The abdomen may be slightly distended, and there may be a little sickness and diarrhœa at the outset. The spleen is not palpable, but in some cases a few rose-spots have been observed which are of a smaller size than the spots in typhoid fever. Pulmonary symptoms may be present from the outset, or appear after the disease has lasted some days. Cough is often frequent and troublesome, but, as a rule, there is little expectoration. Respiration may be rapid, but the pulse-rate remains low. The signs in the lung range from those of a mild bronchitis up to massive bilateral consolidation. Pleuritic signs are very rare. The disease usually lasts from two to three weeks, and the temperature may fall abruptly. Temporary rises of temperature during convalescence are often observed, and there may even be a complete relapse. The mortality is probably one in five. Young people usually recover. In treatment penicillin is usually efficacious but chlortetracycline is the drug of choice.

Precautions in Handling Sick Birds

The petting of birds, allowing them to climb up the arm or on the hea and shoulders, and feeding them mouth to beak are habits full of dang if the bird is sick, has been recently introduced into the aviary, or has ha the opportunity of becoming infected by new arrivals. Overcrowding birds in cages or aviaries should be avoided and strict cleanliness of cag maintained. Persons looking after birds should always wash their hanc after contact with them or anything connected with them. New arrivals i the aviary should be isolated until it is certain that they are not infectec A bird becoming sick should be immediately removed from contact wit healthy birds. Strict precautions should be taken with the carcase of a bin dead from psittacosis. Laboratory workers should protect themselves from inhalation of infected material and from contamination of the conjunctiv (p. 1161). That the most careful scientist exercising all known precaution may become infected at his laboratory bench is shown by the fact that S Samuel Bedson became infected with the disease before the discovery c penicillin and was seriously ill but fortunately recovered. On the othe hand that the trained scientist may sometimes take the most foolhard risks is seen in the patient A.M., Case 26, p. 718, who happily recovere from psittacosis on treatment with penicillin.

Ban on the Importation of Psittacine Birds

The importation of parrots, except under licence, was forbidden from 1930 until 1952. Pressure from the pet trade then ended this prohibition and within a few months infections due to recently imported parrots wer reported from several places. The ban was reimposed, but licences t import, for example, for zoological collections, are still granted on occasion The disease is not confined to the larger parrots. Budgerigars have cause infections in man; and the virus, or a very similar one, has been isolate from fulmar petrels, ducks and pigeons. It has been noticeable that huma infections derived from these birds are on the whole less severe than thos from imported parrots. MacCallum, McDonald and Macrae (1961) in th Virus Reference Laboratory examined a variety of psittacine birds whic had died from causes unknown. They failed to detect the virus in 10 budgerigars, presumably home-bred, but found it in three out of ten parrot of larger species which had been imported under licence. Other worker have reported similar findings, and it is evident that the ban on importatio should remain in force. Now that the sailor no longer returns from th sea with a parrot on his shoulder as a gift for his mother or his sweethear it is unlikely to cause much unhappiness.

Ornithosis in Poultry, Game and Other Birds

Now that the virus of psittacosis has been isolated in non-psittacin birds it would be more logical to use the term *ornithosis*. During an epide mic of pneumonia in the Faroe Islands in 1938, psittacosis was prevalen among fulmar petrels. In this outbreak women were more frequentl affected than men, and it is likely that they inhaled infected dust during the plucking of feathers from birds dead of the disease (Lovell, 1949). The disease is now known to affect pigeons, ducks, turkeys, chickens, grouse, pheasants, canaries and linnets. Investigations in the U.S.A. have shown the growing importance of poultry in the spread of psittacosis. Between 1948 and 1956 in the states of Oregon and Texas more than 600 cases occurred mainly in workers handling turkeys (Laurentz, 1958). In Hungary between 1960 and 1962 there occurred 550 cases of ornithosis among workers engaged in the processing of ducks. The disease occurred mainly in pluckers, killers, bleeders and those working at the wing-plucking machines. But it also affected bricklayers working outside the factory in the path of the effluent from the exhaust ventilation system (Bansági, 1962). The control of the disease in poultry should include examination of all birds before slaughter, elimination of all sick birds, and intensive treatment of infected flocks. Suitable precautions should be instituted in processing plants and compulsory inspection introduced.

Case 25. *Veterinary surgeon—psittacosis after handling sick parrots—recovery.*

J. L., a man aged 38, L.H. Reg. No. 31898/1934, after having treated sick parrots was admitted on the sixth day of an illness which began with headache, shivering, high fever and slight cough.

On examination: temperature 102·5° F., pulse 110. Very ill, with severe headache; no rash. Chest: no dullness, nor alteration in breath sounds, coarse crepitations and rhonchi over both sides of chest, especially at bases. After the tenth day there was no fever, and after the third week he was up and well. The following investigations were carried out:

Sera		Antigens		
		Psittacosis antigen	Ectromelia antigen (control)	Saline
J.L. $\frac{1}{1}$		$+ + + +$	—	—
$\frac{1}{2}$		$+ + + +$	—	—
$\frac{1}{4}$		$+ +$	...	—
N.42 $\frac{1}{1}$	normal human sera each with negative	—	—	—
N.43 $\frac{1}{1}$	Wassermann	—	—	—
P.265 $\frac{1}{4}$	known psittacosis serum	$+ + + +$	—	—

Blood in citrate on sixth day of illness for presence of psittacosis virus: negative.

Sputum collected on ninth day of illness for presence of psittacosis antibody: positive.

Blood collected on eighteenth day of illness for presence of psittacosis antibody: positive.

Case 26. Research worker in bacteriology—psittacosis after handling experimental material from mice—recovery on treatment with penicillin.

(Tasker, 1949.) A. M., a man of 43 years of age, L.H. Reg. No. 54/1948, was admitted to the London Hospital on 14th September 1948. As a medical research worker he was photographing viruses with the electron-microscope. During the previous three months he had handled material obtained from mice infected with psittacosis virus. Contact with the infected material occurred for the last time ten days before the onset of symptoms, when one ultrasonic disintegrator was in frequent use. The apparatus consists essentially of quartz crystal vibrating in oil and throwing up a fountain of oil about 10 cm. high. A plugged test-tube containing crushed infected mouse spleen in buffer is held in the oil fountain. Vibrational energy transmitted through the wall of the test-tube produces violent agitation of the spleen suspension resulting in the rupture of all cells and nuclei within thirty seconds, liberating unaffected virus. If the test-tube is examined in a strong light, a vapour phase can be seen above the suspension of spleen debris. It is highly probable that this contains virus particles. The neck of the tube becomes too hot to touch, and when the cotton-wool plug is removed for pipetting operations, violent convection currents must occur in the air above and inside the tube. It seems likely that infection may have occurred at this operation.

Two weeks before admission he had developed severe coryza. Six days later (eight days before admission) he suffered the sudden onset of marked malaise, shivering and high fever, 103° F., associated with severe headache and vomiting. He went to bed and the symptoms persisted unchanged for forty-eight hours. Then the symptoms suddenly abated and for twelve hours he felt much better. But, *five days before admission*, fever, rigors, headache and vomiting returned. Anorexia was complete. Both mental and physical prostration soon became marked features, and he slept poorly or not at all. He developed slight cough productive of only scanty sputum. *One day before admission* he developed a sore throat.

On admission to hospital, eight days after the onset of the illness, he looked seriously ill, with pale complexion, sunken eyes and hollow cheeks. His lips were crusted with sores, and his tongue was dry, brown and furred. He was not dyspnœic, and lay flat in bed without distress. Temperature, 99°. Pulse, 80. Respiration, 22. The fauces and tonsils were injected, but no exudate was seen. There was tender enlargement of the right tonsillar gland, but other lymphatic glands were normal. Lungs: Bronchial breath sounds were audible in scattered areas over the right lung posteriorly, and there were crepitations on inspiration in this area. Cardiovascular system: Normal. Blood-pressure: 100/70. Abdomen: No splenomegaly. Central Nervous System: Normal, except for the most profound mental prostration. Questions were answered reluctantly, slowly, and with difficulty, but the answers were nevertheless clear and not confused.

Laboratory Investigations

14.9.48. *X-ray of Chest.* Loss of translucency in right lower zone suggesting an inflammatory lesion.

Psittacosis Complement Fixation Test. Positive to a titre of 1/64. The titre rose to the level of 1/256 on 27.9.48.

Blood Culture. Sterile aerobically and anaerobically.

Throat Swab. No hæmolytic streptococci, diphtheria bacilli or Vincent's organisms.

15.9.48. *Blood Count.* Hb. 89 per cent. W.B.C. 5,400 per c.mm. Polymorphs, 84 per cent; eosinophils, 1 per cent; lymphs, 10 per cent; large hyalines, 5 per cent.

Sputum. Many bacteria and some monilia. No virus seen.

21.9.48. *X-ray of Chest.* The lower zone of the right lung field has cleared. An irregular opacity is apparent in the left mid zone.

27.9.48. *X-ray of Chest.* Lung fields clear.

The history of exposure and the clinical features of the illness made the diagnosis of psittacosis sufficiently assured to justify treatment before laboratory confirmation was available. Apart from penicillin, the only drugs used were analgesics to relieve headache and sedatives to ensure sleep. Each dose of penicillin was mixed with 1 ml. of 2 per cent procaine to reduce the discomfort of the injection.

Penicillin therapy was started in the patient's home on 13.9.48, seven days after the onset of the illness. On that day, 1,200,000 units were given in three doses. On 14.9.48, the day of admission to hospital, one dose of 500,000 units and one of 1,000,000 units were given. Thereafter, 1,000,000 units of penicillin were injected daily for $4\frac{1}{2}$ days. The drug was discontinued on 19.9.48, the patient by then having received a total of 11,700,000 units.

Progress. The response to treatment was satisfactory. On 16.9.48, ten days after the onset of the illness and seventy-two hours after penicillin therapy began, fever had disappeared. His mental processes were noticeably clearer and he was sleeping well. On 17.9.48, the signs of consolidation at the base of the right lung were still present, and in addition there was now clinical evidence of left basal pneumonia, without further constitutional symptoms. On 19.9.48 treatment with penicillin was discontinued. On 21.9.48 the clinical findings

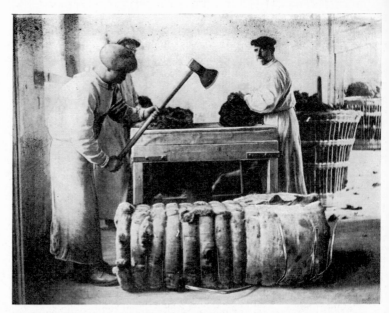

FIG. 245.—Wool-sorters of Bradford. The Man in the foreground is breaking with an Axe the Iron Bands which secure a Bale of Persian Wool. Those in the background are untying the Fleeces

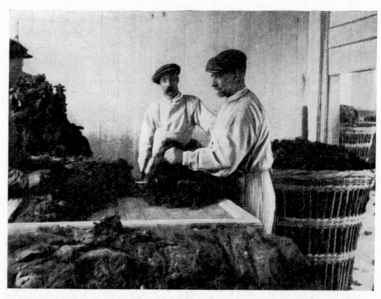

FIG. 246.—Wool-sorters of Bradford. Having untied the Fleece the Workman sorts the Wool into various Baskets. Note the Metal Grille which acts as a Table through which Dust is removed by downward Exhaust Ventilation

were confirmed by X-rays of the lungs, which showed diffuse shadowing in the left mid zone, and some clearing of the right base. Clinical improvement was now rapid, and on 27.9.48 the lungs were normal both clinically and radiologically. The patient was discharged, symptom free, on 1.10.48, twenty-five days after the onset of the illness, and seventeen days after admission to hospital.

ANTHRAX

Anthrax was first recognized as affecting the human subject towards the end of the eighteenth century. It is conveyed to man from horses, cattle, camels, sheep, goats, buffaloes and pigs. In Great Britain, Australia, New Zealand and the United States of America the disease is comparatively rare, but in countries where precautions are not taken to prevent it, as in Russia, Siberia, Turkey, Asia Minor, Iran, Iraq, India, Tibet, China, Japan, Straits Settlements, Egypt, South Africa and Peru, it is common and much infected material is often shipped from their ports.

Viable Spores in Fleeces, Hides and Skins

If an animal dead of anthrax is immediately buried without opening the carcase or removing the skin, there is no risk to man or other animal, for in these circumstances the anthrax bacillus will die in about a week. However, once the blood of an infected animal is allowed to come into contact with air, the bacilli form resistant spores. These can remain alive for years, and any fleece, wool, skin or other part of the carcase upon which blood has escaped will contain them. Such fleeces, hides and skins when dried are the source of dust-containing spores. This dust may come into contact with cuts or even with minute scratches on the skin, or may be inhaled into the lungs.

Exposure Hazards

It is apparent that anthrax may occur in those who come into contact with living animals suffering from the disease, with the carcases of animals that have died of anthrax and with any parts of such carcases whether at the time of death or subsequently, as in the handling of wool, horsehair, bones, bone meal fertilizer, hides or horn. It has even occurred in dock labourers employed in unloading contaminated grain. The occupations concerned include that of butcher, maker of animal charcoal especially bone charcoal, dairy attendant, gardener, slaughterman, dock labourer, wool sorter, wool comber, wool scourer, fellmonger, hair curler, hair sorter, dresser, carpet maker, brush maker and tanner. Sometimes it may be transmitted from one person to another, as at a post-mortem examination, in washing infected clothing or even by unskilful nursing. It occasionally occurs from the bite of a horse fly. Scott (1927) reported the death from anthrax septicæmia of two elephants at the London Zoo. Four of the six men who looked after these animals contracted cutaneous anthrax. Now although elephants in the wild state may die of anthrax and their tusks come on the market it is almost unknown for anthrax to occur in workers either in an ivory market or in the manufacture of ivory billiard balls, knife handles, piano keys, bracelets, or toys. However, in 1947 Seideman and Wheeler reported from Hartford, Connecticut, the death from anthrax bacteriæmia of a man of fifty-nine years of age who had been making piano keys. These he cut from African elephant tusks using an electric saw lubricated with water. Anthrax bacilli were isolated from the ivory. The illness began with a small pimple on the face which became a typical anthrax pustule. Rigors occurred on the fourth day; the cerebro-spinal fluid contained blood and pus and smears revealed anthrax bacilli. Penicillin therapy was begun but the patient died five hours after admission to hospital. It appears that there is no known method of sterilization of elephant tusks which does not alter the physical qualities of the ivory.

Danger of Viable Spores on Glass Slides

A student handled fixed and stained smears made from anthrax cultures and from the blood of a guinea-pig infected with anthrax. Subsequently he developed a typical anthrax lesion on his chin at the site of a cut made during shaving. The infection was mild and he recovered. Each slide used by students in the class was tested for viable anthrax spores by making cultures from them. These were positive for *Bacillus anthracis* on all slides made from cultures, and in some made from the guinea-pig blood. Other anthrax culture smears made some years previously were then examined and *B. anthracis* was grown from most of these. Further experiments have shown that spores of *B. anthracis* in films on slides may remain viable after heating for five to six seconds in a bunsen flame. The dyes and methods of staining commonly used in bacteriological work do not destroy all the spores on glass slides. Viable spores may escape into the atmosphere if spore suspensions of *B. anthracis* are heated in open containers (Soltys, 1948)

Nature and Origin of Wool-sorters' Disease

The first case of anthrax in England was recorded in 1847, soon after the introduction of alpaca and mohair. Many cases appeared subsequently among wool-sorters in Bradford where the condition was called *wool-sorters' disease* by the operatives (fig. 245). The name *maladie de Bradford* is still used in France to describe pulmonary anthrax (fig. 246). The first post-mortem on such a case was done in 1878. In 1879, only three years after Koch had discovered the anthrax bacillus, J. Henry Bell had become convinced that *wool-sorters' disease* was pulmonary anthrax caused by inhaling dust from infected wool (Eurich, 1926).

Frederick William Eurich, 1867–1945

It was F. W. Eurich, physician to the Bradford Royal Infirmary, who was the first to cultivate anthrax bacilli from wool (fig. 247). The achievements of this remarkable man have been recorded by his eldest daughter Margaret Bligh (1960) in her delightful book *Dr. Eurich of Bradford*. In

1905 he was appointed a member of the Anthrax Investigation Board for Bradford and district. Eurich, with limited laboratory facilities and inadequate staff, examined bacteriologically 14,000 samples of wool and hair. His work involved making hundreds of thousands of cultures of anthrax bacilli, and he is known to have conducted many post-mortem examinations on cases in private houses (Messer, 1937). He was able to show that the prevailing idea that dirty or offensive wools were the most dangerous was incorrect. The anthrax bacilli are rapidly killed when putrefaction occurs, but the adherence of blood and serum to the material allowed them to persist in both *clean* fleeces and wool which had been washed and scoured.

Cutaneous Anthrax

The forms of anthrax in man can best be described as external or cutaneous, and internal or pulmonary. Gastro-intestinal anthrax, a variety of the internal form, is exceedingly rare in the British Isles. It is well known in tropical Africa especially where the African native arranges a communal feast upon a dead hippopotamus. Cutaneous anthrax is by far the commonest form of the disease. The term *malignant pustule* is misleading, because the disease is rarely malignant and the lesion never contains pus. Infection usually takes place at some exposed part of the body which has come into contact

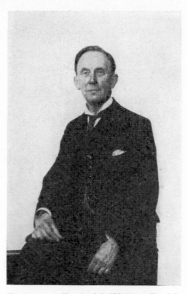

FIG. 247.—Frederick William Eurich, 1867–1945

with infected dust. Seventy-five per cent of cases occur on the head, face or neck, the remainder on the limbs and trunk. The initial lesion is a small red papule which rapidly becomes a vesicle. By the third day browny induration develops, and secondary vesicles surround the initial lesion in a ring. From these bullæ *B. anthracis* can often be cultured. By the fifth day the initial lesion becomes covered by a dry, almost black scab (fig. 248). There is noticeable lack of pain and tenderness although there may be itching. Widespread, intense non-pitting œdema is characteristic. There may be lymphangitis and swelling of lymph glands (Taylor and Carslaw, 1967). The temperature rises to 100° or 102° F. In most cases recovery takes place by separation of the scab and healing of the wound. But death may occur from anthracæmia, the average mortality before the discovery of penicillin being about 11 per cent. Response to treatment by antibiotics is excellent. Incisions into the lesion or the œdema should never be undertaken. Of cases diagnosed and treated early 96 per cent recover. In spite of the intensity of the local reaction almost no scarring occurs.

Pulmonary Anthrax

Pulmonary anthrax can be largely prevented by the provision of adequate exhaust ventilation over the benches on which the work is done.

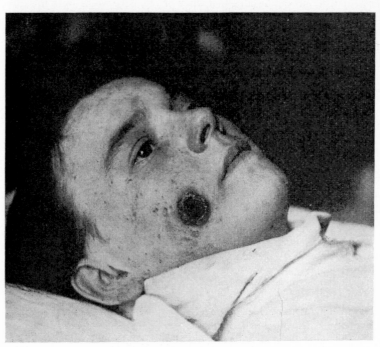

FIG. 248.—Case 27. Anthrax in a Horsehair Sorter, showing the Local Lesion on the Thirteenth Day

The condition is an anthracæmia without an external lesion. Fortunately, only 5 per cent of cases fall into this group. The diagnosis, with rare exceptions, is very difficult clinically. There is fever, rapid respiration, cough and pain in the chest. Death may occur within three days. Eurich (1933) reported twenty-three pulmonary cases all ending fatally. In two the disease was strongly suspected on clinical grounds. The diagnostic history of the remaining twenty-one cases was as follows: in four cases no medical advice was sought; in eight the patients were dying when advice was sought; in four suspicion was aroused only by sudden and unexpected death; in five no suspicion was aroused till collapse occurred. At necropsy extensive effusions often accompanied by hæmorrhages are found in the meninges, pleura and peritoneum. Ecchymoses are common in the mediastinum, heart and omentum.

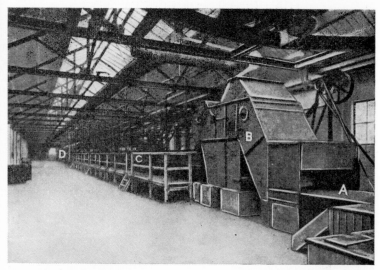

FIG. 249.—The Duckering Machine at the Government Anthrax Disinfecting Station, Liverpool. The Bales are placed on the Platform (A) and the contents are carried automatically into the Bale Opener (B). Here the Wool is teased out under Exhaust Ventilation, of which the Overhead Ducting is seen. It is then automatically transferred to the various Baths for Washing and Scouring (C), and to the Formaldehyde Disinfecting Bath (D).

(By courtesy of Mr. G. E. Duckering)

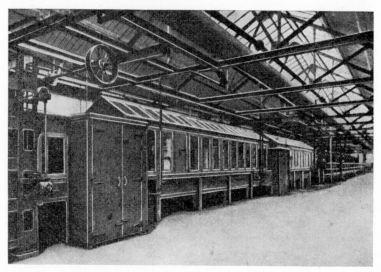

FIG. 250.—Farther along the Duckering Machine the Formaldehyde Disinfecting Bath is seen to be enclosed to prevent the escape of Vapour

(By courtesy of Mr. G. E. Duckering)

Vaccine Treatment of Animals

Since it is difficult to prevent animals all over the world suffering from anthrax, it is necessary to disinfect infected material. An efficient vaccine of living spores of *B. anthracis* is used in South Africa for cattle, sheep and horses, and in Cyprus and Burma for elephants. In many parts of the world the usual precautionary measures as to the disposal of the carcases of

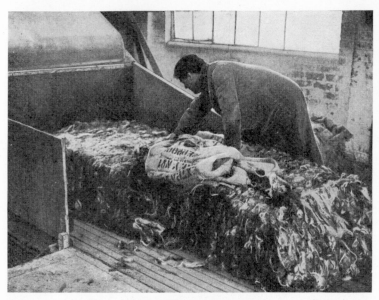

FIG. 251.—The Feeding Table of the Machine. Unhappily the Workman is handling untreated Wool without wearing Gloves
(*By courtesy of Mr. V. D. Nops*)

animals dead of anthrax cannot be assured and, as a result, very large numbers of hides and much hair and wool from animals dead from this disease are imported without warning or precaution into Great Britain to be manufactured into leather articles, hair cloth, carpets, cloths, blankets, rugs, pelts and brushes.

Sterilization of Horsehair by Steam

Disinfection varies according to the material under consideration. For horsehair, steam disinfection is practicable if the temperature does not exceed 230° F. inside the autoclave. The fibres of wool, however, would lose their elasticity and be destroyed for manufacturing purposes by this method. The *Anthrax Prevention Act, 1919*, regulates the importation into the United Kingdom of certain goods likely to be infected with anthrax, and orders made under it apply to goat-hair from any part of the world and to wool and hair coming from Egypt, which it requires to be landed and disinfected at the port of Liverpool. Regulations exempting

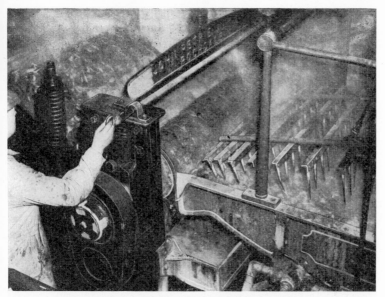

FIG. 252.—The Stainless-steel Prongs attached to a Harrow-like Frame which moves the Wool or Hair slowly through the Troughs

(*By courtesy of Mr. V. D. Nops*)

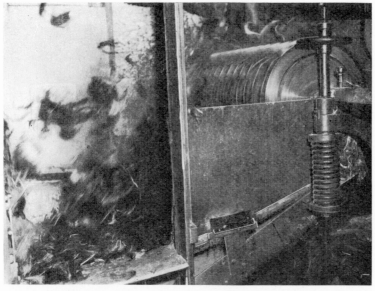

FIG. 253.—Squeeze Roller delivering Wool into a Drying Chamber where it is treated in a Current of Air at a Temperature of 160° F.

(*By courtesy of Mr. V. D. Nops*)

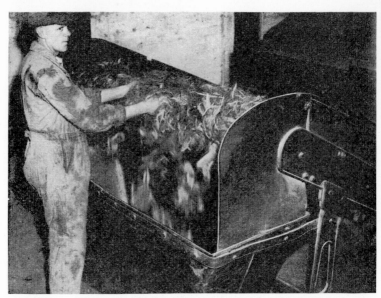

FIG. 254.—Top of the Conveyer Belt or Creeper where the dried, sterilized Wool arrives for Baling. The Workman who handles the Material with Bare Hands is at no risk because all Anthrax Bacilli and Spores have been destroyed

(*By courtesy of Mr. V. D. Nops*)

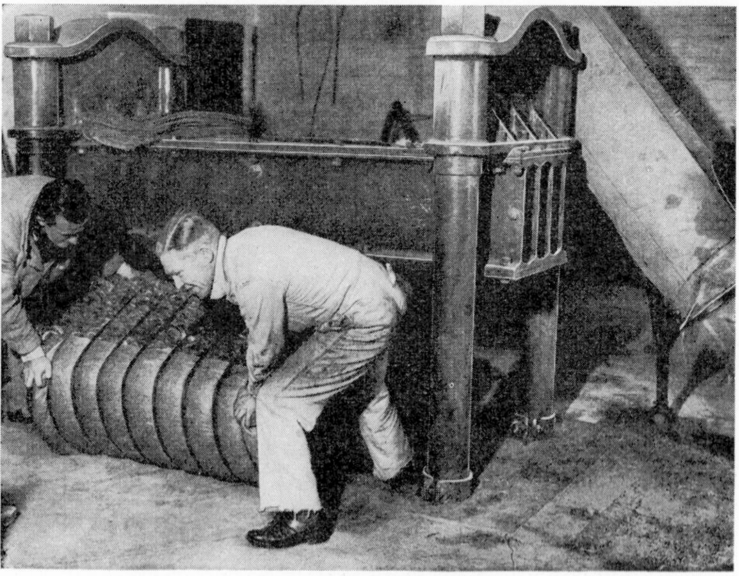

FIG. 255.—Head of the Press which packs the clean Wool or Hair into Bales of 375 pounds

(*By courtesy of Mr. V. D. Nops*)

from treatment certain imported materials have made the legal position complex. It is not surprising, therefore, that cases of anthrax continue to occur in England.

Control of the Importation of Infected Material

There is need for close supervision and attention to detail in the disinfection of wool, since this can be made completely safe. No satisfactory process has been evolved for the treatment of hides and skins without causing damage to the material, but the Government has erected a station in Liverpool to carry out disinfection of the most dangerous kinds of wool and hair. It is hoped that eventually, in all parts of the world, material likely to be contaminated will be disinfected before export in order to prevent infection, not only in transit but also in unpacking and repacking.

The Government Wool Disinfecting Station in Liverpool

During the First World War a method of disinfecting both wool and horsehair was elaborated by Mr. G. E. Duckering, one of H.M. Engineering Inspectors of Factories, and by Dr. F. W. Eurich. This is known as the *Duckering process* (figs. 249, 250). It kills all anthrax in any sample of wool or hair without detriment to the material or harm to the workers. The process is carried out at the Government Wool Disinfecting Station which was set up as an experiment in Liverpool Docks in 1918. The bales are placed on a platform (fig. 251), and the wool or hair is carried automatically into a bale opener which is enclosed and provided with a dust-extracting apparatus. The wool is then moved slowly through a succession of large troughs by stainless-steel prongs attached to a harrow-like frame (fig. 252).

Treatment in Five Troughs

Each batch of hair is treated for ten minutes in each of five troughs. The first contains a 0·5 per cent solution of sodium carbonate in water, and the second a 0·5 per cent solution of soap in water containing a little free sodium hydroxide. Both solutions are kept at a temperature between 102° and 110° F. The material is constantly agitated in the solutions by means of rakes, and between each trough passes through heavy squeeze rollers. This preliminary treatment brings the anthrax spores into a condition in which they are easily killed. The third and fourth troughs both contain a 2 per cent solution of formaldehyde in water at a temperature of from 102° to 105° F. Finally the material is rinsed in clean water at the same temperature to remove excess formaldehyde, passed again through squeeze rollers and dried in a current of air at a temperature of 160° F. (figs. 253, 254). It is then press-packed into bales of 375 pounds (fig. 255).

Protection of Staff of the Anthrax Disinfecting Station

Control of the strength of the solutions and of the temperature is essential to the success of the process, which aims at achieving complete dis-

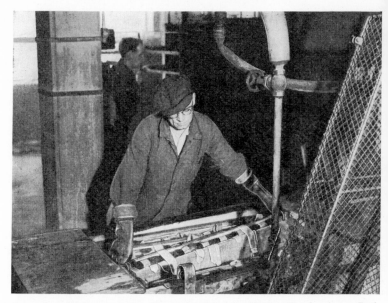

FIG. 256.—Workman putting Trays of Bristles for Shaving Brushes into a Bath of Formaldehyde. Note Protective Clothing, Rubber Gloves and Fan Belt which operates a System of Exhaust Ventilation
(*By courtesy of Mr. V. D. Nops*)

infection without damaging the materials. Routine chemical examination of the solutions and bacteriological examination of materials before and after disinfection ensure that the process is efficient. It is claimed that, in twenty-five years, there has not been a single case of a sample still containing anthrax after being subjected to the *Duckering process*. But, from failure to make use of the protective measures available, three workmen have developed cutaneous anthrax since 1938 while employed at the Liverpool station. Gloves and overalls are provided for the workers and are laundered on the premises (fig. 256). Untreated wool need not come into contact with the skin of the workmen, and dust-extraction apparatus is installed. Unfortunately the men do not always wear their gloves (fig. 251), sometimes fail to use the fork which is provided to feed the machine, and object to the noise made when the exhaust fan is working! (Nops, 1948).

Exhaust Ventilation and Protective Clothing

In factories and workshops where there is a risk of anthrax, dust must be removed by downward exhaust ventilation (fig. 246). It is impossible to remove such dust completely, but in spite of this, cases of internal anthrax are now very rare. Many shipping firms have provided protective gloves for their workmen, but the difficulty of getting the men to wear them is great, and there is some risk that they may harbour infection by dust finding its way into the inside of the glove.

Cautionary Placards and Individual Cards

One vital aspect of prevention is the warning given to working people of the importance of early recognition and prompt treatment. To attain this end, cautionary placards have to be displayed in certain factories by Regulations. These show coloured pictures of the skin lesion in anthrax at various stages. Such notices draw attention to the means by which the disease is communicated, the need for its prompt recognition and for immediate attendance at a hospital. Not only has the worker been warned, but it has been thought advisable to issue a caution to medical practitioners. Anthrax is not a common disease, and it is not surprising that it is overlooked in its early stages. To assist doctors and to ensure the prompt treatment of anthrax, an individual card has been devised by the Factory Department of the Ministry of Labour for workers emdloyed in industries exposing them to risk. Such individual cards when presented to the doctor suggest tactfully to him the possibility of anthrax infection and the need for a more extensive examination.

Treatment of Malignant Pustule

In spite of the implications of the name *malignant pustule*, cutaneous anthrax is a relatively harmless condition (see p. 723). The mortality for all forms of anthrax has been greatly reduced by the use of penicillin, alone or in combination with Sclavo's serum and the sulphonamide drugs. It is not possible to assess the relative vlaue of anti-anthrax serum and other forms of treatment especially as cutaneous anthrax often undergoes spontaneous cure. It is certain that prompt diagnosis and early treatment are the most important factors in increasing the chances of recovery. Sclavo's anti-anthrax serum is given by intravenous injection, 80 millilitres or more on the first day and 60 millilitres on the second if there have been no untoward effects. The serum may be given subcutaneously, but is then less effective. Legge (1934) published figures for the treatment of 800 cases of cutaneous anthrax showing that the mortality could be reduced from 11 per cent to 4 per cent by the use of Sclavo's serum. Such treatment fails completely in cases of pulmonary anthrax, but if the correct diagnosis can be made early in the disease penicillin will save life.

Treatment of Anthrax Bacteriæmia

A case of anthrax meningitis with recovery after treatment with anti-anthrax serum, penicillin and sulphadiazine was reported by Shanahan in 1947. The patient, a man aged fifty-seven, was employed for two weeks as a woolpicker at a carpet factory in Yonkers, New York. He was admitted to hospital with a typical anthrax lesion on the upper lip, which had been present for twenty-four hours. The diagnosis was confirmed bacteriologically. On admission to hospital he was given 100,000 units of penicillin and 100 ml. of anti-anthrax serum intramuscularly. His temperature continued to rise in spite of this and on the next day had reached 102° F. The right submaxillary glands were enlarged, and pain and bulging behind the right eye suggested cavernous sinus thrombosis. Twitching in the arms and feet developed during the night, and he complained of pain in the back of the neck.

Recovery from Anthrax Meningitis

Lumbar puncture showed the cerebrospinal fluid to be clear but, as meningeal involvement was suspected, 30,000 units of penicillin were given intrathecally. Cultures of this specimen of cerebrospinal fluid were negative, but guinea-pig inoculation of the same specimen produced anthrax bacilli in pure culture. Subsequently the cerebrospinal fluid became cloudy, with a cell count of 3,500 cells per c.mm., and a raised protein content. Anthrax bacilli were grown from the second sample of fluid. The patient's temperature was normal on the fifth day of treatment. Except for an attack of serum sickness, he made an uneventful recovery and was able to report for work on the twenty-eighth day. Altogether the patient received 110,000 units of penicillin intrathecally, 4,400,000 units intramuscularly, and the lesion on his lip was covered with a wet penicillin dressing. In addition he was given 500 ml. of anti-anthrax serum, and 28 grams of sulphadiazine.

Cases treated in The London Hospital during Seventy Years

One hundred and twenty cases of anthrax have been treated in The London Hospital between the years 1884 and 1954. One only of these resulted from inhalation of *B. anthracis*, all the others being of the external or cutaneous type (table IV). Analysis of these cases shows that 85 per cent were of occupational origin; 43 per cent worked in the docks and 42 per cent in factories and workshops. Most cases of *malignant pustule* rapidly recovered by separation of the scab and healing of the wound. The average mortality was 10 per cent. Of the twelve who died, there was clear evidence of anthracæmia in nine.

Case 27. Horsehair sorter for four years—anthrax pustule on face— recovery after five weeks.

E. M., girl, aged 19, L.H. Reg. No. 21256/1913. Admitted to the London Hospital under the care of Mr. Robert Milne. *Four years:* employed as a horsehair sorter. *Six days:* minute red pimple on right cheek. *Two days:* rapid increase in size of lesion with discharge of clear fluid. *On examination:* temperature 102° F., pulse 98; raised red lesion 2 cm. diameter on right cheek; row of small vesicles containing clear fluid in edge of lesion (fig. 248). No enlarged glands felt. Anthrax bacilli were found in the lesion. 30 ml. of Sclavo's serum were given on the seventh and again on the eighth day of the illness, and 20 ml. on the thirteenth day. There was no fever after the tenth day. The scab separated in the fourth week and the wound healed in the fifth week.

TABLE IV

Cases of Anthrax in The London Hospital, 1884–1954

120 {	Occupational 102 { Cutaneous 101 / Pulmonary 1	Premises {	Docks	43
			Workshops	42
			Abattoirs	6
			Other	11
		Material Handled {	Animal Hair	33
			Hides and Skins	32
			Wool	13
			Slaughterers	6
			Brushes	5
			Unrecorded	13
		Diagnosis {	Bacteriological	60
			Clinical	42
		Mortality {	Recovery	90
			Death	12
		Site of Skin Lesion {	Face	45
			Neck	37
			Arm	13
			Trunk	4
			Unrecorded	2
	Non-occupational 18 {	Source of Infection unknown 16		
		Infected Shaving Brush 2		

GLANDERS

Glanders is an infectious disease characterized by multiple granulo-matous lesions and caused by *Pfeifferella mallei*. It is primarily a disease of the horse, ass or mule, but most warm-blooded animals, except the ox, pig and white mouse, may be infected by the organism. Carnivora contract the disease by eating infected horseflesh, but there are no records of infection conveyed to man by this means.

Exposure Hazards

In 1189 B.C., at the siege of Troy, a deadly illness spread from mules in the Greek horse-lines to the Greek soldiers. There was great havoc, and funeral pyres burned for days. It is possible that this was an outbreak of glanders, although, of course, there are no clinical details recorded. In the British Isles glanders is now almost extinct, but in the early part of the twentieth century it occurred amongst coachmen, carters, ostlers, grooms, teamsters, stablemen, knackers, shoesmiths, farmers, and the drivers of horse-buses and trams. At times it caused serious localized epidemics among the soldiers of cavalry regiments. In 1948 glanders still affected 5 per cent of all horses in Russia. Cases have occurred in pathologists, veterinary surgeons, butchers, horse-trainers and laboratory workers (p. 1099).

Acute Glanders

Man is infected from the nasal and other secretions of animals by in-halation, ingestion or through abrasions of the skin or mucous membranes.

Very rarely the disease is conveyed from infected human clothing. Commonly a systemic disease develops attacking particularly the nasal mucous membrane and the lungs, but in some cases the lesions are limited to the skin and the condition is then called *farcy*. In its usual form glanders is an acute disease resulting in death. Horses more commonly have chronic glanders from which acute cases develop. The acute disease is characterized by ulceration of the nasal mucosa with a fetid, blood-stained discharge followed rapidly by necrosis of the nasal septum, and ulceration of the mouth, pharynx and larynx.

Farcy Buds along the Lymphatics

The skin of the nose and face becomes red and the lymph glands swollen. A pustular eruption, not unlike malignant smallpox, may extend over the face and limbs. High fever, rigors, vomiting, diarrhœa, with a feeble rapid pulse and dry brown tongue, lead up to delirium, coma and death. In cases where nodules or *farcy buds* form along the lymphatics, the condition is called farcy. These nodules become pustular and rupture forming deep ulcers. The joints may suppurate and abscesses form in the muscles, beneath the periosteum and in the testes. Most of these cases are fatal within ten days. An occasional mild case may terminate in recovery after three weeks.

Cases treated in the London Hospital up to 1903

Five cases of glanders were admitted to the London Hospital between 1893 and 1903, and no case has been admitted since then. All were men four of them had to do with horses and the fifth was a warehouseman. In three cases the onset was acute with generalized pain, shivering and high fever. All three developed purulent swellings, but only one had farcy buds in the skin. *P. mallei* was isolated from the pus in all cases, and in one of them inoculation into a guinea-pig produced typical glanders orchitis. The corresponding patient developed orchitis himself, became delirious and died on the eighteenth day. The other two died on the twelfth day of the illness. Of the two chronic cases, each had multiple subcutaneous abscesses. In one the scrotum was affected. This man became infected through nursing a sick horse, was ill for nearly a year and then recovered. A fatal case was reported in a farmer (figs. 257, 258) by Jacob (1921), and Fawcit (1932) reported a case showing involvement of the lungs.

Chronic Glanders

Chronic glanders differs from the acute disease only in the severity of the lesions (Robins, 1905). The virulence of the organism varies greatly and relative inactivity is common in the chronic form of the disease. Both chronic glanders and chronic farcy are much rarer than the acute forms. In man chronic glanders is a long painful illness with acute exacerbations occurring over many years. Lesions may remain localized but more commonly they involve many parts of the body, forming deep ulcers

n the nose and many
ubcutaneous abscesses.
Gaiger (1913, 1916), a
veterinary surgeon in the
Indian Civil Veterinary
Department, was infected
with *P. mallei* in 1911. His
Illness lasted until 1916
with a remission of only
eight months in the whole
of this time. Multiple
abscesses appeared and
eighty-two operations, including amputation of the
left arm above the elbow,
were necessary. His life was
despaired of on a number
of occasions. Drainage of
abscesses leaves sinuses
which heal slowly and are
intensely painful. Gaiger
writes:

The surgeon who
remarked that glanders
is the most painful

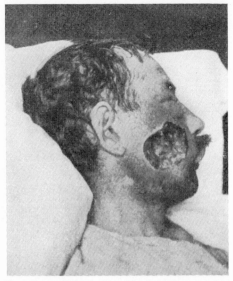

FIG. 257.—Chronic Glanders in a Farmer, aged
51, infected on the Wrist from a Swelling on
the Udder of a Cow. Multiple Skin Lesions
followed by Ulceration continued to spread
for Twelve Months, and one of them destroyed
the Right Side of the Face. Death occurred
from Pyæmia
(*Jacob, F. H. (1921), Brit. J. Derm. and Syph.*, **33**, *39*)

disease which a man can suffer must have been very near the truth.
For many months I endured indescribable torture daily. At one time
as many as sixteen sinuses had plugs removed and fresh ones inserted
daily. The removal of plugs the day after the operation was the most
unspeakable horror.

Diagnosis of Glanders

Diagnosis of human glanders is difficult. A history of contact with
horses may indicate the nature of the illness. In acute cases the incubation
period is from five to six days and early symptoms may suggest pneumonia,
typhoid fever or rheumatic fever. *P. mallei* can be demonstrated easily in the
lesions of acute glanders and during exacerbations in chronic glanders, but
when the lesions in the chronic disease are more or less stationary it may
be extremely difficult to confirm the diagnosis. Cultures should be made
on glycerine agar and potato, and pus from the lesions inoculated into male
guinea-pigs intraperitoneally. The mallein test is reliable in horses, but has
been used less frequently in man. Complement fixation is the most reliable
laboratory test (Burgess, 1936).

Treatment

From personal experience Gaiger (1913, 1916) emphasizes the importance of general treatment and nursing. Large doses of sulphadiazine given

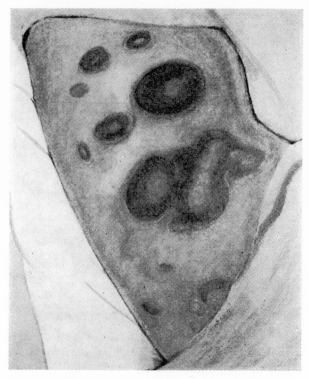

FIG. 258.—Ulcerative Lesions of the Skin of the Trunk in
the Case of Chronic Glanders described in fig. 257
(*Jacob, F. H. (1921), Brit. J. Derm. and Syph.*, **33**, *39*)

for twenty days may be effective. Little is known of the effectiveness of
the modern antibiotics, but the organisms should be tested for sensitivity
and the appropriate substance used. Treatment includes conservative
surgical drainage of abscesses.

WEIL'S DISEASE

The publication by Weil in 1886 of an account of four cases of infectious jaundice led to the recognition of a symptom-complex of fever,
jaundice, enlargement of the liver, the occurrence of hæmorrhages and
occasionally febrile relapses, under the designation of Weil's disease. Since
the causative organism, *Leptospira icterohæmorrhagiæ*, was first demonstrated in Japan by Inada and Ido in 1915, the disease has been recognized in
many different countries, and during the First World War it affected
German, French, Italian and British troops. It has been known variously as
leptospirosis, leptospiral jaundice, spirochætal jaundice, spirochætosis
icterohæmorrhagica, infective hæmorrhagic jaundice and mud fever.

The First or Febrile Stage

The disease can be divided into three stages, the first or febrile stage, the second or toxic stage, and the third or convalescent stage. The first stage lasts approximately one week. The onset of the disease is sudden; it is ushered in by headache, particularly in the occipital region, muscular pains, especially in the legs and back, and nausea and vomiting. Prostration is present in severe cases and meningeal irritation is sometimes seen. Injection of the conjunctivæ and fauces is common. Herpes labialis is sometimes noticed, and it may become hæmorrhagic. Icterus develops between the fourth and seventh days and is present in 50 per cent of cases. The duration of the primary fever is from five to nine days, the temperature varying from 99° to 104° F. A second rise of temperature may occur during the third week of the illness. A moderate leucocytosis ranging from 10,000 to 20,000 is found. Examination of the urine shows albumin and casts. In the early stages of the disease, up to the second day of the jaundice, *L. icterohæmorrhagiæ* can be demonstrated in the blood by culture or guinea-pig inoculation.

The Second or Toxic Stage

The second or toxic stage is characterized by the development of antibodies in the blood and the excretion of *L. icterohæmorrhagiæ* in the urine. By the beginning of the second week the temperature falls to normal by lysis and the jaundice deepens. If no jaundice has developed by this time the patient is considered to be a mild case, and is already nearly free from symptoms. Purpuric hæmorrhages into the skin occur in about 20 per cent of cases; large cutaneous and subcutaneous hæmorrhages indicate a very severe toxæmia and are bad prognostic signs. In more than half the cases epistaxis, hæmoptysis or hæmatemesis are present. During the second week the urinary symptoms are the most marked, and in severe cases the blood urea rises. Usually a steady clinical improvement occurs during the second week. In more severe cases the jaundice deepens and death occurs, often with anuria. The liver is enlarged to palpation in about a third of the cases; the spleen is only rarely felt.

The Third or Convalescent Stage

The third or convalescent stage is characterized by the full development of antibodies in the blood and by the excretion of organisms in the urine. In severe cases jaundice is present for fully three weeks. A second rise of temperature during the third week of the illness occurs in approximately half the cases. It varies from 99° to 102° F. and lasts from five to fourteen days. The apyrexial period between the primary and secondary fever varies from six to fourteen days. Fortunately it may give rise to no subjective symptoms. In the average case convalescence is prolonged, the patient feeling weak and tired for several weeks after getting up. The mortality for England and the continent of Europe is between 5 and 10 per cent, but in Japan it may be as high as 50 per cent.

Criteria of Diagnosis

The diagnosis of Weil's disease may be difficult in the early or pre-icteric stage of the disease, and in those mild cases in which jaundice never develops. The development of jaundice in a patient who a week previously had become suddenly and severely ill with fever, headache, vomiting and muscular pains should, however, warrant the careful consideration of such a diagnosis. In infective hepatitis or in epidemic infectious jaundice, which occurs principally in children, the onset is neither so abrupt nor so severe. Albuminuria is present in practically every case of Weil's disease, and in all patients who are moderately or severely ill, evidence of serious kidney damage is indicated by the presence in the urine of epithelial cells, leucocytes, erythrocytes and casts. Such urinary changes in conjunction with a rise in the blood urea are both of diagnostic and prognostic importance. The final proof of the correctness of the diagnosis must depend in every case on bacteriological and serological tests (Davidson and Smith, 1936).

Exposure Hazards

Weil's disease has a greater incidence and a wider geographical distribution than was formerly recognized. A progressively increasing number of sporadic cases of jaundice where the persons affected have an occupation bringing them in contact with water or slime contaminated by rats is being attributed to this cause. *L. icterohæmorrhagiæ*, which is known to be present in the kidneys of rats in most, if not all, countries, reaches the exterior by way of the urine, and it is from this source that man is infected. There is experimental evidence that the infective organism may pass through the unbroken skin. The incidence of the disease in coal miners, bargemen, sewer labourers, canal workers, workers in ricefields, sugar-cane cutters, fish cleaners, filleters, freshers and curers, fish porters and fishmongers, tripe scrapers, piggery workers, butchers, workers in abattoirs, stablemen, rat catchers and agricultural workers employed in hedging and ditching clearly indicates the necessity for regarding it from the standpoint of an occupational disease.

Among Coal Miners, Bargemen and Abattoir Workers

In Japan coal miners are not infrequently affected. Buchanan (1927) investigated an outbreak of the disease among miners in East Lothian and proved that the fungal slime found on the wooden props and shoring of the mine galleries contained leptospiræ pathogenic to guinea-pigs. A total of thirty-one cases was later reported on the combined clinical and bacteriological findings. The existence of the disease in Scotland among members of the community other than coal miners, particularly those working in rat-infested areas for example, near refuse dumps, piggeries and breweries, was thus proved. In 1935 Swan and McKeon reported twelve cases in coal miners in Northumberland and Durham (fig. 259). Schüffner (1934) states that Weil's disease has become a serious public health problem in Holland. The great majority of the Dutch cases have been infected through

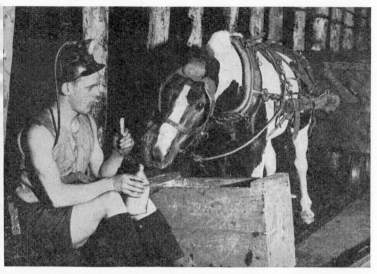

Fig. 259.—Meal-time in a Coal Mine. The use of Pit Ponies helps to keep up Infection of the Miners by *L. icterohæmorrhagiæ* because the Corn used as Fodder attracts Rats

(*By courtesy of Professor I. C. F. Statham*)

anals, either by bathing in swimming-baths to which canal water is admitted, by working in canals or by accidental immersion in them. A higher occupational incidence is reported among bargemen and workers in abattoirs and other rat-infested premises. In Hamburg and Paris cases have been encountered in sewer workers and in other persons coming in contact with water from rat-infested areas.

Among Sewer Workers in London

In 1934 Fairley described a hitherto unrecognized focus of infection among the sewer workers of London, and by means of a clinical inquiry and serological tests was able to show that the disease had been endemic for at least twelve and a half years. It was discovered that labourers engaged in repairing and rebuilding old sewers were particularly affected; among other duties their work consisted in chiselling away and removing old brickwork covered with sewer slime, and this not infrequently led to abrasions of the skin of the hands and the arms. Infected rats have long been known to abound in London sewers, and contact with resulting infected slime was regarded as the source of the disease. In 1935 Alston not only proved the existence of leptospiral jaundice in three London sewer workers, but also isolated virulent *L. icterohæmorrhagiæ* from the slime on the walls of the sewers in which they worked. A case has been described in an English canal worker, who had been standing knee-deep in water to which infected rats had access. His work was to remove with his bare hands old submerged timber (Wolstencroft, 1935).

Among Fish Workers in Aberdeen

From Aberdeen in 1934 Davidson reported twenty-three cases of Weil'
disease, chiefly among fish workers. The patients were mainly employed in
handling white fish, either as filleters, cleaners, curers or as general distribu
tors of raw material in rat-infested premises, the floors of which had be
come covered with slime and offal (fig. 260). In the evening the bulk of the
offal was collected into barrels, which were not removed until the following
morning. As the premises were often rudely constructed, there was little
protection against rats, which infested the whole area in which the business
was conducted. Persons employed in this work had the skin of their hands
frequently broken by their knives, and presumably infection occurred
through the exposed flesh surfaces, or it may have occurred through the
nasal mucosa and upper respiratory tract. A survey was made of 214 cases
of Weil's disease which occurred between 1934 and 1948 in the North
eastern area of Scotland. Of these 86 per cent were fish workers. The
overall case mortality rate was 8·9 per cent (Smith, 1949).

Among Sugar-cane Cutters in Queensland

An outbreak was reported amongst Italians employed as cane cutters
in the Ingham district of Queensland, Australia (Drew, 1934). Jaundice
first appeared in October 1933, and by October 1934 some thirty cases had
been put on record. *L. icterohæmorrhagiæ* was isolated from a human source
and later discovered in the urine of rats which showed a high incidence of
infection. The canefields were heavily infested with these rodents (fig. 261)
and apparently the moist conditions existing after heavy rain were
favourable to the leptospira, for after a prolonged spell of dry weather
fresh cases ceased. Although it is the custom of the men to work bare
footed in the canefields, it seems that the leptospiræ gain access through
the hands. In grasping the cane preparatory to cutting, the hands become
injured with abrasions, and during the course of the disease the axillary
glands become enlarged.

Among Tripe Scrapers and Restaurant Workers

In 1938 Stuart described leptospirosis in a woman employed as a tripe
scraper in the Glasgow Corporation meat market. Evidence was obtained
of the same infection having occurred in four out of twenty-five other tripe
workers in the same tripery. Of fourteen rats caught in the building
eleven showed infection with *L. icterohæmorrhagiæ*. In each of five con
secutive cases of Weil's disease admitted to the London Hospital, the ill
ness could be directly traced to the patient's occupation. Four were London
sewer workers, the fifth was a storekeeper employed in a restaurant, the
infection having occurred after he had cleaned out the trap of a drain with
his bare hands. Proof of the diagnosis was obtained in these cases either by
inoculation of a guinea-pig with the patient's urine, or by tests of the
patient's serum for agglutination and adhesion with *L. icterohæmorrhagiæ*.

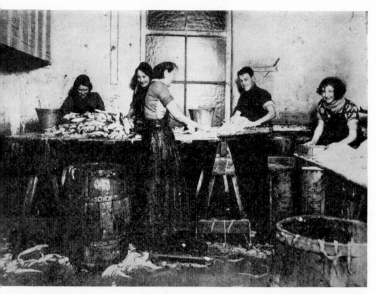

FIG. 260.—Fish Cleaners of Aberdeen at work on crudely constructed Benches. Note Water and Fish Offal on the Floor, conditions favourable to Infestation by Rats and spread of Leptospirosis

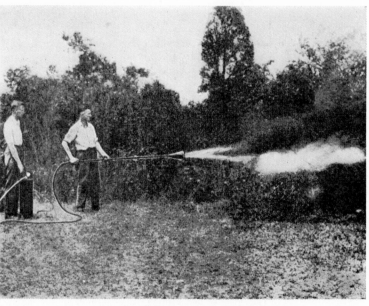

FIG. 261.—Workmen using a Flame-thrower to destroy the Nesting-places of Rats in the Sugar-cane Fields of Queensland, Australia

Human Infections with Canine Leptospirosis

The fact that *L. canicola* as well as *L. icterohæmorrhagiæ* may infec man has led to an interest throughout the world in canine leptospirosis There are on record four human cases of true leptospiral jaundice due t *L. icterohæmorrhagiæ* transmitted directly by dogs (Petersen and Jacobsen 1937). Twenty-two human infections with *L. canicola* have been recorde (Raven, 1941), twelve in Holland, one in Austria, six in Denmark, two i California, and one in Copenhagen. Of the twelve reported from Holland none died and four showed meningitic symptoms. Severe symptoms wer not always recorded and jaundice hardly ever. The serious renal symptom so typical in dogs were not found in the human cases. Most of the patient had a dog and in several cases it was ill. In six of the cases the dog wa shown to be infected with *L. canicola*. Often the dog was only slightly sic and no veterinary surgeon was consulted. Van der Walle (1939) record the recovery of *L. canicola* from the kidneys of a six-year-old foxhoun which had been regarded as healthy.

Preventive Measures

Intensive and systematic destruction of rats should be carried out i infested mines, sewers, docks, ricefields and sugar-cane fields (fig. 261 Much control of Weil's disease could be achieved by cleanliness campaign for removing material soiled by the urine of rats, such as fish offal. Th disease is always found to be associated with wet conditions. In mines i should be controlled by pumping dry those sections which are wet Tohyama (1927) found that in Japan *L. icterohæmorrhagiæ* thrived in th water of the paddyfields, and that coolies working in these fields ofte suffered from Weil's disease. When calcium cyanamide, which readily kill the organism, was used as a fertilizer, none of the coolies became infected whilst in surrounding fields, where ordinary fertilizers were used, larg numbers of workers acquired the disease. In 1931 Taylor and Goyle use the same method to deal with an outbreak of Weil's disease in the Andama Islands. Control of the disease in the case of sewer workers presents diffi culties, and prophylactic immunization would appear to be the best mean available. Each worker should carry an individual card which teaches hin to wash his hands before meals and serves to warn the doctor of th possibility of infection (fig. 262). No man should be employed unless h shows a positive reaction to an agglutination test for leptospiral antibodies A doctor should visit each sewerman who is off sick so that a diagnosis ca be made as early as possible in the disease.

Treatment

In treatment, both antiserum and penicillin must be used as early a possible. Penicillin has a bactericidal and bacteriostatic action on *L. ictero hæmorrhagiæ* (Alston and Broom, 1944). It must be administered withit the first four days of the onset of septicæmia, otherwise its action can avai the patient little, especially if nephritis develops (Smith, 1949).

GREATER LONDON COUNCIL
Department of Public Health Engineering

INSTRUCTIONS TO MEN WORKING IN CONTACT WITH SEWAGE

This card is for YOUR Protection

When you get this card you should

1. Complete the details inside the front cover as soon as possible.
2. Hand the accompanying letter from the Medical Adviser to your Doctor at the earliest opportunity.
3. Complete and detach the tear-off portion of the card and pass it to your Administrative Office.

Whenever you go to your Doctor, or to a hospital, on account of illness or injury always show this card and make sure that those attending you know your occupation.

INSTRUCTIONS TO WORKERS
Precautions against risk of Leptospiral Jaundice

1. After having entered a sewer or after working in contact with sewage or anything, including water, contaminated by sewage, wash your hands and forearms thoroughly with soap and water. If your clothes or boots are contaminated with sewage, wash thoroughly after handling them. It is particularly important to do this before taking any food or drink. Wet protective clothing should be dried as soon as possible.
2. Take immediate action to wash thoroughly any cut, scratch or abrasion of the skin as soon as possible, whether the injury was caused at work or not. Then apply an antiseptic to the wound with a clean piece of cloth or cotton wool, and protect it with a strip of gauze completely covered with adhesive plaster. Keep the wound covered until it is quite healed. Antiseptic, gauze and waterproof plaster are available at your place of work.
3. Further treatment is a matter for your doctor. Visit him, show him this card and tell him the injury occurred in the course of work.
4. Avoid rubbing your nose or mouth with your hands during work.
5. Keep this card in a safe place and whenever you go to your doctor or to a hospital on account of illness, show the card and make sure that those attending you know your occupation.
6. EVERY ACCIDENT AT WORK, HOWEVER TRIVIAL, *MUST* BE REPORTED. MAKE SURE THAT DETAILS ARE ENTERED IN THE NATIONAL INSURANCE (INDUSTRIAL INJURIES) ACCIDENT BOOK No. B.1.510A.

S. H. DAINTY
Acting Director of Public Health Engineering

LEPTOSPIROSIS

Those working in certain occupations (sewer work is one) may very occasionally contact a form of jaundice known as leptospirosis.

The infection sometimes enters through breaks in the skin, so thorough first aid treatment of all wounds is important.

The early stages of this disease may be rather like influenza, so whenever you go to a doctor, you should produce this card so that he can, if necessary, arrange for further examination in hospital and notify the Medical Adviser at County Hall.

(WAT. 5000, Ext. 7555 or 6381)

A. B. STEWART
Medical Adviser

FIG. 262.—Individual Card carried by London Sewermen to warn the Doctor of the possibility of Infection by *L. icterohaemorrhagiae*

Case 28. Sewer flusher for two years—leptospiral jaundice—recovery afte five weeks.

F. W., a man aged 42, L.H. Reg. No. 31966/1933. Two years employed as a flusher in London sewers, wearing waders but n gloves. When using broom, shovel or scraper for cleansing a sewer h sometimes caused abrasions of his hands on projections in the brick work. Fourteen days ago: helped to put down rat poison in the sewer but saw no rats. Five days ago: began to have shivering attack temperature 103° F. Four days: further shivering attacks, sever pain in both shins and in upper abdomen. Two days: vomiting, jaur dice, epistaxis.

On examination: deeply jaundiced man, hæmorrhagic herpes o lips and right side of face, temperature 99° F., pulse 100, tongue dry liver palpable 3 cm. below right costal margin, spleen not felt, no en larged glands. Urine: heavy cloud of albumin, bile, many red cell Injection of blood serum and urine into guinea-pig produced n pathological lesion. Serum collected on fifteenth day of illness fo presence of antibodies for *L. icterohæmorrhagiæ*:

Serum	Agglutination	Adhesion phenomenon
Patient 1/100	+	+
Patient 1/200	+	+
Patient 1/400	±	±
Patient 1/800	—	—
Normal 1/100	—	—
*D.W. 1/100	—	—
*V.W. 1/100	—	—
*B.W. 1/100	—	—
*A.B. 1/100	—	—

* Cases of jaundice in a house epidemic of seven cases.

He was treated by rest in bed, a high-carbohydrate diet, calciur lactate six grams a day, and daily injections of 10 ml. of a 20 per cen solution of calcium gluconate. He was afebrile on the seventh day o the illness, and the jaundice disappeared in the fifth week, when h was discharged well.

ERYSIPELOID OF ROSENBACH

The causal organism of swine erysipelas, *Erysipelothrix rhusiopathiæ* is responsible not only for a major problem in preventive veterinar medicine but also for three forms of infection in man: (1) a mild local ski

ıfection occurring on the finger and well known to doctors working near
sh and meat markets, slaughter-houses and hotel districts; (2) a diffuse
r generalized cutaneous eruption with constitutional symptoms; and (3)
septicæmic form.

Etiology and Pathology

Organisms of the erysipelothrix group were isolated by Koch in 1880
rom mice, and by Leoffler in 1886 from swine. In 1884 Rosenbach applied
he term erysipeloid to the disease as it occurs in man, and in 1886 he iso-
ıted the causative organism and reproduced the disease experimentally.
n 1873 Fox had already reported a similar lesion on the hand of a man
ʌho developed it after trying on boots made of sheepskin. In the same year
Morrant Baker published five cases and called the condition *erythema
erpens*. The bacillus is widely distributed in nature wherever nitrogenous
ompounds are decomposing, and has been recovered from the slime of
sh and from houseflies and horseflesh. In addition to causing severe
rysipelas it is responsible for septicæmia in mice and certain birds, as well
s for the condition known as joint-ills in lambs. In human infections it
as been cultured by ordinary laboratory methods from skin removed
rom the advancing edge of the lesions, but the clinical features are so un-
ıistakable that biopsy is neither necessary nor justifiable.

xposure Hazards

The human disease is widespread in occupations where there is contact
ʌith infected material. In many cases the worker concerned has scratched
r punctured his skin, but in others it seems that the organism has pene-
rated the intact skin. Erysipeloid is especially common among fishermen,
sh cleaners, gutters and picklers, fish porters, fish-box repairers, fish-lorry
rivers ,fish-meal workers, smoke dryers, fishmongers, cooks and house-
ʌives who infect themselves through abrasions of the skin caused by the
pines, fins and bones of fish, especially skate—*fish-handlers' disease*.
Clauder and others (1926) reported "about a thousand cases" among
ommercial fishermen on the eastern seaboard of America. In the Second
World War outbreaks of the disease occurred in factories in Norway
here fish is dried and tinned and cod heads are made into fertilizer. The
elay caused to the fishing boats by forcing them to sail in convoy was
esponsible. In 1943 there were 200 cases in one factory (Bruusgaard,
953). Proctor and Richardson (1954) reported 226 cases among fish
rocessers and trawlermen in Aberdeen.

mong Sealers and Whalers

Erysipeloid occurs in sealers—*seal finger*—and in whalers—*whale
nger*—who scratch their hands on the steel ropes used in their work
Hillebrand, 1953). Anglers may be infected through puncture wounds in
ıe skin made by fish hooks. Sea anglers may be infected through wounds

they receive from the biting parts of fish and from shell-fish, especial
the claws of lobsters and crabs. Although infection is less common in fres
water fish, Stefansky and Grünfeld (1930) reported 200 cases whi
occurred in people dressing golden perch in Odessa.

Among Those handling Meat and Game

Contact with infected meat and game accounts for the high incidence
the disease in abattoir workers, meat porters, butchers and poultere
These workers become infected through small cuts from the knives th
use or through abrasions caused by splinters of bone in beef, mutto
bacon, wild boar, pork—*pork finger*—poultry and rabbit. The hides, pel
bones, fat and milk of infected animals may transmit the infection to ma
Thus kid shoes have been known to convey the disease, and cooks ar
others have developed it after skinning rabbits or handling lard or chees

Among Veterinary Surgeons and Bone-button Workers

An outbreak occurred affecting 210 workers in a bone-button factory
the first ten months of its operation (McGinnis and Spindle, 1934). T
veterinary surgeon becomes accidentally inoculated either by needles
the ragged edges of broken glass ampoules while occupied in vaccinati
animals against swine erysipelas. Greener (1939) recorded a case of fat
septicæmia in a young peacock, and described how the veterinary surge
who performed the necropsy without gloves developed erysipeloid on t
back of the right hand twenty-eight hours later.

Among Those who peel Root Vegetables

Earth contaminated by the manure of infected animals accounts f
cases of erysipeloid in people who peel potatoes and other root vegetable
Infection seldom results from ingestion of infected meat, even when th
comes from animals which have been slaughtered because of swine erysip
las. Nevertheless, Habersang (1926) reported such a case. A butcher dresse
the carcase of a pig which had been slaughtered because of swine erysipela
He ate raw sausage meat which came from this animal and develope
widespread urticaria with the rhomboid pattern characteristic of generalize
swine erysipelas.

The Local Disease

As a rule erysipeloid is an inconsequential disease treated with contem
by the average Billingsgate fish porter. The initial trauma forming the si
of inoculation is usually insufficient to cause bleeding and may be so slig
as to have passed unnoticed. The site involved is nearly always a finger, b
the hand, forearm and face are occasionally affected. The incubation perio
is commonly two or three days, with a variation between one and seve
days. The patient complains of pain and swelling of the affected part, wit
superficial itching or smarting. The pain is often severe and is made wors
by heat, but it is not throbbing as in pyogenic infections. There is often

eeling of tightness and stiffness of the underlying joints. Slight fever occurs
nd sometimes vomiting, but severe constitutional symptoms are absent.

The Physical Signs

Examination reveals an erythematous swelling spreading from the site
f inoculation. The swelling involves both the skin and the subcutaneous
issue, varies in colour from pink to deep purple, is hot and has a well-
efined, slightly raised margin. Tenderness is nothing like so apparent as
1 pyogenic infections, and quite firm palpation of the infected part is well
olerated. The lesion may progress up the edge of the finger into the web
nd then descend the adjoining finger. It commonly spreads to the dorsum
f the hand, but seldom affects the palm. Associated lymphangitis, lympha-
enitis and joint involvement are rare, and when they occur secondary
nfection is responsible. Erysipeloid is a self-limiting condition, subject to
pontaneous remission and ultimate resolution without suppuration. The
hysical signs persist usually for from three to four weeks, and when they
isappear no disability whatsoever remains.

Curative Treatment

In 1944 Heilman and Herrell showed by *in-vitro* and *in-vivo* experi-
1ents that *E. rhusiophathiæ* was sensitive to penicillin. In 1946 Barber and
thers reported five cases which responded to treatment with penicillin,
nd since then many others have been recorded. Injections of aqueous
-enicillin should be given once or twice a day in doses of from 200,000 to
00,000 units. The patient need not stay in bed. No local application is
ecessary. If he so desires, he may rest his arm in a sling. The swelling
apidly subsides and in from three to five days desquamation appears in
he epidermis covering the lesion. Penicillin may then be discontinued
/ithout fear of relapse. Sulphonamides have no influence on the course of
he disease.

The Generalized Form

Sometimes the effects of the disease are more severe and generalized.
Constitutional symptoms occur, including malaise, giddiness, headache,
omiting and fever as high as 104° F. Generalized erythema is followed by
evere urticaria of the skin of the whole body. The wheals measure from 1 to
centimetres in diameter and are rhomboid in shape, hence the expression
iamond skin disease. This is characteristic of generalized swine erysipelas.

The Bacteriæmic Form

Occasionally human cases of the bacteriæmic type of swine erysipelas
ccur. Günther (1912) recorded two fatal cases in veterinary surgeons. In
ne of these the primary infection was in the thumb. This lesion healed but
/as followed after several months by bacteriæmia leading to heart failure and
eath. Necropsy revealed a recent vegetation on the mitral valve. In the
ther case, bacteriæmia with acute endocarditis resulted in death from

heart failure. Russel and Lamb (1940) described the case of a lobst«
fisherman admitted to hospital complaining of malaise, weakness and lo:
of weight of two months' duration. One month previously a non-suppur:
tive erythematous lesion had been present on the upper lip for one wec
but no other cutaneous lesions were observed. He died after one month i
hospital.

Morbid Anatomy

At necropsy the heart was hypertrophied, and small, granular, firm:
adherent vegetations were present on the mitral valve and chordæ tendin:
A bicuspid aortic valve was almost completely destroyed by large, coarse:
granular friable vegetations on the cusps and right commissure, extendin
into each aortic sinus. The endocardium was partly covered by simil:
vegetations which appeared to penetrate the underlying myocardium. Tl
spleen was enlarged and showed a recent infarct. Blood cultures and cu
tures made from endocardial vegetations were positive for *E. rhusiopathic*
It is clear that treatment with penicillin will, in future, save life in this i**
ness.

Preventive Treatment

Prevention of erysipeloid is largely a matter of individual care in pe:
sons who must handle infected material. All such persons should we:
thick rubber gloves covered by cotton gloves which fit tightly over then
When the hands cannot be protected by gloves, frequent inspection f«
small abrasions will reduce the incidence of erysipeloid. Since the adoptio
in bone-button factories of preliminary heating of all bones to 144° F. for n«
less than two hours, the disease has occurred less frequently (Van E
1942). Veterinary surgeons should wear gloves when performing necropsi«
on animals dead of swine erysipelas, and when vaccinating animals again:
this disease. Cultures for such vaccinations must be supplied in vials wit
rubber stoppers, to avoid the risk of skin puncture from the broken poin*
of fused-glass ampoules.

Case 29. Billingsgate fish porter—erysipeloid of Rosenbach following a scrat
with a fish bone—recovery after two weeks.

D. J., a man aged 42, seen in 1949, was referred to hospital by h:
private doctor who had treated him for bronchitis for four months an
wanted further investigations made. The diagnosis was supported b
physical signs and was evidently correct, for there was no evidence «
tuberculosis or other disease of the lungs in X-rays or sputum test:
During routine physical examination a lesion on one of his fingers w:
noticed. In reply to questions he belittled this and dismissed it b
stating that it was a common thing among fish porters. Indeed, th
nurse in the fish market had put a dressing on it and had told him it w:
"only a touch of phosphorus poisoning from the fish!"

Three days previously while packing fish with ice into a box he ha
scratched the ring finger of his left hand with a fish bone. Next day th

finger had become red and the skin irritable and there was slight pain and swelling of the middle knuckle. It was clear from his description that there had been no general and few local symptoms.

On examination: Temperature normal. Pulse 68, regular. The ring finger of the left hand shows redness and slight swelling without tenderness of the skin up to the second joint, the upper margin of the lesion being sharply defined from the normal skin beyond. On the dorsal aspect in the centre of the lesion there is an area 1 by 0·5 cm. where the red colour is intensified, but there is no vesication nor tenderness. The flexor aspect of the finger is unaffected by the inflammation but shows at the base of the middle segment two healing linear abrasions, the larger 3 mm. long, the smaller 1 mm. The proximal inter-phalangeal joint is slightly tender on pressure and on active movement, but there is no limitation of movement nor swelling. There is neither lymphangitis nor any enlargement of lymph nodes.

Scrapings from the area of most intense reddening showed a few polymorphonuclear cells and lymphocytes, but no organisms were seen. In cultures, no growth was obtained. Further search for *Erysipelothrix rhusiopathiæ* by biopsy was clearly unjustified. Seen one week later, the skin lesion was healed but there was slight residual tenderness on manipulation of the proximal inter-phalangeal joint.

ANKYLOSTOMIASIS

The disease, variously known as hookworm disease, ankylostomiasis, ancinariasis, necatoriasis, Egyptian chlorosis, miners' anæmia, tunnel workers' anæmia and brickmakers' anæmia, occurs in tropical and subtropical countries.

History

Hookworm infestation probably existed among the ancient Egyptians, and the clinical disease was described in Italy, Arabia and Brazil long before the parasite was discovered. In 1786 severe anæmia attacked 1,200 coal miners in Schemnitz in Hungary. In 1802 outbreaks occurred in the French coal mines at Anzin, Fresnes and Vieux-condé and in 1820 at Avize, Escarpelle and Graissesac (Patissier, 1822). These were followed by similar outbreaks in the coal mines of Westphalia, as well as in the Cornish tin mines. Happily the coal mines of Great Britain remained free. The doctors at first believed the cause to be contamination of the atmosphere by noxious gases, but the miners blamed the introduction of the steam engine for pumping and winding! In Switzerland, during the construction of the St. Gotthard tunnel in 1880, the high fatality rate of an outbreak of anæmia affecting 10,000 workmen, mainly Italians, called the attention of European workers to the importance of the hookworm as a pathogenic agent. On the completion of the tunnel the returning labourers spread the infestation to the principal mining districts of Hungary, Germany, France, Holland, Belgium, Spain, England and Sicily. Owing to the strict precautions

adopted in 1898, not a single case occurred in tunnelling the Simplon, a
task which lasted seven years.

Incidence

Hookworm disease is especially prevalent in Siam, in South China,
Malaya, the East Indies and Egypt. It was at one time estimated that out of
315 million inhabitants of the Indian subcontinent, 45 million wage earners
were infested. In the districts concerned, all workmen coming in contact
with warm and humid earth are liable to infestation from the larvæ of the
worm; agricultural labourers, planters of coffee, sugar, bananas, cocoa,
tobacco, tea, labourers in ricefields and cottonfields, kitchen gardeners,
peasants, brick workers, pottery workers, tile makers, tunnellers and
miners. The disease is still found in the collieries of Northern France,
Belgium, Hungary and Westphalia, where it is of great industrial importance. It occurs also in the lead mines of Spain (Pacheco, 1928) and in
the sulphur mines of Sicily, Russia and the Balkans. Various mining centres
in the southern states of the U.S.A., in Central America, in India and
Ceylon are affected.

Pathogenesis

The hookworm was first recognized by Dubini of Milan in 1838, but he
did not at that time recognize its pathogenic importance. In 1853 Bilharz
connected the parasite with the extremely severe chlorosis prevalent in
Egypt. In 1882 Perroncito traced the origin of miners' anæmia to the hookworm. Three species of the worm are now known—*Ankylostoma duodenale*,
Ankylostoma braziliense and *Necator americanus* (American murderer). The
adult worm is approximately 1 cm. long. There is no intermediate host, the
ova hatch in the soil and the larvæ gain access through the skin which has
come in contact with damp earth or muddy water. The ova will not hatch
below 60° F., and the optimum temperature for their development is 75° F.
This explains the great prevalence of the disease within a belt 35 degrees
north and south of the Equator. In cold or temperate climates the ova do not
develop outside the warm conditions of deep mines, tunnels or brick-fields

The Route of the Migrating Larvæ

In 1896 Looss accidentally spilled a culture of hookworm larvæ upon
his hand. He noticed that a dermatitis developed at the site, later found
hookworm ova in his fæces, and thus concluded that he had become infested through the skin. In 1911, by experimental studies with *A. caninum*
the dog hookworm, he was able to work out the route of the migrating
larvæ. From the skin they travel through veins to the right side of the heart
and so to the lungs. They are then coughed up in the tracheal mucus and
swallowed. In the alimentary tract male and female hookworms occur in
approximately equal numbers. It is estimated that each female passes 6,000
eggs a day. The ovum develops into a larva in 100 hours. It is stated that
500 worms must be present for six months before symptoms are produced
But when repeated doses of carbon tetrachloride are given until no more

rasites appear in the stools, it is found that some of the most severe cases ve the fewest worms. There is some evidence that ankylostoma is more xic than necator, for, speaking of anæmias of equal severity, more rasites are to be found in American than Egyptian cases.

lechanism of the Anæmia

The ingenious experiments of Wells (1931) suggest that a load of hook-orms much less than 500 can cause anæmia, although it is widely and nphatically maintained that twenty-five hookworms is a light load, im-aterial to man. The experiments of Wells suggest that such a light load ay involve the loss of half an ounce of blood daily. By means of a special imp he has watched the life of hookworms in the opened intestines of gs under anæsthesia. The whole process can be seen when *A. caninum* taches itself near the tip of a villus, and shoulders its way to a deeper and ore vascular hold. The blood vessels of the selected villi dilate, and the okworm œsophagus begins to act as a sucker with a contractile rhythm high as 250 pulsations a minute. This pumping mechanism fills the oral

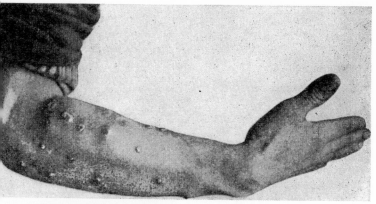

Fig. 263.—Miners' Bunches in a Cornish Tin Miner of 1904
(*Boycott, A. E., and Haldane, J. S.* (*1904*), *Journ. Hygiene*, **4**, *73*)

vity and the œsophagus, first with intestinal epithelium and lymph, and en with blood. This blood the œsophagus passes on to the intestine, iich in turn expels it in droplets per anum. By manœuvring the tails of nging attached worms into the mouths of saline-filled pipettes, by unting a known fraction of the red corpuscles which were expelled into s fluid in a given time and by comparing these with the numbers in the ood of the dog, Wells was able to calculate the amount of blood lost to e host by the activity of each *A. caninum* daily.

mptoms and Signs in the Skin

In the early stages of ankylostomiasis a skin eruption may appear, aracterized by intense itching followed by papular, vesicular and pustular

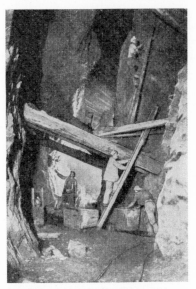

FIG. 264.—Cornish Tin Mines of 1903, showing how the bare Forearms of Miners came in contact with the Rungs of Ladders soiled with contaminated Mud

(Boycott, A. E., and Haldane, J. S. (1903), Journ. Hygiene, 3, 95)

lesions. That this corresponds to in vasion of the skin by the embryo of the parasite has been proved experimentally. It precedes by from two to four months the generalized symptoms of ankylostomiasis. The dermatitis is of much economic importance to the planter. In the case of coolies on plantations, it affects the feet and has been variously known as *coolie itch, ground itch, water itch, water pox, water sore,* and *cow itch.* In the case of Cornish tin miners, Boycott and Haldane (1903) showed that the corresponding lesion occurred on the forearm and was known locally as the *miner's bunches* (fig. 263). The forearms were affected because they were kept bare and came into contact with the rungs of the ladders (fig. 264) which were soiled with mud contaminated by fæces containing the ova of the parasite. Boycott and Haldane worked in the tin mines of

Dolcoath in Cornwall where the parasite, now only of historical interest, is still referred to as *the Dolcoath worm.*

Symptoms and Signs of Anæmia

Within a few months the skin lesion is followed by shortness of breath, weakness, faintness and gastro-intestinal discomfort. In severe cases œdema of the legs with ulceration of the skin may appear. In chronic cases there is stunting of growth and of mental development. The anæmia is of hypochromic type, the hæmoglobin figure being usually 30 per cent, and in severe cases dropping as low as 10 per cent. Eosinophilia is present, the average figure being 10 per cent. Some patients suffering from hookworm anæmia show smooth bald patches devoid of filiform papillæ on the tongue, and soft, cracked,

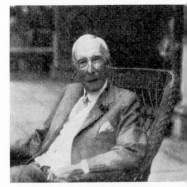

FIG. 265.—John D. Rockefeller on his ninety-first Birthday

(Photograph by F. Ehrenford)

oncave finger-nails, the so-called koilonychia. These are the clinical haracteristics of iron deficiency (Biggam and Ghalioungui, 1934). The liagnosis depends upon the identification of the ova in the fæces.

Preventive Treatment

The Rockefeller Sanitary Commission to Combat Ankylostomiasis (fig. 65) organized in 1909 has waged an energetic and many-sided campaign gainst hookworm. This has been carried out in the United States of America, the West Indies, South America, Asia and Africa. Preventive reatment involves the suitable disposal of excreta, the use of protective foot-ear, education of natives and treatment to diminish the numbers infested. The promiscuous deposition of fæces about huts, villages and fields must be forbidden. Abundant and easily accessible privy accommodation must be provided in coolie lines, and in miners' camps, in native villages and along highways of traffic. In the absence of a more elaborate system of onservancy, pits and trenches will suffice. They may be filled up with arth from time to time, for the embryo soon dies when deprived of air.

Education of the People as to the Transmission of the Disease

Of the many difficulties met, not the least formidable are the social and eligious customs in Mohammedan and Hindu countries. It is manifest hat in devising privies and sanitary regulations the habits and prejudices of the people they are intended to benefit must be taken into account. In Egypt it is difficult to eradicate the disease because of the extensive irriga-ion system, the fact that the natives are too poor to wear boots and that the icefields are so vast that it is usually too far for them to go to special latrines. Education of the public as to the transmission of the disease and the proper use of latrines is as essential as their installation.

Personal Cleanliness and Protective Clothing

Attempts to enforce sanitary regulations are less effective than sanitary nstruction in the home, publicity campaigns and training in the schools. The water supply should be guarded from all possible sources of fæcal ontamination. Drinking-water, unless above suspicion, should be boiled. Where a population can read, the sanitary authorities should issue posters nd leaflets to instruct the people. Personal cleanliness and the use of some orm of foot covering during the wet season are essential. Coolies working n irrigated land should be provided, if possible, with high, well-fitting boots.

Preventive Measures in Mines

In order to prevent the spread of hookworm in mines it is necessary to prevent pollution by human excrement. Closets and pails must be placed t convenient parts of mines, and sanitary overseers must be employed laily for cleansing the sanitary conveniences, stations, drives, cross-cuts, adder-ways and mine workings generally. Well-made boots and gloves fford some protection for miners. A further necessary precaution is the medical examination, including the searching of the stools for ova, of a men applying for employment in mines. One carrier can infest a who mining community.

Wet Methods of Working increase the Hazard

Such measures have practically rid the mines of Australia and Sout Africa of the parasite, and it is no longer found in the tin mines of Corn wall. It must be recognized that wet methods of working increase the hazar of the disease. In 1899 in the coal mines of Westphalia there were 275 case of ankylostomiasis amongst 56,370 miners. In 1900, in order to comba coal-dust explosions, water-spraying was introduced. By 1902 the numbe of cases infested with the worm had risen to 1,355, an increase too great t be regarded as fortuitous (Oliver, 1925).

Curative Treatment

There is evidence that the anæmia is caused by something more than mere loss of blood. Elimination of the worm does not necessarily result i immediate improvement of the anæmia. Equally, treatment by means o large doses of iron, even in the presence of the worm and a defective die may cure the anæmia (Rhoads and others, 1934). Therefore the patien must be removed from exposure, given a well-balanced diet with amp protein and treated with large doses of ferrous sulphate or iron and an monium citrate. Blood transfusion may be necessary in a seriously anæm patient. Later an anthelmintic must be given, preceded and followed by purge.

Use of Tetrachlorethylene and Carbon Tetrachloride

The three most effective substances are tetrachlorethylene, carbo tetrachloride and hexylresorcinol. Oil of chenopodium, although effectiv is not used because of its toxicity, except in combination with carbon tetr chloride and tetrachlorethylene. Tetrachlorethylene is the drug of choi because of its high efficiency, only slightly less than that of carbon tetr chloride, and its low toxicity. A few instances of tetrachlorethylene in toxication, however, have been reported. A single treatment removes fro 77 to 97 per cent of the worms. Carbon tetrachloride is the most effecti drug, a single dose of 3 ml. removing from 91 to 98 per cent of the worr and giving a high percentage of cures. Its relatively high toxicity, how ever, necessitates careful supervision of its administration and therel lessens its value.

Use of Hexylresorcinol for Children

Hexylresorcinol is moderately effective, a single treatment removi about 70 to 75 per cent of the hookworms. It is especially suited for childr and debilitated persons, since it has no untoward or unpleasant effects a treatment may be repeated several times with safety. It is essential realize the practical importance of directing therapy first against the anæm of hookworm disease and secondly against the parasite. Treatment is little value if prevention cannot be accomplished. Nevertheless, curative treatment of infested labourers in Central and South America has increased efficiency as much as 33 per cent and the earning capacity from 15 to 40 per cent.

CYSTICERCOSIS (*Tænia solium*)

Although a chance observation was made more than 350 years ago of numerous vesicles in the dura mater of an epileptic priest (Rumler, 1588), it was not until 1930 that the importance of cysticercosis as a cause of epilepsy was established. The work was done by British Army doctors working under the inspired leadership of Colonel W. P. MacArthur at the Royal Army Medical College, Millbank, London. Cysticercosis is not exclusively an occupational disease, but circumstances peculiar to the life of the private soldier abroad rendered him until 1947 especially liable to suffer from it. In Great Britain no case of the disease is likely to be encountered except in an ex-solider or airman who has served abroad, especially in India. Rarely it is met in an immigrant from Central Europe.

Occurrence of Somatic Tæniasis in Man

In the case of *Tænia solium* man acts usually as definitive host—that is to say, he harbours in his alimentary tract the adult form of the worm. The embryo or bladder worm (*Cysticercus cellulosæ*) is normally developed in the muscles of the pig (fig. 266) and man becomes infested by eating under-cooked measly pork. Pickling and smoking do not kill cysticerci. Both *T. solium* and *C. cellulosæ* are characterized by a scolex surmounted by four suckers and

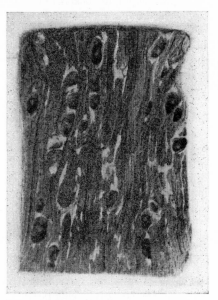

FIG. 266.—Measly Pork. Section of infested Pig Muscle showing Cysticerci, many of them intact with Scolex
(*London Hospital Medical College Museum*)

two rows of hooklets. In certain circumstances man may act as intermediary host, in which case somatic tæniasis occurs, the human tissues becoming invaded by the embryos of the parasite as in the case of the pig.

Indian Native Cooks as Reservoirs of Infestation

Cysticercosis in man is caused by the ingestion of the ova of *T. solium*. Such infestation occurs in countries where sanitation is defective. It is the result of ingestion of food or water contaminated directly by human ex creta or indirectly by flies. Although uncooked food such as lettuce can convey the disease, cooked food also should be suspected. Indeed, a cook especially a native cook in India, acting as a human carrier with unclear hands is the commonest cause of the spread of the disease. Such a possi bility is the more readily understood when it is realized that a single tape worm segment may contain from 30,000 to 50,000 ova. In the majority o cases there is no present evidence nor history of intestinal tæniasis. Never theless, auto-infestation does occur, for 22 per cent of patients give a his tory of tapeworm (Dixon and Lipscomb, 1961).

Geograhical Distribution of the Pork Tapeworm

In the case of the English tapeworm, *Tænia saginata*, man has only rarely been found to act as intermediary host. This parasite is characterized by a scolex with four suckers but no hooklets. Although the occurrence of *Cysticercus bovis* in the human brain and eye has been recorded, the diag noses are uncertain since absence of hooklets occasionally occurs in *C.cellulosæ*. Owing to the high standard of meat inspection in England, and the English habit of eating pork over-cooked, infestation with *C. cellulosæ* is excessively rare in Great Britain. It occurs chiefly in Eastern Europe India, Egypt, Madagascar and South America. The organs and tissues most commonly involved are the brain, meninges, orbit, muscles, heart, liver and lungs. During the first half of the nineteenth century 2 per cent of human necropsies in Berlin showed these cysticerci. Involvement of the fourth ventricle was frequent and led to sudden death. In the twentieth century cysticercosis is a dying disease in Western Europe where it has almost completely disappeared as the result of improvements in sanitation and in meat inspection.

Incidence in Soldiers with Service in India

The work of Colonel W. P. (afterwards Lieutenant-General Sir Wil liam) MacArthur during his appointment as Consulting Physician to the British Army may be said to date from 1929, and he first drew attention to cysticercosis epilepsy in the Annual Report on the Health of the Army for 1930. He gave convincing proof that many soldiers who had served in India, and who developed symptoms that were formerly attributed to idiopathic epilepsy were really victims of cysticercosis (MacArthur, 1934) A follow-up of 450 cases studied by British Army doctors during more than thirty years was published in 1961 by Dixon and Lipscomb. 440 of the patients in their series had lived in India. 444 of the 450 were or had been members of the British Army or Royal Air Force or their families 439 of these had lived in India in the course of their own or their husbands or fathers' Service duty. Thus of the 444 members of the British forces and their families known to have contracted cysticercosis, 439 had resided in India and five had not. Considering the many parts of the world in which British troops were garrisoned, more striking evidence of the relatively high endemicity of India can hardly be adduced. Most of the soldiers infested had served in the plains of the United Provinces and the Punjab, and in Central India and the Deccan; large cities such as Calcutta, Bombay and Madras were very rarely implicated. Since British troops have now ceased to serve in the Indian sub-continent cysticercosis as an occupational disease of our soldiers will disappear.

Three Types of Epileptiform Seizure

Only in 3 per cent of cases does invasion of the muscles give rise to pain, tenderness, muscular weakness, numbness or tingling. In 92 per cent of cases the first symptom is an epileptiform seizure (Dixon and Lipscomb, 1961). Such seizures have nothing to distinguish them from those of idiopathic epilepsy. Patients may suffer attacks of grand mal, petit mal or Jacksonian epilepsy, either singly or in any combination. An extraordinary feature of cysticercosis is that the parasites commonly are present in the body for a period of years before cerebral symptoms become evident. This latency is probably explained by the fact that the living cysticerci in the numbers ordinarily found in the brain are more or less tolerated by the host, but after their death they act as foreign irritants.

Cysticerci in the Muscles

Palpable nodules occur in 54 per cent of cases. They lie mostly in the muscle substance or deep to the skin and subcutaneous tissues attached to the surface of the muscles. They are painless and non-tender, there is no skin reaction over them, and there is no œdema, no hyperæmia and no pigmentation. They are peculiarly dense and of almost cartilaginous hardness; it is difficult to realize by palpation that they are actually tense, thick-walled bladders. The skin and subcutaneous tissues move so freely over them that the impression given is that the cysts themselves are freely movable. Their size depends very much on the length of time they have been present and the tension of the tissues in which they lie. Usually they are ovoid in shape, about a centimetre long and half a centimetre in breadth (fig. 267). They are most easily seen and felt in the upper part of the body, the face, neck, arms, back, chest and abdominal wall. The patient should be examined stripped and in a good light, preferably daylight. He should be asked if he knows of the existence of any nodules. The skin should then be closely scrutinized while he is told to move his muscles in turn. The whole body should be carefully inspected and palpated, at first running the hand lightly over the skin and then with deeper pressure and a kneading motion of the fingers feeling the substance of the muscles. Cases are recorded where the nodules have been mistaken for neurofibromatosis (von Recklinghausen) or multiple subcutaneous gummata, but such mistakes are stupid. The tongue (fig. 268) should always be examined for cysticerci which occur there in 1·8 per cent of cases (Dixon and Lipscomb, 1961).

Intra-ocular Cysticerci

In 1860 Albrecht von Graefe demonstrated with the ophthalmoscope the presence of the cysticercus in the vitreous humour. Where there is an intraocular cyst, a white spot indicates the position of the scolex, which may be seen to move. Intra-ocular cysts are generally subretinal and may cause detachment of the retina, but occasionally they occur in the vitreous or in the anterior chamber (Duke-Elder, 1940). Removal of an intra-ocular cyst without puncture is difficult unless the situation happens to be easily

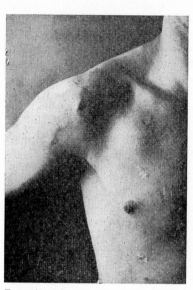 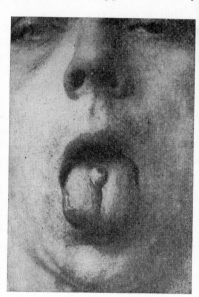

FIG. 267.—Case 30. Two subcutaneous Cysticerci in the substance of the Deltoid Muscle. Note biopsy Scars

FIG. 268.—Case 30. A Cysticercus in the Tongue. A second one was present but is not seen in the Photograph

accessible. Successful removal of an intact subretinal cyst may be effected through a well-placed scleral incision. Other cysts may be found beneath the conjunctiva or in the orbit. They give rise to a local reaction with pain in the orbit when growing and to an intense inflammation if punctured. The death of the parasite may set up a foreign-body reaction and this often leads to iridocyclitis with pupillary occlusion. Cysticerci within the eyeball occur in 1·8 per cent of cases (Dixon and Lipscomb, 1961).

Differential Diagnosis

In addition to epileptic attacks, cerebral cysticercosis may give rise to a wide variety of mental and nervous symptoms including headache, vomiting, hemiparesis, aphasia, delusions and acute mania. The considered diagnoses of patients who eventually were proved to suffer from cysticercosis include melancholia, delusional insanity, dementia præcox and cerebral

umour. Every case of fits occurring in a previously healthy adult who has
ived in a tropical country should be regarded as a probable case of cysti-
:ercosis until it is proved otherwise. Even when full investigation fails to
eveal evidence of the disease, the patient should be kept under observa-
ion for a considerable time, and frequent examination made for subcutane-
•us nodules which may come and go without the patient being aware of
hem.

Findings at Biopsy and Necropsy

Although the history alone may be highly suggestive, the final diag-
1osis in most cases rests in demonstrating *C. cellulosæ* in excised cysts.
such a cyst is an ovoid bladder one centimetre or more in length, opales-
:ent in appearance, containing fluid, and showing the scolex as a central
dark spot. On histological examination it may be possible to demonstrate
vithin the cyst the scolex with four suckers and two rows of hooklets. At
1ecropsy as many as 200 cysticerci have been found in one brain. Many
>f these are found in the leptomeninges and embedded in the grey matter
:lose to the surface (fig. 269). On section the cysts show the interior cystic
:nvelope to be smooth and glistening, and to contain little if any clear fluid.
Attached to this envelope is the invaginated scolex which is a glistening
vhite spherical body about 2 mm. in diameter (fig. 269).

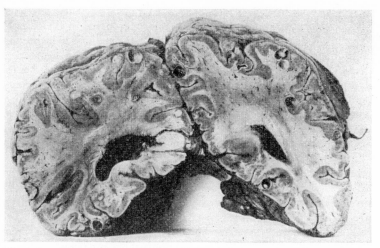

FIG. 269.—Case 30. Section through the Brain showing Cysticerci embedded in
the Grey Matter close to the Surface. In two of the Lesions the invaginated
Scolex is seen as a glistening white Spherical Body about 2 mm. in diameter
(*London Hospital Medical College Museum*)

Radiological Findings

The presence of cysticerci in the body tissues may be demonstrated
adiologically, but since this is rarely possible until at least four or five

years after infestation, radiographs should be repeated at six-monthly or yearly intervals. A radiograph of the skull alone is of value only in 11 per cent of cases. In the 89 per cent of patients in whom the skull shows no abnormality, shadows of cysts can be demonstrated by radiography of the soft parts. Sites where the muscles are thickest, such as the buttocks, thighs and shoulder girdle, will be the most profitable to examine. The older embryos will produce dense elliptical shadows of uniform shape and size (plate VII); younger ones will cast smaller and less definite shadows (plate VI). The radiologist must be prepared to search for suspicious shadows throughout the various films, and to repeat these in doubtful cases. Tattoo marking so frequently seen in soldiers may give rise to misleading shadows, the red pigment, mercuric sulphide, HgS, being the most opaque to X-rays.

Laboratory Tests Available

Serological tests utilizing group reactions to tapeworm antigens are of little value, the positive cases reacting as readily to hydatid antigen as to that prepared from *T. solium*. An eosinophilia in the blood is to be expected during the early stage of infestation, but at the time of diagnosis it is seldom found, the cysticerci being shut off from the general circulation. Examination of the cerebrospinal fluid is of little assistance in making a diagnosis of cysticercosis.

Prevention and Treatment

Imperfect meat hygiene is responsible for the spread of the disease. In regions where cysticercosis is highly enzootic, the methods of inspection in abattoirs, namely additional cuts in diaphragm and shoulder muscles, are inadequate as they may allow infested pig carcasses to be passed over. No person infected with *T. solium* should be employed as cook nor in any other occupation where food is handled. All persons doing such work must be taught to wash their hands after defaecation. In cysticercus epilepsy no treatment has been found effective, and even should some form of chemotherapy be discovered it might well make matters worse by killing off large numbers of parasites at the same time. Anti-convulsant drugs have no effect on the course of the disease, but epanutin helps to control the fits. The large numbers and wide distribution of parasites found in the brain at necropsy do not encourage a resort to operative treatment. Even where cysticerci have been removed from the brain the fits are not relieved, and sometimes operation has been followed by death in status epilepticus. The only indication for surgery is threatened blindness from gross papilloedema which calls for decompression.

Benefit payable by the State

There are, of course, practical advantages in establishing a diagnosis of cysticercosis. In the army, if the disease is contracted abroad, it can be regarded as attributable to military service and therefore a responsibility of the State. Further, the discovery of an organic cause for a supposed idiopathic epilepsy is gratifying, and where the condition progresses so far that the subject becomes certifiable as insane it is a relief to the family to have the dread of familial lunacy removed.

Cases investigated in The London Hospital during forty-five Years

Since 1910 seven patients suffering from cysticercosis have been investigated in The London Hospital. One of these was a man of twenty-eight, an immigrant from Poland who died from acute hydrocephalus due to occlusion of the fourth ventricle by cysticerci. The other six were ex-soldiers who had served in India. Except for the kind collaboration of General MacArthur and Major Dixon, the diagnosis in some of them would have been overlooked. Thus in the following patient (case 30), who was attending my out-patient department, I had made an erroneous diagnosis in 1932 of post-contusional epilepsy until Major Dixon sent for him to attend the Queen Alexandra Military Hospital, Millbank, where he established the diagnosis of cysticercosis. The history and clinical picture in this patient are characteristic, and they emphasize the importance of assuming that every patient with fits who has lived abroad is suffering from cysticercosis, until repeated examination over a period of years has failed to reveal the presence of cysticerci in the tissues either by inspection, palpation or X-ray examination of the whole body.

Prognosis

The prognosis in cysticercosis is considerably better than was at first supposed (Dixon and Lipscomb, 1961). Improvement can take place in patients in whom the outlook for years appeared to be hopeless. Undoubtedly the prognosis in individual cases is difficult. The mortality in a series of 284 cases followed over a period of ten years was 8 per cent. In this series 92 per cent of patients were either unchanged, still improving or free from symptoms, and only 8 per cent were getting worse. It was encouraging to find that 15 per cent had recovered (Dixon and Hargreaves, 1944).

Case 30. Soldier with service in India—onset of epilepsy after five years—Cysticercus cellulosæ found in biopsy of subcutaneous nodule—death from bronchopneumonia; cysticercosis of brain.

(Dixon and Smithers, 1934.) H. A., man aged 30, L.H. Reg. No. 30770/1936. Enlisted in 1923, and proceeded to India in 1926, where he remained for six years. 1929: received knock-out while boxing and fell, hitting the back of his head. He was unconscious for half an hour. Later he received a blow on the head while playing football. He never reported sick, though he states that he suffered from severe headache for one week after the boxing injury. 1931: severe and continuous headache. This persisted for one month, when he had a fit while asleep, fell out of bed, was unconscious for two hours, and bit his tongue. A fortnight later he had two similar fits, both described as typ-

ical epileptiform fits: in one he injured his face and cut his knees and
elbows on the gravel. He was then aged 26 and had served $4\frac{1}{2}$ years in
India. Nov. 1931: well-marked bilateral papillœdema with hæmorrhages; swelling not measurable. Nothing abnormal found in radiographs of skull. He was invalided home with a diagnosis of double optic
neuritis. Feb. 1932: admitted to the London Hospital. "Definite papillœdema, especially upper and inner part of each disc. There is no measurable swelling. About one disc's diameter below the right disc are the
remains of a small hæmorrhage. There are no signs in the maps of the
visual fields"—Mr. C. Goulden. Ventriculography revealed extremely
slight displacement of the third ventricle to the right (Mr. Hugh
Cairns). Blood count: red cells 5,200,000 per c.mm., hæmoglobin 86
per cent (Haldane), colour index 0·82, white cells 8,000 per c.mm.
polymorphs 61 per cent, eosinophils 7·5 per cent, small lymphocytes
12 per cent, large lymphocytes 16 per cent, large hyaline cells 3·5 per
cent. Wassermann reaction negative in blood and cerebrospinal fluid
A diagnosis of cysticercosis was considered but dismissed, as the evidence was insufficient. Feb. 1933: examination by Army Board at
Millbank revealed no evidence of subcutaneous nodules. Feb. 1934
further examination at Millbank showed that he had twenty-eight
firm oval subcutaneous nodules about 1 cm. diam. on his head, face
neck, chest, abdomen, back, arms and legs (fig. 267). There were two
nodules in the tongue (fig. 268). When questioned about them he said
that he had noticed the one on his forehead for a long time, some years at
least, but that he did not know that the other nodules were present
He gave no history of tapeworm. He had had about sixteen major fits
in all, in which he fell down, bit his tongue and was incontinent of
urine or fæces. The fits occurred at any time of the day or night; there
was no aura of any kind. They occurred as a rule every three or four
months. He was a well-nourished man with no evidence of mental
deterioration. Vision 6/6 in each eye. Discs showed secondary optic
atrophy with edges blurred and the cups filled up. There were no
hæmorrhages and no exudate. A subcutaneous nodule was excised and
found to be *Cysticercus cellulosæ*. Radiographs showed cysts in the
muscles of both thighs.

Jan. 1935—He has taken up work as a fish porter and remains well
    except for the occurrence of major fits followed by severe headache
    about every seven weeks.
8 May 1936—Severe vertical headache with focal epilepsy affecting
    first the right side of the face and then the right hand which
    twitched for three minutes. He was admitted to hospital, rolling
    about with pain in which he clasped his head in both hands. He
    remained restless, even with large doses of chloral and bromide.
17 May—Innumerable oval subcutaneous nodules up to 1 cm. diam.
    of cartilaginous hardness palpable all over the body especially in the

head, neck and calves. Papillœdema increasing, temporal and inferior margins of both discs blurred. Plantar responses flexor. Urine: normal. Radiographs showed cysts in both forearms, both thighs and right calf.

Blood count: red cells 5,600,000 per c.mm., hæmoglobin 102 per cent (Haldane), colour index 1·0, white cells 16,400 per c.mm., polymorphs 71·5 per cent, eosinophils 1 per cent, lymphocytes 17·5 per cent, mononuclear cells 10 per cent.

Lumbar puncture: pressure 220 mm. of water; no block c.s.f. 16 lymphocytes per c.mm.; protein 60 mgm. per cent, Wassermann reaction negative.

18 May—Too drowsy to answer questions. On occasions makes violent attacks on male nurses.

24 May—Comatose, but with frequent generalized muscle twitchings. Occasionally maniacal with brief attempts at violence, T. 99°.

30 May—Deep coma, T. 103°, crepitant râles at bases of lungs.

2 June—Died in coma; bronchopneumonia; T. 106°.

Necropsy: Professor Dorothy Russell made the necropsy (L.H. P.M. 198/1936), of which the following is a summary.

Bronchopneumonia. Cysticercosis of brain

Thin coronal slicing of the brain after hardening in formalin disclosed 110 cysts (from 0·5 to just over 1 cm. diam.) distributed fairly uniformly in both cerebral hemispheres, but confined to the cortex or pia-arachnoid (fig. 269), except for occasional ones on the border line between cortex and white matter, and one in ependyma of left frontal horn. Four cysts (from 0·5 to 1·5 cm. diam.) in lumen of fourth ventricle, two of them firmly wedged in opening of Sylvian acqueduct and two in middle and hind end of lumen of ventricle attached to its roof. Four cysts in vermis, two of them under pia-arachnoid, two slightly deeper. A few cysts in basal ganglia. No dilatation of ventricles. No flattening of cerebral convolutions. No abnormality in spinal cord.

All the cysts in the rest of the body were in voluntary muscles, although many of them were just under the superficial sheaths of the muscles and so would be thought clinically to be in dermis or subcutis. One cyst (0·8 cm. diam.) in superficial aspect of muscle of tongue 1 cm. in front of foramen cæcum. A pair of cysts symmetrically situated, one in left and one in right frontalis muscle, one in each sternomastoid, one in right sternohyoid, six in anterior and lateral parts of right chest wall, fewer in left. A few scattered cysts in erector spinæ muscles, one in right and one in left transversus abdominis, two in right and two in left dome of diaphragm, numerous in gluteal muscles. Very numerous cysts of uniform size (from 1·7 × 0·7 cm. to 1·8 × 0·8 cm.) throughout all muscles of thighs and legs, so that practically every slice made through a lower limb muscle revealed several cysts. The lower limb cysts were the largest in the body. The contents of the cysts varied from clear, thin, watery fluid to thick, greyish-yellow fluid or opaque yellow putty-like material; the two latter sorts of contents indicate degeneration and necrosis of the encysted larvæ. No grittiness of calcification appreciated in any cyst.

Purulent bronchiolitis and minute nodules of bronchopneumonic consolidation in collapsed areas in lower lobes. Nothing of importance in other organs. Slightly wasted, moderately muscular man (5 ft. 6 in.; 116 lb. 10 oz.).

Microscopical sections were made of frontal horn, frontal cortex and corpus callosum and sternomastoid, frontalis, sternohyoid, transversus abdominis and biceps femoris muscles and of tongue. An apparently living scolex was found in the frontal cortex and one in frontalis muscle. In all the other cysts examined there was the debris of necrosis and cellular reaction; in this debris in the tongue cyst and those in sternohyoid and transversus abdominis muscles there were the pale ghosts of recently deceased scolices. Around the cysts containing living scolices there were fairly thick reaction capsules of dense fibrous tissue infiltrated with lymphocytes and plasma cells but exceedingly few eosinophil leucocytes. Around the degenerated cysts, such capsules were much thicker and had many large fibroblasts in parts, giving a granulomatous appearance, and also many lymphocytes and plasma cells but no eosinophil leucocytes. In these capsules there were occasionally small patches of calcification.

BIBLIOGRAPHY

Occupational Diseases due to Infections

BÁNSÁGI, J. (1962), *Munkavédelem*, **8**, 7.
BEDSON, S. P., and BLAND, J. O. W. (1932), *Brit. J. exp. Path.*, **13**, 461.
BOYCOTT, J. A. (1964), *Lancet*, **1**, 972.
BREWIS, E. G., NEUBAUER, C., and WESTON HURST, E. (1949), *Lancet*, **1**, 689
CARNE, H. R., WICKHAM, N., WHITTEN, W. K., and LOCKLEY, R. P. (1946), *Australian J. Sci.*, **9**, 73.
CERAM, C. W. (1949), *Götter, Gräber und Gelehrte*, Rowohlt Verlag GmbH. Hamburg-Stuttgart.
COLLETT, R. (1895), *Forh-Vidensk Selsk., Krist.*, **3**, 1.
CONNOLLY, J. H. (1967), Personal communication.
DAUBNEY, R., HUDSON, J. R., and GARNHAM, P. C. (1931), *J. Path. Bact.*, **34**, 545.
DAVENPORT, R. C. (1961), *The Times*, 16 Jan.
DERRICK, E. H. (1937), *Med. J. Aust.*, **2**, 281.
DURAND, P., GIROUD, P., LARRIVE, E., and MESTRALIET, A. (1936), *C.R. Acad. Sci., Paris*, **203**, 830.
JAWETZ, E., KIMURA, S., NICHOLAS, A., THYGESON, P., and HANNA, L. (1955), *Science*, **122**, 1190.
LAURENTZ, F. K. (1958), *Industr. med. and surg.*, **27**, 175.
LIKAR, M., and DANE, D. S. (1958), *Lancet*, **1**, 456.
LOVELL, R. (1949), Personal communication.

MacCallum, F. O., McDonald, J. R., and Macrae, A. D. (1961), *Mon. Bull. Min. Hlth. Lab. Serv.*, **20**, 114.

Milliken, T. G. (1967), Personal communication.

Olin, G. (1938), *Bull. Off. int. Hyg. publ.*, **30**, 2804.

Pearson, A. D. and Barwell, C. F. (1967), *Lond. Hosp. gaz.*, 70, Suppl. vii.

Ross, Constance A. C. (1961), *Lancet*, **2**, 527.

Sanders, M. (1942), *Arch. Ophthal.*, **28**, 581.

Schonell, M. E. and seven others (1966), *Brit. med. J.*, **2**, 148.

Stewart, A., and Hughes, J. P. W. (1949), *Brit. Med. J.* **1**, 926; (1951), *Ibid.*, **1**, 902.

Thiøtta, T. (1931), *Norsk. Mag. Laegevidensk*, **92**, 32.

Anthrax

Annual Report of the Chief Inspector of Factories and Workshops for 1946, H.M.S.O., Cmd. 7299, p. 51.

Bligh, M. (1960), *Dr. Eurich of Bradford*, Clarke, London.

Eurich, F. W. (1926), *Lancet*, **1**, 57; (1933), *Brit. med. J.*, **2**, 50.

Messer, W. (1937), Personai communication.

Nops, V. D. (1948), Personal communication.

Scott, H. H. (1927), *Proc. zool. Soc., Lond.*, Part 1, 179.

Seideman, R. M., and Wheeler, K. M. (1947), *Journ. Amer. med. assoc.*, **135**, 837.

Shanahan, R. H., Griffin, J. R., and von Auersperg, A. P. (1947), *Amer. J. clin. Path.*, **17**, 719.

Soltys, M. A. (1948), *J. Path. Bact.*, **50**, 253.

Taylor, L. and Carslaw, R. W. (1967), *Lancet*, **1**, 1214.

Glanders

Burgess, J. F. (1936), *The Veterinary Record*, **48**, 1034.

Fawcitt, R. (1932), *Brit. J. Radiol.*, n.s., **5**, 717.

Gaiger, S. H. (1913), *J. comp. Path.*, **26**, 223; (1916), *Ibid.*, **29**, 26.

Jacob, F. H. (1921), *Brit. J. Derm.*, **33**, 39.

Robins, G. D. (1905), *Studies from the Royal Victoria Hospital, Montreal*, No. 1, p. 11.

Weil's Disease

Alston, J. M. (1935), *Lancet*, **1**, 806.

Alston, J. M., and Broom, J. C. (1944), *Brit. med. J.*, **2**, 719.

Buchanan, G. (1927), *Med. Res. Counc. Spec. Rep.*, Ser. No. 113.

Davidson, L. S. P., Campbell, R. M., Rae, H. J., and Smith, J. (1934), *Brit. med. J.*, **2**, 1137.

Davidson, L. S. P., and Smith, J. (1936), *Quart. J. Med.*, **5**, 263.

Drew, J. G. (1934), *Brit. med. J.*, **2**, 1142

Fairley, N. H. (1934), *Ibid.*, **2**, 10.

Inada, R., and Ido, Y. (1915), *Tokyo Ijishinshi*, No. 1908.

Petersen, C. B., and Jacobsen, E. (1937), *C.R. Soc. Biol.*, **126**, 797.

Raven, C. (1941), *J. Infect. Dis.*, **69**, 131.

Schüffner, W. (1934), *Trans. R. Soc. trop. Med. Hyg.*, **28**, 7.

Smith, J. (1949), *Brit. J. indust. Med.*, **6**, 213.

Swan, W. G. A., and McKeon, J. A. (1935), *Lancet*, **2**, 570.

Taylor, J., and Goyle, A. N. (1931), *Indian Medical Research Memoirs*, No. 20.

TOHYAMA, Y. (1927), *Sci. Rep. Govt. Inst. Infect. Dis., Tokyo,* **6**, 555.
VAN DER WALLE, N. (1939), *Ned. Tijdschr. Geneesk,* **83**, 740.
WEIL, A. (1886), *Dtsch. Arch. klin. Med.,* **39**, 209.
WOLSTENCROFT, J. (1935), *Lancet,* **1**, 86.

Erysipeloid of Rosenbach

BAKER, W. M. (1873), *St. Bart's Hosp. Rept.,* **9**, 198.
BARBER, M., NELLER, N., and ZOOB, M. (1946), *Lancet,* **1**, 125.
BRUUSGAARD, A. (1953), Personal communication.
FOX, W. T. (1873), *Skin Diseases,* London, p. 108.
GREENER, A. W. (1939), *Brit. J. Derm.,* **51**, 372.
GUNTHER, G. (1912), *Wein. klein Wschr.,* **25**, 1318.
HABERSANG (1926), *Berl. tierärztl. Wschr.,* **42**, 243.
HEILMAN, F. R., and HERRELL, W. E. (1944), *Proc. Mayo Clin.,* **19**, 340.
HILLENBRAND, F. K. M. (1953), *Lancet,* **1**, 680.
KLAUDER, J. V., RIGHTER, L. L., and HARKINS, M. J. (1926), *Arch. Derm Syph., Chicago,* **14**, 662.
McGINNES, G. F., and SPINDLE, F. (1934), *Amer. J. publ. Hlth,* **24**, 32.
PROCTOR, D. M. and RICHARDSON, I. M. (1954), *Brit. J. industr. Med.,* **11**, 175.
ROSENBACH, A. J. F. (1884), *Mikro-Organismen bei den Wund-Infektions-Krankheiten des Menschen, Weisbaden;* (1909), *Z. Hyg. InfektKr.,* **63**, 343.
RUSSEL, W. O., and LAMB, M. E. (1940), *J.A.M.A.,* **114**, 1045.
STEFANSKY, W. K., and GRÜNFELD, A. A. (1930), *Zbl. Bakt.,* **117**, 376.
VAN ES, L. (1942), *Univ. of Nebraska Agricultural Experiment Station, Research Bulletin,* **130**.

Ankylostomiasis

BIGGAM, A. G., and GHALIOUNGUI, P. (1934), *Lancet,* **2**, 299.
BOYCOTT, A. E., and HALDANE, J. S. (1903), *J. Hyg.,* **3**, 95; (1904), *Ibid.* **4**, 73.
LOOSS, A. (1905–11), *The Anatomy and Life History of Agchylostoma duodenale Dubini,* A Monograph, Records Egyptian Govt. School of Med., vols. i–iv.
OLIVER, T. (1925), *Lancet,* **2**, 630.
PACHECO, D. J. (1928), *Med. de los Países cálidos,* **1**, 38.
PATISSIER, P. (1822), *Traité des Maladies des Artisans,* Paris.
RHOADS, C. P., CASTLE, W. B., PAYNE, G. C., and LAWSON, H. A. (1934), *Medicine,* **13**, 317.
WELLS, H. S. (1931), *J. Parasit.,* **17**, 167.

Cysticercosis (*Taenia solium*)

DIXON, H. B. F., and HARGREAVES, W. H. (1944), *Quart. J. Med.,* n.s. **13**, 107.
DIXON, H. B. F., and SMITHERS, D. W. (1934), *Quart. J. Med.,* n.s. **3**, 603. (1934), *J. R. Army Med. Corps.,* **62**, 426; (1935), *Ibid.,* **64**, 227, 300, 375; (1935), *Ibid.,* **65**, 28, 91.
DIXON, H. B. F., and LIPSCOMB, F. M. (1961), *Cysticercosis: An Analysis and Follow-up of 450 Cases,* M.R.C. Spec. Rep. Ser., 299, H.M.S.O.
DUKE-ELDER, W. S. (1940), *Textbook of Ophthalmology,* **3**, 3438, Kimpton, London.
MACARTHUR, W. P. (1934), *Trans. R. Soc. trop. Med. Hyg.,* **27**, 343.
RUMLER, J. U. (1588), *Observationes medicæ,* Obs. **53**, p. 32.

CHAPTER XII

OCCUPATIONAL DISEASES OF THE SKIN AND OCCUPATIONAL CANCER

OCCUPATIONAL DISEASES OF THE SKIN

IN all industrial countries the incidence of occupational dermatitis is high. In Great Britain it accounts for most of the total annual injury benefit for all prescribed diseases or injuries which are not accidents. It is not difficult to appreciate the distress and anxiety among the unfortunate victims, as well as the length of disablement which is likely to result, nor to recognize their lessened security on their return to work. Incapacity from this cause represents so much lost time and waste of health and money, for occupational dermatitis is largely preventable.

History

In the first century A.D., in the sixth book of his *De Re Medicina*, Celsus referred to ulcers of the skin from contact with irritant substances. In 1556, in his *De Re Metallica*, Agricola described in miners ulceration of the skin from contact with corrosive substances. He gave these lesions the graphic title the *black pompholyx*. He also referred to arsenical ulceration of the skin (see p. 333). In 1567, in his monograph on miners' diseases, *Von der Bergsucht*, Paracelsus described ulcers of the skin in metal and salt miners. In 1713, in his *De Morbus Artificum Diatriba*, Ramazzini mentioned the grain itch and attributed the alkali itch to "the sharpness of the lye." He also referred to the cutaneous stigmata of a man's trade (see p. 789).

Ramazzini advocates Cleanliness and Protective Clothing

As preventive treatment he advocated cleanliness and protective clothing. He advised change of occupation for metal workers and the provision of boots and special clothing for those who handled caustic fluids. He deprecated the fact that in his day a bottle of sweet water for drinking was difficult to get and for washing linen quite a luxury. In the golden days of Rome, baths were to be had in every quarter of the town and any tradesman "could remove the sordes and weariness from his body" at nominal cost. In the seventeenth century "owing to the disuse of baths, dirty filth sticks to the workman's skin. Bakers are shut up in the daytime like owls to take their rest, and lice are called the white fleas of millers, because they sleep with their clothes on."

Attempts at Classification

All this work was done long before any logical classification of skin diseases had been attempted. Not until sixty years later did von Plenck in his *Doctrina de Morbis Cutaneis* (1776), which was based on the method of Linnæus, classify diseases of the skin according to the nature of the primary lesion. But medicine is indebted to Robert Willan for the first systematic description of occupational dermatitis. In his *Description and Treatment of Cutaneous Diseases* (1798) he graphically described the *psoriasis palmaris* of shoemakers, the *psoriasis diffusa* of bakers, the dermatoses of metal workers, grocers' itch and washerwomen's eczema.

Beginning of the Modern Period

The modern work on the subject really began after the First World War, when considerable contributions appeared in the literature of France, Germany, the United States of America and other countries. In Great Britain the *Occupational Affections of the Skin* (1934) by Prosser White constitutes an authoritative encyclopædic account of the subject which has a world-wide reputation. Reference should be made to the splendid index of this book whenever the question arises as to whether a particular substance can harm the skin. The American work *Occupational Diseases of the Skin* (1957) by Schwartz, Tulipan and Birmingham is equally thorough and more up to date.

Skin Lesions already Described

Skin lesions produced by diverse chemical substances have been discussed elsewhere in these pages. The effects of inorganic arsenic compounds include arsenic dermatitis, arsenic ulcers, arsenic hyperkeratosis (p. 338) and arsenic cancer (p. 338). The vesicant effects of organic arsenic compounds are described: methyl dichlorarsine (p. 349), ethyl dichlorarsine (p. 349), chlorovinyl dichlorarsine (p. 350), phenyl dichlorarsine (p. 350), diphenyl chlorarsine (p. 350), diphenyl cyanoarsine (p. 351) and phenarsazine chloride (p. 351); and also the vesicant effects or organic mercury compounds: methyl mercury iodide (p. 317), ethyl mercury chloride (p. 317), phenyl mercury acetate (p. 317) and tolyl mercury acetate (p. 317). Effects of other metallic compounds are mercury dermatitis, mercury fulminate dermatitis, fulminate itch, powder holes (p. 312), beryllium dermatitis (p. 432), cement dermatitis, lime dermatitis, lime hole (p. 367), nickel itch, nickel eczema, metal platers' dermatitis, spectacle dermatitis, suspender dermatitis (p. 468), chrome dermatitis, chrome ulcer and chrome hole (p. 455). Organic chemical substances account for TNT dermatitis (p. 547), tetryl dermatitis (p. 570), *para*phenylenediamine dermatitis (p. 571), methyl bromide burns (p. 600), chloronaphthalene acne, chloracne, halowax acne, cable rash, blackhead itch (p. 617), tar warts, tar cancer, pitch cancer (p. 819), anthracene cancer (p. 821), chimney-sweeps' cancer (p. 819), shale oil cancer (p. 819) and mule-spinners' cancer. Asbestos is responsible for asbestos warts (p. 1015), X-rays for X-ray dermatitis (p. 898) and X-ray cancer (p. 899), infections for verruca necrogenica (p. 707) and *Ankylostoma duodenale* for miners' bunches and coolie itch (p. 752).

Causes

The causes can be classified under four headings:

(1) Physical factors—pressure, abrasion, moisture, desiccation, heat, cold, light, X-rays and other rays.

(2) Plant products—leaves, stems, sap, roots, bulbs, flowers, fruits, vegetables, wood dusts, resins and lacquers.

(3) Living agents—bacteria, viruses, fungi, helminth parasites, insects and mites.

(4) Chemical substances—inorganic acids and salts, hydrocarbons, oils, tar, pitch, anthracene and dyes.

Primary Irritants and Sensitizers

In the case of chemical substances two different types of action on the skin are possible. These substances usually act as *primary irritants* when by virtue of their alkalinity or acidity, or from their degreasing, dehydrating, oxidizing or reducing properties, they upset the skin on first exposure of all persons provided there is sufficient concentration and length of exposure. But some chemical substances, usually of complex organic molecular structure, or else simpler substances capable of combining with protein to form complex antigens, give rise to *sensitization dermatitis*. With such substances the first exposure is harmless, but if it is continued or repeated after a variable period of time, sensitization develops and subsequent re-exposure even to minute quantities is followed by dermatitis. It is, of course, possible for a chemical substance to act both as a primary irritant and as a sensitizing substance in the same patient.

Substances and Occupations Involved

The chief causative agents responsible year by year for disability can be classed in the following order: alkalis, sugar, oil, chromium salts, turpentine, dyes, chemical substances, friction, petrol, flour improvers, acids, paraffin, French polish, nickel compounds and rubber antioxidants. Similarly the occupations chiefly involved are as follows: dyers and calico printers, engineers, labourers, metal platers and polishers, bakers and confectioners, cleaners, French polishers, painters, leather workers, chemical workers, tar workers, rubber workers, sugar confectioners, textile workers, oil refiners, printers, sugar refiners, pottery workers, flour workers, biscuit makers, garage hands, gardeners, carpenters, dentists, doctors, florists, dustmen, housewives, nurses, miners, photographers, platers, machine hands and veterinary surgeons. During the six years 1929 to 1934, of 36,634 patients attending the Skin Department at the London Hospital, 961 were found to be suffering from occupational dermatitis (O'Donovan, 1935). The following is an analysis of these cases: alkali (298), fur (77), dyes (23), flour (16), sugar (16), cement (20), lime (5), water (12), plants (8), hops (6), wood (8), chemical substances (8), turpentine (4), formaldehyde (3), methylated spirit (2), oil (8), glue (2), rubber (3), enamel (2), asbestos (1) and tar carcinoma (139).

The Occupational Case History

The elucidation of the cause in a given case often depends upon persuading the patient to describe what he does in his own words, which, if he is a technician, may be far from simple. A man's nominal work does not always indicate his risk. A workman calling himself a fitter may have been exposed for the whole of one day to *para*nitrochlorbenzene (fig. 270) while repairing the plant used to make this substance in a chemical works. A maintenance engineer may one day handle water-pipes, another day a coal conveyer and a third day a still caked with quinine residues. The diagnosis of his skin eruption is made by patch testing, but one only arrives at the need for this by particularity in questioning (O'Donovan, 1952). Know-

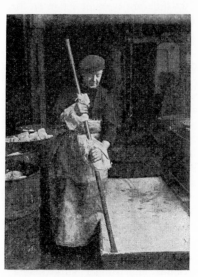

Fig. 270.—Workman breaking up *Para*-nitrochlorbenzene in order to transfer it from the Tray into Drums. He avoids Contact with his Skin and Clothing by gripping the Crowbar with clean Sacking and tying a Sack round his Waist

(*By courtesy of Clayton Aniline Co.*)

ledge of irritants encountered in apparently innocuous occupations is of importance. Thus dermatitis in letterpress printers was traced to the presence of a minute proportion of formaldehyde added to an adhesive paste with the object of checking the growth of moulds. *Apple-sorters' disease* occurs only when a solution of orthophenylates has been used for washing the apples to prevent the growth of moulds (Sealey, 1952). It is unsafe to forget that some men have two occupations and some have hobbies not free from cutaneous hazards.

Type of Lesion

The result of the application of external irritating agents to the skin is the appearance of a reaction varying in all degrees from mere discomfort to itching, smarting or burning, and through stages of redness, punctate or confluent, up to a pustular, scaly, warty or malignant ulcerative reaction. According to White (1934) most occupational dermatoses originate in the stomata, in hair follicles or in the folds of the skin and spread from these sites. In the great majority of the plant dermatoses pinhead vesicles predominate (figs. 271, 276). Sometimes the causal irritant is identified because the dermatitis is associated with some other more characteristic lesion, such as *chrome holes, salt holes* (fig. 272), *soda holes, lime holes* or *powder holes.*

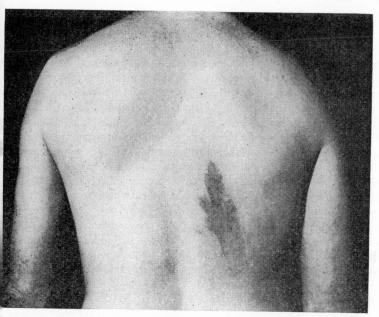

FIG. 271.—Eruption of Pinhead Vesicles after a Chrysanthemum Leaf had been strapped for twenty-four hours to the Skin of a Gardener who complained of Dermatitis of the Hands and Forearms in the Chrysanthemum Season

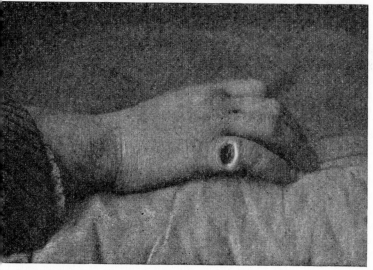

FIG. 272.—Salt Hole in a Yarmouth Fish Cleaner, a woman of 25, whose Hands were constantly soaked in Brine

Site of Origin

Deductions may sometimes be made from the site of origin. For example the dermatoses of lime, sugar, metal and tulip juice have a predilection for, but are not always confined to, the nail areas. It is of some interest to note which hand is first and more affected, for if in a left-handed man the left hand is the first to show a skin lesion and remains throughout the worst part affected and the last to heal, it is difficult to dissociate the left-handed eruption from the left-handed man's occupation (O'Donovan, 1952). It must be recognized that in workers in wet processes, notably dyers, chemical workers and sugar refiners, the feet and legs are often first or alone affected. An irritating dust, as opposed to a liquid, will usually show its effect first on the face and neck, as do certain wood dusts, copra dust and barley. The site of the lesion may be determined by local sweating, on the forehead especially, where caps are worn—namely, in woodworking, flour-packing and dough-mixing. The thighs may be affected from irritation caused by oily overalls and trousers worn by fitters, engineers and metal workers. Oil folliculitis is, of course, easy of recognition, but then it is not strictly a dermatitis (Horner, 1934).

Constitutional Symptoms

When we consider the varied and often deadly effects of plant alkaloids on animal tissues we need not be surprised that constitutional symptoms sometimes accompany dermatitis due to a particular plant. Of the bean family, at least ten members cause dermatitis and most of these contain chemical substances which are systemic poisons. Thus each year in Sardinia many thousands of cases of hæmoglobinuria occur either from ingestion of the horse bean, *Vicia faba*, or from inhalation of the pollen of the plant. It has been known for more than a century that persons with a congenital susceptibility to the effect of hops may be narcotized for some hours merely by placing their hands in a bin of hops (Badham, 1834). When hop-pickers rub an eye with their fingers they are liable to develop smarting pain, lachrymation, conjunctivitis and œdema of the eyelids, a condition known as *hop eye* or *hoppers' eye*.

Rôle of Degreasing Agents

Many cases of trade dermatitis are caused, not by the substances encountered on the job, but by their removal by degreasing agents and other substances harmful to the skin. The worst offenders amongst such cleansers are washing soda, soda ash, chloride of lime, paraffin, petrol, naphtha, turpentine, methylated spirit and trichlorethylene. One such substance commonly used to remove dyes from the skin is a mixture of bleaching powder and soda ash known as *chemic*. Unless all trace of this is removed, preferably under running warm water, it may set up alkali dermatitis. The French polisher likes to use strong aqueous solutions of washing soda to remove the stains from his skin. The stronger the solution used, the quicker does he finish his toilet (fig. 273). Half a pound of washing soda to

, gallon of water is of sufficient strength for his purpose. Painters use
urpentine to clean paint off their skin; cotton-seed oil should be used
nstead (Horner, 1934).

Hazards in the Home

The risk is not confined to industry but extends to the home, where the
domestic worker constantly uses soap and synthetic detergents, and may
have her hands immersed in water for hours at a time; the housewife thus
becomes the victim of *dishpan hands*. In addition, hot alkaline cleansing
solutions are in frequent use, strong solutions of soda, quick chemical

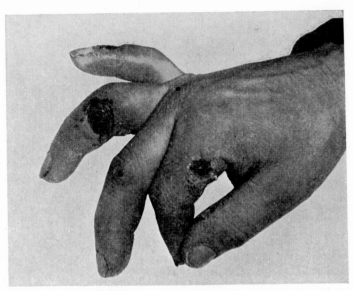

Fig. 273.—Soda Holes in a French Polisher who persistently used strong
Aqueous Solutions of Washing Soda to remove the Stains from his
Skin

cleansers and even chloride of lime are employed to save time, and strong
or dilute acids are used to clean lavatory basins and closet pans. Metal
polishes, furniture polishes and leather preservatives are sold extensively
to the housewife. Quick-drying enamels and paints, varnishes, special
rapid paint renovators, disinfectants, insecticides, artificial plant manures
and storage batteries are in daily use in the home and may all cause
dermatitis (O'Donovan, 1932).

Sensitization Dermatitis

The sensitizers or allergenic chemical substances affect only a small
percentage of people exposed to them; a few of them by sufficient exposure
can produce sensitization in everyone. The tendency to hypersensitivity
may be inherited. A complete list of sensitizing chemical substances would

be a very long one; they include coal-tar products, explosives, photo graphic developers, dye intermediates, dyes, rubber accelerators, insecti cides. oils, resins, synthetic resins and plasticizers. Examples are pheno picric acid, aniline, hydroquinone, crystal violet, hexamethylenetetramine nicotine, tung oil, pine resin, urea formaldehyde and dioctylphthalate In the plastics industry and in the manufacture of paints the epoxy, epoxid or ethoxyline resins are being increasingly used because of their grea binding strength. These resins together with some of their curing agents plasticizers, solvents and diluents can act as severe sensitizers in thei liquid form but become less dangerous when cured (Bourne, (1956) Grandjean, (1957), Calnan, (1958) and Zielhuis (1961)).

Sensitization to Antibiotics

During 1948 nurses, doctors and dispensers handling streptomyci began to be sensitized to this substance, and by 1952 the numbers affecte in some areas caused anxiety. To a less extent penicillin has the sam effect. It seems that something between 1 and 5 per cent of nurses usin; antibiotics become sensitive to them and that a severe degree of sensitiza tion to one antibiotic is frequently associated with sensitization to others. / very early sign seems to be swelling of the eyelids, which, especially in the case of streptomycin, may precede all others. The clear predominance of the hands, arms, face and eyes among the sites affected seems to indicate the importance of local contact. Penicillin is commonly used by herdsmer in the treatment of mastitis of cows and has given rise to sensitizatior dermatitis. Such men are liable also to aureomycin dermatitis arising from sensitivity to this substance present in animal feeding stuffs (Vickers, 1960)

Case 31. A nursing sister—exposure to streptomycin in ward work—œdeme of eyelids and dermatitis affecting upper limbs—treatment by desen sitization.

(Russell, 1953), A. M. J., a single woman aged 25, in Septembei 1947, after handling streptomycin, developed œdema and peeling o the eyelids and of the flexures of the elbows. The rash cleared after avoidance of streptomycin, but recurred in the spring of 1948 after a short re-exposure in which she had given only two injec- tions. In the spring of 1952 there was a further slight recurrence after giving a single injection, and another in November 1952 after checking injections: this became worse after giving some injections.

On examination on 19th December 1952 there was peeling of the eyelids, the left more than the right. Patch-testing was performed with streptomycin 1/1,000,000, 1/100,000, 1/10,000, and 1/1,000, and all tests were negative except the 1/1,000 dilution, which at seventy hours showed slight redness and œdema. The left eye had become swollen about sixty hours after the application of the patch. On re-examination five days after the application there was still marked pinkness and papulation at the 1/1,000 site, but the other test sites were negative. Both eyelids had, however, recently been œdematous and pink. In view of the possibility of some other cause, such as plants, having an influence, patch-testing was also performed using chrysanthemums, with negative results.

Treatment: On 25th September 1953 an intradermal injection of 0·1 mg. of streptomycin was given and on the next day an injection of 0·2 mg. On 27th September erythema and œdema 1 cm. in diameter were noted at the site of the first injection, and this reaction had become more marked after receipt of the second injection. At the site of the second injection there was only a minor response. The eyelids had become sore six hours after the second injection, but this soreness subsided in twenty-four hours.

Subsequent injections were as follows:

Date	Amount (*mg*)	Result
Sept. 28	0·1	
Sept. 30	0·2	No reaction to previous injection
Oct. 2	0·3	No reaction to previous injection
Oct. 4	0·3	Soreness above eyes and old sites flared up
Oct. 8	0·4	No reaction to previous injection
Oct. 9	0·5	No reaction to previous injection
Oct. 11	0·5	Slight reaction to previous injection
Oct. 12	0·6	No reaction to previous injection
Oct. 13	0·6	Slight reaction to previous injection
Oct. 14	0·7	No reaction to previous injection
Oct. 15	0·8	No reaction to previous injection
Oct. 16	0·9	No reaction to previous injection
Oct. 17	1·1	No reaction to previous injection
Oct. 18	1·4	No reaction to previous injection
Oct. 19	1·5	No reaction to previous injection
Oct. 20	1·6	No reaction to previous injection
Oct. 21	1·7	No reaction to previous injection
Oct. 22	1·9	No reaction to previous injection
Oct. 23	2·2	No reaction to previous injection

There was no reaction to this last dose, and the patient was advised deliberately to expose herself to streptomycin, first by checking doses, and secondly by giving injections. She checked two injections without upset and then filled a syringe with streptomycin. Seven hours later there was some moistness and itching of the eyelids, but this subsided rapidly and in her opinion was only half as bad as before. Subsequent further checking caused no reactions.

November 9   Patch-test with 1/1,000 streptomycin
November 11   Above patch negative: 1/500 applied
November 13   Above patches negative: 1/250 applied
November 16   All above patches negative: 1/100 applied
November 18   All patch areas negative

The patient had meanwhile been checking and giving injections, and twenty-one hours previously had deliberately spilled some streptomycin on her fingers and let it dry on, washing her hands three quarters of an hour later. There had been no reaction, although there previously would have been under these circumstances at six hours but on the evening of 18th November there was slight swelling of the eyelids which subsided by next morning. On 19th November the 1/100 patch became red and slightly swollen. This reaction faded within twenty-four hours.

It would appear that this course of intradermal injections diminished the patient's sensitivity tenfold, for a positive reaction was obtained with a dilution of 1/100, comparable in intensity to that previously obtained with a dilution of 1/1,000. Eight weeks after this course of treatment there was a relapse. A second course was begun, starting again with a dose of 0·1 mg. with daily increments of up to 0·3 mg. to a maximum of 5 mg. daily. This second course lasted two months. There were a few reactions on the eyelids. This course was successful and the patient had no trouble except that when she was tired or starting a cold in the head the susceptibility seemed to increase temporarily and the eyelids itched and peeled slightly.

Subsequently when away from work she deliberately exposed herself to streptomycin by having a small bottle on her dressing-table the rubber top being perforated by a large-bore needle. This practice was designed to prevent the loss of immunity which might arise from non-exposure.

Preventive and Curative Treatment

The breakage of ampoules, spillage of solutions, contact with swabs and with the patient's skin can all be avoided by careful technique and by wearing gloves. Air should not be expelled from a filled syringe except into the phial. Industrial experience shows that, in most people, removal from contact at the earliest sign, followed by simple treatment and careful technique thereafter, prevents the development of sensitization and enables a worker to continue her employment. In severe cases desensitization should be carried out, especially where a highly trained nurse would otherwise have to give up her special job (case 31).

The Finger-nails

The various harmful agents which injure the skin are not without their effect on the nails. Electroplaters using nickel salts, and men handling lime, as well as those working with formaldehyde, *formalonychia*, all can be affected by acute ungual eczema. Onychomycosis of brewers due to brewers' mould attacks workers who clean the fermentation vats; the nails present longitudinal fissures with facets and crusty excrescences at the root. Exposure to harmful amounts of radium or X-rays causes the nails to be striated, fissured and brittle (fig. 274). Paronychia occurs in men handling glass wool (p. 1028), in sugar confectioners, in girls who peel and squeeze oranges and lemons, *limonene dermatitis*, and in those who sort nd pack tulip bulbs or gather the crop of tulips in the spring, *tulip fingers*. Mechanical modifications of he nails resulting from various occupations are discussed on p. 799.

Men who rely on their Finger-tips for their Livelihood

Thick, strong finger-nails are a valuable asset to the worker. Congenital hypoplasia, atrophy, extreme thinness, fragility, koilonychia, splitting, separation into layers, detachment from the nail-bed and long-standing infections are serious handicaps to the watchmaker, the jeweller, the engraver, the printer, the weaver and many others who rely on their finger-tips for their livelihood. One particular and peculiar instance illustrates the importance of normal nails. There are expert silk weavers in Japan who use two of their nails finely dented in the fashion of a saw to pull tiny threads in weaving artistic silk fabrics. No fragile, split, splintered or separated nail could be used for this work (Ronchese, 1953).

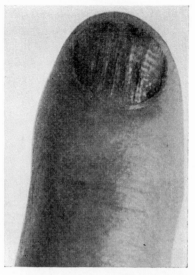

Fig. 274.—Striation, Fissuring and Brittleness of the Nail of the right Forefinger in a Research Technician of 64. The changes started after 21 years' exposure to X-rays and had been present for 3 years. His main work was X-ray Crystallography using a 5-kW tube, 150 milliampères, 35 kV

Effects of Irritant Plants

The plants, vegetables, fruits, wood dusts and resins which produce substances harmful to the skin make a very long list. The workers affected are horticulturists, florists, gardeners, nurserymen, market gardeners, field labourers, pharmacists, perfumers, confectioners, fruit pickers, hop pickers (fig. 275), workers in canning factories and those handling certain insecticides and lacquers. The plants causing dermatitis belong to such Natural Orders as the liliaceæ, primulaceæ, anacardiaceæ, orchidaceæ and irideæ. The vegetables causing trouble are parsnips, celery, asparagus, spinach and haricot beans; the fruits are oranges, lemons, tangerines and tomatoes. Sometimes the origin of a plant dermatitis is not immediately apparent. Thus women shelling peas in Covent Garden market may show severe dermatitis from mayweed, the stinking camomile (*Anthemis cotula*) plucked along with the pea-pods. In some cases the plants are more irritant at certain seasons of the year. Often the poisonous substance remains active even when the plant is dried.

The Family of Liliaceæ

The sap, stems, bulbs, leaves and flower-heads of daffodils, narcissi, jonquils, tulips and hyacinths may act as primary irritants causing painful lesions of the fingers with seasonal recurrence. The condition may remain

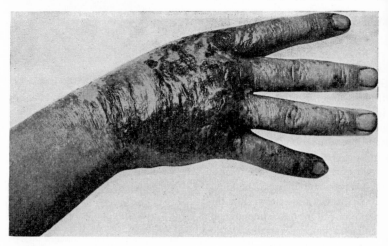

FIG. 275.—Dermatitis in a Hop Picker, a girl of 14. The Vesicles are discrete on the Fingers and confluent on the Hand. There is an Erythematous, Pustular and Scaly Reaction with Shallow Ulceration on the Dorsum of the Hand

localized entirely under and around the finger-nails without affecting the substance of the nail itself—*tulip fingers*. Or it may spread as an itching dermatitis of the hands with desquamation and deep fissures—*lily rash*. In the bulb-growing districts of the Scilly Isles and Cornwall this condition may disable so many workers as to cause serious dislocation of the industry in the early spring. Sorters and packers of tulip and hyacinth bulbs also may be affected.

The Family of Primulaceæ

Of the primrose family, the familiar wild *Primula farinosa* is seen in country districts all over Europe. Its near relative, the cowslip (*Primula veris*), has been known to set up violent dermatitis in cowmen and milkers after the udders of the cow have passed over the plants in dewy grass. *Primula sinensis*, *Primula arendrii*, *Primula mollis* and *Primula contusoides* contain irritants, but the cultivated hot-house *Primula obconica* is the worst of the family and affects 50 per cent of people exposed to it (fig. 276). The poison is a primary irritant and is contained in the glandular hairs which cover all parts of the plant above ground. The rash is composed of numerous closely placed, small, shiny, red, punctiform papules. They are accompanied by much smarting and itching. Occasionally these

ions are associated with large blisters. A gardener, nurseryman,
florist who has shown himself very sensitive to the plant hairs or pollen
P. obconica may be unable ever to work again with this plant or indeed
th others of the same Natural Order.

he Family of Anacardiaceæ

Of all the known plants and woods, the anacardiaceæ cause more
rmatitis than all the other families combined. Happily for Britons, none
the whole group grows in the British Isles. The poison ivy (*Rhus
icodendron*), poison oak (*Rhus
versiloba*), poison sumac, elder
ash (*Rhus vernix*), the Japanese
tree (*Rhus vernifera*), the Indian
arking nut (*Semecarpus anacar-
um*) and the shell of the cashew
t (*Anacardium occidentale*) are
ell-known intense skin irritants.
he leaves of many plants of this
mily are covered with short
arp spines easily seen with a
ns; when these spines are broken
the irritant sap oozes out of the
if. The roots of most of them
e filled with a sticky sap so that
gging in the soil where they grow
n cause dermatitis (Schwartz,
ulipan and Peck, 1947).

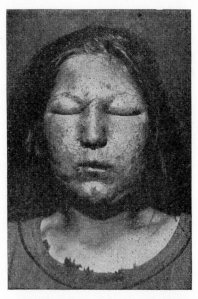

FIG. 276.—Dermatitis from *Primula
obconica* in a girl of 16. There is
itching and burning, with redness,
œdema and close-set Pinhead Vesicles with occasional Pustules

hemical Composition of the Irritant Substances

The active irritants produced
r the anacardiaceæ are polyhydric
nenols related to anacardol; all
e readily destroyed by oxidizing
ents such as potassium permanganate, sodium perborate and hydrogen
roxide. Field workers and others who are going to work where these
ants are likely to be encountered should wear long trousers, long sleeves
d gloves. If for any reason gloves cannot be worn, a barrier cream con-
ining sodium perborate should be used. Of the plants which blister the
in, the stinging nettle (*Urtica dioica*) contains formic acid, and the blister
ant (*Ranunculus acris*), the windflower (*Anemone quinquifolia*) and the
ster flower (*Anemone ulspatilla*) contain anemonine, an acrid alkaloid
lated to cantharidine. The irritating substances in celery, producing
lery itch, and in the peel of oranges and lemons, affecting marmalade
akers, are hydrocarbons of the terpene series (Henry, 1933).

Pyrethrum Dermatitis

Although *Chrysanthemum vulgare* of our English gardens but rare
gives rise to dermatitis in horticulturists, nurserymen and gardeners, oth
varieties of the species are irritant. Pyrethrum is obtained from *Chrysa*
themum pyrethrum and from *Pyrethrum cinerariifolium*, plants which gro
in various parts of Europe, Asia, Africa, Australia and America. Conside
able disability is caused in Europeans who grow these plants on a lar
scale in Kenya. A dermatitis occurs which is severe and incapacitatin
idiosyncrasy is a marked factor and the condition is further aggravate
because the plant irritant causes photosensitivity. Pyrethrum powder
widely used as an ingredient of agricultural and cattle sprays and powde
used to kill flies, mosquitoes, ants and cockroaches. It obstructs the trach
of insects and paralyses their neuromuscular system.

Dalmatian Insect Powder

McCord and others (1921) described eighteen cases of dermatitis whic
occurred among eighty-five workers in a factory manufacturing an insect
cide containing pyrethrum. In *A Blind Hog's Acorns* (1945) Carey McCo
gives a graphic description of how he stumbled upon pyrethrum dermatiti

> One of the opportunities given me by industry for scientific i
> vestigation was concerned with a plant that scarcely may be associate
> with any well-identified industry. The organization bottled castor o
> flavoring extracts and catsup, made peanut butter, patent medicir
> and insecticides, and ground mustard. Self-styled, this plant w
> labeled *Manufacturing Chemists*.
>
> One product was an insecticide in powder form, packaged in sma
> tricornate cardboard bellows. Blown about the habitat of insects, t
> powder was undeniably efficacious. It was prepared in a small sectic
> of the factory, a department employing some eighty-odd worker
> During the summer months many of these men and women develope
> a disturbing skin disease in the elbow folds, at the shoe tops, aroun
> the neck or on the upper eyelids. The work operation was a dusty on
> and it seemed obvious that dust settling on these parts and leache
> out by perspiration was causing the trouble. We who were conductir
> the investigation reached this conclusion immediately, but the manage
> ment scoffed emphatically. "All we're doing is grinding up chrysar
> themum buds," they pointed out. "You can't expect an ordinar
> garden flower to be the cause of all this trouble."
>
> The expectation was not merely sustained, but supported.
>
> Through many decades, much of the romance of Dalmatia h
> been linked with its broad fields of Dalmatian daisies. For years, th
> buds of this variety of chrysanthemum have constituted an outstanc
> ing portion of the province's industry. Prose and poetry have po
> trayed the beauty of this flower, but not divulged is the secret tha

hidden within its petals, is a potent irritant. Although Dalmatia gave name to *Dalmatian Insect Powder*, the world's commercial supplies are in part obtained from Persia, the Caucasus, Montenegro and Japan. California, likewise, has been found to have a climate favorable to the luxurious growth of the plant, and is a notable commercial source.

Lest the uninitiated form the opinion that this material represents only a chemical curiosity, let it be recorded that in so remote a year as 1917, one million five hundred and four thousand pounds were imported into the United States in bales, most likely to have been labeled *Buhach*, since this is its favorite name in many portions of the globe.

Wavering just a little, the management called in its own plant engineer to make installations eliminating some of the dustiness of the operation. Promptly he acquired the disease, which rather crystallized our own belief as to the cause. Unconvinced, a junior member of the management entered the department to give a demonstration of the complete innocuousness of the company's product. He amply coated himself with fine pyrethrum, and promptly developed the worst dermatitis of all. The already afflicted workers concealed their sadistic delight in this instance only a little less than a flock of floating barrage balloons.

This painful approach to conviction proved distressing. Such a state of sensitivity was created in the young official that he confided years later, "All I had to do after that was merely walk into the department, touching nothing, then get my hat and start for the hospital. Time after time every inch of my skin was involved, so that I peeled off even the skin of my palms."

When publication was made concerning the investigation, it was hailed as disclosing a new disease. Fortunately my name was not associated with it, that fashion having long since been discarded. Indeed, just the opposite happened: for years thereafter, within that small group of the brotherhood given to the use of first names, I was dubbed *Pyrethrum McCord*. My name was not attached to the disease, but the disease name was attached to mine.

ffects of Toxic Woods

Carpenters, wood machinists, sawyers, lumberjacks, workers in lumber rds, wood polishers, cabinet makers, shipwrights and furniture manu- cturers often develop dermatitis from contact with wood dust and ccasionally suffer from asthma and other constitutional symptoms (see 1071.) The substances responsible are the sawdust, the sap and the olishings or the oil of the wood. East Indian satinwood (*Chloroxylon ientenia*) produces in cabinet makers a papulovesicular eruption with awny swelling of the skin. The face and upper respiratory tract may be volved and headache and anorexia occur. In 1908 Legge described the fects on workmen of handling ebony (*Diospyrus ebenum*), satin walnut, teak (*Tectona grandis*) and olive wood as well as rosewood (*Dalbergia latifolia*), Cuban sabicu wood, West Indian boxwood and partridge wood.

South African Boxwood

In 1905 the use of South African boxwood (*Gonioma kamassi*) in shuttle making for the Lancashire cotton industry caused widespread disability. It was found that the machinery used in making the wooden shuttles produced a dust, the inhalation of which led to drowsiness in the workmen so that they nearly fell off their benches. A trade-union secretary dispatched pieces of the wood to the Department of Botany in Liverpool University asking Professor Harvey Gibson what it contained to cause such an effect. An alkaloid was discovered in the wood which induced a gradual slowing of the heart-beat. It undoubtedly accounted for the symptoms complained of by the workmen. The condition of these workers was investigated by Hay (1908).

Of the 37 men who had been or were slightly influenced by the wood, 18 complained of headaches, 17 of somnolence, *maziness* or *dofiness*, 14 of running at the nose or a sense of irritation in the nasal passages, 9 of running at the eyes, and in a few instances of the lids being stuck together on awakening in the morning, 6 of sneezing when working the wood, 6 of attacks of coughing, 4 of a sense of tightness across the chest, 3 of some slight dyspnœa, 2 of a loss of appetite, 1 of nausea and vomiting, and 1 of faintness. The men were not all actually suffering from these disabilities when seen by me, but stated that at some time or other they had been so affected when working the South African boxwood (afterwards referred to as the S.A.B.).

It was not at all unusual for men to say that they could taste the wood, that it *clagged up* their throat, and that this was the only thing they noticed.

The headache was of slight intensity and generally of the temporal or frontal type, though it was occasionally occipital or supra-orbital. In some of the men it became evident after one or two hours' work with the S.A.B., whilst in others it only appeared after the wood had been worked two or three days; it persisted while the wood continued to be used and for a day or so longer. In a few instances free watery discharge from the nose relieved the headache.

The somnolence was a very characteristic and common complaint. In the majority of the cases where it was present it was not severe, but in a few it was more troublesome. In fact, one man said he became so sleepy that he could sleep on a clothes line. It usually affected the men after working on the wood for several days, but occasionally it was induced in a much shorter period, i.e. a few hours.

Twenty-three of the men complained of either running of the nose, or of the eyes, or a combination of both. The S.A.B. has very irritating properties, and these are much more noticeable when the mucous membranes are already rendered sensitive by such condition as a coryza, or a bronchitis; for example, 5 men of the 23 said that unless they had a "cold in the head" the S.A.B. did not affect them at all, but given a "cold in the head" it greatly increased the running of the nose, and the cough, etc.

The symptoms resulting from the S.A.B. can be arranged in two groups: (1) those of local irritation, such as running eyes and nose, the congestion of the mucous membrane, and the occasional epistaxis, the cough, and some of the frontal headaches; (2) those of toxæmia resulting from the absorption of the alkaloid present in the dust of the S.A.B. As evidence of this toxæmia we have the somnolence, the headaches, the dyspnœa, expiratory in nature, and the faintness.

In order to deal with this problem Legge (1934) applied local exhaust entilation to the benches of the workmen. This did not entirely suppress he dust, and other types of wood had to be substituted.

Toxic Effects of Iroko

Iroko is a vernacular name and also the British Standard trade name for he wood of *Chlorophora excelsa* Benth. and Hook. f., a tree of East and West Tropical Africa. It has been marketed as African teak or iroko teak, but this designation is incorrect and misleading since the timber is not botanically related to true teak (*Tectona grandis*). Other vernacular names which are used in commerce and may be met with in technical literature re mvule, odum and kambala. Iroko is one of the most widely used utility imbers in Africa and considerable quantities have been exported in recent ears to Europe, where it is used as a substitute for teak. In 1941 Davidson eported an outbreak of allergic dermatitis in men handling a consignment f badly-seasoned iroko logs. The dust from this timber was moister than hat usually associated with more seasoned wood, and tended therefore o adhere more readily to the skin. Of more than fifty men who were ngaged in manipulating this wood in the machine shop nearly all complained of irritation of exposed skin surfaces. Nine complained of more evere symptoms, some within an hour or two of first contact with iroko, ecessitating in the case of three of them complete absence from work for ome weeks and in the others cessation of contact with iroko. The symptoms in these nine cases were more or less alike, but varied in intensity and uration in different individuals. All complained of itching of exposed skin urfaces while some suffered also from intense irritation of covered parts, specially the neck, axillæ, antecubital fossæ, genitalia and backs of the nees. In some cases there was marked œdema of the face with irritation f the conjunctiva and blepharospasm. A few complained of symptoms of cute coryza, with headache and mild pharyngitis, while others complained f chest symptoms—a sense of constriction, retrosternal oppression, dry ugh, and dyspnœa resembling asthma. The symptoms subsided slowly, king up to five weeks to disappear. The affected men were all experienced oodworkers with nothing of note in their previous histories except that two of them had had earlier attacks of dermatitis attributed to teak and had remained sensitive to that wood.

Protection of the Worker against Irritant Woods

Other irritant woods are Oregon pine, East African camphorwood (*Ocotea usambarensis*), balsa wood and coco-bolo, which is made into bowls, handles for cutlery and walking-sticks. Musicians occasionally suffer from dermatitis of the lips from contact with mouthpieces made from grenadilla wood. Cocus wood, or cokus ebony, causes an eczematous eruption both in carpenters who saw it into blocks and in musicians who use flutes made of it. When new woods such as African hardwoods come on to the market, it is proper not only to have samples named by the Forest Products Research Laboratory, Princes Risborough, Bucks., but also to patch-test the skin of the patient with sawdust and shavings. Preventive measures against the harmful effects of toxic woods should include careful attention to dust extraction, the supplying of light-weight respirators, wearing of suitable protective clothing, close-fitting at neck and wrists, and the provision of good washing facilities.

Caterpillar Dermatitis

For perhaps 2,500 years it has been common knowledge that certain caterpillars, especially the hairy ones, can produce a contact dermatitis in man the effects of which are usually trivial. Outbreaks occur from time to time usually in June, when village schoolboys share their finds of caterpillars so plentiful in the hedgerows (Hellier and Warin, 1967). In Europe alone at least 16 species of caterpillar have been responsible for skin eruptions consisting usually of scattered pink papules which may show grouping depending on the main site of contact. The poisonous hairs of the caterpillars are hollow and pierce the skin, injecting some substance as yet unidentified which acts as a primary irritant. Constitutional symptoms have been known to occur from contact with *Megalopyge opercularis* when severe pain, nausea, sweating, headache, fever and shock may arise. Rarely caterpillar hairs involve the eye causing inflammatory changes which at least in one case resulted ultimately in loss of sight. Smith (1966) described the cases of four gardeners who developed dermatitis from the brown tail moth caterpillar (*Euproctis chrysorrhœa*). These caterpillars were on vegetation they were handling, although one of the men had only worked beneath a tree on which there were numerous caterpillars. *Thaumetopœa pinivora*, a caterpillar which feeds on pine trees, has led to outbreaks of severe dermatitis in forest workers in Israel (Katzenellenbogen 1955) and in troops in the Lebanon.

Animal Parasites involving the Skin

Outbreaks of scabies in the camps of soldiers, miners and lumbermen are well known. Prairie camps also can be infested, hence the name *prairie itch*. In soldiers, interdigital burrows are rare and the hands are often quite free from lesions of any kind. Penile lesions are found in the majority of patients, but, rather than suspect syphilis, the doctor must remember that scabies is commonly contracted as a venereal disease. Animal sarcoptes often infest man: burrows are not observed in animal scabies. Victims of the sarcoptes of the horse are either soldiers in mounted units, grooms, coachmen or veterinary students occupied in dissecting horses which have suffered from generalized sarcoptic mange. The sarcoptes of the camel has been transmitted to soldiers in camel corps in Eastern campaigns. Cows with sarcoptic mange can infest farmers and dairymen with the sarcoptes of cattle, hence the name *dairymen's itch*.

Phtheiriasis in Vagrants and Soldiers

Pediculosis corporis is of the highest importance in military campaigns because body lice convey typhus, trench fever and relapsing fever. Happily, impregnation of soldiers' shirts with dicophanum (D.D.T.) is highly effective against this parasite. In tramps and vagrants the combined effects of lice, dirt and constant scratching of the skin give rise to *vagabonds' disease* or phtheiriasis (Greek, φθειριᾶν, louse). The whole of the surface of the body is deeply pigmented, and the epidermis is thickened and covered with scabs and crusts from secondary infection.

Dermatitis caused by Mites

Dermatitis caused by mites is responsible for the names *grain itch*, *barley itch*, *copra itch* and *grocers' itch*. Grain itch occurs in men unloading grain from ships, especially barley and cotton seed. The eruption is caused by *Pediculoides ventricosus*, a parasite which feeds on the grain moth. It attaches itself to man by its claws and apparently introduces an irritant to the skin through its sucking discs. The incubation period is from twelve to sixteen hours. The eruption consists of urticarial wheals, papules, vesicles and pustules on the chest, arms, neck, face and back (fig. 277).

Copra Itch in Dock Workers

Copra itch occurs in dock workers handling copra, the dried kernel of the coconut. The cargo is infested with the mite *Tyroglyphus longior* which transfers itself to the patient and after an incubation period lasting from twenty-four to

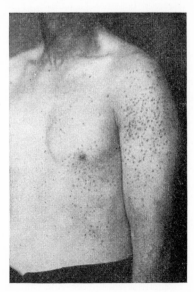

Fig. 277.—Eruption known as Barley Itch in a London Docker

forty-eight hours, gives rise to innumerable intensely itching papules all over the body. This parasite makes no burrow into the skin but dies, leaving its chitinous cover as an irritant. The cheese mite belongs to the same species. It attacks dockers, railway loaders and grocers, hence the name *grocers' itch*.

Mites which attack Grocers

Men handling raw vanilla suffer from an itching eruption thought at one time to be due to a chemical irritant, hence the name *vanillism*. The pruritus has been traced to a mite of the species *Tyroglyphus*. An intensely pruritic skin eruption traced to *Carpoglyphus passularum* in decomposing figs has been named *fig-mite dermatitis*. It affects dock labourers unloading cargoes of figs, and grocers who handle them.

Differential Diagnosis

Long continuance of an alleged occupational dermatitis should make one very suspicious of its cause. The time of onset of symptoms must be ascertained precisely; a skin lesion may be due to the sun during a holiday and not to work. Past treatment must be known, for the present condition may be a dermatitis medicamentosa. Again, the patient may present himself in a phase of urticaria of endogenous origin, or the attack may coincide with a seasonal exacerbation of a long-standing prurigo. If the lesion does not soon heal when the patient is removed from the suspected cause, then the real disease may be an anxiety neurosis with itching as a symptom. Traumatic dermatitis does not recur when the cause is removed and reasonable time has been allowed for it to heal (White, 1934). Cheiro-pompholyx may give rise to difficulty in differential diagnosis. Patients suffering from this condition give a clear history of pinhead irritating water blisters cropping out between the fingers. These lesions may occur in a frail skin, not only as a reaction to chemical substances but also to climatic and emotional stimuli. Certain types of work will increase the severity of an attack of cheiro-pompholyx; water and chemical substances of all kinds will aggravate the irritation, and remorseless scratching will begin, but if it be due to the patient's work, cure on removal will be complete (O'Donovan, 1932).

Treatment

The treatment of occupational dermatitis is largely preventive. It is obviously unwise to employ anyone whose skin shows abnormality. These include young persons and those with frail and thin skins. All persons with hyperidrosis, seborrhœa, xerodermia or a defective peripheral circulation should be rejected. Unfortunately, in certain occupations a moist greasy skin appears to be more easily affected, while a somewhat harsh dry skin remains unaffected, and vice versa.

Periodic Inspection of Exposed Skin

Believing that injury to the skin, whether caused by friction or accidents, is a factor in the production of dermatitis, Bridge (1933) advocated a periodic inspection of exposed parts of the skin so that any injury might be treated. Selection of employees by pre-employment examinations, frequent medical inspections and prompt first-aid treatment are measures of importance in reducing the incidence of occupational dermatitis.

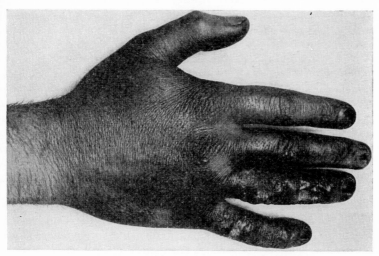

Fig. 278.—Nitric-acid Burn and Argyria in an unskilled workman employed in dissolving Silver in Nitric Acid. He wore a Rubber Glove which was pierced over the Base of the Ring Finger

Instruction in Cleanly Methods of Work

Employees and supervisors should be instructed in the nature of the hazards encountered during work, in cleanly methods of work and how to take care of the skin. Increasing attention to factory hygiene, and particularly to plant design, are of vital importance so as to reduce the chances of irritant materials coming in contact with the skin. Of special preventive measures, the most obvious is protection of the hands by means of gloves. In handling strong acids and alkalis they are essential, but in other operations such as biscuit making, baking, and sugar confectionery, and in certain mechanical operations, they cannot be used.

Improvement of Plant Design

Provision of protective clothing, and carefully chosen barrier creams, are important preventive measures and, although they are often necessary, they should not be relied upon by themselves unless it is impossible to reduce the hazard by improvement of plant design (Jones, 1946). Adequate washing facilities are essential in factories where irritant materials are used,

and it is necessary to stress their strict supervision when once provided
The correct application of barrier substances and the institution of washing
facilities make it possible to eliminate irritant cleansing agents which often
themselves cause skin disease.

Dangers from the Use of Gloves, Boots and Aprons

Protection is not without its own dangers. Rubber gloves may be
pierced and give a false sense of security (fig. 278). It is easy to contaminate
the inside of a glove, and it then holds the harmful substance in close, warm
moist contact with the skin for hours at a stretch. It is necessary to realize
that it takes more trouble and a longer time to teach the worker the proper
use of gloves than to teach a medical student or student nurse an aseptic
habit in donning gloves for use in surgery (O'Donovan, 1952).   A work
man handling mustard gas may burn the skin of his penis for want of
understanding what happens when he touches the outside of his glove a
he removes it to go to the lavatory. Equally, when he comes back he may
introduce the irritant material into the glove. About 1942, patches of
occupational leucodermia were observed on the hands of negro workmen
provided with white rubber gloves. The de-pigmenting agent was
benoquin, the monobenzyl ether of hydroquinone, an antioxidant used
in the processing of the rubber. Sometimes a lathe operator wears a
protective apron with a hole in it and then gets oil folliculitis on the
skin of the abdomen. In wearing rubber high boots, the temperature of
the feet is kept unduly raised so that they may perspire excessively,
causing the skin to become sodden and therefore more liable to disease.

Early Removal from Contact

The early diagnosis of occupational dermatitis is of the utmost im
portance, so that the employed may be removed from contact with the
causative agent. Any other course may lead to intractable skin disease
associated with sensitivity to many agents. In the treatment of the disease
early removal from contact with the irritant substance and protection of
the inflamed skin are cardinal principles. The benefits of rest and hospita
treatment for severe cases are striking. It is sometimes necessary to
transfer the affected person to work not exposing him to risk. Thus
gardener or nurseryman who has shown himself very sensitive to par
ticular plants may be unable ever to work again with these plants.

OCCUPATIONAL STIGMATA

The marks made on the surface of the body in the course of various
occupations include callosities, scars, bursæ, telangiectases, tattoo marks
deformities of the nails, teeth, ears and joints, and colour changes of the
skin and hair. But a man's work may be evident from a simple odour. The
smells speak for themselves and characterize such workers as barmen, fish
porters, fish friers and cheese packers (Ronchese, 1945, 1948).

History

In 1713, in his *De Morbus Artificum Diatriba*, Ramazzini laid stress upon the cutaneous stigmata of a man's trade. His descriptions included the hands of farmers, bricklayers, sailors, bakers and laundry women. Early in the nineteenth century the French clinicians Corvisart, Dupuytren and Trousseau took great pride in announcing the patient's trade or profession at first sight. But in the history of medicine the greatest exponent of stigmata of every sort was Joseph Bell (1837–1911), who emphasized the great value in clinical medicine of taking note of even the slightest peculiarity shown by a patient. In modern times Prosser White (1934) has described in detail the cutaneous stigmata of various occupations.

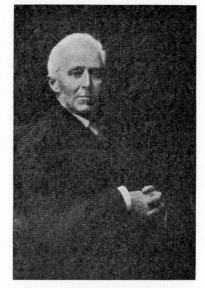

FIG. 279.—Joseph Bell, 1837–1911
(Photograph by Horsburgh

Joseph Bell and Sherlock Holmes

When he was a medical student in Edinburgh, Conan Doyle found the prototype of Sherlock Holmes in his admired chief, Dr. Joseph Bell (fig. 279), whom he served as out-patient clerk. Bell was a surgeon with a wonderful gift of quick perception and rapid deductive reasoning, by which he reached in a flash the truth hidden among tangles. He held that the student must be taught first to observe carefully, and to interest his class in this kind of work he constantly demonstrated how much a practised observer can discover of such matters as the previous history, nationality and occupation of his patient.

> For instance, physiognomy helps you to nationality, accent to district, and, to an educated ear, almost to county. Nearly every handicraft writes its sign-manual on the hands. The scars of the miner differ from those of the quarryman. The carpenter's callosities are not those of the mason. The shoemaker and the tailor are quite different. The soldier and the sailor differ in gait. . . . The subject is endless. The tattoo marks on hand or arm will tell their own tale as to voyages. . . . Carry the same idea of using one's senses accurately and constantly, and you will see that many a surgical case will bring his past history, national, social, and medical, into the consulting-room as the patient walks in.

Joseph Bell describes his Method

Dr. Bell himself related the following incident illustrating his method,

A man walked into the room where I was instructing the students. and his case seemed to be a very simple one. I was talking about what was wrong with him. "Of course, gentlemen," I happened to say, "he has been a soldier in a Highland regiment, and probably a bandsman." I pointed out the swagger in his walk, suggestive of the piper; while his shortness told me that if he had been a soldier it was probably as a bandsman. In fact, he had the whole appearance of a man in one of the Highland regiments. The man turned out to be nothing but a shoe-maker, and said he had never been in the army in his life. This was rather a floorer, but being absolutely certain I was right, and seeing that something was up, I did a pretty cool thing. I told two of the strongest clerks to remove the man to a side room, and to detain him until I came. I went and had him stripped. . . . Under the left breast I instantly detected a little blue "D" branded on his skin. He was a deserter. That was how they used to mark them in the Crimean days and later, although it is not permitted now. Of course, the reason of his evasion was at once clear (Saxby, 1913).

A Student remembers his Clinical Teacher

In 1950 the writer had the privilege to meet in Sydney Dr. Robert Scot Skirving who was in splendid health and practising as a medical consultant at the age of ninety-one. He said that when he was a student in Edinburgh he had often listened to Dr. Joseph Bell who certainly taught in the fashion ascribed to him. He remembered clearly the following case.

A woman with a small child was shown in. Dr. Bell said good morning to her and she said good morning in reply. "What sort of a crossing did ye have fra' Burntisland?" "It was guid." "And had ye a guid walk up Inverleith Row?" "Yes." "And what did ye do with th' other wain?" "I left him with my sister in Leith." "And would ye still be working at the linoleum factory?" "Yes, I am." "You see, gentlemen, when she said good morning to me I noted her Fife accent, and as you know, the nearest town in Fife is Burntisland. You noticed the red clay on the edges of the soles of her shoes, and the only such clay within 20 miles of Edinburgh is in the Botanical Gardens. Inverleith Row borders the gardens and is her nearest way here from Leith. You observed that the coat she carries over her arm is too big for the child who is with her, and therefore she set out from home with two children. Finally she has a dermatitis on the fingers of the right hand which is peculiar to workers in the linoleum factory at Burntisland."

Sherlock Holmes and Dr. Watson

There can be no doubt that this technique inspired some of the more spectacular methods used by Sherlock Holmes, of which the following is an example.

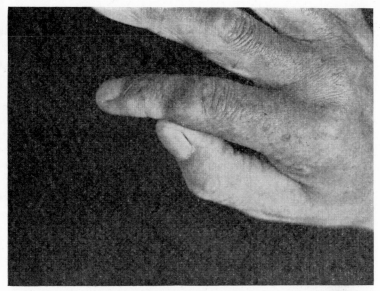

FIG. 280.—Callosity on the Right Forefinger in a Poultry Plucker
(*By courtesy of Dr. A. M. Cooke*)

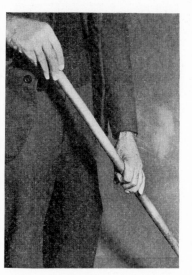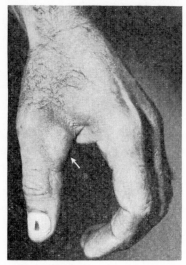

FIG. 281.—Callosity at the Base of the Left Thumb in a Road Sweeper
(*By courtesy of Dr. R. A. J. Asher*)

"But, my dear Holmes, how on earth could you have known that the man was a violinist?" "You know my methods, Watson. Surely you noticed the patch of acneiform dermatitis beneath the angle of the left mandible?"

Callosities on the Hands

Callosities on the hands, especially over the bony prominences of the palm, are common in workmen who use screwdrivers, gimlets, augers and similar instruments. They occur over areas subjected to friction and pressure. In fact, almost every worker who uses a hand tool requiring force in its manipulation develops calluses at the points of greatest pressure. The

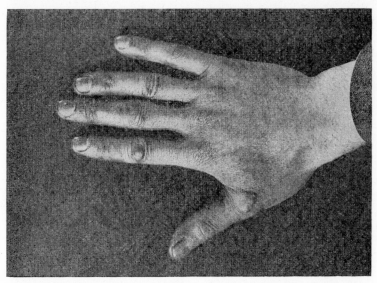

FIG. 282.—Callosities on the Thumb and Fingers in a Tailor's Cutter

areas of hyperkeratosis cause no trouble—in fact, they act as a protection and, in general, the work a man does is facilitated by them and gains in precision. They constitute the trade stigmata of carpenters, cabinet makers, wood machinists, cobblers, painters, varnishers, bakers, locksmiths, furriers, saddlers, poultry pluckers (fig. 280), engravers, ironers, stonemasons, sculptors, weavers, blacksmiths, lamplighters, file cutters, embroiderers, glove makers, photographers, cigarette rollers, acrobats, gymnasts, floor sweepers (fig. 281), stone breakers and lathe workers, and are sometimes described by the men themselves as *segs*.

Distribution of Callosities

They vary slightly in their distribution and may thus be a guide to a man's craft. For example, the cobbler has the palm of the right hand affected owing to the use of the hammer, but the carpenter, in addition to this, has callosities on the thumb and index finger from the use of the plane. Callosities on the thumb and index finger of the right hand occur in tailors and dressmakers from the use of scissors. A single, rounded, well-marked, prominent papilloma on the inner side of the metacarpo-phalangeal joint of the right thumb, and sometimes a thickening of the skin of the middle knuckles of the same hand, form the distinctive marks of the veteran cutter-out in the wholesale fustian trade (fig. 282). These are caused by the pressure and weight of his heavy scissors. The substitution of the electrically driven revolving section knife and the band saw is lessening the frequency and severity of these disfigurements (White, 1934).

Palmar and Interdigital Hyperkeratoses

Interdigital callosities are found in a well-marked form in sugar workers who control the plates of the centrifugal machines used in making cube sugar (Burrows, 1931). In hatters, callosities are found on the thenar eminences and pulps of the fingers from rolling a cylinder with the hands. Deeply indurated calluses are found extending from the thenar and hypothenar eminences to the palmar surfaces of the fingers of felt-hat sizers. In potters the revolving wheel causes horny thickening of the hands. Palmar hyperkeratoses also occur in dry-smokers, who are butchers employed in the removal of the hair from the epidermis of pig carcases. The skin of the fingers and palms of the hands is thickened, the surface being

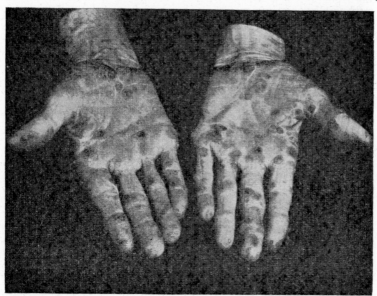

Fig. 283.—Callosities on the Fingers and Palms in a Baker, aged 66, who had baked Bread regularly for 50 years. He could handle Tins much too Hot for a normal Person to hold

(*By courtesy of Dr. D. W. Ryder Richardson*)

indented so numerously with pits and depressions as to give it the appearance of a sponge. It is due to the use of hot water and resin to cause the epidermis to swell and thus to loosen the hairs. The condition disappears when work is abandoned (White, 1934).

Foreign-body Reactions

In certain trades hyperkeratosis of the exposed skin, especially of the fingers, occurs as a foreign-body reaction. It is focal and the warts formed may contain asbestos, cement or fibre-glass according to the work done. Slighter degrees of hyperkeratosis are seen on the tips of the fingers of the left hand in violinists, of both hands in harpists and double bass players, and in the cleft between the finger and thumb in shoemakers and others who habitually pass a strap or cord over this cleft. The span of the hand of pianists, violinists, double-bass players and harpists is more extensive than that of normal persons. Wind-instrument players show a painless, scaly, annular excrescence on the lower lip.

Stigmata affecting the Lower Limbs

Symmetrical, elongated callosities, one in the centre of each shin, occur in house painters and decorators, paper hangers, plasterers, carpenters, electricians, lorry drivers, dustmen and factory-maintenance workers. This distinctive trade stigma results from the continuous pressure of one rung of the ladder on an area practically devoid of subcutaneous fat. Callosities on the thighs occur in men carrying heavy baskets, and in tailors' cutters, packers and bakers, from friction against the bench. Callosities are well known over the patella in people who frequently kneel, on the back of the neck, especially over the seventh cervical spine, in those who carry burdens on their shoulders, and over the upper part of the shoulder and clavicle in bricklayers, stevedores and timber porters. Great thickening of the ball of the foot and heel is seen in those who work barefoot. Waiters, policemen and nurses are liable to flat foot, and ballet dancers and mannequins to

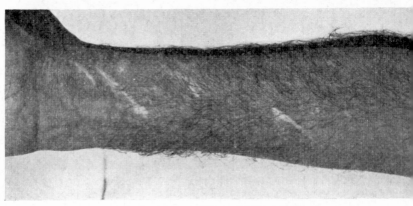

Fig. 284.—Scars of Burns by Liquid Chlorine

pes cavus. Dancers also show shortening and thickening of the tendo
Achillis and callosities on the toes, especially the inner side of the big toe.

Protective Nature of Callosities

The protective nature of callosities on the hands is to be seen in the
case of bakers (fig. 283) and glass blowers. Owing to the constant friction of
the hot blowpipe, which is a length of iron gas piping weighing up to 50 lb.,
and to the use of a mixture of charcoal, pitch and resin to afford a better
grip on its smooth iron surface, these men develop dense callous horny
thickenings on the palms of both hands, more markedly on the left. Many
glass blowers suffer intensely while acquiring the protection of their callosities; once having done so, they are often able to hold live coals without
injury. If they are out of work they may endeavour to keep their hands in
working condition by rolling some object, such as a broom handle, between
the palms or even by pickling the hands in a solution of salt and vinegar.
They do this in order that their hands may not become raw and painful on
resuming work (Kessler, 1931).

Tattoo Marks and Livedo Reticularis

Sometimes tattoo marks are occupational signs. A hammer may indicate a carpenter and a razor a barber. The sailor is liable to be tattooed
with warships, flags, knots and naked women. Telangiectases of the exposed

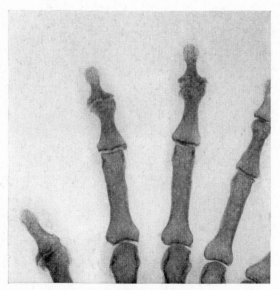

Fig. 285.—Osteo-arthritis of the Fingers in a Dress-
maker aged 65 years. The Condition was of 4 years'
Duration. The terminal Interphalangeal Joints of the
Thumb, Index and Middle Fingers are affected

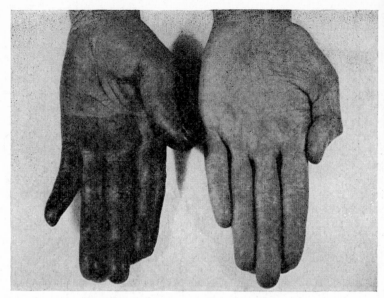

FIG. 286.—Dark brown staining of the Nails and Fingers by Metol in a
Photographer

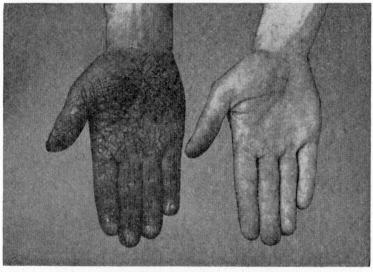

FIG. 287.—Bright red Staining, Thickening and Fissuring of the Skin by Madder
in an Artist's Colour Maker

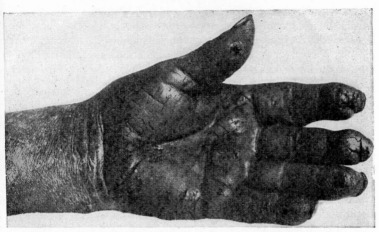

FIG. 288.—Hand of a Galvanizer showing Staining, Thickening, Fissuring and Ulceration of the Skin. In Degreasing, Pickling, Scouring and Plating Metals many Chemical Substances are used. They include Soap, Lime, Potassium Cyanide, strong solutions of Hydrochloric Acid and Nitric Acid and hot aqueous solutions of Potassium Hydroxide

skin develop in farmers, sailors and fishermen. Erythema ab igne giving place to livedo reticularis is a stigma of work done in front of furnaces and other sources of heat by steel workers, foundrymen, optical-glass moulders, attendants of large boilers and others.

Scars of Burns

The casting burns on the dorsum of the foot are examples of stigmata in the foundry worker, and scars of burns are seen on the arms of linotype apprentices and on the feet of the stereotype worker. These are due to the splashings of the molten type-metal and are acquired when they drop the old type and plates into the melting-pot to be refounded. Scars on the hands and forearms are common in chemical-works' labourers. They result from caustic substances such as sodium hydroxide, silver nitrate and liquid chlorine (fig. 284). In spite of gloves and other protective clothing the optical-glass moulder repeatedly burns the knuckles of his hands, the skin of his upper arm and also the dorsa of his feet.

Osteo-arthritis

The constant carrying of heavy loads on the back in dock-labourers and coal-heavers may lead in those so predisposed to osteo-arthritic spondylitis, *labourers' spine*. Veteran tailors, seamstresses and curriers may develop osteo-arthritis in certain digits of the right hand. In tailors both inter-phalangeal joints of the index finger are affected, in seamstresses the corresponding joints of both the index and middle fingers, and in curriers the inter-phalangeal joint of the thumb. After many years the joints show deformity and limitation of movement, and in radiographs (Scott, 1935) the well-known characteristics of osteo-arthritis, including the splayed-out appearance of the base of the terminal phalanx known as Heberden's nodes (fig. 285). Many of these deformities will soon be of historical interest only, owing to the introduction of basting machines in the tailoring trade and of machine methods in place of the shaving-knife of curriers.

Dupuytren's Contracture

Although minor forms of Dupuytren's contracture have been described in upholsterers and oarsmen, there is no sound evidence that occupation or injury has any bearing on the development of this condition. Smith and Masters (1939) investigated 536 men who had worked from two to twenty years in the upholstering trade. The work requires unusual friction and pressure on both palms and yet only 1·1 per cent had Dupuytren's contracture, an incidence no greater than might be expected in any other group of men.

Staining of the Finger-nails and Hands

In 1900 Heller described as occupational stigmata green nails in pea-shellers, red nails in vineyard workers and black nails in feltmakers. At a glance the dark brown staining of the nails and fingers by metol betrays the photographer (fig. 286). In coffee roasters and burnt-sugar workers the

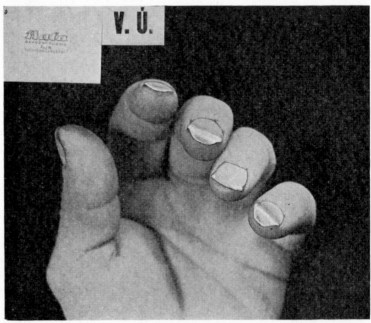

Fig. 289.—Horizontal Angular Deformity of Finger-nails in a man who had been wearing Rubber Gloves which were too small

(*By courtesy of Dr. Jan Roubal*)

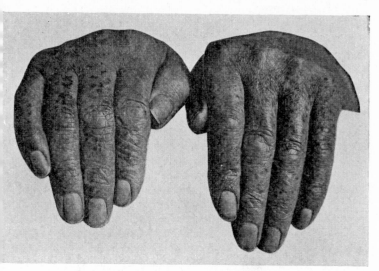

Fig. 290.—Dark blue pigmented scars on the fingers of a millstone dresser due to fine steel chippings which have entered the skin

in of the hands and the nails assume a light brown tint, and in men andling chromates and bichromates they are pale yellow. The shoemaker, ie shoeblack and the man who manufactures silver nitrate have their nails :ained black. Dyers and colour grinders have their hands and nails pig-iented with the various different colours they handle (fig. 287). In occu-ations in which the hands are immersed in brine, leuconychia in the form f white spots may occur. The staining and other changes in the skin and nger-nails of galvanizers (fig. 288) arise in the handling of soap, lime, otassium cyanide and strong acids and alkalis. Furniture polishers show hiny worn-out nails with a reddish discoloration. In men fashioning gold, ilver or aluminium articles, the metal is found under the finger-nails.

Mutilation of the Finger-nails by Trauma

In many trades the nails become mutilated by trauma. This accounts or saw bites, wheel and gear crushes, knife chopping, needle punctures nd chemical burns. File makers and men who use grinding wheels and isks wear down their finger-nails unevenly. In watch and clock makers the ight thumb-nail is short, hard and hypertrophied, from the constant open-ng of watches. The thumb-nails of optical-glass workers become worn way in the shape of a crescent on the lateral edge from picking day by day undreds of glasses from their pitch bed. Girls in munition works who emove cartridges from metal racks show attrition of the lateral free edges f the nails of the third and fourth fingers of each hand. Men wearing ubber gloves which are too small may show horizontal angular deformity f the nails (fig. 289).

Colour Changes of the Skin

Colour changes of the skin sometimes characterize an occupatio. Dyers have their hands pigmented with various different dyestuffs. Th magenta worker not only stains his own clothes, but leaves his trace on th household linen and upholstery. Men handling trinitrotoluene and dinitr benzene show yellow skin, and the skin of the tetryl worker is the colo of apricot. The light-yellow hue of the picric-acid worker is characteristi Those who repeatedly handle tar and asphalt, and workers engaged in th impregnation of railway sleepers with creosote, develop dark brown pi mentation of the exposed skin. Ichthyol turns the skin green, and cadmiu salts turn it black. Indelible blue-black scars occur on the face, arm and trunk of the collier, who works stripped to the waist and soils ever wound with coal dust. The callosities on the feet of stokers may be ta tooed in the same way. Pigmented scars may be seen on the hands, fore arms and faces of iron-stone miners, tin miners, gold miners, millston dressers (fig. 290) and chimney sweeps. Certain employees who chisel th hard steel rollers in flour mills show numerous dark blue spots on th backs of the hands and fingers, due to the fine steel chippings whic have entered the skin and become oxidized. The skin of the hands o workmen who file dinner forks may become tattooed with silver (p. 419)

Stigmata affecting the Hair

A tonsural bald area is commonly seen in Covent Garden porter who carry baskets of fruit on their heads (fig. 291). Exposure to chlorin

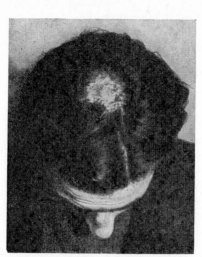

FIG. 291.—Tonsural bald area in a Covent Garden Market Porter

bleaches the hair of the scal and beard. In munition workers trinitrotoluene and dinitroben zene cause bronze-tinted hai picric acid tints the hair olive green in fair people and lea ferrocyanide turns it a reddis colour. In copper smelters burnishers and filers, powdere copper dyes the hair and bear dark green.

Stigmata affecting the Pinn

Gross deformities of the ears commonly known as *cauliflowe ears*, are seen in boxers, wrestler and Rugby football players. The are due to repeated blows an they often begin as a painfu hæmatoma. In a boxer the left ea one is usually affected (fig. 292), the blows causing the deformity being delivered by the opponent's right fist. In addition the nose may be flattened, the eyebrows scarred, the cornea opaque and one or both thumbs dislocated. In wrestlers and Rugby football players both ears are commonly affected. Meat porters who have worked in the cold-storage rooms of Smithfield market and the corresponding dock labourers may show swelling and deformity of the upper part of the pinna on both sides, due to trauma and intense cold which results from continually carrying quarters of frozen beef over the shoulder (Hamill, 1935).

Staining and Abrasion of the Teeth

Workers in copper show teeth which are stained dark green, and those handling cadmium may show a yellow ring on the teeth. Silver produces a greyish-brown stain and nickel a greenish-black stain. Modifications of the teeth by abrasion occur

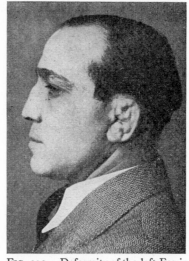

Fig. 292.—Deformity of the left Ear in a professional Boxer

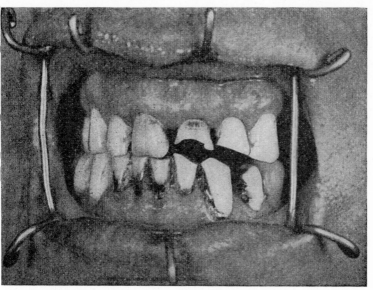

Fig. 293.—Abrasion of Teeth in an Upholsterer who held Iron Nails in his Mouth throughout 12 years

in shoemakers, upholsterers (fig. 293), glass blowers, dress designers, dress makers and seamstresses. They result from holding between the teeth nails, tacks, needles, glass tubes and threads reinforced by metals. The cobbler holds a ready supply of nails, thirty or so, in his mouth and serves them out with his teeth, and the upholsterer does the same with tacks. Hatters' furriers handling nitric acid and mercury in the carroting of rabbit fur show blackening of the enamel of their teeth. Such teeth as remain, generally the lower incisors and canines, show erosion of their cutting edges (Legge, 1934).

Erosion of the Teeth by Acids and Alkalis

Chemical substances attacking the teeth include citric acid, tartaric acid (Elsbury and others, 1951), hydrochloric acid, nitric acid, sulphuric acid, chlorine, chloride of lime and sodium carbonate. In the manufacture of guncotton, workers who dip cotton waste into acid baths are liable to lose the crowns of the mandibular incisors and the cutting edges of the maxillary incisors. Rarely are the canines involved. The chemical substances concerned are sulphuric acid, nitric acid, nitrogen dioxide and nitrogen peroxide (Lynch and Bell, 1947). A similar condition is seen in workers in the forming-rooms of electric-accumulator factories, where a sulphuric-acid mist is produced by the charging process (see p. 592). Whatever the acid concerned, the erosion begins in the incisal third of the teeth and extends on to the labial surface. There is no pitting but always a smooth polished appearance. When the enamel has been destroyed, the dentine is attacked and the pulp chamber shrinks. The condition is quite painless, except in rare cases where the erosion is so rapid that bacterial invasion of the pulp chamber occurs.

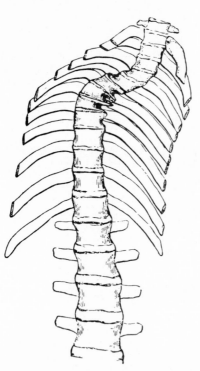

FIG. 294.—Constant carrying of an Excessive Load on the Right Shoulder has caused Scoliosis of the Thoracic Spine with the convexity to the right
(*Lane, W. A.* (1885), *Guy's Hosp. Rep.*, **63**, *321*)

Stigmata affecting the Trunk

When the Industrial Revolution forced upon children and young persons long hours of work

nd the carrying of heavy burdens, postural deformities of the spine were
ommon. In those cases where malnutrition led to rickets the deformities
ere even worse and the limbs were affected too. In 1885 Arbuthnot
ane made detailed investigations of the effects of faulty posture and
howed that the constant bearing of an excessive load on one shoulder
aused scoliosis of the thoracic spine with the convexity to the same
de (fig. 294). Industry is not yet innocent in this respect. In the
ata boot factory at Zlin in Czechoslovakia, Roubal (1947) has described
he work of men who weld the upper to the sole with a special form
f pliers (fig. 295). All day long they perform a twisting movement with
he hand and trunk, and gradually they develop a scoliosis of the thoracic
pine which is present not only in the working position (fig. 296) but
ersists in the erect posture (fig. 297).

OCCUPATIONAL BURSITIS

Chronic bursitis is one of the oldest occupational disabilities known.

Etiology and Pathology

It occurs in those whose work involves pressure, friction or repeated
ight blows over a bursa. Increase of fluid then occurs in the bursal
ac and a local swelling results. The olecranon bursa may be affected in
tudents, bricklayers and miners (miners' elbow), the ischial bursa in
ghtermen, coachmen and weavers (weavers' bottom), the pre-patellar bursa
n housemaids (housemaids' knee), potmen, clergymen and nuns (nuns'
ursitis), and the subacromial bursa
n bricklayers (hodmens' shoulder).
Connective tissue has the capacity
o produce new bursæ if they are
equired on account of oft-repeated
ut unusual types of movement in
he body. Such adventitious bursæ
nay be found over the vertex in
narket-garden   porters   (Covent
Garden hummy), over the seventh
ervical spine in timber porters
humpers' lump) and in fish porters
Billingsgate hump) (fig. 298), over
he upper part of the shoulder and
lavicle in bricklayers, dustmen
dustmen's shoulder) and timber
orters (deal-runners' shoulder),
nd over the external malleolus in
ailors (tailors' ankle).

Symptoms and Signs

Chronic bursitis usually pro-
uces a slowly enlarging, painless

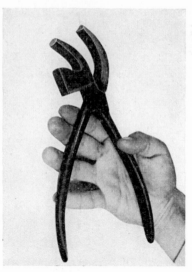

FIG. 295.—Special form of Pliers used
in the Bata Works to weld the Upper
to the Sole of the Boot
(By courtesy of Dr. Jan Roubal)

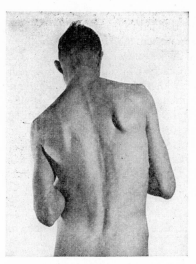 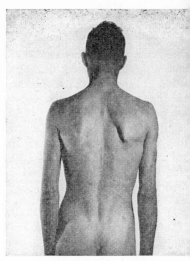

Fig. 296.—Boot Welder in Position adopted while using the Pliers

Fig. 297.—Scoliosis persists in the Erect Posture after Work is over

(By courtesy of Dr. Jan Roubal)

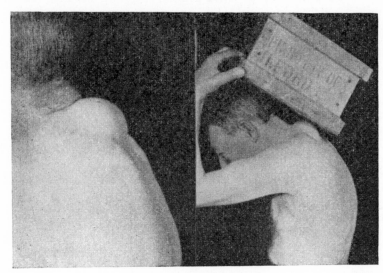

Fig. 298.—Fibro-lipomatous Adventitious Bursa over Lower Cervical Spine (Billingsgate Hump) in a London Fish Porter

(By courtesy of Dr. R. A. J. Asher)

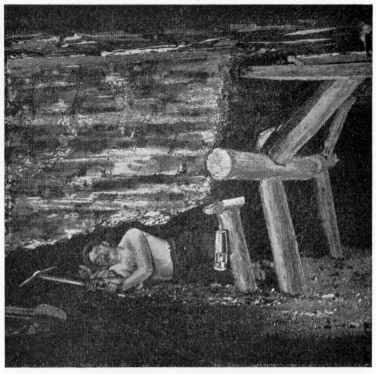

Fig. 299.—Coal Miner bottom-holing or under-cutting by Hand in a thick Seam
(*By courtesy of Professor I. C. F. Statham*)

swelling, and the patient seldom pays much attention to it unless some complication occurs. Contusion of a bursa already distended with fluid may cause either a sudden increase of fluid or bleeding into the sac. In either case there is an acute increase in swelling, accompanied by pain. Where pyogenic infection of a bursa occurs, there is increased swelling accompanied by redness of the overlying skin and acute pain. In some cases of chronic bursitis, a portion of the sac wall may become calcified and then pain is likely to be persistent.

Treatment

A patient with chronic bursitis seldom seeks treatment unless the bursa becomes painful or its size makes it inconvenient or unsightly. Fluid may be aspirated from the distended sac although it usually returns within a few days. When there is an acute infection, incision into the sac with drainage may be indicated. When chronic bursitis continues to be annoying, excision of the sac may be necessary. However, it must be remembered that with the removal of the bursa the normal protection to the underlying bony prominence has also been removed.

The Beat Disorders of Miners

The greatest sufferer from bursitis is the coal miner, who is liable to the so-called beat disorders.

Ætiology and Pathology

The man who works at the coal face is known as the coal-getter. He undercuts the seam of coal by a process known as bottom-holing, in which he lies on his side with his head thrown back and cuts the coal with horizontal swing of the pick (fig. 299). Owing to the constrained attitude necessarily adopted, there is pressure on certain points, and the bursæ over the patella and the olecranon may become enlarged and the surrounding fasciæ thickened. Where mining is mechanized, continued kneeling may be necessary, especially in districts where the seam at the coal face is only 2 feet thick. Thus the highest incidence of beat knee is in cuttermen, prop drawers and conveyer-turners, who have to move about the coal face on their knees (Atkins and Marks, 1952).

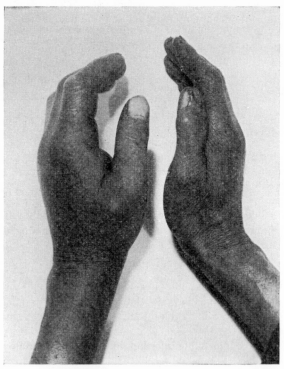

Fig. 300.—Miners' Beat Hand. From the Palm of the left Hand Subcutaneous Cellulitis has spread to the Dorsum, hence the Swelling

(By courtesy of Professor R. C. Browne)

ubcutaneous Cellulitis and Acute Bursitis

The bursæ are liable to get infected, and for this reason the Industrial njuries Act recognizes two types of beat disorder—subcutaneous cellulitis nd acute bursitis. The lesions are legally defined as subcutaneous cellulitis r acute bursitis over the elbow (beat elbow), and subcutaneous cellulitis r acute bursitis arising at or about the knee (beat knee). The subcutaneous ssues of the hands may become thickened owing to the pressure of the ick. Infection of these tissues gives rise to subcutaneous cellulitis of the and (beat hand). Thus the ætiology of beat hand, which is always a ellulitis, differs from that of beat knee and beat elbow (fig. 300). Beat and is not confined to miners; firemen stoking boilers, especially in hips, may suffer from subcutaneous cellulitis of the hand. In the beat isorders, cellulitis commonly arises from the extension of a staphylo-occus infection of a hair follicle into the adjacent subcutaneous tissue. It s unusual to find a cut or abrasion which has afforded entry to the infecting rganism (Atkins and Marks, 1952).

ymptoms and Signs

The symptoms and signs are redness, swelling, heat and pain. At first he skin is unbroken but pits easily (fig. 301). Generally, suppuration ccurs with or without involvement of the adjoining bursæ or tendon heaths. In the case of the knee or elbow the course of the disease is usually enign and without sequelæ, the patient being well in six weeks or even ss. On the contrary, in the case of the hand the infection may involve the ndon sheaths and cause serious disability, sometimes with permanent

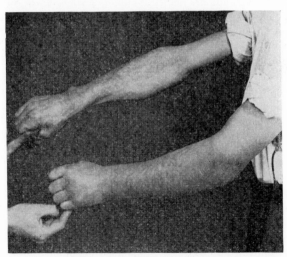

Fig. 301.—Miners' Beat Hand, the same case as in fig. 300. The Subcutaneous Cellulitis has caused considerable Swelling of the Dorsum of the Hand and of the Forearm to the Elbow

(By courtesy of Professor R. C. Browne)

maiming. It follows that an important aim in treatment must be to secu
free movement of the wrist and fingers.

Preventive Treatment

Since the report of Collis and Llewellyn (1924) the incidence of tl
beat disorders in coal miners has increased more than tenfold. Although
was hoped that the increasing use in coal mines of machine cutters wou
greatly reduce the incidence of these conditions, the contrary has occurre
partly because the new methods of mining involve more kneeling. In tl
coalmines of Great Britain the use of knee-pads to reduce trauma, althoug
widespread, has failed to stop the steady increase in the incidence of be
knee. It is probable that pads increase the liability to follicular infectic
because of maceration of the skin beneath them. Coal particles inevitab
accumulate under the pads and reduce protection against trauma. Tl
application of hardening agents to the skin is of doubtful benefit. Supe
vision of men at risk, and especially of those adjudged susceptible, in ord
to detect and treat infection while it is still confined to the neighbourhoc
of the follicle, offers perhaps the most practical approach to the probler
An important therapeutic measure in most cases is temporary transfer
work where there is no kneeling to do.

TRAUMATIC TENOSYNOVITIS

Traumatic tenosynovitis was first observed by Velpeau in 1818, a
was later described by him in his *Anatomie Chirurgicale*, publishedin182
It was noted as early as 1841 that the lesion may lie outside the tendc
sheath, and French authors named it *cellulite peritendineuse*. Troell (191
confirmed these observations and suggested the name *peritendinitis crep
tans*, citing areas such as the tendo Achillis and triceps brachialis whe
tenosynovitis occurs but in which no tendon sheath is present. The loc
histology has been studied by Howard (1937) from biopsy material ol
tained from four acute cases involving the radial extensors at the wrist. I
found both tendon and tendon sheath normal to the naked eye, but tl
musculo-tendinous junction showed a clear jelly-like œdema with dar
coloured muscle exhibiting glycogen depletion and retention of lactic ac
suggesting muscle fatigue and exhaustion. Histological examination r
vealed muscle-fibre destruction with interstitial hæmorrhage and fibr
deposits, which evidently explain the crepitus.

Exposure Hazards

Traumatic tenosynovitis is a frequent cause of incapacity in vario
occupations. As a rule it is due to the constant repetition of stereotype
movements, especially those which involve a grasp between thumb an
fingers accompanied by a quick pronation-supination movement of tl
forearm. Carpenters, upholsterers, linoleum fitters and others who hamm
innumerable nails all day are often affected, as also are tea, tobacco an
food packers and others who repeatedly open and close the lids of box

Blood, 1942). Typists, comptometer workers and sewing-machine operators are liable to the disorder, and so are workers in the motor-car industry
whose job is filing, or assembly work, especially where a spanner is used.
Agricultural workers and gardeners can be affected, especially if they use a
sickle, and the same is true of cane cutters.

Mowers, Hoppers and Harvesters

Employees who have recently returned from holiday or sick-leave are
particularly vulnerable, as are new-comers to a repetitive job—for example,
sedentary workers put to prolonged rowing, soldiers put on to weeding or
harvesting or townsfolk to hop-picking. In the hop gardens of Kent, where
tens of thousands of Londoners are employed as pickers in August and
September, the lesion of traumatic tenosynovitis is known by the erroneous
name *hoppers' gout* or *hop gout* (Smithies, 1929). In 1926 in one section of
these gardens, eighty-seven cases occurred among 25,000 pickers. The
patient complains of pain, limitation of movement and swelling, of fairly
rapid onset. It may occur in the fingers, hand, wrist or forearm and is
unilateral, affecting the right upper limb in right-handed subjects and the
left in those who are left-handed. Although children work in the hop
gardens in large numbers, they are affected only rarely. The swelling, which
is tender, red and tense, corresponds to groups of tendon sheaths. On palpation a fine crepitation is felt like the crunching of crisp snow. After complete rest for a few days all abnormality disappears.

Netting made by Machines

Smiley (1951) has described tenosynovitis in braiders employed by the
Belfast Ropeworks Ltd. This is a modern works which produces not only
ropes with circumferences varying from half an inch to 28 inches, but also
threads, twines and cords of an infinite variety. It has been estimated that
this works has manufactured over half a million different types of product.
It makes netting, including simple netting for tennis courts and also the
more complicated fishing-net which is required in large quantities. Since
the eighteenth century attempts have been made to invent a machine
which could mechanize the process, but success has been only partial. In
1802 the French Government offered a reward of 10,000 francs for a
machine to make netting automatically. Jaquard submitted a model, and
was summoned to Paris by Napoleon who asked: "Are you the man who
pretends to do what God Almighty cannot do—tie a knot in a stretched
string?"

Netting made by Hand

A satisfactory machine is now in operation which can make nets rectangular in shape, but the bulk of netting required is not rectangular, and
the alteration of these rectangles to the required shape and size by tailoring
has proved unsatisfactory. As a result about 300 women and girls are still
engaged in the ancient craft of braiding. While they work, conversation is
impossible, for the shape of the net is determined by the number of meshes

which each worker must therefore count as she braids. On entering a braid
ing room it is impressive to see some hundreds of women standing o
sitting, facing the wall and working in silence. As the net lengthens, i
order to maintain tension, the braider sits on a stool, but after furthe
lengthening she must stand in order to rearrange the net on the steel bar t
which it is fixed. Thus the braider spends her whole working day alter
nately standing or squatting on the stool (fig. 302). The speed at which th
wooden needle moves in the hands of an experienced worker is very grea

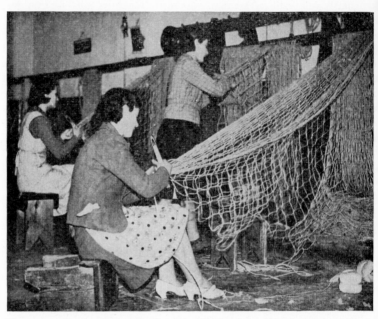

Fig. 302.—The Ancient Craft of braiding Fishing Nets. The Speed of the Work
is very great and the Dexterity gained in a series of complicated Actions of
Flexion, Extension, Pronation and Supination at the Wrist Joint, together with
Flexion and Extension of the Fingers, must be seen to be believed
(*Smiley, J. A.* (*1951*), *Brit· J. industr. Med.*, **8**, *265*)

and varies to some extent according to the material used, but fifty t
seventy meshes per minute is a common rate. The dexterity gained in
series of complicated actions of flexion, extension, pronation and supina
tion at the wrist joint, together with flexion and extension of the fingers
must be seen to be believed. As a result tenosynovitis is common and ma
be regarded as the occupational hazard of the braider.

Braiders of Experience Affected

The condition seldom or never develops in the trainee worker becaus
speed and efficiency develop together rather slowly. Those affected ar
women of experience, who for domestic or other reasons have left th
industry for a time and, returning, attempt to achieve their former speeds

here is also an increase in the incidence of the condition beginning three to five days after the summer holiday. Here the younger workers are just as susceptible as the older. The hand which holds the needle is the one affected. Almost any of the extensor tendons may be involved, but those most commonly affected are the abductor pollicis longus, the extensor pollicis brevis, the radial extensors at the wrist (extensor carpi radialis longior and brevior) and the brachioradialis (supinator longus). These are the common lesions in factory workers in general. Thus Thompson and others (1951) found the tendons of the first four muscles mentioned above to be involved in 77 per cent of a series of 544 patients, most of whom were employed in the manufacture of motor cars.

Factors in the Ætiology

Analysing the ætiology in their series of cases these authors found that five main factors were concerned. In 27 per cent there had been some change of occupation necessitating unaccustomed work; in 21 per cent a return to work after absence; in 15 per cent local strain either single or repetitive; in 13 per cent direct local blunt trauma; and in 10 per cent simple repetitive stereotyped movement associated with intense effort and speed. In 14 per cent of their cases they were unable to find the cause.

Symptoms and Signs

The ulnar extensors of the wrist and the flexors of the wrist and fingers are occasionally affected. Sometimes the peroneal tendons and the extensors and flexors of the toes are involved. The condition is rarely bilateral. There is aching pain, slight fusiform swelling and sometimes local redness and heat without pyrexia. Where the radial extensors of the wrist are affected, the swelling is from 4 to 12 centimetres proximal to the radial styloid in the back of the forearm and well above the upper limit of the tendon sheaths of the wrist. This coincides with the musculo-tendinous junction where, indeed, the actual site of the lesion appears to be. In some cases the tenderness extends well up the forearm into the muscle bellies. Washleather creaking is present and may extend up the forearm almost to the elbow. Crepitus is both palpable and readily audible by stethoscope. During recovery it often disappears before the local swelling and tenderness have subsided.

Treatment

Whatever local treatment is used, rest is essential. Partial immobilization gives better results than rigid immobilization in plaster of Paris. Local heat treatment, especially by short-wave therapy, hastens recovery. Perspex splinting is effective, yielding a relapse rate of 6 per cent and an average recovery period of just over twelve days (Thompson and others, 1951). The detachable perspex splint is heat mouldable, light in weight, clean, impervious to oil and water, and it allows slight movement. Being readily detached, it allows early passive movements to be given every other day.

The splint may be discarded gradually over several days. Some patient
can continue to do their normal work while under treatment, others mus
be given selected work. The prognosis is good, and a patient who has full
recovered seldom relapses on returning to his usual work.

OCCUPATIONAL CANCER

It has long been known that workmen in certain occupations are unduly
liable to develop cancer. Further study has shown that the disease is caused
by prolonged exposure to some substance used in the particular occupation
and that the type of tumour produced is specific for that occupation. The
subject of occupational carcinogenesis in all its aspects has been ably
reviewed by Goldblatt and Goldblatt (1956). They discuss chromium
arsenic, nickel, asbestos, the aromatic amines, beryllium, soot, tar, pitch
and mineral oil.

Clinical Features

Compared with cancer of unknown origin, occupational cancer is a
relatively rare condition, but it is nevertheless interesting and important
The various types of occupational cancer have several characteristic
features in common. They appear only after long exposure in the related
occupation. This latent period varies somewhat, but is usually from ten to
twenty-five years. Workmen who have been exposed for a sufficiently long
period are liable to develop a tumour many years after leaving their work
Their removal from the occupation is therefore no safeguard against the
disease. The average age incidence is earlier than that for cancer in general
and is dependent upon the age at which the men enter the occupation
and on the latent period necessary for the tumour to develop. The
disease is almost invariably pre-
ceded by well-defined precancer-
ous lesions, which are characteristic for each particular occupation
The localization and to a less
extent the histological nature of
the tumours are remarkably constant in any one occupation. Unlike ordinary forms of cancer, the
tumours are frequently multiple.

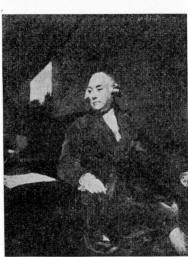

FIG. 303.—Percivall Pott, 1713–88
(*After the portrait by Reynolds*)

History

It is possible that the study of
occupational cancer has led to
greater advances in our knowledge
of the causation and prevention
of tumour formation than any
other line of inquiry. It is true to
say that the sufferings of victims
of occupational cancer initiated

e onslaught on the problem of cancer by chemical technique. Histori-
lly, the study of occupational cancer was begun by Percivall Pott in
'75 (fig. 303), when he drew attention to soot as a cause of scrotal
ncer, and by Butlin in 1892, who showed that pitch, tar and mineral
l similarly affected the same site. In 1915 Yamagiwa and Ichikawa
oduced cancer experimentally by painting the ears of rabbits with coal-
r. In 1922 Leitch produced experimental tumours in mice by applying
:ottish shale-oil to the skin.

hemical Carcinogenesis

Investigation naturally shifted to the chemical identification of the sub-
ance responsible. The application of fluorescence spectroscopy to the
udy of carcinogenic substances proved to be the indispensable technique
hich led to success (fig. 304). Sir Ernest Kennaway became the inspired
ider of a team which discovered the first cancer-producing hydrocarbon
2 : 5 : 6-dibenzanthracene, and then tracked down and isolated 3 : 4-

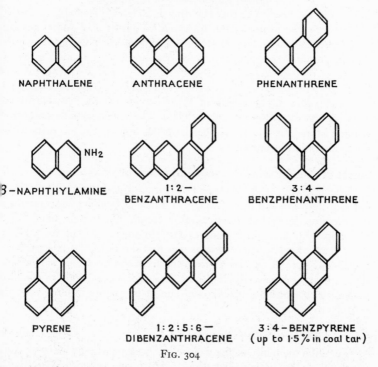

CHEMICAL CARCINOGENESIS
THE POLYCYCLIC HYDROCARBONS

NAPHTHALENE   ANTHRACENE   PHENANTHRENE

β-NAPHTHYLAMINE   1 : 2 —   3 : 4 —
                    BENZANTHRACENE   BENZPHENANTHRENE

PYRENE   1 : 2 : 5 : 6 —   3 : 4 – BENZPYRENE
           DIBENZANTHRACENE   (up to 1·5 % in coal tar)

Fig. 304

nzpyrene from pitch (Kennaway, 1924, 1925; Kennaway and Hieger,
30). Research was then set going on the synthesis and testing of the
drocarbons which were chemical variations of dibenzanthracene. Ben-

zene rings were added and subtracted, alkyl groups were substituted different positions in the nucleus, hexagon rings were replaced by pent gon rings, C was substituted by N and by S, and as a result of all th activity the number of compounds which have been tested for carcinogen activity must now be counted in thousands. In 1943 Berenblum an Schoental isolated 3:4-benzpyrene from Scottish shale oil. The subject chemical carcinogenesis has been reviewed by Hieger (1949).

(a) Cancer of the Lung

The industries concerned in causing or possibly causing cases of canc of the lung are uranium mining at Schneeberg and Jáchymov, the nick industry, the chromate industry, the asbestos industry and the man facture of sheep dip.

Silicosis and Cancer of the Lung in the Schneeberg Miners

In 1531 Paracelsus described the *mala metallorum*, a malady of t lungs which attacked and killed in the prime of life the Schneeberg mine of the Erzgebirge or Ore Mountains which separate Saxony and Bohem In 1556 Agricola ascribed the disease to the inhalation of dust and it w only some 300 years later that Haerting and Hesse (1879) showed the co dition to be due to malignant disease of the lungs. The tumours were first considered to be lymphosarcomata, but have since been shown to true carcinomata arising probably in the bronchi (Schmorl, 1928). T disease of the Schneeberg miners is frequently associated with silicosis condition which is readily detectable during life by X-ray examination a which precedes the development of the carcinoma but by itself produc surprisingly few symptoms (plate XIII). The miners usually suffer from chronic bronchitis which may persist for as long as twenty years witho much alteration in intensity.

Onset of Cancer with Dyspnœa and Loss of Weight

The subsequent development of carcinoma manifests itself by t onset of dyspnœa and loss of weight. Phthisis is relatively uncommon a can therefore be excluded as a causative factor. The tumour tends to gr more slowly than ordinary lung cancer, the men surviving for periods three years or more from the time it is first noticed. This is attributed the altered state of the tissues resulting from the preceding silicosis. T tumours are occasionally multiple (Schmorl, 1928); they commo invade the surrounding tissues and almost invariably produce second growths in other organs.

High Incidence of the Disease

The high incidence of the disease has been proved by an investigati which took place between 1922 and 1926, during which time twenty-c out of 154 miners died and fifteen of these deaths were due to lung can (Rostoski, 1926). In two cases the carcinoma developed ten and sevente years respectively after the men had given up the occupation of mining.

cases of lung cancer were observed among 362 members of the non-mining population of the district. Since 1926 further cases have been reported. The total number of fatalities from lung cancer among Schneeberg miners between 1869 and 1939 was at least 400 (Hueper, 1942). The Schneeberg mines have been worked since the fifteenth century; at first for copper and iron, later for silver and other minerals, and now solely for bismuth, arsenic and cobalt. The dust produced in the drilling of the hard rock is radioactive and is composed of minute particles containing 0·45 per cent arsenic. The air in the mines has been shown to be radioactive.

Cancer of the Lung in the Jáchymov Uranium Miners

On the Bohemian side of the Erzgebirge are the uranium mines of Jáchymov (Joachimstal), made famous in 1898 by Madame Curie when she isolated radium and polonium from the pitchblende found there. Radium chloride is obtained from pitchblende after the extraction of uranium and other bases. Uranium is itself radioactive. Whether arsenic, radium, or cobalt is the carcinogenic agent is at present an unsolved problem but, of course, great suspicion rests upon radium. From a study of data that had been published previously by others, Evans and Goodman (1940) calculated the average radon concentration in the mines of Jáchymov and Schneeberg to be 2,900 pc. per litre. In the review by Lorenz (1944) of available data for these areas reference was made to 336 deaths from lung cancer occurring between 1875 and 1939. This figure represents 43 per cent of all miner deaths. The average duration of underground or radium factory exposure of nine cases from Jáchymov, as described by Pirchan and Sikl (1932), was 17 years (range 13–23); the time between the beginning of work in the mines and death from cancer was from 15 to 43 years (average 25 years); the age at death ranged between 40 and 67 years (average 50 years). The average age at death of 13 cases from Schneeberg described by Rostoski and others (after Lorenz, 1944) was 55 years (range 47–69 years). The commonest histological finding is oat-celled carcinoma of the lung.

Uranium Mines of the Colorado Plateau

In 1950 the U.S. Public Health Service started a survey among the uranium miners of the Colorado Plateau and found an increased incidence of lung cancer (Wagoner and others, 1964). This increase has been attributed to airborne radiation, principally from the radioactive daughter products of radon, but, as in Europe, other agents are still suspect. Buechley (1963) considered that the excess could be satisfactorily explained only by the inhalation of arsenic and not by the inhalation of radioactive products. A team of occupational health workers and epidemiologists from the National Cancer Institute, have now postulated a causal relationship between airborne radioactive substances and lung cancer in the uranium miners of the Colorado Plateau (Wagoner and others, 1965). Their study included 3,415 miners in whom there were 22 deaths from pulmonary

neoplasms compared with six theoretically expected. There was no exces
mortality from neoplasms at sites other than the lung. A dose-respons
relationship between airborne radioactive dust and lung cancer was found
such that the age-standardized incidence increased from three per 10,00
miners at the lowest to 116 in the highest category of cumulative exposure
An association has been shown to exist, but how convincing is the case fo
causation put forward by Wagoner and his associates?

Some Aspects of Association

Sir Austin Bradford Hill (1965) reviewed some aspects of association
which should be especially considered in a study such as this. In th
present instance the strength of the association is dependent on an inci
dence of lung cancer that is four times the theoretically expected incidence
That is not great compared with a ten-fold increase in asbestos workers
a thirty-fold increase in heavy smokers over non-smokers or 150-fol
increase of cancer of the nose (ethmoid) in nickel refiners in Great Britain

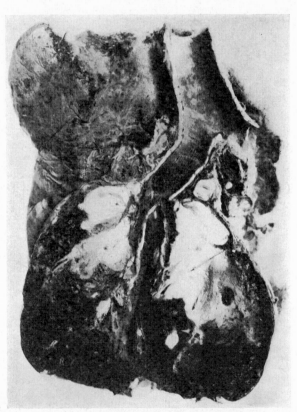

Fig. 305.—Carcinoma of the Lung in a Carpenter of 53,
who had worked for 23 years in the Joachimstal Uranium
Mines and who died six years after he was pensioned
(*By courtesy of Dr. H. Sikl*)

urthermore, the total number of cases of lung cancer in the uranium ainers is small. The authors point to the consistency of the association by eferring to the increased incidence of lung cancer in fluorspar miners also xposed to radon daughter products (de Villiers and Windish, 1964). 'hough it may not be too difficult to show an association between certain nvironmental factors and a particular disease, it may be much more so to ecide that the one is the cause of the other. But results of the survey eported here do add some confirmation to the existing evidence that ae inhalation of radioactive particles is likely to cause some of the lung ancer in uranium miners both in America and in Europe.

ancer of the Lung in Radium Laboratory Workers

Although attempts to reproduce this form of cancer in experimental nimals have failed, there is clinical evidence to support the view that adioactive emanation is responsible for it. Carcinoma of the lung occurs in 1en and women engaged on the purification and production of radioactive ubstances and their compounds, and in technicians working in therapeutic adium laboratories. These cases are apparently of occupational origin and, 1deed, two of the Joachimsthal cases occurred in laboratory workers. Ieitzel (1935) described cases which occurred in commercial and thera-eutic radium laboratories in Germany. A girl chemist in a radium factory 'as suffering from burns to the skin caused by strongly radioactive sub-tances. She continued work with less active material, but died about ten ears later from bronchial carcinoma with metastases. Another chemist vho had worked in a radium plant also died from cancer of the lung.

reventive Measures

Preventive measures include improved systems of ventilation to reduce he inhalation of dust and radium emanation, and the introduction of wet-rilling methods. Shorter hours of work in the mines will reduce the ex-osure to the carcinogenic agent. Frequent holidays, exchange of labourers 'ith other factories and a scheme for early retirement of all mine workers hould be organized. These measures would eliminate the long and con-nuous exposure which appears to be an important factor in the ætiology f lung cancer in the Schneeberg and Jáchymov miners.

he Nickel Industry

A high incidence of cancer of the lung and ethmoid has been reported a men employed in refining nickel from ores containing metallic arsenides.)oll (1958) collected data from the records of deaths held by the medical fficers of health for the districts in which workers at a nickel refinery ved. During 1948–56 the risk of nickel workers dying from carcinoma of 1e nose was 150 times the normal and from carcinoma of the lung 5 times 1e normal. At Clydach works Gwynne Morgan (1958) had records of 31 cases of lung cancer and 61 of cancer of the nose. Such men were not mployed in processes involving the use of metallic nickel or the gas, nickel carbonyl. They were associated with the calcination processes, and it is considered that dust, possibly the heated, calcined dusts, contained the carcinogen. Before 1924 this dust probably contained arsenic from the sulphuric acid used. No deaths from nasal cancer have been recorded from workers engaged after 1924, at which date increased precautions were taken against dust (p. 476).

The Chromate Industry

Reports from Germany and the United States of America suggest that cancer of the lung occurs frequently in workers in the chromate industry. The high incidence is noted particularly in the manufacture of basic chromates from chrome ore, but cases have also occurred in the chrome colour industry in Germany. In a survey of the causes of death in the chromate-producing industry in the United States of America, it was found that death from cancer of the lung occurred among these workers about twenty-five times more frequently than among men of comparable age employed in other industries. The work suggested that men handling monochromates are most likely to be affected. The incidence of lung cancer among workers in the chromates-producing industry in Great Britain is 3·6 times the normal (Bidstrup and Case, 1956) (p. 457).

The Asbestos Industry

Primary carcinoma of the lung in association with pulmonary asbestosis has often been recorded. McCullough, 1959, collected particulars of 360 deaths between 1924 and 1955 in which post-mortem examination had confirmed the presence of asbestosis. In 65 of these (nearly 18 per cent) there was also lung cancer. Doll (1955) concluded that the average risk of cancer of the lung in workers who had been exposed to asbestos dust for twenty years or more was of the order of ten times that experienced by the general population. The majority of the reported series, however, refer to patients in the asbestos textile industry, and some of the findings have been criticized by Braun and Truan (1958), who, in a careful epidemiological survey, found no unusual risk to asbestos miners in the province of Quebec.

Manufacture of Sheep Dip

The statistical work of Hill and Faning (1949) has shown that in a town in England where the principal industry is the manufacture of arsenical sheep dip, the difference between the mortality rates for carcinoma in chemical workers handling arsenic is double that in the rest of the population of the town. This difference is made up almost entirely by carcinoma of the skin and bronchi (p. 340).

(b) Cancer of the Skin

The occupations concerned in causing cancer of the skin include that of chimney sweep, tar, pitch, anthracene and creosote worker, briquette aker, shale-oil worker, gunsmith, oiling coolie, cotton-mule spinner and ttomatic-lathe operator.

ancer of the Skin in Chimney Sweeps

In 1775 Percivall Pott in his description of chimney-sweeps' cancer corded the first observation upon occupational cancer of the skin:

> It is a disease which always makes its first attack on, and its first appearance in, the inferior part of the scrotum, where it produces a superficial, painful, ragged, ill-looking sore, with hard and rising edges: the trade call it soot-wart. I never saw it under the age of puberty, which is, I suppose, one reason why it is generally taken both by patient and surgeon for venereal.

fter a description of its spread to the testicle, spermatic cord and abdoen he goes on:

> The fate of these people seems singularly hard: in their early infancy they are most frequently treated with great brutality, and almost starved with cold and hunger; they are thrust up narrow and sometimes hot chimnies, where they are bruised, burned and almost suffocated, and when they get to puberty become peculiarly liable to a most noisome, painful and fatal disease (p. 141).

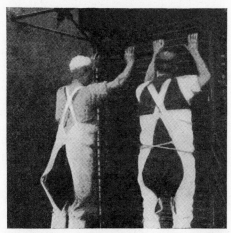

'e now know that soot owes s carcinogenic properties to .r, of which it may contain p to 40 per cent and that the ircinogenic substance reonsible is 3 : 4-benzpyrene.

ffects of Shale Oil, Tar, Pitch and Creosote on the Skin

Those who handle tar, itch, asphalt, creosote and

FIG. 306.—Hydraulic press at one time used in the shale-oil industry. Note unprotected skin of workmen exposed to a carcinogenic oil

ithracene may develop *tar melanosis* of the face, neck, limbs, groins and avel. They are also liable to acne and to papillomata known as *tar mollusca*. 1 1875 Volkmann of Halle published observations on three cases which roved that the constant handling of tar or paraffin over long periods may ad to the development of cancer of the skin. Between 1860 and 1957 iale oil (fig. 306) was distilled from bituminous shale in Linlithgowshire,

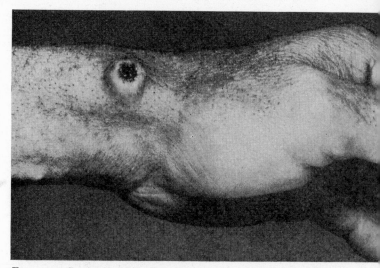

FIG. 307.—Carcinoma of the Skin in a man of 54 who had worked for 15 years in
the Paraffin Department of a Shale-oil Refinery in Scotland
(By courtesy of Dr. Alexander Scott)

and by the year 1876 Joseph Bell had published a paper on the
occurrence of cases of skin cancer
among shale-oil workers. Scott
(1923) described cancer of the skin
mainly affecting the arms among
these refiners of Scottish shale oil
(fig. 307). The serious effect of
pitch dust on patent-fuel workers
in Cardiff, Swansea and Newport
has been studied since 1912. Briquettes are made of coal dust containing about 10 per cent of pitch.
The workers are thus exposed to
pitch dust, which may give rise to
warts, especially on the eyelids, ears,
face and scrotum. Though the warts
are multiple they do not all take on
a malignant character; the scrotum
is often the seat of the malignant
lesion.

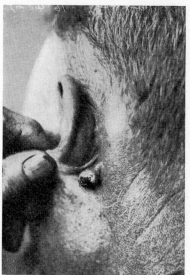

FIG. 308.—Carcinoma of the Skin of
the Face in a man of 63 who had
worked in the tar department of a
Gasworks for 35 years

Multiple Pitch Warts and Tar Carcinomata

Pitch dust causes lachrymation,
all degrees of conjunctivitis and even corneal ulceration. After many

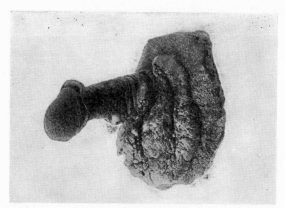

Fig. 309.—Carcinoma of the Scrotum in a man, aged 65, who had worked in the Tar Department of a Gasworks for 42 years. The Fungating Mass of thirteen months' growth was removed surgically, together with the Penis, and found to be a Squamous and Horny Carcinoma
(*London Hospital Medical College Museum*)

ears' work in the tar and pitch department of a gasworks most men ave warts on the exposed skin, but they do not commonly view their ccurrence with any alarm. They know by tradition and experience that the warts may fall off, and a common remedy amongst them is the frequent application through the day of a crystal of washing soda, kept in a pocket and wetted on the tongue before being rubbed across the top of the wart. Other workers go to the nearest pharmacist's shop for the application of glacial acetic acid. Increasing experience of the effects of tar has shown that the cancers of the skin are often multiple. The commonest sites of tar carcinoma are the face (fig. 308), forearms and the scrotum (fig. 309). Ultimately, secondary growths in the lymphatic glands may occur, with a fatal issue (Henry, 1946).

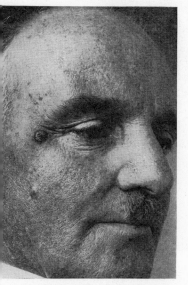

G. 310.—Carcinoma of the Skin in a man of 54 who had been employed for 30 years in creosoting Railway Sleepers

Anthracene and Creosote

Anthracene is a white, crystalline solid obtained from the anthracene

D.O.—27*

oil of coal-tar. The crude anthracene cake of the gasworks contains abou
40 per cent of anthracene and smells strongly of creosote and pheno
Anthracene is used in the manufacture of synthetic dyes and in the pre
paration of anthraquinone. Anthracene oil is used as a preservative fc
wood and is sometimes added to machine oils. Elderly workers in crud
anthracene are liable to carcinomata of the skin, but these cases diffe
from those due to tar in that multiple growths in any one patient ar
rarely found. A plant may run for thirty-five years before a case c
carcinoma develops. Heavy creosote oil is used in wood-preserving. Rai
way sleepers, telegraph poles and piles for piers are all impregnated wit
the oil under pressure to preserve them from insects and fungi. Th
occupation of creosoting timber is a well recognized source of cutaneou
papilloma and carcinoma (fig. 310).

Cancer of the Skin in Cotton-mule Spinners

In 1906 S. R. Wilson, when appointed house surgeon to the Roya
Infirmary, Manchester, noticed that the patients admitted suffering fro
cancer of the scrotum were not chimney sweeps but mule spinners. S
struck was he by the fact that in 1910 he wrote an essay on the subjec
This was submitted for a scholarship, but was not published until twelv

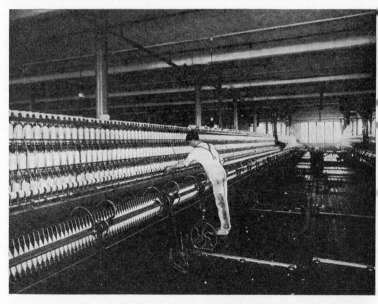

FIG. 311.—Cotton-spinning Mule, showing Horizontal Bar placed some three feet
above the Floor, constantly moist with Lubricating Oil thrown off by the
Spindles. In leaning forward over the Bar to repair Broken Threads the Mule-
spinner gets his Clothing soaked with Oil over a zone some eight inches in
width level with the upper part of the thighs
(By courtesy of Mr. A. H. Southam)

ears later (Southam and Wilson, 1922). Cotton-mule spinning necessitates
requent bending over a horizontal bar, placed some 3 feet above the floor
nd running the length of the spinning machine (fig. 311). It is always
noist with lubricating oil thrown off by the spindles, and frequent contact
vith this bar results in the clothing over the upper part of the thighs
ecoming soaked with oil. The cancer occurs on the scrotum in about 70
er cent of cases (fig. 312), and on the hand, arm (fig. 313), face, leg and
oot in the remainder.

hale Oil responsible for Mule-spinners' Cancer

The oil apparently most potent for its carcinogenic property is shale
il, obtained from the bituminous shale of Scotland. The incidence in
nule spinners is high, and this appears to be the result of a gradual
hange over about 1870 from animal and vegetable to shale oil for pur-
oses of lubrication. The number of mule spinners in England dropped
etween 1933 and 1955 from about 30,000 to 15,000, and 1,989 cases had
een reported by 1955. The average age among mule spinners who con-
ract the disease is fifty-two years. Less than 3 per cent manifest the disease
1 dangerous forms under twenty years' duration of employment, while
he average duration before it occurs is approximately forty years.

Rangoon Oil used by Gun-smiths

Contact with mineral oil outside
he factory must be borne in mind
s a possible source of skin cancer.
n 1926 O'Donovan reported a
ase of a gunsmith aged fifty-five
mployed in reconditioning old
ifles. He had worked for thirty-
ine years wearing clothes saturated
vith oil, mostly rangoon oil and
aseline. Fifteen cutaneous tu-
nours had been removed surgi-
ally. The gravest operation was for
he removal of nearly all his nose.
'our of these tumours were sub-
nitted to histological examination,
nd they were all squamous-celled
arcinomata.

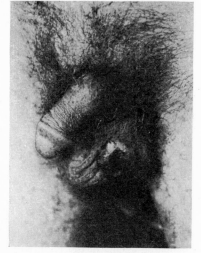

FIG. 312. — Mule-spinners' Cancer. Squamous Carcinoma of Scrotum in a man of 63 who had worked for 54 years in the Mule-room of a Lancashire Cotton Mill

Sumatra Oil as an Anti-malarial Spray

Kingsbury in 1926 reported the
ccurrence of multiple cutaneous carcinomata in a Malay coolie who
ad been employed for three years carrying out extensive anti-malarial oiling

on estates. The patient presented a tumour on the distal phalanx of the right index finger, and two raised nodules on the scrotum, each some three quarters of an inch in diameter and projecting an eighth of an inch. All three tumours proved histologically to be squamous-celled carcinomata

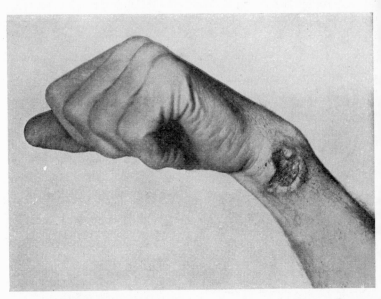

FIG. 313.—Mule-spinners' Cancer. Squamous Carcinomatous Ulcer on Forearm of a man of 56 who had worked for 40 years as a Mule Spinner in Lancashire
(*Legge, T. M.: Industrial Maladies, Oxford Univ. Press, 1934*)

The oil used came from Sumatra, and was sprayed from an atomizer During this process the operator often gets his clothes saturated with oil which collects in the region of the groins and scrotum. Long-continued occupation as an oiling coolie is therefore liable to result in scrotal cancer.

Skin Cancer from Mineral Oil in Engineering

Mineral oils are used in a wide variety of engineering processes—for example as lubricants, as coolants in metal-cutting operations and as quenching agents in the tempering of metals and alloys. The most continuous and widespread skin contamination of workmen is usually to be seen in *bar automatic* shops, where groups of from twenty to a hundred and fifty workmen may all be exposed under similar conditions. The automatic machine tool is designed to conduct a series of operations without removal of the work—for example, upon a long metal bar turning out some such object as a bolt.

Mechanics' Clothing soaked in Oil

These machines frequently work at high speed requiring large amounts of coolant upon the tool edges, and, as they are at present designed, much oil is thrown into the air as a fine spray which eventually settles on machines and floor to form a film. Not only is the operator exposed to this spray, but also in the course of his work he often has to adjust the tool and the metal while the machine is in motion. In spite of the splash-guards which are at present in use, gross skin contamination is usual. Since the machine opera-

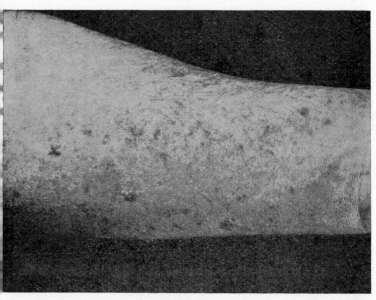

FIG. 314.—Multiple pigmented Hyperkeratoses on Forearm of a Machine Operator exposed for 21 years to Cutting Oils. The worker developed a Scrotal Carcinoma

(Reprinted from the British Journal of Industrial Medicine, 1950, 7, 1, by permission of the Journal and the authors)

tor's clothing soon becomes soaked through with oil, the skin on the thighs and genital regions as well as on the arms becomes very oily. In general, the degree of skin contamination with oil in bar automatic machine shops is very much greater than that to be seen in mule-rooms in the cotton industry.

Oil Folliculitis, Hyperkeratoses and Cancer

Early in their work 80 per cent of these mechanics become afflicted with oil folliculitis; those who have been exposed for many years develop on their arms multiple hyperkeratoses (fig. 314). One case of carcinoma of the scrotum has been described (Cruickshank and Squire, 1950). These authors examined the records of the United Birmingham Hospitals and found that between 1940 and 1949 thirty-four cases of scrotal cancer occurred. Of these, six were in machine operators and six in the workers exposed to oil in the engineering industry; thirteen occurred in workers exposed to tar products; and the remaining nine could not be allocated to any definite category.

Preventive Measures

Men working in the pitch beds of gasworks should be provided with goggles to protect the eyes from conjunctivitis and corneal ulceration. Protective clothing, a double locker system, baths and washing facilities must be provided for workers in pitch, tar, anthracene, creosote and shale oil, and for mule spinners and machine operators exposed to cutting oils. Barrier creams applied before work appear to be of little value. All these workers must be educated as to the danger of their occupation and should also be instructed how to minimize it. Regular periodic medical examination is long overdue. In compensation for death alone the cotton industry must anticipate paying £10,000 a year until it is realized that this sum could be considerably reduced and life spared by timely periodic examination. Voluntary examination is bound to lead to evasion, especially from the desire to conceal a condition situated, as it so often is on the scrotum (Henry, 1947).

Co-operation of Doctor and Engineer

The doctor and the engineer should co-operate in devising apparatus which will prevent contamination of the skin with oil. This has been done for the spinning mule by fitting a device which holds a felt strip in contact with the mule spindle, thus preventing oil-splash (fig. 315). Similar work is called for in the engineering industry where better guarding of lathes is necessary. The guards at present in use frequently have to be removed in the course of adjusting the cutting tool and many workers are careless about their replacement. It is possible that the fitting of automatic spring-back devices would ensure replacement of the guard (Cruickshank and Squire, 1950).

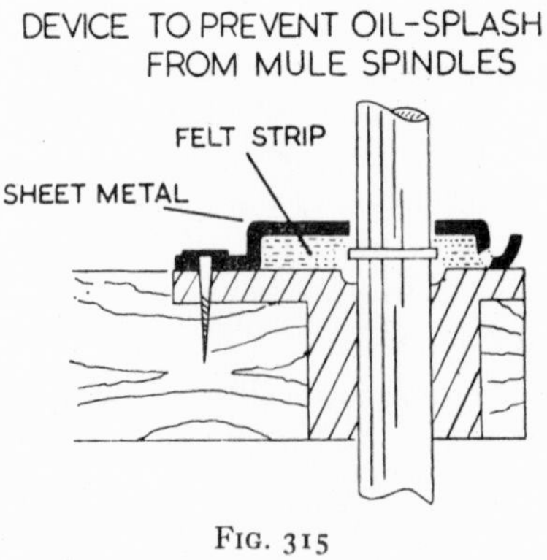

DEVICE TO PREVENT OIL-SPLASH
FROM MULE SPINDLES

FELT STRIP

SHEET METAL

Fig. 315

Commercial Production of Non-carcinogenic Oils

Cancer of the skin in industry will be got rid of in years to come either by the elimination from tar and mineral oils of carcinogenic substances or by their neutralization and destruction. In 1929 Twort and Fulton showed that the car cinogenic activity of certain oils is much reduced or completely removed by extraction with sulphuric acid, by oxidation and by reduction. Later it was found that the method of solvent extraction had the same effect. Modern methods of oil refining are bringing within reach the possibility of the commercial production of non-carcinogenic oils. By agitation of oil distillates in liquid sulphur dioxide, aromatic fractions are extracted from petroleum distillates, leaving an oil which is mainly aliphatic in composition. This process has made practicable the production of non-carcinogenic *white oils* for use in the cotton industry. Much has yet to be learned before analogous developments can be applied economically to engineering oils.

Treatment by Radium or Radon

The prognosis of carcinoma of the skin due to tar or mineral oil is extremely good provided that the patients attend early. In such cases treatment by radon or by flat plates of radium easily removes the whole neoplasm in one application. A large gasworks in London sends all its cases of pitch warts to the Radium Institute. A radon seed containing 1·5 millicuries of radon sheathed in platinum is inserted under the surface of the papule, the needle puncture being sealed with collodion. The local skin reaction is slight, so that patients can continue at work during and after treatment. After five days the seed is expressed. Such patients must be kept under observation for many years in order that further papules may be dealt with as they arise.

(c) Cancer of the Bladder

Workers employed in the manufacture of synthetic dyes as well as those in the rubber and cable industries sometimes suffer from tumours of the bladder. After several years' exposure and then a latent interval lasting up to 20 years the workman develops papillomata of the bladder and finally cancer. It is unfortunate that initially the name *aniline cancer* was given to this disease, for subsequent work has shown that a number of aromatic amines may be responsible but *not* aniline itself. In the case of chemical industry and of the dye industry it is certain that the carcinogenic substances are among the dye intermediates; the finished dyes are harmless. Benzidine has been incriminated on clinical evidence (Scott, 1952), and *beta*-naphthylamine, auramine, magenta and xenylamine both by clinical evidence and by animal experiment. *Alpha*-naphthylamine is probably non-carcinogenic but *alpha*-naphthylamine of commerce frequently contains *beta*-naphthylamine as an impurity.

History

The first cases to be discovered in the dye industry were recorded by Rehn in 1895. At that date the commercial preparation of aniline dyes had been established for some thirty years and had become a flourishing industry, especially in Germany. Rehn discovered three cases of bladder tumour among a group of forty-five men who were engaged in the preparation of fuchsine, and suggested that the condition followed a chronic irritation of the mucous membrane of the bladder by certain chemical compounds excreted in the urine over a period of many years. In 1912 Leuenberger published eighteen similar cases from Basle and offered statistical evidence showing that the incidence of this disease was thirty-three times greater among dye-workers than among the remainder of the male population. In 1920 Curschmann undertook a systematic inquiry into all traceable cases of aniline cancer from German dye factories up to that date and was able to collect 177 cases. In the manufacture of synthetic dyes in Great Britain about forty fatal cases have been recorded. Similar observations have been made in the United States of America, Russia, Austria, Italy and France (Billiard-Duchesne, 1948). The total number of these occupational tumours so far put on record in the various countries is approximately 550, but this does not represent the total incidence (Hueper, 1938). Since 1949 men with malignant tumours of the bladder have been found in two further industries namely rubber manufacture and cable making.

Exposure Hazards

The manufacture of aniline dyes involves the use and production of many chemical substances. For a long time it was not known which substance attacks the bladder, but it seemed, by a process of exclusion, to be an amino- and not a nitro-compound. In 1926 Oppenheimer suggested the name *amino-tumour*. In course of time suspicion fell upon many substances including aniline, *para*-toluidine, xylidines, naphthylamines, fuchsine, benzidine and rosaniline. The difficulties met with in trying to trace the substance responsible are typical of those found in the investigation of all complex industrial processes. In the dye industry it is common to have two distinct processes going on in the same room. Further, in the case of a disease with such a long latent period, the workman may have moved from one factory to another or from one department in the same factory to another, each change bringing new compounds into question. Lastly, the same compounds used in different processes may be attended with very different degrees of danger. Thus, in making benzidine, there may be greater exposure to aniline vapour than in the manufacture of aniline itself (Hamilton, 1925). In rubber manufacture and cable making the carcinogenic substances are antioxidants and hardeners. *Beta*-naphthylamine and an aldol-*alpha*-naphthylamine condensate are the principal substances responsible. The high-risk men are the weighers-out and mixers. In 1966 two rodent operators were found to have carcinoma of the bladder presumed to be due to their having handled the rodenticide ANTU, the active constituent of which is 1-(1-naphthyl)-2-thiourea. This substance may or may not be carcinogenic but it is made from *alpha*-naphthylamine which contains *beta*-naphthylamine as an impurity.

Carcinogenic Substances or Potentiators of Tissues

Goldblatt (1949), in an analysis of 102 cases of tumours of the urinary tract occurring in workers in the dye industry, includes some where exposure has been limited to one compound. Men who have handled only *beta*-naphthylamine, or aniline, or benzidine, have developed tumours. Cases have occurred also where exposure has been to *alpha*-naphthylamine exclusively, but about 4 per cent of the *beta* isomer is usually present as an impurity and may account for these. Bladder tumours occurring in workers exposed to *beta*-naphthylamine alone, or alternatively to more than one compound, are more likely to be malignant from the outset than are those in men exposed only to aniline or benzidine. It seems likely that these compounds are only indirectly responsible for the tumour formation and act as sensitizers or potentiators of the tissue to the true carcinogen. Statistical evidence suggests that magenta and auramine cause bladder tumours in men engaged in their manufacture (Case and Pearson, 1954). So far it has been impossible to determine whether the hazard can be attributed to the intermediates, impurities or the finished dye (Scott and Williams, 1957). The manufacture of 4-amino-diphenyl (xenylamine) as a rubber antioxidant was begun in the U.S.A. in 1935; it has never been manufactured in Great Britain. Its potential dangers were recognized and proof of its carcinogenicity in animals established by Walpole and Williams (1958). In the U.S.A. sixteen cases (22·5 per cent) of bladder tumour have been found among seventy-one workers (Melick, 1958).

Tumours of the Renal Pelvis

In Goldblatt's series only one patient developed a tumour in the pelvis of the kidney. This supports the view that the carcinogen is carried by the urine and not in the blood stream. The patient was a man who began work in the dye industry at the age of twenty-three. From the age of twenty-seven to thirty-four he worked on processes involving exposure to *beta*-naphthylamine. He developed three bladder papillomata which were treated by diathermy. Eight months later he was found to have a fresh papilloma near the left ureteric orifice, and this was successfully treated. He was then free from symptoms for fourteen months. On routine cystoscopy no bladder tumour was present, but on further investigation a diagnosis of a tumour of the pelvis of the right kidney was made. The right kidney and ureter were removed and two papillomata were found in the pelvis of the kidney. In addition, a small papilloma was present at the lower end of the ureter. There was no evidence of malignant change in any of these growths. Macalpine (1947) reported two cases of papilloma of the renal pelvis in dye workers. In one of these the growths were bilateral. Six other cases were recorded in the literature between 1905 and 1947.

Experimental Work on Dogs

Progress towards an explanation of the fundamental causes of these tumours has been slow. Because the dog was the only species known to be susceptible, an individual experiment required up to ten years for its completion. In 1938 Hueper, Wiley and Wolfe succeeded in producing papillomatosis and carcinomatosis of the bladder in dogs by daily subcutaneous and oral treatment with *beta*-naphthylamine (fig. 316). They used from 300 to 450 milligrams of this substance daily for periods of twenty to thirty-two months. The lesions observed on cystoscopic and histological examination of the bladder in twelve of the sixteen dogs thus treated were identical with those seen by these authors in cystoscopic and histological examination of dye workers. In some of the dogs the tumours continued to grow and to become more numerous after the treatment had been discontinued. In one dog the first neoplasms in the bladder were noted several months after exposure had ceased. In necropsies performed upon the dogs, metastatic deposits were not found, although in one case the carcinoma had invaded the subserosa of the bladder.

A Parent Amine produces a Carcinogenic Metabolite

For a long time attempts to find a reason for the unusual localization of the tumours in the bladder epithelium, while all other organs remained apparently normal, failed. It was therefore an important step when Bonser, Clayson and Jull (1951) found that the urine of dogs treated with *beta*-naphthylamine contained a carcinogenic metabolite derived from this substance. This metabolite was a water-soluble *ortho*-hydroxyamine, 2-amino-*l*-naphthol, and its tumour-inducing properties were demonstrated by a new technique of implanting a pellet of the chemical substance suspended in wax into the mouse bladder. A series of experiments then confirmed that the metabolite is carcinogenic, whereas the parent amine is not.

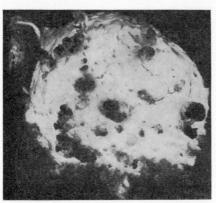

FIG. 316.—Multiple Papillomata and Carcinomata of the Bladder produced experimentally in Dogs by daily Subcutaneous and Oral Treatment with *beta*-naphthylamine

(Hueper, W. C., Wiley, F. H., and Wolfe, A. D. (1938), J industr. hyg., **20**, 69)

Time of Onset after First Exposure

In dye workers the period of exposure is usually twelve years, but tumours have developed in men who had been in the industry from four to forty-eight years. A number of men may work together in a dye factory for thirty years under apparently identical conditions and, although bladder tumours may arise early in some and late in others, the majority remain unaffected. The earlier the age at which the industry is entered, the earlier is death likely to occur if a tumour develops. As to the route of absorption, the respiratory tract as well as the skin is involved. Absorption by inhalation is difficult to control, especially at charging-points, flaking and grinding machines, and drying ovens. Occasionally members of the clerical staff of dye factories have developed bladder tumours, and men working in laundries and repair shops where contaminated materials are handled have also been affected.

Symptoms and Signs

The symptoms and signs of occupational tumour of the bladder do not differ from those of non-occupational origin. There may be a period during which a tumour becomes established in the absence of any external symptoms or signs. Sudden painless hæmaturia may then occur, or epithelial cells or red blood cells may be found on routine microscopic examination of the urine in the absence of symptoms. Cystoscopy reveals either small hæmorrhages in the trigone or multiple papillomata, sometimes benign, sometimes malignant. Macalpine (1929) pointed out that there is often a premonitory period in which the patient suffers from symptoms of cystitis such as increased frequency of micturition with strangury. He has found the cystoscopic picture to differ from that seen in septic cystitis in that the mucosa is more brightly red and shows a tendency to mottling. The morbid anatomy and histology of aniline tumours appear to be identical with what is found in other bladder tumours. Recurrences which are usually fresh tumours at new sites are common. They may occur at any time from months to years after the first incident. The tendency to recurrence persists throughout life and this should be considered in claims for compensation (Goldblatt, 1949). Metastases do occur, but they are less frequent than in other types of neoplasm. It should be noted that a fair number of eye intermediates which are not carcinogenic can cause symptoms such as increased frequency of micturition. *Ortho*-toluidine and 5-chlor-ortho-toluidine are particularly irritating and may cause hæmaturia.

Preventive Measures

Curschmann (1920) observed that the incidence of bladder tumours diminished considerably in the Frankfurt district after the institution of various protective measures in the factories, such as general cleanliness in the workrooms, adequate exhaust ventilation for the removal of vapours, measures designed to diminish the evolution of fume and dust, mechanical transport of chemical products in closed containers and improvements in the personal hygiene of the workmen. Nevertheless, in the dye industry in various parts of the world, bladder tumours still occur in large numbers. Clearly prohibition of the manufacture of certain carcinogens would be the ideal method of prevention. The ethics of the manufacture of such substances has been admirably discussed by Scott (1958). By 1950 *beta*-naphthylamine was universally recognized as highly dangerous. It was found impossible to devise plant for its production and use which afforded adequate protection and yet could be operated at an economic rate. In the United Kingdom it was voluntarily decided to abandon its manufacture. The loss would have been a serious one as *beta*-naphthylamine is extensively used for the manufacture of Tobias acid and similar *beta*-naphthylamine sulphonic acids, which are employed in the synthesis of many azo dyes. Chemists, however, found it possible, but at considerable extra cost, to alter the mode of manufacture so as to produce the Tobias acid by the sulphonation of *beta*-naphthol followed by amidation. The production of the carcinogen was thus avoided. *Beta*-naphthylamine is now no longer made in Great Britain, Germany or Switzerland. The manufacture of rubber antioxidants derived from *alpha*- and *beta*-naphthylamine has also been abandoned in Great Britain. Benzidine and *alpha*-naphthylamine are unfortunately essential intermediate compounds for the manufacture of large ranges of colours used in many industries. No substitutes or alternative methods of making the dyes have yet been devised. Manufacture therefore still continues but is carried out in specially designed plant and under strict medical supervision. Users of these compounds are also warned of their toxicity. Benzidine has also been employed in the rubber industry but its use is now discontinued. During 1957, in order to try to ensure safe working conditions, Scott and Williams (1957) drew up for the Association of British Chemical Manufacturers a *Code of Working Practice Recommended by the British Dyestuffs Industry for the Manufacture and Use of Products Causing Tumours of the Bladder*. This is now accepted as standard practice. In 1967 importation of the carcinogens β-naphthylamine, benzidine, 4-aminodiphenyl, 4-nitrodiphenyl, their salts, and substances containing them was prohibited, except where they are present, as a chemical byproduct, at a concentration of not more than one per cent. From 1950 onwards other associations including the Rubber Manufacturing Employers' Association, the Cable Makers' Association and the Electric Cable Makers' Federation have concerned themselves with the problems of prevention of bladder tumours.

Inadequacy of Follow-up Facilities

Theoretically, while it is the responsiblity of the employer to ensure that the men he employs do not suffer any injury as a result of their employment, it is obviously beyond the competence of every employer to follow up and to determine the cause of illness or death of every man he employs. Undoubtedly, large firms using potentially dangerous new chemicals could carry out this sort of study as a routine on small groups particularly at risk. But for the bulk of the employed population the obligation must fall upon the State. It is for the State to decide whether this recording of illness and matching it with employment records for large sections of the population should be the responsibility of the individual, the Ministry of Labour, the Ministry of Health, the general practitioner or the Registrar General. The big disadvantage of using the

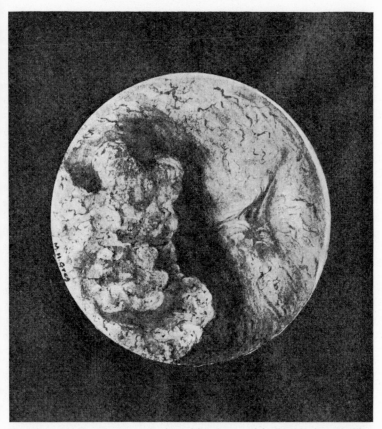

FIG. 317.—Case 32. Cystoscopic view of Carcinoma of the Bladder in an Aniline-dye Works' Technician, a man of 53, who had been exposed to Dye Intermediates for 34 years

(By courtesy of Mr. K. Heritage)

Registrar General's figures for detecting occupational risks is that he records the statement of a relative of the dead man as to his last occupation. This is not only inaccurate but also misleading because it does not record even the principal occupation during the dead man's life-time but may record the one to which he changed just before he retired or died, his end occupation (Elmes, 1966). No record is kept of periods of work in occupations at some time in the past. The occupation responsible for an illness with a long latent interval may therefore be overlooked. Thus in 1964 a man dying of carcinoma of the bladder stated when he was admitted to hospital that he was a lock keeper and formerly a sailmaker. But between 1935 and 1949 he had worked in cable making where he had been exposed to *beta*-naphthylamine, both by skin absorption and by inhalation of the vapour. This problem will never be settled until every man is obliged by law to carry a record card stating the name and date of every job he has ever done together with the name and address of every employer for whom he has worked throughout his life.

Treatment

Workers exposed should be told both of the risk they run and of the nature of the symptoms. Routine examination and centrifugation of the urine should be carried out for red blood cells and exfoliated bladder epithelium. Soon after the first cases were discovered in 1895, facilities were provided in the Höchst factories for cystoscopic examination of every suspicious case. Routine cystoscopy should become universal in the dye industry throughout the world. The strongest argument for the routine use of the cystoscope in aniline dyeworks is that men have remained well for a number of years after cysto-diathermy of a papilloma. Early diagnosis of all cases would ensure removal of every papilloma before it did any harm. Reviewing the treatment and prognosis of 180 patients with occupational tumours of the bladder, Poole-Wilson (1960) records that he used perurethral cystodiathermy in 108 of these. The five-year survival rate was 88 per cent but of course a careful follow-up of these patients is necessary to look for recurrence of the papilloma by repeated cystoscopy. Up to 20 per cent of those who survived five years died later from carcinoma of the bladder. Interstitial irradiation was necessary in 31 and deep x-ray therapy in 21 patients. Cystectomy, partial or total, was required in 17 of the patients. Approximately 9 per cent of the patients developed ureteric or renal lesions and most of these were treated by nephro-ureterectomy.

Case 32. Aniline-dye works' technician—exposure to dye intermediates for thirty-four years—papilloma and carcinoma of the bladder—excision by diathermy.

(Macalpine, 1929; Heritage, 1936.) J. W., a man aged 53. 1895: at the age of 21 first went to work at an aniline-dye works near Manchester. At first he was employed in the drying of sodium naphthionate. 1896: began washing sodium naphthionate with solvent naphtha to remove unchanged *alpha*-naphthylamine. 1910: began to work on the reduction of *alpha*-nitro-naphthalene to *alpha*-naphthylamine by the use of iron turnings and mineral acid. This remained his principal occupation for eighteen years. 1911: admitted to the Manchester Royal Infirmary where suprapubic removal of a vesical papilloma was performed by Mr. Burgess. He remained well after this until 1928 when he came under the care of Mr. Heritage with a four-months' history of recurrent pain with frequency and hæmaturia at the end of micturition. On cystoscopy a tumour was found in the region of the left ureteric orifice (fig. 317). It had the appearance of being more compact and more pink than an ordinary papilloma, and from its nodular tuberose formation it was thought to be carcinomatous. A portion was removed for histological section, and the remainder was excised by diathermy. The mucosa of the bladder was more brightly red than the usual colour in cystitis, and had a tendency to mottling. Histological examination showed a tumour of transitional epithelium, possibly malignant. The patient did not return to the dye works, and remained well for five years. In 1933 he died of lobar pneumonia, and necropsy showed that there was neither recurrence in the bladder nor metastases.

BIBLIOGRAPHY

Occupational Diseases of the Skin

AGRICOLA, G. (1556), *De Re Metallica*, Basel.
BADHAM, J. (1834), *London Med. Gaz.*, **15**, 112.
BOURNE, L. B. (1956), *Trans. Assoc. Industr. Med. Off.*, **6**, 94.
BRIDGE, J. C. (1933), *Brit. med. J.*, **2**, 324.
CALNAN, C. D. (1958), *Trans. St. John's Hosp. Dermatol. Soc.*, London, p. 12.
CELSUS, A. C. (1487), *De Re Medicina*, Florence.
DAVIDSON, J. M. (1941), *Lancet*, **1**, 38.
GRANDJEAN, E. (1957), *Brit. J. industr. Med.*, **14**, 1.
HAY, J. (1908), *Annual Report of the Chief Inspector of Factories and Workshops for 1907*, Cmd. 4166, H.M.S.O., London, p. 266.
HELLIER, F. F., and WARIN, R. P. (1967), *Brit. med. J.*, **2**, 346.
HENRY, S. A. (1933), *Brit. J. Dermol.*, **45**, 301.
HORNER, S. G. (1934), *Lancet*, **2**, 233.
JONES, A. T. (1946), *Brit. J. industr. Med.*, **3**, 83.
KATZENELLENBOGEN, I. (1955), *Dermatologica*, **111**, 99.
LEGGE, T. M. (1908), *Annual Report of the Chief Inspector of Factories and Workshops for 1907*, Cmd. 4166, H.M.S.O., London, p. 248.
McCORD, C. P. (1945), *A Blind Hog's Acorns*, Cloud Inc., Chicago.
O'DONOVAN, W. J. (1932), *Brit. med. J.*, **2**, 292; (1935), Personal communication; (1952), *Trans. assoc. industr. med. off.*, **2**, 34.
PARACELSUS, T. (1567), *Von der Bergsucht*, Dilingen.
VON PLENCK, J. J. (1776), *Doctrina de Morbis Cutaneis*, Vienna.
RAMAZZINI, B. (1713), *De Morbus Artificum Diatriba*, Geneva.
RONCHESE, F. (1953), *Industr. Med. and Surg.*, **22**, 45.
RUSSELL, B. (1953), *Brit. med. J.*, **2**, 1322.
SCHWARTZ, L., TULIPAN, L., and BIRMINGHAM, D. J. (1957), *Occupational Diseases of the Skin*, 3rd ed., Kimpton, London.
SEALEY, L. (1952), *Occup. Hlth.*, **12**, 199.
SMITH, W. D. L. (1966), *Practitioner*, **196**, 690.
SMITHIES, B. M. (1929), *Lancet*, **2**, 494.
VICKERS, H. R. (1960), *Trans. St. John's Hosp. Dermatol. Soc.*, **44**, 1.
WHITE, R. P. (1934), *The Dermatergoses or Occupational Affections of the Skin*, 4th ed., Lewis, London.
WILLAN, R. (1798), *Description and Treatment of Cutaneous Diseases*, London.
ZIELHUIS, R. L. (1961), *Journ. occup. med.*, **3**, 25.

Occupational Stigmata

BELL, J. (1876-7), *Edinb. med. J.*, **22**, 135.
BURROWS, A. (1931), *Proc. R. Soc. Med. (Sect. Dermat.)*, **25**, 216.

ELSBURY, W. B., BROWNE, R. C., and BOYES, J. (1951), *Brit. J. industr. Med.*, **8**, 179.

HAMILL, P. (1935), Personal communication.

HELLER, J. (1900), *Die Krankheiten der Nägel*, Berlin.

KESSLER, H. H. (1931), *Accidental Injuries*, London, p. 643.

LANE, W. A. (1885), *Guy's Hosp. Rep.*, **63**, 321.

LEGGE, Sir T. (1934), *Industrial Maladies*, Oxford.

LYNCH, J. B., and BELL, J. (1947), *Brit. J. industr. Med.*, **4**, 84.

RAMAZZINI, B. (1713), *De Morbus Artificum Diatriba*, Geneva.

RONCHESE, F. (1945), *J. Amer. med. Ass.*, **128**, 925; (1948) *Occupational Marks*, Grune and Stratton, New York; (1953), *Industr. Med. and Surg.*, **22**, 45.

ROUBAL, J. (1947), Personal communication.

SAXBY, J. M. E. (1913), *Joseph Bell*, Edinburgh.

SCOTT, S. G. (1935), *Radiological Atlas of Chronic Rheumatic Arthritis (The Hand)*, Oxford.

SKIRVING, R. S. (1950), Personal communication.

SMITH, K. D., and MASTERS, W. E. (1939), *J. industr. Hyg.*, **21**, 97.

WHITE, R. P. (1934), *The Dermatergoses or Occupational Affections of the Skin*, 4th ed., Lewis, London.

Occupational Bursitis

ATKINS, J. B., and MARKS, J. (1952), *Brit. J. industr. Med.*, **9**, 296.

COLLIS, E. L., and LLEWELLYN, T. L. (1924), *Spec. Rep. Ser. Med. Res. Coun.*, London, No. 89.

Traumatic Tenosynovitis

BLOOD, W. (1942), *Brit. med. J.*, **2**, 468.

HOWARD, N. J. (1937), *J. Bone Jt. Surg.*, **19**, 447.

SMILEY, J. A. (1951), *Brit. J. industr. Med.*, **8**, 265.

SMITHIES, B. M. (1929), *Lancet*, **2**, 494.

THOMPSON, A. R., PLEWES, L. W., and SHAW, E. G. (1951), *Brit. J. industr. Med.*, **8**, 150.

TROELL, A. (1918), *Dtsch. Z. Chir.*, **143**, 125.

Occupational Cancer

BUTLIN, H. T. (1892), *Brit. med. J.*, **1**, 1341; **2**, 1, 66.

GOLDBLATT M. W., and GOLDBLATT, J. (1955), *Occupational Carcinogenesis*, in MEREWETHER, E. R. A., *Industrial Medicine and Hygiene*. Butterworth, London, **3**, 185.

HIEGER, I. (1949), *Brit. J. industr. Med.*, **6**, 1.

KENNAWAY, E. L. (1924), *J. Path. Bact.*, **27**, 233; (1925), *Brit. med. J.*, **2**, 1.

KENNAWAY, E. L., and HIEGER, I. (1930), *Brit. med. J.*, **1**, 1044.

POTT, P. (1775), *Chirurgical Observations relative to the Cataract, the Polypus of the Nose, the Cancer of the Scrotum, the different kind of Ruptures and the Mortification of the Toes and Feet*, London.

YAMAGIWA, K., and ICHIKAWA, K. (1915), *Mitt. med. Fak.*, Tokio, **15**, 295.

(a) Cancer of the Lung

BIDSTRUP, P. L., and CASE, R. A. M. (1956), *Brit. J. industr. Med.*, **13**, 260.

BRAUN, D. C., and TRUAN, T. D. (1958), *Arch. industr. Hlth.*, **17**, 634.

BUECHLEY, R. W. (1963), *Amer. J. publ. Hlth.*, **53**, 1229.

DOLL, R. (1955), *Brit. J. industr. Med.*, **12**, 81; (1958), ibid., **15**, 217.

de VILLIERS, A. J., and WINDISH, J. P. (1964), *Brit. J. industr. Med.*, **21**, 94.

EVANS, R. D., and GOODMAN, C. (1940), *J. industr. Hyg.*, **22**, 89.

HAERTING, F. H., and HESSE, W. (1879), *Vjschr. gerichtl. Med.*, **31**, 102.

HILL, A. B., and FANING, E. L. (1948), *Brit. J. industr. Med.*, **5**, 2.

HILL, Sir A. Bradford (1965), *Proc. Roy. Soc. Med.*, **58**, 295.

HUEPER, W. C. (1942), *Occupational Tumours and Allied Diseases*, Springfield, Illinois.

JACOE, P. W. (1953), *Arch. industr. Hyg.*, **8**, 118.

LORENZ, E. (1944), *J. nat. Cancer Inst.*, **5**, 1.

McCULLOUGH, T. W. (1959), *Ann. Rep. Chief Inspect. Factories on Industrial Health for 1958*, Cmd. 811, H.M.S.O., London.

MORGAN, J. GWYNNE (1958), *Brit. J. industr. Med.*, **15**, 224.

NEITZEL, E. (1935), *Arbeits-med.*, Barth, Leipzig.

OOSTHUIZEN, S. F., PYNE-MERCIER, W. G., FICHARDT, T. and SAVAGE, D. (1958), *Proc. 2nd. U.N. Int. Conf. on Peaceful Uses of Atomic Energy, Geneva*, 1958, **21**, 25, United Nations, Geneva.

PIRCHAN, A., and SIKL, H. (1932), *Amer. J. Cancer*, **16**, 681.

ROSTOSKI and SAUPE (1926), *Z. Krebforsch.*, **23**, 360.

SCHMORL, G. (1928), *International Conference on Cancer*, London, p. 2.

WAGONER, J. K., ARCHER, V. E., CARROLL, B. E., HOLADAY, D. A., and LAWRENCE, P. A. (1964), *J. nat. Cancer Inst.*, **32**, 787.

WAGONER, J. K., ARCHER, V. E., LUNDIN, F. E., HOLADAY, D. A., and LLOYD, J. W. (1965), *New Engl. J. Med.*, **273**, 181.

(b) Cancer of the Skin

BELL, J. (1876–7), *Edinb. med. J.*, **22**, 135.

BERENBLUM, I., and SCHOENTAL, R. (1943), *Brit. J. exp. Path.*, **24**, 232.

CRUICKSHANK, C. N. D., and SQUIRE, J. R. (1950), *Brit. J. industr. Med.*, **7**, 1.

HENRY, S. A. (1946), *Cancer of the Scrotum in Relation to Occupation*, Oxford; (1947), *Brit. med. Bull.*, **4**, 389.

KINGSBURY, A. N. (1926), *Malayan med. J.*, **1**, 11.

LEITCH, A. (1922), *Brit. med. J.*, **2**, 1104.

O'DONOVAN, W. J. (1926), *Lancet*, **2**, 278.

SCOTT, A. (1923), *Eighth Scientific Report, Imperial Cancer Research Fund*, p. 85.

SOUTHAM, A. H., and WILSON, S. R. (1922), *Brit. med. J.*, **2**, 971.

TWORT, C. A., and FULTON, J. D. (1929), *J. Path. Bact.*, **32**, 149.

VON VOLKMANN, R. (1875), *Beitr. z. Chirug.*, Leipzig, p. 370.

(c) Cancer of the Bladder

BILLIARD-DUCHESNE, J. L. (1948), *Arch. Mal. prof.*, **9**, 109.

BONSER, G. M., CLAYSON, D. B., and JULL, J. W. (1951), *Lancet*, **2**, 286.

CASE, R. A. M., and PEARSON, J. T. (1954), *Brit. J. industr. Med.*, **11**, 213.

CURSHMANN, F. (1920), *Zbl. GewHyg.*, **8**, 145.

ELMES, P. C. (1966), *Health Congress of the Royal Society of Health at Blackpool*, April 25, p. 65.

GOLDBLATT, M. W. (1949), *Brit. J. industr. Med.*, **6**, 65.

HAMILTON, A. (1925), *Industrial Poisons in the United States*, Macmillan, New York, p. 493.

HUEPER, W. C. (1938), *Arch. Path.*, **25**, 856.

HUEPER, W. C., WILEY, F. H., and WOLFE, H. D. (1938), *J. industr. Hyg.*, **20**, 69.

JULL, J. W. (1951), *Brit. J. Cancer*, **5**, 328.

LUEUNBERGER, S. G. (1912), *Beitr. klin. Chir.*, **80**, 208.

MACALPINE, J. B. (1929), *Brit. med. J.*, **2**, 794; (1947), *Brit. J. Surg.*, **35**, 137.

MELICK, W. F. (1958), *VII Congr. int. Cancer*, London, p. 73.

OPPENHEIMER, R. (1926), *Verh. dtsch. Ges. Urol.*, 7th Congress, Vienna, p. 348.

POOLE-WILSON, D. S. (1960), *Proc. Roy. Soc. Med.*, London, **53**, 801.

REHN, L. (1895), *Arch. klin. Chir.*, **30**, 588.

SCOTT, T. S. (1952), *Brit. J. industr. Med.*, **9**, 127; (1958), *Trans. Assoc. industr. med. offrs.*, **9**, 57; (1959), M.D. Thesis, Glasgow.

SCOTT, T. S., and WILLIAMS, M. H. C. (1957), *Brit. J. industr. Med.*, **14**, 150.

WALPOLE, A. L., and WILLIAMS, M. H. C. (1958), *Brit. med. Bull*, **14**, 141.

CHAPTER XIII

DISEASES DUE TO PHYSICAL AGENTS

DECOMPRESSION SICKNESS

DECOMPRESSION sickness is a comprehensive title covering caisson disease, compressed-air illness, divers' paralysis and aero-embolism of aviators. It is the name given to the symptoms which appear (i) when workers in compressed air are too rapidly decompressed; (ii) when deep-sea divers or men escaping from sunken submarines come too rapidly to the surface; and (iii) when airmen or air passengers ascend too rapidly to high altitudes.

Structure and Uses of the Caisson

Caisson disease is an industrial hazard encountered in those processes of subaquatic engineering in which compressed air is employed. The work of excavating for the foundations of piers, river bridges, skyscrapers and certain tunnels is carried out in a subaqueous chamber called a caisson. (French, *caisse* from Latin *capsa*, a box or case.) This is essentially a tube of iron or concrete open below and provided with a cutting edge by which it sinks when weighted into mud, sand or moist earth. The working chamber at the bottom is kept clear of water by compressed air, and it is here that the men work. Pressure is produced and maintained by pumps and regulating apparatus. It follows that caisson workers are submitted to a pressure of air which exceeds the hydrostatic pressure of that depth of water in which they work.

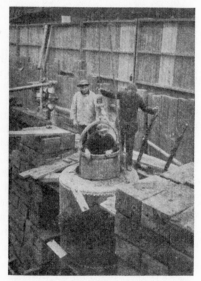

FIG. 318.—Workman about to be lowered in a Bucket into the Air-lock of a Caisson

Descent through Air-locks

Workmen descend to the working-place of the caisson by passing from the normal atmosphere through a series of chambers with airtight doors in which the air pressure is raised by rapid stages until the high pressure of the working-place is reached (fig. 318). They leave through the same chambers, the air pressure being lowered for some space of time in each as they pass through. This process is termed *compression* and *decompression* or *locking in and out*. Caissons are usually worked at a pressure of below 35 lb. per square inch and in six- to eight-hour shifts, but they have been successfully worked at a pressure of 45 lb. per square inch with two-hour shifts, and at 50 lb. per square inch with one-hour shifts.

History of Caisson Disease

Caissons were first employed in England at Rochester in 1851, by Hughes, during the construction of a bridge over the Medway, and shortly afterwards by Brunel at Chepstow and Saltash. At Saltash one man died shortly after coming out of a caisson in which he had been working at a depth of 88 feet and under a pressure of 40 lb. At the St. Louis Bridge, on the Mississippi, 600 men were employed in sinking the foundations. Of these 600 men, 119 suffered from caisson disease, 14 of whom died. At Brooklyn Bridge, New York, there were 110 cases of compressed air illness, with three deaths. The Forth Bridge and the Blackwall Tunnel were the first works using high pressures which were completed without a fatality. No death from caisson disease occurred in the Baker Street and Waterloo Railway tunnel works in London. At the King Edward Bridge, Newcastle upon Tyne, one man died from the effects of caisson disease (Oliver, 1908).

Naked Diving

Diving without appliances is still carried out by men and women who fish in the sea for sponges, pearls, coral, shellfish and edible seaweeds. Under favourable conditions such as those in a swimming-bath of warm water a man can hold his breath and remain submerged for four and a half minutes. In such cases no depth is attained and no work done. The normal type of unassisted naked diving is that practised for thousands of years by the sponge-divers of the Mediterranean and the pearl-divers of India and the Pacific. The naked diver carries a shaped stone which he uses in conjunction with a rope. By holding the stone at a certain angle when diving he is enabled to reach bottom at a chosen spot. Some of these natural divers rub their bodies with oil and plug their ears, or hold a piece of sponge, soaked in oil, in their mouths, but the utility of these precautions is doubtful and the majority of the men disdain them. As a rule, the naked diver does not stay under water more than a minute and a half, or go lower than 75 feet, though much deeper dives have occasionally been made. Cases of bleeding from the nose, ears and mouth are common, and sometimes divers are brought up unconscious. They are, as a rule, short-lived men. In the Tuamotu Archipelago of the South Pacific repeated dives to depths of 120 feet are performed by male pearl divers. Sometimes coming to the surface they are stricken by the bends; if the decompression sickness proves fatal they call it *taravana*.

Sponge and Pearl Fisheries

Today the most important pearl fisheries employing the naked diver are in Ceylon and the Persian Gulf, where several thousand persons are dependent upon the industry for their livelihood. These divers frequently remain below the surface for two minutes at a time. In some parts of Japan there are colonies of naked women pearl-divers who are the acknowledged heads of their families and support both husband and children. The chief sponge fisheries are in the Mediterranean, where the divers, mostly of Greek nationality, all use diving apparatus. There are other fisheries in the Gulf of Florida, in Cuba, the Islands of the Caribbean and on the North African coast. Some of them employ a certain number of naked divers, but in most cases diving apparatus is used. As in the case of the mother-of-pearl shell, the best specimens of sponge are to be found in deep water, the shallow-water fisheries having become practically exhausted through over-fishing (Davis, 1951).

The Diving Women of Korea and Japan

Off the shores of South Korea and southern Japan the bottom of the ocean is rich in shell-fish and edible seaweeds. For at least 1,500 years these foods have been harvested by women divers who support their families by diving daily to reach them. Some 30,000 of these women called ama work four hours a day with intervals of rest away from the water. Childbearing does not interrupt their work. A pregnant diving woman may work up to the day of delivery and afterwards nurse her baby between diving shifts. Operating from a small float at the surface, and naked except for a loincloth, she takes several deep breaths then swims to the bottom, gathers what she can find and swims up to her float again. On occasion she may go as deep as 50 feet but usually she limits her foraging to a depth of 20 feet. Her average dive lasts about 30 seconds of which 15 seconds is spent working on the bottom. When she surfaces she hangs on to the float and rests for about 30 seconds, taking deep breaths, and then dives again. Thus the cycle takes about a minute, and the ama averages about 60 dives an hour. These divers never suffer from decompression sickness. Long experience has taught them the limits of safety and they content themselves with short dives which they can perform again and again for extended periods without danger. Physiological studies of these women show that in training they develop an unusually large vital capacity which fortifies them for diving. Conservation of body heat is assisted by a more generous endowment of subcutaneous fat than exists in the case of men. In addition the ama eats half as much food again as her non-diving sister. But the most surprising finding was that an elevation of the basal rate of metabolism of about 25 per cent was found to be present in the winter months. This arises from the fact that in winter the ama subjects herself to a daily cold stress greater than that of any other group of human beings yet studied (Hong and Rahn, 1967). In recent years the

ama has dwindled in numbers, but her work remains a proud calling an
necessary livelihood. Attempts to introduce self-contained underwate
breathing apparatus (scuba gear) which could at once provide a ten-fol
increase of the food harvest obtained by diving are fiercely resiste
because of the havoc which the women believe would result to the ecc
nomy of hundreds of small villages in terms of unemployment.

Diving with Apparatus

Dress-divers are employed in the construction of harbours, docks, pier
breakwaters and bridges, in recovering sunken ships, cargo and treasure
and in cleaning and repairing the hulls of ships. The diving dress use
consists of a copper helmet attached to a metal corselet, the latter bein
secured watertight to a rubber suit fitting closely every part of the bod
except the hands, which pass through elastic cuffs. The boots are heavil
weighted. Compressed air is supplied by an air-pump on the surfac
through a flexible pipe and is carried through a tube at the back of th
helmet. The exhaled air escapes through a spring valve at the side of th
helmet whenever the inside pressure becomes slightly greater than that c
the surrounding water. For every 33 feet ($5\frac{1}{2}$ fathoms) in depth of water, th
pressure increases by one atmosphere or 15 lb. to a square inch. Thus th
diver is compressed as he slowly descends by an increasing air pressur
from his pump and is decompressed as he ascends much more slowly
The working shifts of divers are much shorter than those of caisso
workers. Divers frequently work at 120 feet (53 lb. per square inch), an
the record depth has been 540 feet (240 lb. per square inch), but to resis
the pressure at such a depth it is best to wear an incompressible metal sui
In 1960 in the Pacific Ocean a ten-ton bathyscaphe of the U.S. Nav
manned by two men reached a depth of 37,800 feet, which is more tha
7 miles. At the bottom the bathyscaphe was subject to a pressure o
16,883 lb. per square inch. The steel gondola housing the crew was built o
six-inch steel, laboratory-tested up to pressures double those met at th
bottom, that is, 16 tons per square inch.

Aero-embolism of Aviators

Decompression sickness of aviators differs from caisson disease only i
its lesser severity. In flying, symptoms may develop at 32,000 feet if th
rate of climb is 2000 feet a minute or more. They may appear after a fe
minutes or only after two or three hours, according to the particula
susceptibility of the individual. Above 37,000 feet any reasonable rate o
climb is very likely to produce symptoms even in the most resistan
individual (Behnke, 1945). It is usually possible in aviation for a man to b
decompressed from one atmosphere to one-quarter of an atmosphere in si
minutes before symptoms of *bends* develop. The symptoms are not severe
although this rate of decompression would correspond, in divers, to a

ascent to the surface in six minutes from a depth of 100 feet after an exposure of five and a half hours. This would result in the most severe form of *bends* and even in the death of the diver if recompression were not undertaken immediately (Rainsford, 1942). Airmen flying above 14,000 feet breathe pure oxygen. Moreover, they tend to develop an alkalosis at altitudes above 10,000 feet owing to hyperventilation occurring in response to anoxæmia. These are conditions which are known to alleviate the symptoms of *bends*, but in themselves are insufficient to explain why pilots do not develop symptoms at altitudes lower than 30,000 feet.

Symptoms and Signs

In caisson workers the onset of symptoms is relatively rapid, in 60 per cent during the first hour, in 35 per cent during the second hour, in 3 per cent during the third hour, and in the remaining 2 per cent after twelve hours (Thorne, 1941). The commonest symptom is dull throbbing pain, gradual in onset, progressive and shifting in character and frequently felt in the joints, or deeply in muscles and bones. Pains of this nature are referred to as *the pressure* or *the bends*. The latter term, established by long usage, arises in the fact that the limb affected is held in a semi-flexed position from which it is found difficult to straighten it. The elbows, wrists, knees and hips are the areas most frequently affected, but the epigastric and lumbar regions may be involved too. Numbness may precede the onset of pain. Skin temperature may fall as the part involved becomes blanched in appearance. Erythema of the skin with pruritus, *the itch* or *prickles*, occurs with regularity if the skin is chilled during decompression. Vertigo, *the staggers*, is a common symptom. The staggering gait may be accompanied by nausea, vomiting, tinnitus and nystagmus.

Asphyxia, Collapse and Death

A type of asphyxia known as *the chokes* or *the chokers* may occur, though it is less frequent than *the bends*. Several hours of complete well-being following decompression may elapse before the appearance of the earliest symptom of *chokes*—namely, a sensation of retrosternal distress felt only during deep inspiration which frequently serves to elicit the cough reflex. This sensation of retrosternal distress may be only transient or it may progress to frank asphyxia. Normal breathing becomes shallow, rapid and then dyspnœic. The skin becomes cyanotic, or ashen grey, cold and clammy. The pulse, at first slow and pounding, becomes thready. Paroxysmal attacks of coughing or true *chokes* may precede loss of consciousness. The picture presented is one of shock and represents a transformation within a period usually of several hours from a state of health and vigour to one of incapacity without any apparent trauma being inflicted upon the individual. It is this condition which not only frequently supervenes in divers when the premonitory symptoms of *bends* are ignored and treatment delayed, but may also be responsible for circulatory collapse and death which occasionally follow too rapid decompression in the low-pressure chamber.

Complications

The complications of decompression sickness are limited to certain lesions of the nervous system, lungs, bones and joints. Paraplegia was a one time so common in divers that it became known as *divers' palsy*. I usually extends as high as the ninth dorsal segmental level, but may reach the cervical region and involve the arms. It comes on rapidly and involves motor sensory and sphincter functions. It may be of any degree of severity, from a slight and transient effect to a complete and permanent loss of the functions of the spinal cord. It occurs with increasing frequency and completeness in proportion to the degree of pressure and the length of exposure to its influence. Hemiplegia or monoplegia of cerebral origin is less commonly seen. Spontaneous pneumothorax is a rare complication of too rapid decompression.

Aseptic Necrosis of Bone

Bone complications have been recorded in caisson workers (Kahlstrom, Burton and Phemister, 1939), and in men who have escaped from sunken submarines (James, 1945). The symptoms of onset are insidious and are

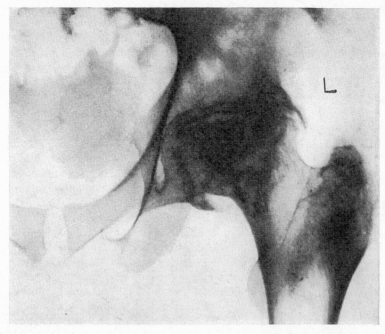

Fig. 319.—Osteo-arthritis of the Hip, the end result of Nitrogen Embolism of the End Arteries supplying the Articular Cartilage of the Head of the Femur. In his younger days the Patient had worked for years in Caissons constructing Tunnels

(*By permission of Surgery, Gynecology and Obstetrics, 1939*, **68**, *129*)

delayed from six months to a year or more following repeated attacks of caisson disease. Various infarcts, possibly due to nitrogen emboli in end arteries of nutrient vessels, lead to aseptic necrosis of areas of bone and sometimes of articular cartilage. The bones of the lower limbs are commonly affected and the joints include hip, knee and shoulder (plates VIII and IX). Where the diaphysis of a bone is involved, the lesion results in an encapsulated calcified area. The joint lesion may lead to persistent pain and ultimately to osteo-arthritis with disablement (fig. 319).

Ætiology and Pathology

Paul Bert (1878), by a remarkable series of experiments, first proved that the cause of compressed-air illness is the effervescence of gas in the body fluids, an effervescence which takes place when a man is rapidly returned to the normal atmospheric pressure. His experiments showed clearly that the illness was due to liberation in the blood and tissues of bubbles of gas consisting almost entirely of nitrogen. The gas bubbles are a mixture of about 82 per cent nitrogen, 16 per cent carbon dioxide and 2 per cent oxygen. Whereas most of the dissolved oxygen in the blood is consumed by the tissues, the nitrogen is inert physiologically and is not utilized; therefore it is customary to speak of the gas bubbles as nitrogen bubbles.

Nitrogen Bubbles in Blood and Tissues

Whether they occur after decompression from high-pressure atmospheres or at high altitude, the nitrogen bubbles are chiefly intravascular and they are held responsible for nearly all the symptoms of decompression sickness. Extravascular nitrogen bubbles occur also in severe instances of decompression from high-pressure atmospheres, but they are restricted to certain lipoid-rich structures, notably the white matter of the spinal cord. It has been shown that nitrogen is much more soluble in fat and oils than in water, and that body fat at blood temperature holds five times as much nitrogen per unit mass as does the blood itself.

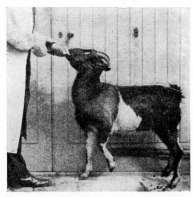

Aero-embolism of Various Tissues

Nitrogen released in the tissues appears to act principally by causing pain in the unyielding tissues such as bone, tendon, fascia, periosteum and nerve sheath. Neural damage due to aero-

Fig. 320.—Paralysis of the Left Fore-paw in a Goat kept in Compressed Air and decompressed too quickly
(*Boycott, A. E., Damant, G. C. C., and Haldane, J. S.* (1908), *J. Hyg.*, **8**, 342)

embolism varies greatly, is nonspecific and unpredictable (fig. 32c
That part of the nervous system which is least vascular—namely, th
four lower dorsal segments of the spinal cord—is the region most con

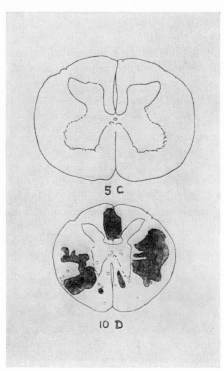

monly affected (fig. 321
Hundreds of bubbles hav
been counted in the spin
cord, and these are muc
more numerous in the whi
than in the grey matter (Bo;
cott, 1907; Boycott, Damai
and Haldane, 1908).

Fatal Distension of th Heart with Gas

In every fatal case whic
has been adequately examine
at necropsy, patches of necr
sis in the dorsal region of th
spinal cord with the usu
secondary degeneration hav
been found. Hæmorrhage
a relatively unimportant fin
ing. Massive escape of nitr
gen bubbles may occur int
the blood stream, and i
rapidly fatal cases the hea
has been found distende
with gas after death. Nitroge
bubbles in the pulmonar
artery and its branches ma
cause death through occlu
ion of the circulation an
asphyxia. Collections of ni
rogen may be found in th
subcutaneous tissues an

FIG. 321.—Spinal Cord of Goat with De-
compression Sickness. The Lower Dorsal
Segments are those most commonly affected.
More Nitrogen Bubbles and therefore
Ischaemia are found in the White Matter
than in the Grey Matter

(Boycott, A. E., Damant, G. C. C., and Haldane J. S
(1908), J. Hyg., 8, 342)

may cause subcutaneous emphysema with palpable crackling. Nitroge
embolism may cause necrosis of the tissues in any part of the body.

Intravascular Agglutination of Red Cells

Swindle (1937) has shown in experimental animals that intravascula
agglutination of red blood cells occurs during decompression. An increas
of carbon dioxide in the air breathed will aggravate this phenomeno
just as it causes an increase in the incidence and severity of decompressio
sickness. Alkalis and oxygen prevent or diminish the erythrocyt
agglutination. The work of End (1938) confirms these findings. Thes
authors suggest, therefore, that the symptoms of decompression sickne:

result from hæmagglutination and circulatory obstruction by cellular emboli. They take the view that bubble formation occurs only in the later stages of severe *bends* as a complicating factor.

Ascent and Descent

The actual ascent and descent of caisson workers, divers and airmen is associated with no worse symptoms than discomfort in the ears from disparity of air pressure in the middle ear, *ear block*. Rupture of the tympanic membrane is rare and may be associated with infection of the middle ear, *aero-otitis media* (Armstrong and Heim, 1937). If air under pressure is trapped in the nasal sinuses there may be pain, *sinus block*. Teeth showing subacute inflammation of the pulp may ache at high altitudes, *aerodontalgia*. Abdominal pain and distension may occur from trapped gases in the intestinal tract.

Length of Exposure

The symptoms resulting from decompression will be severe in direct proportion to the length of exposure to an abnormal pressure and to the rapidity of return to atmospheric pressure. No symptoms occur after short exposures to compressed air such as fifteen minutes at a pressure of 45 lb. per square inch, or two minutes at a pressure of 75 lb. per square inch, even though decompression be as rapid as possible, for these periods are too short to allow of nitrogen saturation of the tissues. It is for this reason that decompression sickness is less common in divers, who for the most part work for a short time only at high pressures, and so much more common in caisson workers who work for many hours at a stretch at a pressure of from 30 to 40 lb. per square inch. Similarly, airmen usually remain above 30,000 feet for too short a time to be affected.

Selection of Workers

The ideal age for compressed-air workers and aviators is between twenty and forty years, since during these years the cardiovascular system is at its greatest efficiency and therefore best able to withstand the hardship involved. There is a wide individual variation in resistance to the effects of pressure. This can be tested by rapid decompression to high altitudes. Some persons develop *bends* at 29,000 feet during one hour exposure. Resistant divers will tolerate 40,000 feet at the rate of 5,000 feet per minute for one hour (Behnke, 1942). All persons with disease of the heart, lungs, kidneys and peripheral vessels should be rejected. Obese men are bad risks because fat deposits act as a gaseous reservoir predisposing to bubble formation. Acute infections of the respiratory passages must temporarily disqualify a man for employment because the infection may involve the Eustachian tubes and the ostia of the sinuses, with the risk that air will be trapped in the middle ear or sinuses with consequent infection or rupture of the tympanum. The workman, airman or air passenger avoids the consequences of unequal pressure on either side of the tympanum by opening the Eustachian tubes with repeated acts of swallowing or yawning. Dental supervision and treatment must be carried out in an endeavour to prevent aerodontalgia.

Preventive Treatment

Symptoms of decompression sickness can always be prevented by adopting suitable limitation of exposure. The malady never arises from compression below 18 lb. to the square inch, or roughly 40 feet of water and those who work at such a pressure may do so for long hours and return to a normal pressure rapidly and without any risk. At higher pressures the working shifts must be shortened as the pressure gets higher. The shift should be not longer than six to eight hours at a pressure of from 30 to 3. lb. per square inch, or 3 atmospheres; two to three hours at a pressure of 45 lb. per square inch, and one hour only at a pressure of 50 lb. per square inch. At higher pressures than this, which are encountered only by divers only a few minutes' exposure is allowed. The regulation must be strictly enforced that no person employed shall consume alcohol whilst in com pressed air.

Slow and Gradual Decompression in Air-locks

Decompression sickness never occurs if the return to the normal atmo spheric pressure be sufficiently slow. In the case of caisson workers a serie of air-locked chambers is provided in which the air pressure is lowered in stages, the men remaining longer and longer at each stage as they approach the normal pressure. The important fact in connexion with decompression is that the absolute pressure can always be halved forthwith without any risk. In the first air-lock on leaving the working face of a caisson, for example, the pressure is at once reduced to one-half that of the working face, and in the remaining air-locks the pressure is reduced by stages until zero is reached. The difficulty and danger is the tendency on the part of the workers to curtail these weary waits in order to get away from work as soon as possible.

Necessity for Strict Supervision

The work of Paton and Walder (1954) on decompression sickness in men constructing a tunnel under the Tyne between 1948 and 1950 em phasizes the necessity for strict supervision at all times. The whole popula tion at risk was investigated. Since only severe cases are reported to the Chief Inspector of Factories, although 350 cases occurred only 3 were notified. A total of 40,000 compressions were carried out, involving 378 men. Of these, 187 experienced symptoms on one or more occasions, and attacks of decompression sickness totalled 350. There was an important correlation between the weekly incidence of bends and the recruitment of new workers; the weekly incidence fell from an initial level of 20 per cent to almost negligible values after months of working in compressed air This decline was due both to acclimatization and to the elimination of the more susceptible workers by natural selection.

Paraplegia in Men who Disregarded the Regulations

Three severe cases of decompression sickness occurred during the two years of work on the tunnel. In two of these cases the patients became paraplegic with incontinence of urine and partial incontinence of fæces; little function had been recovered twelve months and nine months after the onset. In one of these two cases the workman had let himself out through the air-lock normally used for the disposal of rubble from the working site. Fifteen minutes later he noticed numbness and weakness of the legs, and he was immediately taken to the medical lock and recompressed; but this had no effect. The second man developed symptoms during the normal decompression at the end of a working shift, and was immediately transferred to the medical lock for recompression; but again this gave no benefit. The supervision of men working in caissons must be strict and continuous, but it is clear that even when careful precautions are devised they do not wholly eliminate the risk of serious illness.

Admiralty Rules for Divers

In the case of the diver decompression is carried out by raising him to various levels in stages, and letting him remain at each stage a longer and longer period as the surface is approached. The Admiralty rules for divers require that a diver working, say, at 140 feet shall be first raised straightway to a depth of 50 feet where he waits ten minutes, then to 40 feet for ten minutes, 30 feet for twenty minutes, 20 feet for thirty minutes, 10 feet for thirty-five minutes, and then he leaves the water abruptly.

Nitrogen Narcosis

In 1938 End reported a world record dive of 420 feet, using a mixture of helium and oxygen in place of ordinary air. The atmosphere breathed contained 80 per cent helium and 20 per cent oxygen. Behnke (1942) reports two dives made to a sunken submarine at 440 feet. The divers were able to remain on the botton for ten minutes. They felt well although subjected to 14·3 atmospheres pressure, equivalent to 210 lb. per square inch. Dives to such depths are not safe when an atmosphere of air is provided, because a diver breathing air becomes helpless at depths greater than 300 feet. This is due to the effects of absorbed nitrogen on cell function. Symptoms occur which vary from a feeling of hilarity, loss of emotional control and inco-ordination of muscular movements to complete loss of consciousness. The syndrome is known as nitrogen narcosis.

Helium and Oxygen in Deep Diving

Substitution of helium for nitrogen prevents these symptoms from developing even at a depth of 500 feet. It also allows decompression to be undertaken in a shorter time. These advantages are probably due to the lower solubility of helium as compared with nitrogen in both fat and water. An average man when fully saturated with helium holds in his tissues 60 per cent less gas, by volume, than when fully saturated with nitrogen.

When pure oxygen is breathed at one atmosphere, the time necessary for complete desaturation of helium is half that of nitrogen. The time necessary for 50 per cent desaturation is approximately the same for both gases (Behnke, 1938). Hydrogen behaves in a similar way to helium.

Oxygen Poisoning

The increased partial pressure of oxygen in air, or oxygen-helium mixtures, at high pressures may cause symptoms of oxygen poisoning. Those affecting the central nervous system are of practical importance in deep diving. Vague feelings of discomfort and stiffening or twitching of the facial muscles are followed by convulsions in which the muscular contractions may be violent enough to break a bone. Loss of consciousness occurs finally, sometimes without warning. There is considerable variability in the time of onset of such symptoms in different individuals, and in the same individual on different occasions. The percentage of oxygen in the helium oxygen mixture used in the 440-foot dives described by Behnke (1942) was reduced from 21 per cent to 12 per cent at one atmosphere because, at depths of 500 feet, the increase partial pressure of oxygen at the higher percentage may be sufficient to induce unconsciousness.

Prompt Treatment by Surfacing for Fresh Air

All divers using oxygen apparatus should be instructed in the possible warning symptoms that they themselves may feel, and should be taught to come up at once should they occur. The only cure for oxygen poisoning is

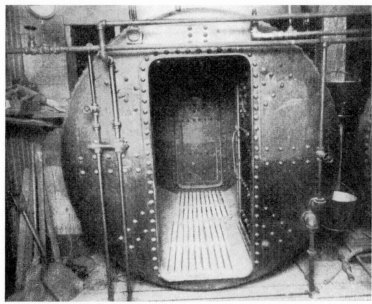

Fig. 322.—Compressed-air Chamber kept on the Site of Tunnelling Operations

o breathe fresh air. The diver's head must be freed from his suit and
he must be made comfortable on deck. Convulsions, if present, will
gradually subside and the diver will go off into a deep sleep for an hour or
two. On waking, although he may suffer a headache and some temporary
loss of memory for twenty-four hours or so, there will be no serious after-
effects.

Sealed Pressure Cabins in Aeroplanes

In commercial aviation passengers should not be flown at altitudes
above 18,000 feet in unsealed cabins, and military flying should be restricted to this level where practicable. Even when using sealed pressure
cabins, altitudes above 30,000 feet should never be exceeded because of the
danger of decompression sickness in the event of cabin failure.

Recompression and Decompression

It was early discovered by the caisson workers themselves that the only
remedy for the malady was to re-enter the high air pressure. A recompression apparatus in the form of a medical air-lock is supplied at all caisson
works and in all ships engaged in deep salvage (fig. 322). On the appearance
of any symptoms the worker is placed in the compressing room and the
pressure is run up to the level at which he has been working, when it is
usual for the symptoms to diminish rapidly or to disappear.

Necessity of Very Slow Decompression

After the recompression the decompression must be carried out very
slowly, for the bubbles once formed in the tissues are not easy to get rid of,
though they may be kept at a small size by the pressure. A patient apparently
at the point of death with cyanosis and coma may completely recover in a
few hours by recompression. When symptoms have appeared, the decompression should take from five to twenty-four hours.

Wearing of Precautionary Metal Labels

Caisson workers and divers should wear on the lapels of their jackets a
metal label clearly inscribed with a notice stating both their occupation and
the address of their place of work (fig. 323). They should sleep and live
close to the medical air-lock in order that they may be near aid during the
first hours following decompression. The paralysis when once established
is to be treated upon ordinary lines. Aseptic necrosis of articular cartilage
may necessitate opening a joint for removal of necrotic material.

Descent of Aeroplanes to Safe Levels

In aviation, recompression fortunately involves only descent to lower
altitudes and higher atmospheric pressures. The descent should be started
as soon as possible after the onset of symptoms and as rapidly as is consistent with the safety of the flight. For mild attacks a descent to about
25,000 feet will generally relieve all the dangerous symptoms, although

pruritus may persist. In a severe attack descent to sea-level or slightly above should be made, and the flight discontinued at the first available landing-point. In crashes following high-altitude flights the possibility of coma or paralysis among the injured being due to decompression sickness should be borne in mind.

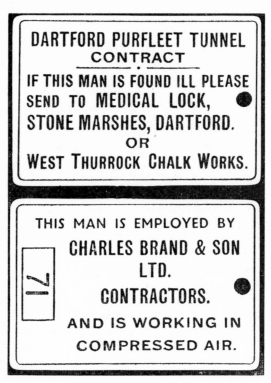

FIG. 323.—Precautionary Metal Tablet worn by a Caisson Worker

The Subject Reviewed

Decompression sickness incident to deep-sea diving and high-altitude ascent has been reviewed by Behnke (1945). A review of the pathological consequences of decompression sickness has been written by Catchpole and Gersh (1947). A comprehensive manual for deep-sea divers and compressed-air workers has been compiled by Sir Robert H. Davis (1951).

HEAT CRAMPS

The occurrence of cramps amongst firemen, furnacemen, metal casters, forge-hammer workers, foundry workers, iron and glass workers, and miners is well known. Workers in the Nevada desert and sugar-cane cutters in North Queensland are liable to be affected (Derrick, 1934).

History

Heat cramps were frequently reported in the stokeholds of warships or merchant ships in the tropics; they were regarded as a form of heat stroke. About 1910 it was common for as many as eighty cases to occur in a year in one ship. As oil-burning steamers increased, the number of cases diminished. It was not in the hot engine-room that the cramps occurred, but in the cooler, better-ventilated stokehold—*stokers' cramp*—where heavy toil provoked profuse sweating (fig. 324). In 1923 Moss pointed out that *miners' cramp* was observed only among the workers in hot mines where the temperature varies between 98° and 102° F.

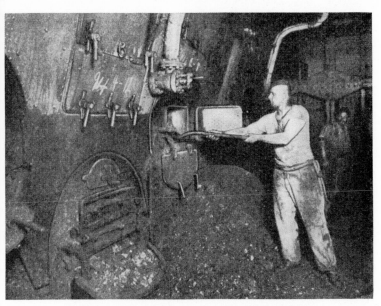

FIG. 324.—Stokehold of a Coal-fired Ship in 1910
(*The Occupational Diseases, W. G. Thompson, New York, 1914*)

Great Heat in Deep Coal Mines

The conditions in such a mine have been described by J. B. S. Haldane (1927).

Perhaps the hottest place in England is about a mile under Salford, where the coal miners work in boots and bathing-drawers, and empty the sweat from their boots at lunch or snapping-time. One man sweated 18 lb. in the course of a shift, and it is probable that even this figure has been exceeded. This sweat contained about an ounce of salt —twice what the average man consumes in all forms per day. The salt loss was instinctively made up above ground by means of bacon, kippers, salted beer and the like. And as long as they did not drink

D.O.—28*

more than a quart of water underground, no harm came to the miners. But a man who has sweated nearly two gallons is thirsty, and coal-dust dries the throat, so this amount was often exceeded and the excess occasionally led to appalling attacks of cramp, often in the stomach, but sometimes in the limbs or back. The victims had taken more water than was needed to adjust the salt concentration in their blood, and the diversion of blood from their kidneys to their muscles and skin was so great that they were unable to excrete the excess. The miners in question were offered a solution of salt in water which was of about the composition of sweat, and would be somewhat unappetising to the average man. They drank it by quarts and asked for more. And now that it has become their regular beverage underground there is no more cramp and far less fatigue. It is almost certain that the cramp of stokers, and of iron and glass workers which is known to be due to excessive water-drinking, could be prevented in the same way.

Symptoms and Signs

Men are generally affected by it during the second half of the shift, and always in the muscles actually being used at the time. Sufferers are usually men of poor physique. The cramps begin generally in the calves and spread to the upper limbs and abdomen. If a man is attacked whilst lifting a full tub on to the rails the cramp may occur in the arms, legs or abdomen. If in the latter the man is put out of action immediately, the contortion of the abdominal muscles being so great as to form a lump the size of a cricket ball. In severe attacks of cramp it may take half a dozen men to hold down a sufferer and straighten out the affected limb. Such treatment produces excessive exhaustion of the sufferer (Brockbank, 1929). In some cases the pain is so severe that the patient states he would rather die than go through another attack. The temperature and pulse are raised little if at all; albuminuria is frequently found (Talbott, 1935).

Ætiology and Pathology

Moss and Haldane showed that miners' cramps are brought about by excessive sweating followed by the drinking of water. The sweating leads to a great loss of water and salt from the body. More than 8 kilograms of sweat, containing 20 grams of sodium chloride, may be lost in a shift by a miner in a hot mine. The urine of a miner with cramps contains no chloride whatever, and his blood chloride content is much reduced. Sweating alone could not bring about this reduction, for sweat contains only about 0·2 per cent sodium chloride, and sweating by itself would tend to concentrate the salt in the blood.

Excess Intake of Water

Thus Talbott, Dill and others (1933) found that exertion in the heat of the Nevada desert for an hour and three-quarters without drinking, concentrated the serum chloride by 4·5 per cent. There must be, in addition, the drinking of more water than is necessary to adjust the salt concentration in the blood. Talbott and Michelson (1933) studied the blood and urine chemistry of patients with heat cramps. Their material was drawn from workers constructing the Hoover dam in the Colorado river basin desert, where the summer climate is extremely hot and dry (fig. 325). They found that the mildest case showed a 2 per cent reduction in serum chloride, and the most severe case a 10 per cent reduction.

Acclimatization at the Hoover Dam

The observations on acclimatization by Dill at the Hoover dam were of much practical importance. Soon after a man first goes into the desert, where sweating is profuse and continued, the percentage of salt in the

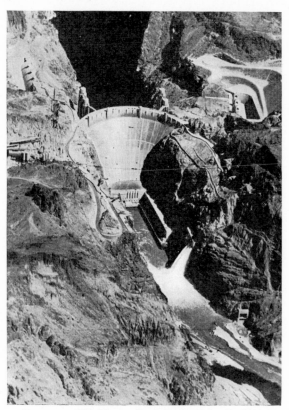

FIG. 325.—The Hoover Dam in the Colorado River
Basin Desert
(*By courtesy of Associated Press of Great Britain, Ltd.*)

sweat falls in the course of a few days to an average of 0·09 per cent. Thus salt is conserved, and heavy work with free sweating becomes possible in a tropical climate without undue salt loss or the necessity for a greatly abnormal salt intake. For example, a man who sweated 10 litres would need to take only about 15 grams of salt. After acclimatization many workers are able to take with their meals all the salt that is necessary. This explains why cramps are not more common.

Treatment

For the unacclimatized, those returning to hot work after a break and those susceptible to cramp, further salt is required. It appears most logical to replace the salt as it is lost, by drinking 0·1 to 0·25 per cent saline solution. The workers on the Hoover dam were recommended to drink milk freely, for it contains 0·3 per cent sodium chloride. The efficacy of sodium chloride in the prevention and treatment of heat cramps has now been widely confirmed by experience among workers in the various occupations concerned. In workers in Great Britain the sodium chloride intake in the diet should normally be 45 to 60 grains (3 to 4 grams) a day. Fatigue and cramps occur in industry mainly amongst workers on hot processes where extensive physical effort is required. In heat waves, however, any worker can be affected, more particularly when ventilation is inadequate (Stewart, 1945).

Tablets for Effervescent Saline Drinks

An effervescent drink can be made up from tablets kept in a suitable container at the place of work. The following tablet is commonly used:

Sodium chloride gr. 5
Potassium citrate gr. $\frac{1}{2}$
Acid sodium phosphate gr. $\frac{1}{2}$
Sodium bicarbonate ⎱
Citric acid |
Tartaric acid ⎰ q.s.
Saccharin |
Oil of lemon ⎰

Each of these tablets when dissolved in half a pint of water makes a pleasant drink with an approximate concentration of 0·1 per cent sodium chloride. In the great majority of workers on hot processes from one to three pints of this mixture per shift will entirely prevent the onset of unpleasant symptoms. Where symptoms have already occurred, this frequently removes them in the most dramatic way. In the prevention of heat symptoms the basic importance of improving working conditions must be emphasized, and it should be remembered that the physical fitness of the worker and the type of clothing he wears are additional factors in determining the onset of symptoms. Saline drinks are only a palliative and where possible the cause of excessive heat at work should be removed.

MINERS' NYSTAGMUS

Nystagmus can occur as an occupational disease affecting miners, sewermen, ceiling plasterers and train despatchers. It has even been de-

scribed in a violinist who was obliged to read his music placed on a high
and badly lighted stand (Kalmus, 1934). It is important only in coal miners,
and is widespread among the coalfields of the British Isles and the continent
of Europe. It would appear to be completely absent in the United States
of America.

Historical Summary

In his book, *The Effects of Arts, Trades and Professions* (1831), Thackrah
makes a statement which evidently refers to miners' nystagmus.

> Their eyes, from the swelling of the lids, appear small, are affected
> with chronic inflammation, and intolerant of full light. Many, after a
> few years' trial, are obliged by the injury which their health has sus-
> tained, and especially by the weakness of their eyes, to leave the mine.

But the first definite accounts of the disease are due to Gillet of Sheffield
and Déconde of Liége (1861). From about 1875, beginning with Taylor, a
number of English, Belgian and German investigators began to apply
themselves to the problem. In England the outstanding investigator was
Simeon Snell, whose monograph, *Miners' Nystagmus* (1892), established
the fact that the disorder is of occupational origin and does cause real
incapacity for work.

Two Divergent Theories of Ætiology

From 1875 on, two divergent theories were proposed to explain the
causation of the disease. The one attributed the nystagmus to the constrained attitude taken by the miner while at work and to the fact that the
line of vision was frequently directed obliquely upward, particularly while
undercutting the seam. The second theory held that defective illumination
was the chief cause; it was upheld by the work of Stassen (1914) in Belgium
and of Collis and Llewellyn (1923) in Great Britain. The Congress of
Ophthalmology, held in Oxford in 1912, was a triumph for the view that
inefficient lighting in coal mines is the real cause of the prevalence of
nystagmus. Statistics show that the frequency of the disease has greatly
increased since it was included under the *Workmen's Compensation Act,*
1907, until by 1930 it was costing the nation about a million pounds a year.
In 1920 new cases certified numbered 2,865, and there were already 4,136
old cases; in 1930 there were 3,066 new cases and 7,572 old cases.

Effect of Inefficient Lighting

Because the presence of methane has acted as a brake to efficient lighting of coal mines in Great Britain the disease is confined to coal miners
who have worked with flame safety-lamps for many years (Fisher, 1949).
In Great Britain measurements have shown that the illumination at the
coal face in naked-light pits is generally from five to ten times as great as that
in safety-lamp pits. Naked-light coal mines, metalliferous mines and slate
mines are practically free from the disease, at least among miners who have
never worked in safety-lamp mines. In the United States of America coal-

face lighting has always been vastly superior to that in Europe. They passed from the naked acetylene flame to the electric cap lamp giving a light from twenty to fifty times brighter than that of the flame safety-lamp. There is no good evidence to suggest that miners' nystagmus is caused by the awkward posture necessitated in coal mining, variations in the temperature and humidity of the pits, infection, or inhalation of carbon monoxide, methane or nitrogen dioxide.

Age Incidence

Miners' nystagmus affects mainly the middle-aged or elderly miner. The average age of onset is forty years and the disorder may take from ten to twenty-five years to develop. In Great Britain most men over fifty who are working in the coal pits under ordinary conditions show signs of it. The majority of miners learn to tolerate the disorder with little or no inconvenience and only a small proportion of those affected actually become incapacitated.

Symptoms and Signs

Of the general symptoms, vertigo is common and may be the determining cause of incapacity. It comes on mainly during work, especially where there is much bending, but it may occur after only slight bending or even on turning sharply to one side or the other. It may be so severe as to make the patient stagger or fall. Headache may occur; it is usually occipital. It may persist long after the other symptoms and signs have disappeared. Some of the symptoms are directly related to the eyes, whereas others are more general. Often there is slowness in dark adaptation, in which the men complain that they take longer than usual to become accustomed to the dim light of the pit. This phenomenon has been wrongly referred to as night blindness. Photophobia is a frequent symptom. The patient may complain of it in connexion with the lamps of other miners in the pit, of the daylight when he comes to the surface and of the headlights of cars at night.

Oscillation of Lights

The symptom of oscillation of lights or of objects looked at is usually described by the patient as spinning of the lights. Though many patients complain pointedly of this symptom, there are others in whom the complaint is not volunteered but can be elicited only by leading questions. In some cases the existence of the oscillation of lights is denied, even while the patient's eyes are clearly seen to oscillate. The explanation of these apparent anomalies probably lies in the degree of tolerance which has been acquired to the oscillation. A person with congenital nystagmus whose eyes have oscillated continuously since infancy perceives no oscillating movement in objects looked at; his cerebral interpretation of the stimuli from his roving eyes is that of a normal image. It appears that miners in whom the disorder has been of slow onset may achieve the same result (Ferguson, 1944). Defective vision is frequently present, more particularly amongst those who complain of objects spinning. Though usually associated with the oscillations, it may persist when the eyes are stationary. It is evidently of psychological origin, for there is no visible retinal lesion to account for it.

The Attributes of a Psychoneurosis

External circumstances, such as prolonged anxiety, the shock of an accident or intercurrent illness, may make the patient rapidly worse and perhaps incapacitate him. In many cases of long standing, psychoneurotic symptoms dominate the picture. They include various combinations of anxiety, insomnia, loss of appetite, irritability, hypochondria, depression, querulousness and resentment. There is usually a preoccupation with discomfort, whether expressed in physical, mental or social terms. The complaints are commonly vague, but expressed with great earnestness, often also with rich prolixity and as though learnt off by heart. On examination, excessive perspiration and tremor of the head and hands are common. Tachycardia may or may not be present; it is found in most cases with psychoneurotic symptoms.

Blepharospasm and Head Tremor

Involuntary movements of the eyelids may occur either in the form of a blepharospasm or of a fibrillary twitching of the eyelids, or both. Such signs are, of course, not uncommonly seen in any type of neurosis secondary to disease of the eye. Head tremor occurs in two forms; the first consists of a rapid rotary movement of the head and is associated with the oscillations; it is, of course, commonly seen also in cases of congenital nystagmus. The second type is a fine rapid vibratory movement which may be coupled with rigidity of the neck and tremors of the hands and, indeed, of the whole body. Sometimes a miner adopts a typical posture with the head thrown back and the cap or hat drawn forward over the eyes. This is a protective reaction to avoid the necessity of elevating the eyes above the horizontal level and to minimize dazzling. Excessive convergence of the eyes is not infrequently present and is accentuated if the eyes are exposed to bright light.

Mechanism of Nystagmus

In order to understand the physical signs of miners' nystagmus it is necessary to inquire into the mechanism of nystagmus in general. The type of movement of the eyeball in nystagmus varies according to the site of the lesion responsible. All forms of nystagmus are due to some interference with the reflex fixation arc. In the case of intracranial lesions farther back than the optic nerve—for example, disseminated sclerosis and labyrinthitis —the nystagmus takes the form of jerky, lateral, pendular movements of both eyes. Such movements are most commonly elicited by horizontal deviation of the eyes, though sometimes by vertical deviation. Lateral nystagmus is made up of two components—a slow jerk from the point of fixation to the point of rest, followed by a more rapid jerk back to the point of fixation. Where the lesion causing nystagmus is in the eye itself, movements of the eyeball are quite different, being undulatory or rotary. Such is the case in congenital nystagmus where reflex fixation has become impaired by a bilateral macular lesion preventing a clear retinal image. The amplitude of the oscillations varies considerably in different cases and is probably related to the extent of the macular defect, but the phases are always equal.

Resemblance to Congenital Nystagmus

The oscillations of miners' nystagmus closely resemble those of congenital nystagmus, and it is not unreasonable to suppose that their origin is similar and that it is therefore due to years of working under conditions which did not permit of sufficient stimulation of the macula by light to support reflex macular fixation. In some cases there may exist a variation in the amplitude, but not the rate, of the oscillations as between the two eyes; in such cases a physical difference between the two eyes, such as a greater error of refraction in the eye with the greater amplitude, is found. Were the interference with macular fixation due to a more central lesion these variations would not occur. The occurrence of miners' nystagmus is paroxysmal and the duration of the paroxysms is variable. In some cases the nystagmus may occur in daylight, even when the patient is at rest; in others, special conditions are necessary before the oscillations become manifest. Thus the oscillations may be induced by diminishing the illumination, by causing the patient to look upwards while keeping the head steady, by stooping or by exercises which involve stooping, especially where the body and arms are used as if handling a pick. In some cases oscillations are not perceptible until after being in the dark for a considerable period, and there is no doubt that cases exist in which oscillations are present only after the man has been continually working underground for some hours.

Differential Diagnosis

Diagnosis is difficult in early cases. A miner complaining of headache and occasional dizziness coming on after some hours of work underground may show none of the physical signs of miners' nystagmus. Such a patient may develop other symptoms and ultimately show visible oscillations. Sometimes it is necessary to keep a man in a dark room for an hour and to get him during this time to imitate shovelling exercises in the dark before the oscillations become manifest. In some cases the amplitude of the oscillations is so fine as to be undetected by the naked eye and to be recognized only by means of an ophthalmoscope focused on the optic disc or retinal vessels. There is really no confusion with congenital nystagmus where the oscillations are continuous and are unaffected by changes in illumination, exercise or posture. Nystagmus accompanying lesions of the central nervous system is readily recognized because it is of the lateral variety. Since vertigo is such a prominent symptom of the condition, it is clear that middle-ear disease and hypertension must be excluded.

Estimation of Incapacity for Work

The majority of miners who develop miners' nystagmus do not stop work, do not complain of the condition and are never seen by medical men because of their eyes. The degree of incapacity must be judged not by the amount of oscillation present, but by the effect on the patient. One man may have more or less continuous oscillations without any apparent ill effects; in other words, he may be as unaware of his oscillations as a person with congenital nystagmus. Another miner may have minimal oscillations yet present all the other signs and symptoms, both ocular and general, to a marked degree. Vertigo is perhaps the most incapacitating of all the symptoms, and it is therefore of the greatest importance in the estimation of incapacity.

Suitable Alternative Work above Ground

A man with nystagmus and marked symptoms should be considered as unfit for work underground. Many such men can perform certain forms of surface work, but work involving stooping should not be included for fear of aggravating the oscillations and the vertigo. Work on the screens is thus not suitable, nor work involving heavy digging nor the filling of trucks or wagons. If vertigo is severe, work amongst moving machinery or traffic also should be excluded. Incredible though it may sound, it is the custom of some medical men to tell their patients that they must never go down the pit again unless they wish to become blind. No man loses his sight from miners' nystagmus, and the first duty of the doctor is to assure the patient that his condition is not incurable and to re-establish the man's confidence in himself by stating most pointedly that blindness never results.

Improved Lighting by Whitening

The reflecting power of coal is small, ranging from about 5 per cent in the case of dull coal to 10 per cent in the case of bright coal. Shale and other rocks met with in coal mines reflect from 20 to 30 per cent, whilst supports and props usually reflect from 10 to 20 per cent. It will be obvious that the lighter the surfaces the more light is usefully employed. Whitewashed surfaces reflect anything from 50 to 60 per cent of the light falling upon them. The *Coal Mines (Lighting) General Regulations, 1947*, enumerate places which are to be whitened:

(*a*) such of the shaft insets and shaft sidings as are regularly used;

(*b*) the top and bottom of every permanent self-acting incline;

(*c*) every siding, landing, passbye, junction, offtake, place at which tubs are regularly coupled or uncoupled or regularly attached to or detached from a haulage rope, and place at which tubs are regularly filled mechanically, except in so far as any such place as aforesaid is within one hundred yards of the face; and

(*d*) every room and place made to house, and containing, any engine, motor, electrical transformer or switchgear.

Preventive Treatment

The provision of better lighting in coal mines has done much towards the eradication of this disease, reducing the number of new cases and alleviating the misery of existing sufferers. Thus in England the number of cases certified as suffering from miners' nystagmus reached its peak in 1922, when 4,092 cases were recorded—that is, 1 out of every 225 miners employed underground. By 1938 the number of cases had fallen to 1,224 or 1 in every 510 employed underground. For various reasons the number rose again during the Second World War to 2,006 in 1943 or about 1 in every 300, but it has since fallen to 641 cases in 1948 or 1 in 830 employed underground. These figures show that progress is being made, and there is hope that with improvement in the quantity and quality of underground lighting we shall see nystagmus entirely eliminated. In the coal miners of Scotland, miners' nystagmus was common a few years ago, but it has become relatively unimportant in recent years owing to improvements in underground lighting.

CATARACT IN INDUSTRY

Cataract may occur in workers in industry as a result of mechanical trauma, electric shock, exposure to heat, light, X-rays, radium and fast neutrons; and possibly from handling substances such as dinitrophenol and dinitro-*ortho*-cresol, which are known in other circumstances to cause it.

Cataract due to Trauma

Traumatic cataract is commonly the result of penetrating injury to the eye in which the lens capsule is ruptured. Total opacity of the lens may occur immediately, or within a few days or weeks of the injury. Sometimes a more localized opacity develops which may become permanent or may gradually regress leaving a clear lens. Less often, contusion of the eyeball without rupture of the lens capsule will lead to cataract. A special form of traumatic cataract develops from trauma to the eye by small pieces of copper from percussion caps or particles of stone or coal from premature blasts. Steel particles from power-driven lathes, drill-presses, punches and shears constitute a further eye hazard. Protection in the form of goggles should be provided wherever there is a risk of penetrating injury to the eye from large or small objects.

Glassblowers' Cataract

A type of cataract with special characteristics occurs in workers exposed to heat and glare for a long period. In glassblowers between the ages of thirty and forty years cataract is five times as common as among persons not exposed to heat and glare (Legge, 1907). The way in which radiant energy acts upon the lens is not fully known. Kuhn (1944) questions the existence of occupational cataract due to radiation as a clinical entity, but there is good evidence against her view. In 1739 Heister noted

he relationship of heat to cataract formation. Meyerhofer (1886) was the
rst to point out that cataract due to heat began in the posterior cortex
f the lens and occurred in the left eye first in right-handed workers.
n 1891 Mr. Alfred Greenwood, the partially blind secretary of the Glass
Bottle Makers of Yorkshire United Trade Protection Society, began to
otice how frequently cataract was named as the cause of incapacity which
rought members on the superannuation funds of the Society. In glass-
ottle making the finisher is exposed for five hours or more each week to
he glare and fierce heat
rom the glory-hole of a
urnace of molten glass at
temperature of about
,500° C. In 1903 Robin-
on described posterior
olar cataract in bottle-
inishers in Sunderland,
ut realized shortly after
hat the condition oc-
urred in men engaged in
ther branches of glass-
vork (fig. 326). He there-
ore called this form of
ataract *glassworkers' cat-*
ract, and described it
ully in 1915. In the Pot-
eries men who fire the
ottle kilns and also the
rit kilns expose one eye
o the glory hole and after
ears at the work are liable
o posterior polar cataract
vhich they call *firemen's*
ye.

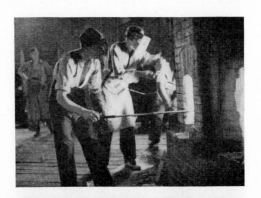

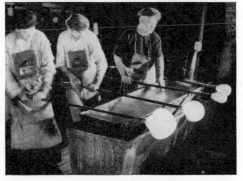

FIG. 326.—Glassblowers' Cataract. In the upper
picture the *Gatherers* are seen exposed to the
Heat and Glare of a Glass Furnace at 1,500° C.
They *gather* the Molten Glass on the end of a
six-foot length of Gas Pipe. When looking
through the *Glory-hole* of the Furnace they
hold the Eye-guard between their Teeth so that
the Window of Green Glass is opposite to their
Eyes. In the lower picture the *Gatherers* are
shaping the Molten Glass and the Eye Guards
are not used

(By courtesy of Mr. Joseph Minton)

Posterior Polar Cataract in Many Trades

Reports followed of
exactly similar changes in
he lens occurring in every
rade where a man was
xposed to radiant energy
or a long period. Grid-
and (1916) described it in
ron puddlers in Wolver-
ampton. Puddling is part of the process to convert pig iron into malle-
ble or wrought iron before rolling can be done. It consists in stirring

about pig iron molten on the bed of a reverberatory furnace unt
the carbon is removed by the action of oxygen circulating through th
furnace. Puddling is done by a bar of iron 10 feet long called a *rabble*
This is introduced through a hole in the bottom of the furnace door an
the metal is stirred for 45 minutes. After removal from the furnac
the white-hot metal is hammered and beaten into various shapes. Th
men exposed to a high degree of infra-red radiation are the *puddler*
shinglers, *furnacemen* and *roughers*. Roberts (1921) described posterio
polar cataract in chain makers in Dudley (fig. 327). Certain types of chai
are still made by hand, the workmen being specially skilled blacksmiths

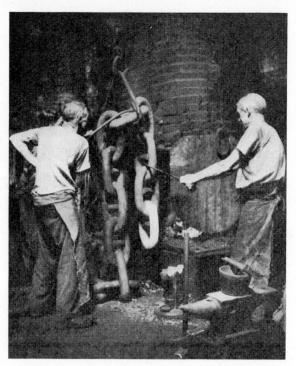

FIG. 327.—Chain Makers at work at Cradley, near
Birmingham
(*By courtesy of the Daily Mirror*)

A piece of rolled iron rod cut to a suitable length is heated and bent int
the shape of a link. The two ends in apposition are heated to a white hea
and welded together on an anvil to complete the link. The hazard to th
unprotected worker comes from gazing during the whole working day
either into the fire to judge when the ends of the link are hot enough t
weld or at the white-hot metal while hammering it on the anvil. Brinto
(1922) described cataract in gold smelters in the Transvaal and Healy
(1929) in tin-plate millmen in Llanelly (fig. 328). Of the 350 tinplat

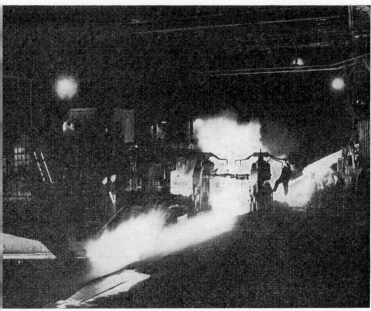

Fig. 328.—Steel-bar Rolling Mill in the Tinplate Industry of South Wales.
The photograph gives some idea of the intense Glare and fierce Heat

illmen over thirty-five examined by Healy, 200 had lenticular opacities.
They developed this only after fifteen years' work in the mill. The inci-
ence increased with every five years' age increment from thirty-five to
ixty years as follows: 17, 18, 34, 62 and 65 per cent. It has been described,
hough rarely, in bakers and laundresses, and Robinson (1915) mentions a
ase of posterior polar cataract occurring in a pet dog which had the habit
f lying with its head on the fender and looking into the fire.

Rôle of Infra-red Radiation

The cause of cataract is still undetermined. The lens opacities in all
ases are due to a change in the lenticular proteins from a colloid to a
articulate condition. This process of coagulation occurs in two stages—
denaturation, a chemical change which alters the proteins to a coagulable
orm, and agglutination, a physical change in which coagula are formed by
occulation of the denatured particles. Only radiation which is absorbed by
. tissue can change its nature. The lens absorbs infra-red rays of wave-
engths between 14,000 and 11,000 A.U., and ultra-violet rays between
.,000 and 2,930 A.U. These rays may act either directly on the lens, or
ndirectly by their influence on the iris and ciliary body they may set up a
disturbance in the metabolism of the lens substance. Experimental evidence suggests that ultra-violet light does not cause lens changes if the
accompanying heat rays are filtered off. Butler (1938) considers that the
damaging rays are not heat rays but those of wavelengths between 7,500

and 10,000 A.U. which lie just below visible red and are emitted from white-hot metal and molten glass.

Chronic Infra-red Radiation Cataract

The fact that the lens changes begin at the posterior pole is attributed by Robinson (1915) and other writers to the concentration at this site of the intense heat and light rays falling on the lens through a contracted pupil. In addition, some of the rays are reflected to this same region from the concave posterior surface of the lens, thus producing a double concentration of heat at the very spot where heat cataract first shows itself. Robinson (1915) gives a detailed description of the characteristics of radiation cataract, and his findings have been confirmed by later observers.

> The opacity first appears at the posterior pole of the lens, immediately under the posterior capsule, and is often irregularly disc-shaped. By oblique illumination it is distinctly brass-coloured. The outline of the disc-like part is well-defined but the opacity is less dense and shades off towards the equator. As the haziness spreads it at first clings closely to the posterior capsule, so that it is saucer-shaped in the earlier stages of the disease, the concavity of the posterior capsule of the lens being easily seen by oblique illumination. By direct examination with a $+$10D lens the central disc is sometimes seen to be not completely opaque, the opacity often presenting an irregular network appearance within an irregular circle, and the surrounding less dense opacity is often like a cobweb. From the posterior pole, the cloudiness and opacity gradually spread to the rest of the cortex, and when the cataract is ripe, the lens has a pearly hue. In later stages of development the cataract cannot be distinguished from the ordinary senile forms.

Characteristic Peeling of Zonular Lamella

Butler (1938) points out that the anterior capsule and cortex are affected as well as the posterior, a fact of medico-legal importance. The zonular lamella of the anterior capsule peels off in large sheets, and this is pathognomonic of ray cataract (fig. 329). Without this change it is difficult to say that posterior polar cataract is of occupational origin. All the other appearances in ray cataract may be seen in senile cataract and cataracta complicata. Butler points out that anyone who went into the witness box and swore that a patient was suffering from a ray cataract when there were no characteristic changes in the anterior capsule would be liable to a very uncomfortable cross-examination from a well-instructed lawyer. Several factors influence the development of occupational cataract due to radiation. The heat exposure varies in different factories and different classes of work. The degree to which the eyes are exposed to glare may vary. Legge (1907) estimated that it takes from seventeen to thirty-five years before a glass-worker becomes disabled by cataracts. Susceptibility also plays a part, for some workers are never affected.

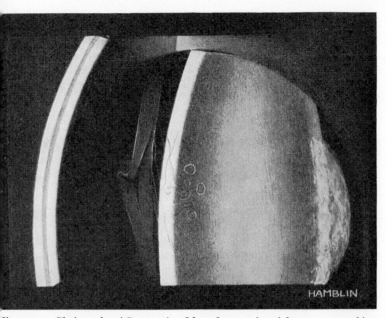

Fig. 329.—Chain-makers' Cataract in a Man of 54 employed for 42 years making Chain Fittings. He worked with the right Hand nearer the Forge. There were Lesions in both Eyes but that on the right side was worse. The Drawing shows the right Eye as seen with a Slit-lamp Microscope. The Posterior Cortical Opacity centrally situated is granular in appearance and shows a Golden Glow in the Slit-lamp Beam. The Opacity in the Anterior Cortex is less dense and shows a few Subcapsular Dots. The Nucleus of the Lens is sclerosed. The Zonular Lamella of the Anterior Capsule of the Lens shows characteristic Exfoliation and Curling

(*By courtesy of Mr. Lloyd Johnstone*)

Manufacture of Glass Bottles by Machinery

Workers exposed to heat and glare should be protected against the development of cataract. The onset of disability is slow and it is therefore difficult to secure co-operation from the individual worker. Where possible, the protection should not depend on this. Bottle-making machines are replacing skilled craftsmen in this industry. The machine automatically sucks up molten glass, blows it and delivers bottles at the rate of forty a minute. The use of these machines has resulted in a great drop in the incidence of cataract among glassworkers. Only twenty-seven cases were notified in the glass industry in Great Britain between 1939 and 1945, and of these only one new case arose in 1945. The position is less satisfactory in the metal industry. For the same period 131 claims for compensation were made, sixteen of these occurring in 1945 (Minton, 1949).

Goggles of Crookes' 217 Glass

Where bottles are still made by hand, and in all industries where there is a risk of prolonged exposure to harmful rays, the eyes of workers should be protected by glass shields or goggles. Physicists have discovered that glass containing metallic oxides can absorb 90 per cent of heat radiation. Such glass is dark green in colour and is more effective than the dark blue which is still commonly used (Minton, 1949). Crookes' 217 glass, containing fused soda flux 96·8 per cent, ferroso-ferric oxide 2·85 per cent and carbon 0·35 per cent, cuts off 96 per cent of heat radiations but transmits 40 per cent of light and is therefore most satisfactory (fig. 330). Advanced cases of cataract can be treated successfully by lens extraction because

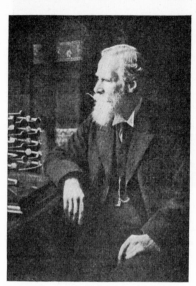

FIG. 330.—Sir William Crookes, 1832–1919

other parts of the eyeball are normal. Iridectomy may be sufficient to restore useful vision in those cases where opacities are present but are not progressive.

Cataract following Electric Shock

A number of cases of cataract occurring after electric shock or lightning-stroke are reported (see p. 1143). Saemisch (1864) first described electrical cataract. His patient was a girl of eighteen years who developed unilateral cataract five months after being struck by lightning. Hess (1888) induced lens changes in animals by means of electric shock produced by a Leyden jar. Desbrières (1905) reported a case of cataract in an electrician aged twenty-six years following an accident which occurred while he was dusting an electric transformer. He suffered an electric shock from a 20,000-volt 30-cycle alternating current source. His burns were predominantly right-sided and only his right eye was affected. Gabriéldès (1935) found twenty-seven cases of electrical cataract reported in the literature. He described another case of a man of thirty-six years of age who developed bilateral cataract eleven months after surviving an electric shock of 5,500 volts.

Characteristics of Electrical Cataract

Clinically electrical cataract may be unilateral, occurring usually on the side of the body on which contact was made, or bilateral (fig. 331). There is often delay of a year or more in the onset of symptoms. Such cataracts may mature rapidly, within a few weeks, or very slowly. In some cases there is spontaneous regression. The opacities are usually situated anteriorly and have been described as a confusion of corkscrew-shaped threads and laces crossing each other in all directions without following the regular run of the lens fibres.

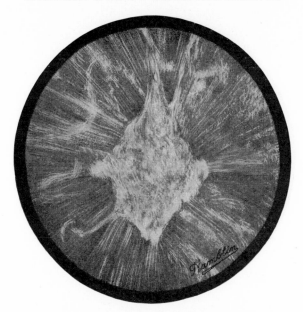

FIG. 331.—Case 33. Cataract in an Electrical Fitter of 38 three months after severe Injury from a High-tension Current. Thickening and Opacity of central part of Anterior Capsule of Lens of right Eye. Cataract appeared later in the left Eye

(*By courtesy of Mr. Joseph Minton*)

ataract due to Ionising Radiations

Radiation cataracts have been widely studied since cataracts were noted cyclotron workers and the Japanese atomic bomb survivors (Voelz, 967). It has been shown that neutrons and X-rays are the most effective ataract-producing forms of ionising radiations (Lerman, 1962). Radiation ataracts are all similar in appearance and structure, irrespective of hether the exposure has been to neutrons, X-rays or γ-rays. The first linical findings are minute opacities which appear in the posterior sub-apsular cortex of the lens. Vacuoles may also be noted at this time, in he same area of the lens. These posterior opacities may progress to form randular opaque discs. Opacities may appear in the anterior surface of he cortex at a later stage but the nucleus of the lens is spared. The clinical ppearance of radiation cataracts is indistinguishable from cataracts aused by other chemical or physical agents, for example chronic infra-red adiation exposure, high voltage electric shocks, or drugs such as dinitro-henol. History of exposure is, therefore, of fundamental importance in rriving at a diagnosis. The radiation dose required to produce lens pacities varies, depending on the quality of the radiation and the dose te. A dose of 500–600 r of 100–250 kV X-rays as an acute single xposure will cause lens opacities in a high proportion of people (fig 332).

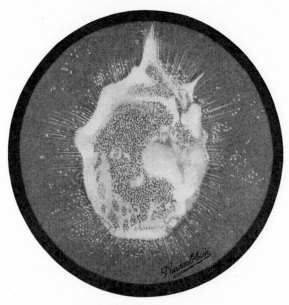

Fig. 332.—Cataract following X-irradiation Therapy for
Sycosis Barbæ in a man of 28. He was exposed to about
500 r over a period of five months. Two years and a half
after the last exposure Vision gradually failed in both
Eyes. The Drawing of the right Eye shows a Plaque-like
Opacity in the Posterior Cortex of the Lens surrounded
by Opaque Powder Dots. The left Eye was affected in a
similar way

(By courtesy of Mr. R. Foster Moore)

Dose fractionation reduces the incidence, for example it has been estimated
by Merrian and Focht (1957) that an exposure of 750–950 r spread over
one to three months will give a 50% chance of causing a progressive
cataract. It is estimated that a dose of only 70–100 rads of fast neutrons
will result in the development of cataracts. The latent interval between
the exposure and the onset of lens opacities varies from one to six years
in cyclotron workers and six months to twelve years following X-ray
exposure. Since X-rays, radium and fast neutrons are being used in
industry on an increasing scale, adequate shielding of plants must be
assured. Treatment of this type of cataract by intracapsular lens extraction
is satisfactory.

Cataract due to Aromatic Nitro-compounds

Certain substances are known to produce cataract in experimental
animals. These include naphthalene, lactose and galactose, thallium and
dinitrophenol. Following the use of dinitrophenol and the related compound dinitro-*ortho*-cresol as slimming agents in the nineteen-thirties, a
number of cases of bilateral cataract were reported among people who had

ken these substances. Horner (1941) collected 177 cases from the literature and estimated that less than 1 per cent of the people who had taken
initrophenol had developed cataract. Symptoms occurred, on an average,
fteen months after the first dose. Neither the duration of treatment nor
the total amount taken plays any part in the liability to the development of
cataract. Individual susceptibility seems to be the determining factor.
Similar cases occurred after taking dinitro-*ortho*-cresol. These were less
frequent, presumably because the use of this substance was less common.

Hazard to Men spraying Cereal Crops

The use of these substances as therapeutic agents ended about 1938,
but in 1940 dinitro-*ortho*-cresol became known in a new rôle. It is a most
effective weed-killer and insecticide. It acts particularly against yellow
charlock and is the most efficient anti-locust substance yet discovered. For
these reasons it is manufactured on a large scale and used for spraying
orchards, cereal crops and locusts in many parts of the world. There have
been no cases of cataract reported yet among persons engaged in the manufacture or spraying of dinitro-*ortho*-cresol, but there is a potential hazard.
Cases of poisoning, resulting in death in some instances, have been reported from England, France, the United States of America and other
countries.

Characteristics of Dinitrophenol Cataract

Horner (1936) states that the earliest change is the appearance in both
lenses of faint grey dust-like opacities just beneath the anterior capsule.
They may be stippled, polychromatic, striate or downy. The anterior
capsule often appears roughened, dry or vacuolated. The posterior subcapsular layers show a peculiar, saucer-shaped granular metallic lustre.
Horner calls this the *cloth of gold reflex*. It may resemble brass filings,
hammered copper or filed steel. The nucleus and remaining lens are clear,
and vision may be normal at this time.

Rapid Progress of Lens Changes

Further changes develop rapidly. The opacities invade the cortex and
finally the nucleus, so that the whole lens becomes silken-grey and then
pearl-like. In later stages segmentation of the lens occurs, with dark, wedge-
like spaces intervening. The lens swells and tension within the eyeball
rises. Glaucoma is a common complication. Spaeth (1936) describes a case
of bilateral cataract in which the lens cortex had liquefied in a young
woman who had taken dinitrophenol for slimming. It would be a wise
precaution to include slit-lamp examination of the lens in the routine tests
made to detect early cases of systemic poisoning in workers manufacturing
or using dinitro-*ortho*-cresol.

Case 33. Electrical fitter—shock from a 6,600-volt source—bilateral cataract.

W. A., a man aged 38, employed as an electrical fitter in a transformer substation (6,600 volts) was under the care of Mr. Joseph
Minton of the Royal Eye Hospital, St. George's Circus, London. He

was repairing switching gear on 27th January 1946. His mate saw an electric flash and smoke, and heard an explosion. The patient was pulled out from the trench unconscious and severely burnt on the right side of the face, the right half of the scalp and the right arm. Three months later he complained of misty vision in the right eye. The vision in his right eye was only sufficient to enable him to count fingers at a distance of 6 feet. There was marked thickening and opacity of the central part of the anterior capsule of the lens (fig. 331). Twenty months after the injury the left lens began to show opacities. Visual acuity in the left eye was 6/9.

OCCUPATIONAL DEAFNESS

Occupational deafness occurs in workers exposed to noise and vibration in many industries. True occupational deafness develops slowly in response to a frequently repeated noise and affects a considerable number of workers engaged on the same work. It must be distinguished from deafness occurring as a result of an accident, such as an explosion, which causes a sudden very intense noise.

Historical Summary

The condition was formerly called *boilermakers' deafness* because it was first recognized among boilermakers, smiths and braziers (fig. 333). Early in the nineteenth century it was noticed that no one obliged to work in the interior of a boiler while riveters are hammering outside escapes impairment of hearing for any length of time. It was clear to everybody that most boilermakers either could not hear at all at a public meeting or heard with difficulty. Fosbroke mentioned the *blacksmiths' deafness* in 1831. Similar deafness occurring in railway workers and weavers was described in the middle of the nineteenth century. In 1907 Wittmarck published a report on the influence of noise on the ear, considered histologically. *Cotton-weavers' deafness* was investigated in Lancashire by Legge and McKelvie (1927). Of 1,011 cotton weavers who had worked from one to sixty-four years, 246 (24·3 per cent) were found to have some degree of deafness. All of these had worked in

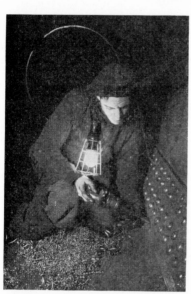

FIG. 333.—Boilermakers' Deafness. The man has crawled into the Steam Drum of a Boiler through the Manhole and is seen caulking a Seam with a Compressed-air Tool. The Noise produced is Indescribable

ιe noise more than ten years, while the number of cases of the disease ιowed a marked increase after twenty years' employment. Modern udies of the problem include the investigation of ship-builders (Larsen, 939), weavers (Kristensen, 1946), aviators and submarine crews.

viation Deafness

Aviation deafness presents the same characteristics as other occupational eafness (Dickson and others, 1942). On analysis, aeroplane engine noise at the low end of the auditory spectrum (110 to 115 decibels), but the eafness is for high tones. This may be due to sound pressure on the basal oil of the cochlea, to sudden pools of noise of high intensity or to a reson- tor action of the external auditory meatus. On the whole, aviation deaf- ess is a minor problem because the effects of noise and pressure of rela- vely short duration are, for the most part, reversible and air crew tend to cover (Campbell, 1945). Individual variation in susceptibility is found. ince the impairment of perception is above the range of the conversational equencies there is no subjective loss of hearing. Air crew should wear eadgear which incorporates ear defenders and telephone equipment. *viation pressure deafness* is a separate condition. It is a low-tone deafness nd is due to blockage of the Eustachian tubes.

ffects of Ultrasonic Vibrations

The jet-engine by its emphasis on the possibilities of ill effects from ltrasonic vibrations has stimulated thought on the physiological effects of ιch vibrations. These are defined as sound-waves at frequencies above ιe upper limit of human hearing. They have a short wave-length, form ɔlatively sharp sound-shadows, can be focused to give intense local ressures, and are attenuated more rapidly as they travel through the air. Vhat effect they have on the ear is not known, nor is there evidence that ny other nerve endings in the body are capable of informing the individual f the presence of ultrasonic radiation. We have little or no exact knowledge f the effects of ultrasonic vibrations on the human body. There is no vidence that air-borne ultrasonics can produce any specific direct effect n the brain or other parts of the nervous system. In the realm of physics ιost of the work has been done in liquids, but little is known of the range, ropagation and transmission of ultrasonic vibrations in gases. Their iological effects seem to be related to the enormous alternating local ressures which are produced in the tissues, and to the local heating effects rising from the absorption of energy dampening the vibrations (Dickson, 954).

)eafness in Sailors in Submarines

Schilling (1942) has investigated the hearing of submarine personnel. Ie finds an acute and chronic deafness with the characteristics already escribed. He ascribes the acute hearing loss to diesel-engine noise, the ffect tending to be cumulative and to become permanent. Every effort should be made to quieten the engines and the crew should wear e defenders.

Deafness independent of Occupation

Other diseases attacking any part of the auditory mechanism may occι in industry and cause deafness. These include the effects of changes : temperature and humidity, bacterial infections, chemical, electrical ar mechanical influences. Nevertheless, most cases are due to noise of loι duration. Deafness which had developed independently may be aggravatε by the effects of occupation. In normal persons there are varying degreε of sensitivity to noise. Larsen (1939) finds that individuals with an heredι tary tendency to deafness are affected after short exposure. Peyser (194: has shown that the normal ear of a person suffering from unilateral eε disease must be regarded as more susceptible than in the case where boι ears are healthy.

Effects in Experimental Animals

In experimental animals exposed to the ordinary noise of factorie histological examination shows that degenerative changes occur in tl organ of Corti and the cells of the spiral ganglion. These changes are mo marked in the basal turn of the cochlea, but their localization depends upo the pitch of the injurious sound, pure tones giving rise to strikingly ci: cumscribed changes. Where vibration contributes to the loss of hearing presumably exerts its effect by bone conduction and the lesions are localizε to the apical turn of the cochlea.

Loss of Perception of High-frequency Tones

There are few reports of the histological study of human cases, bι those available appear to support the experimental evidence. There is son evidence that the type of deafness which develops is different in the case ι exposure to noise from that of exposure to vibration. Exposure to noiε results in loss of perception of the high-frequency tones, while exposure ι vibration causes impaired perception of the low-frequency tones. Obviouslι in most cases both factors play a part.

History of Onset of Deafness

Experimentally and in industrial practice pronounced loss of hearin may occur rapidly—for example, up to 60 decibels in half an hour b exposure to a 4,000-cycle tone at 110 decibels. Most of the hearing los if the average noise level is above 100 decibels, is established during tl first three to four weeks. Subsequent change is gradual but tends to b progressive. The individual susceptibility to the effects of noise varie. Most unaccustomed individuals exposed to a noise of more than 70 decibeι will show temporary changes in the audiogram. In workmen exposed t this level of noise, deafness occurs no more frequently than in the ordinar population. Where the noise level is greater than 100 decibels, most peopι exposed for more than a few weeks show loss of hearing. This is permanenι

ough it may slowly diminish on removal from the noisy occupation. A
nall number of persons so exposed continue to have normal audiograms.

ymptoms and Signs

The worker is frequently unaware of his deafness until it is severe. The
st complaint is commonly that he is unable to carry on a conversation in
hich several persons take part—the so-called *society deafness*. The un-
vareness of loss of hearing is not surprising because irrespective of the
ne predominant in the injurious noise, the earliest defect demonstrated
y the audiometer is confined to a comparatively small area of high-pitched
nes around C_5 (4,096 cycles per second). This is so in all forms of
cupational deafness, and since the speech range lies between 300 and
000 cycles per second, subjective deafness is not normally an early
mptom.

innitus and Vertigo

Tinnitus, variously described as *buzzing, uproar, droning, growling,
nging or whizzing*, occurs in about half the cases but is constant in a much
naller proportion. It is usually bilateral and, in the majority of cases,
riodic and transitory. It is not necessarily related to the degree of deaf-
ss, for this may occur in cases where there is no tinnitus. Vertigo is rare.

aracusis Willisiana

Paracusis Willisiana, which is the ability to hear when exposed to noise
hile in fact showing marked impairment of hearing to functional tests, is
t common. Pain in the ears is rare except in the initial stage of exposure.
eadache and nervousness occur in a few subjects.

coustic After-images

One man employed in a shipyard at Odense stated that he sometimes
perienced at night a precise repetition of the noise with all its different
riations, just like a true reflection, and another that he had the whole
ckyard noise in his ears at night. Larsen has called this condition
oustic after-images.

unctional Tests of Hearing

In the classical case the signs elicited on functional testing of hearing
e a normal range of perception of low tones, with marked lowering of the
per limit for high tones. Hearing of the whispered voice is greatly im-
ired, while the spoken voice is still well heard. Other cases have normal
nits for perception of both low and high tones but show marked reduction
hearing of the whispered voice. Such cases are often unable to hear the
hispered voice at less than 1 metre, the normal distance being more than
metres. This is regarded as a stage in the development of the classical
sease. It is well to remember that such tests are subject to considerable
rsonal error on the part of both examiner and patient.

Audiometric Tests

More accurate assessment of the extent of the loss of hearing, and
detection at an early stage, can be made by audiometric tests. Both air a
bone conduction can be tested over a wide range of frequencies and t
hearing loss measured in decibels. The decibel is a unit of relative pow
commonly used. It is employed especially to express electric or acous
power output, and in the latter sense 1 decibel is approximately t
smallest change of intensity which the normal human ear can dete
It is not an absolute unit, so that measurements of noise-levels or heari
loss are made in relation to a standard.

Defects in Audiograms

In all cases of occupational deafness, audiograms show more
less marked defects confined to a comparatively small range of frequenc
around 4,096 cycles per second (C_5). The sensibility of the ear is great
towards frequencies in this range where changes in intensity and f
quency are most readily appreciated. The perception area for C_5 prese
a special vulnerability whi
decreases towards either si
(fig. 334). This defect in t
audiogram, known as the
dip, is found not only in cas
where there is known i
pairment of hearing, but al
when hearing is apparen
normal. It occurs also
traumatic deafness such
that following an explosic
in deafness due to to:
causes such as alcohol, qui
ine, cocaine and carbon
sulphide, in syphilis, aft
cerebral concussion and
the deafness associated wi
retinitis pigmentosa. T

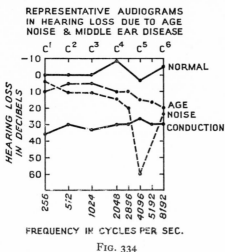

REPRESENTATIVE AUDIOGRAMS
IN HEARING LOSS DUE TO AGE
NOISE & MIDDLE EAR DISEASE

FIG. 334

audiogram, however, differs distinctly from that found in senile deafn
and deafness due to middle-ear disease. In senile deafness it shows
gradual loss of acuity for the higher frequencies, and in middle-ear de
ness there is a loss of from 30 to 40 decibels at all frequencies.

The Education of the Public

The education of the public both in industrial and ordinary life to
awareness of noise and methods of noise control is long overdue. It
accepted that noise produces significant deafness, that it contributes
fatigue and in some circumstances lowers work output. In a few trad
nearly all workers suffer varying degrees of deafness, and heavy for

perators are so universally affected that partial deafness is recognized as
ome proof of experience in the trade. Methods of noise abatement are no
onger technically mysterious nor is there need for so much noise so con-
tantly to be endured.

Use of Pre-employment Audiograms

Since occupational deafness, once established, is a permanent disability,
: is imperative that every effort should be made to keep the noise below a
armful level. This lies somewhere between 70 and 100 decibels. There are
oo few immune individuals to employ only these. Pre-employment audio-
rams should be done on all workmen who will be exposed to a noise-level
f more than 100 decibels. This should be repeated after one month's
mployment, and again after six months. If impairment of perception of
requencies below 3,000 cycles per second has increased at either time, the
ndividual should be removed to a quieter occupation.

Use of Ear Defenders

Many types of ear defenders have been designed. Their efficiency to
educe a given noise to below the harmful level can be tested by means of
he audiometer. Ear defenders of various sorts afford considerable pro-
ection from noise, but too often the workmen are unwilling to co-operate
y wearing them constantly. It is therefore desirable to use methods of
oise reduction which do not depend on the co-operation of the workmen.
hus on the looms weaving heavy linen canvases in Belfast, noise can be
educed by cupping both ends of the shuttle with rubber.

Improvements in Architectural Design

Much unnecessary noise is tolerated in spite of efficient methods of
oise control. Carey McCord (1943) writes:

In the average factory with mechanical operations the noise level
is approximately 90 decibels, or 10,000,000,000 times the least perceptible sound and 100,000 times the sound of ordinary conversation.
Holes in walls, such as for the previous passage of pipes, permit the
passage of much unwanted sound. Even a keyhole may transmit sound
energy sufficient to warrant suppression. Under these circumstances a
constriction of the sound stream takes place so that more energy passes
through than might be expected.

Acoustic Treatment of Walls and Ceilings

Improvements in architectural design can do much to lessen noise.
Many factories are so constructed as to accentuate reverberation—that is,
he reflection of a sound wave from the walls, ceiling, floor and furnishings
ntil the sound energy is dissipated. Two structural features which will
ssist are a design of wall structure to prevent transmission of sound from
xteriors and between rooms, and sufficient absorption within rooms to
educe reverberation time to a minimum. Acoustic treatment of walls and
eilings has little effect in reducing low-frequency reverberation and is

seldom practicable in industry. It has, however, been done effectively in
police pistol-squad training alley in the United States of America.

Change in Design of Noisy Machines

In industry it may be possible to change a method of operation from
noisy to a quieter one. The replacement of riveting by welding is an
example of this. Where change in design of a noisy machine is not practicable, it should be isolated so that its noise is not transmitted through the
whole factory. Operatives working such a machine should wear adequate
ear defenders. Complete silence is disturbing rather than welcome, a low
background noise level of 20–30 decibels being desirable. Music during
work may be advantageous in some circumstances, but where a job has its
own rhythm the varying tempo of music may wholly upset this. Production
may be reduced and accidents result indirectly.

OCCUPATIONAL CRAMPS

The term occupational cramps is used for a group of psychoneuroses
in which certain symptoms are excited by the attempt to perform a customary act involving an often-repeated muscular action. The necessary
co-ordination of movement breaks down, and spasm, tremor, pain, weakness and loss of control occur in the muscles accustomed to perform
harmoniously the regular act concerned. These psychoneuroses are also
known as craft palsies, occupational palsies and professional spasms.

Numerous Occupations Involved

The hands are affected in writers, telegraphists, cotton twisters, tailors
drapers, seamstresses, sailmakers, knitters, hairdressers, ironers, bowler
metal workers, hammermen, turners, engravers, goldbeaters, cabinet
makers, sawyers, locksmiths, tinsmiths, nailmakers, masons, painters
enamellers, compositors, watchmakers, shoemakers, saddlers, sailors
fencers, diamond cutters, money counters, letter sorters, cigarette rollers
cigar makers, pianists, organists, violinists, violoncellists, harpists, flautists
drummers, orchestra conductors, typists, comptometer workers, waiters
florists, artificial-flower makers, folders of newspapers and milkers of
cows. Rarely the lower limbs are affected as in dancers, sewing-machine
workers, knife sharpenters and tradesmen's tricyclists. Identical spasms of
the muscles of the head and neck are still rarer. Cramp of the tongue in
clarinet players and of the lips in trumpet players have been described
(Kalmus, 1934).

Complex Rapid Repetitive Movements

Most of these occupations involve rapid, repetitive movements of short
range, either by one or by both hands. The movements concerned are complex and are perfected by education and practice. They necessitate a high
degree of precision and co-ordination, and they may involve as many as ten
repetitive movements a second. The first manifestations of the disorder are
likely to make their appearance when the worker is called upon to exceed

certain level of performance. There may therefore be an associated anxiety on the part of the individual to get the work done in time and up to standard. Symptoms may appear after physical or psychological events which lower the patient's normal level of efficiency.

Causative Factors both Physical and Psychological

No structural change in the cerebral cortex, nervous system or muscles has ever been demonstrated. By careful and detailed clinical interview it is possible in many cases to elicit the presence of psychoneurotic symptoms. Opinion has gradually moved away from the conception of the disorder as being due to physical fatigue of muscle or nerve towards the view that it is primarily a disorder of behaviour. The causative factors are no doubt multiple and both physical and psychological in nature. They result in the breakdown of the smooth execution of a stereotyped movement and ultimately lead to the setting up of a faulty habit closely akin to a tic.

Writers' Cramp in 1713

In his description of the *Diseases of scribes and notaries* Ramazzini (1713) states:

That there was a far greater number of scribes and notaries among the ancients than there is in our day because of the invention of the art of printing, is certain; nevertheless, everyone knows that in every city and town there are many persons who support themselves and their families solely by writing. Incessant driving of the pen over paper causes intense fatigue of the hand and the whole arm because of the continuous and almost tonic strain on the muscles and tendons, which in course of time results in failure of power in the right hand. An acquaintance of mine, a notary by profession, still living, used to spend his whole life continually engaged in writing, and he made a good deal of money by it; first he began to complain of intense fatigue in the whole arm, but no remedy could relieve this, and finally the whole right arm became completely paralyzed. In order to offset this infirmity he began to train himself to write with the left hand, but it was not very long before it too was attacked by the same malady. But what tortures these workers most acutely is the intense and incessant application of the mind, for in such work as this the whole brain, its nerves and fibres, must be kept constantly on the stretch; hence ensues loss of tonus. From this result headaches, heavy colds, sore throats, and fluxes to the eyes from keeping them fixed on the paper; those who suffer most from these ailments are book-keepers and accountants, as they are called, for example those who hire themselves to work for merchants. Also we must reckon in the same category the private secretaries of princes. For weakness of the arm and right hand it will be beneficial to apply rubbing but it should be rather gentle and done with oil of sweet almonds to which you can add a small portion of brandy to strengthen the part affected. In winter they must take care not to let the hands grow numb from excessive cold, so they must be protected by good thick gloves.

Writers' Cramp in 1890

Writers' cramp was described by Sir Charles Bell in the year 1830 it has also been called writing neurosis, scriveners' palsy and graphospasm The description of this condition by Gowers (1893) is a classic. It occurs in men twice as frequently as women, and 83 per cent of the cases are between twenty and fifty years of age. Occasionally more than one member of a family is involved. Nervous individuals are especially liable and anxiety is an important predisposing factor. Local disease or injury of the limb may precipitate symptoms.

The chief agent in the production of the malady is the act of writing, which has usually been excessive in degree. Hence the affection occurs chiefly among those who earn their living by writing, and clerks furnish the majority of cases. But it now and then occurs in persons who have not done an excessive amount of writing; and in such cases a powerful predisposing cause, such as anxiety or neuralgia, may commonly be traced. The occurrence of the disease is influenced less by the amount than by the manner of writing. There are in writing two chief elements: the way in which the pen is held, and the way in which the movements are effected. The mode in which the pen is held is comparatively unimportant; it is the mode in which the pen is moved that chiefly determines the occurrence of the disease.

Four Different Methods of Writing

Gowers recognized that lawyers' clerks are especially affected by reason of their cramped position and that the condition is unknown in shorthand writers. He described four methods of writing:

(1) The hand resting on the little finger; movement of the pen by the fingers and the thumb.

(2) The hand resting on the wrist; lateral movement assisted by the abductors of the wrist.

(3) The middle of the forearm used as a fulcrum.

(4) The arm moved freely from the shoulder; the fingers scarcely move He found that cramp occurred especially in the first two groups; writers using the last method are immune.

The best and only free method is to write from the upper arm and shoulder, with no fixation of the arm; the forearm, wrist and little finger rest on the table so as to take some of the weight of the limb from the shoulder-muscles, but both wrist and forearm move along the table as the writing progresses from left to right. In this way the pen can be held lightly; very little of the movement is effected by the small muscles of the hand; the fingers scarcely alter their position except when a stroke is carried far above or below the line; and even for this a movement of the fingers is not always necessary. No styl can be considered free unless it is easy to write a whole line across a page of foolscap without once breaking contact between the pen and the paper.

The Spastic Type of the Disease

Most commonly the presenting symptom is motor spasm, but besides the spastic type there are also tremulous and neuralgic types of the disease. The paralytic type with simple inability to write is extremely rare. The onset is gradual.

After writing for some time the patient finds something unusual about his writing; the pen does not move quite as he intended it to do; a stroke now and again is irregular, extends too high or too low; a slight involuntary movement causes an unintended mark. He finds that he is grasping the pen too tightly, and cannot help doing so; that the fingers do not keep in their accustomed place; and the first finger has a tendency to slip off the pen, so that this gets between the first and second finger. He endeavours to mend matters by taking a firmer hold, but this seems to increase the difficulty, and he finds that he writes slowly, as if a weight were attached to the hand. The hand feels strangely tired, and an aching pain in the finger or thumb or first metacarpal bone, or in the wrist or forearm, makes it still more difficult for him to go on writing. These symptoms may continue, with only slight impairment of the power of writing, for weeks or months, but they occur after writing for a shorter time; they increase in degree, and now and then there is distinct spasm, which cannot be controlled. The first finger or the thumb tends to become flexed at the middle joint, so that its tip moves up the pen, or, less commonly, the fingers become extended, so that the pen is not pressed against the paper with sufficient force, and may even drop from the hand, or the thumb may become extended across the pen. The characters of the writing become still more irregular, the down-strokes are too thick, the point of the pen may be driven through the paper, and in its irregularity of form and force the writing resembles that done in a jolting carriage.

Involvement of the Whole Hand and the Forearm

Rarely the chief spasm is in the fourth finger, or in the third and fourth fingers, and pain may be felt in the long flexors of these fingers, and the ulnar flexors of the wrist. Sometimes the whole hand seems to get stiff, and its movements slow; in such cases there is a tendency for the letters that are formed to become smaller and smaller as the writing proceeds, until they are illegible. As the spasm increases in degree, it extends in range, and involves more of the muscles of the forearm. There is a tendency for the wrist to become flexed, or extended, or supinated, and in the effort to prevent the disturbing movement, the opponents contract strongly, until at last all the muscles of the forearm may be in such energetic spasm as to render movement of the pen impossible. Various devices are at first employed to counteract the spasm. The mode of holding the pen is changed; it is held between the first two fingers, or fixed in a piece of cork, which is grasped by the hand, and the movements in writing are effected by the upper arm or the patient fixes the right hand by the help of the other, placing, for instance, some fingers of the left hand between the two last fingers of the right. For a time these devices give a little help but the spasm gradually increases in degree, and overcomes the fixing help, or it spreads to the muscles of the upper arm.

Symptoms, Signs and Course of Writers' Cramp

Occasionally the onset is acute. Other delicate movements are not affected until late in the disorder, and it is striking how, asked to unlace his shoe with the affected hand, the patient performs this act to perfection. Power in the hand may be slightly impaired; wasting is exceptional. The electrical reactions are only slightly disturbed, if at all. Sensory symptoms are usually prominent and rarely absent. A sense of fatigue in the hand is followed by spasm and dull pain, occasionally with local tenderness. The pain may be referred along the course of nerves; paræsthesiæ may affect the fingers. The symptoms continue with the attempts to write. The sensory symptoms spread more than the motor. In about 50 per cent of those who have learnt to write with the other hand, symptoms appear for a second time and may progress more rapidly in the second arm than in the first. Rarely the legs are affected at the same time as the arms.

The Attributes of a Psychoneurosis

No anatomical changes are known. Clearly the condition is one of central and not of local origin, since local weakness is only found to a degree comparable with spasm. The theory of central origin is supported by involvement of the opposite hand. That the pain starts from the skin where the grasp of the pen is unduly firm, but spreads beyond this point, is evidence in favour of a central origin. The majority of patients are nervous subjects; in showing the signs and symptoms of pathological anxiety they reveal the psychoneurotic personality.

Diagnosis and Prognosis

The limitation of symptoms to the act of writing is diagnostic. Distinction must most often be made from painful and paralytic affections of the hand, including gradual hemiplegia, disseminated sclerosis, cervical tabes, radial palsy and even torsion dystonia at its onset. Simple pain from excessive writing must also be distinguished. The prognosis is poor when the disorder is more established, if there are no extraneous causes other than writing and if complete rest from writing is impossible.

Treatment of Writers' Cramp

Writing should be taught with free movements from the shoulder. It is also desirable that those who experience any difficulty or discomfort in writing should at once change their style for the freer mode. To make a person realize the characteristics of the free method, I have found the following expedient useful. Let him first draw a line across a sheet of paper; for this, the arm must be moved as a whole from the shoulder. Then let him make the line wavy, next increase the wavy character, and then slightly slope the waves, so as at last to make the line a series of m's—m m m m. These are letters, and the transition to other letters will then be easy. As I have already said, the object to be aimed at is to write in such a manner that it shall be easy to form an entire line of words without once lifting the pen from the paper. The hand should grasp the pen lightly, and move as a whole. The comfort and ease experienced when this method is acquired are very remarkable.

Treatment, to be effective, must be early. Rest may relieve the symptoms within a month, but in well-established cases six months will be required Facility in writing with the unaffected hand is not difficult to acquire. A typewriter may be recommended for recalcitrant cases. Where there is pain, sedatives internally and locally are certainly of service. Electricity is of little use, but massage and exercises often relieve the spasm and pain.

Telegraphists' Cramp

The discovery by Faraday in 1831 of electro-magnetic induction made possible the electric telegraph. In 1844 Samuel F. B. Morse sent a telegraph message over a wire from Baltimore to Washington. By the year 1860 his instruments were in use in most countries of the world. Lord Kelvin laid the first transatlantic cable in 1866. The use of the Morse key soon led to a new type of occupational disability called telegraphists' cramp, and this became well known by the year 1880. The Morse key is a clumsy brass instrument, the knob of which is depressed by hand in a series of rapid movements which make and break the circuit in such a way as to transmit the dots and dashes of the Morse code. In the 1911 *Report of the Departmental Committee on Telegraphists' Cramp* various objective factors—such as types of keys, length of service, hours of work and bad style—were reviewed and found not to be necessary antecedents of the disability. Even the physiological signs of cramp were shown to be indeterminate, as there might, or might not, be a visible spasm, and the disability in its objective manifestations could be specific to one letter, or selective for certain muscular activities, or associated with general muscular weakness.

The Attributes of a Psychoneurosis

The chief objective fact in regard to cramp is that people engaged in telegraphic sending sometimes suddenly, sometimes gradually, become unable to control the movements required for using the Morse key. This would suggest some muscular difficulty due to the cumulative effect of the work, or to an initial weakness, or to the introduction of some new factor. The muscular difficulty alone, however, is not disabling, as many telegraphists carry on in spite of it. Scattered throughout the *Report* in connexion with each suggested cause are references to neurasthenic telegraphists, cramp subjects, nervous instability, personal factors, temperamental factors, highly strung disposition, nervous temperament, nervous condition and neurasthenic temperament. As in the case of writers' cramp these attributes are clearly those of the psychoneurotic person who shows pathological anxiety.

Three Different Clinical Types

Patients with telegraphists' cramp do not all show the same symptoms. At least three types are known:

(1) There are those suffering from a general disability to use the arm after many years of sending; not only is the use of the telegraphic key or a pencil interfered with, but also most other actions which demand the use of the arm. The holding of a cup, or of a needle for sewing or knitting, is difficult or impossible; a glass if taken up may be dropped; even the handle of a spade cannot be grasped. This disability may or may not be accompanied by pain, which may be localized in the wrist or may be general.

(2) There are those who can neither send nor write but who can use the arm for other occupations—for example, they can play the piano, use a spade and are quite efficient if the larger muscles are brought into action. This group comprises very many individual variants—from ability to use the arm for anything except telegraphic work, through various grades of inability, to total disability as described in the previous section.

(3) Others again are all right, having no pain, and no muscular disability except for the sending of a particular letter or group of letters. Particular combinations of dots and dashes prove stumbling blocks. Some have difficulty in letters involving a sequence of dots, particularly at the end of a word; others find that having got the key down they cannot get it up again quickly enough for the formation of dots—in other words, the key seems *sticky*.

A Type of Sending which is difficult to Read

If one particular letter were always the cause of the trouble the remedy would be easier, but there are few letters of the alphabet that have not been given as difficulties. While certain sequences are likely to be more difficult if there is any loss of control, some of them have probably a purely individual significance. Sometimes the onset is quite sudden; the telegraphist has a feeling, which comes upon him without warning, that he is not going to be able to send a particular letter; the letter then seems to stand out in relief from all the others and is anticipated with dread and greeted with panic. His state is reflected in a style of sending which the telegraphist at the other end of the wire has difficulty in reading. The receiver then protests, so that to the initial painful mental state is added the objective effects of inefficient work.

Cases where Recovery is Spontaneous

The sufferer feels innocent and may react with antagonism to those around him, or recognize his inefficiency but still feel he is powerless to alter it. Even if this state were the invariable sequence, a remedy would be relatively simple—namely, to accept such initial difficulties and take the telegraphist off. There are, however, many subjects who have admitted that they have had occasional difficulty with certain words and sequences, but that it has passed away; the mechanism of this passing away is obscure, but it probably involves improvement in general health, absence of the fear of cramp and temperamental stability. The fear of cramp is very real to many telegraphists and probably plays no small part in determining the attack, which, without this, might be temporary muscular tiredness, relieved by rest.

Treatment of Telegraphists' Cramp

Mild cases recover when prolonged rest is ordered. In many of the severe cases nothing short of an entire change of employment will cure the condition. The disappearance of anxiety naturally has a good influence on the prognosis. The problem was largely solved by mechanization in the form of the tape machine. Automatic recording systems which are essentially letter-printing instruments came into extensive use about 1880. The teleprinter is an electrically operated typewriter with a standard keyboard. It has replaced the Morse key almost universally. The extended use of the telephone also has helped the situation. In places where the pressure of telegraphic work is slight only, as in isolated country post-offices, the messages are relayed by telephone to the nearest telegraph station.

Cotton-twisters' Cramp

In 1920 Bridge described a form of occupational cramp in the Lancashire cotton trade which may suddenly attack twisters of many years' experience. In joining the threads of a warp, the weaving of which has been completed, to the threads of a new warp the two ends are twisted between the flexed left thumb and the dorsum of the left index finger. An experienced man may join 2,000 ends in one hour, each warp having between 2,000 and 2,500 threads. The symptoms are pain, cramp and loss of power in the affected muscles, and about 50 per cent of the patients show wasting of the thenar eminence. It is a disability causing much loss of earning power in the men affected, and anxiety makes it worse. Treatment by massage and exercises, though alleviating the condition, will not permanently cure it. In severe cases an entire change of employment will be found necessary.

EFFECTS OF VIBRATING TOOLS

There are two main varieties of vibrating tools—namely, piston-operated compressed-air tools and rotating tools operated by electric motors or air turbines.

Uses and Names

Pneumatic tools were first used in French mines as early as 1839, bu they were not employed extensively in other industries until 1883. The are now used for hammering and ramming metals; splitting and shapin blocks of stone; fixing parquet flooring; breaking ground; making concret roads; pounding and lasting leather; cutting, dressing, chipping, grooving engraving, chasing, scaling and scouring metals; perforating wood, ston or metal; piercing holes in mining, quarrying and well sinking; and rivetin in locomotive workshops, shipbuilding (fig. 335) and the construction c aeroplanes. In the various trades the tools have different names such a air hammer, compressed-air chisel, compressed-air drill, Jack hammer, pneu matic chisel, pneumatic drill, pneumatic hammer, pneumatic tool, pounding up machine, riveting gun, riveting tool and stone-cutters' hammer.

Oscillations of the Piston

The tools, which vary in weight from 3 to 30 lb., are operated by reciprocating piston. The air as it passes through the distribution box c the instrument sets up a loud and disagreeable noise, and the rapid chang of direction which it undergoes inside the box, together with the oscil lations of the piston, sets up a rapid vibration of the tool which is trans mitted to the body of the workman. Pneumatic drills work in simila fashion, but they have an addition; mechanism which translates th reciprocating movement to a rotar one.

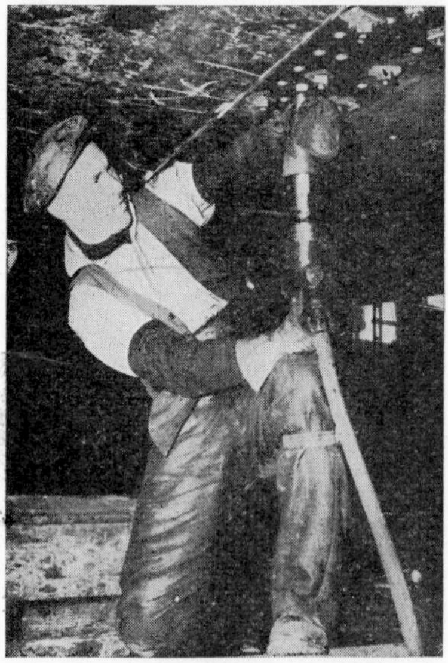

Light, Medium and Heavy Tools

The to-and-fro movement c the piston varies from 250 to 6,00 strokes per minute. In general, tl heavier the tool the slower is th vibration rate. Heavy tools are use in mines, quarries and in roa making. In shipbuilding and re pairing and in boiler shop medium-sized tools are used fe hot riveting and cold copper stayin and caulking. In foundries, mediun sized tools with a chisel are use for dressing or fettling metal cas ings, and tools of comparab weight are used by stonemasons fe dressing stone. Much lighter too

FIG. 335.—Workman using Compressed-
air Riveting Tool in Shipbuilding
(*By courtesy of The Listener*)

are used in the motor-car and aircraft industries and for riveting tanl

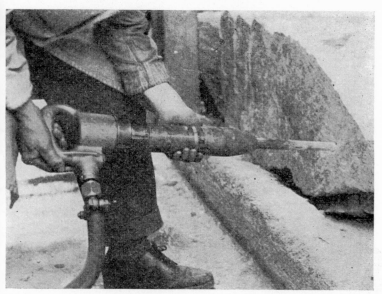

Fig. 336.—Compressed-air Drill without axial Water Feed. Note Method of holding Tool

and cisterns. Tools of about 4 lb. in weight are used in the scaling of boiler tubes.

Method of Holding the Tool

The worker holds the tool with both hands; he supports it with the left hand and holds the trigger with the right (fig. 336). A glove is worn on the left hand to protect it from the heat engendered by the friction set up by the movement of the piston and chisel, but as a rule no glove is worn on the right hand. If the tool is working well, air escapes only through the exhaust, which can be directed away from the man's hands. Sometimes, however, there is a leak and the right hand is exposed to a stream of cold air.

Occupational Disorder of Four Types

Four types of occupational disorder due to the handling of vibrating tools can be recognized:

(1) *Small areas of decalcification seen in X-rays of the bones of the carpus.* These are quite commonly found in pneumatic-tool workers. In the series studied by Hunter, McLaughlin and Perry (1945) they were found in 119 out of 286 men. They are not specific to pneumatic-tool workers; there is reason to think they can occur in anyone engaged on heavy manual work. They are symptomless and do not predispose to fracture or any other complication.

(2) *Injury to the soft tissues of the hands.* This includes injury to the palmar aponeurosis, and perhaps the onset of Dupuytren's contracture; the formation of adventitious bursæ and even chronic bursitis in the palm; atrophy of palmar muscles, and injury to the ulnar nerve. These injuries are much less common than the other effects of vibration.

(3) *Osteoarthritis of the joints of the arms.* The elbows are more commonly affected than the wrist, and the wrists more commonly than the shoulders. This specific form of arthritis has been compensatable in Germany since 1929, and between 1929 and 1935 1,448 cases were notified and 398 were paid compensation. It is not compensatable in Great Britain.

(4) *Vascular disturbance,* namely, the Raynaud phenomenon. This disorder is the most common of the four types. Hunter, McLaughlin and Perry (1945) found that fully half of a group of 286 pneumatic-tool workers were affected, and Agate and Druett (1946) that more than two-thirds of another group of similar size were affected.

The Thesis of Maurice Raynaud, 1862

It is now recognized that Maurice Raynaud included amongst the cases he described in his thesis of 1862 examples of several different diseases in which the same manifestations had appeared. At the present time it is usually accepted that the term Raynaud's disease shall be used only for a distinct but rare symmetrical vascular disorder of unknown ætiology which is found mostly in young women; similarly that the Raynaud phenomenon shall apply to a symptom or sign—namely, intermittent pallor or cyanosis of the extremities. Hutchinson (1901) advocated the use of the latter term and suggested it should be qualified whenever the ætiology was known. The colour changes of the Raynaud phenomenon do occur in cases of Raynaud's disease itself, but are also to be seen in such conditions as hereditary cold fingers, certain cases of cervical rib and pneumatic-hammer disease amongst others (Hunt, 1936).

Definition of the Raynaud Phenomenon

The clinical definition of the Raynaud phenomenon given by Hunt will be used here, in spite of the opinion of Allen and others (1946) that it is too narrow for all purposes. Hunt defined the Raynaud phenomenon as

> Intermittent pallor or cyanosis of the extremities precipitated by exposure to cold, without clinical evidence of blockage of the large peripheral vessels and with nutritional lesions, if present at all, limited to the skin.

Synonyms used to describe the Disability

The following synonyms are to be found in the accounts already published: dead hand (Telford and others, 1945; Biden-Steele and King 1947); dead fingers; white fingers (Hamilton and others, 1918); pneumatic hammer disease (Mills, 1942); pseudo-Raynaud's disease (Brocklehurst 1945); traumatic vasospastic disease of the hand (Gurjian and Walker

1945). The first three of these are graphic but are wanting in accuracy: they may have unfortunate mental associations for the sufferers and their use cannot be defended. The term pseudo-Raynaud's disease seems to add nothing to an understanding of the disease and can have no more claim to be used than the name Raynaud's disease itself, which has been excluded by definition.

The Raynaud Phenomenon of Occupational Origin

Biden-Steele and King (1947) appeal for the abandonment of both Raynaud's disease and the Raynaud phenomenon on the ground that legal confusion may be caused; but these authors themselves confuse the meanings of the two terms and have only suggested dead hand as an alternative. Traumatic vasospastic disease defines the probable ætiology and disorder of function, but has been used by only one author. The name pneumatic-hammer disease, at one time specific, must be considered outmoded in the light of later experiences. The Raynaud phenomenon is a widely accepted descriptive term, and it is suggested that all vascular disorders of the type under review might best be included within the single diagnosis of *the Raynaud phenomenon of occupational origin*, at least until the factors in their causation are all understood. In nearly every case vibration will be found to be the principal factor.

Historical Summary

The discovery of the occupational disease dates back to 1911, when Loriga reported the first case of a vascular lesion attributable to the use of pneumatic tools. In 1918 Alice Hamilton found it amongst Indiana stone-cutters who used pneumatic chisels; in 1930 Maria Seyring found the same state of affairs in a group of German foundry workers. Middleton (1930) saw the phenomenon in boot and shoe operatives who used pounding-up machines which set up tremendous vibration. Such machines have been abolished in England, but they are still in use in certain countries. Several other outbreaks were detected between 1936 and 1945 in groups of workers using pneumatic hammers. Some of the tools were small, others fairly large. No outbreaks have been reported in men who use the largest road or rock drills, but this does not mean that no cases have occurred.

Tools which Vibrate without Hammering

Up to 1945 the disability had been confined to workers who had used tools delivering hammer-like blows. Since that date rotating tools operated by electric motors have come into general use (figs. 337, 338). In 1945 there was a serious outbreak in an engineering works in Manchester where a simple portable rotary metal-grinding tool was in use (fig. 339). Furthermore, thirty-two cases were discovered amongst thirty-seven men and women who were grinding small iron castings against carborundum wheels (Agate, Druett and Tombleson, 1946). Here they were holding in their fingers the castings and not the tools; nevertheless the vibration was

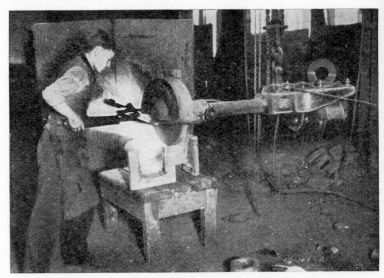

Fig. 337.—High-speed Swing-frame Grinder working at a thousand revolutions per minute on a Steel Casting. Note Direct Electrical Drive eliminating Rope or Belt

(By courtesy of Pneulec, Ltd)

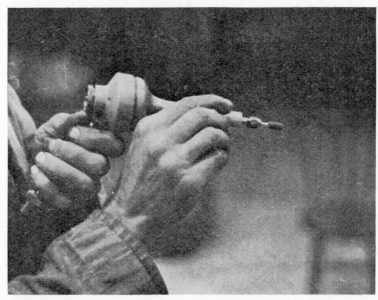

Fig. 338.—Electrically Driven Portable Tool comprising a Cutter mounted on a Flexible Cable on the principle of a Dental Drill. Note Method of holding Tool

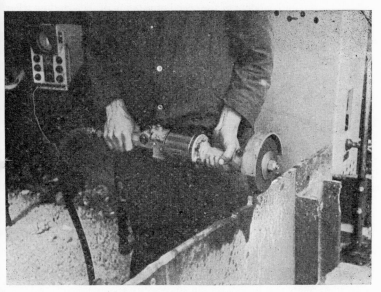

FIG. 339.—Carborundum Wheel operated by Compressed Air and used to grind
Steel. Note Method of holding Tool
(By courtesy of Mr. Treve Holman)

ntense. Even in metal-beating the worker can suffer vascular disorders in
he hand that holds the sheet metal.

Frequency in Beats per Minute

Thus it appears that vibration, however generated, can cause disease if
t impinges directly upon the hand or fingers. There has been much argument about the type of vibration which will cause disease. This vibration
was always described in terms of beats per minute, because most of the
tools implicated were hammer-like. Even in 1918 Leake, who worked with
Alice Hamilton, recorded the vibration of stone-cutters' hammers by a
mechanical device, which was the only method then available. He thought
that 3,500 beats per minute was the dangerous frequency. Since then
various workers have claimed that tool speeds of from 2,000 to 36,000 per
minute were the dangerous ones. Thus Hunter and others (1945) found
that vibration rates of from 2,000 to 3,000 per minute were the worst.
Most of these estimates were made by inference, not experiment. When,
however, tools other than hammers were blamed, difficulties arose because
beats per minute was no longer a sensible measurement.

Frequency in Revolutions per Minute

In the case of rotary tools, revolutions per minute was the unit used,
but even this would not do for grinders of castings, whose exposure to
vibrations was for at most a second at a time repeated thousands of times

a day and quite independent of the speed of rotation of the grinding wheel. In addition to the vibration, other factors were blamed. One was the cold exhaust air from pneumatic tools; but it was soon observed that the exhaust usually played on the hand which was less affected or even entirely unaffected. The second was the hardness of the materials upon which the tools were worked; this factor can be dismissed because hardness merely alters the character of the vibration and then not appreciably.

The Fundamental and its Various Harmonics

Vibration is never a pure quantity: it is always made up of a fundamental oscillation or note and a series of harmonics of progressively greater speed and smaller displacement. To describe a vibration it is necessary to specify the fundamental, its various harmonics, and the frequency and amplitude of each harmonic. The result is a vibration spectrum. By reducing them to such spectra, it is possible to compare the regular vibrations from a pneumatic hammer with the apparently bizarre disturbance set up by the grinding operations of a rotary tool.

Frequency and Amplitude of the Harmonics

In 1946 Agate and Druett set out to measure vibrations in terms of the frequency and amplitude of all the various harmonics. They needed a device which could be used at the factory bench, which would take hundreds of instantaneous readings to cover all the many methods of using tools and which would give a permanent record for purposes of comparison. Only an electrical method could serve. A piezo-electrical crystal was used to pick up vibrations. Certain crystals of Rochelle salt generate an electrical response when bent or shaken. In these experiments the response from such a crystal was analysed electrically in an acoustic spectrometer.

Use of the Acoustic Spectrometer

Finally the spectrum was presented as a number of vertical lines on a cathode-ray tube screen, each vertical line corresponded to a frequency, its length being proportional to the amplitude at that frequency. The picture was photographed, the length of the lines was measured, calculations were made and the spectrum was finally shown in tabular form. The frequencies are stated in cycles per second and the amplitudes in millimetres or microns. Fortunately, the method fulfilled all the requirements and it was used for experiments in several factories.

Frequency in Cycles per Second

It was found that many different tools and mechanical processes produced similar vibration spectra. The spectra of machines already known to have caused Raynaud's phenomenon showed points in common. So, by comparing spectra from various tools and the incidence or complete absence of disease clinically, it was possible to find out which were the most dangerous types of vibration. These appeared to be at frequencies of from

40 to 125 cycles per second, especially if the amplitudes in this range exceeded 100 microns. Any process generating this kind of vibration in contact with the hands will probably produce disease sooner or later. The grinding of castings certainly produces vibration in this range. Some very high-speed tools, driven by air turbines, produce spectra in which all the vibration is above 600 cycles per second and is small in amplitude. Vascular disease from the use of these tools has not been recorded but they do sometimes cause subjective symptoms such as pain and numbness.

An Outbreak of the Disorder in Manchester

In 1949 Agate investigated an outbreak of the Raynaud phenomenon of occupational origin in Manchester. In the aero-engine factory concerned there were some 300 people polishing or scurfing duralumin and steel castings by means of a portable tool comprising a cutter or grinding wheel mounted on a flexible cable on the principle of the dental drill (fig. 338). These people used either felt buffs about 3 inches in diameter dressed with emery, silicon-carbide stones $1\frac{1}{2}$ inches in diameter or spiral-toothed steel cutters which could remove as much as $\frac{1}{4}$ inch of duralumin at a cut. The vibration set up was considerable. These workers held the metal handpiece of the tool in such a way that the left hand was in front nearest the cutting head, and this hand did most of the work. Left-handed men usually used it with the position of their hands reversed.

Cyanosis used as an Index of Severity

In 1945, when they were first seen, 66 per cent of the group of 278 men and women using this tool had already become affected by vascular disturbances, after an average of 23·5 months at the work. Without question the disease was directly attributable to occupation. Most of these people were affected soonest, and most severely, in the left hand, the hand nearest the cutting head. The other hand was often involved six months later. The ring and middle fingers suffered worst, but in many cases even the thumb did not escape. The attacks came on in cold weather, often when the worker was getting up in the morning or bicycling to work. In the factory it was warm, and attacks were quite uncommon; consequently a man's work was seldom interrupted. Cyanosis followed the blanching in many cases, but often there was a period of six months during which the only colour change noticed was the blanching. More than one-third of the 278 workers had cyanosis during their attack, and since this was most frequently seen in those who were most severely affected, it was possible to use it as an index of severity.

No Safeguard to stop working with Vibrating Tools

The same 278 workers were followed up by correspondence two and a half years later, the factory having closed down in the interval. Not all of them replied, and some were never reached because they had left the district. Nevertheless, it was possible to estimate that between 77 and 90 per cent of those who originally used this tool had become subject to attacks of the Raynaud phenomenon. This incidence is remarkably high for an occupational disease. In only one case had spontaneous cure occurred. In half of the cases the disease seemed to be stationary; certainly there had been no improvement since they had changed their occupation. In over 40 per cent there was a distinct worsening of the condition—that is to say, more fingers were affected, attacks came more frequently and cyanosis was more pronounced. About a dozen men had contracted the disease after they had ceased to do this kind of work. It is therefore no safeguard to stop working with vibrating tools, and even if exposure is limited to one year the disease may still follow. Once having developed, it shows more tendency to progress than to regress. Fortunately, gangrene and other serious complications are very rare if, indeed, they occur at all.

Disability beginning only with the Next Job

This outbreak raises interesting side issues. At first these men and women complained of their disease and were anxious for the future, but they did not claim the slightest disability, for attacks so seldom came on in the warmth of the workshops. Nevertheless, they were expecting to lose their jobs because the Second World War was coming to an end. Another group of workers—namely, the grinders of castings already mentioned— were just as severely affected but did not regard their symptoms as being important. On the other hand, they saw no danger of losing their jobs. When the Manchester factory closed down, the outlook for the sufferers from the Raynaud phenomenon was not good. They were unable to get any other metal-polishing work and were obliged to go back to their prewar jobs. Those who were in textile trades or who took outdoor jobs were often handicapped in their new work. Here, therefore, is a new form of disability which arises in the course of one job but only becomes disabling during the next. It never causes the loss of a whole day's work, yet in the course of a week, especially in winter, it can result in much loss of time and efficiency.

Flanging and Clinching of Motor-car Doors

A type of disability which has been observed in the motor-body building industry deserves further investigation (Reynard, 1952). During seven years in a works employing 10,000 people, three men using pneumatic piston-operated hammers in the flanging and clinching of the panels of motor-car doors have suffered considerable loss of faculty. This consists of pain, a persistent cramping sensation, paræsthesiæ, apparent loss of muscular power and even permanent flexion of the fingers. The hypoalgesia to pin-prick and cotton-wool touch is present only during the colour change. One of the three men hit the ulnar fingers of his hand while working but did not know it until he saw blood. When fresh men take up this job of flanging and clinching motor-car doors it is possible to postpone the onset of the Raynaud phenomenon by providing them with a left-hand cotton glove fitted with a rubber insert.

Effect of Protective Devices

Apart from comparing various tools and processes, it was possible by the use of the acoustic spectrometer to study the various conditions of working and to judge the effect of protective devices. Also it was easy to say which of several methods of doing grinding work was the least harmful. It was disappointing to find that absorbent materials such as rubber and felt were ineffective, for they did not reduce the vibration by more than one-third (Agate and Druett, 1946). In order to postpone as long as possible the onset of the disability, gloves padded at suitable points with absorbent materials should be worn at work. Equally it is advisable for all men liable to attacks of the Raynaud phenomenon to wear thick woollen gloves when exposed to cold, as in bicycling to work. But there can be no real solution to the problem short of an entirely new design of portable tool or, indeed, of the complete mechanization of grinding methods.

Case 34. Copper stayer—using pneumatic hammer for six and a half years—Raynaud phenomenon of both hands.

(Hunter, McLaughlin and Perry, 1945.) A. B., a man aged 40. Twelve and a half years before examination he started work as a copper stayer using a hammer weighing $12\frac{1}{4}$ lb. with a frequency of 2,300 vibrations a minute. He also wore a glove on the left hand. After he had been working for two years he noticed his fingers would go white. The first one involved was the index finger on the left hand: the whiteness was associated with paræsthesiæ. Gradually the right hand became involved and soon all the fingers on both hands would go white. He found the hands very awkward to use and had difficulty in doing up buttons. It often took two hours for the sensation to return. At the start the syndrome occurred only in winter, but after four years it occurred in summer as well. After six and a half years' work with the hammer he had to give up this work on account of the symptoms, and is now working as a labourer in the boiler shop.

Case 35. Caulker—using pneumatic chisel for four years—Raynaud phenomenon of both hands.

(Hunter, McLaughlin and Perry, 1945.) I. C., a man aged 29, for fourteen years had worked as a caulker with a tool having a vibration frequency of 2,850 per minute, and weighing $11\frac{1}{4}$ lb. After he had used the caulking chisel for four years he started to have white numb fingers: first the left index finger and then spreading to involve all the fingers. The syndrome usually appeared soon after he started work, but it sometimes occurred on Sundays when he was not working. After warming or rubbing for fifteen minutes the circulation returned. After he was questioned, he washed his hands in cold water on a hot August afternoon and it was observed that all his fingers went completely white, with a sharp line of demarcation where they joined the hand. Sensation to pin-prick and light touch was much impaired in these fingers. The phenomenon took fifteen minutes to disappear.

Effects of Ionizing Radiation

Ionizing radiations are those capable of producing ionization. This is a process by which atoms or molecules lose or gain electrons resulting in the production of electrically charged particles (ions). Ionization is accompanied by a transfer of energy to the material in which the ions are formed. The ionizing radiations which will be discussed in this section are alpha and beta particles, protons, neutrons, X-rays and γ-rays. Of these, X- and γ-rays are electromagnetic radiations similar to and propagated like light waves and radio waves; the rest are material particles of atomic or sub-atomic size. The biological effects of ionizing radiations will depend on the magnitude of the dose and also upon a number of additional factors, namely whether the radiation is to the whole body or only to parts of the body, its energy and hence whether the radiation is penetrating or superficial, and finally, whether it is radiation from an external source or from radioactive materials deposited in tissues—internal radiation. These effects will also vary depending on whether the radiation is received acutely or accumulated over a period of time, that is the dose rate. The attention of doctors and physicists was first called to X-ray injuries in 1896, to the harmful effects of radium in 1900 and to those of uranium fission products in 1944. It was not until the detonation of the atomic bombs over Hiroshima and Nagasaki that the effects of total body irradiation were fully appreciated. It is therefore logical to describe such effects in chronological order under the three corresponding headings.

(a) Injuries from X-rays

The subject of injuries from X-rays and radium was reviewed in detail by Rolleston in 1930 and by Colwell and Russ in 1934. Wilhelm C. Röntgen discovered X-rays in November 1895. Within three months of his announcement of the discovery it became known that T. A. Edison and W. J. Morton had suffered from conjunctivitis after some hours of exposure to X-irradiation.

Erythema and Necrosis of the Skin

Within a year erythema, swelling and necrosis of the skin, alopecia and chronic radio-dermatitis were reported. In 1897 D. Walsh first directed attention to the acute constitutional symptoms by describing colicky abdominal pain and diarrhœa in an X-ray worker, in whom the symptoms disappeared after the abdomen was protected by lead. The literature of the accidents and bad effects of X-rays has since become extensive. In 1902 Codman collected 171 cases of accidental X-ray burns, less than half of which were serious and about one-third of which occurred in X-ray workers. More than two-thirds of these injuries appeared within two years of the first use of X-rays. In 1902 Frieben recorded cancer following chronic ulceration of the skin caused by X-rays. By 1911 Hesse was able to collect ninety-four such cases, of which fifty-four occurred in medical men or technicians, and in 1914 Feygin tabulated 104 cases of malignant disease caused by X-irradiation.

The First Case of Cataract

The first case of cataract resulting from exposure to X-rays was reported by Paton in 1909. The patient was a lady who had had thirty-eight
exposures to X-rays for lupus of the cheeks. Her sight began to fail nine
months after the completion of treatment, and two years later she was
able to count fingers only. The main opacity in the lens was a greyish-
white granular plaque probably lying against the posterior capsule.
Normal acuity of vision was restored by removal of the cataract. (See also
pp. 862–72.)

The First Fatality

The first death to be recognized as due to the action of X-rays occurred
as recently as 1914 in a radiologist, Emilio Tiraboschi of Bergamo. He had
worked for fourteen years with X-rays and had taken no precautions. For
several years he had had a radio-dermatitis of the left hand and of the right
side of the face. In the last three years of his life he lost his strength and
became pale. Finally he bled from the gums, and necropsy revealed aplastic
anæmia together with atrophy of the testes (Faber, 1923). In 1922 Ledoux-
Lebard estimated that one hundred radiologists had died from malignant
disease due to their occupation. Deaths among radiologists exposed to
X-rays before the importance of adequate protection was realized unfortunately still occur. So far the victims have been research workers,
radiologists, laboratory assistants, technicians and nurses.

Beginning of Industrial Radiography

Cases of industrial origin occurred later, because the use of X-rays in
industry began later. At first industrial workers, unlike professional
workers, were often ignorant as to the possible dangers of the apparatus
they used, so that with respect to the use of X-rays industry lagged behind
medicine. Fortunately, however, the lamentable history of the pioneers in
the medical field has not been repeated. The human experiments have been
made, the tragic results of carelessness demonstrated and the measures
necessary for adequate protection are known and available to anyone who
cares to learn them.

Uses of X-rays in Industry

The possible uses of X-rays in industry are many and varied. They may
be used for the detection of welding defects, of cracks and blowholes in
castings, of defects in alloys from faulty mixture, of corrosion in cables or
gas cylinders and of defects in reinforced concrete. Rubber heels may be
examined by the fluoroscope to see if the metal plate is in the centre. X-rays
are also used to sort fresh eggs from stale, to reveal mineral adulterants in
vegetable foods and weevils in grain. For the examination of metals and
all thick specimens, very penetrating rays must be used and protection of
the worker is then a major problem.

Acute X-ray Burns

Injuries which follow a short single exposure, or perhaps several exposures, may vary enormously in intensity. In mild cases there is simply a transient reddening, lasting a few days and followed by scaling and loss of hair. If the burn is deeper, blisters appear which may be serous or purulent and the condition resembles that following a scald but is less acute in character and slower to heal. Sometimes the process, instead of disappearing in a few weeks, penetrates to the deeper layers of the skin and to the subcutaneous tissues with the formation of a leathery slough surrounded by a brawny indurated swelling with ill-defined limits. The process is exceedingly slow and obstinate, and has a tendency to progress and to resist treatment in a remarkable way. It is at times very painful. In March 1899 Dr. J. Weldon, of Willimantic, Connecticut, exposed himself for an X-ray picture of the hip joint for forty-five minutes with the Crookes tube but five inches from the skin of the groin. A most intractable burn resulted, necessitating a severe operation and producing disability for a year and a half (Cassidy, 1900).

Chronic X-ray Dermatitis

The clinical aspects of chronic X-ray dermatitis in radiologists were described in 1904 by F. Hall-Edwards, himself an unfortunate victim of the disease. The change in the hands begins round the base of the nails as an acute erythema and gradually increases. Transverse and longitudinal ridges appear on the nails, which become brittle, assume a characteristic dirty-brown appearance, tend to separate from the matrix and eventually thicken and form shapeless masses. The skin becomes uniformly red and atrophied; small warts appear, increase in size and number and, when situated over the knuckles, crack and cause much pain. Later the dry thickened skin shows telangiectases, absence of hair, paronychia and ulcers which are slow to heal and prone to break down. The hair follicles and the sebaceous and sweat glands completely disappear in cases of long standing. The freedom of the palms of the hands may be due to the naturally thicker skin there, but the greater liability to exposure of the backs of the hands and fingers is probably the more important factor. The lesions are as a rule slowly progressive (fig. 340).

Post-irradiation Telangiectases

Post-irradiation telangiectases, which have been regarded as compensatory for obliteration of the vessels in the corium, usually appear within two years, and sometimes in the absence of an initial erythema; in some instances the interval between irradiation and the appearance of telangiectases is prolonged, even to fifteen years. If exposure is continued, the lesions may progress to involve the tendon sheaths and joints. There may be intense pain, of which the severity is out of proportion to the size of the lesions; it is caused by the exposure of nerve endings.

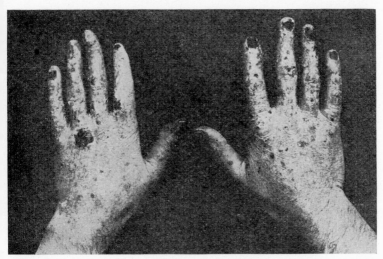

FIG. 340.—Case 36. X-ray Dermatitis and Carcinoma of Dorsum of the left Hand in a pioneer X-ray Technician. He had begun work eight years previously, in 1898. He died of Carcinomatosis 36 years later

Squamous-celled Carcinoma of the Skin

Squamous-celled carcinoma is almost always the form of malignant disease which has followed excessive X-ray exposure and long-continued X-ray dermatitis in man. Although most often seen in radiologists and manufacturers of X-ray apparatus, X-ray carcinoma may, of course, also occur in patients who have undergone treatment by X-irradiation. In 1914 Feygin collected six cases of this kind. One of the earliest victims of X-ray carcinoma was a man engaged in the manufacture of X-ray lamps (Frieben, 1902). The interval between the onset of chronic X-ray dermatitis and the appearance of malignant disease varies from three to twenty-seven years. The average of thirty-five cases was seven years (Feygin). The age incidence from thirty-five to fifty is comparatively early, that of ordinary carcinoma of the skin being between fifty-five and fifty-eight. The most frequent site of the growth, which is not uncommonly multiple, is on the backs of the hands and fingers (fig. 341), and the hand more exposed appears to be the one more severely affected—the left in radiologists and the right in those engaged in the manufacture of apparatus (Feygin). Among radiologists, carcinoma usually develops in an ulcer, less often in keratotic areas. The predominating symptom is pain, which may be constant and very severe. It has been ascribed to invasion of the terminations of nerves by the growth, and to a neuritis.

Basal-celled Carcinoma of the Skin

Occasionally basal-celled carcinoma occurs as the result of X-irradiation. In one case a basal-celled carcinoma of the scalp appeared eighteen

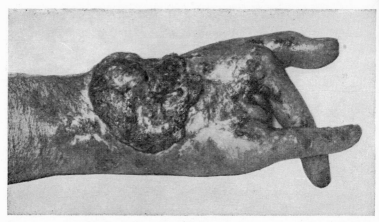

Fig. 341.—Carcinoma of Dorsum of right Hand in a man aged 57 who had begun work 27 years previously in the manufacture of X-ray Apparatus

years after epilation for ringworm (Burrows, 1928). A case has also been recorded of multiple basal-celled carcinomata on the trunk of a radiographer (O'Donovan, 1927). This man, H. J. Suggars, learned the arts of radiography and photography in Dr. Sequeira's department at the London Hospital. In his early professional days, from 1902 onwards, he made a constant practice of demonstrating his heart to students and visitors. It is interesting to record that his photographic work has achieved much recognition and has provided clinical illustrations for the published works of London Hospital men over many years.

Treatment of X-ray Carcinoma

X-ray carcinoma was at one time treated by radium or by diathermocoagulation. H. Bordier, a victim of the disease, claimed that radium aggravates the dermatitis, as occurred in the case of his teacher, J. Bergonié of Bordeaux. Bordier strongly recommended the employment of diathermo-coagulation under a local anæsthetic, and J. Nicholas, who was himself treated in this way, confirmed the benefit obtained by this method. Experience shows that where isolated lesions have been treated by a radium mould the necrosis risk is high. There is no doubt that most of the cases should be treated by surgical excision and skin grafting. It is particularly important to follow them up carefully for the development of secondary carcinoma—for example, in the epitrochlear and axillary lymph glands.

Ill Effects of Deep X-ray Therapy

Constitutional symptoms became prominent only after the introduction of deep X-ray therapy, in which massive doses of deep penetrating rays were given. In 1923 A. E. Barclay gave the following description of his own symptoms. After twelve years' work and much screen examination with

inadequate protection during the First World War, he began to have painless attacks of profuse diarrhœa, at first without other symptoms but later
attended by initial malaise, nausea, vomiting and, on a few occasions, by
the passage of intestinal casts. Eventually it became necessary for him to
give up work and the symptoms then ceased after three weeks. Return to
work was followed by an attack twenty days later, and on eight occasions
such an interval of from eighteen to twenty days was definitely established.
He then adopted the most efficient means of protection known—a lead
apron to cover the abdomen—and remained free from further attacks.

Severe Constitutional Symptoms

Severe constitutional symptoms may occur. They are nausea, uncontrollable vomiting, sometimes with hæmatemesis, diarrhœa with the passage
of blood, abdominal pain and distension, fever up to 104° F., restlessness,
profound prostration, progressive cardiac failure, small rapid pulse and
dyspnœa. When death has occurred it has usually taken place about the
fourth day from the onset. Both animal experiments and post-mortem
studies of human victims show that the application of X-rays to the abdomen may result in necrosis of the intestinal mucosa.

Fibrous Atrophy of the Testes

As long ago as 1905 unsuspected sterility was found in eighteen persons
who had for various periods been exposed to X-rays (Brown and Osgood).
As acute degenerative changes are known to follow vigorous irradiation in
almost all the organs of the body, the development of chronic fibrosis is to
be anticipated as a further result. In two of the famous radiologists who
died from X-ray injuries—E. Tiraboschi and S. Nordentoft—necropsy
revealed fibrous atrophy of the testes (Faber, 1923).

Anæmia due to X-irradiation

Changes in the blood in X-ray workers were early noted, and have been
extensively studied. The lymphocytes are first increased in number by
small doses of X-rays, then diminished. The red cells also may be increased
at first, but anæmia sets in later and may attain a very extreme degree. In
cases that recover, the anæmia is slower to disappear than is the leucopenia.
E. Tiraboschi died of a profound refractory anæmia (Faber, 1923). The
possibility of exposure to radium should always be excluded before attributing true aplastic anæmia in an X-ray worker to X-irradiation.

Death Roll of X-ray Workers

Many difficulties are encountered in tracing which doctors, nurses and
technicians have lost their lives as a result of their work with X-rays.
Detailed study of this melancholy subject shows that more than once a
man disfigured by X-ray injuries has lived to old age and has died of some
independent condition. There is good evidence that the following have lost

their lives as a result of their work with X-rays: H. E. Albers-Schönberg
L. G. Allen, E. F. Ascheim, F. H. Baetjer, B. E.Baker, J. Bauer, R. Blackall,
I. Bruce, E. W. Caldwell, H. Cox, C. M. Dally, J. M. Davidson, W. J
Dodd, C. G. Dyke, L. M. Early, W. C. Egelhoff, H. Fowler, W. W. Fray
W. C. Fuchs, S. C. Glidden, H. Green, F. J. Hall-Edwards, E. H. Harnack
W. Hillier, G. Holden, G. Holzknecht, C. Infroit, M. K. Kassabian, W
Krauss, C. L. Leonard, A. Leray, C. R. C. Lyster, R. H. Machlett, F
Mann, S. Melville, J. T. Morehouse, L. B. Morrison, R. Morton, S
Nordentoft, F. H. Orton, G. F. Parker, G. A. Pirie, J. T. Pitkin, Radiguet,
G. E. Richards, J. R. Riddell, F. le R. Satterlee, I. Sims, J. W. L. Spence,
H. J. Suggars, F. H. Swett, B. F. Thomas, E. Tiraboschi, R. V. Wagner,
T. L. Wagner, L. A. Weigel, C. A. Wilcox, J. C. Williams, E. E. Wilson
and J. Young (Meyer, 1937).

History of Protection of the X-ray Worker

Methods to protect the X-ray worker from injury have been worked
out all too slowly (fig. 342). Within the first few months after their
discovery it was found that X-rays were stopped more effectively by
lead than by any other common metal. Hence lead for protection
came into early use. Transparent lead-glass windows in tube containers
were first used about 1900. At that time the need for protecting both
operator and patient during radiographic exposure was great, because
low voltages were used with consequent long exposures to a very soft

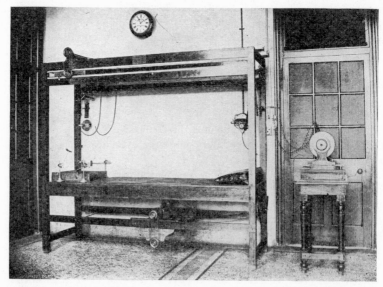

FIG. 342.—X-ray Couch installed in the London Hospital in 1903. It was fitted
with two X-ray Bulbs and was often used for hours on end. There was no
Protection for the Workers

nd easily absorbed radiation (fig. 43). For example, to radiograph he spine required exposures up o one hour. That the radiologist was not more frequently affected by he scattered radiation was due to he fact that during the long exposure he might retire to another oom to see other patients (fig. 344). bout 1903 there appeared a multitude of protective devices to e worn by the radiologist, including apron, jacket, gloves and oggles (fig. 345). This type of rotection gradually reached its eak about 1914, when the more laborate devices gave place to neans of protection which were uilt into the apparatus (fig. 346). he protective materials used include lead, lead glass, lead rubber ig. 347), lead plastics, and building

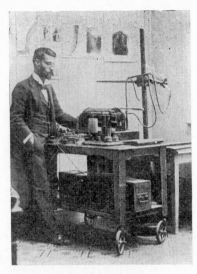

FIG. 343.—X-ray Equipment of 1903. The Lack of Protection led to the Death of the Technician in the picture (see case 36)

materials impregnated with barium salts (fig. 348). When installing an ndustrial X-ray set, advice must be taken regarding the thickness of ead, barium concrete or brick necessary to protect the worker.

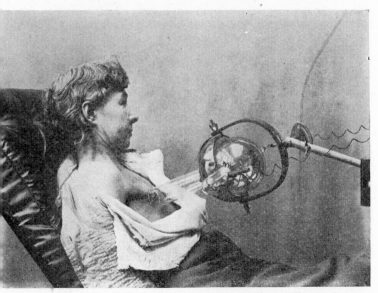

FIG. 344.—Unprotected X-ray Tube used for X-irradiation Therapy in 1903

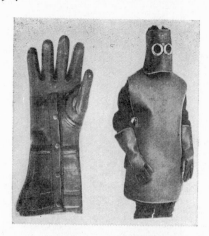

FIG. 345.—Massive Protective Equipment of Leaded Rubber and Glass used in 1910

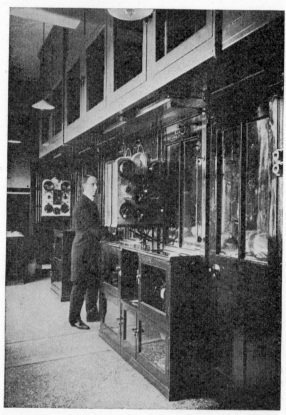

FIG. 346.—Technician protected by Leaded Glass built into the Equipment of an X-ray Room in 1912

International Commission on Radiological Units

The first British X-ray Units Committee was set up in 1925 under the chairmanship of Sir William Bragg at the time of the formation of the International Commission on Radiological Units (ICRU) by the first International Congress of Radiology in London. Largely as a result of the work of the British Committee the roentgen was established as a unit of dose, when the ICRU met in 1928 in Stockholm.

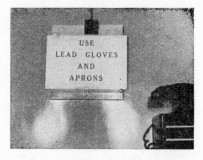

FIG. 347.—Notice of Warning to Radiologists and Technicians in a Hospital

The committee subsequently became the British Committee on Radiological Units and played an important part in the revision of the definition of the roentgen, including its applicability to gamma rays, and also, under the chairmanship of Dr. L. H. Gray, it helped to establish the rad as the unit of absorbed dose. The following units are in general use at the present time:

Roentgen (r)—the Unit of Exposure

The ionization produced in air by X or gamma radiation is taken as a measure of exposure; it is calculated by dividing the sum of the electrical charge on all ions of one sign produced by X or gamma irradiation in a small volume of air, by the mass of that volume. The unit of exposure is the roentgen (r) and 1 roentgen = $2 \cdot 58 \times 10^{-4}$ coulombs/kg. An exposure of 1 roentgen corresponds to an energy absorption of $86 \cdot 9$ ergs/g. in air or about 93 ergs/g. in soft tissue.

Rad (rad)—the Unit of Absorbed Dose

When ionizing radiation irradiates matter, the absorbed dose is found by dividing the energy imparted to a small volume of matter, by the mass of that volume. The unit of absorbed dose is the rad and 1 rad = 100 ergs/g. Absorbed dose differs from exposure in that it is influenced by the material to which the dose is imparted.

Rem (rem)—the Dose Equivalent and Quality Factor (QF.s)

When exposed persons are irradiated the effects in the living tissue depend on a number of modifying factors, besides the amount of the absorbed dose. For example, the effects differ according to the kind of radiation. For determining permissible doses for radiological protection purposes a modifying factor, termed the Quality Factor, is used to take account of the kind of radiation and so obtain from the absorbed dose a quantity, termed the dose equivalent, which is expressed in rems. This enables the effects of the irradiation incurred to be expressed on a common scale. The unit of dose equivalent is the rem and is such that apart from other possible modifying factors: Dose Equivalent (rem) = Absorbe Dose (rad) × Quality Factor (QF). The values recommended for use i many cases of radiological protection work are:

Kind of Radiation	Quality Facto.
X-rays, gamma rays, electrons and beta rays of maximum energy greater than 30 KeV	1·0
Beta rays and electrons of maximum energy not greater than 30 KeV	1·7
Thermal neutrons	3·0
Fast neutrons and protons up to 10 MeV	10
Naturally occurring alpha particles	Compare with 0·1 μ CiRa, otherwise 10
Heavy recoil nuclei	20

It follows that for small doses of X and γ rays and β rays of maximui energy greater than 30 KeV, an exposure of 1 r gives a dose of 1 rad whic is equal to 1 rem. There are exceptions to these values, for example whe the lens of the eye is concerned, the QF for fast neutrons is taken as 30 in stead of 10. These figures are quoted to illustrate the numerical variatio of the quality factor according to the type of radiation.

Curie (Ci)—the Unit of Radioactivity

The unit of radioactivity is the curie (Ci) and 1 curie = $3·7 \times 10^1$ atomic disintegrations per second. The curie was originally defined a the radioactivity of 1 gram of radium. Until 1962 the factor used to conver rads to rems was termed the RBE—the relative biological effectiveness this term presented a number of problems for use in the field of radiatio protection and the term RBE is now used in radiobiology only (ICR. publication 6, 1964).

International Commission on Radiological Protection

All procedures aimed at protecting the individual against radiatio injury embody as a principle some means of controlling the dose to th individual to a predetermined maximum permissible quantity. Th definition of a maximum permissible dose (MPD) is, therefore, of funda mental importance. This is done on an international basis by a voluntar organization, the International Commission on Radiological Protectio (ICRP). The ICRP was formed in 1928 under the auspices of the Secon International Congress of Radiology then meeting in Stockholm. Th formation of an international protection committee was discussed at th First Congress in London in 1925 by the British X-ray and Radiu Protection Committee. During the Second Congress the British Com mittee submitted proposals for establishing an international protectio committee and this was done. The committee was named the Internationa

-ray and Radium Protection hairman from 1928 to 1937 was ᴊational Physical Laboratory. It ᴉight be remarked, with some ᴉterest in view of later events, that t the time of its formation the roblem of radiation protection was ᴏt considered to be as important ᴉr as serious as that of radiation nits. The Committee held its ᴉitial meeting in 1928 for the urpose of adopting some interim rotection regulations. Until that ᴉme, the only recommendations ᴉere those prepared a few years ᴉarlier by the British Committee. ᴉhe first recommendations of the ᴉnternational Committee were very ᴉimilar to these early British pro- ᴏsals, and until 1950 its recom- ᴉendations were patterned around ᴉem.

Committee (Taylor, 1958). The Dr. G. W. Kaye, then of the

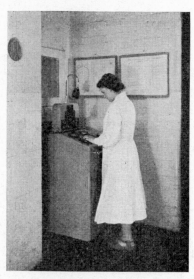

Fɪɢ. 348.—Operator protected from X-irradiation by Leaded Glass and Interlocking Barium Bricks
(*By courtesy of Kodak, Ltd.*)

ᴊaximum Permissible Dose

The first MPD was defined as ᴉ1 erythema dose per year (that is ᴉbout 100 r/year). The roentgen was adopted as the unit of dose in 1928 ᴉnd the maximum permissible dose defined as 0·2 r/day in 1934 (that is ᴉbout 80 r/year). In 1950 the MPD for external radiation was reduced to ᴉ·3 r/week (that is 15 r/year) and adopted the values recommended by the ᴉnited States National Commission on Radiological Protection (NCRP) ᴏr internally deposited radionuclides. The NCRP had been very active ᴉince 1935 and had recommended a reduction in the MPD in 1935 and ᴉgain in 1947. It also considered the problem of the genetic effects of ᴉadiation in 1935 and again in 1947. The present MPD recommended by ᴉCRP (ICRP 9, 1966) for external radiation of the whole body is 5 rems ᴉer annum for persons occupationally exposed to ionizing radiation. It ᴉecommends that the maximum dose in any one quarter of a year should ᴉot exceed half the annual dose (that is 2·5 rems). The maximum per- ᴉissible doses in one year as recommended by ICRP, both for whole ᴉody radiation and for parts of the body, are as follows:

Gonads and red bone-marrow (and, in the case of uniform irradiation, the whole body)	5 rems
Skin; thyroid; bone	30 rems
Hands and forearms; feet and ankles	75 rems
All other organs	15 rems

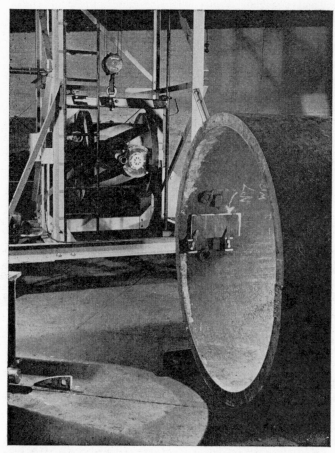

Fig. 349.—Taking an X-ray of a longitudinal boiler seam using a multi-curie cobalt-60 source. The cassette is held in position by magnetic clamps on the inside of the drum. Welds in steel plate up to $4\frac{1}{2}''$ in thickness require the utilization of the high energy gamma emissions of cobalt-60 to obtain satisfactory radiographs.

(*Reproduced by courtesy of Mr. B. G. Litting from* X Ray Focus, *published by Ilford, Ltd.*)

These are maximum recommended doses for irradiation from controlled sources. It may sometimes be necessary to provide flexibility for the control of persons receiving small accidental additional doses involving exposure of the whole body, where the gonads and the red bone-marrow are the critical organs. In such cases it will be justifiable to permit the quarterly quota to be repeated in each quarter of the year, provided that the total dose accumulated at any age over 18 years does not exceed $5(N-18)$, where N is the age in years. This would allow for an accumulation of a dose of 5 rems per annum for each year of work beginning at the

ge of 18 years, but prevents the exposure of young workers from exceed-
ng the specified MPD.

rotection of Women of Reproductive Age

It is also recommended that the employment of women of reproductive
ige should be limited to conditions where the dose to the abdomen does
ot exceed 1·3 rems in a quarter, corresponding to a maximum of 5 rems
er annum delivered at an even rate. Under these conditions the dose to
n embryo during the critical first two months of organogenesis would
ot exceed 1 rem. For pregnant women it is recommended that the dose
f radiation to the abdomen and hence to the fœtus should not exceed
 rem from the time the pregnancy is diagnosed. In addition to irradiation
rom an external source, radionuclides absorbed into the body may be
etained and concentrated in specific organs where they give rise to intense
ocal irradiation of these organs. For example, radioactive iodine is retained
n the thyroid gland; radium, strontium and the transuranic elements,
otably plutonium, are concentrated in bone. The ICRP has listed the
naximum permissible body burden (MPBB) of all radionuclides and also
he maximum permissible concentration (MPC) of these nuclides in air
nd water; for example, for Radium 226 the MPBB is 0·1 μCi, for Pluton-
um 239 the MPBB is 0·04 μCi, for Strontium 90 the MPBB is 2 μCi. In all
hese examples the critical organ is bone (ICRP 2, 1959). The maximum
ermissible dose to the individual includes the sum of doses from both
xternal and internal radiation.

*ase 36. Pioneer X-ray technician—carcinoma of skin of hands—multiple
amputations—death from carcinomatosis with involvement of the mediastinum.*

E. H. H., a man aged 67. 1898: pioneer X-ray worker at the London
Hospital. 1899: X-ray dermatitis with thickening and brown discoloration of the finger-nails and paronychia. There was a great deal of pain
and many operations were performed for removal of the nails and scraping of the matrices. 1902: multiple papillomata; histological sections
showed no malignant changes. 1903: at the time for the opening of the
present London Hospital out-patient building a couch was installed (fig.
342) and fitted with two X-ray bulbs without protection for the workers
(figs. 343, 344). This couch was used for hours together, looking for needles in the hand and coins in the œsophagus. Sometimes
more than one case would be operated upon in the same day under
screening. 1906: squamous carcinoma on dorsum of left hand at
base of ring finger (fig. 340). 1907: squamous carcinomata, some of
them with ulceration, on four digits. No enlargement of glands.
Many of these carcinomata were locally excised and skin grafts
used to cover the wounds. 1908: retired from X-ray work, having
had twelve operations at which six digits were amputated. 1909:
amputation through left forearm and removal of left axillary glands.
No secondary deposits were found in the glands. 1921: removal of

three further digits from right hand, leaving only the thumb. 193〈
carcinomatous ulcer, 2 by 1 centimetres, on dorsum of right hand ov〈
first metacarpal; it increased in size in spite of radium treatmen〈
Amputation through lower third of right forearm; histological se〈
tions showed squamous-celled and horny carcinoma of the skin of th〈
ulnar side of the hand. A small squamous-celled carcinoma, 1 cent〈
metre diameter, was excised from the skin over the cricoid cartilag〈
1942: death from carcinomatosis with involvement of the mediastinun〈

(b) Injuries from Radioactive Substances

Radium was isolated by the Curies in 1898 (fig. 350). Its local effec〈
on the skin and subcutaneous tissues soon claimed attention. The la〈
effects of internally deposited radi〈
active materials in man were studi〈
from 1925 onwards, especially 〈
Martland. This aspect of the su〈
ject was reviewed by Aub, Evan〈
Hempelmann and Martland in 195〈

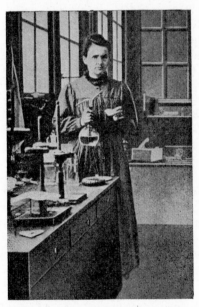

Radium Dermatitis

Dermatitis due to the effects 〈
radium was first reported in Octob〈
1900 by Walkoff. In December 〈
the same year Giesel published 〈
account of the skin lesion caused 〈
exposing his arm for two hours t〈
celluloid capsule containing radiu〈
bromide. In the following ye〈
Henri Becquerel, the discoverer 〈
radioactivity, and Pierre Cur〈
described their own experience〈
Becquerel had carried an i〈
sufficiently protected tube of radiu〈
salts in his waistcoat pocket for s〈
hours; after a week the skin becan〈
red and eleven days later it ulcerate〈

Fig. 350.—Marie Curie in her Laboratory at the Sorbonne

Curie repeated Giesel's experiment, keeping radium chloride in conta〈
with his skin for ten hours, and in three weeks' time an ulcer appeare〈
Dermatitis has since been reported in a number of persons engaged 〈
making radium preparations and less often in medical men.

Deaths from Aplastic Anæmia

In 1921 Mottram commented that even though there were many mo〈
X-ray workers than radium workers, the gamma rays of radium appear〈
to have a greater tendency than X-rays to cause aplastic anæmia and th〈
this impression received support from the experimental evidence that t〈
penetrative gamma rays of radium reached the bone marrow more readi〈

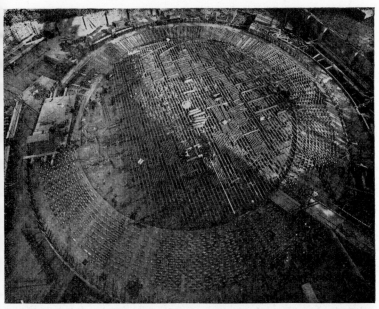

Fig 351.—Pre-stressed concrete pressure vessel under construction at Oldbury Nuclear Power Station. The concrete ring shows the beginning of the construction of the 15ft. thick concrete walls of the pressure vessel. The ring of stubs standing out at an angle from the surface of the concrete are the ducts through which cables will later be threaded to pre-stress the vessel. Some idea of the depth of biological shielding can be gained from the comparative size of the man on the platform to the left.

(*By courtesy of the Central Electricity Generating Board*)

han do X-rays. Examination of the workers in the London Radium Institute where radium applicators are prepared and tested, and also of hospital attendants who apply them, revealed a low white-cell count in over half (Mottram and Clarke, 1920). In the workers definitely exposed to radium the red-cell count was low as compared with employees not so exposed. Three fatal cases of aplastic anæmia occurred in this Institute, one in a nurse and two in laboratory assistants. At that time this anæmia was sometimes referred to as *anæmia radiotoxica*.

Leukæmia following Exposure to Radium

Weil and Lacassagne (1925) reported the cases of two chemical engineers working with radium and thorium-X. One of them died of aplastic anæmia and the other, although exposed to the same form of radiation, died of typical myeloid leukæmia. In 1930 Rolleston pointed out that attractive as it might be to suppose that small doses of X-rays or radium exert a stimulating action on the bone marrow, this idea was speculative and it was safer to be content with the view that the occurrence of leukæmia in workers with radium and X-rays was a coincidence. Nevertheless Marie Curie died of leukæmia and so did her daughter. Irène Joliot-Curie died in

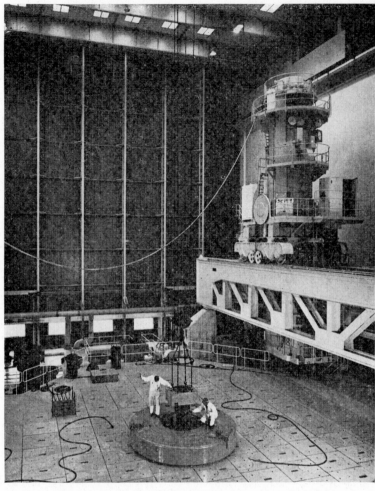

FIG. 352.—Reactor No. 2 at Bradwell Nuclear Power Station showing the cap area of the graphite pile. The plant operators are fixing the chute headbox on the standpipe prior to bringing the charging machine (top right) into position for refuelling.

(*By courtesy of the Central Electricity Generating Board*)

1956 fifteen years after a laboratory accident in which a capsule of polonium exploded on her bench.

Exposure Hazards

Though medical practice is now almost safe so far as X-irradiation concerned, matters are very different in the case of radium. There is n doubt that many people in Great Britain, and in other countries too, are affected by handling radium, mostly by the gamma rays. Their penetratin

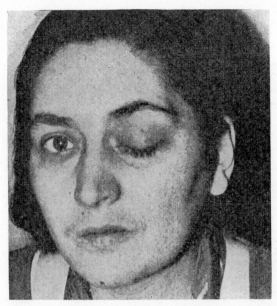

FIG. 353.—Dial Painter who died of Carcinoma of the
Paranasal Sinuses 14 years after leaving Dial Painting
(*By courtesy of Professor J. C. Aub and the Williams and Wilkins
Co., Baltimore*)

power is so great that it is not practicable to protect completely those who
handle radium. The British X-ray and Radium Protection Committee has
had investigations made in the radium centres throughout Great Britain
from 1930 onwards, and it has not been an uncommon thing to find one or
more of the radium personnel showing signs of too much radiation. In the
case of people who carry radium about, the weight of lead they can bear to
carry only partly protects them. The surgeon handling radium is also ill-
protected. In the case of a man using 120 milligrams of radium for
treatment of carcinoma of the cervix uteri, repeated three times, protection
is very difficult, as each time he has to handle the radium closely and carefully (Russ, 1935).

The Painting of Luminous Dials

The first use of radium salts in industry was for the manufacture of
luminous paint to apply to the figures of clocks and watches and to
certain important parts of the machinery of aeroplanes. This became
known as the *luminizing industry*. An interesting but rare form of industrial
risk from the swallowing of radioactive substances in this work was found
to occur at two factories, one in New Jersey and the other in Connecticut
(Flinn, 1927). Twenty deaths occurred: sixteen of girls employed in
painting luminous dials and four of chemists or physicists. In the New
Jersey works forty-eight cases, of which eighteen were fatal, occurred

among some 800 workers who were employed there from 1917 to 1924. Most of the cases occurred from four to seven years after the girls had left the works. The ill effects included severe anæmia, sometimes aplastic in

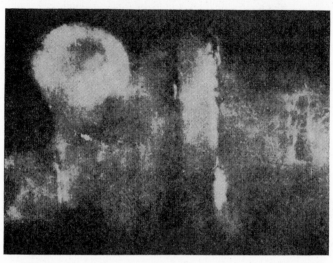

Fig. 354.—Auto-radiograph of the Head and Shaft of the Humerus in a Dial Painter who had used Mesothorium Paint and had pointed the Brush with the Lips. The picture was obtained by placing the Dried Bones on a Photographic Film which was kept in the dark for seven days

type, necrosis of the jaw, spontaneous fracture and sarcoma of bone. The results of an injury into this occupation in the United States of America were summarized by Martland in 1931.

Paints containing Radium 226, Mesothorium and Radiothorium

Paints consisting of crystalline phosphorescent zinc sulphide rendered permanently luminous by the addition of a very small proportion of insoluble sulphates of radium, mesothorium and radiothorium came into use about 1908. The girls affected introduced the paint into their mouths through the habit of pointing the brush between their lips, and swallowed it for periods of from four or more years between 1916 and 1923 (fig. 355). The insoluble radioactive materials became deposited in the body to such an extent that even during life radioactive emanations could be detected in the expired air. After death the bones were found to be the main tissue in which the materials had accumulated. The anæmia resulted from the continuous bombardment of the hæmatogenous marrow by alpha particles, and it is emphasized that these changes were quite different from those due to external irradiation with beta and gamma rays only. The necrosis of the jaw is similar to that produced by phosphorus and is attributed to infection supervening upon changes in the bones.

utoradiographs of Bones and Teeth

Radioactivity in the bones and eth could be demonstrated by utophotography. Dental films in ark-paper envelopes when rapped to the bones showed hotographic impressions in from ourteen to thirty days. The outnes of metal clips and coins placed etween the bone and the surface f the film were clearly visible. hese autoradiographs were produced by beta and gamma rays oming from deposits in the bones, ie alpha rays being screened and ltered out by the paper covering ie dental film. The bones when laced directly on photographic lates or films produced photoraphic impressions in as short a eriod as three days. After seven lays' exposure the irregular disribution of the radioactive deposits ould be plainly ascertained (fig.

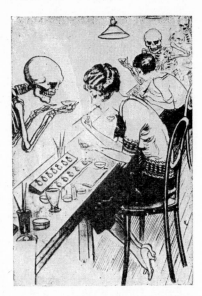

FIG. 355.—Cartoon in a New York Newspaper showing the Figure of Death holding a Dish of Mesothorium Paint which the Dial Painter applies to the Watch Face, meanwhile pointing the Brush with her Lips

54). Bones incinerated to a white ash and given thirty days in which to egain their equilibrium, when placed on photographic films produced hotographic impressions in from two to three days' exposure (Martland nd Humphries, 1929).

Death of a Research Chemist

Dr. S. A. von Sochocky, research chemist and technical director of the ompany in which the New Jersey cases occurred, died of aplastic anæmia n 1928 (Martland, 1929). The luminous paint used by the girls in the actory was made according to a formula which he had worked out. From 913 to 1921 he personally extracted about 30 grams of radium from the re and was exposed continually to heavy penetrative radiation. He was xposed also to the inhalation of radioactive dust in the crystallizing aboratory and on four occasions to explosions of tubes containing high oncentrations of radium and mesothorium. He had an extensive radium lermatitis of the fingers of both hands and later developed necrosis of the aw with buccal lesions. In 1925 he devised methods of measuring the mounts of radioactivity in the bones at necropsy. At this time he tested is own expired air and found larger amounts of emanation than in any of he factory girls examined. He thus realized the hopelessness of his own ondition.

Treatment by repeated Blood Transfusion

He was in a fair state of health and able to do his work until August 1928, when he became weak, pale and dyspnœic. Blood examination showed red cells 1,720,000 per cubic millimetre, hæmoglobin 28 per cent, white cells 4,000 per cubic millimetre, with polymorphs 48 per cent. Later the white-cell count dropped below 2,000 with scarcely any granular cells. The blood platelets dropped to less than 40,000 per cubic millimetre. Ultimately he was kept alive by thirteen blood transfusions varying from 450 to 900 cubic centimetres and given every fourth day. Except for a fine purpuric eruption over the extremities which appeared in crops, there was no bleeding until the last. He died with hæmoptysis, hæmaturia, retinal hæmorrhages and terminal bronchopneumonia. Necropsy showed radioactive deposits in the lungs, the portal of entry having evidently been the respiratory tract.

Radiation Osteitis and Sarcoma of Bone

In certain cases anæmia and necrosis of the jaw did not occur, but after a number of years generalized changes in the bones developed with deformities and sometimes spontaneous fracture, a condition known as radiation osteitis. In addition to the thirteen deaths from intractable anæmia and two from necrosis of the jaw, one girl died in 1924 from a sarcoma of the femur and another girl in 1927 from a sarcoma of the scapula. The painting of dials was prohibited in 1924. Since no further cases of anæmia had developed by 1929, there seemed reason to hope that the danger was over. Nevertheless, in the following two years three more deaths occurred from osteogenic sarcoma. By 1952 there had been fourteen deaths from sarcoma of bone, which had appeared on an average twenty-three years after cessation of exposure to the luminous paint. In many cases the patients were still excreting radium ten or twenty years after they had ceased to absorb it. Nearly all those who stored more than 0·7 micrograms of radium suffered from bone disease. Radiation osteitis had crippled two patients by causing repeated spontaneous fractures of both femora (Aub and others, 1952).

Carcinoma of the Mastoid and Paranasal Sinuses

In three cases death occurred from carcinoma of the paranasal sinuses fourteen, thirty-three and thirty-four years respectively after exposure. All showed intractable facial neuralgia with anæsthesia dolorosa. In one case ptosis of the left eyelid was gradually followed by total ophthalmoplegia (fig. 353). Although invasion of the base of the skull and the cranial cavity occurred in all cases, none had either involvement of regional lymphatic glands or visceral metastases. In one of the cases necropsy showed an epidural abscess and in the second an abscess of the left temporal lobe. In none of these cases was it possible to determine the exact origin of the original tumour because of the extensive destruction of the base of the skull emporal bone and surrounding tissues (Aub and others, 1952). The pithelium of the mastoid air cells may be affected in the same way. Thus Iasterlik and others (1964) described seven cases, most of them lumin-zers, who had carcinomas of the mastoid air cells. In none of these patients vas there a previous history of chronic middle ear disease. It is likely that nese tumours of the sinuses of the skull arise at these sites because of the nique anatomical relationship of a thin layer of epithelial and connective ssue in close relation to bone. The total thickness of the epithelium and onnective tissue structures at these sites is only about 50 to 100 microns. 'he radioactive decay of radium gives rise to energetic alpha and beta articles; these alpha particles have a mean path in bone of about 50 iicrons, the beta particles have an even longer path. In the mastoids and aranasal sinuses the epithelium is continually irradiated by the intensely nizing alpha and beta particles in the underlying bone: in addition, idon, the first decay product, which is also an alpha particle emitter, aving the chemical properties of a noble gas, can diffuse into the air ells and by direct contact with the epithelium give rise to intense radiation.

lutonium 239 and Radium 226 the Deadliest Poisons Known

It is interesting that the watch-dial industry has revealed a carcinogenic gent hitherto unknown—namely, continuous bombardment by the alpha article. This agent is quite different from all other known carcinogenic gents, and although its action is continuous, there is the usual prolonged eriod before malignancy manifests itself. The alpha particle can be held esponsible because over 92 per cent of the radiation coming from the ones is alpha, and only 8 per cent

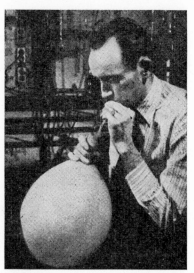

eta and gamma. The total amount f radioactive material in the de-osit necessary to produce fatal esults is extremely small; 0·01 iilligram distributed over the vhole skeleton is sufficient to pro-uce death years after it has been igested. We know that plutonium 39 is the most deadly poison ever olated. It is three times as toxic as idium. Before the discovery of nese two substances tetanus toxin eld the record with a lethal dose f 0·22 milligram.

one-seeking Isotopes

The luminizing industry has nown us how radium 226 and meso-norium become concentrated in one if they enter the body. Iamilton (1947) has pointed out

FIG. 356.—Method of sampling ex-haled air for radon in a man exposed to radium

D.O.—30*

that a large number of radioactive products of uranium fission are
also selectively retained in the skeleton. Thus uranium, thorium
plutonium 239 and the isotopes of yttrium are bone-seeking (Vaughan
and Tutt, 1953), and the isotopes of strontium are, *par excellence*
producers of bone tumours (Brues, 1949). An X-ray of the skull of a dial
painter, a woman aged 74, taken 40 years after exposure to the luminous
paint had ceased is reproduced as Plate VI. The calvaria shows areas of
bone resorption (Hasterlik and Finkel, 1965). The body burden of radium
in 1962 was 1·44 μCi. Since some of these elements have extremely long
half-lives and are excreted very slowly, they will irradiate both bone and
bone marrow continuously for many years.

Effect of Alpha Particles

The alpha particles, consisting of the nuclei of helium atoms, are shot
out with great force, travel at a high speed and possess an enormous
momentum on account of their mass which is much greater than that of
beta rays. They collide with other atoms with powerful impact, disrupting
them and producing molecular chemical changes. Thus alpha particles
decompose water into hydrogen, oxygen and hydrogen peroxide, and hydrochloric acid into hydrogen and chlorine, expending locally over one
thousand times as much energy as beta rays and acting in a manner corre-
spondingly more destructive of human tissues.

Deadly Hazard of pointing the Brush with the Lips

It is obvious that ingestion or inhalation of radioactive materials in
industry is highly dangerous and that all occupations involving the handling of such substances should be strictly controlled and supervised. Outside New Jersey and Connecticut, the practice of pointing the brush with
the lips is unknown. The International Labour Office found by inquiry
from watch factories in Switzerland, France, Germany, Austria, Britain
and Belgium that the painting in those countries is done with a style
which is not sucked, and that no ill effects have been observed. In Great
Britain the number of workers in this trade in 1925 was less than ten. The
paint contained 0·0375 milligram of radium bromide per gram of zinc
sulphide. Out of seven British women engaged in luminous painting for
periods of one to ten years, two showed a relative diminution in the
number of polymorphonuclear leucocytes and one showed leucopenia with
21 per cent of polymorphonuclear leucocytes (Legge, 1925).

Protective Measures in the Luminizing Industry

When the luminizing industry rapidly expanded during the Second
World War, special preventive measures were introduced to protect the
workers in Great Britain and the United States of America. Operatives
called luminizers, apply luminous paint containing 70 micrograms of
radioactive substance per gram to aeroplane or watch dials, compasses
gun sights and electrical instruments. The potential hazards in this occu-

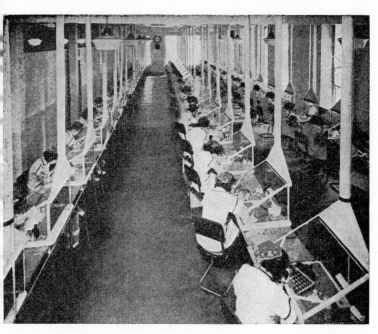

FIG. 357.—Radium dial-painting room where the hands and figures of instruments were luminized. The bench of each worker was provided with a glass cabinet connected to a system of exhaust ventilation. Stylets were used instead of brushes so that nothing could be conveyed to the mouth
(Evans, R. D. (1933), Journ. industr. Hyg., 25, 253)

ation are irradiation by alpha particles and beta and gamma rays, inalation of emanations of radon from the luminous compound, and inalation or ingestion of radioactive dust. A glass screen placed between the luminizer and the work protected operatives from external irradiation (fig. 57), and the risk of inhalation was reduced to a minimum by adequate exaust ventilation. The worker wore a rubber apron and protective gown. The use of brushes to apply the luminous paint was prohibited, and pens or olid applicators were used. Thus the risk of ingestion from pointing the rush with the lips according to the habit of the New Jersey and Connecticut victims was eliminated. Frequent washing of the hands was necessary to remove contaminating powder. Inhalation of radioactive dust was ontrolled as far as possible by daily washing of walls and benches, but ltra-violet illumination frequently revealed fine particles of luminous ust which came from small splashes of paint on the benches. Workers ad to wear beta- and gamma-ray sensitive photographic films, and tests f the expired air for radon were repeatedly made. After the Second Vorld War luminizing was carried out in dry boxes (fig. 358). In addition ecords have to be kept for a minimum period of 30 years after cessation f employment.

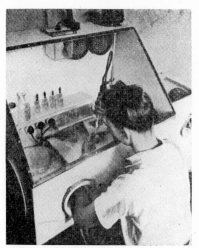

FIG. 358.—Dry Box in use to protect a worker from Radioactive Substances. The operator, working with his Hands in Rubber Gloves let into the Walls of the Dry Box is measuring a Minute Quantity of Active Solution by means of a Micro-pipette
(*By courtesy AERE, Harwell*)

Alternatives to Radium 226 as Luminizing Substance

Ever since the first reports of the tragic consequences which befell the early luminizers there has been continuing apprehension about the effects on workers of using paint containing Radium 226 for luminizing watches, clocks and instrument dials. In addition, in 1960 the Medical Research Council pointed out the potential somatic and genetic effects of the penetrating γ-rays of radium on members of the general public. For this reason alternative materials have been tried in which radium has been replaced by radio nuclides which are not gamma emitters. It was suggested that Strontium 90 should be used, but this was unacceptable because the high specific activity which would be necessary to give adequate luminizing properties in the paint meant that appreciable doses would be delivered by the energetic β radiation. In addition Sr 90 was considered too hazardous a material to handle in factories; this decision was taken too late to prevent a number of Swiss and Czechoslovakian luminizers from receiving appreciable body burdens of Sr 90 (Müller and others, 1961). The second alternative suggested was tritium incorporated in a chemically inert molecule such as polystyrene. It was hoped that the very low energies of the β radiation would cause no hazard to the public and, since tritium is chemically inert, it was thought it would not present an occupational hazard. Unfortunately, during the manufacturing process tritiated water is formed and this is readily metabolized and mixes with the body water. More recently promethium 137 has been suggested as a further alternative since it is a low energy β emitter and is poorly absorbed from the gut. Vennart (1967) reported the experience gained in the United Kingdom of monitoring luminizers handling radium paint and tritiated paint and also considered the possible problems arising from the use of promethium 147. Vennart enumerates three principles when handling unsealed radioactive materials stressing the necessity: (i) to maintain a high standard of containment of the material; (ii) to measure environmental contamination to demonstrate that the containment is efficient (this requires continuous monitoring), and (iii) to estimate the radiation doses received by personnel either from external or internal radiation. Whereas tritium and promethium 147 are far less hazardous materials than radium, it is necessary

) monitor the urine and fæces of workers in the former, whereas radon
reath measurements and total body γ spectrometry can be used in the
atter. Biological monitoring is never popular with workmen and it has
een demonstrated that radium luminizing can be effectively controlled.
t would appear, therefore, that the alternatives to radium which are
vailable at the present time may pose new problems unless their intro-
uction is accompanied by plans for the protection of the workers.

Routine Clinical and Blood Examination

As a result of the Statutory Order in Council (1942) which brought
he occupation of luminizing under the medical supervision of the Factory
)epartment, Browning (1949) made routine clinical and blood examinations
f luminizers at regular intervals and continued to do so up to four years
fter exposure had ceased. She found no clinical abnormality and no
vidence of depression of hæmopoiesis. There was, in fact, stimulation of
vhite-blood cell formation resulting in a high normal total white-cell
ount, relative lymphocytosis and the presence of abnormal cells. These
vere apparently young forms of the large monocyte, and stimulation of the
ells of the reticulo-endothelial sytem would explain the abnormal find-
ıgs. She found that the effects on the blood had completely disappeared
ı from one to four years after exposure. Of 470 exposed persons examined
·y Vennart and others (1964) none of the 227 employed exclusively as
ɪminizers since 1942 was found with more than half the maximum
·ermissible body burden (MPBB) of radium.

Cancer of the Lung and Radiation Fibrosis

Carcinoma of the lung in laboratory workers handling radioactive sub-
tances is recorded (see p. 817). Pulmonary fibrosis causing death also
ccurs (Hueper, 1942). This develops after much shorter exposure than is
ɪsual in the case of neoplastic change. A chemist, who had been working
or two years in a plant where radium was prepared, noticed difficulty in
·reathing. There were no changes in the X-ray appearances of the lungs at
his time, but nodular shadows developed within two years and the man
lied shortly afterwards. Necropsy showed marked fibrosis of the lungs. A
voman working in the same plant for five years died two years later from
he same cause (Teleky, 1937).

Origin of the Welsbach Gas Mantle

In 1818 Berzelius discovered a new earth which he named thoria, after
he Scandinavian god Thor. The principal source of thorium is monazite,
vhich, although essentially a cerium lanthanum phosphate, always contains
horium. In 1880 Dr. Carl Auer, Baron von Welsbach, began to work in
'ienna on the rare earth elements. His researches were in chemistry and
vere considered ultra-academic. However, in using spectrum analysis, he
lipped strips of cotton into solutions of rare earth compounds and found
hat the Bunsen flame burned away the cotton and left behind the oxides of

the rare earths, in the form of a skeleton of the cotton thread keeping it
exact shape and remaining coherent instead of falling to powder. This wa
the origin of the Welsbach gas mantle which was patented in 1884.

Health Record of Gas-mantle Makers

In 1891 Auer discovered that the light emitted by an incandescent ga
mantle of thorium dioxide increases to a maximum when nine parts pe
thousand of cerium dioxide are added. Today traces of aluminium and beryl
lium salts are added for toughening purposes. Mantles are made b
weaving a hose in ramie fibre or artificial silk and soaking this hose in
solution of thorium and cerium nitrates. The mantle is then dried, th
fibre is burnt away in a flame and the skeleton of mixed oxides remaining i
dipped in collodion to make it strong enough for packing. Marie Curi
discovered in 1898 that thorium has feeble radioactive properties. It emit
alpha particles, and mesothorium emits beta and gamma rays. A certai
number of chemists, technicians and workmen exposed to thorium com
pounds for periods of up to forty years in the gas-mantle industry have bee
examined and found to be healthy men with normal blood counts, an
with normal bones as seen in X-rays, neither did their exhaled breat
contain radioactive substances. There is certainly a case for a long-tern
follow-up of all the workers in this industry, and until this has bee
carried out we cannot be certain that commercial thorium compounds ar
harmless.

Dangers from the Use of Thorotrast

Thorotrast is a colloidal suspension of 232 thorium dioxide. Its us
for diagnostic or other purposes was largely discontinued in 1947 follow
ing a report of its carcinogenic properties (MacMahon and others, 1947)
Prior to that date it had been employed for 17 years in hepatolienography
retrograde pyelography and arteriography; its elimination from the bod
is insignificant. In the diagnostic procedures mentioned it may be in
definitely retained in the liver, renal pelvis or subarachnoid space. Betwee
1930 and 1952 in Portugal, with a population of about 8 million, 2,37
individuals are known to have received thorotrast. In a follow-up of thes
patients Horta and others (1965) have been able to trace 1,107 of whon
699 had died. Eighty-one had granulomata at the injection site and in 8 o
these it was the cause of death. Cirrhosis of the liver occurred in 42 patient
and in 17 this was fatal. Eight patients died of leukæmia and 6 of aplasti
anæmia. Twenty-two patients died of hepatic insufficiency from a specia
primary sarcoma of the liver, hæmangioendothelioma. This tumour is vir
tually thorotrast-specific. The latent periods between thorotrast adminis
tration and disease onset for these conditions varied from 2 years to 2
years with a mean of 17 years. In an investigation of 35 patients who ha
received intra-arterial thorotrast 11 or more years previously, Langland
and Williamson (1967) reported the presence of Howell-Jolly bodies in th
red cells of the peripheral blood in 34 of these patients. Since none of then

ad undergone splenectomy and in all other respects the blood was normal,
t was suggested that these rare peripheral blood changes were due to
progressive loss of splenic function due to the effect of radiation. Chromosome aberrations in the peripheral blood were found by Fischer and others
1966) in 19 out of 20 patients given thorotrast 19 to 27 years previously.
Since the thorotrast method has been in general use for little more than
twenty years, further deaths will yet occur (Berenbaum and Birch, 1953).
Clearly its use as a radiological contrast medium stands utterly condemned.

(c) Injuries from Fission Products

The splitting of the nucleus of uranium 235 by bombardment with
neutrons was reported in 1939. The nucleus splits by the process known
as nuclear fission. The reaction is accompanied by the release of an enormous amount of energy, and the production of two radioactive fragments
fission products, from each atom undergoing fission. It is apparent that
the sudden release of energy of this nature and magnitude is highly
dangerous to life. Many atomic bombs have been exploded; large groups
of people are concerned with the processing of intensely radioactive
materials; cyclotrons and other instruments for the production of sub-
atomic particles with high energy are increasing in size and number, and
the use of radioactive elements for diagnostic, therapeutic and scientific
purposes has become widespread.

Historical Summary

In 1934 Curie and Joliot found that certain atoms showed artificial
radioactivity after bombardment with alpha particles (helium nuclei)
emitted by polonium, and following this discovery a wide range of new
radioactive isotopes has been obtained by bombarding stable nuclei with
certain fundamental particles, particularly deuterons and neutrons. These
particles have been produced by the cyclotron or the uranium pile. In the
cyclotron, which was developed by E. O. Lawrence in California, deuterons
and other charged particles can be given enormous velocities. The particles are subjected to a moderate voltage and guided round in a spiral path
by a strong magnetic field. The voltage is altered in such a way that the
particles are accelerated each time they make one half-circle and they move
with higher velocities in circles of increasing radius. When they reach the
outer edge of the apparatus they are deflected by an electric field to form
an emergent beam.

A Self-sustaining Chain Reaction

Neutrons may be obtained by bombarding beryllium or lithium with
fast deuterons from the cyclotron. Neutrons from the uranium pile are
formed in the fission reaction discovered by Hahn and Strassman in 1939.
The rare isotope of uranium U 235 is split on absorption of a slow neutron
into nuclei. At each fission a number of fast neutrons are liberated and, if

the mass of fissile material is great enough to ensure that more than one of these neutrons produces further fission, a self-sustaining chain reaction is initiated. In the uranium pile which was put into operation for the first time at the University of Chicago in 1942 uranium is embedded in graphite to slow down the neutrons, and the reaction is controlled by cadmium rods by which neutrons are strongly absorbed. When neutrons are absorbed by Uranium 238, reactions occur which lead to the formation of neptunium and plutonium. Plutonium 239 is three times as toxic as radium. It undergoes fission in a fashion similar to Uranium 235.

Effects of Atomic Bombs

The effects of massive doses of radiation in man were first seen on a large scale in 1945 when atomic bombs were dropped on Hiroshima and Nagasaki and some 25,000 people died. The atomic bomb generated vast amounts of heat and ionizing radiation within about one second. People within 500 metres of the explosion appeared to have been instantly burned to death. At much greater distances those in the open received severe flash burns, although quite thin layers of clothing were able to afford considerable protection. Naturally the blast effects were the most devastating and destructive of life and property. Disruption of electric and gas systems led to death from fire and to burns of all degrees of severity (Le Roy, 1947). People who died from radiation injury were troubled by nausea and vomiting on the day of the bombing. Those receiving doses greater than 600 r had initial radiation sickness rapidly followed by prostration and intractable diarrhœa and they died within ten days. If the dose was somewhat smaller the initial vomiting was followed by a period free from clinical symptoms, but after two or three weeks the patients became seriously ill and about half of them subsequently died. Diarrhœa was one of the earliest symptoms, and epilation and purpura preceded death. In those who lived more than two weeks, sepsis was a common feature (Oughterson and others, 1951).

Criticality Accidents

Within twelve months of the bombing of Hiroshima and Nagasaki two criticality accidents had occurred at the Los Alamos Scientific Laboratory in the USA. As a result of these accidents, ten men were exposed to bursts of penetrating ionizing radiation. Two died as a result, and clinically demonstrable abnormalities were found in the remainder. The term *critical mass* or *critical assembly* refers to a situation when there is just sufficient fissionable material present and in the correct configuration for a chain reaction to be maintained. A criticality accident is, therefore, one in which sufficient quantities of fissionable material come together accidentally, resulting in a significant emission of neutrons and ionizing radiation. Such a release may last for very brief time intervals or if the assembly is only just critical, several successive bursts of radiation may ɔccur. A nuclear explosion is one in which *supercritical* masses of fission-able material are brought together deliberately and in a predetermined configuration in order to give an extremely rapid release of energy. Since 1945 there has been a number of incidents at atomic energy establishments where persons have been exposed to massive doses of ionizing radiation. In all but one of these major radiation accidents, the exposure was due to a criticality accident.

The Y12 Accident at Oakridge

The accident at the Oakridge National Laboratory, Tennessee, in June 1958 occurred when an enriched uranium solution, that is, natural uranium in which the proportion of ^{235}U had been artificially increased, accidentally entered a large metal container producing a critical geometry. Eight workers in the neighbourhood were exposed for less than one minute; five of these men received a dose in excess of 200 rads. The area of the laboratory in which this accident occurred was called the Y12 plant and this incident is frequently referred to as the Y12 accident. In October 1958 at Vinca, Jugoslavia, an unshielded experimental nuclear reactor consisting of rods of natural uranium immersed in a moderator of heavy water went out of control when the quantity of heavy water present became suddenly increased. The reaction was not immediately detected and six persons present were exposed for several minutes, receiving a dose of mixed gamma and neutron radiation in excess of 300 rads (Pendic, 1961).

The Third Los Alamos Accident

The third Los Alamos criticality accident in December 1958 is of particular interest because of the extremely high dose of radiation received by one man who died within 34 hours of the incident (Shipman, 1961). In March 1960 nine men were exposed to high doses of X-rays from an unshielded klystron tube at a military establishment in Lockport. This is the one incident giving rise to the acute radiation syndrome which was not due to a criticality accident. In December 1965 a research worker at the Centre for Nuclear Studies at Mol in Belgium received a massive dose of whole body radiation as a result of working near to a critical assembly. This latter case is referred to in detail below. In all criticality accidents the radiation is a complex combination of neutrons and gamma rays of many different energies. Whilst it is possible to reproduce and analyse the type of radiation produced, it is very difficult to determine precisely the amount of radiation absorbed by the patients. The difficulties are exemplified by the different results of the studies and assessments of the dose received by the victims of the Vinca and Y12 accidents. The acute radiation syndrome is an acute illness resulting from excessive exposure of the whole body or substantial parts of the body to penetrating ionizing radiation. The severity of the symptoms depends essentially on the size of the dose and to a lesser extent on the susceptibility of the individual. Cases which have resulted in death within hours or weeks have been described (Hempelmann and others, 1952; Shipman, 1961) while less severe exposures giving rise to a well defined sequence of symptoms and signs and resulting apparently in complete recovery have also been reported (Vinca, Y12, and Mol). It was not until the detonation of the atomic bombs over Hiroshima and Nagasaki that the effects of total body irradiation were fully appreciated.

Reactions to Whole Body Radiation

The type and severity of reactions to different doses of whole body radiation are summarized below:

Up to 25 r No symptoms, no abnormal findings apart from a transient lymphopenia immediately after exposure. Some chromosome aberrations may be detected in cultures of leucocytes.

25 to 50 r A few susceptible persons might complain of nausea, but it is extremely unlikely that anyone would be incapacitated. Abnormal chromosomes would be present in the leucocytes of most people receiving this dose.

100 *r* Even at this dosage the majority of people would remain free of symptoms. An appreciable number would show a reduction in the total leucocyte count, with a marked lymphopenia. The platelets would be affected. All persons would show chromosome aberrations. Those more susceptible would suffer from nausea and possibly vomiting. There is no means of identifying the more susceptible people beforehand, although it is believed that persons whose total white cell counts are on the lower limits of normal suffer more severe reactions during the course of radiotherapy.

200 *r* The majority of persons receiving a radiation dose of this order will show symptoms and signs of the acute radiation syndrome. The interval between exposure and the onset of symptoms is an important indication of the severity of the illness. The shorter the interval the more severe the reaction. Doses in excess of 200 r give rise to increasingly severe symptoms and recovery would be rare following doses in excess of 600 r. The median lethal dose to man is probably about 500 r.

500 to 1,000 r Symptoms would become evident within one hour of exposure. Intensive treatment in special units can save an appreciable number of patients. Immediate removal to such a unit is therefore vital. Doses in excess of 1,000 r are lethal in almost all cases. Symptoms will begin almost at once and certainly within half an hour. Treatment is palliative only.

Methods of Dose Assessment

Owing to the complex nature of the radiation produced in a criticality incident, there is almost always considerable difficulty in deciding the dose which has been received by exposed persons. The radiations consist of neutrons with a wide range of energies, and also γ rays of varying energies. The method of assessing the dose of radiation received by an individual is based on the activation of stable isotopes in the vicinity. Fortunately the human body with its approximately uniform distribution of ^{23}Na is an excellent fast neutron flux detector. The reaction ^{23}Na (n γ) $\rightarrow$ ^{24}Na takes place and ^{24}Na is easily detected because of its high energy γ emission with a half life of 14·8 hours. For a given neutron energy spectrum the fast neutron dose is proportional to the ratio ^{24}Na/^{23}Na in the body. From this information an assessment of both the neutron and γ dose to the individual can be made. It is usual to try to reproduce the conditions of a criticality accident and to expose plastic phantoms to the radiation and then measure the activation products in the phantoms.

The Acute Radiation Syndrome

The symptoms and signs which make up the acute radiation syndrome occur in four well defined phases. There is usually a short interval between exposure and the onset of symptoms, which, depending on the size of the dose, is measured in seconds or hours. The most consistent and disabling symptom of the second phase is intractable and almost continuous nausea and vomiting which may be accompanied by diarrhœa and abdominal pain. This phase usually persists for from 24 to 72 hours and there may in addition be headache, erythema of the skin and conjunctivitis. These symptoms subside and are then followed by a quiescent phase during which the patient feels reasonably well. During this time there may be loss of hair and a fine desquamation of the skin which was previously erythematous. Finally there is a period of severe hæmatological damage when there is aplasia of the bone marrow affecting all the formed elements of the blood, giving rise to agranulocytosis and hæmorrhagic disturbances during which the resistance to infection is virtually non-existent. It is during this fourth phase that stringent nursing care is necessary to avoid secondary infections, and the judicious use of antibiotics. Bone marrow transfusions have been used for the treatment of casualties during this phase of the acute radiation syndrome. The indications for this latter form of treatment will be discussed later.

Symptoms and Signs in a Fatal Case

The time interval between exposure and the onset of symptoms provides a reliable clinical indication of the size of the dose and the severity of the ensuing illness. In the fatal case described by Shipman (1961) the patient was found by a colleague to be ataxic and disorientated within 30 seconds of the accident. His face was flushed and he was almost unconscious within five minutes. On admission to hospital 25 minutes after the accident the patient was semi-conscious but disorientated, all visible areas of skin were of a dusky purplish colour, he had severe conjunctivitis and he was obviously suffering from severe abdominal pain. He had frequent attacks of retching, and shortly after admission suffered a severe attack of watery diarrhœa. He died within 34 hours of the incident, having received the highest recorded dose of mixed neutron and gamma radiation. The total dose to the head was in the region of 10,000 rads, with 12,000 rads to the upper abdomen; it was calculated that the average total body dose was in the range of 3,900 to 4,900 rads. Even in this case, a period of comparative tranquility occurred, beginning within 5 hours and lasting approximately 24 hours, during which time the patient was relatively free from symptoms. His condition suddenly deteriorated 30 hours after the accident and he died from cardiac arrest four hours later. The cardiac muscle had been the main target and received about 12,000 rads of ionizing radiation.

Symptoms and Signs in Less Severe Cases

In the criticality accidents at Vinca and Oakridge (Y12) the radiation dose received by the patients presenting symptoms of the acute radiation syndrome varied between about 240 rads and 640 rads whole body radiation. The Jugoslav patients probably received higher doses than the American. Severe nausea and vomiting began during the first hour in three of the Vinca casualties believed to have been exposed to over 500 rads and during the second hour in the two whose dose was 420 and 500 rads respectively. The sixth patient, who had received a dose of 350 rads, had slight nausea but no vomiting. These symptoms persisted for 24 hours and then gradually improved during the following 2 to 3 days. Of the five patients involved in the Y12 accident, three had nausea and vomiting within 2 to 4 hours and one became nauseated after about five hours, but did not vomit. These symptoms had subsided within 24 hours, but recurred to a lesser extent for a brief period 48 hours later. At this time, the fifth patient had transient nausea for the first time. The doses in these patients were estimated to be in the range 230 to 365 rads. Facial erythema and conjunctivitis were observed in all the Vinca patients 8 to 10 hours after the accident. All the patients improved considerably and there followed a period of about three weeks during which time they felt quite well. Loss of hair became evident at the beginning of the third week, on the 14th day in the more severely affected Vinca patients, and on the 17th day in the Y12 patients. Alopecia was almost complete in four of the Vinca patients. Regrowth of hair began at about three months and was complete within about six months of the accident. The symptoms during the critical third phase were typical of severe bone marrow depression. In the Jugoslav patients purpura and epistaxis occurred. In the one woman exposed there was menorrhagia. Transfusions of blood and platelets were required. Four of the five surviving Jugoslav patients were treated by marrow transfusion, but there is some doubt about its efficacy.

Hæmatological Changes during the first 2 months after Irradiation

Within 2 to 3 hours of exposure a leucocytosis involving the poly-morphonuclear cells and an absolute lymphopenia is seen. The lymphocyte count remains at a low level for the remainder of the illness and well into the convalescent period. The leucocytosis subsides after about 48 hours and, whereas abnormally large and symmetrical neutrophils are seen, the total number of cells present remains fairly constant and at a normal level. From about the 14th day the leucocyte count falls gradually until between the 21st and the 40th day when it reaches very low levels, corresponding to the most critical period in the condition of the patient. The platelets remain within normal limits until about the 14th day, when there is a rapid and severe reduction in the platelet count. Hæmorrhagic reactions in the form of epistaxis, gingival bleeding, purpura, and menorrhagia in women, occur at about the time when the platelet count is at its lowest level, from about the 14th to the 21st day. The red cells show little change until about the fourth week when a severe anæmia may occur. There is a marked reduction in the reticulocytes immediately after irradiation and these cells virtually disappear from the peripheral blood, particularly dur-ing the critical third phase of the illness. Within the first few hours after irradiation, abnormal cells appear in the peripheral blood; many of these appear to be degenerating and artificial white blood cells of various types which are difficult to identify. Within a few days abnormal monocytes, many with irregular or lobulated nuclei make their appearance and persist for many weeks. Abnormal lymphocytes with fissured or bilobed nuclei also appear at these times. Giant granulocytes were seen in all five of the Y12 patients. These large cells appeared within 3 to 4 days, but they had disappeared from the peripheral blood within five weeks of the accident. There is an initial reduction in the degree of cellularity of the bone marrow during the first few days after irradiation. This hypoplastic state of the bone marrow gradually becomes more marked and by the fourth week it may be completely aplastic, depending on the dose of radiation. It has been shown by Stewart (1958) that a dose of 300 r of penetrating external radiation is sufficient to cause complete acellularity of the marrow.

The Effects of a Criticality Accident

In December 1965 a research worker was involved in a criticality accident at the Centre for Nuclear Studies at Mol in Belgium. He had been exposed to a whole body dose of over 500 r of mixed γ rays and neutrons. In addition he received a localized dose of approximately 5,000 rads to his left foot and leg. He was admitted to the Curie Hospital in Paris on the same day for investigation and treatment (Jammet and others, 1966). Special attention was paid to the assessment of the dose to the bone marrow since this was vitally important in deciding the course of treatment. The course of the illness was dominated at first by the hæmatological changes and 8 weeks later by the symptoms from the heavy dose localized to the foot. There were the usual four phases; nausea and vomiting which began within two hours but were followed by apparent recovery within 24 hours. Then occurred the latent phase which lasted 3 weeks, followed by the critical third phase coinciding with the extreme changes in the peripheral blood and blood-forming tissues. This started on the 21st day with severe headache, high fever, collapse, and a dulling of the mental processes. Despite a marked improvement in the blood picture during the fifth week the pyrexia remained until the seventh week. Erythema of the skin first appeared on the seventh day. It progressed to ulceration of some parts, notably the scrotum, by the 14th day. Loss of hair was first noticed after 14 days, and was most marked during the fourth week; it began to grow again during the fifth week. Detailed blood examinations were carried out daily and the results were similar to those seen in previous cases of the acute radiation syndrome. The early lymphopenia, most marked after 48 hours when there were only 130 lymphocytes per cmm., was accompanied by an initial polymorphonuclear leucocytosis, when the total white cell count was 18,500 per cmm. after 6 hours. Over the period of two months of the acute illness, almost one litre of blood was removed for purposes of investigation. During the early phase multiple bone marrow aspirations were undertaken at numerous sites in a search for evidence of viable blood-forming tissue. On the 15th day cellular bone marrow containing 6% of stem cells was found in the cervical spine following marrow puncture at the level of the sixth cervical vertebra. On the basis of this finding it was decided that the patient could survive by his own blood-forming tissue and that marrow transfusion was contra-indicated.

Treatment of the Acute Radiation Syndrome

The general principles of treatment of the acute radiation syndrome are dictated by the condition of the patient in the various phases of the progress of the illness. In the first 24 hours, treatment is aimed at counteracting the initial shock, the pyrexia and the nausea and vomiting. Great care is necessary to avoid any drugs which have a potentially depressing effect on the bone marrow, so that most of the analgesics, antipyretics and antibiotics are contra-indicated. Following the initial phase the patient remains reasonably free from symptoms. Full use must be made of the time available during this phase to carry out investigations which will decide the course of treatment during the critical third phase. In this patient it was evident from the absence of cellular bone marrow at all sites other than the neck that there had been widespread heavy irradiation of the whole body. The estimate of the dose to the marrow suggested an overall effective dose of 400 rads, with doses of over 500 rads to the lower part of the trunk. It was clear that the risk of overwhelming infection both from external and internal sources would be extreme.

Nursing by Triple Barrier Isolation

The patient was completely isolated in a specially designed and constructed triple barrier installation. This consisted of an antechamber

terilized by the use of antiseptics and ultra-violet light, together with an
nner sterile chamber fed with compressed and filtered air. Inside this
chamber a plastic caisson had been constructed which was also provided
vith compressed air. It had an air lock for feeding, and another for the
access of the medical and nursing staff. All materials, including drugs and
food, going into the antechamber were sterilized. Not only were visitors
prohibited but also nursing and medical staff arranged to enter and to stay
as little time as possible. The bedclothes were sterilized and the internal
walls of the caisson cleaned each day with antiseptics. The patient had the
whole of his skin carefully cleaned for at least an hour each day with an
antiseptic solution. Special attention was paid to the cleansing of the mouth,
nose, eyes, ears, urinary meatus and anus. One problem was the elimination of endogenous infection, and broad spectrum antibiotics were given
systematically in an attempt to control the intestinal bacterial flora. The
atmosphere of the antechamber, of the sterile chamber and of the isolation
caisson was tested bacteriologically every day by sampling on Petri dishes.
In addition the surfaces were tested by swabbing. All the samples taken
from the skin, mucous membranes, urine and fæces were cultured and
tested for sensitivity to antibiotics. Also swabs were taken from the nasopharynx of all the medical and nursing staff.

Maintenance of Morale

Every effort must be made to maintain the patient's morale and for this
reason radio and television sets were installed and he was able to talk at a
distance with members of his family. Reading was prohibited because it
was not possible to guarantee sterility of the reading matter. The patient
was under direct television observation and his temperature, respiration,
pulse rate, blood pressure, E.C.G. and E.E.G. were recorded by remote
control. The critical third phase of the illness started on the 21st day and
the patient had a temperature of up to 104°F for four weeks. No anti-
pyretic drugs were used; the fever was controlled by lowering the temperature of the caisson and by covering the patient with ice. Despite three
negative blood cultures antibiotics based on the cultures and sensitivities
obtained during the latent phase were given. Two broad spectrum antibiotics in large doses were given for the four weeks during which the fever
lasted. During this phase of the illness the granulocytes were greatly
reduced, reaching a figure of 14 per cmm. on the 21st day. The platelets
remained below 50,000 per cmm. from the 14th to the 31st day. Since
there was evidence of viable bone marrow in the cervical spine it was
decided that marrow transfusions were contra-indicated because of the
hazard of immunological reactions. Arrangements had been made, however, to obtain suitable marrow for transfusion in case it became necessary. For this reason, blood transfusions were delayed until there was some
evidence of recovery of marrow function or until other indications
appeared, for example evidence of hæmorrhage pointing to the need for
platelet transfusion, or an uncontrollable septicæmia indicating the need

for the transfusion of granulocytes. In the fifth week transfusion of packed red cells became necessary because of signs of cardiac ischæmia. The patient first showed signs of recovery during the fifth week, but required supportive treatment for a further two weeks.

Treatment of a Local Complication

The recovery from the acute radiation syndrome was complicated by the development of the localized lesion of the left foot which had received a dose of about 5,000 rads. The skin of the foot became erythematous at the end of the first week and a primary blister appeared at the end of the second week. The blistering became more severe, so that by the sixth week the full thickness of the epidermis sloughed off leaving the dermis of the whole lower surface of the foot bare as far as the heel. The foot remained necrotic and gradually became extremely painful, eventually necessitating a high thigh amputation of the left leg 26 weeks after the accident. Following this operation the patient remained well.

Chronic Effects of Radiation

The long-term or chronic effects of exposure to radiation are four in number; the increased incidence of malignant disease, the overall reduction in the life span and developmental abnormalities, the somatic effects, and fourthly the genetic effects of ionizing radiations.

Increased Incidence of Malignant Disease

Exposure to ionizing radiations from various sources has been shown to cause an increased incidence of all forms of malignant disease. This has been demonstrated by animal experiments and by the study of a number of human groups exposed to radiation for a variety of reasons. Court-Brown and Doll (1957) demonstrated the increased incidence of myeloid leukæmia in patients suffering from ankylosing spondylitis who were treated by high voltage X-ray therapy. Thyroid carcinomata occur with increased frequency in persons whose thymus glands were irradiated in infancy (Simpson and Hempelmann, 1957, Pifer and others, 1963). In one series of childhood carcinomas studied by Winship and Rosvoll (1961) a history of previous X-ray therapy for enlarged thymus, hypertrophied tonsils and adenoids, or vascular nævi of the neck was obtained in 80% of 277 children specifically questioned about radiation exposure. Studies of the mortality among radiologists in the United States of America showed an increased incidence of myeloid leukæmia compared with the general population (Warren, 1956). In a later paper (Warren and Lombard, 1966) attention was drawn to the fact that the age distribution of the disease was different from that to be expected in the general population. In radiologists the incidence of leukæmia was considerably higher in those over the age of 40 years. The major source of information about the effects of external radiation comes from these three groups and from the survivors of the bombing of Hiroshima and Nagasaki. In this latter group an increased

ncidence of leukæmia was apparent in the years immediately following the
ombing, but in addition an increased incidence of all malignant diseases
as since become apparent (Harada and others, 1963). Tissues are also
rradiated as the result of the deposition of radioactive materials following
bsorption by inhalation or ingestion. Again, the main source of experience
elating to human exposure arises from early therapeutic procedures and
ccupational exposure involving radium and thorium. The widespread
arenteral administration of radium and thorium, particularly in the
Jnited States of America in the 1920's and 30's, has provided a large
umber of cases for the study of the long-term effects of the deposition of
hese materials in the skeleton. Evans (1966) estimated that several thous-
nd people were treated by parenteral radium or mesothorium. Two other
ccupationally exposed groups have been studied; the first includes
adium chemists and technicians, and the second the well known category
f radium dial painters or luminizers (see p. 913). Since 1941 the recom-
nended maximum permissible body burden (MPBB) of radium in the
keleton is 0·1 μCi. The radiographically demonstrable long-term effects
f radium deposited in the skeleton varies from patchy areas of bone re-
orption and sclerosis with coarsening of trabeculation to widespread large
unched-out areas in the flat or long bones, together with areas of bone
clerosis. Advanced changes include large areas of aseptic necrosis with
athological fracture and sarcomatous changes. Cases of carcinoma of the
aranasal and mastoid air sinuses occurring in workers in the luminizing
ndustry have already been described (p. 916). Myeloid leukæmia does not
ppear to occur with increased frequency in these persons, but aplastic
næmia frequently occurs as a terminal event.

Effects on the Life Span

It is suggested that radiation exposure reduces the life span of people
nd animals for reasons other than the production of cancer. Such an
ffect has been demonstrated in mice given doses of over 200 rads. There
s no clear evidence that this effect occurs at low doses. However, a study
y Warren (1956) of the mortality data in American radiologists showed
hat the average age at death was less than that for other physicians for all
he principal disease groups. In a later paper, Warren and Lombard (1966)
howed that these differences started to diminish in 1935 and that they
ad disappeared by 1960, and they suggested that this was because ex-
osures had been kept below the recommended maximum permissible
lose. A comparison of the mortality among members of the Radiological
Society of North America from 1915–1958, with members of the American
Academy of Ophthalmology and Otolaryngology, and members of the
American College of Physicians, supported the view that prolonged
exposure to relatively small doses of radiation may have an effect on
nortality from causes other than cancer (Seltser and Sartwell, 1964). A
study of British radiologists showed that apart from skin cancer and
eukæmia their experience compared favourably with other groups in the

medical profession and with other men in the same social and economic class (Court-Brown and Doll, 1958). A study of the survivors of Hiroshima and Nagasaki also provides some suggestive evidence. An expert group set up under the auspices of the International Commission on Radiological Protection concluded that the sum of the present evidence on this question was inconclusive (ICRP 8, 1966).

Developmental Abnormalities

Children exposed in utero to radiation at Hiroshima and Nagasaki have been examined at various times and in all, 12 children were found with mental retardation and microcephaly. All embryos irradiated at 7–15 weeks and within 1,200 metres of the hypocentre were affected and 4 out of 22 exposed at a range of 12–1,500 metres (18%) were also affected. Of 37 embryos exposed at a range of 1,500–2,000 metres none was affected. Other abnormalities included three cases of strabismus and two of congenital dislocation of the hips all with microcephaly as well as two cases of mongolism (ICRP 8, 1966). It is doubtful whether the radiation doses received in the course of diagnostic radiography, apart from pelvimetry, or from background radiation are sufficient to give rise to the severe developmental abnormalities referred to above. Later in pregnancy, irradiation gives rise to malignant disease and it is suggested that a dose of as little as 1 rad to the fœtus is sufficient to double the incidence of leukæmia in childhood (Upton, 1961).

Genetic Effects

The assessment of the genetic risks of radiation is more difficult than is that of the somatic risks. This difficulty is due to a number of factors, including the extremely varied nature of genetic damage and the fact that injuries may be seen only in subsequent generations. All the estimates of the genetic effects of radiation on man depend on the results of animal experiments, and there is some justification for the assumption that all the harmful mutations seen in laboratory animals can occur in man. No attempt will be made to discuss the genetic effects of ionizing radiation except to point out that there has, in general, been little change during the past ten years in the theoretical considerations of the mechanism of genetic damage (ICRP 8, 1966).

Chromosomal Aberrations

There has been considerable interest for many years in the possibility of developing a biological method of estimating radiation dosage as opposed to physical methods. It was believed at one time that the urinary excretion of specific metabolic products, notably beta-amino-*iso*-butyric acid (BAIBA) would be directly proportional to radiation dosage, but it has now been almost universally accepted that this is not the case. A more promising biological method of assessing radiation dosages of moderate degree has been the quantitative studies of chromosome aberrations in

rculating leucocytes. Court-Brown, Buckton and McLean (1965) studied
e chromosomal changes in 78 patients who had received deep X-ray
erapy for ankylosing spondylitis and 42 men exposed in their occupation
ionizing radiations. They found that there was an increased frequency
chromosomal aberrations in the small lymphocytes. They suggested that
is technique could be developed as a means of measuring the exposure to
w doses of radiation. There is an undoubted need for a reliable method
measuring the radiation dose received by individuals, as opposed to the
ysical methods which rely on the assessment of whole body dose, from
e effects of radiation on a small piece of photographic film worn on one
rt of the body.

adiation Exposure of the Population

In the countries of Western Europe and North America the main
uses of the increase in the radiation burden to the population are prob-
ly medical diagnostic and therapeutic procedures. The benefits of these
rocedures far outweigh the theoretical considerations and fears about
diation hazards. The precautions taken in modern medical practice
drian Committee, 1966) have considerably reduced any potential
angers. In comparison, industrial uses of radiation have given rise only
a small addition to the total radiation dose received by the general
opulation. This could increase following the wider industrial uses of
diation and the rapidly expanding nuclear power programme. At the
resent time, there are 3,500 MW of installed electrical capacity in the
K derived entirely from nuclear power; this will have reached 15,000
W by 1975.

adiation Protection of Workers

Persons occupationally exposed may receive a dose from external
diation or from internally deposited radioactive materials. External
diation from a sealed source or from a reactor may be attenuated either
y appropriate shielding or by distance. In some circumstances, having
duced the radiation levels, the dose to an individual may be kept to a
redetermined permissible one by controlling the time spent by a worker
a any given area. Statutory regulations, safety rules and codes of practice
ave been drawn up specifying this type of working procedure. These
recautions are supplemented by monitoring the individual and thus con-
rming that the dose received does not exceed a permitted maximum. As
ith other industrial poisons the deposition of radioactive materials in
arious tissues may arise following their inhalation, ingestion or passage
rough the skin. Appropriate safety rules, regulations and codes of prac-
ce specify safe methods of working, and individuals are monitored before
aving their place of work. The amount of many radioactive materials
tained in the body may be assessed by examination of activity in urine
r fæces, or by the use of a total body gamma spectrometer.

Some Industrial Applications

Unsealed or open sources of radioactive materials are used in man different ways; these include luminous compounds and paints and als tracer materials. They have an obvious place in research laboratories an for this reason the Factory Department has sponsored a special Code of Practice for use in Research Establishments. This code of practice cover procedures for protecting the research workers and also makes recom mendations which parallel the requirements of the Factories (Sealed Sources) Regulations. Industrial radiography forms a vital part of the process of quality control in manufacturing industries and also in nor destructive testing in the light and heavy engineering industries. I radiography high voltage X-ray machines are used, as also are a variety of sealed sources which vary in power from a few curies to large kilo-cur sources for the radiography of heavy castings (fig. 349). The isotopes mos commonly used as sealed sources are iridium 192, cobalt 60 and caesiun 137. All sealed sources are stored and transported in specially designe pots of lead and steel to prevent irradiation of personnel. The source themselves are manipulated by the use of long handled tools in order t take advantage of the effect of distance. Since 1956 nuclear energy has bee used as a source of power for the generation of electricity (see fig. 352) an in the United Kingdom nuclear power stations with a capacity of ove 1,000 MW are already nearing completion and others of later design wit an output of 2,500 MW of electricity are projected. It is in this field of development that the really massive concrete shields are built around th reactors and since their function is to protect people against the effect of ionizing radiation this is referred to as the biological shield. The thicknes of concrete forming this shield may be 15 feet (fig. 351).

Monitoring Devices

In order to measure the dose of radiation received by a worker thre personal monitoring devices are in common use.

(*a*) **The Film Badge.** Ionizing radiations blacken photographic film The degree of blackening is a measure of the amount of radiation to whic the film has been exposed. The film badge in general use in this countr (fig. 359) consists of a plastic holder with a number of filters so that i addition to measuring the total dose, it is possible to assess the quality an energies of the radiation to which the film has been exposed. The film i developed under controlled conditions and the degree of blackenin measured. This gives an accurate and permanent record of the dos received. Additional film badges can be worn on various parts of the bod to determine whether doses of radiation have been received uniformly. A film badge service is provided for industry by the Radiological Protectio Service who assess over 440,000 films per annum. In addition, large user such as the Central Electricity Generating Board and the UK Atomi Energy Authority have their own film badge laboratory service.

(b) **Quartz-fibre Electrometer (QFE).** This instrument is similar in appearance to a fountain pen. When held up to the light and viewed in the same way as one looks through a telescope, a scale is seen marked off from 0 to 500 millirads (Fig. 359). The scale can be varied depending on the use for which they are intended, for example in civil defence work the scale can be 0 to 50 r. The QFE works on the same principle as the gold-leaf electroscope. It is charged from a small battery and the quartz fibre moves to the zero mark. On exposure to ionizing radiation the chamber is discharged by leakage and the fibre moves across the scale until it reaches the 500 mrad mark. The great advantage of this instrument is that it gives an immediate indication of the dose received and is ideally suited to control the exposure of workers carrying out a specific task in radiation areas of known dose rate. It has a number

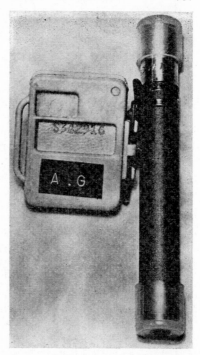

FIG. 359.—Film badge and quartz-fibre electrometer (QFE)
(By courtesy of the Central Electricity Generating Board)

of disadvantages in that it does not give a permanent record, it is less reliable and less accurate than the film badge, and since it operates by leakage of the electrical charge it may indicate that a dose has been received, when in fact this has not been the case. It will also be discharged following a fall or physical blow.

(c) **Thermo-luminescent Device (TLD).** Lithium fluoride has the unusual property of emitting light when heated in a controlled manner following exposure to ionizing radiations. The amount of light emitted is proportional to the amount of ionizing radiation it has absorbed. A dispensing device is used to deliver a fixed amount of lithium fluoride which is then sealed in a plastic container and can be worn by radiation workers before undertaking specific tasks. This is extremely useful in controlling the dose to parts of the body, particularly the hands and tips of the fingers when fine manipulative movements are required during the handling of irradiated equipment. The lithium fluoride is expensive but only small quantities are used at a time and it can be re-used after heating. In addition, instruments which measure the dose rate in any given situation are used particularly for routine surveys or for specific surveys prior to starting work. Equipment for atmosphere sampling is necessary in areas

where air-borne contamination by radioactive materials is suspecte
(fig. 362).

Air and Surface Contamination of Workplaces

In ideal situations the accidental spillage of radioactive materials causin
contamination of workplaces will result in the institution of decontamin
tion procedures to clean up the affected area. This may not always I
possible owing to the type of operations taking place in a specific area,
which case it is better to accept permanently a certain level of contamin
tion and require persons who work there to take special precautions. Sue
an area must be separated from uncontaminated areas, and barriers wi
change room facilities must be set up so that people may don protecti
clothing. This may vary from simply putting on overshoes and white coa
to a complete change of clothing, depending on the level of contaminatio
Facilities must be provided for washing and monitoring on leaving tl
area (fig. 365). Eating, drinking, smoking and taking of snuff are forbidde
In addition it may be advisable to take samples of urine or fæces from tl
workers for radiochemical analysis. In the event of an accidental spilla
or release of radioactive materials, it may be necessary to investiga
personnel suspected of absorbing quantities of radioactive materials in
total body γ spectrometer. This is a complex piece of equipment where tl
radioactivity present in the body is measured in an environment which
shielded from all external sources. Only isotopes which emit γ rays can I
measured. It follows that this apparatus is not suitable for the investig
tion of men suspected of absorbing pure α emitters such as plutonium 2
or pure β emitters such as Strontium 90. The only method available f
assessing body contents of these isotopes is by examining urine and fæc
and occasionally blood.

Barriers and Protective Clothing

Protection against external radiation, as has already been pointed ou
is based upon either the use of shielding or by distance. Shielding mater
consists of appropriate thicknesses of lead, steel or concrete, the choice
material depending on the prevailing conditions. The intensity of radi
tion at any given point is inversely proportional to the square of the di
tance of the source from that point. For this reason there is an enormo
reduction in the dose of radiation if long handled tools are used to mo
radiation sources from place to place. Having reduced the radiation lev
to manageable proportions, the dose to an individual can be controlled |
limiting the time spent by the individual in an area of known dose rat
Manipulations, including the machining of highly radioactive metals, a
carried out in heavily shielded facilities or caves, the operators carryi
out the manipulative process by the use of remotely controlled equipmei
Windows consisting of perspex or glass tanks filled with a saturat
aqueous solution of zinc bromide allow for direct visual control of t
process in complete safety (fig. 363). Smaller operations such as t

illing of glass bottles with radioactive isotopes is carried out by a technician who operates remote handling equipment from behind a lead brick wall looking through a lead glass window (fig. 364). Contamination of working surfaces or the atmosphere will require the use of protective clothing. In severe cases it will be necessary to wear complete suits made of PVC or other impervious material, carrying their own air supply under pressure (fig. 360). In these suits workers carry their own environment and are, therefore, able to work in complete safety. Entry and exit to and from working areas of this category must be carefully controlled; the exterior of the suit is decontaminated before the worker starts to undress, and he will require assistance to dress and undress. Washing and monitoring facilities are provided. Biological monitoring by the examination of urine and faeces may be required on occasions, for example if it is suspected that absorption of radioactive materials has occurred, or if the impervious clothing has been torn whilst working in contaminated areas.

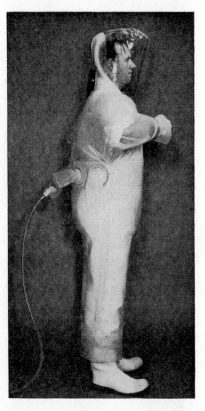

Fig. 360.—PVC pressurised suit developed for use in the UKAEA. It is used to protect men who have to enter areas of high radioactive contamination. It shows the air inlet tube and exhaust vents

(*By courtesy of the UKAEA*)

The Health Physics Team

A new profession has grown up with the requirement for radiation protection in industry and research, the profession of health physics. Health physicists are responsible for advising management on procedures for the protection of occupationally exposed persons including the design of equipment and for laboratory or factory layout. They give advice on the means of preventing exposure from external radiation and from absorption of radioactive materials in contaminated areas (fig. 361). They are responsible for organizing radiation monitoring services and also for the development of instruments to be used in radiation measurement (fig. 362). Their duties and responsibilities are analogous to those of industrial hygienists in conventional industries.

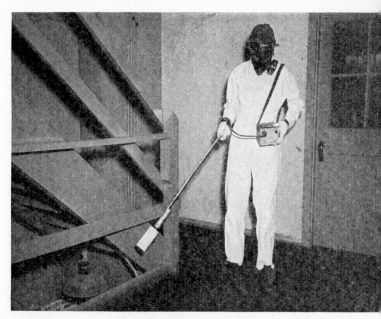

FIG. 361.—Technician wearing Protective Clothing searches for Radioactive
Material with a portable Geiger Counter
(*By courtesy of Monsanto Chemical Co.*)

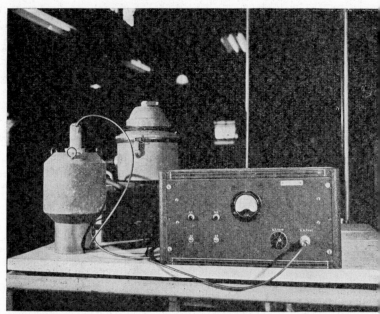

FIG. 362.—Stationary Instruments used to measure and record the Level of Radiation in the General Environment
(*By courtesy of Monsanto Chemical Co.*)

iting of Nuclear Establishments

The siting of nuclear power stations has remained under the direct
ontrol of the Government; the present policy has been described by
riffiths and Gausden (1964). The stations are built in sparsely populated
reas and arrangements are made to ensure that no developments occur

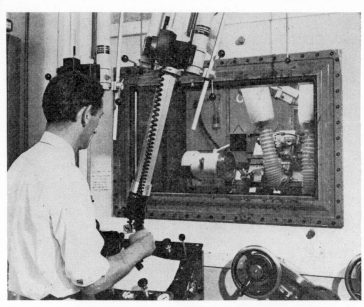

Fig. 363.—Technician in complete safety operating remote handling equipment. Cutting, grinding and milling machines are used with great precision
to cut intensely radioactive fuel elements removed from nuclear reactors
for investigations at the CEGB nuclear laboratories at Berkeley. Direct
vision is possible through a window which consists of a tank 8 to 12 feet
thick filled with a saturated aqueous solution of zinc bromide
(By courtesy of the Central Electricity Generating Board)

their immediate neighbourhood without the knowledge of the res-
onsible Government department. Planning permission could be refused
it appeared likely that the siting criteria would be violated. In the un-
kely event of an accident involving the release of fission products, it is
bvious that it would be easier to evacuate tens of people rather than
undreds or thousands from specified areas which could become affected.
s the design of stations becomes more advanced and more extensive
perating experience is gained, it is likely that these stringent siting criteria
ill be relaxed.

mergency Plans

Before discussing the principles embodied in emergency plans drawn
p for nuclear power stations in Great Britain, it would be of interest to
iscuss the nature of any potential accident. No hazard to public health

could arise unless radioactive materials were released from a reactor. I
the reactors operated by the Central Electricity Generating Board whe:
natural uranium metal is used as a nuclear fuel, the immediate risk follov
ing the release of fresh fission products is the inhalation of radioactiv
iodine. The iodine isotopes are present in great abundance, they a.
volatile and in addition they are selectively concentrated in the thyroi
The relative quantities of the isotopes of greatest biological interest r
leased during the accident to No. 1 Pile at Windscale in 1957 are listed
Table V (Loutit and others, 1960). ^{132}Te decays to ^{132}I; the thyroid glar

TABLE V

Radioactive Materials Released in the Windscale Accident 1957

Iodine 131	.	.	.	.	20,000 Curies
Tellurium 132		.	.	.	12,000 Curies
Caesium 137		.	.	.	600 Curies
Strontium 89		.	.	.	80 Curies
Strontium 90		.	.	.	2 Curies

is, therefore, the critical organ for accidents in which fresh fission pr
ducts are released to the atmosphere. Calculations and recommendation
that define emergency dose levels refer to a specific dose to the thyroid
infants aged 6 to 12 months—the most susceptible member of the popul.
tion (M.R.C. 1959). The other isotopes which could cause concern a
those of strontium and caesium. The problem presented by these isotop
is less acute because there are less of them present, they are less volati
and on assimilation they are not concentrated in one small organ. In
emergency any procedure that reduces the hazard to the thyroid will

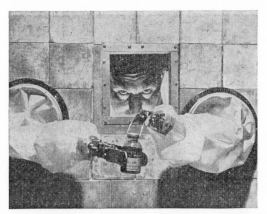

FIG. 364.—Remote handling of radioactive isotopes
from behind a lead brick wall looking through a
lead glass window

(*By courtesy of the Radio-Chemical Centre, Amersham*)

great value. Small doses of stable iodide in the form of potassium iodide ken at the time of absorption of radioactive iodine reduces the potential >se to the thyroid by a factor of at least 10 (Adams and Bonnell, 1962): .e administration of the stable iodide within 2 to 4 hours of absorption of ⁴I gives a worthwhile reduction in thyroid dose (Pochin and Burnaby,)62). This fact has been made use of in all emergency plans at nuclear tablishments in the United ingdom and elsewhere, and ocks of potassium iodide tablets e readily available for immediate stribution to those members of e general public who may be at sk. At this stage of an emergency very effort is made to gain time . order to mobilize vehicles and ersonnel and prepare reception ntres in case it becomes necessary arrange temporary evacuation residents. The time gained by ie distribution of stable iodide ould also allow for a better sessment of an accident and educe the occasions when evacua-on may have seemed advisable. 'he deposition of radioactive iaterials downwind of the affected actor poses different problems. f immediate concern is the ppearance of radioactive iodine,

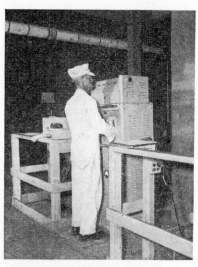

Fig. 365.—Worker testing his Hands for Contamination by Radioactive Substances before leaving Work
(By courtesy of Monsanto Chemical Co.)

rontium and cæsium in milk. It may, therefore, be necessary to ban the ile and consumption of milk and local food products.

adioactive Waste

There are two major sources of highly radioactive waste products hich occur during the operation of a nuclear reactor. One is due to wear id tear of essential equipment within the reactor, such as control rods, hich have to be replaced from time to time. This type of waste product stored on site in specially designed and constructed vaults. The materials e highly radioactive, the quantities are small and storage is therefore the ifest and simplest method of disposal. The other source, by far the more nportant, is the irradiated fuel elements. The reactors are constantly fuelled at a slow and controlled rate so that the fuel elements in the entral part of the reactor core are replaced over periods of up to three and half years. Elements in the more peripheral part of the reactor core may ot be replaced for up to 5 years. Certain types of the magnox alloy case : sheath which assist in transferring heat to the carbon dioxide in its

passage along the fuel channels, are removed and stored on site again
specially designed vaults. The uranium fuel elements with the magn
sheath are stored on site, when first removed from the reactor, in cooli

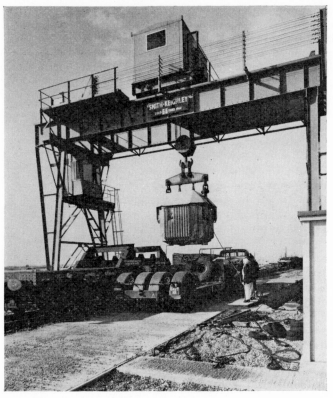

FIG. 366.—A 50-ton steel flask of spent fuel from Dungeness Nuclear
Power Station having arrived by road at a railway siding is being
lifted by crane on to a train wagon for its journey by rail to the
UKAEA factory at Windscale for processing
(*By courtesy of the Central Electricity Generating Board*)

ponds for a period of up to three months (120 days). The cooling period
chosen to provide a reasonable time for the shorter-lived and hence m
highly radioactive isotopes to decay. This reduces the hazard in t
handling and transport of the elements. Having "cooled" for the requis
period of time the fuel is removed from the pond and placed in specia
designed fuel flasks and conveyed first by road and then by rail to t
UKAEA factory at Windscale for processing (fig. 366).

Transport of Radioactive Materials

The transport of radioactive materials should comply with the reco
mendations of the International Atomic Energy Agency Safe Transp

egulations (1967). These Regulations lay down three standards of packing: (i) standard industrial package, (ii) Type A package which is proof ainst the minor mishaps incidental to transport, and (iii) Type B package nich has been shown by rigorous testing to be highly resistant to serious cidents. The transport flasks used to transport used nuclear fuel are ade of mild steel and weigh up to 50 tons (fig. 366). They contain approximately 2·5 tons of irradiated fuel. During the rail journey across untry, joint plans for dealing with a transport emergency have been awn up by the electricity and transport authorities (Bonnell, 1965).

K. Nuclear Legislation

Eight Acts of Parliament dealing with atomic energy and radioactive bstances have been passed since 1946.

The Atomic Energy Act, 1946 transferred responsibility for atomic ergy from the Department of Scientific and Industrial Research to the inistry of Supply and set up the Atomic Energy Research Establishment Harwell and the Radio-Chemical Centre at Amersham.

The Radioactive Substances Act, 1948 empowered the government to ntrol the use of radioactive substances and irradiating apparatus in edicine, industry and research and in the transport of such substances d apparatus. It provided for the setting up of the Radioactive Substances dvisory Committee, now called the Inter-departmental Committee on tomic Health and Safety. The Ministry of Health was the responsible vernment department.

The Atomic Energy Authority Act, 1954 established the Atomic Energy uthority. Amongst other requirements a duty was placed on the Authority prevent injury or damage by radioactivity and unauthorized discharge radioactive waste from its premises.

The Nuclear Installations (Licensing and Insurance) Act, 1959 empowered the Ministry of Power to control, by the granting of site licences, e building and operation of nuclear power reactors for electricity generan or for research purposes; it imposed an absolute liability on licensees, respective of negligence, for personal injury to any person and/or damage third party property attributable to ionizing radiations emitted from eir installations including nuclear fuel in transit. The Act required ensees to provide cover by insurance or other approved means up to a aximum of £5,000,000 for one site, £10,000,000 for two or more during specified cover period, and laid down a special limitation period of thirty ars during which actions for damages had to be instituted. The Act also nned production of plutonium and enriched uranium by anyone other an the United Kingdom Atomic Energy Authority or the Government cept for permitted research and development and empowered the inister to set up a Nuclear Installations Inspectorate.

adioactive Substances Act, 1960

The main purpose of this Act is to protect the public from ionizing diations from radioactive waste by instituting a central control for the

accumulation and disposal of such waste. It made permanent the tem
porary provisions relating to the discharge of radioactive waste in th
Atomic Energy Authority Act, 1954 and of the Nuclear Installation
(Licensing and Insurance) Act, 1959. Premises where radioactive materi;
is kept or used must be registered by the user with the Ministry of Housin
and Local Government and except when national security is involved th
Minister is required to send a copy of the certificate of registration to th
local authority in whose area the registered premises are situated.

The Electricity (Amendment) Act, 1961 empowered the Central Elec
tricity Generating Board to produce in their nuclear reactors radioisotope
for sale.

The Nuclear Installations (Amendment) Act, 1965 extended the scop
of the 1959 Act and thus enabled the United Kingdom to ratify the Paris
Brussels and Vienna conventions on third party liability in the field c
nuclear energy. The main provision extended the absolute liability impose
by the 1959 Act to nuclear matter in transit.

The Nuclear Installations Act, 1965 consolidated the two previou
Nuclear Installations Acts. A site licence must be obtained from th
Minister of Power before installing or operating any plant for the produc
tion or use of atomic energy. Conditions specifying the operational limit
are attached to the licence and these must be posted on the site where the
can conveniently be read by those employed on the site. In general it is th
conditions attached to a licence which regulate the application of radio
logical safety principles on the site. A licensee must ensure that ionizin;
radiations from any source on site do not cause injury to any person o
damage to the property of any person other than the licensee. A Chic
Inspector of Nuclear Installations, with a staff of inspectors, has bee;
appointed by the Minister to ensure that the provisions of the Act ar
complied with. It is of interest that this Act allows the Minister at hi
discretion to charge a licensee for that part of the costs incurred by th
Minister which are attributable to the licensee's nuclear installation.

The Ionizing Radiations (Sealed Sources) Regulations 1961 were mad
by the Minister of Labour under the Factories Acts. These Regulation
are for the protection of people employed in factories and other places t
which the Factories Acts apply, in which sealed sources are stored o
used. They do not apply to nuclear fuel elements or plant used for th
production of atomic energy by a fission process. They do, however, appl
to sealed sources used on sites licensed under the Nuclear Installation;
Act, 1965. Sealed sources are defined as "any radioactive substances seale
in a container (otherwise than solely for the purpose of storage, transpor
or disposal) or bonded solely within material including the immediat
container or the bonding." These Regulations also cover ionizing radia
tions emitted from a machine or apparatus including X-ray apparatus use
for industrial radiography. The Regulations require that persons must b
instructed in the hazards involved in their work and of the precautions t
be observed. A competent person must be appointed to exercise specia

pervision. Persons, who must be over the age of 18, who work with
nizing radiations and who are exposed to a dose rate of above 0·75 milli-
ds in air per hour are termed *classified workers*. Classified workers must
: medically examined each 14 months and must wear a film badge which
ust be processed in an approved laboratory. A Health Register, record-
g the results of medical and blood examinations and a Radiation Dose
cord and Transfer Record, recording the results of film badge develop-
ent must be kept and retained for 30 years from the last entry on the
ealth Register. Sealed sources are to conform to specified standards of
nstruction and the containers must be coloured orange. Precautions must
: instituted if sealed sources are damaged or lost, and facts reported
thin 24 hours. The particulars and whereabouts of all sealed sources must
: entered in a register which must be kept up-to-date daily. Detailed
ecautions are specified for radiography, the testing of X-ray tubes and
ts and irradiation of materials. These processes are to be carried out,
herever practicable, within a walled enclosure which provides adequate
ielding (fig. 349). These walled enclosures must be fitted with safety
vices and warning signals. Where a walled enclosure is not practicable,
diography may be conducted inside a suitably marked area. The maxi-
um permissible radiation doses for classified and other workers are
ecified. These doses conform to, but are not identical with, the recom-
endations of the International Commission on Radiological Protection.
hen a worker has been exposed in the past to an unknown dose of
diation it must be assumed that the maximum permissible dose has
en accumulated during the period concerned.

The Ionizing Regulations (Unsealed Radioactive Substances) Regulations,
67. In 1967 the Minister of Labour made available for comment new
aft regulations for the management of unsealed radioactive substances
factories. For the most part, the regulations will apply to situations
here the total activity of the unsealed substance exceeds 1, 10, or 100 μCi
he exact limit depending on whether the radionuclide is of high, medium,
low toxicity), to certain luminizing compounds (for example, radium-
tivated compounds of activity greater than 10 μCi), and to objects, such
apparatus, where contamination exceeds 10^{-4} or 10^{-3} μCi per sq. cm.,
pending on the type of emission and on the toxicity.

BIBLIOGRAPHY

ecompression Sickness

RMSTRONG, H. G., and HEIM, J. W. (1937), *J. Amer. med. Ass.*, **109**, 417.
EHNKE, A. R. (1942), *U.S. Nav. med. Bull.*, **40**, 65; (1945), *Medicine,
Baltimore*, **24**, 381.
EHNKE, A. R., and YARBOROUGH, O. D. (1938), *U.S. Nav. med. Bull.*, **36**,
542.
ERT, P. (1878), *La Pression Barometrique*, Paris.
OYCOTT, A. E. (1907–8), *Quart. J. Med.*, **1**, 348.

BOYCOTT, A. E., DAMANT, G. C. C., and HALDANE, J. S. (1908), *J. Hyg.*, **8** 342.

CATCHPOLE, H. R., and GERSH, I. (1947), *Physiol. Rev.*, **27**, 360.

DAVIS, SIR R. H. (1951), *Deep Diving and Submarine Operations*, The Saint Catherine Press, London.

END, E. (1938), *J. industr. Hyg.*, **20**, 511.

HILL, L. E. (1912), *Caisson Sickness and the Physiology of Work in Compressed Air*, London.

HONG, S. K. and RAHN, H. (1967), *The Scientific American*, **216**, 34.

JAMES, C. C. M. (1945), *Lancet*, **2**, 6.

KAHLSTROM, S. C., BURTON, C. C., and PHEMISTER, D. B. (1939), *Surg Gynæc. and Obstet.*, **68**, 129.

OLIVER, T. (1908), *Diseases of Occupation*, Methuen, London, p. 94.

PATON, W. D. M., and WALDER, D. N. (1954), *Compressed Air Illness.* Spec. Rep. Ser. Med. Res. Counc., No. 281, H.M.S.O., London.

RAINSFORD, S. G. (1942), *J. R. Nav. med. Serv.*, **28**, 326.

SWINDLE, P. F. (1937), *Amer. J. Physiol.*, **120**, 59.

THORNE, I. J. (1941), *J. Amer. med. Ass.*, **117**, 585.

Heat Cramps

BROCKBANK, E. M. (1929), *Brit. med. J.*, **1**, 65.

DERRICK, E. H. (1934), *Med. J. Austr.*, **2**, 612.

HALDANE, J. B. S. (1927), *Possible Worlds and Other Essays*, Chatto & Windus, London, p. 77.

MOSS, K. N. (1923), *Proc. R. Soc.*, *B*, **95**, 181.

STEWART, D. (1945), *Brit. J. industr. Med.*, **2**, 102.

TALBOTT, J. H. (1935), *Medicine*, **14**, 323.

TALBOTT, J. H., EDWARDS, H. T., DILL, D. B., and DRASTICH, L. (1933) *Amer. J. Trop. Med.*, **13**, 381.

TALBOTT, J. H., and MICHELSON, J. (1933), *J. clin. Invest.*, **12**, 533.

Miners' Nystagmus

COLLIS, E. L., and LLEWELLYN, T. D. L. (1923), *Second Report of the Miners Nystagmus Committee*, H.M.S.O., London.

FERGUSON, W. J. W. (1944), *Industrial Medicine*, edited by Sir Humphrey Rolleston and Alan A. Moncrieff, Eyre & Spottiswoode, London, p. 52.

FISHER, S. W. (1949), *Proc. Ninth Internat. Congr. Industr. Med., London* Wright, Bristol, p. 235.

KALMUS, E. (1934), *Occupation and Health*, I.L.O., Geneva, **2**, 473.

LLEWELLYN, T. D. L. (1922), *First Report of the Miners' Nystagmus Committee*, Med. Res. Counc. Rept. No. 65.

SNELL, S. (1892), *Miners' Nystagmus*, London.

STASSEN, M. (1914), *La fatigue de l'appareil visuel chez les ouvriers mineurs* Liége.

TAYLOR, C. B. (1875), *Lancet*, **1**, 821.

Cataract in Industry

BRINTON, A. G. (1922), *Brit. J. Ophthal.*, **6**, 269.

BUTLER, T. H. (1938), *Trans. Ophth. Soc. U.K.*, **57** (Part 2), 412.

CRIDLAND, B. (1921), *Brit. J. Ophthal.*, **5**, 193.
DESBRIÈRES, et al. (1905), *Ann. d'Ocul.*, **133**, 118.
GABRIÉLDÈS, A. (1935), *Arch. d'Ophth*, **52**, 394.
HEALY, J. J. (1921), *Brit. J. Ophthal.*, **5**, 194.
HEISTER (1739), *Institutiones Chirurgicæ*, Amsterdam, p. 598.
HESS, C. (1888), *Ber. d. internat. Ophthalmologen Kongress (7th)*, p. 308.
HORNER, W. D. (1941), *Trans. Amer. Ophth. Soc.*, **77**, 405; (1936), *Arch. Ophth.* n.s., **16**, 447.
KUHN, H. S. (1944), *Industrial Ophthalmology*, C. V. Mosby Co., St. Louis.
LEGGE, T. M. (1907), *Home Office Report on Cataract in Glassworkers*, H.M.S.O., London.
LERMAN, S. (1962), *New York J. med.*, **62**, 3075.
MERRIAN, G. and FOCHT, E. (1957), *Amer. J. Roentgenol.*, **77**, 759.
MEYERHOFER, W. (1886), *Klin. Monatsbl. f. Augen.*, **24**, 49.
MINTON, J. (1949), *Brit. med. J.*, **1**, 393.
ROBERTS, B.H.St.C. (1921), *Brit. J. Ophthal.*, **5**, 210.
ROBINSON, W. (1903), *Brit. med. J.*, **1**, 191; (1915), *Ophthalmoscope*, **13**, 545.
SAEMISCH, Th. (1864), *Klin. Monatsbl. f. Augen.*, **2**, 22.
SPAETH, E. B. (1936), *Amer. J. Ophthal.*, **19**, 321.
VOELZ, G. L. (1967), *J. occup. med.*, **9**, 286.

Occupational Deafness

CAMPBELL, P. A. (1945), *Arch. Oto. Laryng.*, **41**, 319.
DICKSON, E. D. D. (1942), *F. Larying. and Otol.*, **57**, 483; (1954) *Intense Sound and Ultra-sound*, in MEREWETHER, E. R. A., *Industrial Medicine and Hygiene*, Butterworth, London, **2**, 335.
DICKSON, E. D. D., EWING, A. W. G., and LITTLER, T. S. (1939), *Ibid.*, **54**, 531.
FOSBROKE, J. (1831), *Lancet*, **1**, 645.
KRISTENSEN, H. K. (1946), *Acta Oto. Laryng.*, **34**, 157.
LARSEN, B. (1939), *Ibid.*, Suppt., p. 36.
LEGGE, T. M., and MCKELVIE, W. B. (1927), *Annual Report of the Chief Inspector of Factories and Workshops*, H.M.S.O., London, p. 108.
MCCORD, C., and GOODELL, J. D. (1943), *J. Amer. med. Ass.*, **123**, 476.
MACLAREN, W. R., and CHANEY, A. L. (1947), *Industr. Med.*, **16**, 109.
PEYSER, A. (1942), *Acta Oto. Laryng.*, **31**, 351.
SCHILLING, C. W., and EVERLEY, J. A. (1942), *U.S. Nav. med. Bull.*, **40**, 12.
WITTMARCK, K. (1907), *Zeitschr. für Ophthal.*, **54**, 37.

Occupational Cramps

BRIDGE, J. C. (1920), *Annual Report of the Chief Inspector of Factories and Workshops for 1919*, H.M.S.O., Cmd. 941, p. 69.
CRITCHLEY, M. (1954), *Proc. Roy. Soc. Med.*, **47**, 593.
GOWERS, W. R. (1893), *A Manual of Diseases of the Nervous System*, 2nd ed., London, p. 710.
KALMUS, E. (1934), *Occupation and Health*, I.L.O., Geneva, **2**, 473.
LIVERSEDGE, L. A., and SYLVESTER, J. D. (1955), *Lancet*, **1**, 1147.
RAMAZZINI, B. (1713), *De morbus artificum diatriba.*, Transl. by Wilmer Cave Wright, Chicago, 1940.

Effects of Vibrating Tools

AGATE, J. N. (1949), *Brit. J. industr. Med.*, **6**, 144.

AGATE, J. N., and DRUETT, H. A. (1946), *Ibid.*, **3**, 159.

AGATE, J. N., DRUETT, H. A., and TOMBLESON, J. B. L. (1946), *Ibid.*, **3**, 167

ALLEN, E. V., BARKER, N. W., and HINES, E. A. (1946), *Peripheral Vascula Diseases*, W. B. Saunders Co., Philadelphia.

BIDEN-STEELE, K., and KING, F. H. (1947), *Med. Pr.*, **218**, 144.

BROCKLEHURST, T. (1945), *Ibid.*, **213**, 10.

GURDJIAN, E. S., and WALKER, L. W. (1945), *J. Amer. med. Ass.*, **129**, 668

HAMILTON, A., LEAKE, J. P., and others (1918), *U.S. Department of Labor Bureau of Labor Statistics*, Bulletin No. 236.

HUNT, J. H. (1936), *Quart. J. Med.*, n.s., **5**, 399.

HUNTER, D., McLAUGHLIN, A. I. G., and PERRY, K. M. A. (1945), *Brit. J industr. Med.*, **2**, 10.

HUTCHINSON, J. (1901), (Abstract) *Med. Pr.*, **72**, 403.

LEWIS, T., and PICKERING, G. W. (1934), *Clin. Sci.*, **1**, 327.

LORIGA, G. (1911), Quoted by TELEKY, L., *Occupation and Health Supple ment*, I.L.O., Geneva, 1938.

MIDDLETON, E. L. (1930), *Annual Report of the Chief Inspector of Factorie and Workshops*, H.M.S.O., London, p. 119.

MILLS, J. H. (1942), *Northwest Med.*, **41**, 282.

RAYNAUD, M. (1862), Thesis on *Local Asphyxia and Symmetrical Gangren of the Extremities*, Trans. BARLOW, T. (1888), in *Selected Monographs* New Sydenham Soc., London.

REYNARD, W. A. (1952), Personal communication.

SEYRING, M. (1930), *Arch. Gewerbepath. Gewerbehyg.*, **1**, 359.

TELFORD, E. D., McCANN, M. B., and MacCORMACK, D. H. (1945), *Lancet* **2**, 359.

EFFECTS OF IONIZING RADIATION

(a) Injuries from X-rays

BARCLAY, A. E. (1923), *J. Röntgen Soc.*, **12**, 9.

BERGONIÉ, J. (1916), *Compt. rend. Acad. d. Sc.*, **162**, 613.

BORDIER, H. (1926), *J. belg. de radiol.*, **15**, 409.

BROWN, F. T., and OSGOOD, A. T. (1905), *Amer. J. Surg.*, **18**, 179.

BURROWS, A. (1931), *Proc. R. Soc. Med.* (Sect. Dermat.), **25**, 216.

CASSIDY, P. (1900), *New York med. Record*, **57**, 180.

CODMAN, E. A. (1902), *Philad. med. J.*, **9**, 438, 499.

COLWELL, H. A., and RUSS, S. (1934), *X-ray and Radium Injuries*, Oxfor University Press, London.

FABER, K. (1923), *Acta Radiol.*, **2**, 110.

FEYGIN, S. (1913–14), *Thèse de Paris*, No. 265.

FRIEBEN, —— (1902), *Aertzl. Verein.*, Hamburg, Quoted by Flaskamp.

HALL-EDWARDS, F. (1904), *Brit. med. J.*, **2**, 993.

HESSE, O. (1911), *Fortsch. a. d. Geb. Röntgenstrahl.*, **7**, 82.

LEDOUS-LEBARD, R. (1922), *Paris méd.*, **12**, 299.

MEYER, H. (1937), *Ehrenbuch der Röntgenologen und Radiologen aller Nationen* Urban und Schwarzenberg, Berlin und Wien.

NICHOLAS, J. (1930), *Compt. rend. Acad. d. Sc.*, **190**, 659.

O'DONOVAN, W. J. (1927), *Proc. R. Soc. Med.* (Sect. Dermat.), **21**, 1.
PATON, L. (1909), *Trans. Ophth. Soc. U.K.*, **29**, 37.
ROLLESTON, H. (1930), *Quart. J. Med.*, **23**, 101.
WALSH, D. (1897), *Brit. med. J.*, **2**, 272.

(b) Injuries from Radioactive Substances

AUB, J. C., EVANS, R. D., HEMPELMANN, L. H., and MARTLAND, H. S. (1952), *Medicine*, Baltimore, **31**, 221.
BECQUEREL, H., and CURIE, P. (1901), *Compt. rend. Acad. d. Sc.*, **133**, 1289.
BERENBAUM, M. C., and BIRCH, C. A. (1953), *Lancet*, **2**, 852.
BROWNING, E. (1949), *Brit. med. J.*, **1**, 428.
BRUES, A. M. (1949), *J. clin. Invest.*, **28**, 1286.
FISCHER, P., GOLOB, E, KUNZ-MÜHL, E., BENHAIM, A., DUDLEY, R. A., MÜLLNER, T., PARR, R. M., and VETTER, H. (1966), *Radiation Research*, **29**, 505.
FLINN, F. B. (1927), *Laryngoscope*, **37**, 341.
GIESEL, F. (1900), *Ber. d. deutsch. chem. Gesellsch.*, **33**, 3569.
HAMILTON, J. G. (1947), *Radiology*, **49**, 325.
HASTERLIK, R. J., and FINKEL, A. J. (1965), *Med. Clinics. N. Amer.*, **49**, 285.
HASTERLIK, R. J., FINKEL, A. J., and MILLER, C. E. (1964), *Ann. New York Acad. Sci.*, **114**, 832.
HORTA, J. LA S., ABBATT, J. D., DA MOTTA, L. C., and RORIZ, M. L. (1965), *Lancet*, **2**, 201.
HUEPER, W. C. (1942), *Occupational Tumours and Allied Diseases*, Thomas, Springfield, Ill., p. 456.
LANGLANDS, A. O., and WILLIAMSON, E. (1967), *Brit. med. J.*, **2**, 206.
LEGGE, T. (1925), *Annual Report of the Chief Inspector of Factories and Workshops for 1925*, H.M.S.O., Cmd. 2714, London, p. 63.
MACMAHON, H. E., MURPHY, A. S., and BATES, M. I. (1947), *Amer. J. Path.*, **23**, 585.
MARTLAND, H. S. (1929), *J. Amer. med. Ass.*, **92**, 466, 552; (1931), *Amer. J. Cancer*, **15**, 2435.
MARTLAND, H. S., and HUMPHRIES, R. E. (1929), *Arch. Path.*, **7**, 406.
MOTTRAM, J. C. (1921), *Arch. Radiol. and Electrother.*, **25**, 194, 197.
MOTTRAM, J. C., and CLARKE, J. R. (1920), *Ibid.*, **24**, 345.
MÜLLER, J., DAVID, A., REJSKOVA, M., and BREZIKOVA, D. (1961), *Lancet*, **2**, 129.
ROLLESTON, H. (1930-1), *Quart. J. Med.*, **23**, 101.
RUSS, S. (1935), Personal communication.
TELEKY, L. (1937), *J. industr. Hyg.*, **19**, 73,
VAUGHAN, J., and TUTT, M. (1953), *Lancet*, **2**, 856.
VENNART, J. (1967), *Health Physics*, **13**, 959.
VENNART, J., MAYCOCK, G., GODFREY, B. E., and DAVIES, B. L. (1964), *Symposium on Assessment of Radioactive Body Burdens in Man*, IAEA, ILO, WHO, Heidelberg.
WEIL, P. E., and LACASSAGNE, A. (1925), *Bull. Acad. de. méd.*, **93**, 237.

(c) Injuries from Fission Products

ADAMS, C. A., and BONNELL, J. A. (1962), *Health Physics*, **1**, 127.
BIELSCHOWSKI, F. (1955), *Brit. J. Cancer*, **9**, 80.
BONNELL, J. A. (1965), *Roy. Soc. Hlth. Journ.*, **85**, 347.

CONRAD, R. A., RALL, J. E., and SUTOW, W. W. (1966), *New England J. of Med.*, **274**, 1391.

COURT-BROWN, W. M., BUCKTON, K. E., and McLEAN, A. S. (1965), *Lancet*, **1**, 1239.

COURT-BROWN, W. M., and DOLL, R. (1957), *Medical Research Council Special Report Series No. 295*, HMSO, London; (1958), *Brit. med. J.*, **2**, 181; (1965), *Brit. med. J.*, **2**, 1327.

Diagnosis and Treatment of Acute Radiation Injury, WHO, Geneva, 1961.

The Evaluation of Risks from Radiation. ICRP Publication 8. Pergamon Press, Oxford (1966).

EVANS, R. D. (1966), *Brit. J. Radiol.*, **39**, 881.

Final Report of the Committee on Radiological Hazards to Patients (1966) (Adrian Committee), HMSO, London.

GRIFFITHS, T., and GAUSDEN, R. (1964), *Third International Conference on the Peaceful Uses of Atomic Energy*, Geneva.

HARADA, J., IDE, M., ISHIDA, M., and TROUP, G. M. (1963), *Atomic Bomb Casualty Commission Technical Report*, 23–63, Hiroshima.

HEMPELMANN, L. H., LISCO, H., and HOFFMAN, J. G. (1952), *Ann. intern. Med.*, **36**, 279.

JAMMET, H. P., GONGORA, R., LE GO, R., MARBLE, G., and FAES, M. (1966) First International Radiation Protection Association Congress, Rome.

LE ROY, G. V. (1947), *J. Amer. med. Assoc.*, **134**, 1143.

LOUTIT, J. F., MARLEY, W. G., and RUSSELL, R. S. (1960), MRC Appendix H. *The Hazards to Man of Nuclear and Allied Radiation*, H.M.S.O. London.

Medical Research Council (1959), *Brit. med. J.*, **1**, 967.

Medical Research Council (1960), *The Hazards to Man of Nuclear and Allied Radiation*. Cmnd. 1226, H.M.S.O., London.

MUTCH, N. (1931), *Lancet*, **2**, 1013.

OUGHTERSON, A. W., LEROY, G. V., LIEBOW, A. A., HAMMOND, E. C. BARNETT, H. L., ROSENBAUM, J. D., and SCHNEIDER, B. A. (1951), *Medical Effects of Atomic Bombs*, Oak Ridge, Tenn. Office of Air Surgeon, N.P. 3037, U.S. Atomic Energy Commission Tech. Information Service.

PENDIC, B. (1961), *Diagnosis and Treatment of Acute Radiation Injury*, p. 67 WHO, Geneva.

PENNA FRANCA, E., ALMEIDA, J. C., BECKER, J., EMMERICH, M., PETROW, H. DREW, R. T., and EISENBUD, M. (1965), *Health Physics*, **11**, 699.

PIFER, J. W., TOYOOKA, E. T., MURRAY, R. W., AMES, W. R., and HEMPEL-MANN, L. H. (1963), *J. Nat. Cancer Inst.*, **31**, 1333.

POCHIN, E. E. (1964), *Proc. Roy. Soc. Med.*, **57**, 564.

POCHIN, E. E., and BURNABY, C. F. (1962), *Health Physics*, **1**, 125.

A Programme of Nuclear Power: Cmnd. 9389, H.M.S.O., London (1955).

Recommendations of the International Commission on Radiological Protection ICRP Publication 2, Pergamon Press, Oxford (1959); *Ibid.*, Publication 6 (1964); *Ibid.*, Publication 9 (1966).

SELTSER, R. and SARTWELL, P. E. (1964), *J. Amer. Med. Ass.*, **190**, 1046.

SHIPMAN, T. L. (1961), *Diagnosis and Treatment of Acute Radiation Injury* p. 113, WHO, Geneva.

SIMPSON, C. L., and HEMPELMANN, L. H. (1957), *Cancer*, **10**, 42.

STEWART, J. W. (1958), *Proceedings of the Seventh International Congress of the Society of Hæmatology*, Rome.

TAYLOR, L. S. (1958), *Health Physics*, **1**, 97.
United Nations Scientific Committee on the Effects of Atomic Radiation. Report to General Assembly, New York (1962).
UPTON, A. C. (1961), *Cancer Research*, **21**, 717.
VENNART, J. (1967), Personal communication.
WARREN, S. (1956), *J. Amer. Med. Ass.*, **162**, 464.
WARREN, S., and LOMBARD, O. M. (1966), *Arch. Envir. Hlth.*, **13**, 415.
WINSHIP, T., and ROSVOLL, R. V. (1961), *Cancer*, **14**, 734.

CHAPTER XIV

THE PNEUMOCONIOSES

The pneumonokonioses (Greek, πνεύμων lung; κόνις dust) or, more shortly, pneumoconioses constitute a group of lung diseases which result from the inhalation of dust in certain occupations.

SILICOSIS

Silicosis (Latin, *silex*, flint) is the most important disease of this group and is defined as a pathological condition of the lungs due to the inhalation of particulate matter containing free or uncombined silica, silicon dioxide, SiO_2. It is important to distinguish between silica in the free state as SiO_2 and in the combined state as the various silicates.

Silicosis and Pneumoconiosis not Synonymous

Silicosis and pneumoconiosis must not be used as synonymous terms. Logically one could classify the pneumoconioses as pneumoconiosis due to silica, pneumoconiosis due to asbestos, pneumoconiosis of coal miners and so on, but such a method would be too cumbersome. Legal considerations make it important that the term silicosis be reserved for that condition caused by the inhalation of uncombined silica, the special characters of which render it capable of being identified when it occurs in typical form. Dusts other than uncombined silica produce pneumoconioses, but these do not present the characters which are possessed by silicosis in its typical form.

Great Prevalence of Silicosis

Silicosis is widespread throughout the world. It is prevalent in many industries, and of all the pneumoconioses it claims the largest number of victims, either alone or with tuberculosis with which it is frequently allied. Silicosis has been known as dust consumption, ganister disease, grinders' asthma, grinders' consumption, grinders' rot, grit consumption, masons' disease, miners' asthma, miners' phthisis, potters' rot, sewer disease, rock tuberculosis, stone-hewers' phthisis and stonemason's disease. Stone-workers' lung is sometimes referred to as chalicosis and slateworkers' lung as schistosis. The origin of these terms is obvious. Recognition of silicosis depends in a given case on a knowledge of the occupational history, on the clinical and the radiological examination, and in fatal cases on the necropsy findings.

Prehistoric Flint Implements

How early in the history of mankind silicosis appeared is a subject for interesting conjecture. It probably existed in the palæolithic period, for prehistoric man manufactured flint implements extensively. In 1915 Collis pointed out that the flint-knappers of the village of Brandon in Suffolk suffered a high mortality from phthisis induced by flint dust generated in their work (see p. 970). Probability suggests, therefore, that the starting-point of human progress was associated with at least one form of silicosis. Hippocrates in his *Epidemics* speaks of the metal digger as a man who breathes with difficulty, and Pliny mentions the use of respirators to avoid dust inhalation.

A Substance like Sand in the Lungs

We have seen (p. 25) how in the sixteenth century Joachimsthal in Bohemia was the greatest mining area in Central Europe. It was here that Agricola (1556) strongly advocated the ventilation of mines, for he knew that dust entering the lungs caused disease associated with dyspnœa, and he spoke of corrosive dusts which ulcerated the lungs, producing consumption. He relates that in the Carpathian mountains there were women who had married seven husbands, all of whom were brought to an early grave by the dust disease of the mines. But the first account of the pathology of what we now call silicosis came from Holland. In 1672 in his *Anatome corporis humani* Isbrand van Diemerbroeck (1609–74), professor of medicine in Utrecht, described how several stone cutters died of asthma, and he found at necropsy that to cut their lungs was like cutting a mass of sand. Ramazzini (1713) describes how stone cutters breathe in small splinters and turn asthmatic and consumptive.

Starting-point of Modern Studies

The starting-point of the study of silicosis in modern times was a paper by Johnstone in 1796, calling attention to the high mortality among needle pointers at Redditch. Arnold Knight was apparently the first to write of silicosis in Sheffield. In 1819 he propounded the view that criminals should be employed for the process of dry grinding. This proposal was immediately denounced. The period just after this date seems to have been the time when grinders' asthma became notorious, about the time that the water power of Sheffield, which originally had made the industry possible, was changed to steam power. Immediately there was a great increase in the amount and severity of silicosis. We have seen (p. 122) how Thackrah (1831) knew of Knight's work describing the deadly effects of the dry grinding of forks in Sheffield. But he knew much more than this, for he made it his business to survey many industries. We have seen (p. 122) that he knew of the danger from sandstone dust in mining and of the harmlessness of limestone dust. He had noted that bricklayers and limeworkers were long-lived and that sandstone masons usually died before they reached the age of forty. In men employed in grinding he recognized the association of dust inhalation and tuberculosis. He had noticed, too, that pulmonary disease was prevalent amongst men filing iron castings to remove burnt-on sand.

Fate of the Sheffield Cutlery Grinders

In 1843, Calvert Holland described the conditions of work amongst Sheffield grinders. He showed how grinding was always performed on a dry stone, in a room in which there were usually about ten people at work and the dust rose in clouds pervading the atmosphere in which they were confined (fig. 367). He discovered on examination that among ninety-seven men, about thirty were suffering in varying degree from the grinders' asthma. He obtained records of sixty-one persons who had died between 1825 and 1840. Thirty-five of these were under thirty years of age.

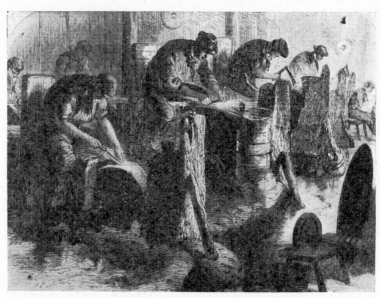

Fig. 367.—Table-blade grinding in Sheffield (1886). The underground Workshop was known as a Hull or Stye. It was estimated at the time that the Conditions of Work robbed the Men of 25 years of Life
(*By courtesy of The Illustrated London News*)

In *The Vital Statistics of Sheffield* (1843) G. Calvert Holland, who was physician to the Sheffield General Infirmary, wrote:

> The analysis of the trade of fork grinding will present a vivid but painful picture of the condition of an extensive class of artisans in this town. It is perhaps more destructive to human life than any pursuit in the united empire. Wet grinding is generally confined to saws, scythes and edge-tools; the dry to an extensive class of small articles, such as razors, scissors, pen and pocket knives, forks and needles. Fork-grinding is always performed on a dry stone, and in this consists the peculiarly destructive character of the branch. In the room in which it is carried on there are generally from eight to ten individuals at work

and the dust which is created, composed of the fine particles of stone and metal, rises in clouds and pervades the atmosphere to which they are confined.

The dust, which is thus every moment inhaled, gradually undermines the vigour of the constitution, and produces permanent disease of the lungs, accompanied by difficulty of breathing, cough, and a wasting of the animal frame, often at the early age of twenty-five. Such is the destructive tendency of the occupation, that grinders in other departments frequently refuse to work in the same room, and many sick clubs have an especial rule against the admission of dry grinders generally, as they would draw largely on the funds from frequent and long-continued sickness. In 1,000 deaths of persons above 20 years of age, the proportion between 20 and 29 years, in England and Wales, is annually 160, in Sheffield, 184; but among the fork-grinders, the proportion is the appalling number 475; so that between these two periods, three in this trade die to one in the kingdom generally.

Between the ages of 30 and 39, a still greater disparity presents itself. In the kingdom, 136 only in the 1,000 die annually between these two periods. In Sheffield, 164; but in the fork-grinding branch, 410; so that between 20 and 40 years of age, in this trade, 885 perish out of the 1,000; while in the kingdom at large, only 296. Another step in the analysis, and we perceive that between 40 and 49, in the kingdom, 126 die; in this town, 155; and in this branch, 115, which completes the 1,000. They are all killed off. For in carrying forward the inquiry we observe that between 50 and 59, in the kingdom, 127 die; and in Sheffield, 155; but among the fork-grinders, there is not a single individual left. After this period of life, there are remaining in the kingdom, of the 1,000, 441; and in the town, 339; but none in this branch of manufacture.

Grinders' asthma in its advanced stages admits neither of cure nor of any material alleviation. In the early stages the only efficient remedy is the withdrawal from the influence of the exciting cause; but how is this to be effected by men who depend from day to day upon their labour, and whose industry from early life has been confined to one particular branch? Here then, is the melancholy truth that nearly one-third of this class of artisans, in addition to the poverty and wretchedness common to the whole, is in a state of actual disease— and disease which no art can cure. Fiction can add no colour or touches to a picture like this. Truth transcends the gaudy embellishments of imagination. The distempered fancy has here no room to exercise her powers.

Further evidence of the wretched state of the fork-grinders—and the remark applies with great truth to grinders generally—is the low state of education among them. Of the 197 men and boys, 109 can read only, and 69 can write. Thus, in a Christian country—a country that expends vast wealth in attempting to educate and enlighten the dark heathen—one-half of an important body of human beings, near this source of benevolence and comprehensive charity, actually cannot read, and about two-thirds cannot write! The inability to work, and yet the necessity to labour, creates a degree of wretchedness and suffering easier to imagine than describe. But the wretchedness is not confined to the individual. A wife and increasing family are involved in the accumulated evils. Poverty, yoked with disease, embitters and shortens life in a thousand forms, but all forms of misery. We do not hesitate to assert that this is a picture of wretchedness, which has no parallel in the annals of any country, or in the records of any trade.

The Work of Greenhow and Peacock

Two other great Englishmen figure in the history of the pneumoconioses —namely, T. B. Peacock and E. H. Greenhow. Peacock, a physician on the staff of St. Thomas's Hospital, first established between 1860 and 1866 the existence of miners' disease as an entity and distinguished it clinically from pulmonary tuberculosis. Greenhow (1860, 1861), who was physician to the Middlesex Hospital, carried out the first large field investigation into the dusty industries such as the potteries, metal trades, cutlery making, tin and copper mining, coal mining, lead mining, cotton, flax, silk and woollen manufacture, hosiery and lace making, glove making and agriculture. In the *Transactions of the Pathological Society of London* (1860–66) are to be

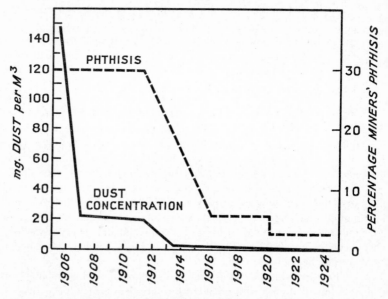

FIG. 368.—Conditions of work in the Gold Mines of the Witwatersrand. The Incidence of Miners' Phthisis began to fall steeply about seven years after the Dust Concentration was significantly reduced

(*After Mavrogordato*)

und excellent clinical and pathological descriptions by both these doctors f the disease which was later to be called silicosis by Visconti in 1870. They ven found the dust of free silica in the lungs and examined it under olarized light.

World-wide Interest in Silicosis

In 1885 Arnold published a monograph on dust inhalation, pointing ut that dust particles may be found in the liver, spleen and bone marrow, s well as in the lungs. The work of J. S. Haldane in tin miners (1904), Hay n granite workers (1909) and Wheatley (1911) in sandstone-quarry workers, nd the report of a Commission on Miners' Phthisis in South Africa (1912) pened the twentieth century (fig. 368), the early part of which has been

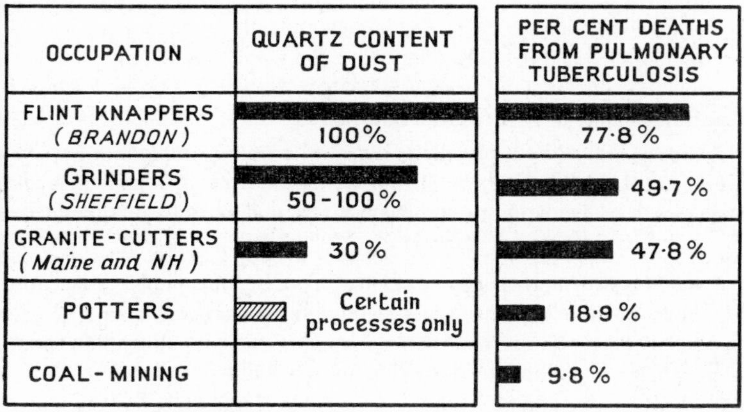

OCCUPATION	QUARTZ CONTENT OF DUST	PER CENT DEATHS FROM PULMONARY TUBERCULOSIS
FLINT KNAPPERS (BRANDON)	100%	77·8%
GRINDERS (SHEFFIELD)	50-100%	49·7%
GRANITE-CUTTERS (Maine and NH)	30%	47·8%
POTTERS	Certain processes only	18·9%
COAL-MINING		9·8%

FIG. 369.—Relationship of Deaths from Tuberculosis to Quartz Content of Dust
(After Collis)

notable for a gradually extending and now world-wide interest in the ubject (fig. 369).

Mechanization increases the Dust Hazard

By this time mechanization of industry had come to stay, and with ncreased speed of production there was, of course, more dust. On this ubject McLaughlin (1953) wrote:

With the turn of the century a new interest began to be taken in the problem, not only in this country, but also in other parts of the world. It is significant that about the same time there was a quickening of the tempo of life in general. The horse began to give way to the motor car, and soon there came the first aeroplane. Then, too, there was the telegraph and the telephone and all those "comforts" of present-day life which give us little or no time to think. In the factories

and in the mines there was a speeding-up of output. Hand labour
began to be replaced by the machine. In the cotton industry the change
had come a little earlier. But the air-hammer or the pneumatic tool
began to be used more extensively in the early part of the century for
such jobs as mining, quarrying and the cleaning of castings in
foundries. There is also the spray gun, which is used to spray paint,
glazes, metals and asbestos, and was introduced with the idea of
speeding up the work. This, from a health point of view, is a dangerous
instrument, because it is very difficult to control the spray and to
prevent its inhalation by the workers.

If there is one thing certain about increased speed of production in
industry, it is that a dusty process will become more dusty; and that
there will be a greater incidence of the dust diseases, if attention is not
given at the same time to increased control of dust. But quite often the
efforts at dust control are inadequate and do not keep pace with the
increased speed of production.

Mechanization of Mines and Foundries

Silicosis and silico-tuberculosis did not become a problem in hæmatite
mining until the introduction of the pneumatic drill. Stewart and Faulds
(1934) say that hæmatite mining has been carried on in Cumberland since
the time of the Roman occupation.

> It was formerly considered a healthy trade, but evidence is accumu-
> lating to show that in this respect a definite change for the worse has
> taken place. The miners themselves believe that the trouble started
> with the introduction of the dry mechanical drill in 1913.

Previously the ore had been obtained by the old hammer and jumper
method. Mechanical cutting and conveying of coal was introduced into the
coal mines of Great Britain early in the present century. The change from
hand-cutting of coal led to an increased dustiness of the air in the mines
not only at the coal face but generally throughout the workings. In 1950
H.M. Chief Inspector of Mines wrote:

> There is no doubt that one result of the adoption of many of the
> present methods of machine mining is that the production of dust in
> mines has increased in recent years and is still increasing. If we are to
> get rid of the scourge of pneumoconiosis, this process must be re-
> versed (Bryan, 1950).

McCallum (1952) also thinks that mechanized coal-getting has increased
the prevalence of pneumoconiosis in the Durham coalfield, and that
future developments in the coalfield will intensify dust production and the
risks of pneumoconiosis unless dust-suppression methods are considerably
extended. The use of the pneumatic tools in place of hand methods for the
fettling of steel castings has also increased the risk of silicosis in this
occupation (McLaughlin and others, 1950).

Symptoms and Signs

Silicosis is generally divided into first, second and third stages, or slight, moderate and severe degrees. South Africa and Ontario speak of ante-primary, primary and secondary stages, terms of importance in connexion with their compensation laws. The first stage, the so-called simple silicosis, supervenes in a workman who has been employed in an industrial process involving exposure to siliceous dusts for a period of many years. The changes can occur from a few months after exposure to over sixty years. Commonly they are found half-way between these extremes. The onset of symptoms is marked by dyspnœa on exertion, slight at first, and later increasing in severity. Throughout the illness dyspnœa remains the most important symptom. Slight cough may be present from the first. It is usually unproductive or with scanty sputum. The general condition of the patient is unimpaired. Physical signs in the chest are slight. Diminished expansion is scarcely, if at all, present. Dullness can rarely be demonstrated, and in older subjects there may be areas of hyper-resonance due to emphysema. There is no alteration of the breath sounds, and there are no added sounds. In this stage, impairment of working capacity may be slight or absent. In the second stage, dyspnœa and cough become established and further physical signs appear. There is diminished expansion of the chest, patchy dullness, sometimes with bronchial breath sounds, and scattered rhonchi, especially at the bases. There is always some degree of impairment of working capacity. In the third stage, dyspnœa leads to total incapacity. Right heart hypertrophy and then failure may supervene.

Radiographic Appearances

In the first stage of silicosis the radiograph shows the presence of discrete nodular shadows, circular, and at the most 2 millimetres in diameter. They may be partially distributed throughout the films, more widespread, or even generalized, but they remain discrete (plate X). Sometimes they are, in part, obscured by emphysema (plate XI). In the second stage the whole of both lung fields are occupied by nodular shadows, and there is some coalescence to form more or less dense opacities. In the third stage the radiographs indicate areas of massive consolidation. It is sometimes necessary to differentiate the X-ray findings from those of chronic miliary tuberculosis, sarcoidosis, berylliosis (plate I), miliary carcinomatosis, siderosis, and the hæmosiderosis of chronic heart failure (plate XIV).

Pulmonary Tuberculosis Supervenes

Pulmonary tuberculosis may be present in any stage of silicosis. It may alter the symptoms, physical signs, radiological appearances and the whole course of the disease (plate XII). It is the most frequent accompaniment of silicosis. Since tuberculosis of the lungs may simulate silicosis in radiographs, no diagnosis should ever be made exclusively on radiographic appearances.

Morbid Anatomy

At necropsy the lungs are generally large and retain their shape o removal from the thorax. Pleural adhesions are nearly always present an they may be extensive at the bases. On parts of the lung not covered b thickened pleura, the surface is studded over with pale grey nodules, eac of which is felt to protrude above the general surface and to be part of nodule which extends into the lung substance.

Silicotic Nodules

The cut surface of the lung shows excess of pigmentation throughou but the striking and distinctive feature is the presence of numerous roun

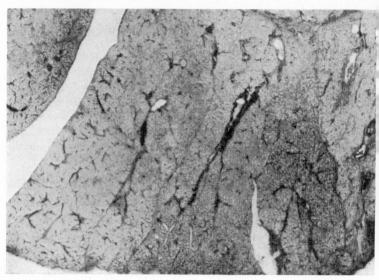

Fig. 370.—Large Tissue Section of Normal Lung, natural size

nodules. These are dense, tough and black or grey in colour (fig. 371) Each nodule is from 2 to 5 millimetres in diameter, but several may b aggregated together to form large composite nodules, or many may b united in a massive fibrosis. In long-standing cases, individual nodules ma be thrown into sharp relief by emphysema of the surrounding lung. Th centres of the nodules may undergo calcareous change. In cases wher exposure to dust has been intense and the course of the disease relativel rapid, the nodules may be so crowded together that practically no norma lung tissue can be seen. This condition is likely to occur in occupations such as sand-blasting, where there has been exposure to dust containing very high proportion of free silica. Histologically, the silicotic nodule is mass of concentrically laminated dense fibrous tissue.

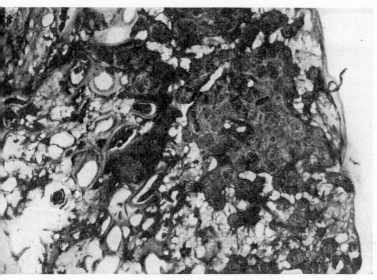

Fig. 371.—Large Tissue Section of Lung, natural size, showing Silicotic Nodules, both Individual and Confluent

Massive Fibrosis

Discrete masses of fibrous tissue, rounded or oval in shape, may be found centrally or peripherally situated in the lung, usually about the middle zones. The masses are nearly always bilateral and may be multiple, and frequently more extensive in one lung. In these cases the remaining parts of the lungs usually show discrete nodules. It is possible that the massive fibrosis is inflammatory in origin. Certainly the interlobar fissures are frequently obliterated by adhesions, and bands of fibrous tissue may extend from the periphery into the substance of the lung.

The Cuirass Form

There is a second form of distribution met with following exposure to very high concentrations of free silica dust. It is known as the cuirass form. In it there is a layer of fibrosis extending from the pleura to a distance of a centimetre or more into the lung substance, and frequently over its whole extent, and with nodules of denser fibrosis embedded in it.

Tuberculosis as a Complication

The presence of tuberculosis may render the diagnosis of silicosis at necropsy very difficult. Either the tuberculosis may be completely obscured by the silicotic process, or the silicosis may be obscured by the changes produced by tuberculosis, which may have left no unaltered silicotic tissue. In the first instance, the presence of tuberculosis may be determined only after the finding of tubercle bacilli in the lung or a positive result to animal inoculation. In the second instance, great difficulty ma be found in establishing a diagnosis of silicosis.

Changes in Lymphatic Glands

Changes in the lymphatic glands are important in the diagnosis c silicosis. The tracheo-bronchial groups are usually affected early in th course of the disease. At first enlarged, they are found in more advance cases of the disease, hard and, on section, dark-grey or black, often showin several concentrically arranged systems of nodular fibrosis. Parts of the cu surface may show white points or bands of fibrous tissue, or the whole c the gland structure may be replaced by fibrous tissue. Some glands in group may be more affected than others, and several stages in the replace ment of the glandular tissue by nodules may be seen. The lymphatic gland may show foci of tuberculosis, while tuberculous lesions are not apparer in extensively silicotic lungs.

Absence of Predisposition to Cancer

Considerable difference of opinion exists on the question whether th presence of silicosis has any influence in predisposing the affected lungs t develop cancer. The two diseases are certainly found together. From statistical study Kennaway found no occupation involving exposure to an kind of dust in which there was any very high incidence of cancer of th lung or larynx. It must be concluded that on the evidence at present avai able there is no justification for any statement that the presence of silicos predisposes to cancer in the affected lungs.

Properties of Dusts and Fumes

In order to understand the dust diseases it is necessary to know a goo deal about the chemical and physical properties of dusts and fumes, th behaviour of dust clouds and the reaction between them and the tissues c the respiratory tract. The nature of gases and vapours has already bee discussed (see p. 643). Unlike gases and vapours, both dusts and fumes ar composed of particles which, when airborne, can be inhaled into the lung Fumes consist of material in such fine particulate form as to resemble gase but which condense to solids at room temperature. Dusts, on the othe hand, consist of larger particulate matter suspended in air. It must b realized that these definitions are not rigid and that they merely indicat somewhat roughly different stages of attenuation of matter.

Particle Size of Dusts and Fumes

While dusts have been classified as particles or aggregates of particle from 150 microns to one micron in diameter, fumes from one micron t 0·2 micron in size, and smokes as particles less than 0·3 micron in diamete size alone represents at best only a rough separation of these three classe The mode of formation must also be considered. Thus dusts ordinaril result from vigorous mechanized attrition, blasting, grinding, drilling ubbing, crushing, hammering and sawing. In general they have the same hemical composition as the substances from which they are derived; they ave not been altered chemically by the process of subdivision. Fumes and mokes are formed and carried into the air usually as the result of chemical eaction, or some physio-chemical change, or the sudden dispersion of a hemically active substance by release of pressure or by explosion.

umes and Smokes

In industry, fumes are usually the oxides formed from hot or boiling netals. Thus lead fume produced in the smelting of lead is lead oxide, and inc fume from molten brass is zinc oxide, the particle size being between ·1 and 1·0 microns. In electric welding, iron oxide coming hot from the velding arc is a fume, but when it is in the form of rust knocked off an iron irder it is a dust. Smokes from burning carbonaceous fuel like coal, oil and vood contain droplets as well as dry particles. Tobacco smoke is typical of he wet smokes and is composed of minute tarry droplets of particle size bout 0·25 microns (Drinker and Hatch, 1954).

ogs and Mists

Mists are represented by atmospheric fogs and are essentially tiny iquid droplets, often microscopic in size, condensed about solid particles uch as carbon, as a nucleus. They are composed mainly of water, and their article size is of no particular importance, except that the particles must be n the microscopic range if they are to travel any distance. We have already een (p. 561) the importance of the drift of mist in agricultural spraying vhere the weed-killers used are poisonous to man. Another example of nterest in industrial toxicology is the mist entrained from the acid baths n chromium plating (p. 455).

Size of Vegetable Particles

No fine particles can float for long in still air unless their particle size is vell under 10 microns. The diameter of a red blood corpuscle is 7·2 nicrons, a white blood cell about 16 microns and a pollen grain of the ommon ragwort, *Senecio jacobæa*, about 20 microns. A person with 1ormal eyes can easily see an object 50 microns in diameter or pick up a hiny fibre of quartz 20 microns in diameter. Animal and vegetable dusts ncluding pollen grains can be air-floated, and if inhaled can produce hay ever and asthma in susceptible persons. Particles of this size become rapped in the nose and upper respiratory passages.

ize of Lung Alveolus

It is incorrect to assert that in occupational medicine we are concerned olely with dusts in the range 0·5 to 5·0 microns. In the sputum of men xposed in dusty occupations, in the ashed lung specimens of men who ave died of silicosis, and in the lungs of animals which have been dusted xperimentally, the most representative dust particle found measures about

1 micron in diameter. It is often assumed that anything larger than 3 microns in diameter cannot get into the alveoli of the lungs. But these structures measure up to 100 microns across and there seems to be no reason why particles much larger than 3 microns cannot get into them. Surely the factor which limits the size of dust particles found in the lungs is the diameter of the lymphatic channels and not the alveoli (McLaughlin, 1953).

Defence Mechanisms of the Body against Dust

Healthy lungs can deal with a certain quantity of dust or fume without becoming damaged. The defence mechanisms of the body against dust are briefly: (*a*) the vibrissæ of the nose, which act as a partial filter for the larger particles; (*b*) the mucous secretions of the nose and the upper respiratory passages, in which a large proportion of the particles is trapped and then expelled by (*c*) the wave-like action of the cilia of the nasal and bronchial epithelium. Below the respiratory bronchioles, where there are no cilia, (*d*) the phagocytes come into play. They engulf the dust particles and take them up to the area of ciliary action, or into the lung lymphatics. There is some doubt whether or not dust is taken into the lung parenchyma by phagocytic action, but the fact remains that dust does get into the lungs, whatever may be the exact method of locomotion.

Amount and Type of Dust Inhaled

The concentration of dust which can be inhaled without danger varies according to the nature of the dust and also to the length of time it is breathed. Again, the intermittent exposure to high concentrations of dust may be more dangerous than exposure to lower concentrations over a longer period. The harder the job is, the more deeply will a man have to breathe, and in consequence he will breathe more dust. In tunnelling through siliceous rocks for hydro-electric schemes in the Alps of France, Switzerland or other high mountains, the dyspnœa brought on by the high altitude increases the quantity of dust inhaled.

Individual Susceptibility

Individuals, too, vary greatly in their capacity to deal with dusts, and of two men who have been working at the same job for the same length of time one may get a disease of the lungs and the other may be unaffected. The reasons for the differences in individual reaction to dust are not accurately known, but it is likely that they depend on anatomical, physiological and biochemical variations from one person to another. It is known, however, that previous damage to the lungs is a factor which leads to the retention of dust in them. In any case, there are instances where people have spent many years in the dusty trades and have died from causes other than the dust diseases. On the other hand, many thousands have died as a direct result of the inhalation of dust.

Action of Silica on Lung Tissue

Although in silicotic lungs van Diemerbroeck (1672), Peacock (1860) and Greenhow (1865) all showed the presence of hard gritty material and isolated what they called *sand* from the ashed tissue, the manner in which this material exerts its effect on pulmonary tissue remained a matter for speculation.

The Mechanical Theory of Silicosis

It was first thought that the fine particles of stone dust cut and lacerated the tissues with which they came into contact. As viewed under the microscope the mineral particles certainly showed sharp edges and points, but it was nevertheless difficult to believe that such extremely fine material could cause trauma. As a consequence, doubts were early expressed as to the validity of this *mechanical theory* of silicosis. Two crucial experiments turned the attention of investigators to an alternative hypothesis. The first of these was by Gardner, who in 1923 brought convincing evidence against the mechanical theory by demonstrating that the dust of silicon carbide, which is extremely hard and has just as sharp edges as stone dust, failed to produce the typical fibrous reaction which powdered quartz dust would cause when placed in the lungs of animals. These classic experiments of Gardner's marked the beginning of the modern theories and investigations of silicosis. The second investigation which threw doubt upon the mechanical theory of silicosis was that of Gye and Purdy (1922). These workers produced in the lungs of mice treated with amorphous silica a lesion characterized by acute inflammation and necrosis, and in the liver a condition of necrosis by the injection of colloidal silicic acid. This work pointed to the possibility that stone dust might be harmful to the lungs, not because it was hard and sharp but because it produced a soluble substance which was toxic to the tissues. Policard (1933) showed that cells poisoned with silicic acid do not disintegrate and disappear as do other cells, but tend to preserve their structure in a fashion which suggests mummification.

The Chemical Theory of Silicosis

Kettle (1932) demonstrated that quartz particles which readily produced silicosis in animals would no longer do so if they were first coated with a layer of iron oxide, which did not alter their sharpness but which effectively prevented any part of their substance from going into solution. Thus the *chemical theory* or *solubility theory* of silicosis supposes that the fine particles of stone dust which get into the lungs are pathogenic, not because they produce microscopic trauma but because something of a toxic nature dissolves from their surfaces. This toxic substance is thought to be silicic acid, and it might be supposed that the pathogenicity of any stone dust would bear a direct relation to the rate at which it will release silicic acid into solution. Broadly speaking, this is usually the case (King and Belt, 1938). Quartz and flint, which dissolve to the extent of about 10 milligrams of silica per 100 millilitres of blood plasma, are the most patho-genic of the mineral dusts, and shale and mica dusts which dissolve to the extent of only about 1 to 2 milligrams of silica per 100 millilitres are among the least pathogenic.

Rôle of Silicic-acid Polymers

Nevertheless King (1947) was careful to emphasize some anomalies which are not easily explained by the simple solubility theory. Thus cement, which releases high concentrations of silicic acid in the body, is relatively harmless. The work of Holt and Osborne (1953) and of Holt and Yates (1954) suggests that the rôle of silicic acid in silicotic tissue is analogous to that of the muco-polysaccharides of high molecular weight which are present in normal fibrous tissue, and that only highly poly-merized silicic acids are capable of producing fibrosis. Ortho-silicic acid is formed at the surface of quartz particles at a low pH and, when neutralized by the tissues, the silicate ion must pass through the region of pH 5·5 to 6 in which polymerization is most rapid. Cement dust also dissolves to pro-duce a high concentration of silicic acid, but at an alkaline pH, so that in diffusing away from the dust particle the silicate ion is brought to the pH of the plasma without passing through the pH range in which rapid poly-merization occurs. Consequently, in the case of cement, large polymers (polysilicic acid) are not formed, and this may explain the relatively harm-less nature of cement dust.

The Immunological Theory of Silicosis

Even the complex solubility theory fails to account for some recently observed experimental facts, notably that with pure silica the toxicity is not necessarily proportional to solubility. Sakabe and others (1960) showed convincingly that prolonged grinding of quartz powder reduced its toxic effect on the intraperitoneal monocytes of rats despite an initial increase in solubility due to the formation around the basic crystal of a substance akin to amorphous silica. Pernis, Clerici and Bhezzi (1958) and Curran and Rowsell (1958) showed that capsules containing quartz and fitted with a membrane to allow the diffusion of interstitial fluids into and silica solu-tions out of the capsule failed to produce tissue reactions when implanted subcutaneously into rats and mice, despite a loss of silica from the capsules. This type of experiment demonstrates the necessity for contact between the tissues and the essential quartz crystal, as does the increase in toxicity of crystalline silica following washing with hydrofluoric acid or sodium hydroxide solution to remove the surface layer. Seifert (1958), Antweiler and Hirsch (1957) and other workers have demonstrated the deposition of protein on quartz crystals, and suggest that this is caused by the crystal lattice of crystalline silica, so giving the *matrix theory of silicosis*. Antweiler and Hirsch further suggest an immunological reaction, the quartz coated with protein being the antigen which produces homologous antibodies. A different immunological approach is that suggested by Vigliani and Pernis

(1960), following their investigations into the nature of the silicotic hyaline substance. They suggest that "the silica dust modifies the macrophages which have phagocytosed it in such a way that these set free substances, probably polysaccharides, which activate the reticulo-endothial system and are auto-antigenic." Thus the present concept of the action of silica is that of a biological action of the silica crystal itself, as opposed to polysilicic acids, setting in train an auto-immunological action. Whether quartz is antigenic or transforms proteins into auto-antigens, or whether quartz is simply an immunological adjuvant is a matter for further investigation.

The Occupations in which Silicosis Occurs

In reviewing these occupations it is found that in all of them the workers are exposed to the risk of inhalation of dust of uncombined silica, SiO_2, in the form of quartz, or the chalcedonic forms as flint, chert and Tripoli, and occasionally in an amorphous form as in kieselguhr and Neuburg chalk. The free silica may be the only constituent of the dust as, for example, in sandblasting with quartzose sand and in crushing flint, or it may occur in the dust mixed with other substances, either naturally, like the quartz in granite, or artificially like the ground flint in earthenware pottery. The characteristics of the diseases which result from exposure to pure silica and mixed dusts vary in a way which appears to bear a definite relationship to the mineralogical composition of the dust.

(1) The Gun-flint Industry

The flint-knapping industry in East Anglia represents the only survival in any civilized country of the most ancient industry of mankind. Progress in the design of firearms has of course reduced it to small proportions. Today it employs only a few part-time workers. At Grimes' Graves, Norfolk, three miles north-east of Brandon, Suffolk, across the Little Ouse which forms the county boundary, are to be seen the remains of extensive pits in the chalk sunk to the depth of 20 to 60 feet and numbering 254 in all. Through passages radiating in all directions neolithic man mined flint which occurs here in bands in the chalk. It is estimated that he was already making flint tools and weapons in this district as long ago as 6000 B.C. In these mine-workings numerous deer antlers which had been used as picks were found, and the flint miners of today use steel picks similar in shape to the deer-horn picks of their prehistoric ancestors (fig. 372). Flint-lock firearms were introduced about the year 1695. The percussion cap superseded the gun-flint in 1835. Today the flint is mined at Lingheath, south of Brandon, at a depth of about 30 feet and the large nodules are brought to the surface by hand.

Operations and Processes

The nodules (fig. 373) are conveyed to wooden sheds where the flints are shaped. The flint worker rests the nodule on a thick leather knee-pad and strikes it with a quartering hammer (fig. 374). The quarters are then

worked up on the pad into suitable cores, and from these flakes are struck
off with a flaking hammer. Operations are now transferred to the heavy
wooden knapping block. In a hole in the block is a steel stake which is
packed round with leather and is thus firmly held, not in contact with the
wood, but in such a manner that it possesses the resilience when struck
which is necessary to the proper knapping of flint.

The Art of Flint Knapping

The flake is held in loose contact with the front edge of the stake and is
struck a light blow with the knapping hammer. It is fractured by the
resulting upward blow on the underside of the flake due to the rebound of
the stake. In this way both ends of the flake are removed, leaving the central
portion which, after trimming, is the completed gun flint. This is thrown

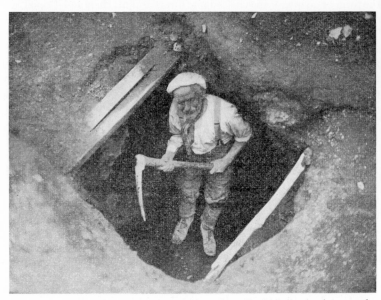

Fig. 372.—Flint Miner of Brandon with an Iron Tool similar in shape to the
Deer-horn Pick of his Prehistoric Ancestors
(*By courtesy of the Daily Mirror*)

into one or other of the receptacles standing on the block, according to its
size and quality. Often three or four gun flints can be made from one flake.
The art is one which requires a very high degree of skill. Gun flints are
made to standard sizes as judged by the trained eye of the skilled knapper.
These are known as wall piece, long dane, fowling, musket, carbine, horse
pistol, single pistol, and pocket pistol, and they vary from pieces $\frac{1}{2}$ inch to
inch in diameter. They are square, flat on one side and with bevelled edge
on the other side, the faces showing the typical conchoidal fracture of
flint (fig. 375).

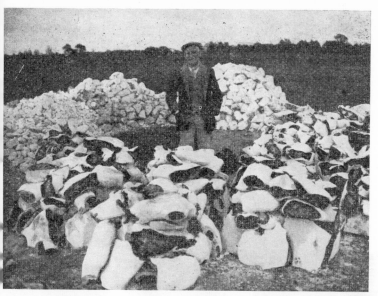

FIG. 373.—Large Nodules of Flint which have been brought to the Surface by Hand

(By courtesy of the Daily Mirror)

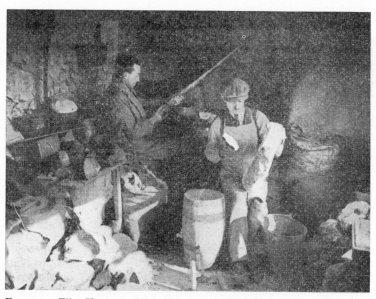

FIG. 374.—Flint Knapper of Brandon at work in his Shack. Resting a Nodule on his thick Leather Knee-pad he is about to strike it with his Quartering Hammer. Note the absence of Ventilation

(By courtesy of the Daily Mirror)

A Dying Industry

The flints are packed in small sacks of 200 and are exported for barterin with natives of Africa. Until the year 1835, when the percussion cap super seded the gun-flint, the bulk of flints used in the British Army were supplie by the Brandon workers. Flints were also exported to other countries, an there is no doubt that Napoleon's soldiers at Waterloo shot down Englis soldiers with firearms provided with Brandon flints. In 1800 the industr employed 200 men. In 1846 there were about 100 workers. In the nin

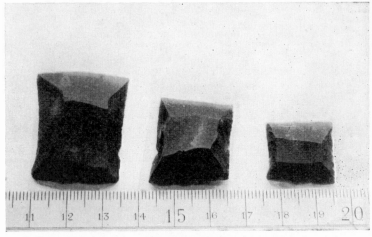

Fig. 375.—Bevelled Flints, actual size, as used for the Flint Locks of Guns, Pistols and Lighters
(*London Hospital Medical College Museum*)

years prior to 1889 sixty million flints were manufactured (Bridge, 1933 In 1896 there were about eighteen workers and in 1911 only twelve. B 1931 the industry was rapidly dying and only a few part-time worker remained to make a few gun flints for the old flint-lock firearms which ar still used in some parts of Asia and Africa.

Characters of the Dust

The flint knappers generated by their hammering a large amount fine flint dust. Middleton (1930) took samples of atmospheric dust breathing level of two men knapping flints. The counts gave up to 1,31 particles per millilitre with 2 per cent of particles over 2 microns in siz Most of the particles were under one micron in diameter. They worked ill-ventilated sheds and undoubtedly they had silicosis and suffered a hig mortality from phthisis. A similar state of affairs was described in 183 among the population of Meusnes in France when the gun-flint industr was introduced (Collis, 1915).

Methods of Prevention

As the workers maintain that the flint must be dry for proper working, water cannot be employed. Localized exhaust draught would be too costly for this decadent and precarious industry, in which no mechanical power is used. Respirators, standardized to protect against this very fine dust, would be difficult to attain, but at least partial protection might be afforded in this way and, together with the intermittency of the work and the possibility of working in the open air, as is done in summer, sufficient relief from exposure might be attained to carry the worker through his life without a disabling degree of silicosis (Middleton, 1930).

(2) The Sandstone Industry

The sandstone quarrying, mining and dressing industry represents perhaps the most widespread of all silicosis-producing industries in Great Britain. To a great extent, processes in cutting, shaping, dressing and crushing of the stone are carried out near the places where it is got from the quarry or mine.

Distribution

The sandstone-producing districts are the northern, central and south-western counties of England and the south and east of Scotland. Chepstow Castle and Liverpool Cathedral (fig. 376) are built of red sandstone, and Bristol Cathedral and Furness Abbey are part sandstone and part limestone. Early in the nineteenth century a good deal of Edinburgh was built in Craigleith sandstone, the supply of which is now exhausted. The famous pennant stone from the Forest of Dean is grey sandstone, that from Yorkshire is mostly brown, and a beautiful red sandstone is quarried in Corsehill,

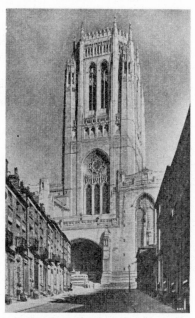

Fig. 376.—The Tower and South Porch of Liverpool Cathedral
(Photograph by Photochrom Co., Ltd.)

Dumfries (see p. 220). Other quarries are in or near Elgin, Alnwick, St. Bees, Carlisle, Penrith, Lancaster, Bolton, Bacup, Darley Dale and Matlock. Sandstone is found in many countries of the world; the Union Building in Pretoria is of local sandstone.

Characters of the Dust

Sandstones are sedimentary siliceous rocks containing from 75 to 95 per cent of free silica and consisting more or less of quartz grains mixed

with other minerals, and held together by a cement of varying compositi
and proportion. The composition, amount and hardness of the cement a
important factors in determining the dangerous characters of the dust pi
duced. In Great Britain about 12,000 men are employed on the process
in quarries, and in addition there are about 20,000 sandstone maso
employed in builders' and sculptors' yards throughout the country.

Operations and Processes

The workers include rock-getters who work at the stone face in quar
or mine; quarrymen or stone cutters who rough-hew the blocks; maso
who shape and carve the stone to dimensions and patterns; plane
sawyers and turners who operate stone-cutting machines; drillers wi
pneumatic hand tools; crushermen, labourers and cranemen; and builde
fixers, wallers or wallstone dressers who frequently do some dressing of t
stone. The action of wind has the most important beneficial influence f
workers employed in the open. Unfortunately, the worker is not alwa
able to stand to windward of the point of origin of the dust produced
neighbouring workers.

Work of Stonemasons in Closed Sheds

The stonemasons most particularly exposed to dangerous dust are t
banker mason, banker hand and banker hewer. Such men working
closed or partly closed sheds are liable to be exposed to dust produced
their neighbours as well as by their own work. Danger is increased by t
practice of brushing the dry dust and debris from the surface of the sto
and by blowing with the mouth while carving. Wetting the surface of t
stone by rain has some influence in diminishing dust, more especially
getting the stone from the quarry, but it has little effect in reducing t
fine dust given off by the action of a cutting tool.

Work at Stone-crushing Plants

Stone-crushing plants are frequently found in quarry sites for using
rubble to make road material. At the crushers, elevators and screens, den
clouds of dust are frequently given off and travel for considerable di
tances, so that though few workers may be employed on the crusher-hou
plant, many may be subjected to the dust produced by it.

Incidence of Silicosis

In 1929 Sutherland and Bryson investigated the occurrence of silico
in sandstone workers in England. They examined clinically 454 worke
and of these 266 were selected for radiological examination. Judged
X-rays, 112 of these men had silicosis. The workers most affected are t
stone masons and after them the quarrymen, rock-getters, planers a
wallstone dressers. Men who dig tunnels, sewers and graves in sandsto
may be affected too. The disease appeared to become more common aft
forty years of age, and after twenty years in the industry.

(3) The Granite Industry

The granite industry assumed importance in Great Britain after the destruction by fire of the wooden town of Aberdeen in 1741. The present Granite City was planned and gradually built up of stones fashioned in the local quarries. Although the art of polishing granite stones for ornamental purposes was carried out in ancient Egypt, it became a lost art until it reappeared in Scotland about 1820. Since that date the city of Aberdeen has become the centre of the monumental granite trade, and the building and monumental sections of the industry have flourished side by side (Mair, 1951). Today, more than 80 per cent of the granite used for the manufacture of monuments in Aberdeen is imported from Norway, Sweden and Finland.

Distribution

Granites and allied rocks of igneous origin are found in many parts of the world. They are characterized by a crystalline structure and a certain hardness or toughness which demands special methods for quarrying them and adapting them for use. True granites are found in the west and north of Scotland and in Cornwall, Devon and the Lake District of England. Other igneous rocks resembling granite are distributed in many parts of Great Britain.

Characters of the Dust

True granite consists of orthoclase feldspar, quartz and mica. The chemical composition is distinctly acid, there being from 65 to 75 per cent of silica. In intermediate rocks—for example, the syenites (p. 225) and diorites—the silica percentage varies from 55 to 60; while in the basic rocks, dolorite and gabbro, the silica content is from 45 to 55 per cent.

Operations and Processes

The occupations in the granite industry may be classified as follows:

(i) *Labourers* are unskilled workers employed in removing overburden, or loading and filling granite, and they may assist in blocking, getting or drilling.

(ii) *Getters* are skilled quarrymen who get the granite from the quarry face and roughly square it into blocks of suitable size. The group includes blockers and rockmen.

(iii) *Drillers* include workmen employed in using all forms of drills, including hand drills, steam drills, and wet and dry air drills.

(iv) *Settmakers* shape the setts or stone blocks for road material by means of hand hammers. They work in a shelter or open shed.

(v) *Kerb-dressers* are sometimes referred to as masons, particularly in Leicestershire.

(vi) *Crushermen* include all workmen employed in crushing mills a[i]
in concrete works. The group includes breakermen, screenmen, oile[i]
labourers about the mill and loaders.

(vii) *Building masons* are skilled workmen engaged in cutting a[i]
dressing granite in builders' yards. Some of these work only with ha[i]
tools, and others use pneumatic tools. The use of the pneumatic tool var[i]
considerably in different districts. In Cornwall it is used to a comparativ[e]

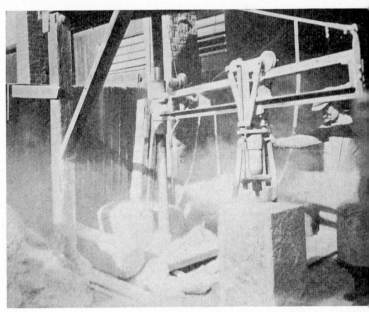

FIG. 377.—Dunter used for smoothing Granite. Note extensive Dust Clou[d]
produced in spite of the arrangement for providing localised Exhaust Ventilatio[n]

slight extent. In Aberdeen the pneumatic tool was found to be more
evidence among building masons. These pneumatic tools may be
cutting or surfacing. Building masons work in open sheds.

(viii) *Monumental operatives* or monumental masons. This group
cludes squarers, duntermen, finishers and turners working in monumen[t]
yards. The squarer uses a hand chisel and a pneumatic cutter. The dunt[er]
man is employed in operating the pneumatic dunter or surfacing mach[ine]
(fig. 377). The finishers use the pneumatic tool almost exclusively for th[eir]
work. Turners work with a power-driven lathe. The squarers can work[in]
a shed by themselves or in the same shed as finishers. The duntermen w[ork]
in widely open sheds in the yard. Turners are, as a rule, in the same sh[ed]
as the polishers.

(ix) *Polishers* are employed in monumental yards. Polishing is a [wet]
process; it may be done by hand but, as a rule, machinery is used.

cidence of Silicosis

In 1929 Sutherland, Bryson and Keating investigated clinically 494 orkers in granite, of whom 211 were examined radiologically. Judged by -rays, thirty-six of these men had silicosis. Examination of the radio-aphs in the positive cases classed as silicosis shows that the prevalent pe of the shadows indicating fibrotic changes is somewhat different from at found in workers exposed to silica dust in other industries. In the diographs of granite workers there are usually the increased hilar, linear d reticular shadows, but instead of the discrete, dense nodules found to a eater or less extent over the whole of both lungs, there is a diffuse, cloudy woolly effect with more or less definite fine or very fine nodules occur-ng in areas irregularly placed over the lungs. In the whole series the diograph showing the most discrete nodules of the silicotic type is in the se of a man who worked for nine years as a driller on granite, but had en employed for eighteen years as a tin miner underground. Amongst e other cases, who had been almost exclusively employed on granite, ere appears to be some relationship between the composition of the rock d the character of the fibrosis, as shown on the radiograph.

ifferent Type of Fibrosis

Clinical evidence of fibrosis, as distinguished from radiological evidence silicosis, was found in 260 cases, or 52·6 per cent of the 494 workmen amined; but X-rays showed silicosis in 17 per cent only. Comparing the sults of the medical examinations in the sandstone industry and the anite industry, the proportion of cases of fibrosis amongst sandstone orkers was 59 per cent of those examined, compared with 52·6 per cent in e case of granite workers. The proportion of cases of silicosis in sandstone orkers was 42 per cent of those radiologically examined, and 17 per cent the case of the granite workers. If fibrosis of the lungs, diagnosed by nical examination, be regarded as representing a slighter or earlier in-lvement of the same character as silicosis, then it would seem that anites and the igneous rocks of granite type produce less injury to the ngs than do the sandstone. Having regard to the appearances of the diographs in the two series of workers, there is a probability of a difference character of the types of fibrosis produced by the two kinds of dust, and is probability is increased by the proportion of cases of fibrosis in the anite series showing an approximation to that found in the sandstone ries, while the proportion of silicosis cases remains far behind (Middle-n, 1930).

(4) The Pottery Industry

We have seen (p. 65) how the Potteries began before there were canals railways, and how an export trade was established using packhorses and iles for the transport of raw materials and finished goods. Today the orth Staffordshire Potteries consist of the towns of Tunstall, Burslem,

Hanley, Stoke, Fenton and Longton, federated in the County Borough c Stoke-on-Trent. Before 1939 they gave work to 67,000 persons, of whor 55 per cent were women and girls. Among these, nearly 35,000 were em ployed in general earthenware, more than 10,000 in china, just over 18,00 in tiles, nearly 6,000 in sanitary earthenware and sanitary fireclay, abou 4,000 in electrical porcelain and just over 2,000 in Rockingham and je (Meiklejohn, 1946).

Calcined Flints for Chinaware

In 1720 John Astbury introduced finely powdered calcined flint int the body of his chinaware so as to produce on firing a remarkably whit and hard product. In 1865 in her *Life of Josiah Wedgwood*, Eliza Meteyar states that at first the flint, being used but sparingly, was kept in cellars an private rooms, and when reduced to powder in large iron mortars it wa passed through hair sieves. This process was slow and extremely injuriou as, in spite of every precaution, the dust was inhaled by the workmen an produced lung diseases of various kinds. She relates in detail how a painte employed in the potteries was struck by overhearing the story of the fata effects of the flint. It occurred to him that the crushing could be performe by millstones under water, and the adoption of this method led to a con siderable reduction in the amount of dust. Unfortunately, in the manufac ture of ceramics in certain circumstances the dry method for the milling c flint is still employed.

Branches of the Industry

The industry includes several distinct branches, sub-division bein determined by the nature of the article being manufactured and th materials entering into the composition of the ware. The principal division are: earthenware, tiles, sanitary earthenware and electrical fittings; china jet and Rockingham; sanitary fireclay; stone-ware; and coarse ware. Th occurrence of silicosis is especially associated with the first two groups— namely, earthenware and china—and the others will not be further con sidered.

Earthenware

In the manufacture of earthenware, the ingredients—ball clay, chin clay, china stone, feldspar and flint in a ground state—are mixed togethe in the form of liquid slip, from which excess water is removed by pressing The resulting composite body is made into the consistence convenient fo the manufacture of the various articles. So long as it remains moist it i harmless, but in the process of manufacture fragments fall on benches an floors or adhere to the clothing of the workers, become dry and give rise t dust. After the article has been made in the plastic form, partly dried, it i frequently smoothed on a revolving disc and fettled, to remove irregulari ties of surface and edges. The articles are then placed in fire-clay saggaı with some sand and fired in the oven. On removal from the oven th

osely adherent sand is brushed off. Subsequent processes of decoration
ıd glazing are not associated with the occurrence of silicosis.

hinaware

English china is made from calcined bone, china clay and china stone,
ıt it contains no added flint. The processes of making the articles are
ɪnilar, in general, to those employed for earthenware, but the articles
·quire much more support in the process of firing than do earthenware
ticles, and until 1937 to provide this support they were placed in finely
ɔwdered flint. The flint was prepared by calcining and subsequently
ushing it in the dry state. When the saggars of china ware were taken
ɔm the oven, the flint, which was used in placing the ware, was removed
ʏ women in a series of processes known as scouring.

ıcidence of Silicosis

Finally, after the ware was decorated and glazed, blemishes were re-
ɪoved by polishers, who frequently used finely powdered flint mixed
ith water as a finishing abrasive, on a rapidly revolving wheel. It will be
en that the exposure to flint dust in the pottery industry occurred in the
ɪocesses of the preparation of the flint by grinding; in the manufacture
˙ general earthenware, earthenware tiles, sanitary earthenware and
ectrical fittings, amongst those manipulating the earthenware body in the
astic and semi-dry states; in the manufacture of china, those employed
placing the biscuit ware in powdered flint and in removing the flint
ɔm it after firing; and in polishing the finished ware with the use of flint.
he serious morbidity and mortality from silicosis among china biscuit-
are placers and oddmen and china biscuit warehouse workers, when
.nt was the placing medium for the biscuit firing, have been fully recorded
ʏ Arlidge (1892), Sutherland and Bryson (1926), Middleton (1938), and
íeiklejohn (1949). So alarming was the hazard that ceramic chemists
ıd practical potters urgently strove to discover a safe placing medium,
hich could be used as a substitute for flint (see p. 997).

(5) Gold Mining

The prevalence of silicosis in certain gold mines has been of immense
ɪnportance to the industry, and the researches which have been carried out
ith a view to preventing the disease and providing compensation for in-
ıred workmen have contributed greatly to the sum of present-day know-
dge on the subject. This applies to important goldfields in several
ɔuntries, including those in the Transvaal and Ontario. In 1902 attention
as drawn for the first time to the disease known as *miners' phthisis* (fig.
58). Careful inquiry at that time showed that out of 1,377 men who had
een employed on rock drills in the Witwatersrand prior to the Boer War,
25 were known to have died from miners' phthisis between October
899 and January 1902, an annual death-rate of 73 per 1,000. Medical
χaminations of all white miners, of whom there were over 21,000 em-

ployed in 1934–5, are made twice a year. Miners have been recruited from other countries for work in gold mines and many of them return to their own country if they become disabled by silicosis. During each of the six years, 1930 to 1935, an average of twenty gold miners from South Africa died from silicosis in England.

(6) Tin Mining

Objects made of tin have often been found in tombs of Ancient Egypt. At some early date the Phœnicians obtained tin from England. The Greeks called the metal κασσίτερος and Pliny stated that it came from the *insulæ cassiterides*. In other words, the Romans went to the tin islands to exploit the Cornish mines. *Tinstone* or *cassiterite* is the sole source of commercial tin. It is stannic oxide (SnO_2) contaminated with copper pyrites ($CuFeS_2$), arsenical pyrites and other metallic sulphides. We have seen (pp. 5, 159) how the fortuitous association of tin and copper minerals in parts of Cornwall led to the manufacture of bronze at an early date. In the Cornish tin mines the mother rock is granite. The *Report on the Health of Cornish Miners* (1904) refers to the high mortality from respiratory disease among rock-drillers in the mines. Out of 142 deaths of rock-drill men, 120 were certified as from various forms of phthisis or *miners' disease*, and thirteen from other respiratory diseases. The majority of these rock-drillers had worked in other countries and ninety of them had worked drills in the Transvaal. There is no doubt, however, that silicosis has been caused by working in the tin mines of Cornwall, for thirty-eight of the rock-drillers referred to in the *Report* had worked in Cornwall alone.

Modern methods of dust suppression have greatly reduced the incidence of silicosis in this industry. The dust risk is greatest in the operations of drilling, shot-firing, and the shovelling of ore into trams. Although dust may be found lying thick upon ledges in the walls of the stope cavities, the amount of this redispersed into the air is probably insignificant save at the time of shot-firing. The disturbing of dust on the floor of levels by the feet of the men as they move about does not occur in the Cornish mines owing to the constantly wet state of the floor. When work has been done in an improper manner the atmosphere is comparable in appearance to that in a bath-room full of water-vapour. The measures employed to combat dust are natural ventilation, wet rock-drilling, mist-projectors and hand-operated water-sprays for directing water on the piles of broken ore before and during shovelling. The work is done in two shifts daily and shot-firing is done only at the end of a shift. During shot-firing all the men leave the mine, with the exception of the drillers, who withdraw to a safe distance upstream in the air-current, and wait to count their shots as they explode. Having done this they also leave the mine, which is then blown through with compressed air for not less than two hours and remains empty for not less than three hours. The familiarity of the skilled miner with dust is apt to result in carelessness. The penalty for offence, moreover, has not the immediate and dramatic quality which breach of the regulations is apt o produce in a coal mine, and close supervision of the miners is difficult because they work in pairs in widely scattered working-places. It is desirable that education in this respect should be authoritative, imaginatively planned, and continuous through the man's working life (Hale, 1946). Benign pneumoconiosis resulting from the inhalation of stannic oxide dust is described on p. 1053.

(7) Hæmatite Iron-ore Mining

Ferric oxide (Fe$_2$O$_3$) is widely distributed in nature as *red hæmatite*, from the Greek αἷμα, blood. Compact massive forms occur and include a reniform variety known as *kidney ore*. Much hæmatite occurs in an earthy form when it is termed soft red ore. The term *brown hæmatite* covers a class of hydrated oxides which may be represented by the general formula Fe$_2$O$_3$.nH$_2$O. The innocent effects on the lungs of the inhalation of iron oxide dusts are described on pp. 993–5. But the case for the hæmatite miner is different because he has to blast and excavate hæmatite deposited in detrital quartz.

We have seen (pp. 8 and 908) that hæmatite mining has been carried on in Cumberland since the Roman occupation. With the introduction of the dry pneumatic drill in 1913 the incidence of silicosis rapidly increased. During the six-year period, 1930 to 1935, forty-eight hæmatite miners were certified in England as having died from silicosis. No case was certified during the year 1930, and the numbers for the subsequent years were 10, 7, 6, 13 and 12 respectively. Until about 1930 silicosis had not been generally regarded as an occupational risk in this industry. At that time it was pointed out that the Cumberland and Lancashire group of iron-ore miners had a higher mortality rate than the rest of the ironstone group for phthisis and other respiratory diseases, while the maximum incidence for phthisis was at a later period. Since that time a form of pulmonary fibrosis, frequently accompanied by tuberculosis, has been proved to exist in this industry. The change in the outlook may have been brought about by a change in methods of working. About 1913 hand-drilling was replaced by machine-drilling and with it more frequent blasting was made possible.

The dust to which hæmatite iron-ore miners are exposed differs from that with which other workers come into contact who suffer from silicosis, and in view of this important point in the ætiology of the disease, it may be well to consider certain geological data. Much of the hæmatite deposits of Great Britain are precipitates from ferruginous solutions which must have been in most cases charged with CO$_2$, and such solutions would carry dissolved silica, which would be simultaneously precipitated with the iron, generally in the form of finely divided quartz. Also, in cases where the calcium carbonate of calcareous rocks has been replaced by iron compounds, all the insoluble siliceous constituents of the original calcareous rock will find their place in the newly formed iron ore.

Thus a siliceous limestone will give place to a siliceous iron-ore, in which the silica is mainly in the form of detrital quartz. Further, quartzose rocks may form one side of a lode of ore and these have often to be blasted and cut in order to work the ore-deposit. Insoluble residue of better-class ores amounts to 5 or 7 per cent, but rises to 15 per cent, mostly in the form of free silica, and in lower-grade ores the insoluble residue and free silica may rise to much higher figures. Some ore bodies may have definitely siliceous courses and the bounding wall of a lode may be highly siliceous (Middleton, 1938).

In the Cumberland mines in the years prior to 1935 the atmosphere underground was in a constant state of heavy pollution with hæmatite dust. The number of particles was never less than 4–5 millions per ml. Craw (1947) divided the radiographic changes in the miners' lungs into reticulation, nodulation and massive shadows. The reaction of the lung to mixed hæmatite and silica dust is usually mild and very slow. In the class known as X-ray reticulation the dust lies inert in the lungs yet is highly radiopaque and therefore throws a dense shadow. He introduced improved ventilation together with the Wetherill apparatus, a mist-projector producing a vapour-mist of minute particles of water containing one per cent of castor oil (fig. 395). In operation the holes in the rock face are first charged with explosive, the shot-firer then lights the fuses and on the way out he turns on the compressed air to set the atomizer in operation.

Craw introduced his new regime in 1935. Dust allaying by the mist projector diminished the dust content of the air to an average of 2,500 particles per ml. Medical control consists in selecting only fit men for work, radiographs of the chest being taken before admission and periodically thereafter. Uncomplicated pneumoconiosis or X-ray reticulation is not in itself an incapacitating condition. The single disabling and death-causing factor is infection, usually tuberculosis. Elimination of infected miners together with proper selection of new workers, and engineering control led to very great improvement in the first ten-year period.

(8) Coal Mining

In 1920 Middleton, working as a tuberculosis officer, recorded the toll of silicosis among men driving hard-headings in South Wales coal mines. Almost simultaneously the doctors of Radstock in the Somerset coalfield noticed a chronic lung disease in miners employed in *branching*. This work involves machine drilling in driving roads through highly siliceous sandstones called Pennant rock, grit or flag and known locally as *greys*. In 1924 one of these men died and the lungs at necropsy showed silicosis. In 1925 twelve of these rock-drillers were examined by X-rays; all but one were found to be suffering from silicosis, the one case being doubtful (Fisher 1935). A local study of the problem by Kemp and Wilson (1946) has confirmed the serious incidence of silicosis among Somerset miners engaged in drilling and blasting in Pennant rock.

Only a small percentage of coal miners develop classical silicosis. The processes underground in a coal mine which may involve exposure to silica dust are:

(i) *Ripping:* taking down the roof or top of a roadway, to make height.

(ii) *Brushing:* ripping or blasting of the roof and using the debris for building stone packs.

(iii) *Driving a hard-heading:* which is a drift, tunnel or roadway driven in rock or through hard measures.

(iv) *Driving a cross-measure drift:* which is driving a roadway in such a direction as is necessary to form a travelling road from stratum to stratum.

More than sixty names have been given to variants of this job (see p. 219). Hand drills and compressed-air percussive drills are used. The dusts met with in these processes are mainly those evolved from clift, bind or shale, which may contain as much as from 40 to 60 per cent free silica and rock, bastard rock or sandstone, in which the free silica may range from 60 to 85 per cent.

(9) Graphite Mining

The name graphite is derived from the Greek γράφειν (I write), and because in early days it was mistaken for lead it was called plumbago and black lead. Approximately 12 per cent of the world's graphite is used in pencils and crayons, whereas 60 per cent is employed in foundries and in making graphite crucibles for metallurgical purposes. Finely powdered graphite finds extensive use as a lubricant either alone or more commonly with grease. Graphite occurs in various parts of the world, always in association with quartz. Formerly, for many years Ceylon and Madagascar dominated the graphite market and they still have a virtual monopoly of high-grade crystalline graphite for crucibles.

Harding and Oliver (1949) found that samples of graphite from Ceylon, S.W. Africa and Korea contained from 3·6 to 10 per cent free silica; Parmeggiani (1949) states that in Italian graphite from Pinerolo free silica is about 11 per cent. The clinical, radiological and pathological findings in workers exposed to dust of graphite have been described by Dunner (1945), Dassanayake (1948), Gloyne, Marshall and Hoyle (1949), Dunner and Bagnall (1949) and Harding and Oliver (1949). The radiological evidence of pulmonary changes often preceded subjective symptoms, and occurred after ten to fifteen years or more; it included scattered nodular shadows, and rounded conglomerate masses which varied in shape and size and, in some cases, were seen to contain cavities; their presence was confirmed by necropsy. The clinical picture was that of a slowly developing silicosis, whereas the radiological and pathological findings more closely resembled those of pneumoconiosis of coal miners; copious black graphite-containing liquid was found in the lungs, with numbers of *graphite bodies* resembling asbestosis bodies in general form. The large amount of carbon probably acted by upsetting the expulsive power of the lungs and thus allowed the quartz to exert prolonged localized action.

(10) The Slate Quarrying and Dressing Industry

This industry is concerned with quarrying or mining the rock and making and shaping slates for roofing and other structural work. The large blocks of slate are conveyed to the mills, where they are sawn to sizes with power-driven saws cutting across the grain. The blocks are then split with chisel and mallet and cut to required sizes by hand or machine. Slate is the typical cleaved rock. The most important constituents quanti-tatively are silica, free as quartz, and combined as silicates of aluminium, iron, alkalis and other bases. In Penrhyn slates, quartz exists to the extent of from 35 to 43 per cent, while the total silica (free and combined) is from 58 to 63 per cent. Silicosis in slate-workers is sometimes referred to as slate-workers' lung or schistosis.

(11) Millstone Dressing

This is an occupation in which a comparatively small number of persons are employed. It consists in dressing the millstones for the grinding of corn in distilleries, corn and fodder mills, and for grinding chocolate in chocolate factories. The process is carried on in many districts throughout Britain where the mills exist. The persons employed may be specially skilled men

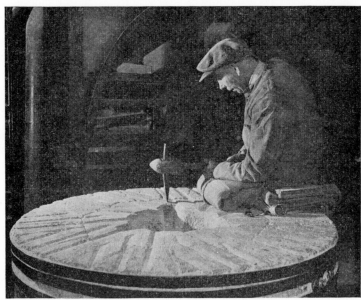

Fig. 378.—Workman dressing a millstone with an adze-shaped steel tool which he is using to chip radial grooves in the stone
(*By courtesy of John Pound & Son, Ltd., John's Lane Distillery, Dublin*)

who have learned the trade and are solely employed on the process, or the work may be done as a part-time occupation. The corn mills consist of two circular stones placed horizontally. They may be composed of any hard stone, but are usually a hard quartzite grit, chert or buhrstone, a chalcedonic form of silica, or artificial stones. Dressing of the stones is done with an adze-shaped steel tool, by chipping along the ridges which run radially from the centre (fig. 378). During chipping, a slight cloud of fine dust

·ises (Middleton, 1930). In the milling of wheat flour the introduction of
·teel rollers about the year 1877 removed the need for fashioning mill-
·tones from natural silica rock thus reducing considerably the number of
·nen who ran the risk of silicosis (p. 984). We have already mentioned the
·tigmata at one time commonly seen on the hands of the millstone dresser,
·amely dark blue pigmented scars due to fine steel chippings which had
·ntered the skin (p. 799).

(12) The Grinding of Metals

The processes which cause silicosis in the grinding of metals are con-
·ined to those in which grindstones composed of natural sandstone are used.
·he industries in which metal-grinding is an important process can be
·livided broadly into (i) the cutlery and edge-tool trades, and (ii) the
·nachinery, general engineering and foundry works.

Grinding may be done wet or dry and the metal being ground may be
·noved by hand or by mechanical power on a machine. In wet grinding,

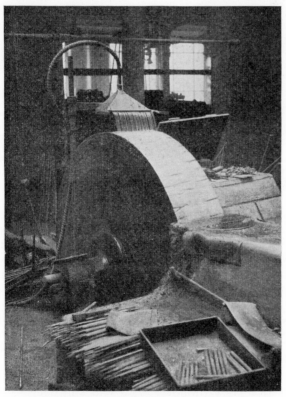

Fig. 379.—Dust Suppression at hacking and rodding a
Grindstone. Note the continuous Stream of Water
(By courtesy of Messrs. Platt Bros. & Co., Ltd.)

water is laid on from a tap or spray above the stone and is drained away
beneath it (fig. 379). Wet grinding is done by machines, especially in the
manufacture of files, saws and machine-knives, when the metal being
ground is fixed to a part of the machine which moves under or across the
revolving grindstone. The processes of dressing the grinding surface of the
grindstone are very important from the health point of view, on account of
the high concentrations of dust given off (fig. 380). Dust is produced by

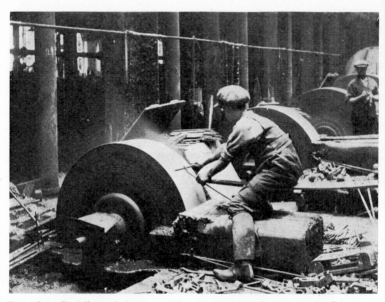

Fig. 380.—Rodding a Grindstone. Note the Cloud of Dust from the Sandstone
Wheel as the workman smoothes its Surface by bearing down upon it with a
Rod of Steel

(*By courtesy of Messrs. Platt Bros. & Co., Ltd.*)

attrition of the grindstone in all processes in the grinding of metal and it
varies in amount with the consistence of the stone, the hardness of the
metal, the shape of the article being ground and the amount of force
exerted (fig. 381).

The grinding of metals on sandstone wheels has been recognized for
generations as a cause of silicosis and an increased mortality from tuberculosis. A decline in the number of deaths has occurred from two causes:
(i) the change from sandstone to artificial abrasive wheels, and (ii) the
effect of stringent preventive measures in the grinding rooms. At the
coming into force of the Workmen's Compensation (Silicosis) Scheme for
the grinding of metals industry on 1st July 1927, there was a widespread
departure from the use of sandstone wheels and a corresponding adoption
of the artificial abrasive. Artificial abrasive wheels are composed of carborundum (silicon carbide, SiC) or some form of aluminium oxide, and contain
only a small proportion of silica or none at all.

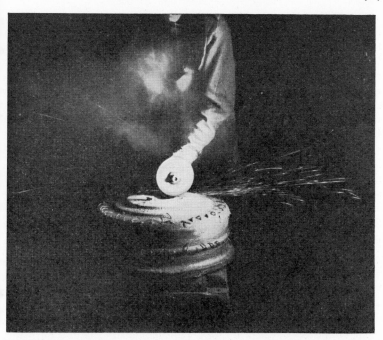

Fig. 381.—The workman is cleaning a Casting with a Portable Grinding Wheel. Sparks visible to the Naked Eye suggest that Dust is scattered laterally away from his Face. Photography using the Tyndall Beam shows a Vortex of Dust above the Wheel revolving in the same direction and travelling towards his Nose and Mouth

(By courtesy of Dr. A. I. G. McLaughlin, Mr. W. B. Lawrie and the British Institute of Foundrymen)

(13) Iron and Steel Foundries

The founding of metal is an ancient craft, so ancient that, under the weight of tradition, both employers and workers have regarded the hot, dusty, and dangerous conditions as inevitable; and industrial countries made no campaigns for better working conditions until about 1930. Metal castings vary in weight from less than an ounce to many tons. There are therefore widely varying types of foundries known as light, heavy and jobbing foundries. Some of these are mechanized. In Great Britain steel foundries are concentrated in Sheffield, Lancashire, Middlesbrough, South Wales and on the Clyde. Iron casting is mainly done in Falkirk, Birmingham and the Black Country. Foundries in the South of England handle chiefly non-ferrous metals. Foundry work employs large numbers of men. Its importance is seen in the motto adopted by the University of Birmingham Metallurgical Society: *The hand that wields the ladle rules the world.*

Processes involved in making a casting

Founding depends on the construction of complicated sand moulds which, with careful treatment, can be inverted and will stand up to the stream of liquid metal without being distorted. Sand used for moulding may be *naturally bonded*, in which case it holds together because it contains clay. *Synthetic moulding sands* are mixtures of silica sand with a *binder* such as ball clay, china clay or dextrin. In founding a *pattern* of the casting is first made, usually in wood. A mould is then made by ramming sand round the pattern so that when this is removed an impression of it remains in the sand. Molten metal is then poured into this impression and when it cools it forms a solid casting with the same shape as the pattern. If a hollow casting is required a sand *core* is prepared with its external surface conforming to the internal shape desired in the casting. The core is then placed in the impression left in the mould by the pattern so that the molten metal fills the space between the core and the mould. These cores are frequently made of oil-bonded sand and are baked to give them strength and rigidity. A complicated large mould may have over a hundred loose core pieces and take many days to make.

Foundry or Moulding Shop

Moulding sand used in foundries is generally excavated from quarries. There are excellent supplies of naturally bonded sand near Mansfield, Wolverhampton, Erith and Leighton Buzzard. The sand mixtures for moulds or cores are prepared either by hand or in a special sand preparation plant. The *moulders* make the moulds on a bench if the castings are small, on the foundry floor if they are medium in size and in a pit if they are very big. The moulding of the sand is done in a pair of *moulding boxes* which are rigid frames, generally of cast iron, for carrying and supporting the sand. A channel or *runner* must be cut through the sand in the one half of the mould so that liquid metal can be poured down this runner and flow into the cavity. One or more channels called *risers* must also be made, so that the cast metal fills the cavity in the mould and rises up the riser which also provides an outlet for gases. When the metal has solidified and the two halves of the mould have been separated, the casting remains attached to a neck of metal representing the runner which is subsequently cut off. After the metal in the moulds has been allowed to cool the moulding sand and cores are knocked or shaken away from the casting by the *knock-out*, the dustiest of all foundry operations.

Parting Powders and Silica Washes

In particular cases the moulder, as a final treatment, dusts the mould with a parting-powder which may consist of silica flour. A bench moulder may make as many as 150 boxes in a shift and because the parting-powder may be dusted twice on each box he may be enveloped during the shift in 300 dust clouds each having a high free silica content (McLaughlin and others, 1950). The most important forms of silica used for parting-powders are Tripoli and Neuberg chalk. Tripoli is generally regarded as a chalcedonic variety of silica, and contains about 97 per cent of silica. The substance generally known by the name is imported from Seneca, Missouri, and is of two kinds, which differ in their mode of origin but resemble each ther in composition. The name comes from Tripoli in North Africa, where the product is a true diatomite. Silicosis with tuberculosis has occurred from exposure to dust of Tripoli in England in men who had been employed for periods of ten years or more mixing ingredients in the manufacture of parting-sand. In foundries in the United States of America, as late as 1930, one could see a silica wash being used to face the moulds in steel foundries and observe this wash being applied with a spray gun. All persons in the immediate vicinity were then showered with a mist, of which the essential ingredients were water and fine silica made from ground flint, one of the most deadly silicosis producers known (Clark and Drinker, 1935).

Fettling Shop

In foundry work *fettling* or *dressing* means cleaning. The term *chipping* is applied to the use of tools to remove rough edges of metal from castings. The removal of adherent moulding sand and core sand is called *stripping*, *roughing-off* or *mucking-off*; it is done with hand tools or portable pneumatic tools. Small castings are cleaned and smoothed by *rumbling* in a revolving barrel in which they are tumbled against each other and some abrading agent. Abrasive blasting is carried out in chambers or cabinets making use of *sandblasting* or *shotblasting* by compressed air, or of the *wheel abrading machine*. After the castings are blasted they are sent to the fettlers or dressers who use *pneumatic chisels* as well as hammers, chisels and brushes to remove the burnt-on moulding sand and the rough edges of metal. Some castings are smoothed by *grinding* with *abrasive wheels* of carborundum, emery or alumina. In special cases the *hydroblast* is used for cleaning castings (see p. 1002).

Dusty Processes in Foundries

The main dust-producing processes in foundry work are those connected with the removal of the moulds and core sands from castings and their subsequent cleaning and dressing. Moulding and core-making are not particularly dusty jobs because the moulding materials are damp when handled. The preparation of sand, the application of parting-powders and the cleaning of moulds and metal plates with jets of compressed air are all dusty jobs. The knockout of castings and the dismantling and rebuilding of furnace linings and ladles also produce much dust. But the jobs in the fettling shop cause the finest dust so that fettling work with pneumatic chisels, sandblasting, shotblasting, wheelabrator work, portable grinder work, rumbling and stripping are all dangerous jobs so far as dust diseases of the lungs are concerned.

Steel Fettlers compensated for Silicosis

Macklin and Middleton (1923) carried out the first large-scale investigation into the chest condition of foundry workers in England. During a general enquiry directed especially into the health of metal grinders using sandstone wheels, they included in the survey examinations of 201 dressers of steel castings and found that 22·8 per cent had pulmonary fibrosis. Their work was done without the help of radiological and bacteriological examinations, their conclusions being made from clinical studies. In comparison, 73 per cent of a group of 495 wet sandstone grinders showed pulmonary fibrosis; the fettling of castings was therefore shown to be a less unhealthy job. It should be noted that at this time fettling was done mainly with hand tools; pneumatic tools came into more general use later. When the silicosis compensation schemes came to be formulated steel dressers, but not iron dressers, were scheduled as a group entitled to compensation for silicosis.

Higher Incidence of Lung Disease amongst workers in Steel

There are three reasons why the incidence of dust diseases of the lungs is higher in steel than in iron foundry workers. The melting point of steel is approximately 1600° C. as opposed to 1100° C. for iron. Therefore there is a greater tendency for the metal to penetrate the sand mould and cause *burning-on* of the moulding sand on steel than on iron castings. The *burnt-on* sand is difficult to remove and pneumatic chisels are used to clean steel castings, whereas hand tools usually suffice in iron fettling shops. The pneumatic tool breaks up the sand granules into freshly-fractured small particles which, when inhaled, are more active in producing silicosis. Finally, the mixtures used for making moulds for steel castings contain more free silica than moulds for iron castings. Steel moulding sand contains up to 99 per cent of free silica, whereas iron moulding-sands rarely have more than 80 per cent and usually have less.

Mixed Dust Pneumoconiosis in Iron Fettlers

Until 1943 the known cases of pneumoconiosis in iron foundry workers were few and they were not at first included in the compensation schemes. The difficulty about bringing them under such a scheme was partly due to the fact that hitherto the classical silicotic nodule had dominated the study of the pathology of the industrial diseases of the lungs. Any case in which classical silicotic lesions were not found could not be diagnosed as silicosis and hence was not eligible for compensation. But the inhalation of mixed dusts containing free silica and other dusts such as iron oxide tends to retard the development of classical silicosis. New pathological studies culminating in the work of McLaughlin and others (1950) showed that the main lesion in the lungs of iron foundry workers, particularly iron fettlers or dressers, was another type of nodule with a linear and radial pattern as opposed to the whorled arrangement of fibres in the classical silicotic nodule. To this type of lesion Harding, Gloyne and McLaughlin applied the term *mixed dust pneumoconiosis* or *mixed dust fibrosis*. The survey directed by Dr. A. I. G. McLaughlin was a concerted effort by employers, trade unions, Government departments, statisticians, pathologists, radiologists, clinicians and engineers. The investigation included the results of clinical and radiographic examinations of 3,059 workers in 19 foundries, an analysis of the records of lung disease in foundry workers in the files of the Factory Department and the Silicosis Medical Board, pathological investigations of the lungs of 64 foundry workers and dust surveys in three foundries. As a result of this work, under the *Iron and Steel Foundries Regulations, 1953,* which became fully operative in 1956, iron foundry workers are protected by special regulations and paid benefit if they develop pneumoconiosis.

(14) Amorphous Forms of Silica

We have seen that amorphous forms of silica are used as parting-powders in foundry work, but in addition to this they are used as polishing compositions and also in the manufacture of steel.

Neuberg chalk is a natural deposit of siliceous material occurring at Neuberg on the Danube. The composition varies somewhat in different localities and the silica content is sometimes given as from 65 to 86 per cent. Besides free silica it contains from 7 to 8 per cent kaolin, and traces of iron and magnesium. There are indications that silicosis has followed exposure to the dust. In one factory six of the men employed on a process in which this material was used for periods from three and a half years to seventeen years had died of tuberculosis or silicosis with tuberculosis. Following this experience, examinations were made and early signs of silicosis were found in three men. In another factory one or two of the men who had been employed ten and twelve years on the process showed early signs of silicosis.

Diatomite (kieselguhr, diatomaceous earth) is composed of minute siliceous skeletons of aquatic plants of marine or fresh-water origin. When pure it contains up to 96 per cent of silica, but it may contain alumina, iron, lime, magnesia and alkalis, reducing the silica content to about 75 per cent. It is used as a mild abrasive or polishing medium, as filtering material and for insulating purposes. Where men handled a diatomaceous deposit in Santa Barbara County, California, which yielded, when dry, a silica content of 85 per cent, much dust was produced in conveying, grinding, drying and bagging. Clinical and radiological examinations were made of 108 men, and silicosis was found in 81 (68·5 per cent); very early in 15, early in 45, moderately advanced in 15, and advanced in 6.

In a process in the manufacture of steel, in which a number of men had been exposed to dust of kieselguhr for six years, in Great Britain, radiographic examination showed more fibrosis than usual, with very early indications of a modified form of nodulation in some of them (Middleton, 1938).

(15) Flint Crushing

Flint, a chalcedonic form of silica, is crushed for making chicken grit, sandblasting grit, abrasive papers and brake-sand for tramcars. The flints may be first calcined, in order to make the material more friable and whiter, before crushing. High concentrations of dust are produced at the crushing and screening processes and it is an extremely difficult problem to control and dispose of it. Sand becomes dangerous when it is dried and manipulated in such a way as to give rise to fine particles of quartz dust. This occurs in sieving dried sand for sandblasting, for facing bricks, in the manufacture of glass and other products, and in mixing dried sand with other substances.

(16) Silica Milling and the Manufacture of Abrasive Soaps

These processes may be carried on in the same factory, but more usually silica milling is done in one factory and the ground material is supplied to manufacturers of abrasive soaps. The silica may be quartzite rock containing over 90 per cent of silica, or crystalline quartz, or quartz-sand. It is dried, crushed and ground to a fine powder by machinery, which is totally enclosed and provided with exhaust draught to remove dust. In the manufacture of abrasive soaps, ground silica is mixed with powdered soap and anhydrous sodium carbonate. Dust is produced in the processes of mixing, sieving and packing the powders. About 1928, numerous firms who had no knowledge of the dangers of exposure to the dust and were inadequately provided with protective measures became engaged in this manufacture. This resulted in the occurrence at one factory of three or four cases of respiratory disease which was regarded as an acute form of silicosis. The manufacture began in England in 1910, but was not important in quantity until 1921, and in 1928 it was given up owing to the death of workers attributed to the inhalation of the dust (Middleton, 1938).

(17) Refractory Products

This industry has a special interest in relation to silicosis, because it was the first to which the Workmen's Compensation (Silicosis) Act, 1919, was applied. It is engaged in the manufacture of refractory materials which contain over 80 per cent of total silica and are used in the construction of furnaces, flues and crucibles.

It is a small industry; some 3,000 workers are employed in Britain. The processes include the quarrying or mining of the raw material, usually a sandstone of the coal measures called ganister, which occurs in open quarries and in mines, or, in some localities, sands or pocket-clays are used. The raw material, which contains usually from 92 to 98 per cent of silica, is crushed, mixed with suitable bonding substances, and made into silica bricks, silica cement, steel-moulders' composition and similar products for use as refractories in the manufacture of metals, especially steel or steel castings, and in the construction of gas-retorts and flues. Mechanization is improving conditions in the manufacturing processes, from the health point of view, especially with the use of continuous kilns which the workers do not enter.

(18) Sandblasting

This is the process of projecting sand or other grit, by means of compressed air or steam, or by the centrifugal action of a wheel against a surface. It was introduced about 1904 and is used:

(i) In metal works to remove adherent sand and irregularities from castings.

(ii) To produce, on clean metal, a surface suitable for subsequent treatment by coating with enamel or another metal.

(iii) For etching glass and treating other non-metallic articles.

(iv) For removing paint from, and otherwise cleaning, large surfaces, as of ships and buildings.

Sandblasting of metal articles can be carried out in various ways. For large articles the operator works in a specially constructed room, and he is protected by special clothing and a helmet which is supplied with pure air under pressure (fig. 382). The dusty air is removed from the room by exhaust draught. Smaller articles are treated in a closed cabinet, the worker passing his arms through guarded holes to direct the abrasive while watching the process through a glass panel. Other types of apparatus are the mechanical turntable and revolving barrel, in which the sandblast is directed from a fixed point and close application of the worker is not necessary. Wheel abrading machines vary in design, but in all of them a rapidly revolving wheel projects the abrasive against the casting. Such machines are operated outside the blasting enclosure.

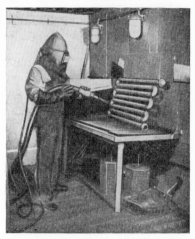

FIG. 382.—Sandblasting Cabinet, open only for purposes of Photography. Note Air Line to Helmet

(Johnstone, R. T. (1948), Occupational Medicine and Industrial Hygiene, The C. V. Mosby Company)

The dust hazard is from the abrasive when this consists of quartzose sand, crushed flint, quartz, quartzite or granite. On hygienic grounds, metal grit and certain other non-siliceous abrasives have now replaced the siliceous material to a considerable extent, and where these are used on clean metal no siliceous dust is produced; when they are used for cleaning metal castings, however, dust is produced from the adherent moulding sand, which is highly siliceous (see p. 999).

There is no doubt that sandblasting, and to a lesser extent shotblasting, is a dangerous occupation if adequate precautions are not taken. Risks are incurred by workers by faulty or careless methods, or through defects in the appliances, which require constant attention for maintenance. Silicosis is found amongst sandblasters in various parts of the world, and the same features—a short period of employment and rapid course of the disease—characterize all the cases. In 1936 Merewether surveyed the silicosis risk in sand and shotblasters in Great Britain, and showed statistically that the average duration of employment of sandblasters who

ultimately died of silicosis was 10·3 years as compared with 40·1 years
which was the average duration of employment of all fatal cases of
silicosis irrespective of the causative occupation. Of course the men
themselves are aware of the hazard. Thus in 1934 in a works in Coventry
they put up a notice:

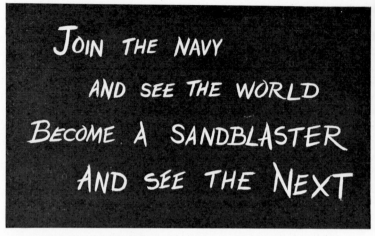

JOIN THE NAVY

AND SEE THE WORLD

BECOME A SANDBLASTER

AND SEE THE NEXT

FIG. 383.—Notice chalked up in a foundry in Coventry in 1934

Prevention of Silicosis

In order to be certain that people will not get silicosis, it is clear that
harmful dust must not get into the air which they breathe. But this presents
great difficulties because many factory processes and most types of mining
are inherently dusty. Nevertheless, dust clouds *can* be controlled, sometimes partially and sometimes completely.

No Room for Complacency

All silicosis is man-made. On the subject of its prevention there is no
room for complacency, because the figures for deaths are going up every
year. Thus in 1956 in Switzerland at an altitude of 7,500 ft. in the Alps of
the Canton Valais quartz dust was still producing silicosis amongst tunnellers working on the vast hydro-electric scheme known as La Grande
Dixence (fig. 384). While it is true that dust suppression by wet rock-
drilling was applied in the larger tunnels there were many small tunnels
where all the drilling was done dry. Why? Things like this still happen in
spite of the fact that at no time in history has more attention been given to
the problem by doctors, engineers, chemists, physicists and others; by
organizations and individuals; and by employers and trade unions. The
practical details of dust control are largely in the domain of the engineers.
But the problem is primarily one of health, and it is the business and the
duty of doctors to lead the campaign and to inspire the engineers, if
necessary, to greater efforts (McLaughlin, 1953).

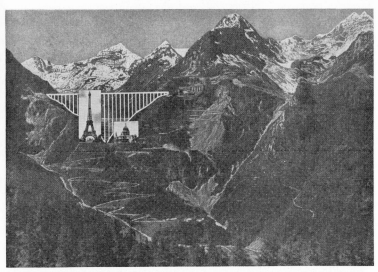

FIG. 384.—La Grande Dixence, a hydro-electric scheme in the Valais Alps of Switzerland. The concrete dam is 932 feet high, that is nearly three times the height of St. Paul's Cathedral (365 ft.) and 52 ft. less than the height of the Eiffel Tower (984 ft.)

Basic Principles of Prevention

Not only can dust be controlled, but in some instances the process can be altered so that no dust is formed. Again, it is possible, occasionally, to replace the substance which gives rise to the dangerous dust by another which is non-toxic or at least not so harmful. But in this event the process will still be dusty if dust control is not applied. There are some jobs in which it has not been possible, up to the present time, to control the dust, and in these it is necessary for the workers to be protected by dust respirators or by breathing apparatus. The basic principles of the prevention of silicosis can be considered under the four headings: (i) replacement of the harmful material by a less toxic one; (ii) dust suppression or control; (iii) personal protection of the worker, and (iv) medical examination.

(1) Replacement or Substitution

In England today, in spite of the tradition to build in dolomite or limestone (p. 357) which goes back 350 years to Inigo Jones, we still build some of our cathedrals and other buildings in sandstone. Now it is very difficult to provide satisfactory protection against silicosis for sandstone banker masons. For the building of Liverpool Cathedral (fig. 376) the red sandstone of the Woolton quarries should have been left in the ground and dolomite brought into the Mersey from Portland Bill just as it was brought into the Thames to build the new Waterloo Bridge. For both limestone and dolomite afford superb and beautiful building stones the shaping of which produces only innocent dust. Grasping this point

Queen Juliana of the Netherlands passed a law in 1951 making it difficu᷈ or impossible for builders in Holland to obtain a licence to use sandstor᷈ in building (fig. 385). Though the principle of replacing a harmf᷈ material by a less dangerous one is of the first importance, it is not alway᷈ practicable to put it into operation. For instance, coal gives rise to eno᷈ mous amounts of dust, but is indispensable. But when the material givin᷈

STAATSBLAD

VAN HET

KONINKRIJK DER NEDERLANDEN

No. 443 BESLUIT *van 4 October 1951 tot vaststel- ling van een algemene maatregel van bestuur, ais bedoeld in de Silicosewet (Zandsteenbesluit).*

WIJ JULIANA, BIJ DE GRATIE GODS, KONINGIN DER NEDERLANDEN, PRINSES VAN ORANJE NASSAU, ENZ., ENZ., ENZ.

FIG. 385.—Regulation signed by Queen Juliana of the Netherlands restricting the use of sandstone for builders in Holland

rise to a dangerous dust can be replaced, then the danger can be eliminate᷈ Thus limestone, $CaCO_3$, has replaced kieselguhr, SiO_2, for use in the slo᷈ cooling of steel ingots, and zircon, $ZrSiO_4$, can be used instead of silic᷈ flour for mould paints in foundries. There are at least four industries i᷈ which the principle of replacement has been applied on a large scale— namely, flour milling, metal grinding, the pottery industry and sand᷈ blasting.

Flour Milling and Metal Grinding

The first of these is flour milling. About the year 1877 the introductio᷈ of steel rollers for milling corn removed the need for fashioning millstone᷈ from natural silica rock (see p. 984). The second is the grinding industry᷈ For many years grinding wheels made of natural sandstone were used i᷈ the cutlery, edge tools and other trades. In fact, the natural abrasives— hard, gritty materials, most of them siliceous rocks—have been used i᷈ various forms for sharpening, grinding and polishing for 3,500 years. Thes᷈ substances were at one time quarried in vast amounts—for example Grindstone City, Michigan, in the years between 1835 and 1929 produce᷈ 25,000 tons of natural silica stones each year.

Discovery of Synthetic Abrasives

And then in 1891 Edward G. Acheson, of Monongahela, Pennsylvania᷈ made the first synthetic abrasive, silicon carbide, SiC. Seeking to syn᷈ thesize diamond, he was heating clay and coke in an electric arc. H᷈ obtained a product as hard as the natural abrasive corundum, Al_2O_3, an᷈ wrongly thought that what he had produced was a compound of carbo᷈ ith corundum, hence *carborundum*, a misnomer adopted as a trade name or silicon carbide. It has a hardness of 13, compared with 15 for diamond and 10·5 for sandstone. The method of manufacture is simple; sand, coke and sawdust being fused in the heat of the electric arc. Cheap hydro-electric power played its part, especially at Niagara. In 1899 fused alumina, Al_2O_3, or *synthetic emery*, was added to the manufactured abrasives. By 945 the United States of America was making 30,000 tons a year of artificial abrasives.

Reduction of Silicosis among Grinders and Foundrymen

Since about 1923 sandstone wheels have gradually been replaced by wheels made of carborundum, emery or alumina, so that now sandstone is barely used for any grinding or polishing job. Though it is not certain that the dust of silicon carbide is completely harmless, it is so much harder than sandstone that it gives off much less dust. The number of cases of silicosis among grinders has been dropping year by year and, with the exception of those who grind castings on which there is burnt-on sand, there should be no cases of silicosis among grinders by about 1975. A new ceramic material silicon nitride, Si_3N_4, was introduced in 1964 to make cores for the casting of turbine blades for jet aircraft. It is fair to assume that this substance will not cause silicosis in workmen making or handling it.

The Pottery Industry

Another instance in which it has been possible to replace a siliceous substance by a less harmful one is to be found in the pottery industry fig. 386). In the placing of biscuit ware in the saggars so that they can be fired in ovens, it used to be the practice to embed the china articles in ground flint, which is nearly pure free silica (see p. 978). The incidence of silicosis amongst this group of pottery workers was high, but since about 937 calcined alumina, Al_2O_3 has been used to replace flint both for placing china ware and for polishing articles of pottery (fig. 387). Since then the number of cases has been getting less. The introduction of this safe substitute for powdered flint has been regarded as one of the major achievements in the prevention of silicosis. Indeed Plant (1939) a leading china manufacturer and humanitarian, described 1937 as the *annus mirabilis* of the Potteries. In 1957 the Mass Radiography Service at Stoke-on-Trent examined 97 biscuit placers and oddmen at the china factories in north Staffordshire; 87 of these men, exposed to alumina only, showed no radiographic evidence of pneumoconiosis; the other 10 who did show such evidence had been exposed also to other dusts known to cause pneumoconiosis (Meiklejohn and Posner, 1957).

Sandblasting and Shotblasting

A fourth example of replacement is seen in the process known as abrasive blasting. In this job a stream of abrasive material is blown under high pressure at articles to clean them. It is used, for example, in the foundry industry to clean castings; it is also used to etch glass and to smooth the

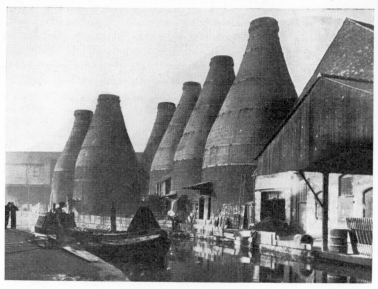

FIG. 386.—The Potteries
(Reproduced by permission of the Sunday Times

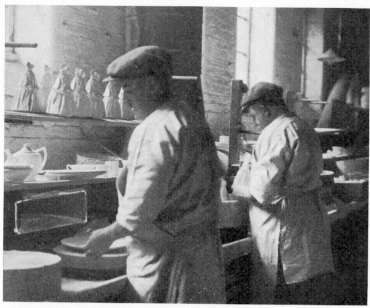

FIG. 387.—China Biscuit placing in the Potteries. The workman is seen placing a
Plate in a Bed of Alumina which is a safe Substitute for Powdered Flint. Note
the Exhaust Ventilation locally applied
(By courtesy of Messrs. Doulton, Ltd.)

urfaces of metal before it is painted or enamelled. About 1904 sand was
introduced as an abrasive, and though the number of workers was small,
he incidence of silicosis and tuberculosis was high and the disease came
n quickly (see p. 993). Since about 1920 sand for blasting has been
lmost entirely replaced by other abrasives such as steel grit or shot and
alcined alumina, aluminium oxide grit. The use of sand in blasting opera-
ions is now prohibited by the *Blasting (Castings and Other Articles)
Special Regulations, 1949.*

(2) Dust Suppression or Control

Ventilation may be either local or general.

General Ventilation

General ventilation is usually obtained by having open doors and
windows, but this practice is not popular in cold weather and it puts up the
ost of heating the workrooms. Air-conditioning is being adopted in some
industries with good results. For this type of ventilation, in which filtered
air is blown into the room and extracted by fans, the doors and windows
should be kept closed. Where there are furnaces or ovens in a workshop,
advantage is taken of the upward currents of air caused by the heat. In
these rooms the incoming air is brought in low down in the walls and the
outgoing air is extracted through the roof. By contrast, in rooms in which
here are no hot processes, the air currents are reversed. For example, in a
room in which castings are cleaned, the air is blown in high up, either
through the roof or the walls, and the air exits are placed low down.

Local Exhaust Ventilation

When dangerous dust is given off, general ventilation is not enough
because it allows the dust, even though it may be diluted, to get into the
workers' breathing area. In these cases local exhaust ventilation should be
installed. This consists of a hood, placed as near as possible to the source of
he dust, and a duct leading from the hood to a fan which creates a current
of air to draw away the dust. It may be taken to a dust collector or be discharged to the outside air. Exhaust ventilation has been applied to many
industrial processes, but it is never really satisfactory unless it is combined
with enclosure of the process. An example of this is the chemical fume cupboard, and the principle can be and has been adopted in many industrial
processes with excellent results.

Changing the Process

This can be illustrated by the experiments now being made to avoid the
use of the pneumatic tool for the fettling of castings. Attempts are being
made to burn off the sand adhering to the castings with a very hot flame
produced by acetylene, air and a fluxing powder. Though iron oxide is
given off in the fume, no harmful dust is evolved, and altogether it is a
promising development. Another way to avoid the use of the pneumatic
tool is to put the casting into an annealing furnace, in which a great deal of

the burnt-on sand is removed from the casting. However, the fundamental method of tackling this problem is to control the technique of moulding and casting in such a way that the casting comes clean away from the mould so that the use of the pneumatic tool or any other method of cleaning is not necessary. In one foundry, where clean castings are the rule, there has been no case of silicosis for about ten years. This is the ideal way of getting rid of a health risk, but so far it has not been possible to apply it generally (McLaughlin, 1953).

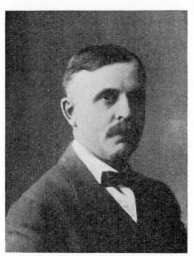

FIG. 388.—John G. Leyner
(Holman. T. (1947), Brit. J. industr. Med., 4, 1)

Isolating the Process

If the dusty process can be isolated from other parts of the factory, the number of people exposed to the risk can be reduced. In some foundries all processes, from sand preparation and core-making to the final cleaning of the castings, are carried out in one large workroom. The dangerous dust created in fettling becomes distributed through the workroom and affects to some degree all groups of workers. If the coremakers who handle damp sand work in a separate room, they in-

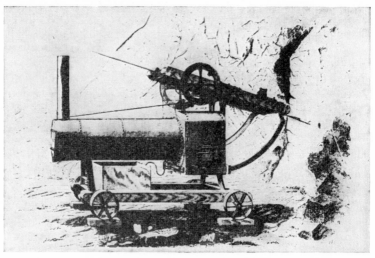

FIG. 389.—The first Percussive Rock Drill, made by Couch in Philadelphia
in 1849
(Holman, T. (1947), Brit. J. industr. Med., 4, 1)

hale little or no dangerous dust. In general, the best policy is to isolate as far as possible all dusty processes, and to protect the workers engaged in them by good general and local ventilation together with personal protective methods. A less satisfactory way, but one which is better than nothing, is to operate a dusty process at night when the other workers have gone home. In some foundries the *knockout*, that is stripping the castings away from the sand moulds, is done at night.

Wet Rock Drilling

Water, foam and oil may be used for allaying dust. In hard-rock mining, wet drilling is widely used. John G. Leyner, of Denver, Colorado, has been called the outstanding mechanical genius of rock drilling (fig. 388). In 1897 he brought to practical success the principle of the pneumatic-hammer drill (figs. 389, 390). A blast of air was blown through a hollow drill-steel to remove rock cuttings from the hole. This produced so much dust that the drill became known as the *widow maker*, and miners refused to use it. In 1898 Leyner obtained a patent on the commingling of air and water in the drill-steel (fig. 391). This is the principle of the axial water feed and is the basis of all wet rock drilling (Holman, 1947). The adoption of the method had to wait upon the invention of suitable steel alloys, but by 1920 it was in use all over the world. As an engineering device it cools the drill and clears the chips of rock most efficiently from the hole: happily it also suppresses dust (figs. 392, 393).

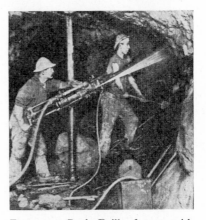

FIG. 390.—Rock Drill of 1902 with Water Spray
(*Holman, T. (1947), Brit. J. industr. Med.*, **4**, *1*)

The Dryductor and the Mist Projector

Where wet drilling proves impossible or objectionable, foam-drilling equipment can be used. By means of compressed air a viscous foam is forced through the drill-steel from a closed vessel. Although the foam traps the dust, the method has the defect that when the bubbles burst they may release dust particles. Since the tungsten-carbide bit need not be cooled and will last for 300 feet of drilling as against 10 feet in the case of steel-alloy drills, a new drill called the *Holman dryductor* has been perfected which sucks the dust back through the axial channel in the drill steel and ejects it into a dust collector (Holman, 1954). Near the rock face after shot-firing (fig. 394), a mist projector is used to allay dust (fig. 395). It is really an atomizer using compressed air and spraying a mixture of castor oil and water in which the proportion of oil to water is about 1 in 100. After shot-firing nobody may enter the area until eight hours have elapsed for the dust to settle (fig. 396).

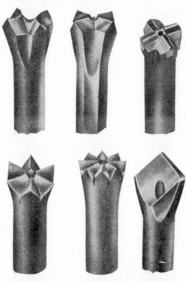

FIG. 391.—Various Patterns of Hollow Drill-steels. The most efficient Bit (top right) is of cemented Tungsten Carbide

(*By courtesy of Mr. Treve Holman*)

The Hydro-blast for cleaning Castings

An apparatus used to clean certain types of casting, and the safest yet devised, is known as the hydro-blast. A high-velocity jet of sand and water is projected on to the castings, thereby removing moulding material, cores and scale. The velocity of the water as it leaves the hydro-blast gun is in excess of 3 miles per minute (fig. 397). It can be readily understood that this apparatus has greatly improved the cleaning of castings and much reduced the dust in the atmosphere of fettling shops where it has been installed. When it was first introduced it was hoped that it would take the burnt-on sand away from the castings and so avoid the use of dusty methods of fettling or cleaning. Unhappily, this hope has not been realized, because the cleaning has to be completed in the shotblast or wheelabrator chambers or even with pneumatic tools.

Inefficiency of Wet Methods

New methods of dust control by water are devised from time to time. Thus the *First Report of the Joint Standing Committee on Conditions in Iron Foundries, 1956*, describes in particular a new type of wet decoring bar for use in foundry work. But although wet methods for dust suppression are a great deal better than nothing it should be pointed out that water is not as efficient as good exhaust ventilation in controlling dust. The finest particles are not brought down by water; indeed, they may actually be held in suspension by droplets in the air. Investigations have shown that in wet grinding, for instance, there may be more dust present in the air than when the grinding is done dry under efficient exhaust ventilation. If the damp dust is not removed, it will become dry and contaminate the air of the workroom. The addition to water of wetting agents which lower the surface tension of the droplets should theoretically help to engulf and control the dust particles more easily. They have been tried in some instances, but not with conspicuous success. The use of water is therefore not the ideal method of dust control and may give a false sense of security

Electrostatic Precipitation

Dust particles can be removed from a space containing air or gas by creating an electric field in it, thereby giving each particle a negative charge

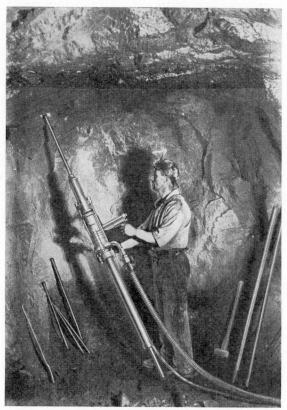

FIG. 392.—Wet Rock Drilling in a Cornish Tin Mine. Overhead Stoper using Drill with axial Water Feed. Note naked Flame of Candle fixed to his Helmet with Clay

(By courtesy of Mr. Treve Holman)

of electricity. The particles will then adhere to positively charged plates at the sides of the space. The method is used in Great Britain to clean certain chimney effluents and also coal gas, but it has not been applied to dusty factory processes except occasionally in dust collectors. In the gold mines of the Transvaal it is used successfully on a fairly large scale to control the airborne dust. After a high initial capital outlay, the running costs are low.

Good Housekeeping

Factories should be kept in a tidy state, and the floors, walls and rafters should be cleaned regularly. Accumulations of dust on the rafters and

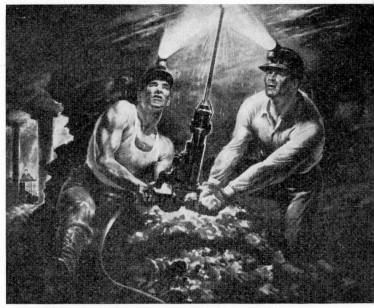

FIG. 393.—Overhead-stoping with a Compressed-air Drill operated by
two Miners
(*Drawing by Herman Giesen*)

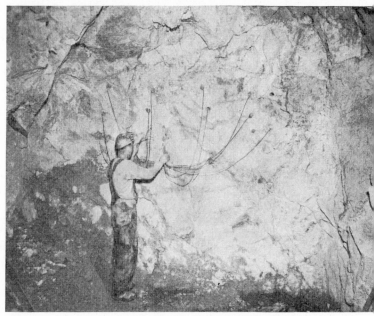

FIG. 394.—Shot-firer gathers the Wires attached to Detonators in Charges
inserted into a dozen Holes drilled into the Rock Face

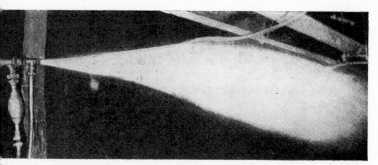

FIG. 395.—Mist Projector in operation in the Hæmatite Mines in Cumberland
(*By courtesy of Dr. John Craw*)

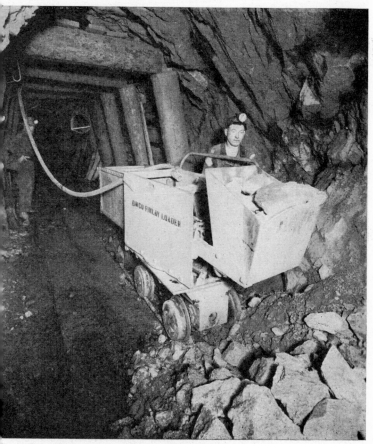

FIG. 396.—Eight hours after Shot-firing a Miner removes the Rock with a
Mechanical Loader
(*By courtesy of Anaconda Copper Mines, Inc.*)

ledges can be a source of airborne dust, especially when there is vibrating machinery in the workroom. Dust should not be allowed to accumulate on the floor of the workroom, because it is easily kicked up to become air borne. It should be removed daily by vacuum cleaning rather than by sweeping. Attention to these matters will reduce greatly the amount of dangerous dust in the air of the workroom.

(3) Personal Protection of the Worker

Where it is found impossible to control the dust completely, the worker must wear either a dust mask or an air-line breathing apparatus. A respirator must never be used as a lazy excuse for avoiding dust control.

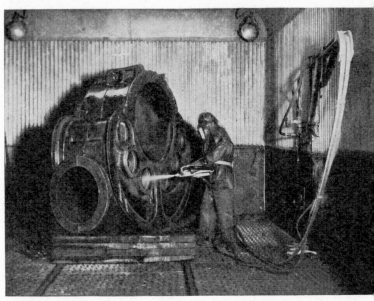

Fig. 397.—Workman cleaning a Turbine Casting. The Hydro-blast Gun is not turned on full otherwise he would be leaning forward to resist the Force of the Blast. Note Waterproof Clothing and Air-line to Helmet

Dust Masks

A dust mask is a filtering device for removing particulate impurities from inspired air. It does not remove gaseous impurities, and its use by mistake as a gas mask could lead to a fatal result. The dust mask protects the nose and mouth. It is made of some light, durable material such as rubber, plastic or aluminium. The edge of the facepiece is lined with soft rubber and may be fitted with renewable cloth facings. The filter medium may be paper, wool, cotton, wool-asbestos, glass wool or various combinations of these substances. The filter is usually renewable (Drinker and Hatch, 1954). Dust respirators are most suitable for tem orary use where there are short periods of exposure to dust, for example, when asbestos dust collectors are being cleaned out. It is almost impossible for a man to do a heavy job continuously when breathing against the resistance of the filter of the respirator.

Air-line Breathing Apparatus

If an air line has to be used, it is better to have it attached to a helmet as in the *breathing apparatus* illustrated in fig. 382. This apparatus can be used to protect people who have to go into a dangerous atmosphere, whether the contaminant is dust, fume or gas. A constant stream of warm clean air under slight positive pressure is blown into the top of the helmet, over the face and out at the sides. This type of helmet is used by shotblasters, and if it is maintained properly and not taken off before the worker is out of the dangerous atmosphere, it gives excellent protection.

(4) Medical Examination

Medical examination is used in the prophylaxis of silicosis in two ways: the initial examination of applicants for employment in an occupation with a silicosis risk, and the periodical medical examination of workers engaged in such occupations. The object of the initial examination is to prevent workmen whose respiratory physique is defective, through malformation or disease, from entering the dangerous industry. The periodical examinations enable silicosis to be detected at an early stage so that the workmen concerned can be transferred to other work. The examinations are also a means of discovering men with pulmonary tuberculosis who not only expose themselves to additional risk by remaining in the dusty occupation, but are possible sources of infection to their fellow workers who, following exposure to siliceous dust, have been rendered more liable to develop tuberculosis. In addition, these examinations provide cumulative evidence of the changes in the workmen's condition. But X-ray examination does not prevent a man from contracting silicosis. It does help to get him out of a dusty industry before the damage to his lungs has gone too far. X-ray and other examinations can also indicate in which part of the job the danger lies, and as such they are valuable because greater attention can be given to dust control in the dangerous job. It is not fair to the workers, however, to use X-ray surveys deliberately in order to save the time and trouble of the engineers whose business it is to control dust clouds wherever they arise.

Treatment of Silicosis

Since 1930 researches have been carried out upon the effects of various substances as antidotal dusts in the case of patients suffering from silicosis. As a result of such work there is a danger that efforts to control the dust clouds in the work-places might be relaxed. Clearly it is better to spend money in suppressing the dust at its source than in providing an antidote after it has got into the lungs.

Antidotal Dusts in Experimental Animals

In 1932 Kettle showed that if silica dust particles were coated with iron oxide they did not cause fibrosis in the lungs of animals. Iron may therefore be regarded as an antidote to silica. No practical application has been made of this observation, but a great deal of attention has been paid to another antidotal dust—namely, aluminium. It was first tried in laboratory animals in Canada (Denny and others, 1939) and the United States of America (Gardner and others, 1944), and it was found that both aluminium powder and hydrated alumina gave the animals a measure of protection from the onset of silicosis. This observation has been confirmed in this country by King and others (1950). It was also found by Gardner that hydrated alumina increased the susceptibility of the animals to tuberculosis.

Treatment of Patients with Aluminium Dust

We shall see (p. 1055) that aluminium, in some forms at least, can cause fibrosis of the lungs. Meanwhile, aluminium is being used in some industries in an attempt to protect the workers against silicosis. Before beginning work they pass through an aluminium-dusting chamber and breathe a daily dose of the powder (fig. 398). Aluminium inhalation in the treatment of established silicosis in pottery workers has been given an extensive trial by Kennedy (1956). By the pairing of 120 volunteers satisfactory controls were provided. The treatment was given over a period of three and a half years and the condition of the patients was assessed each year up to five years. The results were unequivocal; there were no important differences in the behaviour of the two groups; there was no retrogression of the radiological picture and no evidence that aluminium inhalation favoured the development of pulmonary tuberculosis (see p. 1058).

Inhalation of Spray charged with Calcium Salts

In Germany the effect of an electrically charged spray of calcium salts in solution is being tried as an antidote (Rosenthal, 1952). The droplets measure about 0·01 microns and it is claimed that they penetrate deeply into the lungs to combine with the silica and form calcium silicate which is said not to damage the lung tissues. There are now six calcium-inhalation chambers at the Ruhr coal mines, one in a porcelain works and another in an electric insulator factory. It is still too early to say whether or not the method will be successful (McLaughlin, 1953).

ASBESTOS AND OTHER FIBROUS SILICATES

The question as to whether silicates are toxic when inhaled has been much debated since Jones (1933) put forward the view that sericite, a potassium aluminium silicate, is the cause of much industrial silicosis. His view has received but little support. Certain silicates are noxious, and the chief of these is the group of fibrous mineral silicates known as asbestos. To a less extent talc produces a fibrous reaction in the lungs; sillimanite and glass wool seem to be harmless.

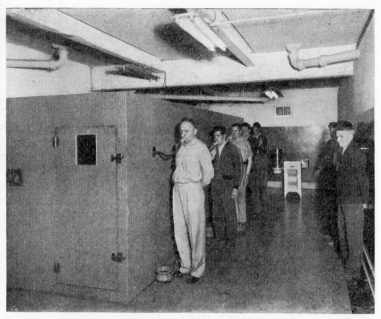

FIG. 398.—Patients with Silicosis at Timmins, Ontario, breathing Aluminium Powder from an Experimental Treatment Chamber
(*By courtesy of Dr. H. W. Jacob*)

(*a*) Asbestos

Asbestos is the name given to a series of minerals composed of silicates of magnesium and iron. It is sometimes referred to as earth flax, stone flax or mountain cork. It is silky and fibrous in form, and this fibrous structure determines many of the characteristics of *asbestosis*, the disease caused by inhalation of the dust. Asbestosis is a more serious disease even than silicosis. In addition to this asbestos workers face the risk of cancer of the lung and of mesothelioma of the pleura and peritoneum both of which are of course fatal diseases.

History of Asbestos

On a small scale, asbestos was made into cloth at least 2,000 years ago. Herodotus (450 B.C.) relates how the Romans mined it in the Italian Alps and Ural Mountains, using it for enshrouding corpses before cremation to permit of easy collection of the ashes for burial. They named it *amianthus*, meaning without miasma, undefiled or incorruptible. Pliny (A.D. 50) refers not only to difficulties in the weaving of asbestos, but also to the use of respirators to avoid the inhalation of dust. Strabo (30 B.C.) and Plutarch (A.D. 70) refer to the wicks of the lamps of the vestal virgins as *asbesta*, the unquenchable, inextinguishable or inconsumable. It is stated that Charlemagne possessed a tablecloth made of it, which was cleansed by passage through fire. However, although the occurrence of asbestos is widespread throughout the world, it is only since about 1890 that it has been used for industrial purposes. In 1880 the annual world production was only 500 tons, a figure which had risen to 200,000 tons by 1920 and nearly 3,500,000 tons by 1967.

Sources and Varieties

Canada produces 65 per cent of the world's asbestos. The remainder comes from Italy, Cyprus, Finland, Russia, South Africa, Australia, New Zealand, the United States of America and Peru. The term asbestos is a collective name applied in commerce to a variety of silicate minerals which differ from each other in chemical composition and physical properties but resemble one another in their finely fibrous nature and flexibility. Their value depends on the facility with which they can be split into long and short flexible fibres, their resistance to acids and their insulating properties with respect to heat and electricity. Most of the asbestos in commerce is fibrous serpentine, especially chrysotile, $3MgO.2SiO_2.2H_2O$. This has the longest and strongest fibres and can be spun. Asbestos is derived also from the hornblende (amphibole) group of minerals, of which the most important are crocidolite and amosite. These consist of fibres too short for spinning, but more stable chemically and more resistant to acid and heat than chrysotile. The hornblende varieties contain less magnesium and usually more aluminium and iron, crocidolite being mainly a silicate of iron, $NaFe(SiO_3)_2FeSiO_3$. It is also known as *blue asbestos*, an allusion to its prevalent colour, and as *Cape blue*, because formerly it was mined only in Cape Province, South Africa. Amosite, $(MgFe)O.SiO_2$, which occurs in workable quantities only in the Union of South Africa, is named from the initial letters of Asbestos Mine of South Africa, the title of the mine where it was first worked. Other varieties are actinolite, $CaO.3(MgFe)O.4SiO$ and tremolite, $CaO.3MgO.4SiO_2$.

Uses

Capable of being spun into yarn and woven into cloth or of mixing with cement, rubber, resin, plastics or graphite, it provides the engineering, automobile, shipbuilding, electrical, building, chemical and other trades with a variety of useful products. These include a wide range of insulation products for pipe lagging, as well as flat and corrugated cement sheets for building work, and also roofing shingles, cements, tiles and fireproof paints. Wool-asbestos fibre is even used in the filter pads of certain types of respirator! From modest beginnings in a small disused Austrian paper mill in 1893 the asbestos-cement industry has constantly expanded so that by 1967 it was estimated that over 100,000 people were employed in it. In 1912 an Italian engineer built the first machine for making seamless asbestos-cement pipes. In 50 years the demand for such pipes for use in domestic installations, water mains and sewerage has greatly expanded in at least 40 countries. In brake linings and clutch facings the asbestos usually reinforced with wire threads. Asbestos is made into acid-resisting filtering cloth, linings for chemical pans, valve packings, gaskets, jointing and lagging material for steam pipes, and is used for coating the bulkheads of ships and marine piers. Long-fibred asbestos, which can be spun and woven into textiles, is used for fire-fighting suits, firemen's helmets, sheets and ropes, theatre safety curtains, boiler mattresses and for the coverings of welding rods where it acts as a flux. Domestic uses include plastic floor tiles, linoleum, ironing boards, oven cloths, table and cooking mats. In 1966 tests were being made with asbestos-asphalt for road surfacing. The labour force in many of these industries is highly mobile and distributed over a large number of small units. In addition there is a vast number of "do it yourself" enthusiasts who may be exposed intermittently to highly concentrated asbestos dust.

Mining

In South Africa asbestos is obtained from both open cast and deep mines. Drilling and explosives are used when the host rock is hard and mechanical excavation when it is softer. The crude ore is milled to remove the host rock and the fibrous asbestos is partially teazed out before it is packed into bags. Where labour is cheap some of the separation of rock from fibre is done by hand with a cobbing hammer (fig. 399) usually by men but sometimes by women often accompanied by their babies. Until recently large amounts of asbestos fibre escaped into the air from the mines and mills so that not only the miners and millers but the whole population of the mining towns and the surrounding countryside have been exposed. From the air a cloud of asbestos dust can be seen over the small mining townships. It was customary to transport asbestos from the mines to the factories in jute bags. Sometimes a boy who did this using a donkey wagon would sleep on the asbestos bags during part of the journey. This exposure of a whole series of transport workers could be eliminated by using sealed impervious bags.

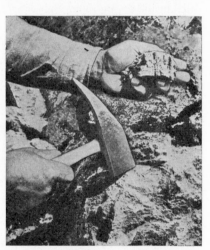

FIG. 399.—Cobbing hammer used in asbestos mining in Canada
(*By courtesy of Canadian Johns-Manville Co., Ltd., Asbestos, Que.*)

Work in Factories

For the manufacture of asbestos textiles raw asbestos in crude and fibre form is imported into Great Britain and stored in sacks in open sheds.

The sacks are carried to a rotary mill and opened, two or three at a time by hand. The crushing process is dusty. The material then passes by vacuum suction into a closed-in machine which delivers flocculent, soft fibrous material, free from grit. For the manufacture of yarn and cloth cotton is often incorporated with the fibre before carding. The carding machine consists of large, fast-running cylinders, covered with innumerable minute wire points to ensure that the fibres are laid parallel. From the end of this machine the material is received as a sliver or rope. Stripping the carding machines (fig. 400) and cleaning the cylinders with a wire brush was a very dusty occupation before modern types of exhaust ventilation were applied locally. Spinning, doubling and weaving follow the process of carding. Dry weaving is usually practised, for wet weaving has the disadvantage of rusting certain fittings on the machinery. For non textiles, such as mill-boards, a wet process is employed. Fibred asbestos is mixed with clay, cement and water, and run through a series of sedimentation tanks to secure the finest of the pulp. This passes along the machine as an emulsion, becoming drier and more doughy on its way, until it is eventually rolled out upon a cylinder. From this it is cut, removed and dried in the drying-room. Subsequent operations, such as sawing, grinding, turning and polishing, give rise to much dust. Insulating mattresses are made almost entirely by hand from lengths of asbestos cloth, and are

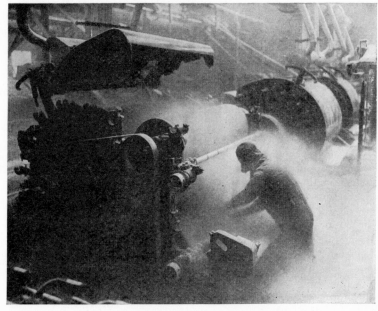

FIG. 400.—Stripping an Asbestos-carding Machine before a modern type of Exhaust Ventilation was applied locally

(*By courtesy of British Belting and Asbestos, Ltd.*)

lled with fibred asbestos by hand, scoop or shovel, levelled by beating
nd finished by sewing.

Jse of Asbestos Goods

The products of asbestos factories are used in the manufacture of
vorkshops, houses, power units, ships, cars and domestic stoves, by a
ariety of skilled tradesmen with their helpers. These men sometimes use
owdered material which they mix with water and apply on the spot
vhilst the mixture is wet, or they use prefabricated blocks or mattresses
vhich require cutting, sawing or shaping to make them fit. The materials
re usually rough-finished when they leave the factory and release some
ust when handled by storemen and transport workers. Hot water pipes
f copper and other metals are insulated by covering them with asbestos.
•team pipes are similarly treated with asbestos, wire and cement. The job
s known as pipe-lagging and it is carried out in shipbuilding, in factory
onstruction and in private houses. At one time the asbestos was applied
vet but now prefabricated materials shaped to the job are used dry, the
vorkman sawing them up to the required lengths as he goes on with his
vork. It follows that the new method produces dust whereas the old
method did not. Building workers, interior decorators and many others
lso use asbestos materials. Electricians, plumbers, fitters and painters
may work in confined spaces and may create dust cutting or drilling these
materials in the course of their work. Most asbestos materials are coated
vith paint or sandwiched between other substances so that they do not
•resent a continuing risk until the building or installation is demolished.
3ut asbestos roofing and brake linings unhappily cause some general
tmospheric pollution, and certain uses such as the lining of ducts for air
onditioning with soft asbestos, and the use of unsealed ceiling tiles cause
ontinuous pollution of the air of office and factory buildings where people
vork all day.

Asbestos in Fire Protection

In 1903 the Paris Métro, as a result of a fire in which 83 people died,
hanged from cast iron brake blocks to asbestos-resin blocks. The fire had
•een started by metallic dust, causing a short circuit. Asbestos-resin brake
•locks have been used by the London Underground for this and other
easons ever since. In 1932 when the *Queen Mary* was being built, mock
abins were constructed and ignited to test different materials, and it was
hen that asbestos-based board established its supremacy in fire protection.
Today asbestos insulation board is increasingly used for compartment
valls where large numbers of people congregate, for example in offices,
tores, schools, hospitals and multi-storey flats. Asbestos-cement sheets,
videly employed for side-cladding and roofing are weather-proof and will
esist the surface spread of flame. Asbestos textiles are used for furnace
ire curtains and other types of fire shield, of which the theatre fire safety
urtain is one. Wherever workers are exposed to great heat or to the risk

of hot metal splashes the use of protective clothing is desirable. For this purpose aluminized asbestos textile materials have been developed. In a major fire steel girders prove surprisingly vulnerable and their distortion may cause the collapse of floors. Their resistance to fire can be enhanced by treating them with asbestos spray. This forms a homogeneous coating and has the advantage of adding but little weight (Brown, 1967).

Historical Summary

The dangers of asbestos remained for long unsuspected. They came to light with a somewhat disconcerting suddenness. The first case of asbestosis known in Great Britain was observed in 1900 and described by Murray in 1907. The man had worked on a carding machine for fourteen years and was the last survivor of ten men who had worked in the card room, the others all having died about the age of thirty with lung disease. He died in Charing Cross Hospital at the age of thirty-four, and necropsy revealed extensive diffuse pulmonary fibrosis. Although the lungs were found to contain asbestos bodies, a diagnosis was made of typical fibroid phthisis. Difficulties of certification delayed further action and cases of asbestosis continued to occur. Special attention was drawn to the disease by Cooke (1924). But it was the case published by Sieler in 1928 which seemed to establish an unequivocal relationship between asbestos and pulmonary fibrosis which precipitated the inquiry leading to the Report of Merewether and Price (1930). Reports of a heavy incidence of asbestosis were then made in some German factories, especially in Dresden (Krüger and others, 1931) and Berlin (Gerbis and Ucko, 1932). In Great Britain the report by Merewether and Price led to safety measures being adopted in factories and to the workers being kept under medical surveillance. But although improvements in dust control were effective in most of the asbestos textile factories new cases are still being diagnosed by the Panels of the Ministry of Social Security. Furthermore we now know that many people with asbestosis or mesothelioma had contact with asbestos only outside industry either through living near a mine or a factory or through dusty clothes being brought home from work. The story of mesothelioma of the pleura and peritoneum is related on p. 1019.

Thirty Cases in One London Factory

Between 1930 and 1934 thirty-seven workers in asbestos all from one factory attended the Out-patient Department of the London Hospital; twenty-five were women and twelve were men. Of these, thirty were judged to be suffering from asbestosis. Seven of these died; and in four necropsy showed that the asbestosis was complicated by pulmonary tuberculosis. Many had worked in more than one department of the same factory but the principal occupations in order of frequency were as follows: spinner, weaver, disintegrator, mixer, mattress maker, card cleaner, storekeeper, slab maker, presser and machinist. The average length of exposure before the onset of symptoms was seven years. Of the patients who died, one was a weaver who had been exposed for eighteen months and another a storekeeper who had been at work for nineteen years. In many cases there was a long interval between removal from exposure and the onset of symptoms: the longest such interval was eight years.

Symptoms

The presenting symptom was dyspnœa. This was early, conspicuous and always out of proportion to the signs found in the chest. It was nearly always associated with non-productive cough, as many as eighteen cases having little or no sputum. Hæmoptysis never occurred in the absence of pulmonary tuberculosis: it was found in three cases. In sixteen cases pain occurred between the shoulders, under the scapula or behind the sternum; it was never more than slight. In two cases a diagnosis of acute pleurisy had been made during the period of employment in asbestos, but in no case had a pleural effusion occurred. A history of laryngitis was obtained in three cases and of conjunctivitis in two. Warts on the fingers had been present at one time in thirteen cases and had subsequently disappeared. It is amosite, a heavier and thicker fibre than chrysotile, which may, in some operations, penetrate the skin and form a *corn* or *wart*. Histologically the lesion shows extreme keratosis (Alden and Howell, 1944).

Physical Signs

The patients were usually well nourished. Clubbing of the fingers was present in six cases. Cyanosis was occasionally noticed, but was only slight. Examination of the chest showed limitation of the respiratory excursion on both sides. The percussion note was never seriously impaired, but slight dullness was sometimes found at the bases. The breath sounds were vesicular, and auscultation sometimes revealed scattered, medium, crepitant râles, often with a metallic tone, and situated especially at the bases. Added sounds were absent on repeated examination in ten cases. For obvious reasons the condition is not unilateral, and therefore displacement of the heart and other mediastinal structures was not found. The tubercle bacillus was found in the sputum of five of the above thirty cases, and four of these died.

Asbestos Bodies in the Sputum

Thirteen cases showed asbestos bodies in the sputum. These are golden-yellow structures of elongated bead-like form, often with bulbous ends (Cooke and Hill, 1927). The appearance of fully formed bodies has been compared to beads on a necklace. The beads vary in size and make up an irregularly segmented body. These bodies have been found to vary in length from 20 to over 200 microns. An asbestos fibre forms the central core in each body (Gloyne, 1929). They are best seen with an oil immersion lens, and show up clearly without staining as golden-yellow structures (fig. 401). They can be stained by hæmatoxylin. The demonstration of asbestos bodies in the sputum has not proved to be a useful diagnostic technique

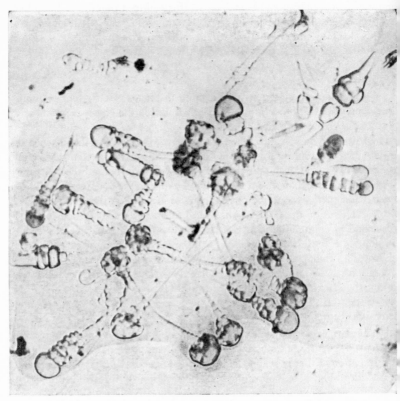

FIG. 401.—Asbestos bodies in the sputum magnified 1,000 diameters

because so many patients in industrial communities have some asbestos in their lungs which are otherwise normal. Therefore the presence of asbestos bodies in the sputum indicates that the patient has been exposed to asbestos dust at some time in the past only, and as a solitary positive finding is certainly not an indication of asbestosis. In fact, one London Hospital patient with sputum due to broncho-pneumonia apparently released asbestos bodies more readily at the height of the illness, the numbers in the sputum diminishing as the inflammatory condition resolved.

Asbestos Bodies in the Lungs at Necropsy

In a case of asbestosis necropsy may show large numbers of asbestos bodies in the lung sections both in alveolar spaces and within the thickened alveolar walls. They are readily demonstrated in smears of fluid scraped from the cut surface of the lung. In asbestosis the presence of asbestos bodies may be demonstrated in the hilar lymph nodes also. It is important to emphasize that asbestos bodies are seen more often in the absence of asbestosis. In many of these cases the number of asbestos bodies is small;

as a result they are less readily demonstrated, but by examining thick unstained sections of lung their identification is facilitated. These sections are thirty microns in thickness, being approximately six times as thick as standard sections; in addition to visualizing a greater volume of lung parenchyma there is less likelihood of asbestos bodies being knocked out of the sections when the paraffin blocks are cut. At The London Hospital it has been possible to identify asbestos bodies in the lungs in 30 to 40 per cent of routine adult necropsies. Lungs of such cases may contain only one or two asbestos bodies per section; generally there is a negative occupational history, but many of these patients have lived and worked in the East End of London for many years. Since other structures may superficially resemble asbestos bodies it is valuable to identify them with greater certainty. The heat resistant property of asbestos is utilized when sections of lung are incinerated by heating to 600° C. which effectively removes the lung parenchyma. Surprisingly the characteristic shell of the asbestos body remains intact so that these structures are still readily recognizable. In fact, since the incineration removes the carbon deposits in the lung too, many more asbestos bodies are revealed in the post-incineration specimens (Smith, 1967).

Radiographic Appearances

The fibrosis in asbestosis is much more diffuse than that due to silica. In silicosis it occurs in the form of numerous more or less isolated foci, but in asbestosis as a fine network throughout the lungs. In radiographs it is so fine as to resemble ground glass or fine cobweb (plate XVI). Homogeneous opacities of this nature are seen at both bases, and may later become more obvious as a fine punctate stippling. The inter-lobar pleura is usually thickened, and there is a shaggy outline to the heart shadow. Ultimately the fine punctate mottling can be observed to have spread beyond the limits of the lower zone to the middle and even the upper zone, but the apices usually remain free. This fine, diffuse, punctate mottling stands out in definite contrast to the nodulation seen in silicosis. In fact, in advanced asbestosis the degree of shadowing present would have little significance if seen in silicosis (Timmermans, 1931).

Pleural Plaques

Pleural plaques are frequently present in asbestosis. They may be nodular or smooth and are composed of very firm, white hyaline material which may be focally calcified. They have a characteristic distribution and are usually confined to the parietal pleura. The usual sites are the central tendons of the diaphragms and in parallel lines over the ribs of the postero-lateral chest wall, but plaques may be present also behind the sternum just lateral to the mid-line. Plaques, with the same distribution, are more commonly seen in patients without asbestosis. However, examination of thick, unstained lung sections reveals small numbers of asbestos bodies in over 80 per cent of these cases. On microscopy pleural plaques are composed of hyaline, acellular fibrous tissue arranged parallel to the pleural surface; they often contain variable sized foci of calcification which when extensive may be visible on chest X-ray. Films such as these may be misinterpreted unless the possible presence of calcified plaques is borne in mind (Hourihane, Lessof and Richardson, 1966).

Respiratory Function Tests

These tests are of little value in the detection of early asbestosis in the individual case unless serial readings over previous years are available. The pattern of functional impairment includes low total lung volume, low vital capacity without evidence of airways obstruction, low pulmonary compliance and low diffusing capacity. The extent of the diffusion defect is the best estimate of disability. Williams and Hugh Jones (1960) reported abnormalities in diffusing capacity for carbon monoxide, before X-ray changes had occurred in factory workers. However other workers have found this test less sensitive than X-rays of the chest in the early detection of asbestosis.

Prognosis

Broadly speaking, the length of time which may elapse between exposure to the dust and a fatal termination is only one-half of that in silicosis. In other words, in asbestosis the fibrosis develops more rapidly. With continued exposure to high concentrations of dust, the fibrosis may be fully developed in seven years, and may cause death after about twelve years' exposure as compared with thirty-five years for all cases of silicosis. The shortest length of exposure to asbestos dust which has ultimately caused death is eighteen months. Since about 1930, as conditions in the factories improved, and tuberculosis declined, the onset of asbestosis became delayed so that now it requires an average of 17 years' exposure to develop. It must be remembered that the existence of a clinically recognizable degree of asbestos fibrosis in any individual is an additional adverse factor in the prognosis of any acute infection of the lungs such as pneumonia or broncho-pneumonia.

Pathology of Asbestosis

At necropsy pleural adhesions are extensive and dense, and there are often thick subpleural plaques of fibrous tissue. Large areas of the lung are tough owing to the presence of fibrous tissue; emphysema is extensive but usually localized to the lower and apical parts of the lungs. There are two views regarding the mode of development of asbestosis. According to the one, the action of the dust is chemical; the other view supposes that the asbestos fibres act mechanically. Experiments carried out at the Saranac laboratories do not support the chemical theory, since aluminium hydroxide which neutralizes the toxic action of quartz does not prevent asbestosis. Moreover, asbestos fibres shorter than 20 microns were found to be relatively innocuous, whereas if the action were chemical an increase in potency would have been expected with reduction in particle size below 5 microns, as in the case of silica. A comparison of the effect of asbestos fibres 15 microns long with those 2·5 microns long (King and others, 1946) showed that rabbits receiving the long fibres developed a nodular reticulin formation comparable with experimental silicotic nodules; animals receiving the short fibres developed a diffuse interstitial reticulin formation.

Incidence of Associated Pulmonary Tuberculosis

Precise information as to the incidence of pulmonary tuberculosis amongst asbestos workers cannot be obtained, but the Factory Department figures for 1935 suggest a less close association between asbestosis and tuberculosis than is the case with silicosis and tuberculosis. Thus among 702 deaths from silicosis the disease was accompanied by tuberculosis in 56 per cent, whereas among eighty-two deaths from asbestosis only 36 per cent showed associated tuberculosis. Later, with the decline of tuberculosis, these percentage figures both for asbestosis and silicosis have become less.

Association with Carcinoma of the Lung

The first recorded case of carcinoma of the lung associated with asbestos was described by Lynch and Smith (1935). By 1955, according to Doll, a total of 61 cases had been reported. We have already seen (p. 818) that Doll (1955) reached the conclusion that asbestos workers faced a risk of cancer of the lung ten times as great as that in the general population; and that McCullough (1959) collected particulars of a series of 365 patients with asbestosis among whom 18 per cent had cancer of the lung. But the carcinogenic effects of asbestos are evidently not confined to the lungs. for Keal (1960) found a high incidence of peritoneal carcinoma in women with asbestosis. He showed that during the period 1948–58, twenty-three women were admitted to The London Hospital with asbestosis; fifteen of these had subsequently died, four with carcinoma of the lung, nine with carcinomatosis peritonei; of the latter, one was certainly ovarian in origin, and this was possibly the primary site in four others, but in the remaining two no primary site could be found.

Mesothelioma of the Pleura and Peritoneum

The idea of an association between mesothelioma and exposure to asbestos came from Cape Province, South Africa and was suggested by Wagner, Sleggs and Marchand in 1960. They found their cases in the asbestos hills west of Kimberley where communities tend to cluster round the mine workings. Schools have been built close to mounds of asbestos on which children played. There was asbestos dust in the air, in houses and in the streets. Within three years they collected 120 patients with mesothelioma, nearly all of whom had evidence of exposure to crocidolite often non-occupational. By contrast, there are no reported cases from the vicinity of amosite workings. They recorded 31 cases of diffuse pleural mesothelioma. Histological proof of asbestosis was present in eight of these cases. Prior to this work only occasional cases of this condition had been associated with asbestosis. In 1946 Wyers published the first case of mesothelioma of the pleura to be diagnosed in an asbestos worker in Great Britain. Up to February 1965 the total number of cases diagnosed in the British Isles was 160 (Gilson, 1966). In contrast to the average latent interval of twenty years between the first exposure to asbestos and the development of carcinoma of the lung, the interval between the first exposure and the onset of symptoms from mesothelioma may vary from between 25 and 50 years with an average of 33 years. While some patients give a story of continuous exposure to asbestos over many years, a significant proportion give a history of only transient exposure sometimes amounting to a few weeks only, many years before. Such patients may show little or no evidence of fibrosis of the lungs but do show large or small quantities of asbestos bodies in the lung parenchyma. Some of these latter cases show identical amounts of asbestos in the lung to that observed in many patients living in the East End of London. This raises the question of whether minor degrees of community contamination by asbestos are capable of giving rise to mesothelioma.

Exposure in Factory, Shipyard and Community

Hourihane (1964) examined tissues and records of 83 cases of mesothelioma from the files of the pathology department of the London Hospital. Fifty-six of these were pleural, and 27 peritoneal tumours. Occupational and residential histories were obtained from the relatives of 76 of these cases by Newhouse and Thompson (1965). Forty out of 76 gave a history of occupational or domestic exposure to asbestos. Only 9 of 76 control patients suffering from other diseases gave such a history. Among those with *no* evidence of occupational or domestic exposure, one-third lived within half a mile of a large asbestos factory. Seventeen cases of mesothelioma were investigated in the Merseyside area. Exposure to asbestos was confirmed in 14. Eleven patients gave clear histories of handling asbestos as laggers, boiler makers and ship repairers. Two female patients had been sorters of used sacking (Owen, 1964). Mesothelioma occurs with equal frequency in the two sexes, which is in contrast to the striking male preponderance in carcinoma of the lung. The condition is invariably fatal in months rather than years.

Symptoms and Signs of Mesothelioma

The principal symptom is dyspnœa, usually rapidly increasing, and it may be associated with pain in the chest, cough and hæmoptysis. The signs are those of pleural effusion usually with complete collapse of the lung. The fluid removed is straw-clooured and sometimes bloodstained. Cytological examination shows malignant cells. Metastases are rare but they may occur as generalized lymphadenopathy, small nodules in the subcutaneous tissues over neck and chest or nodules on the tongue.

X-rays of the chest show massive thickening of the pleura and sometimes a tumour which quickly increases. The fluid of course is seen and sometimes a loculated effusion is present. Thickening of the oblique fissure may be seen. Ultimately the pleural cavity becomes obliterated. A progressively enlarging mediastinal tumour is common. Thoracoscopy usually shows tumour nodules on the thickened pleura with the lung collapsed and immobile. Thoracoscopic pleural biopsy should be used as a method of diagnosis.

Morbid Anatomy of Mesothelioma

Mesothelioma is an uncommon primary tumour of the serosal surfaces and may occur in the pleura, peritoneum or pericardium. The pleural and peritoneal tumours, either alone or together, are the most frequent, although all or any combination of the three may occur. Pleural mesotheliomas are massive white tumours which tend to surround the lung spreading to involve both the fissures and main pleural space and to cause collapse. Peritoneal tumours usually involve all surfaces of the abdominal cavity. Usually the distribution of tumour is uneven, with a main mass perhaps involving the greater omentum and with discrete or confluent nodules elsewhere. Persistently recurring effusion or ascites may occur. Lymph node metastases are common but discrete metastases within parenchymatous organs are not seen. The liver may be closely invested by tumour with distortion and even erosion of its capsule, but all the tumour seen is in continuity with that in the peritoneal cavity. Mesotheliomas tend to show a mixed histological picture consisting of epithelial patterns in some areas and spindle-cell fibromatous tumour in others.

Preventive Measures

In asbestos mining wet rock drilling is imperative. Hand cobbing should be replaced by crushing in enclosed machines. Asbestos must not be dumped carelessly about the mine workings and towns. Transport must be carried out by the use of strong impervious bags. In the factories of Great Britain legislation has been effective in controlling the severity of the disease but cases do still occur. In factories and textile mills the principle of locally applied exhaust ventilation must be enforced to prevent the escape of asbestos dust into the air of any room in which work is done. Hand cleaning of the cylinders of carding machines is prohibited while any other person is present, nor may it be done by hand strickles or other hand tools. Those cleaning cylinders, filling insulating mattresses and entering chambers containing loose asbestos should be provided with an efficient apparatus by means of which they can breathe air free from dust. Suppression of dust in the cleaning of carding machines is best ensured by the use of a revolving brush fitted with a cover and connected to a portable vacuum cleaner (fig. 403). By the use of closed-in machines, handling should be reduced to a minimum. In one factory, spinning frames have been totally enclosed in *perspex* with an ingenious device which permits

easy access to bobbins (Wyers, 1949). Education of the worker must aim
at a high standard of good housekeeping (fig. 402). Workers exposed to
asbestos dust such as those in shipbuilding, ship-breaking and pipe
lagging and those handling asbestos as stevedores and asbestos-cement
workers should wear efficient dust masks at such times as their

DO NOT USE AIR HOSE

TO CLEAN YOUR CLOTHES

FIG. 402.—Notice in use in an asbestos factory in Canada
(*By courtesy of Canadian Johns-Manville Co., Ltd., Matheson, Ont.*)

work produces dust. Since mesothelioma seems to be associated in some
cases with very small exposures to asbestos a system of control by licence of
the import and use of what is probably the most dangerous form of
asbestos, crocidolite or blue asbestos, has been advocated. In 1967 British
Rail announced that asbestos was no longer used as insulation in railway
carriages because of possible danger to men in the workshops where
panelling was removed, and glass fibre was used instead. The British

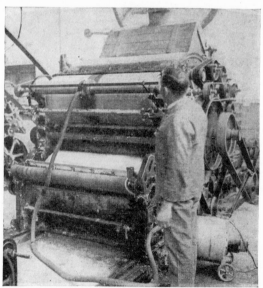

FIG. 403.—Portable Vacuum Apparatus for cleaning
Asbestos Carding Machine. Note the Revolving Brush
fitted with a Cover and connected to a Vacuum Cleaner
(*Report on Conferences concerning Methods for Suppressing Dust in
Asbestos Textile Factories, 1931*)

sbestos Industry has proposed that all asbestos fibre shipped to Great
ritain shall be packed in dustproof bags, and that all blue asbestos shall
 addition be shipped on pallets which can be handled mechanically.

ipping of Asbestos Waste

In July 1966 at Buxworth, Derbyshire, a local enquiry by the Ministry
f Housing and Local Government revealed that a firm using asbestos in
he manufacture of brake linings and clutch facings had dumped its waste
 disused quarries for about 40 years. At first there were no houses in the
mmediate vicinity of the quarry used, tipping was done from open lorries
nd the dust was not bagged. In July 1964 space in the first quarry had
ecome exhausted and tipping was transferred to another quarry only 60
ards from the nearest house. By July 1966 contractors were tipping 230
ons monthly and the conditions under which this was done were totally
nsatisfactory. Asbestos dust formed 25 per cent of the material dumped
nd although this was bagged, sometimes a bag would fall from a lorry and
emain on the ground split open and uncovered. The manufacturing firm
ad disclaimed responsibility for the waste once it had left their gates.
lthough public health inspectors had visited the site regularly the
uisance persisted. From what we now know of the etiology of meso-
helioma, it is clear that uncontrolled tipping of asbestos waste such as
appened in the village of Buxworth should be sternly repressed.

raft Asbestos Regulations, 1968

These long-awaited draft regulations, to supersede those of 1931, have
een issued and circulated to interested parties for criticism. They will
ow apply to all factories, building operations, civil engineering work,
hipbuilding and ship-repairing; and particularly to lagging and delagging,
which are known to be dangerous operations not previously covered. Any
rocess in which asbestos dust is liable to be given off to a dangerous extent
will be carried out either under an exhaust draught which will effectively
revent the escape of asbestos dust into the air of the workplace or in some
qually safe way. If this is not possible, workers must be given protective
lothing and approved respiratory-protective equipment. Any person
ndertaking a process in which crocidolite is used will have to notify the
istrict inspector of factories. But the Factories Act cannot protect private
sers. We know that inhalation of dust from such activities as sawing or
anding material containing asbestos presents the hazard of malignant
mesothelioma outside as well as inside industrial situations. It seems not
unreasonable, therefore, to insist that materials containing asbestos should
be clearly marked to show this, so that adequate precautions can be taken
by the users. For instance, amateur handymen sawing materials containing
asbestos could easily wear a lightweight dust mask, and either work out of
doors or in a well ventilated room. Meanwhile many doctors have asked
whether the properties of asbestos are as unique as the salesmanship of
the asbestos companies appears to indicate. There are many other mineral

fibres such as glass wool, rock wool or slag wool, which have usef
inherent fire-proofing properties but not the fibrogenic or carcinogen
effects on the lungs. Is it certain that the properties of asbestos justify tl
risks of asbestosis, carcinoma of the lung and mesothelioma which a
entailed by its use?

Case 37. Asbestos spinner—exposure to asbestos dust for five years—asbestos

A. R., a woman, aged 27, had worked from 1924 to 1929 in tl
spinning department of an asbestos works where the protection fro
dust was poor. In 1928 she suffered from a dry cough, and in 19
from shortness of breath and occasional pain in the right side of tl
chest on breathing.

On examination: five warts on fingers, the largest 3 by 1 mm. N
clubbing of fingers. Dyspnœa, but no cyanosis. Apex beat not di
placed, and heart sounds normal. There was diminished movement
the base of the right lung, with slight dullness, diminished breat
sounds and extensive creaking pleuritic sounds. A few crepitations
both bases. No sputum. X-ray showed the heart to be normal
situated, and there were fine homogeneous opacities resemblin
ground glass at the bases of both lungs. In 1935 the shortness
breath was worse; there was a dry cough. On examination there we
no warts on the fingers, and the physical signs in the chest were ur
changed.

Case 38. Asbestos carder and weaver—exposure to asbestos dust for three yea
—latent interval of twenty-five years—death from compression paraplegi
secondary carcinoma of spine; primary carcinoma of lung; asbestosis.

M. C., a married woman, aged 43, L.H. Reg. No. 41149/1947.

1919–22: between the ages of fifteen and eighteen she worked
carder and weaver in an asbestos factory. It is not known whether sh
cleaned the carding machines with a steel handbrush, but this metho
was in use at the time. She gave up the work owing to shortness
breath.

25 years: she had frequent brief attacks of breathlessness some
times with cough but was not disabled.

16 years: at the age of twenty-seven she married, and later had on
miscarriage but no further pregnancy. She remained active, doing a
the duties of a housewife.

Four months: sudden onset of aching pain in the back of the nec
without any apparent precipitating factor. The pain radiated to bot
shoulders and to both sides of the chest, was continuous and sever
enough to interfere with sleep. It remained for some time practicall
unchanged, but had gradually increased in severity during six week

Three weeks: she felt unsteady on getting out of bed in the mornin
and since then she had become progressively weaker and more un

steady on her legs. There were occasional involuntary movements of the legs, usually flexion of the knees with plantar flexion of the ankles. Occasional paræsthesiæ of the legs. Hesitancy of micturition. Bowels open regularly.

On examination: temperature 99° F. Pulse 112. Respiration 22. A nervous distressed woman, in considerable pain. Furred moist tongue. No pallor. No enlarged lymph glands or œdema. Regular pulse. Apex beat 1 inch lateral to mid-clavicular line. Blood-pressure 120/90. Heart sounds normal. There was some impairment of resonance and diminution of breath sounds with coarse crepitations at the bases of both lungs. The abdomen, including digital examination of rectum and vagina, showed nothing abnormal. Nervous system: an anxious but co-operative lady. Cranial nerves normal. Upper limbs normal. Lower limbs—approximately symmetrical spastic paralysis with brisk reflexes, ankle clonus and extensor plantar responses. Abdominal reflexes absent, and some weakness of lower trunk musculature. Loss of sensation to pin-prick, postural sense and vibration up to the level of D6.

Investigations: catheter urine: trace of albumin; deposit; calcium oxalate crystals; culture sterile. Blood count: hæmoglobin 89 per cent, red blood cells 4,720,000 per c.mm., colour index 0·94, platelets 255,000 per c.mm., white blood cells and differential count normal. Cerebrospinal fluid: clear, colourless fluid, under normal pressure, rising unevenly on jugular compression to 300 mm., and falling similarly; no increase in cells, protein 500 mgm. per cent, Lange 111,211, Wassermann reaction negative. X-ray of chest: lung markings heavy throughout, excessive fine interlacing shadows at bases, no nodulation. X-ray of spine—the body of D4 is smaller than its neighbours, especially in vertical height, and is mottled. The pedicles are not visible.

Progress: while in hospital the pain continued without much alteration. In the middle of the second week she suddenly developed severe pain in the left chest, became dyspnœic, collapsed, pale and cyanosed. Some relief was obtained from morphine and oxygen. This was followed by fever up to 101·8° F., with rapid respiration rate and two further attacks of chest pain. Electrocardiogram at this time showed absent Q and inverted T in lead 3 with right axis deviation, the rate being 180. She became steadily weaker and died 2½ weeks after admission.

Necropsy: Professor Dorothy Russell made the necropsy (L.H.P.M. 282/1947), of which the following is a summary.

Secondary carcinoma of thoracic vertebræ invading epidural space. Primary carcinoma of lung. Asbestosis.

Dark greyish-black reticular fibrosis throughout both lungs, especially lower lobes and right middle lobe, with conspicuous sub-

pleural fibrosis (0·5 cm. deep). Area (3 × 3 × 2 cm.) of pale gre
carcinoma beneath pleura of mesial aspect of left upper lobe. Clea
yellow pleural effusion, left (3 oz.). A few fibrous pleural adhesion
over posterior surface of left lung and mesial aspect of right uppe
lobe. Secondary carcinoma of hilar glands, most marked right, an
one in superior mediastinum. Secondary carcinoma of greater part c
bodies of 2nd to 4th thoracic vertebræ. Collar of growth encirclin
dura over 4th and 5th thoracic segments. Patchy softening of spina
cord at this level. Nodule (1 cm. diam.) of secondary carcinoma i
mesial surface of left parietal cortex. Secondary carcinoma in supra
clavicular glands. Swollen red pulp in spleen. A well-nourished
edentulous woman.

Microscopic. Lungs: conspicuous anastomosing bands of dens
fibrosis containing numerous asbestos bodies, often in clumps, an
associated with foreign body giant-cells. Similar zone beneath pleur
of lower lobes; less marked and interrupted over middle lobe. Con
gestion and emphysema of residual lung tissue; many macrophage
and occasional asbestos bodies in alveolar spaces. *Left upper lobe*
similar changes, together with ill-defined, infiltrating tubular
columnar-celled and polygonal trabecular carcinoma beneath mesia
pleura, apparently arising from bronchus. *Gland from right hilum*
focus of secondary polygonal-celled carcinoma; anthracosis and a fev
collections of asbestos bodies. *Right and left supraclavicular glands*
extensive secondary carcinoma. *Fifth thoracic segment with dura:* ex
tensive secondary carcinoma of epidural tissues, not penetrating dura
Permeation of many veins. Engorgement of pial veins. Ill-defined
wedges of ischæmic softening in both lateral columns of spinal cor
extending into crossed pyramidal tracts, and a few smaller similar foc
in anterior and posterior columns. *Thoracic vertebræ 2–3 with inter*
vertebral disc: extensive osteoclastic and osteoplastic secondary carci
noma of spongiosa and periosteum. Considerable necrosis of medullar
tissue. *Left parietal cerebrum:* nodule of secondary carcinoma i
superficial cortex. *Spleen:* slight myeloid reaction in pulp.

(b) Talc

Talc is a hydrated magnesium silicate, $3MgO.4SiO_2.H_2O$. The pures
deposits occur in association with dolomite and magnesian limestone, wher
the talc owes its origin to the hydration of the magnesium silicate mineral
which were formed during the earlier metamorphism of the carbonat
rocks. Talc mining is carried out mainly in the United States of Americ
and Manchuria. The largest deposit in Europe is on the northern slope o
the Pyrenees.

Uses

Talc is the first mineral man encounters upon entering the world, for i
is the main constituent of talcum powder and of toilet powders in general
It is soft and has a greasy feel, and on that account the massive impur

ubstance has been called *steatite* or *soapstone*. This is the *French chalk* used
y tailors for marking cloth. Perhaps 90 per cent of all the talc produced is
marketed in the form of an impalpable powder. Nearly half the total output
s used in the manufacture of paint and distemper. In ceramics, talc is used
or the manufacture of tiles, electrical porcelain, table-ware and refractories.
Nearly 25 per cent of talc production goes into the manufacture of paper in
which the mineral serves for filling and glazing better than kaolin. It is
widely used as a dusting agent for rubber tyres, rubber gloves, furs and for
packing parachutes to prevent rotting from moisture. Workmen who
handle it for such purposes often call it *pounce*.

Pneumoconiosis in Talc Mining and Milling

In New York State, disabling pneumoconiosis occurred in 14·5 per cent
of the workers in the talc mining and milling industry. The dust contained
ine, straight, needle-like fibres. The talc fibrosis was associated with an
increased susceptibility to tuberculosis (Siegal and others, 1943). Marked
radiological changes were found in nine out of thirty-four men employed
in a talc mill in Norway for periods lasting from seven to twenty-four years;
there was less disablement than would have been expected from the X-ray
appearances (Bruusgaard and Skjelbred-Knudsen, 1949).

A Case proved by Necropsy

The first case of this type proved by necropsy to occur in Great Britain
was published by McLaughlin and others in 1949. The man was fifty-one
years of age and had worked in a rubber-tyre factory since he left school at
fourteen years of age. The only industrial dust to which he was exposed
was that of talc. For two years he had complained of increasing dyspnœa,
which was partly due to heart failure arising from rheumatic carditis with
aortic incompetence. The X-ray film showed nodular shadows distributed
over both lung fields. At necropsy, throughout the lungs there were grey
nodules which had coalesced in some places, especially in the lower lobes.
Microscopically the nodules showed whorling, but this had not the typical
appearance of silicosis. Within the nodules were fibre-like structures from
10 to 90 microns in length, arranged singly and in clumps; the non-fibrous
particles apparently had been eliminated. Some of the fibre-like structures
were similar to asbestos bodies, and the appearances suggested that talc
pneumoconiosis and asbestosis are similar diseases and that the former may
be caused only by the fibrous varieties of talc. Asbestos is more actively
fibrogenic than talc, and this might be due to the higher proportion of
fibres in asbestos.

(c) Sericite

Sericite is of geological rather than commercial importance. It is a
variety of the mica known as muscovite, $K_2O.3Al_2O_3.6SiO_2.2H_2O$. It occurs
as minute shreds or in very thin veins and is a secondary mineral formed by
hydrothermal alteration of silicates such as the felspars. It forms acicular
crystals and has been suggested as a cause of pulmonary disease by Mavrogordato (1926), Badham (1927) and Jones (1933). Since it occurs in many

rocks in association with quartz it is not surprising that it has been found in the lungs of miners with silicosis. It is a residual material only and has not by itself been found to cause progressive fibrosis of the lungs, possibly because the fibrous particles are too small to have the effect caused by asbestos.

(d) Sillimanite

Until about 1920 the minerals of the sillimanite group were almost unknown outside the geological world, but now they are in great demand for making high-grade refractories. They are all aluminium silicates capable of withstanding high temperatures. Andalusite comes from California and the Transvaal; kyanite and sillimanite are mined in India. Porcelain made from them is characterized by its high melting-point, low coefficient of expansion, resistance to shock and low electrical conductivity, properties which render the porcelain eminently suitable for sparking-plugs, laboratory ware, thermo-couple tubing and special refractory bricks used in electric and forging furnaces and cement kilns.

Sillimanite Pneumoconiosis

Sillimanite presents a fibrous crystalline form in the raw state and when calcined, but, unlike asbestos, the fibrous form is lost when it is crushed. When fused in a furnace at 1,545° C., sillimanite is converted partly or wholly into mullite. Gärtner (1947) suggested that this fact may be related to the histological changes, with the formation of small irregular nodules, found in a portion of lung of a furnace worker, and reported by Gärtner and van Marwyck (1947). In the examination of sixteen workers exposed to dust of calcined sillimanite, Henry and Middleton (1936) found radiographic changes but no disability, and no signs or symptoms which could be related to the dust exposure.

(e) Glass Wool

Fibrous glass, *fibre glass* or *glass wool*, is a manufactured silicate used in industry for sound and heat insulation, air filtration, as a filter in resin-bonded laminates, and as an inert base for textile manufacture or packing processes. Inhalation of fibre glass dust does not cause pneumoconiosis. Schepers (1959) showed in three animal species that the dust, when inhaled, behaves as a biologically inert substance. In dust produced by the machining of plastic materials containing a glass wool filler the working atmosphere may contain particles of glass wool from about 3 to 20 μ in length. These particles may be inhaled by the workmen but despite their physical similarity to asbestos particles there is no evidence that fibrosis of the lungs results or that *fibre glass bodies* similar to *asbestos bodies* are produced (Gardner, 1942). The spicules of fibre glass, or glass wool may, however, cause irritation of the skin, conjunctivæ and upper respiratory tract. Implantation of splinters of glass wool in the region of the nail fold of the finger may produce paronychia sometimes with secondary malformation of the nail (McKenna, Smith and Maclean, 1958). Away from the nail fold fibres of spun glass wool may produce warts on the ingers. The particles will penetrate normal clothing but woollen under-clothing may provide some protection, as may barrier creams for the exposed skin. The skin irritation disappears following a bath and a change of clothing. Glass wool does not itself cause dermatitis. However, oils used as lubricants in the manipulation of the fibre may cause oil folliculitis. Likewise in the plastics industry an epoxy resin may be added to the resins used as binders for the glass fibre filling material. Should dermatitis then occur it is caused not by the glass fibre but by the epoxy resin.

NON-FIBROUS SILICATES

In the absence of quartz and of fibrous structure, silicate minerals appear to produce radiographic changes accompanied by symptoms which are less severe than might be expected from the radiographic signs. The amount of change depends on the concentration of dust and the period of exposure.

(a) Mica

Micas are complex aluminium silicates combined with either potassium, magnesium or iron. The more common are muscovite, $K_2O.3Al_2O_3$. $5SiO_2.2H_2O$, biotite, $(KH_2)_2MgFe)_2(AlFe)_2(SiO_4)_3$, and phlogopite, $KH)_3Mg_3Al(SiO_4)_3$.

Sources

Muscovite, or white mica, is transparent and colourless in thin sheets, and is distinguished by its highly perfect cleavage. It is not decomposed by sulphuric acid. The name is derived from Muscovy in Russia, where the mineral was in early use as window glass. In commercial deposits the crystals vary from a few inches to a foot or so in diameter and up to two inches in thickness. They are referred to as *books* of mica because they can be cleaved into sheets almost as easily as separating the pages of a book. India supplies 70 per cent of the world total of sheet mica. Large quantities of muscovite are mined in the United States of America, but only a small percentage is of sheet-quality, the rest being used as ground mica. Phlogopite, or amber mica, is mined in Canada and Madagascar. It is difficult to differentiate from muscovite, except that it is decomposed by sulphuric acid. Biotite varies in colour, being either brown, black or dark green, and even in thin sheets, in contrast to muscovite, it has a smoky colour and is spotted with impurities. For this reason it is rarely used in sheet form but is employed as ground mica.

Uses

Owing to its transparency and heat resistance, muscovite is used for the chimneys of oil-lamps, for peep-holes in stove doors, ovens, furnaces and optical lanterns, and is then often termed isinglass stone, after isinglass, which is a semi-transparent form of gelatin. No other mineral has better cleavage, flexibility or elasticity; it is possible to roll a sheet of muscovite a thousandth of an inch in thickness into a cylinder a quarter of an inch in diameter, and its elasticity would enable the sheet to flatten out again quite easily. Its high resistance to the passage of electricity is so great that no substitute, artificial or natural, has proved equally satisfactory, so that in the electrical industry it is as important as copper, and now ranks as one of the essential minerals in modern civilization.

Mica is employed in industry either as sheet or as powdered mica. It has been estimated that 90 per cent of the production of sheet mica is used in the electrical industry. For condensers, as insulating material between the segments of commutators of generators and dynamos and for telephones, only the highest-quality mica is employed; and the increased demand since about 1925 for use in wireless apparatus and in motor-car and aeroplane engines has been spectacular. Phlogopite is more suitable than muscovite for separating the segments of a commutator, because it wears more evenly and at about the same rate as the metal bars; and the best grades of phlogopite, such as those produced in Canada, are used extensively in aeroplane sparking-plugs.

Mica which is unsuitable for use as sheets, and the parts of sheet trimmed off, is marketed as scrap or ground mica. About two-thirds of all such mica is utilized in the roofing trade as a backing for rolled asphalt roofing and shingles to prevent sticking, and to a lesser extent as a decorative surface for these materials. Some scrap mica is mixed with shellac and moulded for use in electrical insulation. Approximately 10 per cent of ground mica is employed to give lustre to decorated wallpaper and to produce the glistening *Jack Frost* effect on Christmas trees and Christmas cards. It is also used in paints, as a filler in rubber and as a dusting medium to prevent rubber tyres and rubber goods from adhering to the moulds in which they are shaped. Among miscellaneous uses for ground mica are to give a finish to stucco and concrete; in the making of artificial stone slabs and blocks; for lubrication in axle grease and as a dry lubricant.

Mica Pneumoconiosis

In an examination of fifty-seven men exposed to mica dust for periods lasting from eighteen to forty-six years Dreesen and others (1940) found ten cases of pneumoconiosis. The dust was generated by grinding hand-sorted mica and contained practically no free silica. Radiological examination of 456 men who had spent more than half their working life in mica dust showed changes in the lungs in 9·4 per cent of cases, a figure almost double that in a comparable group with no exposure to mica. Vestal and others (1943) found similar X-ray changes in seventy-nine workers handling mica containing no free silica.

(b) Fuller's Earth

Fuller's earth is so named from its use at one time as an absorbent of the grease in wool and cloth, a process called *fulling*. It is a non-plastic clay which disintegrates to a fine powder when placed in water. The composition varies; it usually contains up to 90 per cent of montmorillonite, an aluminium silicate, together with traces of quartz.

ources

It is found at Nutfield, Surrey, at Midford near Bath and at Bala, Jorth Wales, and also in Saxony, in California and in eight other states of he United States of America. It is either mined or dug in the open accord-1g to local circumstances. It is then ground to a fine powder and made 1to a slurry with water which is allowed to carry off the coarser particles. After consolidation the finer particles are dried, broken into lumps and acked for transport.

Jses

Although the use of fuller's earth for cleansing wool and cloth has reatly decreased, the demand for the material is greater than ever. It is ow used for the filtration of mineral oils, for soap, cleansing preparations, igments for wallpapers and toilet requisites.

Hazard to the Worker

Radiographic examination of five men exposed to the dust of fuller's arth for periods from four to thirty-nine years showed in three men, mployed from four to nineteen years, films within normal limits; two others, employed thirty-five and thirty-nine years respectively, had signs of fine punctate mottling and some coalescence. One of these men died, at he age of fifty-six, after chest symptoms for some years and disablement or eighteen months. A necropsy was made by Gloyne (Campbell and Gloyne, 1942), who described the condition found as soft patchy pneumo-oniosis without massive fibrosis and with none of the hard nodular character associated with silicosis. From microscopic examination of a por-ion of one of the lungs Belt described small black rubbery lesions, each of which appeared to represent the cut end of a small blood vessel or bronchus; here was no silicotic nodulation or massive fibrosis, and no tuberculosis Middleton, 1940). The persistence of the pulmonary changes which follow mpregnation by dust is shown in a case reported by Tonning (1949). This patient, when a young man, had been employed for about fifteen years in he same fuller's-earth works as that in which the above cases occurred; he had gone to Canada and, after various employments, with no exposure to dust, died there at the age of seventy-nine of pneumonia following an operation for cancer of the lip. The pathological changes found in the lungs resembled those found in Belt's English case (Middleton, 1940).

(c) Kaolin

China clay is so called because samples of it were originally obtained in the eighteenth century from China. Kaolin is a corruption of the Chinese word *Kau-ling*, the *high ridge* to the east of *King-te-chen* which for cen-turies has been the chief centre in China for the manufacture of pottery. China clay was discovered in Cornwall near St. Austell in 1750 and soon afterwards Josiah Wedgwood began shipping it from Fowey to the Potteries. The wastes excavated from the pits are eight times the volume of the useful china clay and huge white cones of this material are now to be seen glistening across the countryside.

Sources and Chemical Composition

All the china-clay deposits of the world are the product of the de
composition of feldspars in granitic rocks. Feldspar is sodium or potassium
aluminium silicate, $K_2O.Al_2O_3.6SiO_2$, and the potash is leached out b
downward percolating waters containing carbon dioxide and other sub
stances, especially organic acids. The residue is china clay, $Al_2O_3.SiO_2.2H_2O$
an hydrated aluminium silicate, together with quartz, mica and othe
minerals from the granite. The clay is sluiced out of vast craters in th
rock with high pressure hoses. The china clays of Cornwall and Devonshir
have the advantage of being pure white. Those of Czechoslovakia, Ger
many, Japan and the United States of America may have a yellowish ting
and this colour has to be disguised by the addition of blue dyes which the
interfere with the usefulness of subsequent products. It is not surprising
therefore, that of all the raw materials exported by Great Britain china cla
ranks second in tonnage after coal.

Uses

In the manufacture of paper, china clay is the chief filler in the pulp
producing the body of the paper and the smooth surface. Newsprint con
tains 10 per cent of its weight of china clay. Used in ceramics, it is a
essential constituent of the bodies and glazes of cups, saucers and plates. I
is used as a filler in the rubber industry, for paints, as a stiffener for textil
fabrics, for wall-plasters and in white Portland cement. For pharmaceutica
purposes *Kaolinum Leve, B.P.* is used in the treatment of cholera and foo
poisoning to absorb the toxins of the cholera vibrio and of Salmonell
organisms. *Cataplasma Kaolini, B.P.* is often used in place of the linsee
poultice.

The Worker remains in Good Health

Men quarrying and mining kaolin suffer no harm. Experiments hav
been carried out to test its toxicity. Two types of kaolin, from coal measure
and china-clay deposits, were tested by intratracheal insufflation in rats b
King, Harrison and Nagelschmidt (1948). The kaolins produced only
very mild reticulin reaction in the lungs; a specimen of ignited kaoli
which contained amorphous silica in the form of a glass produced slight
more reticulinosis but not fibrous silicosis.

PNEUMOCONIOSIS OF COAL MINERS

We have seen (p. 982) that only a small percentage of coal miner
develop classical silicosis, and that the mining occupations involving ex
posure to silica dust include ripping, brushing, driving a hard heading an
driving a cross-measure drift. But there is a very much commoner diseas
of coal miners working at the coal face resulting from the inhalation of
mixed dust of coal together with a relatively small proportion of free silica
This pneumoconiosis of coal workers occurs in all countries where coal i
mined, and it is found also in trimmers of coal cargoes in ships. In Grea
Britain it accounts for more deaths than do all other forms of pneumo
coniosis combined, and since 1930 it has constituted the greatest medical an

cial problem in all industry. The distribution of the disease in Great
ritain shows a preponderance in the South Wales coalfield.

Historical Summary

The history of lung diseases of coal miners in Great Britain from 1800
1952 has been reviewed in detail by Meiklejohn (1951, 1952). According
Bremner (1869) the earliest documents in which coal mining in Great
ritain is mentioned are *The Saxon Chronicle of Peterborough* (852), and
shop Pudsey's *Boldon Book* (1180). Newcastle coal is first alluded to in a
aarter granted to the inhabitants of that town in 1234, and the first men-
on of coal in Scotland occurs in a charter granted in 1291 to the Abbot
d Convent of Dunfermline. We have seen (p. 55) how a shortage of
ood about the year 1578 during the reign of Elizabeth I led to an ex-
ansion of coal mining, with the corresponding alteration of domestic
earths and furnace fires to suit sea coal.

oal Miners' Consumptions and Phthisicks

It was not long before chest disease in coal miners gave rise to com-
ent. In his *Fumifugium, or the inconvenience of the Aer and Smoak of
ondon dissipated* (1661) John Evelyn wrote:

> Newcastle Cole as an expert Physician affirms, causeth consump-
> tions, phthisicks and the indisposition of the lungs, not only by the
> suffocating aboundance of smoak, but also by its virulency, for all
> subterrany fuel hath a kind of virulent or arsenical vapour rising from
> it; which, as it speedily destroys those who dig it in the mines, so does
> it, by little and little, those who use it here above them.

Ielanosis of the Lungs

Early in the nineteenth century the morbid anatomists of Paris de-
ribed melanosis of the lungs. In his *Traité de L'Auscultation Médiate*
819) Laennec clearly differentiates secondary melanotic carcinoma of the
angs and the black pulmonary matter deposited in coal-miners' lungs. But
ae first author to record in print that the disease arises out of employment
a coal mines was Gregory (1831); his patient was a Dalkeith collier who
ad worked in the coalpits for twelve years. Various opinions were at that
me held as to the causation of the disease, but in the main it was attributed
ther to the effects of blasting with gunpowder or to the inhalation of
mp-black or soot from the oil-lamps of the miners.

lack Spit and Phthisis Melanotica

In 1833 Marshall of Cambuslang near Glasgow published details of
aree men, all of whom had worked about fifty years as coal miners. In two
f the patients the chest symptoms culminated in the expectoration of
aaterial as black as printers' ink. This *black spit* corresponded to a necropsy
icture of lungs with jet-black nodules and cavities, the expectoration in-
reasing in quantity as the destruction of the lung advanced. Marshall re-
cted all previous views as to the origin of the black material and stated
aat the inhalation of fine coal dust and its deposition in the substance of

the lung was the cause of *spurious melanosis* or *phthisis melanotica*. He con
sidered that though there was an individual predisposition to the diseas
the main factor in its causation was the excessive dustiness of certain mine
where there were hard dry seams and much pick work.

Anthracosis of Colliers

The word *anthracosis* was first used for the disease in colliers b
Thomas Stratton of North Shields in 1837. It was at this time that th
Thomsons of Edinburgh, father and son (1837, 1838), published thei
classic inquiry into the subject. The tubercle bacillus was unknown t
them, but they clearly differentiated between phthisis and tuberculou
phthisis and between those patients who died with anasarca and thos
with hectic fever. They had, of course, no X-rays, but their descriptions o
pathological changes were minute and accurate and closely correlated wit
the clinical findings. They recognized the nodulation of the lungs of ston
workers as opposed to the massive black agglomerations in the lungs c
men who worked at the coal face. From necropsies on men killed i
accidents they learned that lungs which were universally jet black with coa
were compatible with health and full work.

Supposed Decline in the Disease

The generic name *pneumonokoniosis* was introduced by Zenker in 186(
and in 1874 Proust invented the shorter form *pneumoconiosis anthracosic*
The idea that coal dust may possess the property of hindering the develop
ment of pulmonary tuberculosis and of arresting its progress originated wit
Hirt (1871) of Breslau. Arlidge (1892) did not subscribe to this view; h
believed that large fibrotic masses could break down without the presenc
of tuberculosis. Meanwhile, the discovery by Koch in 1882 of the tuberc
bacillus had enabled medical men to distinguish with certainty betwee
phthisis and tuberculous phthisis. As the nineteenth century drew to it
close doctors all over Great Britain had satisfied themselves that anthra
cosis of colliers had for all practical purposes ceased to exist as a medic
problem. This happy state of affairs, so they thought, had been achieved i
fifty years by improved ventilation and improved sanitary conditions i
coal mines together with shorter working hours. In the Milroy Lectures o
1915 Collis said—

> Miners' asthma, common though it used to be, has passed un
> observed from our midst, and conjectures as to its character an
> causation are idle.

Mechanization in Coal Mines

Whether such opinions were correct or not we cannot now be sure, bu
mechanical methods of mining were soon to change people's views of th
effects of coal dust inhaled into the lungs. Late in the nineteenth centur
many patents were granted for coal-cutting machines. In 1913 only 8 pe
cent of coal in Great Britain was machine-cut (fig. 404); by 1950 th
figures had increased to 80 per cent. The earliest machine worked like

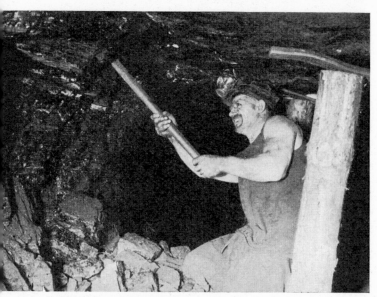

FIG. 404.—Miner hand-cleaning at the Coal Face
(*By courtesy of the National Coal Board*)

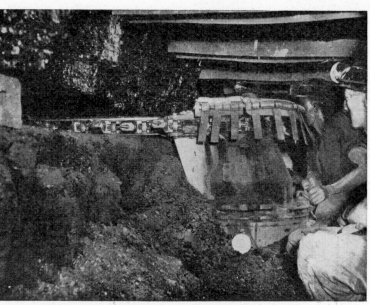

FIG. 405.—Chain Coal Cutter middle-cutting Coal-seam
(*By courtesy of Professor I. C. F. Statham*)

circular saw and was called a *disc machine*. Since 1920 the most widely use
type of machine is the *chain machine*. It depends for its action upon
traversing band saw represented by the chain which carries a series o
cutter picks. In 1938 only 140 disc machines were in use in our coal mine
whereas 6,005 chain machines were operating. Since that year 95 per cen
of the coal-cutters have been of the chain type (fig. 405). With th
mechanical cutting and conveying of coal there was a great increase of dus
and by 1930 the lung diseases of coal miners were again compelling atten
tion, particularly in South Wales.

John Scott Haldane (1860–1936)

By his important studies on the chemical regulation of respiration J. S
Haldane of Edinburgh gained an international reputation as a physiologis
(fig. 406). He devised the standard apparatus and methods common
used in gas analysis, gasometry of the blood and estimation of th
basal rate of metabolism. In addition to his academic appointment a
professor of physiology at Oxford, he acted as honorary director of th
Mining Research Laboratory of the University of Birmingham. His investi
gations of factory ventilation and mine explosions, his work on the physic

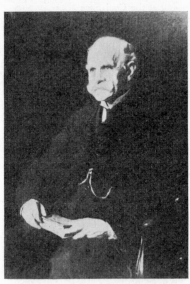

and physiology of deep diving an
his discovery of hookworm in th
Cornish tin mines (p. 752) hav
been of great moment to industria
hygiene. He was mainly responsibl
for the introduction of stone-dust
ing in coal mines as a means of con
trolling underground explosions
His work among metalliferou
miners, particularly Cornish ti
miners, led him to study the cell
storage and expulsion of dusts an
the retention in the lungs of siliceou
dusts. His work on silicosis in miner
in metalliferous mines emphasize
the particular liability of such me
to die of tuberculosis.

Ill-informed Complacency o Medical Men

Fig. 406.—John Scott Haldane,
1860–1936
(*By courtesy of Mr. A. Shaw*)

But coal miners show a lo
death-rate from pulmonary tuber
culosis, and this fact led to the acceptance of the view that silicosis was rar
among them. The declaration by Haldane (1923) that—

the inhalation of coal dust causes no danger to life but on the contrar
gives even protection against the development of tuberculosis,

was largely responsible for the fact that mining engineers made no attempt to reduce the concentration of air-borne coal dust at a time when the introduction of mechanized methods of mining was causing an increased concentration of coal dust. Of this situation Fletcher (1948) has said—

> It must be admitted that medical men by their ill-informed complacency have a heavy load of responsibility to bear for the present high incidence of pneumoconiosis among coal miners.

Improved Methods of Chest Radiography

This period of complacency was closed chiefly by the increasing use of radiography in the diagnosis of chest disease. Cases of definite silicosis in coal miners who had carried out drilling in rock were first reported in South Wales in 1926 by Tattersall. Soon after this, in South Wales, tuberculosis officers of the Welsh National Memorial Association and private radiologists, in particular Harper (1934) in Ammanford, began to observe radiological pictures similar to silicosis in coal miners who would have been diagnosed clinically as cases of chronic bronchitis, and even in apparently healthy miners. In 1930 Cummins and Sladden in a classical paper published a detailed account of the pathology of such cases, showing that they had a kind of silicosis modified by what was regarded as an accumulation of coal dust due to lymphatic blockage by silicotic fibrosis. It was at this time that the technique of chest radiography became perfected as we know it today. In consequence, from 1930 onwards, knowledge of the dust diseases of the lungs was acquired at a greatly accelerated pace.

Exposure of Anthracite Miners in Spakes

Haldane (1935) maintained that coal miners developed bronchitis because of the excessive pulmonary ventilation occasioned by their strenuous work, and that consequently inhaled coal dust was not normally eliminated from their lungs and accumulated to cause a benign type of fibrosis which was not silicotic. Jones (1936) added the suggestion that bronchitis was especially common among anthracite miners because of the method used to bring them to the surface. Entry to and exit from many anthracite pits in South Wales is by drift, a slope negotiated in trams of open cars called *spakes*. In winter the ride is cold and long drawn out, giving maximum exposure to cold air of men who had become hot from heavy muscular work. Examined by X-rays, these men had lung shadows which in Johannesburg gold miners would have meant a sentence of death. And so with the advent of modern chest radiography Haldane found himself in violent collision with clinicians and radiologists.

Mounting Number of Anomalous Cases in South Wales

Meanwhile the Registrar-General's figures for the occupational mortality statistics for the years 1930–2 were published. They showed that respiratory diseases were on the increase in coal miners; they were not benefiting from public health measures to the same extent as other groups.

By 1935 certifications among coal miners by the Silicosis Medical Board focused attention on the progressively mounting number of cases occurring almost entirely in South Wales, especially in the anthracite area around Swansea. In 1936 Dr. Charles L. Sutherland, Chief Medical Officer of the Silicosis Medical Board, directed the attention of the Home Secretary and of the members of the Industrial Pulmonary Diseases Committee of the Medical Research Council to the fact that, in the previous three years, claims for compensation on account of silicosis by coal miners had increased by 70 per cent and these were almost entirely in South Wales. There was also a vast number of men whose cases were of anomalous types and who failed to obtain compensation.

Pathological Significance of Coal Dust

The situation was a most unhappy one and called for immediate scientific investigation. In 1936 the Medical Research Council undertook to investigate the problem of chronic pulmonary disease among coal miners, with particular reference to conditions in the South Wales coalfield. The inquiry which was set up extended over the years 1936–42 and consisted of a medical survey and pathological and environmental studies Hart and Aslett (1942) confirmed that hard-heading workers driving through siliceous rock were subject to silicosis, but that they were few and provided only a small fraction of all the cases of lung disease. The bulk of cases occurred in colliers working at the coal face and to a less extent among other underground workers. Similar lung changes were found amongst surface workers on the screens and coal trimmers at the docks. It was this observation which underlined the importance of coal dust and not rock dust as the causative agent in pneumoconiosis of coal workers.

Reticulation the Earliest Sign in X-rays

According to Hart and Aslett (1942) the pathological changes in the lungs were reflected by radiographic appearances which they classified as (a) reticulation, (b) nodulation, (c) coalescent nodulation, (d) massive shadows and (e) multiple fluffy shadows. Nodulation and massive shadows were already well recognized as features of silicosis. They introduced the term *reticulation* to denote the radiographic appearances in which the lung fields were diffusely altered by delicate shadows like a net of very fine mesh It was the earliest radiological sign of any abnormal changes in the lungs and was the commonest X-ray abnormality amongst the younger colliers in all mines whatever the type of coal.

Pneumoconiosis of Coal Workers

Even when reticulation was not accompanied by clinical disability, its presence still implied the risk of the later progression to consolidation with its more serious accompaniments. Yet this condition could not rightly be designated silicosis. Thus Hart and Aslett had defined a new concept which led to fresh legal definitions and demanded a new name. They uggested *pneumokoniosis of coal miners,* which the Committee on Industrial ʼulmonary Disease later altered to *pneumokoniosis of coal workers* so as to nclude workers engaged in any operation underground in coal mines, in creen workers at collieries and in coal trimmers at docks.

The Cardiff Pneumoconiosis Research Unit

The next step in the investigation of this complex problem was the ːstablishment in Cardiff in 1945 of the Pneumoconiosis Research Unit ınder the direction of Dr. Charles M. Fletcher. As a result of extensive ʼesearches Fletcher and his colleagues have made many useful contribuːions to the subject. One of many lines of investigation they have pursued ːoncerns the study of disability in the miner by physiological methods. ʌpart from its intrinsic interest, this study has two important practical ıspects derived from the fact that the degree of radiological abnormality in ıny case does not give an accurate indication of the severity of the associated ʼespiratory disability: first, there is the need to provide some objective method of disability assessment for purposes of compensation and job ɛelection; secondly, there is need for a means of diagnosis in certain cases ɩn whose X-ray films focal emphysema may have obscured the underlying ɛoal nodulation.

Radiographic Appearances

The Unit have agreed that it is impossible radiographically to identify ɛither the presence or the extent of focal emphysema (see p. 1042). They have concluded that the radiographic appearances may be divided into two main forms: simple pneumoconiosis and progressive massive fibrosis, ɛorresponding with the pathological distinction made by Gough. Fletcher ʻ(1948) points out the confusion which has arisen from the use of the term *reticulation* and from the description of its appearance as being that of a network.

Whatever may be the merits of the word *reticulation* to describe the characteristic pattern of early coal-miners' pneumoconiosis, there is no doubt that in practice its use may give rise to some misunderstanding. Hart and Aslett were forced by circumstances to use a portable X-ray set for their radiography and were therefore unable to achieve a high degree of definition in their films. In the Pneumoconiosis Research Unit we have been fortunate in having a fine-focus rotating anode tube, and we have used ordinary films and high-definition screens. With this technique we find that the most characteristic and almost universal change in the disease is a fine mottling whose main components are usually less than 1 mm. in diameter but may reach twice that size.

Pin-head Mottling

For this appearance we have, for the time being, used the term *pin-head mottling*. In the earliest stages it appears alongside and between exaggerated lung markings, but later it may become so intense that it obscures the normal markings completely. It is uncommon for this pin-head mottling to remain in a pure form. Frequently it is associated with a coarser mottling, through which it can still be distinguished, so that a film is often seen which appears nodular when viewed at a distance of a few feet but in which, on closer scrutiny, the nodules can be seen to be composed of aggregates of pin-head mottling. These granular nodules may be distinguished from a more homogeneous type of nodule which we see particularly in cases resembling classical silicosis with a history of heavy exposure to rock dust or in cases where we suspect a complicating tuberculosis.

Coarser Nodular Shadows

The commonest type of film is one in which there is a mixture of pin-head mottling with rather coarser nodular shadows of irregular shape and size. We are not inclined to use the word *network* to describe any of these appearances. We do not suggest that at present the term *reticulation* should be abandoned. It has proved useful in emphasizing the differences between the early stages of coal-miners' pneumoconiosis and those of classical silicosis, and it can only be supplanted by some better term as a result of wide agreement among workers in the field of pneumoconiosis. Moreover, it may be that, with further advances in radiographic technique, further modifications in terminology may become necessary.

Progressive Massive Fibrosis

This nodulation in due course may coalesce so that conglomerate shadows develop. These may be symmetrical, resembling *angel's wings*, or they may be massive, homogeneous, smooth, rounded shadows, well-defined and commonly in the upper zones (plate XV). Following melanoptysis a central translucent area develops within a massive shadow indicating the presence of a cavity which may show a fluid level. They are accompanied by some degree of simple pneumoconiosis and by basal emphysema. The combination of simple pneumoconiosis with progressive massive fibrosis has been called *complicated pneumoconiosis*.

Clinical Varieties of the Disease

Coal-miners' pneumoconiosis presents three different clinical pictures. There is the pure coal-dust disease, non-progressive and benign unless focal emphysema develops, when it may be fatal. In this respect it is a more serious condition than the second disease, the classical non-infective silicosis of rock workers, in which focal emphysema is much less prominent. In coal miners these two diseases are often indistinguishably combined. Then there is a third disease process, due to the interaction between some infective process, often tuberculosis, and the dust ensnared in the lung. The fundamental similarity of coal-miners' pneumoconiosis to pure siliosis is close. Fletcher (1948) believes the differences must be due, as Cummins (1934) maintained, to some action of the coal dust in the lung in subduing the toxic effects of tuberculosis both generally and locally, so that it is not clinically apparent, and so that the bacilli only occasionally escape from their fibrous prison to spread throughout the lung or appear in the sputum. The clinical differences between coal-miners' pneumoconiosis and silicosis are chiefly that the coal miner with his focal emphysema and his anthraco-silico-tuberculosis is more breathless than ill and his death is like that of a chronic bronchitic with emphysema and right heart failure. He has, as Cummins has emphasized, miners' dyspnœa or miners' asthma. On the other hand, the silicotic with silico-tuberculosis is more often ill as well as dyspnœic. He has miners' phthisis, and dies of clinically recognizable tuberculosis.

Clinical Course

The clinical course of the illness may cover many years. Sometimes the patient has no symptoms, although routine X-rays show abnormalities in the lungs. And then for a long time the only prominent symptom is dyspnœa. As the disease progresses this gets worse and cough may appear. In 1955 Gilson and Hugh-Jones published the results of a detailed investigation of the breathlessness relating its severity to the radiographic changes. In simple pneumoconiosis it is age rather than the extent of the disease which is important in predicting the degree of disability. In complicated pneumoconiosis breathlessness is nearly always severe; it increases with radiological abnormality; and it is augmented by increasing age. The excessive feeling of breathlessness on exertion results primarily from a diminution of the maximum ventilatory capacity of the lungs, and only to a relatively small extent from increase in the ventilation required for exercise. *Melanoptysis*, the coughing up of coal-black sputum, sometimes occurs and continues on and off for years. The chest becomes barrel-shaped and there may be clubbing of the fingers. Hyper-resonance appears at the bases, and here the breath sounds become diminished. When bronchitis supervenes there will be coarse crepitations throughout the lungs. The progress of the disease is often accompanied by a rising erythrocyte sedimentation-rate. The ultimate clinical picture depends upon whether right heart failure or silico-tuberculosis supervenes.

Pathology of Simple Pneumoconiosis

In the simple state the dust is found throughout the lungs in the form of black foci measuring up to about 5 millimetres in diameter. The dust collects around the small bronchioles and their accompanying arteries, having been brought there from the alveoli by phagocytes. For the most part the dust remains within these cells, the general shape of which is preserved, although the nuclei are obscured. Reticulin fibres develop in the foci of dust (Belt and Ferris, 1942). Fibrosis may not proceed beyond this stage or there may be the development of collagen. The latter does not

develop to the same extent as in classical silicosis, nor does it have
the concentric disposition, but runs irregularly or radially. The foci
have a crenated edge with the processes extending into the unaffected
tissues.

Pathology of Focal Emphysema

In and around the coal foci the air-spaces become dilated, giving a char
acteristic appearance described as focal emphysema. This emphysema has
also been described in classical silicosis, but it is very much more severe in
the coal worker, and in the latter the emphysematous spaces may enlarge and
become confluent (Gough, 1947, 1949). They can be demonstrated to per
fection by the new technique of large tissue sections (fig. 407). The focal
emphysema appears to be due to some mechanical disturbance within the
secondary lobules of the lung, as in these units the emphysema starts
around the bronchioles and extends outward towards the interlobular
septa. In focal emphysema there are no bullæ projecting from the surface
of the lung, so that the condition can be distinguished from ordinary
bullous emphysema. Williams (1944) observed that there was interference
with the lumen of the terminal bronchioles, causing partial obstruction
with trapping of air and consequent development of emphysema. Hepple
ston (1947) considers that the development of focal emphysema in coal
workers can be explained by the accumulated dust acting mechanically, the
foci of coal dust interfering with the function of the respiratory bronchioles
He also considers that shrinkage of the dust foci contributes to the
development of surrounding emphysema.

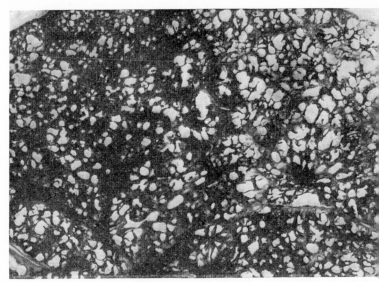

FIG. 407.—Large Tissue Section of Lung, natural size, showing the Multi-
focal Emphysema of Coal Workers' Pneumoconiosis

Relationship to the Rank of Coal

King and Nagelschmidt (1945) regard coal-miners' pneumoconiosis as a form of silicosis and they contend that the small amount of quartz in the dust is the pathogenic agent, although their chemical analysis of coal-miners' lungs does not give conclusive support to this view. King (1945) found that the dust from the Welsh coal mines has a low silica solubility, and Hicks and Nagelschmidt (1943) failed to find any marked relationship between the silica content of the dust in the various Welsh coal mines and the incidence of the disease. Reverting to the hypothesis of Hart and Aslett (1942) they suggest that the latter may be related to the rank of coal in the different mines; by *rank* is meant the amount of volatile material present. In the South Wales coalfield the character and rank of coal change gradually from north-west to south-east. The highest rank of anthracite with about 5 per cent of volatile matter is found in the north-west, and, proceeding towards the south-east, the volatile content steadily increases, the coal changing in character to lower-rank anthracite, steam coal, and finally in the south-eastern and eastern parts of the coalfield to bituminous coal with up to 36 per cent of volatile matter. The incidence of lung disease is higher in the anthracite and steam-coal areas than in the bituminous areas.

Harmful Effect of Coal not restricted to Silica Content

The opposing theories of mechanical and chemical action of the dust in coal-miners' lungs may be reconciled by accepting that each is in part correct, as is suggested by the following experiments. King and his co-workers (1948), treating rats by intratracheal injections of coal mixed with quartz, found that the mixtures produced more fibrosis than quartz alone, and they conclude that a small amount of quartz in the presence of a large amount of coal will bring about greater pathological results than the probable sum of the two components used separately. No difference was found between bituminous and anthracite coals, either when given alone or when mixed with quartz, and it is suggested that perhaps the coal dust blocks the lymphatic channels so that the quartz remains longer in the lung. These results support the conclusion that the harmful effect of coal is not restricted to its silica content. The practical result of such a view is that all dusts in the coal mine should be regarded as harmful and should be suppressed.

Identical Lung Disease in Coal Trimmers working in Ships

We have seen that Hart and Aslett found pneumoconiosis in coal trimmers who worked only in ships (fig. 408). In 1940 Gough investigated the pathology of this condition and demonstrated focal emphysema identical with that in men working at the coal face. This proves conclusively that the dust of commercial coal is noxious. In the past it has been argued that the respiratory disease in coal miners may be due to nitrogen-dioxide fumes from the explosives used in getting the coal, or to severe chilling when

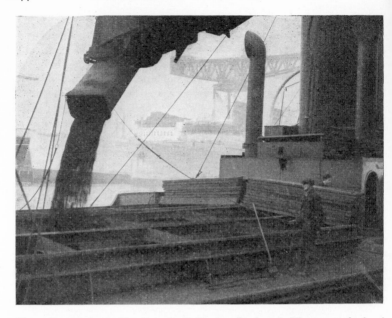

FIG. 408.—Mechanical loading of a Collier in a Dockyard. The men who level the Cargo in the Holds of the Ship are called Coal Trimmers

leaving the working-place on the long journeys underground against the incoming air. The occurrence of an identical form of the disease in men loading coal into ships shows that cold and nitrogen dioxide can be at the most only contributory factors and that the essential cause is the inhalation of dust.

Infective Variety of Coal-workers' Pneumoconiosis

The condition described above as simple pneumoconiosis seems to be due to the action of dust alone, but superimposed upon it there is frequently a fibrosis which appears to be due to the combined action of tuberculosis and dust. This fibrosis occurs in the form of circumscribed masses most frequently in the upper and posterior parts of the lungs, sometimes unilateral, usually bilateral. The fibrous masses are black and may be several inches in diameter, and are firm and rubbery in consistency (fig. 409). The centres of the masses often contain black inky fluid in which are crystals of cholesterol; in some cases the fluid is expectorated, leaving ragged cavities. These cavities appear to be formed by necrosis due to obliterative endarteritis.

Massive Fibrosis due to Tuberculosis

In about 40 per cent of cases of massive fibrosis, tubercle bacilli can be demonstrated in the lesions post-mortem by culture or animal inoculation,

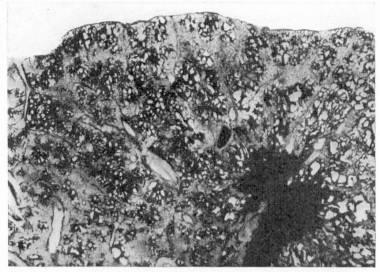

FIG. 409.—Large Tissue Section of Lung, natural size, showing the Black Areas of Massive Fibrosis in Coal Workers' Pneumoconiosis

and in those cases where no bacilli are found it is assumed that the infection has died out. In the past, tuberculosis has been regarded as of low incidence in coal workers, but the form of tuberculous reaction which occurs does not usually give rise to caseation or to the usual symptoms of open tuberculosis. There is greater formation of fibrous tissue, the progress is very slow and the ill effects are principally on the pulmonary circulation, causing right heart hypertrophy and death from congestive heart failure. In a smaller percentage of cases the tuberculosis spreads more acutely, and in these there is caseation and bronchopneumonic spread of the infection. Another cause of death is pulmonary arterial thrombosis. This begins in a branch of the artery in relation to an area of massive fibrosis, and the thrombus spreads towards the hilum of the lung.

Hazard of Right Heart Failure

In summarizing the outstanding differences between the pathology of coal-workers' pneumoconiosis and classical silicosis, emphasis is placed first on the more severe focal emphysema in the coal-worker's lung, and secondly on the somewhat different effects of tuberculosis in the two conditions. In classical silicosis the open type of tuberculosis is a common terminal event, although heart failure from massive fibrosis also occurs; in coal workers, massive fibrosis leading to heart failure is the usual occurrence, whereas open tuberculosis is a less common complication.

Rheumatoid Pneumoconiosis (Caplan's Syndrome)

The quantity and nature of dust in the working environment are the prime factors in the hazard of pneumoconiosis, but there is also a host factor as some individuals are more susceptible than others working under identical conditions. The explanation of one cause of increased susceptibility was made in 1953 by Dr. A. Caplan of the Pneumoconiosis Panel in Cardiff. He noted that coal miners who suffer from rheumatoid arthritis are particularly liable to develop in X-rays of the chest large nodular lesions if they are exposed to dust. The large circumscribed nodules which may develop rapidly in the lungs can be distinguished from the pneumoconiosis of non-rheumatoid subjects. The dust in some way renders the lungs vulnerable to the rheumatoid process, perhaps by the formation of abnormal collagen. Following the original cases in coal miners in Wales similar examples have been seen in coal workers in other parts of Great Britain and in other European countries. In Belgium Clerens (1953) described two cases from the same factory in women exposed to a pure silica hazard. From Holland van der Meer (1954) reported one case in a man who had worked as a diamond and metal polisher and also as a sandblaster. Cases of the rheumatoid pneumoconiosis syndrome have been observed in Great Britain in workers exposed to dust in the potteries, brass and iron foundries and sandblasting (Caplan, Cowen and Gough, 1958). A case was reported by Campbell (1958) in a boiler-scaler and another by Rickards and Barrett (1958) in an asbestos worker.

Radiological Features of Rheumatoid Pneumoconiosis

X-rays show multiple, well-defined round opacities 0·5 to 5 cm. in diameter distributed throughout both lung fields. The opacities often appear with a suddenness that is not usually observed in the development of ordinary progressive massive fibrosis. In many cases the background of simple pneumoconiosis is slight and indeed it may be absent. The opacities may appear before, coincident with or after the onset of arthritis, and there is no apparent relationship between the severity of the arthritis and the extent and type of the radiological changes. In some cases the opacities increase in size and number and crops of fresh lesions may appear at intervals of a few months. In other cases a few round opacities are localized to one or more areas of the lung fields and remain stationary. Cavitation or calcification of the lesions is fairly common, and in many instances they ultimately become incorporated in the progressive massive fibrosis (Caplan, Cowen and Gough, 1958).

Rheumatoid Granulomata occasioned by Dust

A detailed pathological study of the syndrome has been made by Gough, Rivers and Seal (1955). They described the lung lesions in sixteen coal workers, from material obtained at necropsy and biopsy, as having a characteristic appearance and distinguishable from progressive massive fibrosis and the classical silicotic nodule. Macroscopically the lesions show a characteristic concentric arrangement of lighter and darker layers. The pale areas are grey in some instances and yellow in others. Liquefaction tends to occur in the pale areas leaving clefts. In some cases the nodules

ιre densely calcified. The histological criteria upon which diagnosis should
ϸe made are a central area of necrotic collagen, outside which is a zone of
ιctive inflammation consisting of a cellular infiltration of macrophages and
ʾrequently also of polymorphonuclear leucocytes. In this zone collagen is
ϸeing destroyed. In sections stained with hæmatoxylin and eosin the
ιntense blue of the inflammatory zone contrasts with the pink of the central
ιecrotic collagen. Some of the macrophages in the inflammatory zone con-
ain dust. When these macrophages die and disintegrate the dust is
leposited and this accounts for the dark concentric rings seen in the
ιodules. The inflammatory zone may involve the whole or only part of the
ϲircumference of a nodule. Multinuclear giant cells are present in some
ιnstances, and these lie in a zone of fibroblasts outside the zone of inflam-
ιatory cells. The fibroblasts are arranged in the style of a palisade outside
ϲhe circumference of which is a zone of collagen. Endarteritis is present in
ʋessels at the periphery of the nodules, and in the lumen of the vessels
ϲhere are more lymphocytes and plasma cells than are seen in the endar-
ϲeritis usually present in pneumoconiosis. In North America these lesions
ʰave been mistaken for fungus granuloma, particularly histoplasmosis.
However, they contain no fungi and the histological picture they present
ιs undoubtedly a combination of dust effect and rheumatoid granuloma
ΐGough, 1958).

Periodic Radiographic Examination of Coal Workers

The course of the disease under various environmental conditions is of
considerable importance in prognosis and in deciding whether or not a
patient may safely continue in his occupation. On the average, young men
with quite advanced simple pneumoconiosis are not seriously disabled.
Men with progressive massive fibrosis on the other hand are usually much
disabled and their disability increases both with age and the radiological
degree of the progressive massive fibrosis. Simple pneumoconiosis, judged
radiologically, does not progress as such in the absence of further inhalation
of coal dust, but once massive fibrosis has started it is nearly always progressive whether or not dust exposure ceases. It has therefore been argued
that if men could be removed from the danger before the critical stage is
reached, their future health would be safeguarded. To fulfil this desirable
purpose, a system of periodic radiographic examinations of coal workers
was advocated (Fletcher, 1948; Cochrane and others, 1951).

National Coal Board Medical Service

Under the National Coal Board there is a comprehensive full-time
occupational health service covering every coalpit in Great Britain (p. 210).
This service is assisted by a staff of nurses (p. 210) and collaborates with
H.M. Inspectors of Mines (p. 209), who ensure the observance of mining
regulations. Under the *Coal Mines (Medical Examinations) General Regulations, 1952*, it is provided that all persons entering employment in or about
coal mines shall be medically examined. By 1953 in some coalfields the

examination included a radiograph of the chest. Since the beginning of 1959 a regulation has been in force making radiographic examination of the chest universal throughout the coal mines of Great Britain (p. 210).

Neglect of Airborne Coal Dust

After the passing of the *Coal Mines Act* in 1911 the use of some device to prevent the escape of rock dust into the air during drilling became obligatory, but no attempts were made to suppress coal dust. In 1938 the

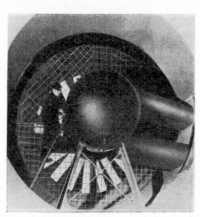

Royal Commission for Safety in Coal Mines discussed suppression of coal dust only as a means of reducing the danger from explosions. Research into the problem was, however, advised, and the British Coalowners' Research Associations and the Safety in Mines Research Board began to investigate the problem. In South Wales, as the results of the Medical Research Council's investigations came to be known, serious attention began to be paid to the prevention and suppression of coal dust under-

FIG. 410.—Centrifugal Fan in a Coal Mine. It can circulate up to 400,000 cubic feet of Air per minute

ground, by the Mines Inspectorate, the Monmouthshire and South Wales Coal Owners' Association and by the Amalgamated Anthracite Company, who set up their own Silicosis Research Committee.

Methods of Dust Suppression

Six main methods are used to protect the coal miner against airborne dust.

(i) *Ventilation* is essential in reducing dust concentration (fig. 410). It has been particularly important in the South Wales anthracite mines, where, owing to the methods of working the coal in common use and owing to the rather haphazard development of the mines from shallow surface workings, poor ventilation was formerly one of the main reasons for the high dust concentrations.

(ii) *Wet Cutting* is achieved by directing two jets of water on the chain of the coal-cutter at the points where it enters and leaves the coal (fig. 411). The usual quantity of water is 5 gallons per yard of advance on the coal face. Of course, this treatment has a very beneficial effect during the subsequent loading on to conveyers. Dry cutting should be forbidden.

(iii) *Wet Drilling* is carried out with compressed-air drills, in which the water passes under pressure through a hollow drill-steel and is directed on to its cutting edge. Dry drilling should be forbidden (fig. 412).

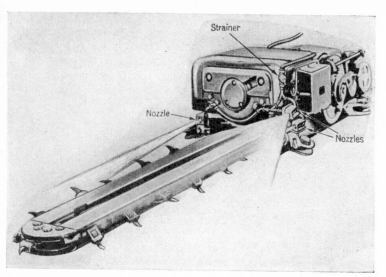

FIG. 411.—Jeffrey 35B Shortwall Mining Machine with Spray Equipment to
allay Dust during undercutting
(*By courtesy of Professor I. C. F. Statham*)

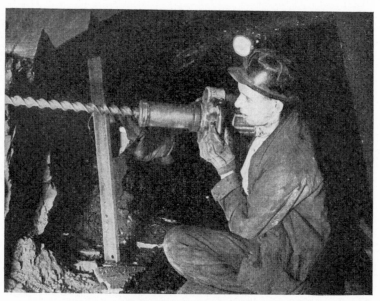

FIG. 412.—Drilling Shot-holes at the Coal Face
(*By courtesy of the National Coal Board*)

(iv) *Water Infusion* is carried out on coal faces which are not undercut At intervals of 12 feet along the face a series of 7-foot holes is drilled. A tube with an expansible rubber collar is inserted into each hole and 1 gallons of water at 100 lb. pressure are forced in, a small meter being use to indicate the quantity. The water spreads through the cleavage planes i the coal and wets the loose dust which is always present in the joints an seams.

(v) *Hand Spraying* is the wetting down with water of the coal fac before the coal is pulled down, and of the loose coal before it is loaded, o before it is transferred from one conveyer to another, or from a conveyo into trams.

(vi) *Dust Masks.* There are certain mining methods in which the pro duction of heavy dust clouds will be unavoidable—for instance, shot firing. It will then be necessary for men to wear respirators. Unfortunately no efficient respirator has yet been devised which men are willing to wea consistently. In the design of respirators, filtration efficiency has been give priority over wearability, despite the obvious fact that an efficient mask i the pocket is of much less use than an inefficient mask on the face. In thi field of investigation the biological approach is needed, giving first attentio to the convenience of the man, if necessary at the expense of perfec filtration efficiency (Fletcher, 1948).

The rest of England is still behind South Wales in the application o these methods. Dust Prevention Committees have been set up in ever division of the British coalfields and the fruit of their labours is anxiousl awaited.

Need for fully trained Dust-suppression Officers

Fletcher (1948) emphasizes that it is the doctor's rôle not to ask ove how many miles of coal face measures of dust prevention are officiall being applied; he must ask, rather, how far dust levels are in fact bein reduced.

A further rôle for the doctor as a human biologist is to insist tha dust-suppression measures should not only be mechanically and physic ally effective, but that the men who have to operate them should fin them convenient and acceptable in use, and that they should by policy of education come fully to appreciate their need. Sprays tha are ill-adjusted may wet the men more than the coal and will be turne off. Excessive use of water in any method may cause unpleasan working conditions. Men are always unwilling to accept measures fo their own safety that are inconvenient and require care and attention Perhaps the most urgent needs today in the field of dust suppressio are that more attention should be paid to the human factor, that i every piece of mining machinery automatic dust-suppression device should be incorporated by the manufacturers, and that there shoul be *fully trained* dust-suppression officers in every pit.

Non-pathogenic Inorganic Dusts

The dusts of the compounds of certain metals, among them calcium, iron, tin and barium, seem to be inert when inhaled. The resulting conditions are sometimes referred to as the *benign pneumoconioses*. The particles, provided they are small enough to enter the alveoli, are engulfed in phagocytes, some of which are coughed up, while others are deposited in the aggregations of lymphoid tissue at the bifurcations of the bronchioles. They are capable of lying there for years without inducing any deposition of fibrous tissue or other reaction, but because they are relatively opaque to X-rays they may produce changes in the X-ray film which then must be distinguished from those of silicosis. The density of the X-ray shadows increases with the atomic weight of the element in the compound concerned as follows: calcium 40·08, iron 55·85, tin 118·70 and barium 137·36.

(*a*) Calcium

We have seen (p. 360) that the dusts of limestone, marble, lime, cement and gypsum are harmless to the lungs, producing at the most nonprogressive arborescent shadows in X-rays of the chest but no symptoms or disability and no fibrosis of the lungs.

(*b*) Iron

In 1866 Zenker ascribed fibrosis of the lungs to the inhalation of iron dust and named the condition *siderosis*. For many years this was considered to be the first of the pneumoconioses. But both the cases he had examined had pulmonary tuberculosis and such fibrosis as he found in the lungs may well have resulted from infection with the tubercle bacillus. We now know that inhalation of iron or iron oxide causes no fibrous reaction in the lung tissue. The disease at first called siderosis in knife grinders and needle finishers is, in fact, *sidero-silicosis*, and is produced not by the iron in the tissues, for this is inert, but by the free silica arising as a dust from the sandstone wheel used for grinding.

Welders' Siderosis or Iron-oxide Lung

Today opportunities for inhaling iron-oxide dust occur in many occupations, including welding and silver finishing. The heat of the electric arc or the oxy-acetylene torch melts and boils the metal being welded, iron coming off as a blue-grey fume and oxidizing almost immediately to iron oxide in minute particles. Welders who have spent years at this work, particularly if they have performed substantial amounts of welding inside boilers, tanks and other ill-ventilated spaces, may be found on X-ray examination to show reticulation or nodulation. But this does not necessarily mean fibrosis of the lungs nor, indeed, disease of any sort, and many a worker has passed through a very unhappy period after being told he was suffering from silicosis when, in fact, he was merely exhibiting a dusting or tattooing of his lungs with iron oxide.

The Worker remains in Good Health

The condition called *welders' siderosis* or *iron-oxide lung* was first described by Doig and McLaughlin in 1936. They emphasized that the X-ray changes occurred in men who were apparently in good health. Further experience by clinical examinations of some hundreds of welders has shown that the condition is benign and unaccompanied by symptoms, abnormal physical signs or diminished capacity for work. Some welders with dust reticulation have remained well and continued at work without disability up to fourteen years. The X-ray changes are not associated with dyspnœa or clinical evidence of fibrosis. Chest expansion is good and tolerance for exercise is normal. These findings have been confirmed by numerous investigators, not only in welders (Lanza, 1945) but also in other workers exposed to iron oxide, such as silver finishers (Barrie and Harding, 1947).

Non-progressive X-ray Changes

The X-ray picture may be identical with that of silicosis, and examination of a single X-ray film does not supply evidence of the inert nature of the condition. Serial X-rays taken over a period of years, particularly after exposure to welding has ceased, may, however, give supporting evidence. X-ray changes in silicosis are permanent; if they change it is for the worse, indicating a progression of the process, and such a change is unfortunately common. Improvement in the X-ray appearances has not been described nor is it to be expected in a disease characterized by the laying down of a considerable amount of fibrous tissue. On the other hand, Doig and McLaughlin (1948) have described two welders in whom the X-ray appearances changed for the better, and, indeed, in one case the picture returned to normal some years after giving up welding. Such an observation is only compatible with a condition in which the dust lies amongst normal tissue and is not shut in by fibrous tissue or associated with other changes of a permanent nature.

No Fibrosis of Lungs at Necropsy

There is only one report in the literature of a post-mortem examination of a welder who showed X-ray changes of the dust-inhalation type during life (Enzer and Sander, 1938). This is illustrated by excellent photomicrographs showing no fibrosis round the collections of dust, which were found to give the Prussian-blue reaction. The man's death was not related to his occupation or his lung condition, but was the result of an accident. In successive papers McLaughlin and others (1945), Barrie and Harding (1947) and Harding (1948) describe the post-mortem findings in five silver finishers using as an abrasive *jewellers' rouge* which is finely divided ferric oxide, Fe_2O_3. The X-rays of these men had shown the typical changes of

ust-deposition in the lungs. In the first four cases there was no fibrosis
ound the deposits of iron oxide. In the fifth case there was a minimal amount
f fibrosis of the reticulation type, not at all like that produced by silica.
Harding thinks that in this case individual susceptibility may have been of
nportance, but there is always the possibility that the iron dust at some
eriod in the forty years of the man's working life may have contained silica
r some other constituent capable of producing fibrosis. Indeed, it is not
mpossible that he may have used sand as the polishing medium at one
ime (Doig, 1949). Histological examination disclosed iron oxide and silver
n the lungs; the former was in phagocytic cells along the course of the
ymphatics and had produced no interstitial fibrosis. The silver dust was
leposited in the elastic tissue of the alveolar walls and the small pulmonary
essels. In two cases there was marked emphysema, but the authors were
lot prepared to associate this with the silver impregnation of the alveolar
valls.

Experimental and Statistical Evidence

Further evidence of the inert behaviour of iron oxide has been obtained
rom animal experiments. Harding, Grout and Lloyd Davies (1947) pro-
luced X-ray changes in the lungs of rats exposed to iron-oxide dust, but
examination of the tissues showed no fibrotic or other reaction. Finally,
here is statistical evidence. The Registrar-General's *Supplementary Report on Occupational Mortality*, 1931, shows that of the 11,542 welders in
England and Wales in that year there were only 123 deaths compared with
161 expected on the basis of age-rates for all males. In welders in the
Kaiser shipyards in Oregon, Collen (1947) describes the incidence of
pneumonia in welders, showing that the incidence, death-rates and case
fatality-rates were similar to those of all other shipyard workers and that
:here was no difference in the severity, the number of days required for
treatment or the incidence of complications. It seems clear that iron oxide,
inhaled into the lungs in amounts sufficient to give rise to changes in the
X-ray film, lies inert in the tissues for years without giving rise to pulmonary fibrosis or other permanent change.

(c) Tin

Tin is much more radio-opaque than iron and therefore deposits in the
lungs cause particularly dense shadows, a condition known as *stannosis*.
Pendergrass and Pryde (1948) reproduce an excellent X-ray of this type,
the subject being a man aged forty-five years who had bagged tin oxide for
fifteen years. He had no disability, the X-ray abnormality being discovered
during a routine survey of all the work-people. Barták and Tomečka (1948)
also consider that tin oxide, although producing radiographic changes,
does not produce ill-effects clinically. These authors in 1939 examined one
worker in an enamel factory who consulted a doctor on account of asthma
which had suddenly become worse. He was forty-nine years of age and for
eighteen years had had charge of a furnace in which pure tin was burned

to tin oxide. The atmosphere in which he worked was loaded with the du of the oxide. There were no abnormal physical signs, but the X-ra picture of the lungs showed scattered dense punctate shadows. Of sixtee co-workers at the same factory, six showed the same X-ray picture. Thes men had been exposed to the dust of tin oxide for periods from six month to twenty-five years. The remaining ten workers had been employed at th furnace only occasionally; their real work was in the same room as th furnace, but 6 metres away from it. None of them had symptoms, an X-ray pictures of their chests were normal. A year later (1940) the patier with stannosis was found to have carcinoma of the stomach, of which h died in 1942.

At a time when only 13 cases had ever been reported and none i Great Britain, Robertson and Whitaker (1955) examined 215 workers i a dirty, manually operated tin refinery on Merseyside and showed tha 121 of these showed the X-ray changes of pneumoconiosis although non had ever had any symptoms or signs whatsoever. Without doubt they ha been exposed, most of them heavily, either to the dust or to the fume o stannous oxide for periods varying between 3 and 41 years. Detailed lun function studies showed no abnormality in any one of them. Robertso (1960) obtained two necropsies; in one of these the patient was a man of 8 who had worked for 40 years as a furnaceman in tin refining and had the retired for 20 years. He had never had symptoms of any respiratory disease and even one year before he died no abnormal physical signs were t be found in his chest. X-rays had shown the punctate mottling of pneumo coniosis. Histological examination showed groups of alveoli filled wit dust cells, but no fibrosis could be detected even on reticulin staining After incineration of the lung some of the dust particles were found t measure only 0·1 micron in diameter, which is what might be expecte from breathing the fume of tin oxide from a furnace for 40 years. Analysi showed that the total amount of stannous oxide for both lungs was 6· grams. The figure for silica was negligible. Robertson's work confirm the view not only that pneumoconiosis due to stannous oxide is benig and symptomless, but also that this oxide reaching the alveolar tissues o the lungs is entirely innocuous and may lie there quite inert setting up n reaction at all even after 60 years.

(d) Barium

Baritosis is a type of benign pneumoconiosis first described by Arrigon (1933) among the baryta miners of Valsassina in Italy. It occurs particularl in the grinders and packers, and results from the inhalation of finely groun particles of barium sulphate. In the men concerned there was no respiratory incapacity, and abnormal physical signs were slight or absent. The onl evidence of its presence was the demonstration by X-rays of small sharpl circumscribed nodules evenly distributed throughout the lung fields. I 1953 Pendergrass and Greening described a case of baritosis in a man wh had worked for twenty years in the grinding department of a lithopone plant

Analysis of the ground material showed 97 per cent barium sulphate and 3 per cent silica. Analysis of the air-floated dust sample revealed barium 49·1 per cent and silica 2·1 per cent. Wearing a respirator, the man had been exposed for one and a half hours a day to dust of which the particle count was 6,000,000,000 particles per cubic foot of air. At the age of seventy-one, and twelve years after the detection of the baritosis, he had a sudden severe attack of retrosternal pain and died of a large infarct of the heart. At necropsy the lungs showed uniformly scattered black firm fibrous nodules from 1 to 3 millimetres in diameter. Barium sulphate was detected in the lung by chemical analysis, spectrographic examination and X-ray diffraction. There were about twenty other workers exposed to the same hazard, but of the group only this man and one other showed changes in the lungs.

Pathogenic Inorganic Dusts

Various non-siliceous dusts are capable of producing pulmonary lesions, the most important of these being aluminium, beryllium and silicon carbide. We have seen already how manganese (p. 464), cadmium (p. 447) and vanadium (p. 497) can give rise to chemical pneumonitis.

(a) Aluminium

In the Second World War exposure of workmen in Germany to the inhalation of aluminium dust and of others in Canada to the fumes from bauxite smelting gave rise to a condition known as *aluminosis* or *aluminium lung*. Examination of material from the German cases showed that there was undoubtedly a pneumoconiosis, so that aluminium must be regarded as a toxic substance under certain conditions of exposure. In the Second World War powdered metallic aluminium was used extensively in making explosives, incendiary mixtures and paints. The powder was made by two processes: either it was blown, when the particles were covered with a thin film of alumina, or it was stamped, when they were covered with a thin film of stearine. The fact that German workers were affected in this industry rather than those of other countries may have been due to the omission of lubricants in the stamping process or perhaps to the increase in the amount of dust in the atmosphere in consequence of war conditions.

Symptoms and Signs

Describing the investigation of 700 workers in Germany, Goralewski (1939, 1940, 1941 and 1943) gives details of various types of disease attributed to aluminium. The aluminium powder to which the workers had been exposed contained about four milliards of particles per grain of dust, but the size was not stated. The development of the illness was rapid and appeared to bear no relation to the length of exposure to aluminium. They complained of dry cough with pain on breathing, shortness of breath, poor appetite, and gnawing abdominal pain. Spontaneous pneumothorax was described in four workers. Blood counts showed a relative lymphocytosis with an eosinophilia up to 10 per cent. In 78 per cent of the cases the sedimentation-rate was within normal limits, and the vital capacity was decreased in twenty-seven instances. Radiographs showed focal shadows in the apical region with an increase of normal bronchial markings in the upper and middle thirds of the lung, giving a reticular appearance which at a later stage tended to increase and become confluent.

A Colloidal Aluminium-hydroxide Complex

Histological examination of the lung of a patient who died revealed coarse, branching, hyaline, collagenous fibres which enclosed phagocytes containing fine and coarsely granular particles distinguished by jagged outline from carbon particles. Jager and Jager (1941) suggested that while aluminium powder is highly resistant to aerial oxidation, it is freely soluble in sodium chloride solution, giving sodium aluminate and aluminium chloride in equilibrium. A colloidal aluminium-hydroxide complex results if the sodium and chlor ions are allowed to diffuse away, and if protein is also present it is co-precipitated round the partly dissolved aluminium particles. Jager and Jager think it is this complex which causes the lung changes. Koelsch (1942), however, believes that the disease was a consequence of the unsatisfactory ventilation of workrooms resulting from the blackout imposed by the war.

Pneumoconiosis in Bauxite Smelters (Shaver's Disease)

In connexion with aluminium, another form of pneumoconiosis was described in Canada (Shaver and Riddell, 1947; Shaver, 1948) as occurring in men exposed to the fumes arising in the process of making the abrasive *corundum*, Al_2O_3, a form of artificial emery. This is done in a works at Niagara by heating bauxite, an ore containing approximately 80 per cent Al_2O_3 and up to 7 per cent silica, with iron and coke in the electric arc at 2,000° C. The men affected were bin men, furnace feeders and overhead crane men. Between 1941 and 1943 visible fume came off from the kettles in which the bauxite was being fused. In 1943, production was accelerated, thus giving rise to a greater dose of fume per man. There were 13 deaths from pneumothorax. One man had 8 pneumothoraces and he is the only man seriously affected who still lives (Riddell, 1954). Silicotic nodules did not develop, but there was diffuse fibrosis and the formation of emphysematous bullæ which often ruptured and sometimes fused together to form larger cavities. The ætiology of the fibrosis of the lung is uncertain, as the noxious atmosphere contained 32·3 per cent silicon dioxide and 56 per cent aluminium oxide, the silica being almost entirely in amorphous form (Pratt, 1950). The particles were from 0·02 to 0·5 microns in diameter, a particle size which has in the past been regarded as of little significance (Hatch, 1950). In order to render silica insoluble by means of alumina the latter must be of a type which readily takes up water and becomes adsorbed on the silica particles. The alumina in the fume at the Niagara works was not of that type (Irwin, 1950). Meanwhile, tuberculosis has not developed in the lungs of the survivors, and Riddell (1954) believes that the disease is aluminosis and not silicosis.

xposure in Men grinding Duralumin Propellers

Hunter, Milton and Perry (1944) studied the effect of dust on the lungs
f grinders of duralumin aeroplane propellers. The grinders were exposed
> a mixture of aluminium dust arising from the propellers, and alumina,
.l₂O₃, from the alundum grinding wheels (fig. 413). The average concen-
-ation of aluminium dust close to the operator's mouth was found to be 3
uilligrams per cubic metre of air, of which the particle size in 1 milligram was
etween 2 and 7 microns, the remaining 2 milligrams consisting of larger
articles. The alumina particles were mostly of less than 1 micron diameter.
'he health of these workers, as shown by their records for sick absence
uring the preceding year, was better than that of those in a machine shop
elonging to the same company. None gave any history of spontaneous
neumothorax, and no abnormality was found in their blood counts.
.adiographs were taken of the chests of ninety-two workers; in seven
istances there were shadows in the peripheral part of the lung which were
ifferent from those usually found in this situation. These shadows are
robably of little significance, but attention is drawn to them since it is
onceivable that they are shadows caused by concretions of aluminium
ust as described by Belt and King in their rats. Nevertheless, the men
·orked for long periods in the dust without any obvious effect on their
ealth. Sixty-two of the workers were under forty, and thirty over forty:
wenty-eight of them had been on the job for more than seven years, a
urther nine for more than five years, and thirty-one for more than two

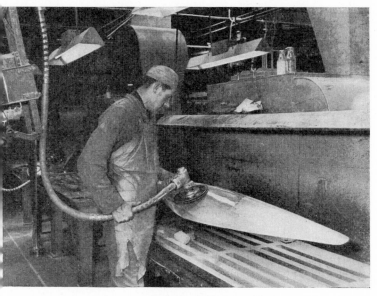

FIG. 413.—Duralumin Propeller Grinder at work
By courtesy of the De Havilland Aircraft Co.)

years. In the German cases the changes were not related to length of time on the job.

Inhalation of Aluminium Powder in the Treatment of Silicosis

Crombie, Blaisdell and McPherson (1944) investigated 125 workers employed in the Pittsburgh stamp mills of the Aluminum Company of America. The workers here had been exposed to aluminium dust for periods ranging from six to twenty-three years, and their health was found to be as good as the 3,000 other workers in the plant. Radiographs of the chests of all the men taken each year for three years showed no abnormalities that could be attributed to the inhalation of dust. They then treated thirty-four silicotic miners by the daily inhalation of fine aluminium powder freshly ground from small aluminium pellets in a specially constructed mill. Daily treatment began with five-minute inhalations, which were gradually increased to thirty minutes (fig. 398). Some of the men received 300 treatments, but the majority only 200. Out of the thirty-four cases thus treated, clinical improvement in nineteen was manifested by lessening or disappearance of shortness of breath, cough, pain in the chest and fatigue. In fifteen cases the condition became stationary, and remained so in spite of continuous employment in silica dust throughout the treatment. The progress of the disease was assessed by means of tests of respiratory function, repeated at three-monthly intervals. Crombie and his colleagues drew the conclusion that the inhalation of finely particulate aluminium powder is not harmful to human lungs. The work of Kennedy (1956) leaves no doubt that the use of aluminium powder in the treatment of man has no effect on established silicosis (see p. 1008). Denny, Robson and Irwin (1939) exposed eight rabbits to metallic aluminium dust of particle size below 5 microns and showed that no fibrosis was produced, but Belt and King (1943) repeated these experiments in rats and showed that the rats' lungs treated the particles as foreign bodies and formed small concretions with fibrous tissue round them.

(b) Beryllium

The toxicity of beryllium and its compounds is discussed on p. 417. Since the inhalation of certain beryllium compounds can produce pulmonary lesions, these must be regarded as within the definition of pneumoconiosis. Two types of pulmonary disease are described. The first is acute chemical pneumonitis, with onset during exposure to the dust, and is characterized by cough, blood-stained sputum, retrosternal pain, dyspnœa, cyanosis, anorexia, loss of weight and prostration; resolution may occur within a few weeks or months or, rarely, chronic granulomatosis may follow. In the chronic type, anorexia, loss of weight and weakness are early symptoms; cough, extreme dyspnœa, œdema of extremities and cardiac failure develop; mortality is high, and many of those patients who survive suffer permanently from pulmonary distress.

Beryllium has been found in many organs and tissues, suggesting that

e disease is systemic. It is of some interest to mention an analogy with
ica; besides pulmonary lesions, certain compounds of beryllium cause
ronic cutaneous lesions when implanted in the tissues (see p. 432);
milarly, a condition called *pseudotuberculoma silicoticum* has been de-
ribed by Shattock (1917), and by Faulds (1935), who described two such
ses, in which quartz-containing material was introduced into the skin
d subcutaneous tissue by accidental injury.

(c) Silicon Carbide

Silicon carbide (carborundum) has been regarded as harmless since the
assical experiments of Gardner (1923) showed that it produced no fibrosis
 the lungs in experimental animals. Since carborundum is harder than
artz this work refutes rather convincingly the mechanical theory of
licosis—namely, that it is the hardness or sharpness of particles that
uses damage in the lung. It would be ironical if it were now to be found
at carborundum produces pneumoconiosis in man. Yet Smith and Perina
948) found nodular shadows by X-ray examination in workers exposed to
e dust of silicon carbide and alumina. Bruusgaard (1949) found definite
diographic changes in ten out of thirty-two workers exposed exclusively
 the dust of silicon carbide. These authors suggest that the question of
athogenicity of this substance will need to be reconsidered, and further
vestigation, including post-mortem studies, will be necessary before the
osition can be clarified. It may be mentioned, however, that Gardner
938) found in experimental animals that silicon carbide, together with
berculous infection, could produce a fibrotic reaction, and this may
rhaps explain the human cases.

DUSTS OF VEGETABLE ORIGIN

Vegetable dusts encountered in various occupations include the dusts of
agasse, carob flour (locust bean gum), cork, cotton, derris, flax, flour,
ain, gum arabic, hay, hemp, jute, linseed, malt, nuts, paprika, sisal,
raw, tamarind seed, tea, tobacco and wood. Pollen and fungus spores
e often large enough to be trapped in the nose and upper respiratory
assages (p. 1075). Many of these produce inhalant allergy; asthma, hay
ver and urticaria. Dusts of particle size small enough to reach the alveoli
ometimes produce acute and chronic bronchitis, chronic emphysema,
d even bronchopneumonia, fibroid lung and bronchiectasis.

McNair and Middleton (1924) showed that the handling of grain in
ulk causes liberation of an irritating dust consisting of the hairs from the
ush of wheat and rye grains, and from the paleæ and awns of barley and
ats; the dust also contains mould spores, débris and mineral matter.

bsence of Silica Hazard

In many cases it is not known whether the noxious agent lies in the
egetable matter itself—for instance, some protein, which is toxic—or
hether it lies in the impurities. In the case of chronic disease silica has
een considered, for free silica derived from soil is a universal contaminant

of vegetable material. The amount present, however, is small, generall
about 2 per cent or less, and particle size so great that it is most unlikel
that silica plays any part in the production of lung disease from vegetabl
dust.

Bacteria and Fungi

The biological contaminants are more important. Vegetable mat:ei
especially if it is wet or rotting, may contain a high content of bacteria
and spores and mycelia of fungi, some of which are known to be pathogenic
Thus the mycological examination of cotton dust has revealed fungi of th
genera *Alternaria, Mucor, Rhizopus, Fusarium, Sporotrichum, Aspergillu*
Gladosporium and *Penicillium.* Viable counts of such fungi may reac
figures as high as 400 millions per gram (Furness and Maitland, 1952
When such masses of fungi exist in the dust inhaled, they naturally appea
in the sputum, but this is no proof that the lung disease under consider
ation is of mycotic origin.

Fungus Allergens

In certain occupations inhalant allergic symptoms occur fron
sensitization to fungus spores or mould spores. The men affected are doc
workers unloading grain, lumbermen debarking trees infested wit]
Cryptostroma corticale, dealers in second-hand furniture and gardener
handling tomato plants infested with *Cladosporium.* However a differen
form of allergy, with symptoms unlike those of bronchial asthma, affectin
the alveolar tissue of the lung was identified and described by Pepys (1963
and later given the name *extrinsic allergic alveolitis* (p. 1075). The allergen
concerned are often minute fungus spores, but animal as well as vegetabl
dusts can produce the lung lesions. The spores concerned in this proces
are about one micron in diameter, a size which makes it likely for aero
dynamic reasons, that they would penetrate deeply into the respirator
tract. This may be the reason for the appearance of reactions in the peri
pheral part of the broncho-pulmonary tree, rather than in the bronch
which are characteristic of this group of illnesses.

Cotton Dust

Four conditions affecting the respiratory system are described in worker
exposed to cotton dust in different parts of the world. These are mill feve
byssinosis, weavers' cough and an acute illness occurring among peop]
who handle low-grade stained cotton. Of these, byssinosis is the mos
serious. It is principally a disease of Lancashire, where the cotton-spinnin
industry is concentrated in towns like Oldham, Rochdale, Bury and Boltor
It is a progressive condition resulting in total disablement if exposure t
cotton dust continues after symptoms first appear. No specific cause ha
been found for mill fever, byssinosis or weavers' cough. The endotoxin o
Aerobacter cloacæ has been held responsible for the symptoms in an acut
illness of workers handling contaminated cotton in the United States c
America.

Processes in the Cotton Textile Industry

The processes used in the manufacture of cotton yarn and cloth are
ginning, baling, bale breaking, bale opening, scutching, carding, spinning,
weaving and finishing.

Cotton Ginning

Cotton ginning, or separation of the lint from the seed, is performed in
the field in order to save unnecessary transport of the seed, which forms
about two-thirds of the weight of the harvested crop. The modern gin-
neries in America are almost automatic, the whole operation being carried
out by pneumatic suction so that the cotton is hardly touched by hand.
From the gin the lint is carried pneumatically into a chamber where it is
compressed into bales, which are then bound with steel strips.

Processes in the Cotton Mill

Cotton is imported into England chiefly from Egypt, India and the
United States of America. Arrived in Lancashire, the bales are taken to the
cotton mills. The functions of the processes in the mill are as follows:

(i) to divide up and clean the compressed cotton from the bale;

(ii) to form the fibres into a rope or sliver which can be attentuated
until it is thin enough to form threads;

(iii) to comb out the fibres and set them parallel by drawing them
between carding cylinders;

(iv) to insert sufficient twist into the material to make a firm thread;

(v) to finish and prepare the yarn;

(vi) to divide the warp or horizontal threads of the fabric so that the
weft or cross-threads may be interwoven between them;

(vii) to insert the weft or cross-threads;

(viii) to beat up the last inserted weft thread to the fabric proper, and

(ix) to finish the cloth by smoothing, stiffening and glazing.

The Hazard of Dust Exposure

From what follows it will be seen that although the processes in the
cotton chamber, the blowing room and the card room are dusty, the subsequent processes of spinning, weaving and finishing are free from dust. To
understand how respiratory disorders arise in the industry, one must
concentrate upon what happens in the card room.

The Hopper Bale Opener

The raw cotton arrives in bales, tightly compressed and containing particles of leaf and seed coat, cotton hairs, fragments of mould and fine sand.
In the process of cleaning it passes through the cotton chamber, the blowing
room and the card room. In the cotton chambers the bales are broken and
the tightly compressed cotton is pulled off in layers and hand-fed by the
cotton feeder into a machine known as a hopper bale opener. It then passes
into the blowing room, where it is dealt with successively by hopper
openers, hopper feeders, porcupine openers and finisher scutchers.

The Blowing Room

The purpose of all these machines is to open out the compressed cotto
to spread it well and, by a beating action aided by powerful currents of ai
to free it from a high percentage of its impurities and at the same tim
ensure adequate mixing of the different qualities of cotton. With the e
ception of the cotton feeder tending the hopper bale opener, all machin
are enclosed in dust-proof covers. The machines, however, have to I
hand-cleaned and, as this is a particularly dusty job, the operatives engage
on the work are suitably clothed and wear respirators. Operatives in tl
cotton chamber and blowing room do not show a high incidence
respiratory disorders.

The Card Room

Emerging from the blowing room, the cotton passes to the card roor
Not only does the carding process arrange the cotton fibres in parall
order, but also it carries out the final cleansing process by eliminating su
impurities as have survived the previous operations. The name *cardi*
comes from the Latin, *carduus*, a thistle, since the dried bracts of thistl
were originally used for the job. The hooked prickles of *Dipsacus fullonur*
the fuller's teasel, are still used for dressing cloth, their action being
raise a smooth nap on the material treated. For this purpose the drie
teasel heads are mounted close together on a wooden frame known as
teasel frame. In cotton carding at a later date the thistle heads were r
placed by wire brushes operated by hand. Today the combing action
mechanized.

The Carding Engine

The carding engine consists of a horizontal metal cylinder fitted wit
sharp-pointed steel-wire teeth, 300 or so to the square inch. The rotatir
cylinder carries the cotton fibres upwards until they meet the flats. Thes
are iron bars 2 inches wide, covered with wire teeth similar to those on tl
cylinder but pointing the opposite way. The flats move in the same directio
as the carding cylinder but at a much slower rate. By this means the fibr
are combed into line with each other in a wide mat or lap and short lengtl
are removed. Women working in the card room, the engine-head tenter
slubber-tenters and intermediate tenters are rarely affected by respirato
disorders. The strippers and grinders, the operatives in charge of th
carding engines, are the principal sufferers. In men over thirty-five yea
of age working in the Lancashire cotton industry, chronic bronchitis an
emphysema are found in 20 per cent of weavers, but in 80 per cent o
strippers and grinders (Schilling and Goodman, 1951).

Stripping and Grinding

Usually each stripper and grinder is in charge of sixteen carding engine
Each engine is cleaned four times a day by a vacuum process, and twic
weekly it is brush-stripped. This is done by another form of metalli
combing cylinder or brush. The brush-stripping is necessary because th

vacuum process fails to clean sufficiently deeply between the teeth of the machine, and the evidence is very strong that the atmosphere in the immediate vicinity of the carding engine contains the injurious substance causing byssinosis (Gill, 1947). In time the teeth of the carding cylinder become blunted and distorted in shape and have to be cleaned by a process known as stripping, and then reshaped and sharpened by grinding them by means of a revolving cylinder covered with emery. The men employed at this work are known as strippers and grinders. In the past the stripping of carding engines was a very dusty job and can still be so if proper precautions are not taken (fig. 414). It is not surprising that chronic lung disease in these men became known as *strippers' and grinders' asthma*.

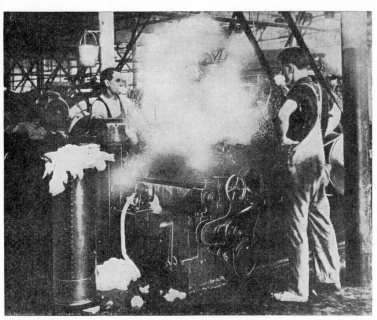

FIG. 414.—Cotton-carding Engine, showing Dust Cloud from stripping the Cylinder in the days before Exhaust Ventilation was applied locally to the Stripping-brush

(*From Legge, T. M., Industrial Maladies, Oxford Univ. Press, 1934*

Mill Fever

Almost all workers suffer from *mill fever*, or *cotton cold*, when they begin to work in the cotton mills. The term *mill fever* was first used by Arlidge in 1892 to describe a condition occurring on exposure to flax dust. This curious illness has been given many names, according to the dust producing it—*hackling fever* and *flax fever* in flax mills, *combers' fever* in hemp mills, *grain fever* in grain porters and *malt fever* in maltmen. It is uncertain whether an attack caused by one dust confers immunity to some other vegetable dusts, but Doig (1949) records that he knew several workers who had experienced mill fever from jute and who suffered no illness or discomfort on later working in flax mills. *Mill fever* differs from *Monday fever*, with which it is sometimes confused. The latter condition occurs only after exposure of more than ten years to cotton dust, and is the first stage of byssinosis.

Mill fever occurs among cotton workers who have not previously been exposed to the dust. Tolerance is developed usually within a few days, though symptoms may reappear following an absence from work for a time as short as two to four weeks. Oliver (1902) wrote:

> Workers when exposed to the dust for the first time complain of dryness of the throat and suffer from what is called *mill fever*. The indisposition lasts for two or three days; the patients complain of headache, with a sense of feeling ill all over, accompanied by a slight rise of temperature.

A short, slight, dry cough is common and attacks of sneezing sometimes occur. In a few cases an urticarial rash appears on the forearms, especially in women operatives (Gill, 1947). A visitor to the card room frequently has an attack of *mill fever* within the next twelve hours. The new employee may develop symptoms during the first working day, but more commonly the symptoms develop after he gets home in the evening. The temperature may rise as high as 100° to 103° F., but it is invariably normal again by next morning. Headache, malaise and exhaustion accompany the fever, and occasionally nose-bleeding, nausea and vomiting occur. These symptoms may reappear each night for the first few days, or even weeks, of exposure, but most workers become acclimatized within the first month. Severe cases and complications are unknown. Exposure to a higher concentration of dust than that to which the worker has become accustomed may result in a recurrence of *mill fever*.

Byssinosis

The word *byssinosis* is derived from the Greek word βύσσος, meaning *fine linen* or *fine flax*. The disease has been known to exist among cotton workers for nearly a hundred years. It was, and still is, known in the cotton trade as *strippers'* or *grinders' asthma*, or the *cotton card-room asthma*. It was mentioned by Greenhow in 1860 in a report to the Privy Council in London and it was described in detail in 1863 by Jesse Leach, factory surgeon, who found it prevalent in the mills of Heywood and district. Cases of byssinosis still occur among the cotton spinners of Lancashire (Schilling, 1959) and also among the hemp spinners (Smiley, 1951) and flax spinners (Smiley, 1961) of Belfast. In the spinning mills of Northern Ireland the workers both in flax and in hemp call the condition *pouce* or *poucey chest*. Three stages are recognized in the development of the disease.

The First Stage

The first of these is commonly called *Monday feeling* or *Monday fever* by card-room operatives (Prausnitz, 1936). The symptoms begin after long exposure to cotton dust, and commonly occur in workers who suffered

om *mill fever* on beginning work in the cotton industry. The worker may
ave been quite well for ten years or more except for slight cough. Sud-
enly the cough becomes aggravated and exceedingly irritating, or the
orker has attacks of tightness in the chest and breathlessness. These
tacks usually happen on Monday, and the man is well for the rest of the
eek. This condition may persist without getting any worse, until the
orker leaves the industry.

he Second Stage

In the second stage the symptoms extend over more days in the week
d finally become permanent. Removal from exposure to cotton dust
uring the first stage of byssinosis will result in complete cure, but symp-
ms recur suddenly and with great severity if work at the mill is resumed.
exposure continues, attacks of bronchitis or asthma follow. These are
no way different from the bronchitis and asthma of the general popula-
on. Intervals of absence from work become necessary, and these increase
frequency and duration. Even at this stage recovery can occur, at least
the extent of making the individual fit for some job, if exposure to
tton dust is ended.

he Third Stage

But many men who reach the second stage do not leave the industry,
d pass into the third stage of disabling byssinosis. The symptoms of
ghtness of the chest and dyspnœa are so distressing that the worker has to
ave the cotton industry. Though he will have some relief when he is away
om cotton dust, the dyspnœa remains as a permanent disability. The
isease progresses to chronic bronchitis with emphysema. Cough with
uco-purulent sputum is present, but there is no fibrosis and therefore
aracteristic X-ray findings are absent. Post-mortem examination reveals
lvanced emphysema (Shaw Dunn and Sheehan, 1932). Thus, there are
changes which distinguish byssinosis from the chronic bronchitis and
nphysema occurring in persons not exposed to cotton dust.

iagnosis and Prognosis

The rate at which the disease progresses depends upon the amount of
ust inhaled and on the susceptibility of the individual. Dust-control
ethods are helping to reduce the incidence and severity of the illness.
iagnosis depends on a history of long exposure to cotton dust, together
ith the symptoms and signs of chronic bronchitis and emphysema.

tiology of Byssinosis

The exact mode of action of the cotton dust is not known. The natural
story of the disease suggests that there is an allergen in cotton dust which
nsitizes the bronchial mucous membrane and produces bronchospasm
d possibly swelling of the mucous membrane. After prolonged exposure,
is leads to emphysema. But the work of Furness and Maitland (1952)
es not confirm this hypothesis. They prepared different extracts of cotton

dust and did skin tests on men with mild and severe symptoms of byssinosi and on men who had worked in cotton card rooms without symptoms, an on others who had never worked in a cotton mill. Those who had a whea and flare type of reaction were equally distributed between all these group: This reaction probably indicates hypersensitivity to cotton dust, but it doe not indicate a hypersensitivity specific to byssinosis.

The Morbidity and Mortality Rates

The morbidity and mortality rates of men working in the cotton industr emphasize how serious the effects of exposure to fine cotton dust can b Bradford Hill (1930) compared the sickness experience of strippers an grinders with that of warehousemen and ring-room spinners in the perio 1923–7. He showed that after the age of thirty sickness due to respirator disease was for the strippers and grinders three times as high as for tho: working in the same industry but not in the dusty rooms. Death-rates fro respiratory disease in the triennium 1930–2 were equally striking. Fe strippers and grinders over fifty-five the respiratory mortality was at lea three times as great as for men working in other parts of the cotton mi But the respiratory mortality of strippers and grinders declined appreciab between 1920 and 1930. This was no doubt to some extent due to the re cession in the trade at this time and the consequent reduction in the tin spent in the mills; but in the previous decade attempts had been made wit some success to enclose the stripping brush and to remove the dust t exhaust ventilation. This, no doubt, also had a beneficial effect on th death-rate.

Weavers' Cough

From time to time outbreaks of an acute respiratory illness varying severity from a dry cough, *weavers' cough*, to severe asthma have occurre in cotton-weaving sheds.

Ætiology

No one ætiological factor explains the various outbreaks, but the du liberated from the size applied to cotton yarns is evidently responsibl sometimes because it has become mildewed and therefore contains mou allergens (p. 1060), and at other times because it contains a particular veg table allergen such as the dust of the kernel of tamarind seed, which is tl seed of the tree, *Tamarindus indica*. In addition it is of course possible both cases that finely divided vegetable dust either from the cotton from the size or both is inhaled, swells up, and results in multiple sm; areas of atelectasis prone to become secondarily infected (p. 1059). Such condition would be analogous to the self-limited bronchiolitis of bagas shredders known as bagassosis (p. 1079).

Sizing and Weaving

The application of a size to the warp threads is a necessary prelimina to weaving in order to give the yarn power to withstand the friction in t

om. In the past several substances have been used, usually of a starchy
.aracter. Sago, farina, maize, potato starch, and carob flour (locust bean
.m) are commonly used materials but research is constantly going on to
.scover better sizing agents. Improvements in finishing, such as crease
.sistance, very often depend upon the size used and the ease and complete-
.ss of its removal. About one-twentieth of the size applied leaves the warp
.ring weaving. An unknown quantity remains suspended in the atmos-
.ere but most falls on the floor, together with short fibre, forming a
.ffy deposit called, in north-east Lancashire, *dawn*.

utbreaks due to Mildewed Yarn

In 1913 Collis described an outbreak of an unusual cough among
.eavers in north-east Lancashire. The condition was associated with con-
.riction of the chest, an irritating cough, purulent sputum, dyspnœa on
.fort, and asthmatic attacks. The material woven was cotton, sized with a
.ixture of flour (derived from wheat, sago or potatoes), tallow, china
.ay, and water without any preservative. Just before the onset of the
.ness the warp threads developed a mildew while on the looms. When
.y threads were substituted the symptoms disappeared. A recurrence of
.ildew on the yarn led to a reappearance of symptoms. In another mill
.here there was a sharp division of mildewed and unaffected warps only
.e weavers working on the former became affected. Collis concluded that
.e illness was due to mildew. Again in Lancashire, Bridge (1924) and
.iddleton (1926) described similar attacks of weavers' cough due to
.ildew. The air over the looms using the affected yarn was found to con-
.in many fragments of mycelia and conidia, and examination of the dust
.d of the yarn revealed the presence of various fungi, including penicil-
.m, aspergillus, mucor and others.

n Outbreak of Weavers' Cough in Italy

In 1954 in Italy Vigliani, Parmeggiani and Sassi (1954) described an
.idemic of bronchial asthma among the weavers of a large cotton factory.
. this instance the cotton yarn was sized with carob flour (locust bean
.m) and potato starch. Fifty per cent of the weavers had been affected
.ith a dry cough, scanty sputum, dyspnœa and rasping in the throat.
.ymptoms were worse on Mondays. On examination 105 weavers were
.fected with bronchial asthma, twenty-seven of them severely. In the
.ight cases the attacks lasted for two or three months while the more
.vere cases lasted for five to six months. It was assumed that the epidemic
.as similar in origin to those described by Collis but investigations carried
.t towards the end of the epidemic did not disclose any particular abun-
.nce of moulds. Indeed, the atmospheric contamination of bacteria and
.ngi was greater in the spinning and weaving preparation departments,
.hich were not affected by the epidemic. Skin tests with mould extracts
.ere negative except for *Aerobacter aerogenes* which gave a positive
.action in 46 per cent of the controls, in 76 per cent of the moderate and

slight cases, and in 100 per cent of those severely affected. The organism however, was either very scarce or absent in samples of the yarn and dust from the weaving department. It was considered that as the bacteriological and immunological investigations had been delayed until the epidemic was abating no conclusions could be reached concerning the cause of the epidemic.

An Outbreak Associated with Tamarind Seed Powder

In India, about 1952, tamarind seed powder entirely replaced starch for the sizing of jute and to some extent also of cotton yarns. Its use conserves the food starches and is held to have certain advantages over starch from the standpoint both of weaving and of finishing. Laboratory and mill trials in Lancashire carried out by the British Cotton Industry Research Association demonstrated that tamarind seed kernel powder was a practicable sizing adhesive for spun viscose rayon cloth. In 1957 Murray Dingwall-Fordyce and Lane recorded an outbreak in a large weaving shed where 180 men and 208 women worked on looms weaving rayon cloth. The firm had begun using tamarind size in October 1955 and by January 1956 the workers began to show symptoms. These varied from a dry cough to an acute and severe respiratory distress sometimes with purulent sputum. The effect was not produced on first exposure; a minimum period of at least two weeks was required apparently for sensitization. Of all those exposed, 84 per cent of the women and 63 per cent of the men were affected. Further evidence that the reaction was indeed due to the tararind size was the demonstration that four volunteer workers who had had an illness in the mill reacted violently to the inhalation of the tamarind size and not to a starch powder. On the other hand four persons who had never been exposed to tamarind were unaffected by a few doses of the powder, but after a number of doses, varying in different individuals, reacted to a amount of powder that had not previously caused any effect (Tuffnell and Dingwall-Fordyce, 1957).

Acute Respiratory Illness from Contaminated Cotton

In 1941 an acute illness among people handling dusty, low-grade stained cotton broke out in the United States of America (Neal, Schneiter and Caminita, 1942). This illness is a distinct clinical entity not connected with byssinosis. Sudden outbreaks occurred among rural mattress makers and among workers in one cotton mill and several cotton-seed processing plants. Schemes for rural mattress making were designed to reduce the cotton surplus and to benefit farm workers. Poor families who wished make mattresses for home use were supplied with 50 lb. of cotton and yards of cotton ticking for each mattress. They gathered at a central depot to make their mattresses, and contact with the cotton was limited to the time allowed each family to make its quota of mattresses.

Symptoms and Signs

The illness occurred among workers exposed to high dust concentrations. The dust was produced in opening the bales, carding the cotton, filling and closing the mattresses, and finally beating them. Dust concentrations were particularly heavy when low-grade stained cotton was used. Symptoms began within the first six hours of exposure, with fatigue and generalized aching. Anorexia, headache, nausea and vomiting followed. The vomiting persisted for from six to nine hours. Rigors, with a temperature of 102° F., and headache occurred. Many people complained of abdominal pain or cramp and a sense of retrosternal discomfort which prevented them from taking a deep breath. Symptoms lasted from two to five days.

Etiology

This disease has been attributed to the effects of the endotoxin of *Aerobacter cloacæ* (Neal and others, 1942; Schneiter and others, 1942). Samples of cotton from all sources where outbreaks occurred were heavily contaminated with this organism almost to the exclusion of other bacteria. Its abundance in this cotton was associated with particular climatic circumstances and undue exposure of the cotton to contamination from the soil. The clinical symptoms were reproduced experimentally in human beings by the inhalation of dust from the cotton and by the inhalation of mist from cell-free culture filtrates of *A. cloacæ*. Although the clinical picture is similar to that of weavers' cough in Lancashire, there is no proof that these two conditions are related nor can a relationship with mill fever, byssinosis or bagassosis be established.

Control of Dust in Cotton Mills

It was not until 1908 that attempts to control the dust in cotton mills were made. Obviously the ideal method is to ensure that the cotton dust does not escape into the atmosphere. This has not yet been found possible. Considerable improvements have been achieved by the introduction of dust covers and exhaust fans for machines in the cotton chamber and blowing rooms. Unfortunately, even in the best equipped mills, at least one-third of the trash is carried into the card room in the laps; it is this third which is eliminated in the carding process. The sliver emerging from the carding engine is almost dust-free.

Oiling the Cotton

In spite of constant experimental work designed to make the atmosphere free from dust, particularly in the vicinity of the carding engines, no completely satisfactory method of dust suppression has yet been evolved. In some mills 1 per cent mineral oil is sprayed on the cotton in the hopper bale breaker. This treatment helps to reduce the dust and does not interfere with the quality of the yarn, since most of the oil is absorbed before this stage is reached. The modern flat carding engine is not totally en-

closed. Attempts to do this have been made by completely hooding th
whole of the top of the carding engine and exhausting by means of a fan
The air, drawn through the hood, is then filtered before re-entering th
room.

Exhaust Suction and Air Conditioning

The under-space of the carding engine is completely sealed off, and t
clean under the engine the stripper and grinder has only to pull a smal
lever; the entire collection of dust is then swept away by the creation of
vacuum. According to Gill (1947) this arrangement has greatly reduced th
amount of dust in the atmosphere; 3·66 lb. was extracted from the hood
of twelve carding engines, through which 11,400 lb. of cotton had passe
in forty-four hours. These figures do not include the weight of debris fron
underneath the carding engine. Many mills have insufficient air space, with
the machinery crowded into too small an area. Greater air space means
greater dilution of the dust. Improved air conditioning, in conjunctio
with improved dust extraction, is necessary. Air conditioning must in
clude a correctly controlled temperature, the right humidity and adequat
air movement. These are also the best conditions for the cotton fibre. Bu
the engineering problems involved are complex and the British Cotto
Industry Research Association at the Shirley Institute, Didsbury, Lanca
shire, is continuously employed in researches on the subject.

Need for Periodical Medical Examination

A careful selection of operatives for the card room, and regular examina
tion of existing workers, offer the best protection. All intending card-roon
operatives should be medically examined before engagement, and ever
effort should be made to exclude those likely to be susceptible to th
disease. Any operative who gives a personal or a family history of asthma
bronchitis, hay fever, eczema or recurrent urticarial attacks should be ex
cluded from the card room. The general build and shape of the thoraci
cage should be noted, and also the type of respiration. Mouth breathers ar
bad subjects. Malformation of the nasal bones, deflected septum, nasa
polypi, enlarged tonsils and extensive adenoid vegetations are all contra
indications for work in the card room. A chest expansion below 3 inches i
suspect. All operatives are urged to practise nasal inspiration and to wea
protective respirators.

Need for Improved Engineering Control

In spite of all the improvements introduced, a substantial number o
men employed in the more dusty mills spinning the coarser grades o
cotton were found by Schilling and others (1952) to be suffering fron
byssinosis. Of 131 men over the age of thirty-five with at least ten years
exposure in card and blowing rooms, 45 had no symptoms, 52 were in th
first stage of the disease, and 16 and 15 in the second and third stage
respectively. Schilling (1952) points out that there could be a more effectiv

control of the disease if medical supervision and engineering control of dust were combined. There is at present no system of periodical medical examination of card-room workers. If there were, the incidence and severity of the disease found would indicate both the mills where improved methods of dust control were needed, and the men who were getting progressively worse and who should be encouraged to leave the industry or work in the less dusty mills.

Allergy to Wood Dusts

Bronchial asthma due to allergy to a particular wood dust has often been noted. Dermatitis, as well as running of the eyes and nose, also may occur (p. 781). Usually only those isolated workmen who are unduly sensitive are affected, but sometimes small outbreaks occur. Thus in 1905 the use of South African boxwood (*Gonioma kamassi*) in shuttle making in Lancashire caused a great deal of disability. Out of 112 men seen, thirty-four experienced difficulty in breathing, but there were other toxic symptoms as well (see p. 782). In 1936 Bridge described the effects of bronchial spasm in men handling mansonia wood (*Sterculiacea altissima*). In 1941 Davidson reported nine cases of asthma, coryza, conjunctivitis and dermatitis in men exposed to sawdust from iroko wood (*Chlorophora excelsa*). Doig (1949) recorded two small outbreaks of asthma in factories where Western red cedar (*Thuja plicata*) was handled. Thirteen men were known to have suffered from *cedar poisoning*; one of them was still working and still allergic to the wood after eleven years, another had been free from symptoms for two years since his retirement from work. In British Columbia, Canada, cedar poisoning occurs as asthma, dermatitis or both. It is seen in carpenters making window sashes of the local cedar wood and in men firing household furnaces with cedar sawdust. It is rare in loggers (Strong, 1954).

Effects of Tobacco Dust

In factories, tobacco dust affects especially beginners, causing irritation of the eyelids and conjunctiva with lachrymation. The dust or juice from the leaves may cause dermatitis on the back of the hands and face. The genitalia may become affected where the dust is conveyed by unwashed hands. Acute nicotine poisoning with insomnia, headache, watering of the eyes, nausea, vomiting and tachycardia may occur. One fatal case took place in a workman employed in steeping tobacco in water. Gardeners and vine growers have been affected after using insecticidal sprays containing nicotine. Where a solution containing nicotine comes in contact with the skin, the use of hot water to remove it must be avoided, otherwise absorption will be facilitated. Chronic poisoning in tobacco workers is rare. It takes the form of tobacco amblyopia with colour scotomata in the visual fields due to degeneration of ganglion cells of the retina, especially in the macular area. Optic atrophy with partial blindness may follow. Its occurrence in non-smokers has been many times confirmed. The occurrence of attacks of asthma in cigarette cutters has been recognized for many years, but the condition is less common since the industry has been mechanized. At the necropsy on two women workers Zenker observed brown patches on the pulmonary parenchyma and on the hilar glands as well. He attributed these lesions to the action of tobacco and called the condition *tobaccosis*. In a study of the tobacco drying and stemming industry, McCormick, Smith and Marsh (1948) found that dust liberated in the processes contained from 22 to 58 per cent of free silica, and that the particles were of respirable size.

Printers' Asthma

Gums have come into increasing use in industry and, in the various reports on sensitivity to different gums, acacia, or gum arabic (*Acacia senegal* Willd.), sterculia or karaya gum (*Sterculia urens* Roxb.), and tragacanth or gum dragon (*Astragalus gummifer* Labill) have been the three most common allergens, in the order listed (Brown and Crepea 1947). Bohner and others (1941), in the United States of America, were the first to describe a group of printers with asthma due to sensitivity to gum acacia. They reported ten cases and reviewed the literature of isolated reports of sensitivity to inhaled acacia. In Canada, Sprague (1942) reported a further case of asthma in a printer sensitive to inhaled acacia. Fowler (1952) described thirty-two cases of *printers' asthma* in men exposed to a spray, made of gum acacia and *iso*propyl alcohol, which is used in colour-printing. This spray is thrown over each sheet and the gum forms a barrier between successive sheets on which the colour-print is still wet. Colour from one sheet is thus prevented from passing on to the back of the next sheet added to the pile. With many spray machines working, the mist can be seen spreading from one printing-machine to the next. The first patient attended a hospital complaining of asthma which he believed was due to the spray fluid to which he was exposed at work. A few weeks later thirty-one further printers were examined. They came in response to a letter sent to London printing chapels asking members who thought they were affected by the spray fluid to attend for examination. The average duration of exposure before asthma developed was 4·8 years, but the period of exposure was half as long for the six printers who had a past or family history of allergy. In one firm 19 per cent of the printers had asthma and a further 30 per cent had early symptoms of asthma due to sensitization to the spray. This industrial hazard can be eradicated by the substitution of dextrose for gum acacia in the spray fluid or by using chalk as a dust.

Effects of Grain Dust

Many observers have from time to time reported a high incidence of respiratory disease among men who handle grain; for example, grain porters, dock labourers, threshers, millers and maltsters, all of whom may be exposed to high concentrations of grain dust during their work.

Grain Sifting

In his description entitled *Diseases of sifters and measurers of grain,* Ramazzini (1713) states:

All kinds of grain, and in particular wheat, whether they are stored in pits and trenches as in Tuscany, or in granaries and barns with roofs as is done in the whole country on both sides of the Po, always have mixed in with them a very fine dust; not only the dust that they pick up from the threshing-floor, in the threshing, but also another less innocent sort which is shed from the grain itself when it is kept for long. Inasmuch as the seeds of cereals are full of volatile salt, and so much of it that unless they are well dried in the summer sun before being stored they become overheated and very soon crumble to dust, it follows that fine particles are continually dropping from the skin with which the grain is coated; besides these there is the residual dust and decay caused by the grubs, borers and weevils that consume the grain and by other such corn pests and their excrements. Hence, whenever it is necessary to sift wheat and barley or other kinds of grain to be ground in the mill, or to measure it when corn-merchants convey it hither and thither, the men who sift and measure are so plagued by this kind of dust that when the work is finished they heap a thousand curses on their calling. The throat, lungs, and eyes are keenly aware of serious damage; the throat is choked and dried up with dust, the pulmonary passages become coated with crust formed by dust, and the result is a dry and obstinate cough; the eyes are much inflamed and watery; and almost all who make a living by sifting or measuring grain are short of breath and cachectic and rarely reach old age; in fact, they are very liable to lapse into orthopnœa and finally dropsy. The dust moreover is so irritating that it excites intense itching over the whole body, of the sort that is sometimes observed in nettlerash.

Dusty Cargoes

Today large seaports with modern equipment handle cargoes of grain by suction methods. Smaller ports are not so equipped, and in any case suction is not suitable for every type of grain cargo. In many seaports dock labourers are called upon to spend at least a third to half of their time working grain and seed ships under conditions creating incredible amounts of dust. The dustiness of a grain cargo will vary not only with the particular grain or seed being handled, but also with its place of origin. Thus dockers in Antwerp complain that grain from the Black Sea is the most dusty. The port of Hull imports wheat from Canada, Australia and India, maize from South Africa, South America, Australia and Russia, barley from Turkey, Morocco and Russia, oats from Russia, millet from India, linseed from South America and Russia, rape seed from Africa and India and cotton seed from Egypt (West, 1951).

Filthy Working Conditions

Usually cargoes of grain or seed are carried loose in the holds in bulk. Only occasionally is the grain found bagged on arrival, and then no dust problem arises. The apparatus found to cause the greatest amount of dust is the elevator fitted with hoppers. Very often unloading is carried out by the age-old method of shovelling the grain or seed into wicker baskets which are then hoisted over the sides of the ships into trucks or lighters. Sometimes a grain ship is unloaded by the more modern method of buckets passing on an endless belt into a silo. With the method of shovel and basket the dockers find themselves working farther and farther down in the hold as unloading proceeds. Here the conditions are very dusty indeed and the men become filthy and caked with dust. The grain works into their clothes and boots and the dust hangs on their eyebrows and eyelashes. Various methods of keeping the dust from the ears and nostrils are used, such as an old stocking worn round the nose and mouth.

Symptoms and Signs

A person who is not used to it, on going down into the hold of a ship where grain is being unloaded immediately experiences irritation of the upper respiratory tract with sneezing, cough and a burning sensation in the mucous membranes of nose and pharynx. This lasts all the time he is in the dust-laden atmosphere and even persists after he gets back into the fresh air, sometimes for several hours. As to the docker, the presenting symptom is shortness of breath while he is actually on the job. Only rarely does he complain of cough and expectoration. But nothing is known as to the physical signs, if any, which may occur in these men. Do they suffer unduly from bronchitis, asthma or chronic emphysema? What radiological changes, if any, are to be found in their lungs? Although they are no longer a casual labour force, we have only a vague picture of their health and we do not know how it compares with that of other sections of the working community. A survey of this problem by clinical and radiological methods badly needs to be done.

Ætiology and Pathology

As long ago as 285 B.C. in his *Historia Plantarum*, the earliest extant Greek herbal, Theophrastus of Eresos raises the question why the dust from wheat is more irritating than that from other kinds of grain. Grain dust consists of husk particles, cellulose hairs and spikes, starch granules, moulds and 5 per cent of mineral particles.

The hairs differ according to the grain concerned. They are generally thick, strong and sharp, and therefore they can penetrate into the mucosa of the upper air passages. Those from wheat are long and stout and, according to the dockers themselves, wheat dust seems to be the most irritating even when the grain is clean and healthy. Maize has finer hairs, and maize cargoes cause less severe symptoms. McNair and Middleton (1924) investigated grain dusts, making forty-three dust counts with Owens' dust ounter. Of these, twenty-four were found to contain from 190 to 3,880 airs per 500 millilitres of air with an average of 932. The most usual igure was 1,050 hairs in wheat dust and 1,147 in barley dust.

In the wheat-flour mills of Kansas City, asthma occurs in some of the men exposed to the dusts arising from the first cleaning of the wheat grain. The minute hairs of the grain have been held responsible. Injection of nfinitesimal amounts of wheat-hair extract gives rise to severe local reactions and to asthma in sensitive millers (Duke, 1935).

From time to time fungi growing on mouldy grain have been found in he sputum of workmen. Thus in 1928 *Aspergillus fumigatus* and *Mucor mucedo* were held responsible for a small outbreak of respiratory disease in men who shovelled barley in a French malting-house. Such outbreaks raise he old question as to whether the fungi are pathogenic or merely saprophytic. The need for systematic mycological studies in the occupations where grain dusts are encountered is apparent.

EXTRINSIC ALLERGIC ALVEOLITIS

Respiratory disorders due to dusts of vegetable fibres were first described by Ramazzini (1713) in flax and silk workers in Italy. Since this many similar conditions have been recognized, the best known being farmers' lung and bagassosis. In recent years farmers' lung has come to be recognized as a not infrequent condition occurring in agricultural workers exposed to the dust arising from disturbing mouldy hay and other vegetable matter, and to be due to hypersensitivity to an antigen present in the dust of mouldy hay and other mouldy forage. The exact nature of this antigen was for long a subject of speculation, but the work of Pepys (1963) showed that the antigens involved were the spores of thermophilic actinomycetes growing in the heated hay, chiefly *Micropolyspora fæni*, and rarely *Micromonospora vulgaris*. On an average these spores measure one micron in diameter so that when they are inhaled they penetrate into the alveoli of the lungs. A farmer exposing himself to the dust of mouldy hay may retain in his lung 750,000 spores per minute. By means of agar-gel diffusion and immunoelectrophoresis it was demonstrated that the serum of the majority of patients suffering from farmers' lung contained precipitins to these organisms. In farmers' lung the subject develops constitutional and respiratory symptoms, usually three to six hours after exposure to the offending dust. The symptoms are unlike those of bronchial asthma; thus there is no wheeze, there is no eosinophilia, skin allergy tests are negative, chest radiographs show a diffuse miliary mottling, pulmonary function tests demonstrate an alveolar block diffusion defect, and lung biopsy reveals granulomata resembling those of sarcoidosis.

Many organic dusts of vegetable and animal origin cause allergic alveolitis. These include maple-bark disease due to the fungus *Cryptostroma corticale*, lung disease due to the grain weevil *Sitophilus granarius*, bird-fanciers' lung and duck fever (feather-pickers' disease) due to avian antigens, as well as mushroom-workers' lung and pituitary snuff-takers' lung due to porcine and bovine posterior pituitary powder. Other similar diseases in which precipitins have either not yet been found or not certainly identified include suberosis due to cork dust, paprika-splitters' lung, smallpox-handlers' lung, the chronic lung disease of New Guinea natives attributed to dust from thatched roofs and a similar disease in palm-kernel plantation workers. Perhaps also broken wind of horses and fog-fever of cattle belong to this group.

Farmers' Lung

Agriculture is one of the largest industries in Great Britain, employing about 800,000 persons. In rural areas, especially where there is a high rainfall, the workers are liable to lung disease arising from the handling of mouldy hay and straw. The condition which has been called *farmers' lung* was first mentioned by Campbell (1932). His original account concerned 5 farm workers in Cumberland. It was clearly described by Fawcitt (1938) in Westmorland and Cumberland, but it exists in other agricultural districts, including Lancashire, Wales, Lincolnshire and Devonshire. Fuller (1953) collected 32 cases from the Devonshire area in eight years, and Williams and Mulhall (1956) 10 cases from Radnor and North Breconshire. Sweeney (1952) found cases in north-west Ireland. In 1958 in the U.S.A. Frank reported 27 cases and Dickie and Rankin 32 cases. In 1961 Staines and Forman reported the results of a postal inquiry conducted on behalf of the research organization of the Royal College of General Practitioners, London. General practitioners and consultants reported to them 444 cases, forming a larger series than any previously described. The criteria for diagnosis were quite broad and it is therefore possible that conditions other than farmers' lung were included. The relation of farmers' lung to the inhalation of the dust of mouldy hay or straw remained for many years unquestioned, but the commonly held view that it was a true pulmonary mycosis was based only on the occupational history of the patient and the cultivation of moulds from his sputum. It is noteworthy that the single necropsy in the series of cases described by Fawcitt (1936) revealed no sign of pulmonary mycosis. An analogous condition has been reported from Scandinavia, where nine cases of *threshers' lung* were described in workers exposed to the dust of mouldy wheat (Törnell, 1946). This author reported marked improvement after treatment with potassium iodide. Hoffman (1946) reported a similar disease occurring in the canton of Appenzell in Switzerland during the harvest of 1945. The crops of barley and oats had stood out in wet weather and were dried for only half a day before threshing. They were infected with a fungus of the genus *Ascomycetes*.

Exposure Hazard

Hay becomes mouldy when it has lain wet in the field after cutting. The extra moisture encourages the growth of various moulds, and when the hay s handled, large amounts of spore-bearing dust may be inhaled. The cow-man puts out fresh hay for the cattle each day, and when this is being done t is impossible to see across the cowshed for dust. The same thing happens during the threshing of ricks of oats, wheat and barley which have been harvested in bad weather. The greatest risk is to members of mobile threshing teams, who may be repeatedly exposed.

Symptoms and Signs

The usual history is that a farmer after working continuously for a time with mouldy hay develops a short, dry cough, with little or no expectoration. He may also suffer from general malaise, weakness and slight fever, but the outstanding feature is distressing dyspnœa provoked by any physical exertion. Moist sounds may be heard in the lungs, but radiographs of the chest are normal. The acute illness is so short that the patient does not always consult a doctor. Removal from exposure to the dust of mouldy hay is followed by rapid recovery, which is complete and permanent if further exposure is avoided.

Subacute Phase

The subacute phase, however, is more incapacitating and often brings the patient to hospital or chest clinic. The man gives a history of repeated exposure to mouldy hay or straw during the previous two or three months. He complains of increasing breathlessness, with a short, dry cough and bouts of fever in the evenings after exposure. Often he is cyanosed, but there is no bronchospasm or other evidence of asthma. Physical signs include patches of dullness and crepitations. The erythrocyte sedimentation rate is increased. X-ray examination of the chest shows a fine alveolar mottling, with evidence of compensatory emphysema. The symptoms clear up in a month or two after the patient has been removed from contact with the dust, but the radiographic appearances remain abnormal for three or four months.

Chronic Phase

With successive seasonal recurrences the disease tends to become chronic. Fortunately, such cases are rare. The cough becomes more productive, the sputum is muco-purulent and slight hæmoptysis may occur. Physical weakness is marked, and so great is the dyspnœa, even after slight exertion, that the man becomes incapacitated for work. The dullness to percussion is now more extensive and added sounds are found over wider areas. Radiographs show increase in the density of the mottling, patches of opacity due to coalescent areas of fibrosis, increase in the hilar and perihilar shadows, marked restriction of the movements of the diaphragm and considerable areas of emphysema. This stage of pulmonary fibrosis with emphysema and sometimes bronchiectasis is irreversible. It is indistinguishable from what is seen in the final stages of byssinosis and bagassosis.

Ætiology and Pathology

Duncan (1945) examined specimens of sputum from cases of supposed farmers' lung and found mould spores often present. From one specimen alone he cultivated six different species of *Aspergillus*, as well as other moulds. He is in no doubt that the fungal elements in the sputum represent recently inhaled matter, and he finds it significant that fungal conidia are scarce or absent in the sputum of patients who have been removed for ever a short time from exposure to hay dust. He points out that the rapid clinical improvement brought about by a change from the dust-laden atmosphere does not suggest a progressive mycosis. It remained for Pepys (1963) to point out that the minute spores of *Micropolyspora fæni* present in countless millions when mouldy hay is disturbed are inhaled by the farmer and the farm labourer, reach the alveoli and produce allergy of the Arthus (Aŕtoos) type. Instead of the well-known immediate hyper-sensitivity response with wheezing, tightness in the chest and a change in the forced expiratory volume, there is a delayed reponse with systemic upset and a change in the transfer factor. The serum of the majority of patients suffering from farmers' lung contains precipitins either to *Micropolyspora fæni* or to *Micromonospora vulgaris*.

Preventive Treatment

In cowsheds, barns and stackyards and in places where threshing machines are in use, a systematic plan using wet methods for dust suppres-sion should be carried out. All workers unstacking or tossing mouldy hay should wear light-weight dust masks for the occasion. Schemes for mechanization of farm work should embody the means to minimize the escape of vegetable dust into the working environment. The risk to the farm worker of dust disease of the lungs is greatly reduced by the use of the combine harvester, when the corn is threshed as soon as it is cut and is therefore free from moulds and spores. In 1965 farmers' lung was added to the list of prescribed diseases under the *National Insurance (Industrial Injuries) Act, 1965*.

Broken Wind of Horses

Stall-fed horses are exposed to a much greater degree than farm workers to inhalation of dust of mouldy hay. In consequence of this they develop a disease known as *heaves*, or *broken wind of horses*. The ætiology of this condition is disputed, but it seems not to occur in pastured animals. It is an affection of horses in advanced and middle age. It is rare before the age of five years and its frequency increases with age. It frequently follows some kind of pneumonia.

Symptoms and Signs

It may be preceded by chronic cough, an annoying defect which may disappear in the summer and reappear in the winter months. The symptoms consist of wheezing, a peculiar hollow cough and the fact of being too easily fatigued. The symptoms are aggravated by heavy exertion, inclement weather and bad working conditions. The principal physical sign is a double expiratory movement of the flanks brought about by the use of the abdominal muscles in an effort to overcome the effect of loss of elasticity of the lungs. A horse is tested for broken wind by pulling it up suddenly after galloping, when a broken-winded horse will be recognized by the cough and double respiration (Lovell, 1952).

Morbid Anatomy

In broken wind of horses the main pathological change is hypertrophic vesicular emphysema. At necropsy, on opening the thorax the lungs are over-distended and marked on the surface by deep imprints of the ribs. Air bullæ under the pleura are often present where the breakdown of alveolar walls is extensive. Right heart hypertrophy occurs in advanced cases. Although chronic bronchiolitis is a constant finding, no adequate mycological or bacteriological studies have been made of the disease. Presumably it is of the same nature as farmers' lung.

Preventive Treatment

Broken wind of horses has become prevalent only since timothy hay, red clover, alfalfa and cultivated grasses have been introduced as feeding stuffs. The claim is made that it can be prevented if the hay is wetted sufficiently to suppress dust from rising and being inhaled.

Fog Fever in Cattle

Fog fever in cattle has some resemblance to farmers' lung, but the pathological changes may be rather more complex. Characteristically it is seen in beasts brought on to a lush second growth of grass in early autumn; the word *fog* refers to this grass (as in *Yorkshire fog* or *Holcus lanatus*) and not to any atmospheric opacity.

Bagassosis

Bagasse is a word of French origin indicating the cellulose fibre of sugar-cane after the sugar has been extracted. It is used for making boarding for the interior decoration of buildings and for thermal insulation. The sugar-cane which is used for this purpose is grown in Louisiana and the bagasse is shipped to Great Britain in bales. Inhalation of dust from certain consignments has caused a disease of the respiratory system known as *bagassosis*. It was first recognized in Louisiana in 1937; an outbreak occurred in England in 1940; and in 1959 the disease occurred at a newly established paper mill in Arecibo, Puerto Rico (Buechner, 1961).

Fungi of Twenty Species

When samples of bagasse are examined, innumerable fungi are found to be present and the dust arising from bagasse in a badly conducted factory may contain as many as 240 million fungal spores per gram. These consist of the uncultivable teliospores of fungi of the order *Pucciniales* (rusts), as well as the conidia of many species of saprophytic fungi. About twenty different species have been isolated in culture, including *Pæcilomyces varioti, Aspergillus fumigatus, A. niger, A. terreus, A. candida, Trichoderma lignorum, Monilia sitophilia,* and species of *Penicillium, Mucor* and *Rhizopus.* Amorphous silica forms only 1 to 2 per cent of the bagasse, and quartz 0·1 per cent, many of the quartz particles being from 20 to 30 microns in diameter. It is most improbable therefore that exposure to bagasse dust could lead to silicosis.

Dust Hazard from Shredding Machine

A febrile illness affecting the lungs of workers exposed to the dust of bagasse has been described in the United States of America, England, Mexico and Puerto Rico. In England the disease arose in workers on a machine called the shredder. which broke up the bales of bagasse (Hunter and Perry, 1946). In England before 1940 the bales were broken in a soak pit by a wet process causing no dust. During the Second World War in order to save shipping space the material in the bales was packed more tightly. In order to open such bales it became necessary to use the shredder, which produced heavy clouds of dust. In the factory concerned the shredder was housed in a separate building and no hazard existed in the main buildings away from this machine.

Symptoms and Signs

Out of twenty-one men exposed to the dust in a period of fifteen months, ten (47·5 per cent) developed a characteristic acute respiratory illness. Symptoms usually began after the men had been working on the machine for eight weeks. The disease manifested itself as an acute febrile illness with extreme shortness of breath, cough with scanty, black, stringy sputum, and occasional hæmoptysis. Signs were scattered throughout both lungs, and radiographs showed miliary shadows throughout the lung fields. The appearances were therefore those of an acute bronchiolitis. The symptoms gradually improved over a period of six weeks, at the end of which time radiographs showed the lung fields to be clear. One patient in 1941 died after twenty-five days' illness, but unfortunately no necropsy was performed. These cases afford strong evidence that a specific disease, manifesting itself by acute bronchiolitis, collapse and broncho-pneumonia, has occurred in the lungs of men handling bagasse.

Complete Occupational History

In 1943 all the workers in the factory were interviewed and occupational histories taken. It was found that out of 163 men employed, twenty-two had worked in coal mines, and of these, nineteen showed radiographic evidence of either reticulation, nodulation or massive shadows, a complicating factor not considered in certain reports on the disease. In 1944 further radiographs were made, and these revealed a man who had worked on the shredder for a year and who showed in his chest the radiographic changes already described. He had a cough and was short of breath.

Ætiology and Pathology

Between bagassosis, farmers' lung, broken wind of horses and fog fever in cattle certain resemblances can be picked out. Schneiter and others (1948) put forward the view that it is due to the endotoxin of *Aerobacter cloacæ*. But Pepys has identified precipitins to extracts of bagasse dust in the majority of sera of patients with bagassosis. The hypersensitivity response in the alveolar tissue is that of granuloma formation. In two of the patients described by Hunter and Perry (1946) the condition did not resolve, and they developed a fibrosis of the lungs with cough and sputum and great shortness of breath. Radiographs showed thick bands of fibrous tissue traversing the lung fields so as to simulate cavities. One of these men died, and at necropsy he was found to have chronic bronchiolitis and bronchiectasis, but no large cavities were found.

Absence of Evidence of Pulmonary Mycosis

The disease is not a true pulmonary mycosis, though it is possible that fungi play a rôle in breaking down the bagasse fibre into a very fine vegetable dust. *Aspergillus* is present in all specimens of bagasse dust and it can be grown from the sputum of men exposed to this dust. This fungus had been present in the sputum of the man who died, but, of course, this is no proof that it was the cause of his illness. Indeed, the post-mortem material from the lung showed no evidence of *Aspergillus*, and histological examination in no way suggested a disease of fungal origin. On the other hand, administration of bagasse to rabbits produced pneumonic lesions from which *Aspergillus* was isolated, whereas bagasse which had been autoclaved caused only a foreign-body giant-cell reaction and slight fibrosis (Gerstl and others, 1949).

Preventive Treatment

Resumption of wet methods of working prevented further outbreaks of the disease in the English factory. When the bales were again broken in the soak pit no appreciable dust was produced. In the Puerto Rico outbreak in a paper mill further cases were prevented by mechanization of the debaling process. In 1965, under the heading Farmers' Lung, bagassosis was added to the list of prescribed diseases under the *National Insurance (Industrial Injuries) Act, 1965*.

Paprika-splitters' Lung

The red-pepper industry of Eastern Europe dates back to the sixteenth century, when the Turkish invaders introduced the paprika plant which they grew for medicinal purposes. In modern times the species *Capsicum annuum longum* has been cultivated in the region of Szeged, and this town is the centre of the Hungarian red-pepper industry. Other centres along the

Danubian plain include Horgoš in Yugoslavia. The fruit of the plant when dry is deep red and is four inches long, one inch broad at the stalk and tapers to a point.

Exposure Hazard

Women called splitters cut open the fruit with a knife and strip out a series of thin pale ribs which line it longitudinally. The ribs are discarded before grinding because they contain too much of the pungent principle capsaicin. Fruits picked late in the season are often infested with the mould *Mucor stolonifer*, the colonies of which are removed along with the ribs by the women splitters. The air of the workroom is then clouded by spores and mycelia which settle everywhere as a fine dust. In 1931 a disease of the splitters, *paprika splitters' lung*, was described. Workers grinding the split fruits and those handling the finished pepper do not suffer from it.

Symptoms and Signs

A proportion of the splitters, especially those who have been many years at the job, suffer from loss of weight, poor appetite, poor sleep and even hæmoptysis. There is slight fever, and signs of bronchitis develop. In its chronic form the disease presents with cough, fetid expectoration, and apical dullness and cavities in the lungs. X-rays confirm the presence of consolidation and the cavities show in bronchograms (fig. 415).

Ætiology and Pathology

Necropsy shows extensive fibrosis of the lungs with bronchiectasis, and right heart failure. It is not clear what part the fungus plays in the ætiology of the disease, but, of course, the

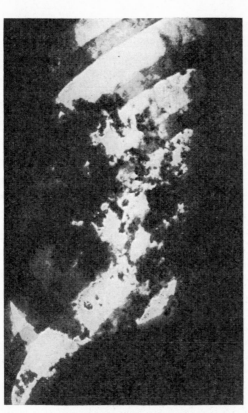

Fig. 415.—Bronchogram showing Bronchiectasis in a Paprika Splitter
(*von Kováts, F.* (1937), *Acta med. Szeged*, **8**, *1*)

presence of its spores in the sputum and in the bronchi after death does not prove it is more than a saprophyte. Although generations of women had followed this occupation, using the same method for eighty years, neither employers, workers nor doctors became aware of its existence until 1931.

Preventive Treatment

It was at first sought to prevent the disease by the use of cotton-wool respirators, but these had little success. Ultimately the chief botanist of the Paprika Research Institute in Szeged succeeded in cultivating a variety of the plant in which the fruit had ribs containing much less capsaicin. Since it is possible to obtain first-class red pepper by grinding this fruit whole, there is now no risk to the worker of inhaling the fungus spores for, indeed, the paprika splitter is no longer needed (Von Kováts, 1937). This example of the application of research in horticulture to the protection of the worker is unique.

Maple-Bark Disease

Maple-bark disease was first described in 1932 in men engaged in peeling bark from maple logs. It is caused by the fungus *Cryptostroma corticale* which causes black areas up to 2 cm. diam. beneath the bark. In 1952 this fungus caused an epiphytotic which destroyed a large number of sycamore trees in Surrey. In 1962 in Marshfield, Wisconsin, Emanuel and others investigated the cases of five men employed in the wood room of a paper mill where such logs were cut in order to convert them into paper pulp. The patients had cough, expectoration, night sweats and loss of weight. On examination no evidence of bronchospasm was found but there were moist crepitant râles in the lower two-thirds of both lung fields. Pulmonary function studies were not particularly helpful in the diagnosis of the disease; the principal abnormality is a diffusion defect. X-rays of the chest show a diffuse reticulo-nodular parenchymal infiltrate involving the lower two-thirds of both lungs. Two of the patients showed areas of confluent broncho-pneumonia. Biopsy of the lung showed chronic interstitial pneumonitis, and the histological appearances were those of fibrosis of alveolar walls with granulomata showing multinuclear giant cells and spores of *C. corticale*. In four of the five cases such spores were cultured from the lung. The disease is a hypersensitivity reaction to these spores and does not represent a true infection since the spores do not grow at body temperature. Antigenic extracts of the spores gave positive agar-gel diffusion tests showing precipitating antibodies. Such immunological studies are essential in diagnosis, for the signs and symptoms of this disease cannot be differentiated from those produced by other types of interstitial pneumonia. The five patients were all severely disabled but ultimately got quite well.

DUSTS OF ANIMAL ORIGIN

Although Ramazzini (1713) suspected that 'small fragments of dead silkworms as well as brukes (locust larvæ) and caterpillars possess some sort of noxious and corrosive acrimony injurious to the lungs' it was not until 1940 that the scales, pellicles and fæcal dust of beetles and other insects were recognized as an important cause of inhalant allergic symptoms in some men who handle these creatures. Reports as to the harmful effects of other animal dusts have been scanty. Animal dusts include those of bone, feathers, fur, hair, horn, ivory, leather, silk and wool. Although such dusts contain virtually no silica, it should be pointed out that both bone and horn are sometimes shaped by the use of sandstone grinding wheels, the dust from which could in time produce silicosis. Occasionally animal dusts may carry infections, especially anthrax. Pulmonary anthrax at one time occurred from inhaling the dust of infected wool (p. 722). The crushing of bones from anthrax-infected animals may carry a similar risk, especially when sun-dried bones are used (p. 721). The manufacture and use of bone, hide, and horn fertilizers have all occasionally caused anthrax in man. We now know that some animal dusts can produce extrinsic allergic alveolitis.

Lung Disease due to the Grain Weevil

In his description entitled *Diseases of dressers of flax and hemp and carders of silk rolls* Ramazzini (1713) states:

After the cocoons of the silkworms have been steeped in warm water they are unrolled and drawn into very fine threads and wound on reels, and from this process a number of coarse filaments are left over mingled with fragments of dead silkworms. Of this compound the women make what are called silk rolls, dry them in the sun, and hand them over to special workers who comb them into threads with very fine combs. Now the men who comb these rolls are attacked by a terrible cough and serious difficulty of respiration; few indeed of these workmen grow old at this occupation. But the injurious effects of working over this stuff are caused wholly by the small fragments of dead silkworms that are scattered all through the silk rolls. It is worth mentioning that, when this little insect is alive and feeding on mulberry leaves, if its excrements are thrown out for some days in a heap and stick where they are till they putrefy and then someone stirs them up, they give off so foul a smell that they infest the whole neighbourhood; hence in some cities it is expressly forbidden to throw this sort of filth into the public streets, and it must be taken outside the city walls. This insect, then, like many others of the same class, e.g. brukes and caterpillars which like silkworms wrap themselves in cocoons and have been known to devour whole woods, possesses some sort of noxious and corrosive acrimony injurious to the lungs. I know a whole family in Modena that had made a good deal of money at this business, but they all died miserably worn down by consumption; they had been employed continuously at this trade, and the doctors held it responsible for their cruel fate.

In 1940 Wittich postulated that asthma in grain handlers working in mill dust could be due to the grain becoming contaminated by insects, and he was the first to describe allergic rhinitis and asthma due to the Mexican bean weevil (*Zabrotes subfasciatus* Boh) in bean sorters. In 1941 Sheldon and Johnston reported a case of hypersensitivity to beetles. Dermestid beetles used for removing the flesh from zoological specimens caused rhinorrhœa and bronchial asthma in a museum curator. Entomologists, technicians and other laboratory workers employed in anti-locust research may develop locust sensitivity presenting as urticaria, allergic rhinitis or asthma. It is especially important to protect them from the fæcal dust of the insects; cleaning the cages in which locusts are bred distributes a cloud of fine locust fæcal dust (Frankland, 1953). The same effects can be brought about by emanations such as scales and pellicles arising from cockroaches, bees, May-flies and caddis flies as well as from certain beetles and water-fleas (Brown, 1944). The grain weevil (*Sitophilus granarius*), like other insects, easily gives rise to inhalant allergic symptoms as well as to the Arthus phenomenon. Further, precipitating antibodies have been found in the serum of patients affected (Lunn and Hughes, 1967). The condition is therefore analogous to farmers' lung, and if the patient is not removed from exposure, the lungs will become involved. Laboratory workers may become so sensitive to weevil dust that they have to abandon the work altogether. Those less seriously affected may be able to carry on by using an extractor fan and wearing a mask. It is possible that certain cases of asthma in grain-handlers, silo-workers and bakers are due to infestation of grain and flour by the grain-weevil (Frankland and Lunn, 1965). This has been described by Lunn (1966) as *millworkers' asthma*.

Feather-Pickers' Disease

In workshops handling feathers there seems to be a direct relationship between the dustiness of a process and complaints by workers of cough and a feeling of tightness in the chest (Bridge, 1934). This subject needs further investigation by clinical and radiological methods. In France certain workers who clean, sort and prepare duck and goose feathers have been found to suffer from *feather-pickers' disease* or *duck fever* (Plessner, 1959). They handle not only raw feathers of local origin but also feathers imported from China. The Chinese feathers produce more dust and this seems to be more potent in producing symptoms than does dust from French feathers. The symptoms appear toward the end of the first working day and consist of fatigue, general malaise, nausea and headache, accompanied by distressing paroxysmal cough and dyspnœa, rigors and fever up to 103° F. After a few hours profuse sweating terminates the attack. The disorder is mild and seldom compels cessation of work. After exposure for three or four days in succession a certain tolerance develops but two or three years usually elapse before the workers become immune to contact with feathers. The men cannot be persuaded to wear masks and the solution of the problem is to mechanize all the processes involved.

Bird-Breeders' (Fanciers') Lung

In 1966 Hargreave, Pepys and others showed that budgerigar and pigeon excreta contained antigens the inhalation of which in some people could cause a disease resembling farmers' lung. Fever, shivering, malaise and loss of weight are accompanied by cough and dyspnœa crepitant râles, evidence of impaired carbon monoxide transfer and decreased lung compliance. In seven affected pigeon fanciers and five affected budgerigar fanciers precipitins were present against antigens in the avian excreta and serum proteins. Skin tests gave, in all except two cases, dual reactions consisting of an immediate wheal followed after three to four hours by an extensive, œdematous reaction, regarded as being of the Arthus type. A strong immunological response, consisting of the appearance of precipitins, results from the entry of the organic, avian antigens through the respiratory tract and the evidence suggests that the clinical manifestations are the result of a precipitin mediated hypersensitivity reaction.

Smallpox-Handlers' Lung

Over many years doctors have observed from time to time cases of pneumonia in successfully vaccinated smallpox contacts. Howat and Arnott (1944) had this experience while serving in the war in the Middle East. A patient with smallpox was admitted to their ward on the fourth day of the illness and died on the twelfth day with confluent lesions. Five medical officers who examined him and two orderlies who nursed him became ill with fever up to 104°F. and headache but no catarrhal symptoms. In the chest there were migratory crepitant râles. X-rays of the chest showed areas of fine diffuse mottling with multiple scattered shadows up to eight millimetres in diameter. All seven men recovered completely. In 1962 in the Rhondda Valley of Wales there was a comparatively serious outbreak of malignant smallpox started by an immigrant Pakistani. There were fifty-four cases with 17 deaths. An illness of contact occurred in the nursing staff (Evans and Foreman, 1963). Thirty-two nurses, all successfully vaccinated, the majority repeatedly, were affected. Nine to twelve days after contact they suffered from malaise, frontal headache, shivering, sweating and general aching especially lumbar backache lasting four days, but they had no catarrhal symptoms. Dry cough followed and scanty crepitations were heard in the chest. Fever up to 103°F. persisted for ten days and there was slight exertional dyspnœa for eight weeks. Of the twelve nurses who showed major symptoms six had X-ray abnormalities in the lungs, namely scattered opacities up to five millimetres across. All thirty-two nurses were completely well in the third week. Since routine bed making during the scaling stage of smallpox produces clouds of scale dust it seems probable that allergy with the Arthus reaction was the cause of the illness.

BIBLIOGRAPHY

ALDEN, H. S., and HOWELL, W. M. (1944), *Arch. Dermat. Syph.*, **49**, 312.

ANTWEILER, H., and HIRSCH, E. (1957), *Z. Immun Forsch.*, **114**, 378.

ARLIDGE, J. J. (1892), *The Hygiene, Diseases and Mortality of Occupations*, Percival, London.

ARNOLD, J. (1885), *Staubinhalation und Staubmetastase*, Berlin.

ARRIGONI, A. (1933), *Med. d. Lavoro*, **24**, 461.

BADHAM, C. (1927), *Rep. Dir. publ. Hlth. N.S.W.*, p. 105.

BARRIE, H. F., and HARDING, H. E. (1947), *Brit. J. industr. Med.*, **4**, 225.

BARTAK, F., and TOMECKA, M. (1949), *Proc. Ninth Intern. Cong. Industr. Med., London*, Wright, Bristol, p. 744.

BELT, T. H., and FERRIS, A. A. (1942), *Med. Research Counc. Spec. Rep. Series*, No. 243.

BOHNER, C. B., SHELDON, J. M., and TRENIS, J. W. (1941), *J. Allergy*, **12**, 290.

BRAUN, D. C., and TRUAN, T. D. (1958), *Arch. industr. Hlth.*, **17**, 634.

BREMNER, D. (1869), *The Industries of Scotland*, Edinburgh.

BRIDGE, J. C. (1924), *Annual Report of the Chief Inspector of Factories*, p. 80; (1933), *Ibid.*, p. 48; (1934), *Ibid.*, p. 66; (1936), *Ibid.*, p. 56.

BROWN, E. A. (1944), *Annals of Allergy*, **2**, 235.

BROWN, E. B., and CREPEA, S. B. (1947), *J. Allergy*, **18**, 214.

BROWN, M. (1967), *The Times*, 28 Nov.

BRUUSGAARD, A. (1949), *Proc. Ninth Intern. Cong. Industr. Med., London*, Wright, Bristol, p. 676.

BRYAN, A. M. (1950), *Report of Inspector of Mines for 1948*, H.M.S.O., London.

BUECHNER, H. A. (1961), *Industr. med., and Surg.*, **30**, 294.

CAMPBELL, A. H., and GLOYNE, S. R. (1942), *J. Path. Bact.*, **54**, 75.

CAMPBELL, J. A. (1958), *Thorax*, **13**, 177.

CAMPBELL, J. M. (1932), *Brit. med. J.*, **2**, 1143.

CAPLAN, A. (1953), *Thorax*, **8**, 29.

CAPLAN, A., COWEN, E. D. H., and GOUGH, J. (1958), *Ibid.*, **13**, 181.

CLARK, W. I., and DRINKER, P. (1935), *Industrial Medicine*, Nat. Med. Book Co., Inc., New York.

CLERENS, J. (1953), *Arch. belges méd. Soc.*, **11**, 336.

COCHRANE, A. L., FLETCHER, C. M., GILSON, J. C., and HUGH-JONES, P. (1951), *Brit. J. industr. Med.*, **8**, 53.

COLLEN, M. F. (1947), *J. industr. Hyg.*, **29**, 113.

COLLIS, E. L. (1913), *Annual Report of the Chief Inspector of Factories*, p. 150; (1915), *Public Health*, **28**, 252.

COOKE, W. E. (1924), *Brit. med. J.*, **2**, 147.

COOKE, W. E., and HILL, C. F. (1927), *J. R. micr. Soc.*, **47**, 232.

CRAW, J. (1947), *Silicosis Pneumokoniosis and Dust Suppression in Mines*, Proc. Confer. held in London, Inst. Mining Engineers and Inst. of Mining and Metallurgy, London, p. 68.

CUMMINS, S. L. (1934), *Amer. Rev. Tuberc.*, **29**, 17.

CUMMINS, S. L., and SLADDEN, A. F. S. (1930), *J. Path. Bact.*, **33**, 1095.

CURRAN, R. C., and ROWSELL, E. V. (1958), *Ibid.*, **76**, 561.

DASSANAYAKE, W. L. P. (1948), *Brit. J. industr. Med.*, **5**, 141.

DAVIDSON., J. M. (1941), *Lancet*, **1**, 38.

DENNY, J. J., ROBSON, W. D., and IRWIN, D. A. (1939), *Canad. med. Ass. J.*, **40**, 213.

DICKIE, H. A., and RANKIN, J. (1958), *J. Amer. med. Ass.*, **167**, 1069.

VAN DIEMERBROECK, I. (1672), *Anatome corporis humani*, Utrecht, **2**, 13.

DOIG, A. T. (1949), *Post Grad. med. J.*, **25**, 639.

DOIG, A. T., and McLAUGHLIN, A. I. G. (1936), *Lancet*, **1**, 771; (1948), *Ibid.*, **1**, 789.

DOLL, R. (1955), *Brit. J. industr. Med.*, **12**, 81.

DREESSEN, W. C., DALLAVALLE, J. M., EDWARDS, T. L., and SAYERS, R. R. (1940), *Publ. Hlth. Bull.*, Wash., No. 250, p. 42.

DRINKER, P., and HATCH, T. (1954), *Industrial Dust*, Second Edition, McGraw-Hill Book Co., Inc., New York.

DUKE, W. W. (1935), *J. Amer. med. Ass.*, **105**, 957.

DUNCAN, J. T. (1943), *Brit. med. J.*, **2**, 715.

DUNNER, L. (1945), *Brit. J. Radiol.*, **18**, 33.

DUNNER, L., and BAGNALL, D. J. T. (1949), *Ibid.*, **22**, 573.

EMANUEL, D. A., WENZEL, F. J., and LAWSON, B. R. (1966), *New Engl. J. Med.*, **274**, 1413.

ENZER, M., and SANDER, O. A. (1938), *J. industr. Hyg.*, **20**, 333.

FAULDS, J. S. (1935), *J. Path. Bact.*, **41**, 129.

FAWCITT, R. (1936), *Brit. J. Radiol.*, **9**, 172; (1938), *Ibid.*, **11**, 378.

FISHER, S. W. (1935), *Trans. instn. min. engrs.*, Lond., **88**, 377, 409.

FLETCHER, C. M. (1948), *Brit. med. J.*, **1**, 1015, 1065.

FLETCHER, C. M., and OLDHAM, P. D. (1949), *Brit. J. industr. Med.*, **6**, 168; (1951), *Ibid.*, **8**, 138.

FOWLER, P. B. S. (1952), *Lancet*, **2**, 755.

FRANK, R. C. (1958), *Amer. J. Roentgenol.*, **79**, 189.

FRANKLAND, A. W. (1953), *Annals of Allergy*, **11**, 445.

FRANKLAND, A. W., and LUNN, J. A. (1965), *Brit. J. industr. Med.*, **22**, 157.

FULLER, G. J. (1953), *Thorax*, **8**, 59.

FURNESS, G., and MAITLAND, H. B. (1952), *Brit. J. industr. Med.*, **9**, 138.

GARDNER, L. U. (1923), *Amer. Rev. Tuberc.*, **7**, 344; (1938), *Silicosis and Asbestosis*, edit. A. J. Lanza.

GARDNER, L. U., DWORSKI, M., and DELAHANT, A. B. (1944), *J. industr. Hyg.*, **26**, 211.

GÄRTNER, H. (1947), *Z. inn. Med.*, **2**, 761.

GÄRTNER, H., and VAN MARWYCK, C., (1947), *Dtsch. med. Wschr.*, **72**, 708.

GERBIS, H., and UCKO (1932), *Ibid.*, **58**, 285.

GERSTL, B., TAGER, M., and SZCSEPANIAK, L. W. (1949), *Proc. Soc. exp. Biol.*, **70**, 697.

GILL, G. I. C. (1947), *Brit. J. industr. Med.*, **4**, 48.

GILSON, J. C. (1966), *Trans. Soc. Gcc. Med.*, **16**, 62.

GILSON, J. C., and HUGH-JONES, P. (1955), *Lung Function in Coalworkers' Pneumoconiosis*, Medical Research Council, Spec. Rep. Ser. No. 290, H.M.S.O., London.

GLOYNE, S. R. (1929), *Tubercle*, **10**, 404.

GLOYNE, S. R., MARSHALL, G., and HOYLE, C. (1949), *Thorax*, **4**, 31.

GOUGH, J. (1940), *J. Path. Bact.*, **51**, 277; (1947), *Occup. Med.*, **4**, 86; (1949), *Post Grad. Med. J.*, **25**, 611; (1958), *Middlesex Hosp. Journ.*, **58**, 144.

GOUGH, J., RIVERS, D., and SEAL, R. M. E. (1955), *Thorax*, **10**, 9.

GREENHOW, E. H. (1860), *Report of the M.O. of the Privy Council*, Third Report, H.M.S.O., London; (1861), *Trans. path. Soc. Lond.*, **12**, 36;

(1862), *Report of the M.O. Local Govt. Bd.*; (1865), *Trans. path. Soc. Lond.*, **16**, 59; (1866), *Ibid.*, **17**, 24.

GREGORY, J. C. (1831), *Edinb. med. J.*, **36**, 389.

GYE, W. E., and PURDY, W. J. (1922), *Brit. J. exp. Path.*, **3**, 75.

HALDANE, J. S. (1915), *The Effects of Inhaling Dusts Applicable for Stone-dusting in Coal Mines*. Seventh Report of the Explosives in Mines Committee, Cmd. 8122, H.M.S.O., London.

HALDANE, J. S., MARTIN, J. S., and THOMAS, R. A. (1904), *Report on the Health of Cornish Miners*, Cmd. 2091, H.M.S.O., London.

HALE, L. W. (1946), *Thorax*, **1**, 71.

HARDING, H. E. (1948), *Brit. J. industr. Med.*, **5**, 70.

HARDING, H. E., GROUT, J. L. A., LLOYD DAVIES, T. A. (1947), *Ibid.*, **5**, 70.

HARDING, H. E., and OLIVER, G. B. (1949), *Ibid.*, **6**, 91.

HARGREAVE, F. E., PEPYS, J., LONGBOTTOM, J. L., and WRAITH, D. C. (1966), *Lancet*, **1**, 445.

HARPER, A. (1934), *Brit. med. J.*, **1**, 920.

HART, P. d'A., and ASLETT, E. A. (1942), *Med. Research Counc. Spec. Rep. Series*, No. 243, London.

HATCH, T. F. (1950), *Pneumoconiosis: 6th Saranac Symposium*, edit. A. J. Vorwald.

HAY, M. (1909), *Ann. Rep. Med. Off. Health*, Aberdeen.

HENRY, S. A., and MIDDLETON, E. L. (1936), *Lancet*, **2**, 59.

HEPPLESTON, A. G. (1947), *J. Path. Bact.*, **59**, 453.

HICKS, D., and NAGELSCHMIDT, G. (1943), *Med. Res. Counc. Spec. Rep. Series*, No. 244.

HILL, A. B. (1930), *Report of the Industrial Health Research Board*, No. 59, H.M.S.O., London.

HIRT, L. (1871), *Die Krankheiten der Arbeiter*, Breslau.

HOFFMANN, W. (1946), *Schweiz. med. Wschr.*, **76**, 988.

HOLLAND, G. C. (1843), *The Vital Statistics of Sheffield*, Tyas, London.

HOLMAN, A. T. (1947), *Brit. J. industr. Med.*, **4**, 1; (1954), Personal communication.

HOLT, P. F., and OSBORNE, S. G. (1953), *Brit. J. industr. Med.*, **10**, 152.

HOLT, P. F., and YATES, D. M. (1954), *Brit. J. exp. Path.*, **35**, 52.

HOURIHANE, D. O'B. (1964), *Thorax*, **19**, 268.

HOURIHANE, D. O'B., LESSOF, L., and RICHARDSON, P. C. (1966), *Brit. med. J.*, **1**, 1069.

HOWAT, H. T., and ARNOTT, W. M. (1944), *Lancet*, **2**, 312.

HUGH-JONES, P. (1951), *Brit. J. industr. Med.*, **8**, 53.

HUNTER, D., MILTON, R., PERRY, K. M. A., and THOMPSON, D. R. (1944), *Ibid.*, **1**, 159.

HUNTER, D., and PERRY, K. M. A. (1946), *Ibid.*, **3**, 64.

INTERNATIONAL LABOUR OFFICE (1959), International Classification of Radiographs of the Pneumoconioses, *Occup. Safety and Health*, **9**, No. 2, Geneva.

IRWIN, D. A. (1950), *Pneumoconiosis: 6th Saranac Symposium*, edit. A. J. Vorwald.

JONES, T. D. (1936), *Proc. S. Wales Inst. Engrs.*, **52**, 157.

JONES, W. R. (1933), *J. Hyg., Camb.*, **33**, 307.

KEAL, E. E. (1960), *Lancet*, **2**, 1211.

KEMP, F. H., and WILSON, D. C. (1946), *Ibid.*, **1**, 172.

KENNEDY, M. C. S. (1956), *Brit. J. industr. Med.*, **13**, 85.

KETTLE, E. H. (1932), *J. Path. Bact.*, **35**, 395.

KING, E. J. (1945), *Med. Res. Counc. Spec. Rep. Series*, No. 250; (1947) *Occup. med.*, **4**, 26.

KING, E. J., and BELT, T. H. (1938), *Physiol. Rev.*, **18**, 329.

KING, E. J., CLEGG, J. W., and RAE, V. M. (1946), *Thorax*, **1**, 188.

KING, E. J., HARRISON, C. V., and RAY, S. C. (1948), *Proc. Ninth Intern Cong. Industr. Med., London*, Wright, Bristol.

KING, E. J., and NAGELSCHMIDT, G. (1945), *Med. Res. Counc. Spec. Rep Series*, No. 250.

KING, E. J., WRIGHT, B. M., RAY, S. C., and HARRISON, C. V. (1950) *Brit. J. industr. Med.*, **7**, 27.

VON KOVÁTS, F. (1937), *Die Lungenerkrankung der Paprikaspalter, Acta med Szeged*, Budapest, **8**, 1.

KRÜGER, E., ROSTOSKI, O., and SAUPE, E. (1931), *Arch. Gewerbepath Gewerbehyg.*, **2**, 558.

LAENNEC, R. T. H. (1819), *Traité de l'auscultation médiate*, Paris.

LANZA, A. J. (1945), *J. Mo. med. Ass.*, **42**, 765 (from *Occ. Med.*, 1946, **1**, 193)

LEACH, J. (1863), *Lancet*, **2**, 648.

LOVELL, R. (1952), Personal communication.

LUNN, J. A. (1966), *Brit. J. industr. Med.*, **23**, 149.

LUNN, J. A., and HUGHES, D. T. D. (1967), *Brit. J. industr. Med.*, **24**, 158.

LYNCH, K. M., and SMITH, W. A. (1935), *Amer. J. Cancer*, **24**, 56.

McCALLUM, R. I. (1952), *Brit. J. industr. Med.*, **9**, 99.

McCORMICK, W. E., SMITH, M., and MARSH, S. P. (1948), *J. industr. Hyg.* **30**, 43.

McCULLOUGH, T. W. (1959), *Ann. Rep. of the Chief Inspector of Factorie on Industr. Hlth. for 1958*, Cmd. 811, H.M.S.O., London.

McKENNA, W. B., SMITH, J. F. F., and MACLEAN, D. A. (1958), *Brit. J industr. Med.*, **15**, 47.

McLAUGHLIN, A. I. G., GROUP, J. L. A., BARRIE, H. F., and HARDING, H. E (1945), *Ibid.*, **1**, 337.

McLAUGHLIN, A. I. G., and others (1950), *Industrial Lung Diseases of Iron and Steel Foundry Workers*, H.M.S.O., London.

McNAIR, L. C., and MIDDLETON, E. L. (1925), *Annual Report of the Chie Inspector of Factories and Workshops for 1924*, H.M.S.O., Cmd. 2437, p. 103

MACKLIN, E. L., and MIDDLETON, E. L. (1923), *Report on Grinding o Metals and Cleaning of Castings*, Home Office, H.M.S.O., London.

MAIR, A. (1951), *Edinb. med. J.*, **58**, 457.

MARSHALL, W. (1833), *Lancet*, **2**, 271.

MAVROGORDATO, A. (1926), *Publ. S. Afr. Inst. med. Res.*, **3**, 18.

VAN MECHELEN, V., and McLAUGHLIN, A. I. G. (1962), *Ann. Occup. Hyg.* **4**, 237.

MEER, C. van der (1954), *Ned. Geneesk.*, **98**, 3539.

MEIKLEJOHN, A. (1949), *Brit. J. industr Med.*, **6**, 230; *Ibid.*, **8**, 127; (1952) *Ibid.*, **9**, 93, 208.

MEIKLEJOHN, A., and POSNER, E. (1957), *Brit. J. industr. Med.*, **14**, 229.

MEREWETHER, E. R. A. (1936), *Tubercle*, **17**, 385.

MEREWETHER, E. R. A., and PRICE, C. W. (1930), *Report on Effects of As bestos Dust on the Lungs and Dust Suppression in the Asbestos Industry* H.M.S.O., London.

MIDDLETON, E. L. (1920), *Tubercle*, **1**, 257; (1926), *J. industr. Hyg.*, **8**, 428; (1930), *Silicosis, Records of the Internat. Conference held at Johannesburg*, I.L.O., Geneva, King, London, p. 384; (1938), *Silicosis, Occupation and Health*, Suppl. of Jan, 1938; (1940), *Proc. Internat. Confer. on Silicosis, Geneva, 1938*, I.L.O. Studies and Reports, ser. F. (Industr. Hyg.), No. 17, p. 134, Ling, London.

MORRIS EVANS, W. H., and FOREMAN, H. M. (1963), *Proc. roy. soc. med.*, **56**, 274.

MURRAY, M. (1907), *Departmental Comm. on Compens. for Industr. Dis.*, Cmd. 3495, p. 14, Cmd. 3496, p. 127, H.M.S.O., London.

MURRAY, R., DINGWALL-FORDYCE, I., and LANE, R. E. (1957), *Brit. J. industr. Med.*, **14**, 105.

NEAL, P. A., SCHNEITER, R., and CAMINITA, B. H. (1942), *J. Amer. Med. Ass.*, **119**, 1074.

NEWHOUSE, M. L., and THOMPSON, H. (1965), *Brit. J. industr. Med.*, **22**, 261.

OWEN, W. G. (1964), *Brit. med. J.*, **2**, 214.

OLIVER, T. (1902), *Dangerous Trades*, Murray, London.

PARMEGGIANI, L. (1949), *Rass. Med. industr.*, **18**, 93.

PEACOCK, T. B. (1860), *Med.-chir. Trans.*, **26**, 214; (1861), *Trans. path. Soc. Lond.*, **12**, 36; (1865), *Ibid.*, **16**, 57.

PENDERGRASS, E. P., and GREENING, R. R. (1934), *J. Path. Bact.*, **39**, 233.

PENDERGRASS, E. P., and PRYDE, A. W. (1948), *J. industr. Hyg.*, **30**, 119.

PEPYS, J., JENKINS, P. A., FESTENSTEIN, G. N., GREGORY, P. H., LACEY, M. E., and SKINNER, F. A. (1963), *Lancet*, **2**, 607.

PERNIS, B., CLERICI, E., and BHEZZI, I. (1958), *Med. d. Lavoro*, **49**, 672.

PLANT, H. J. (1939), *Trans. Brit. Ceramic Soc.*, **38**, 476.

PLESSNER, M. M. (1959), *Arch. med. prof.*, **21**, 67.

POLICARD, A. (1933), *Pr. méd.*, **41**, 89.

PRATT, P. C. (1950), *Pneumoconiosis: 6th Saranac Symposium*, edit. A. J. Vorwald.

PRAUSNITZ, C. (1936), *Med. Res. Counc. Spec. Rep.*, Series No. 312, London.

PROUST, A. (1874), *Bull. Acad. Méd.*, Paris, **3**, 624.

RAMAZZINI, B. (1713), *De Morbus Artificum Diatriba*. Transl. by Wilmer Cave Wright, Chicago, 1940.

RICKARDS, A. G., and BARRETT, G. M. (1958), *Thorax*, **13**, 185.,

RIDDELL, A. R. (1954), Personal communication.

ROBERTSON, A. J., in KING, E. J., and FLETCHER, C. M. (1960), *A Symposium on Industrial Pulmonary Diseases*, J. & A. Churchill, London, p. 168.

ROBERTSON, A. J., and WHITAKER, P. H. (1955), *J. fac. Radiol.*, **6**, 224.

ROSENTHAL, E. (1952), *Elect. Rev.*, Lond., **151**, 121.

SAKABE, H., KAWAI, K., KOSHI, K., SODA, R., HAMADA, A., SHIMAZU. M., and HAYASHI, H. (1960), *Bull. Nat. Inst. industr. Hlth.*, **4**, 1.

SCHEPERS, G. W. H. (1959), *Amer. industr. hyg. Assoc.*, **20**, 73.

SCHILLING, R. S. F. (1952), *Proc. R. Soc. Med.*, **45**, 601; (1959), *J. occup. Med.*, **1**, 33.

SCHILLING, R. S. F., and GOODMAN, N. M. (1951), *Brit. J. indust. Med.*, **8**, 77.

SCHILLING, R. S. F., GOODMAN, N. M., and O'SULLIVAN, J. G. (1952), *Ibid.*, **9**, 146.

SCHNEITER, R., NEAL, P. A., and CAMINITA, B. H. (1942), *Amer. J. publ. Hlth.*, **32**, 1345.

SCHNEITER, R., REINHART, W. H., and CAMINITA, B. H. (1948), *J. industr Hyg.*, **30**, 238.

SEIFERT, H. (1958), *Staub*, **18**, 201.

SEILER, H. E. (1928), *Brit. med. J.*, **2**, 982.

SHATTOCK, S. G. (1917), *Proc. R. Soc. Med.*, **10**, Sect. Path., 6.

SHAVER, C. G. (1948), *Radiology*, **50**, 760.

SHAVER, C. G., and RIDDELL, A. R. (1947), *J. mdustr. Hyg.*, **29**, 145.

SHAW DUNN, J., and SHEEHAN, H. L. (1932), *Report of Departmental Committee on Dust in Card Rooms*, Home Office, H.M.S.O., London.

SHELDON, J. A., and JOHNSTON, J. H. (1941), *Journ. of Allergy*, **12**, 493.

SMILEY, J. A. (1951), *Brit. J. industr. Med.*, **8**, 265; (1961), *ibid.*, **18**, 1.

SMITH, A. R., and PERINA, A. E. (1949), *N.Y. Dept. of Labour Monthly Review*, **28**, No. 8.

SMITH, P. G. (1967), *The London Hospital Gazette*, **70**, Suppl., ii.

SPRAGUE, P. H. (1942), *Canad. med. Ass. J.*, **47**, 253.

STAINES, F. H., and FORMAN, J. A. S. (1961), *J. Coll. gen. Practit.*, **4**, 351.

STEWART, M. J. (1947), *Proc. R. Soc. Med.*, **40**, 781.

STRATTON, T. (1937), *Edinb. med. J.*, **49**, 490.

STRONG, G. F. (1954), Personal communication.

SUTHERLAND, C. L., and BRYSON, S. (1926), *Report on the Incidence of Silicosis in the Pottery Industry*, H.M.S.O., London; (1929), *Report on the Recurrence of Silicosis among Sandstone Workers*, H.M.S.O., London.

SUTHERLAND, C. L., BRYSON, S., and KEATING, N. (1930), *Report on the Occurrence of Silicosis among Granite Workers*, H.M.S.O., London.

SWEENEY, P. J. (1952), *Ulster med. J.*, **21**, 150.

TATTERSALL, N. (1926), *J. industr. Hyg.*, **8**, 466.

THOMSON, J. B. (1858), *Edinb. med. J.*, **4**, 226.

THOMSON, W. (1837), *Med.-chir. Trans.*, **20**, 230; (1838), *Ibid.*, **21**, 340.

TIMMERMANS, F. D. (1931), *Zbl. GewHyg.*, **8**, 280, 307.

TONNING, H. O. (1949), *J. industr. Hyg.*, **31**, 41.

TÖRNELL, E. (1946), *Acta. med. scand.*, **125**, 191.

TUFFNELL, P. G. and DINGWALL-FORDYCE, I. (1957), *Brit. J. industr. Med.*, **14**, 250.

VESTAL, T. F., WINSTEAD, J. A., and JOLIET, P. V. (1943), *Industr. med.*, **12**, 11.

VIGLIANI, E. C., PARMEGGIANI, L., and SASSI, C. (1954), *Med. d. Lavoro*, **45**, 349.

VIGLIANI, E. C., and PERNIS, B. (1959), *J. occup. Med.*, **1**, 319.

WAGNER, J. C., SLEGGS, C. A., and MARCHAND, P. (1960), *Brit. J. industr Med.*, **17**, 260.

WEST, R. (1951), *Trans. assoc. industr. med. off.*, **1**, 153.

WHEATLEY, J. (1911), *Report on the Prevalence of Lung Disease amongst Workers at Grinshill Quarries*, County Medical Officer for Shropshire.

WILLIAMS, D. I., and MULHALL, P. P. (1956), *Brit. med. J.*, **2**, 216.

WILLIAMS, E. (1944), *Rep. Advisory Committee on Pneumokoniosis*, H.M.S.O., London.

WILLIAMS, R., and HUGH-JONES, P. (1960), *Thorax*, **15**, 109.

WITTICH, F. W. (1940), *Lancet*, **60**, 418.

WYERS, H. (1946), Thesis presented to the University of Glasgow for the degree of Doctor of Medicine; (1949), *Post Grad. Med. J.*, **25**, 631.

ZENKER, F. A. (1866), *Dtsch. Arch. klin. Med.*, **2**, 116.

CHAPTER XV

ACCIDENTS

ONLY doctors see the full consequences of accidents, with their wastage of life and working efficiency, the disruption of family life and the tragic effects on the individual (fig. 416). It is up to us as a profession to give more thought to the prevention of accidents and to make our views public. In the United States of America in 1953 accidents from all causes brought death or disabling injuries to one out of every sixteen persons in the nation; deaths from accident totalled 95,000. Industry is, of course, responsible for a high proportion of this total. In industry, as well as factory

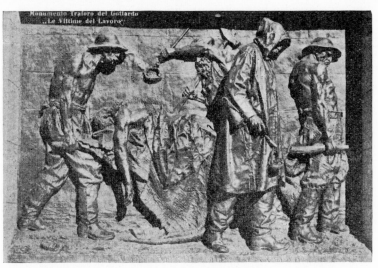

FIG. 416.—Swiss Memorial to the men who died in driving the St. Gotthard Tunnel

accidents, we must consider also accidents in mines, quarries and sewers, at docks, wharves and railway sidings; and also firedamp and dust explosions in coal mines, dust explosions in factories, accidents in agricultural work, electrical injuries, accidents in chemical laboratories, hazards of pharmaceutical work; accidental infections in bacteriological laboratories and attacks by animals, reptiles, insects and fish.

ACCIDENTS IN FACTORIES

In the causation of accidents in factories we have to consider factors such as temperature, ventilation, lighting, fatigue, speed of production,

experience, age and, above all, human factors, especially carelessness and
inattention. In Great Britain the law has provided for the protection of the
worker since the passing of the *Factory Act, 1844. The Factories Act, 1937*
requires all accidents or mishaps, resulting in death of the workman or an ab
sence from work for more than three days, to be reported to the Factory In
spector, who then either visits the works or takes other appropriate action

Dangerous Occurrences

Dangerous Occurrences (Sect. 65 of the Factories Act, 1937), and *The*
Dangerous Occurrences (Notification) Regulations, 1947, must be notified to
the Factory Inspector. Such dangers include bursting of a revolving vessel
wheel, grindstone or grinding wheel moved by mechanical power; collapse
or failure of a crane, derrick, winch, hoist or other appliance (used for
goods or persons), or the overturning of a crane; explosion or fire due to
ignition of dust, gas, vapour or celluloid, causing damage resulting in stoppage of work for five hours; electrical short-circuit or failure of electrical
plant, etc., attended by explosion or fire, involving stoppage of work for
five hours; explosion or fire in a room in which persons are employed and
involving stoppage of work for twenty-four hours; and explosion of a
receiver or container used for storage at a pressure of gas (or gases including air), liquid or solid.

The Bursting of a Revolving Grindstone

The horrible effects of the bursting of a revolving grindstone have been
described by Charles Reade in his novel *Put Yourself in His Place* (1870)

> "I'm an old Saw."
> "Well, then, all the better, for you can tell me, and please do: have
> you ever actually known fatal accidents from this cause?"
> "I have known the light grinders very much shaken by a breaking
> stone, and away from work a month after it. And, working among
> saw-grinders, who use heavy stones, and stand over them in working.
> I've seen—— Billy, go and look at thy shilling, in the yard, and see
> which is the brightest, it or the moon. Is he gone? I've seen three men
> die within a few yards of me. One, the stone flew in two pieces; a frag-
> ment, weighing about four hundredweight, I should say, struck him
> on the breast, and killed him on place; he never spoke. I've forgotten
> his very name. Another; the stone went clean out of the window, but
> it kicked the grinder backwards among the machinery, and his head
> was crushed like an eggshell. But the worst of all was poor Billy's
> father. He had been warned against his stone; but he said he would
> run it out. Well, his little boy, that is, Billy, had just brought him in
> his tea, and was standing beside him, when the stone went like a
> pistol-shot, and snapped the horsing chains like thread; a piece struck
> the wall, and did no harm, only made a hole; but the bigger half went
> clean up to the ceiling, and then fell plumb down again; the grinder
> he was knocked stupid-like, and had fallen forward on his broken

horsing; the grindstone fell right on him, and, ah,—— I saw the son covered with the father's blood."

He shuddered visibly, at the recollection. "Ay," said he, "the man a corpse, and the lad an idiot. One faulty stone did that, within four yards of me, in a moment of time."

"Good heavens!"

"I was grinding at the next stone but one. He was taken, and I was left. It might just as well have been the other way. No saw-grinder can make sure, when he gets on his horsing, that he will come off it alive!"

The defect in this grindstone was not so serious but that the stone might perhaps have been ground out with fair treatment; but, by fixing a small pulley-wheel, Simmons had caused it to rotate at furious speed. This tried it too hard, and it flew in two pieces, just as the grinder was pressing down a heavy saw on it with all his force.

One piece, weighing about five hundredweight, tore the horsing chains out of the floor, and went clean through the window (smashing the woodwork), out of the yard, and was descending on Little's head; but he heard the crash and saw it coming; he ran yelling out of the way, and dragged Bayne with him. The other fragment went straight up to the ceiling, and broke a heavy joist as if it had been a cane; then fell down again plump, and would have destroyed the grinder on the spot, had he been there; but the tremendous shock had sent him flying clean over the splatter-board, and he fell on his stomach on the wheel-band of the next grindstone, and so close to the drum, that, before any one could recover the shock and seize him, the band drew him on to the drum, and the drum, which was drawing away from the window, pounded him against the wall, with cruel thuds.

One ran and screamed to stop the power, another to cut the big wheelbands. All this took several seconds; and here seconds were torn flesh and broken bones. Just as Little darted into the room, pale with his own narrow escape, and awe-stricken at the cries of horror within, the other grinders succeeded in dragging out, from between the wall and the drum, a bag of broken bones and blood and grease, which, a minute before, was Ned Simmons, and was talking over a deed of violence to be done.

The others carried him and laid him on a horsing; and there they still supported his head and his broken limbs, sick with horror.

The man's face was white, and his eyes stared, and his body quivered. They sprinkled him with water.

Then he muttered, "All right. I'm not much hurt.—— Ay, but I am, though. I'm done for!"

The Causes of Accidents

Accidents in factories can be classified as due to the handling of goods, power-driven machinery and lifting machinery, to persons falling and blows by a falling body, the use of hand tools, stepping on or striking against objects, to burns from molten metal, and to transport. Of the fatal accidents, nearly a third are due to falls, sometimes from a height, but often

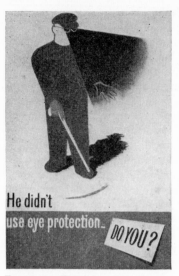

while walking on the level. Many of these mishaps are attributable to lack of suitable appliances, such as ladders or the wearing of unsuitable shoes especially by women. Slippery floors and imperfectly guarded gaps in the floor or walls lead to many accidental falls. The mishandling of goods is responsible for over a quarter of the non-fatal accidents and is often associated with faulty supervision, or with the employment of persons who lack the necessary experience, strength or agility to do the work safely. Accidents continue to occur frequently through falls through roofs made of fragile material such as asbestos sheeting or glass. Such accidents are often due to carelessness, and entail a high mortality, about 20 per cent. Many accidents on building sites and in engineering construction can be traced to faulty methods of stacking and

He didn't
use eye protection..
DO YOU?

FIG. 417.—Gruesome Warning to workmen of the Need for the Protection of the Eyes in Industry
(*Royal Society for the Prevention of Accidents*)

storing materials; here, as in factories, there is need for greater study of good housekeeping.

Accidents to the Eyes

In Great Britain on an average each year some 7,000 accidents to the

NEVER PUT A WET STICK

LADLE OR BAR

INTO MOLTEN METAL

FIG. 418.—Notice in use in a zinc smelter in Canada
(*By courtesy of Cominco, Trail, B.C.*)

eyes are reported to the Factory Department and it is estimated that nearly 250,000 lesser eye injuries occur which are not reported. For certain processes, especially in the chemical industry, the provision and use of goggles is compulsory, and in a number of other processes they have been introduced by voluntary action on the part of the employers or adopted by he workers themselves (fig. 417). The processes mainly responsible for hese accidents are the grinding, glazing and polishing of metal articles; he pouring, stirring and carrying of molten metal (figs. 418, 419, 420, 421); iveting, dressing castings, chipping metal articles (fig. 422), smithing fig. 423), metal working by machinery and stone dressing. The provision

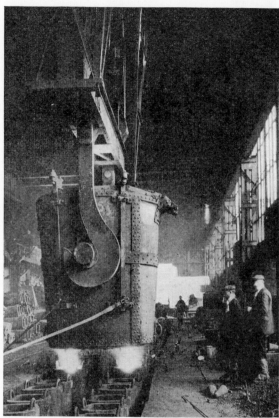

FIG. 419.—When Molten Steel is run into Containers, these must be absolutely dry to avoid Explosion
(*Crown Copyright: Central Office of Information*)

f an adjustable transparent screen between the worker and his work is an lternative which has been found successful (fig. 424). Where possible, rrangements should be made for the repair of goggles at the actual place f work. Unhappily the goggles service man (fig. 425) is an economic ossibility only in firms employing large numbers of men.

Photophthalmia

As a serious industrial problem photophthalmia is of importance only n electric arc welding and in gas welding by means of oxy-hydrogen, oxy-

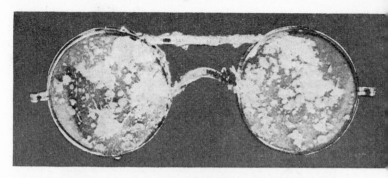

FIG. 420.—Goggles which saved a workman's Eyes, although his Face was burnt when an Explosion occurred from the sudden formation of Water Vapour when Molten Steel was run into a wet Container

coal gas and oxy-acetylene torches. For this reason it is often referred to as *arc eye, arc flash* or *electric arc welders' eye-flash*. Although experience welders are rarely affected their mates and even passers-by often are les fortunate. It may also arise from gazing at the intense glare of molten steel, from the examination of furnaces and hearths in power plants, from the failure to screen the arc lamps in cinema studios and from exposure to the arcs formed by electrical apparatus equipped with ineffective switch gear. Its occurrence in certain case of electric shock is described on p. 1084. Beyond the momentary glare and dazzle there is no immediate effect of exposure to intense ultra-violet radiation. A few hours later, however, the victim may observe coloured rings around lights; these arise from œdema of the corneal epithelium. This symptom may be followed by pain and a feeling as of grit in the eyes excessive secretion of tears and intolerance to light. Fear of blindness may lead to emotional upset. The eyes become suffused and there may be marked spasm of the eyelids. The injury responds to simple treatment such as eye drops of liquid paraffin. In all occupations presenting this hazard goggles, eye shields, visors or screens of Crookes' glass (fig. 426) must be provided and properly used.

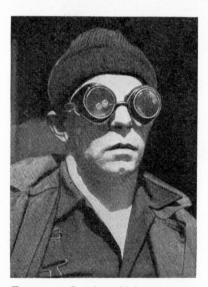

FIG. 421.—Goggles which saved the Eye of a workman when Molten Lead was spattered on the Glass during Soldering
(*By courtesy of Consolidated Edison Co., Inc.*)

Factors predisposing to Accidents

We can accept (Vernon, 1936) without further discussion that the occurrence of accidents is influenced by such factors as hours of work, speed of output, temperature and lighting, the inexperience or youth of the workers and the injudicious use of alcohol. However well machinery may be guarded by law, a reduction of not more than 10 per cent in the accident-rate can be looked for by the provision of safeguards alone. Psychological factors

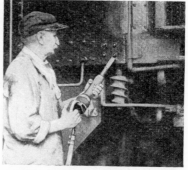

FIG. 422.—Removing the Heads of Rivets by means of a Compressed-air Chisel. Note the absence of Goggles

in the causation of accidents have been systematically studied in England since 1917 under the direction of what was at first the Industrial Fatigue Research Board and is now called the Industrial Health Research Board. The important fact that a minority of workers is responsible for more than their proper share of accidents, if not actually a discovery of the Board's investigators, was first established by them upon a statistical basis (Greenwood and Woods, 1919; Newbold, 1926; and Farmer, Chambers and Kirk, 1933).

Industrial Fatigue

Industrial fatigue is not the simple physico-chemical phenomenon seen in a nerve-muscle preparation; psychological factors such as boredom, lack of incentives to work, and the presence of opportunities for divided attention may reduce the workers' efficiency and must therefore be recognized and studied. Many changes have taken place in industry since the replacement of man-power by machines. With the reduction of working hours from ten to eight, excessive muscular fatigue is less important, and we are now concerned

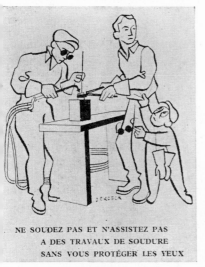

NE SOUDEZ PAS ET N'ASSISTEZ PAS
A DES TRAVAUX DE SOUDURE
SANS VOUS PROTÉGER LES YEUX

FIG. 423.—Poster warning Welders to wear Goggles
(*By courtesy of L'Association des Industriels de Belgique*)

more with the workers' mental and nervous reactions to their environment. Accidents which were formerly charged against fatigue are now attributed to the personal equation. A predisposition to cause accidents

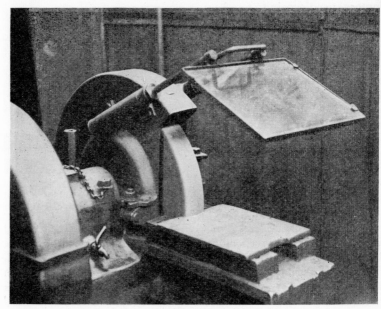

FIG. 424.—Adjustable Screen of thick Plate Glass to protect the Eyes of workmen grinding Metal Objects on the Wheel
(*Royal Society for the Prevention of Accidents*)

may result from lack of training or from an abnormal attitude toward
the work. Noise should receive attention, because it leads to nervousness
and a feeling of weariness similar to that produced by muscular fatigue

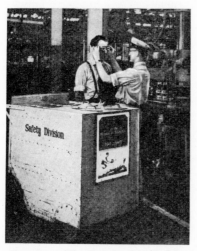

FIG. 425.—The Goggles Service Man

Rest Periods reanimate Interest

The benefit of rest periods lie
chiefly in the reanimation of interest. In addition, the change in
posture or occupation involved permits the blood to circulate more
freely to those parts of the body
which were not receiving their
proper supply in a cramped position
at the machine or bench. The mental
and nervous reactions of workers to
their environment as causes of
fatigue and so of accidents will
increase in importance with the
passing of time. No matter how
well working conditions may be
controlled, such factors as the
home life and psychological make-

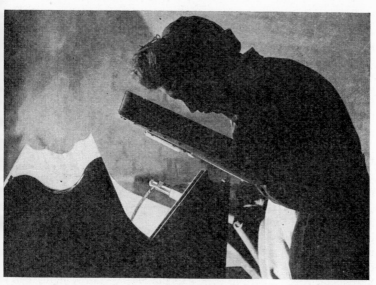

Fig. 426.—Screen of Crookes' Glass to protect the Eyes against Electric Arc
Welders' Eye-flash

p of the individual worker will remain and become increasingly more
nportant.

Accident Proneness

An examination of almost any large collection of accident statistics
hows that accidents are very unevenly distributed among those exposed
⟩ risk. With equal exposure to risk, roughly three-quarters of recorded
ccidents happen to one-quarter of the people exposed. This phenomenon
; known as *accident proneness*, a term coined by Farmer (1932) and now
₁ world-wide use. The probable number of persons who are accident-
rone ranges from 10 to 25 per cent of the total. In considering the psycho-
enesis of accidents Jung (1928) said:

> Accidents of every sort, in greater number than the public would
> ever guess, are of psychological origin. Ranging from insignificant
> mishaps like stumbling, bumping oneself, burning the fingers, etc., to
> automobile accidents and catastrophies in the mountains, instances
> may be found of psychological causation.

Jnfortunately, few firms subject their new employees to psychological
ests before assigning them to one occupation or another. Even in the
bsence of such tests it would be possible to sift them roughly by putting
₁em for a time on occupations free from major risks, and only after they
ave shown themselves to be reasonably free from accident proneness to
ransfer them to more dangerous occupations. Accident proneness is
reatly influenced by the mental attitude of the subjects. The accident-

prone are apt to be insubordinate, temperamentally excitable and to sho
a tendency to get flustered in an emergency. These and other defects
personality indicate a lack of aptitude on the part of the subjects for the
occupation. But whenever we are considering how to prevent acciden
we must avoid the danger of laying too much blame on abnormalities
temperament and personality. Let us beware lest the concept of tl
accident-prone person be stretched beyond the limits within which it ca
be a fruitful idea. We should indeed be guilty of a grave error if for ar
reason we discouraged the manufacture of safe machinery.

Detection of Accident Proneness

It would clearly be desirable to devise means by which accident pron
ness can be detected before exposure to industrial hazards. It was foun
(Farmer and Chambers, 1929) that accident proneness was general
associated with some impairment of neuro-muscular control, and th
certain psychological tests, particularly the use of the Pursuit Meter and
the McDougall-Schuster Dotting Machine, could be used to measure suc
control, as it affected attention, muscular precision and co-ordination
movement. A bad record in these tests did not necessarily imply that tl
subject would show a high susceptibility to accident, but some very sig
nificant associations were established. Thus, in a group of 1,800 er
gineering apprentices subjected to these tests, whose records at work we
afterwards examined, it was found that, if they were arranged in order
proficiency at these tests, the quarter fraction at the bottom of the li
subsequently sustained accidents at work at a rate which was two ar
a half times as high as that in the remaining three-quarters of the group. It
clear that if this quarter had been put into some less dangerous occupatio
the incidence of accidents in the whole group would have been great
diminished. There are no large-scale records available to show the effect
the early detection of accident-prone workers and their transfer to saf
jobs, but this procedure has been put into operation in a few firms.

Simple Tests for Accident Proneness

Turning to the individual, the problem is more complex. Divid
attention may be due to emotional influences such as injustices imagin
or real, quarrels with colleagues or at home, and love affairs. Simple tes
for accident proneness can be illustrated by quoting the case of mot
drivers. The National Institute of Industrial Psychology devised a seri
of tests for the purpose of directly measuring certain qualities regarded
essential for safe and efficient motor driving. Reaction time, resistance
distraction, vigilance, judgement of speed, judgement of spatial relatio
ships, confidence, road behaviour, vision—these and other qualities a
given separate marking, the final judgement resting upon the sum of tl
reactions. This method is satisfactory up to a point, for those who con
out badly in the tests are shown by their records to be liable to an exce
of accidents.

Inadequacy of the Tests

But the disadvantage of such tests is that they cannot reproduce the conditions of long-distance driving—they are too transverse; what is required is something more longitudinal. As in the case of intelligence tests, they are adequate only for the short period of the test, not for longer periods when the attention is less held. In the competent motor driver we find a fluid state of mind which diminishes fatigue. He is watching all the time not only his own road but side roads, and his judgement is continually operating. This includes judgement of the speed of vehicles coming towards him both in front and behind. His psychological make-up is important; the too-careful driver may be almost as bad as the reckless driver. When motor drivers are interviewed, the accident-prone driver can often be picked out. A single bad habit in driving, susceptibility to a small dose of alcohol, wilful road-hogging, loss of sleep, family worries, lack of correct instruction are all known causes. It is claimed that psycho-physiological selection before training has reduced the proportion of unsuitable trainees for the buses of Paris from 20 per cent to 3·4 per cent. Psychoneurotic inhibitions or impulses easily predispose to accidents, especially in motor driving. Some men have an impulse to speed and to charge at an oncoming vehicle, and have to give up driving. Some drivers when interviewed will admit the existence of an impulse which makes it impossible for them to drive behind another car when they cannot see the road ahead of it. They are thus impelled to draw out and try to pass.

The Method of Clinical Interview

Such impulses and inhibitions can now be detected by the method of clinical interview. Here a knowledge of disease and symptomatology is, of course, necessary in order that the clues given by the patient may be followed up. An interviewer seeking for nervous symptoms or temperamental qualities must know what to look for and how to look for it. The use of the method shows that about 20 per cent of the working population suffer from nervous symptoms which interfere with happiness and efficiency. Preventable accidents thus constitute a problem of human behaviour, and in feeling our way to an understanding of the behaviour problems concerned we are reaching out to new means for the prevention of accidents.

Individual Accident Susceptibility in Miners

An advance in the understanding of individual accident susceptibility was made by Whitfield (1954). He analysed information on underground *compensation accidents* in relation to individual working records at a Nottinghamshire colliery employing approximately 2,000 men. By classifying the accidents and the shifts worked according to occupation and place of work it was possible to calculate the accident risk per shift for moderately homogeneous working groups. From these figures an expected total of accidents could be computed for each miner and compared with the actual number experienced. The results indicated clearly that there were individual differences in accident susceptibility among coal-miners which persisted for several years, but that these were not readily attributable the age of the worker nor to inherited tendencies. A detailed investigation was therefore made of three small samples of the miners. One was composed of men who had experienced many more accidents than we expected, the accident-prone group. Each individual was then matched by age and normal mining occupation, with two others who had experienced, respectively, about as many accidents as were expected and fewer accidents than were expected.

Accident Proneness by Age Groups

Thirty-two of these triads were examined by interview and a series tests; the panel which tested each triad did not know which member belonged to which accident category. Among the tests used were measurements of visual and auditory acuities, performance tests of perceptual cognitive and memory functions, and tests of motor control and coordination. It was found that the younger accident-prone men were markedly deficient in the perceptual-cognitive tests, while the older accident-prone men were markedly deficient in motor control and co-ordination. Whitfield suggests that the younger accident-prone man is unable to appreciate the demands of a hazardous situation or to decide what response should be made, although capable of making the response, whereas the older accident-prone individual fails to produce an adequate response, even though the hazard has been perceived and an appropriate course of action initiated. If this is so, it is easy to understand why those naturally deficient in motor ability when young should become accident prone as their motor ability slowly deteriorates with age. It is not so easy to see why young accident-prone miners should apparently cease to be so. Some, presumably, die young; the rest perhaps leave the industry for less hazardous occupations, or, while remaining in coal-mining, adjust themselves to a reduced level of activity.

The So-called Traumatic Neurosis

The idea that the onset of the symptoms of a psychoneurosis could determined by trauma dates back to the nineteenth century when the terms *railway spine*, *railway brain* and *traumatic neurasthenia* all came into being. After injury in a railway accident a patient might have persistent pain the back accompanied by extravagant subjective symptoms whereas the objective signs were but few and slight. It was noticeable that such patient never showed improvement until his claim was legally settled, but that immediately after such settlement all the symptoms cleared up without treatment. Since, in hysteria, the precipitating factor for the onset symptoms is usually a situation, emotionally charged, out of which the patient's symptoms will bring him more or less overt, but unacknowledged, gain the case of such a patient was termed *litigation hysteria*, less accurately, *compensation neurosis*. And indeed even before the dawn

e twentieth century it became clear that all the symptoms at first claimed
be due to a blow on the head or the spine were found sometimes to
cur in men with lead poisoning, while they awaited settlement of their
aims for compensation (p. 261).

rcumstances in which Trauma is followed by Neurosis

Do all accidents physical or emotional give rise to the *accident neurosis*
traumatic neurosis? It is common knowledge that they do not. For
ample, we do not see the symptoms of traumatic neurosis after accidents
d injuries sustained at sports and games or in the domestic scene. Foot-
ll players, huntsmen riding to hounds, steeplechase jockeys, skiers and
aters and the housewife in her home do not present with traumatic
uroses ensuing upon injury. One must conclude therefore that some non-
edical factor operates to determine the development of the neurosis. It
not the fright, anxiety or trauma that engender the neurosis, but the
vantage that the victim may gain by making someone else responsible
r the accident. It should be understood that the subject is unaware
at his symptoms arose and are sustained as purposive phenomena.

ploitation for Gain engenders Neurosis

It is not the misadventure, but its exploitation for gain that engenders
d maintains the traumatic neurosis, and trauma appears rather as the
portunity than the essential causal factor in this neurosis. As thus briefly
ated this may seem a harsh doctrine but it is plainly indicated in the
itings of Freud (1922) and is convincingly expounded by Ross (1937)
d must surely be the conclusion of all who have had experience of such
tients. The expression *compensation neurosis* is an explicit recognition of
is point of view, while the non-occurrence of the traumatic neurosis in
uations where no question of compensation arises, implies that this
ctor is the indispensable one, and that trauma by itself is not adequate to
d to this neurosis.

mptoms of the Traumatic Neurosis

The symptoms include headache, described usually as *terrible* or
onizing, attacks of dizziness on stooping or exertion, defects of memory
d of concentration, sleeplessness, intolerance of noises pleasant or
pleasant, irritability, restlessness, an inability to settle to any activity or
deed to sit still. For such a patient all the ordinary natural pleasures are
oiled. What the family of such a person endures may well be imagined,
e spouse of the victim being commonly the worst sufferer from his or
r moroseness and irritability. It seems that these last complaints come
m the boredom of prolonged idleness, but since, when a claim for
mpensation is in process, a lightening of his sufferings may appear dis-
vantageous, it is reluctantly admitted, when at all.

ctors Perpetuating the Symptoms

This view of the ætiology and nature of the traumatic neurosis implies
at the doctor under whose care the subject first comes may have a con-

siderable influence in preventing or in inducing and perpetuating it. Man
such patients attend their doctors' surgeries for months and more, receiv
ing certificates of unfitness and prescriptions for phenobarbitone or tran
quillizers, and never admitting to improvement, yet not showing an
objective signs of inability to engage in regular gainful occupation. I
agree that the management and disposal of these patients is difficult, an
that, if signed off, they will resort to other doctors, is not to allow ourselve
to feel any satisfaction with what is surely a most deplorable state o
affairs. Finally, the frequently interminable processes of negotiation, an
of offer and refusal that go on between lawyers engaged on the two side
when a claim for damages or compensation is in question, gravely aggra
vate the situation and tend to demoralize the victim in his prolonge
idleness. The traumatic neurosis is a constant drain on manpower an
upon the resources of industry. It involves heavy expense in litigation
sick pay, public assistance and compensation, and unfortunately it leads
much domestic discord and wretchedness (Walshe, 1958). Further wor
on this subject is to be found in the publications of the Medical Researc
Council's Industrial Psychology Research Unit, London.

Treatment of the Traumatic Neurosis

It is common knowledge that this illness does not respond effective
to any form of therapy. The physiotherapy departments of hospitals a
full of the victims of trivial injuries, really suffering from this neurosi
and occupying the time of too many therapists, and all in vain. Ever
resource of modern therapeutics and of psychiatry is lavished upon ther
and in the files of these patients there seldom lacks at least one medic
report stating that "this patient will not improve until his claim has bee
settled." We may well ask what is the nature of this illness which is n
expected to respond to any form of treatment, but which is widely expecte
to clear up when, as a result of a court decision or an agreement betwee
solicitors, some form of compensation is awarded? If, subsequently,
does clear up, it does so without treatment. Unfortunately if litigation
too long drawn out even settlement does not remove the symptoms. Th
doctor is sometimes able to shorten the legal proceedings, and it is h
clear duty to demand of his colleagues of the law that they remember th
expeditious settlement is, in the claimant's interests, of the first impo
tance. Roffey Park Rehabilitation Centre, near Horsham, Sussex, has 1
beds for neurotic patients. It is vital to remember that prolonged idlene
may do such a patient great harm.

PREVENTION OF ACCIDENTS

On the subject of the prevention of accidents in industry the
is no room for complacency; in 1960 the figures rose by 9 per cent
190,266, the highest total for ten years. In that year there were 675 fat
accidents, compared with 589 in 1959 (McCullough, 1961). The Minist
of Labour commenting on these figures described the continuing rise
accidents as a *major disaster*.

Severity of Accidents on Construction Work

Unhappily, constructional work continues to claim a high proportion of deaths: one in seventy-six accidents in 1960 was fatal, as compared with an average of one in 282 for all processes subject to the Factories Acts. This is evidence of the special severity of accidents on construction work and of the consequent need for the highest standards of safety. But safety in the working environment aimed at the prevention of accidents is a responsibility which *must* be shouldered by management. When bulldozers on construction sites run over workmen and kill them *management should be blamed* rather than the foreman. In firms such as Imperial Chemical Industries, Ltd., where such a discipline exists, a workman is *less* liable to an accident at work than in his own home. Therefore the safety engineers of I.C.I. are busy waging a campaign for greater safety in the homes of employees (Hunter, 1961). Unhappily the reliance on voluntary efforts from management still goes on. In his Annual Report for 1966 the Chief Inspector of Factories notes the 'disturbing' rise in fatal accidents, and goes on to say that safety consciousness is not a matter for legislation but for education!

An Organized System of Prevention

To protect a machine by mechanical guards is a simple and obvious procedure, but teaching good housekeeping and safe conduct in workplaces is a slow process of education both of workers and supervisors. Safety regulations are restricted to general indications and cannot provide for particular cases. There must be organized a system of prevention considered from the human aspect with provision for individual selection of workers on entering industry and periodical medical supervision. This is especially important in those trades which expose the workers to special causes of fatigue and to sustained attention. All this is very much the concern of the doctor and it is admitted that medical officers in industry have not paid sufficient attention to the prevention of accidents.

Industrial Health and Safety Centre

The Regulations under the Factories Acts have reduced the workers' liability to accidents, and, in order still further to forward the work, the Factory Department of the Ministry of Labour maintains in Horseferry Road, London, the *Industrial Health and Safety Centre* where various types of safety devices can be seen and studied. During 1950 there were slightly more than 12,000 visitors to the Centre; most of them were in organized parties numbering from six to fifty persons. More than half these parties came from factory groups, trade schools, technical schools, medical schools and universities. In 1951 one group comprised all seventy members of the safety committee of a large factory in Birmingham, while another consisted of fifty-five doctors taking a post-graduate course in public health. Each year some hundreds of people come by appointment to discuss problems regarding existing machinery and future extensions to plant and factories.

Fencing of Machinery

Transmission machinery is responsible for many accidents of the most serious kind. They are caused by the workers coming into contact with the revolving shafting or other moving parts of machinery while engaged in oiling bearings, adjusting belts, cleaning shafting, executing repairs or performing other work in the vicinity. The danger of revolving shafting cannot be overestimated.

Revolving Shafting and Moving Belts

If loose clothing, such as an apron, a coat end, a wide or ragged sleeve, or a rag in the hand of a cleaner, comes into contact with the shaft, it may wrap

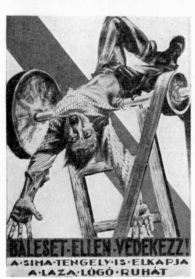

FIG. 427.—Hungarian Poster which gives Gruesome Warning to workmen against the Dangers of Revolving Shafts
(*By courtesy of Népjóléti Minisztérium, Budapest*)

round the shaft in a moment and, before the wearer is aware of what is happening, he may be caught, whirled round and killed or terribly injured. Such accidents can and do occur even with smooth shafting; the contrary view often expressed is contradicted by experience (fig. 427). Moving belts are also responsible for many accidents, in some of which the worker is caught and carried round the shaft (fig. 428). Every kind of transmission machinery is a potential cause of accidents, and it is required by the Factory Acts that all such machinery be securely fenced or be in such a position or of such construction as to be equally safe. Whenever possible, machines should be driven directly by a motor or engine so as to eliminate transmission machinery.

Guards for Power Presses

Machine tools are responsible for numbers of accidents. Many of them are due to the absence of efficient guards upon dangerous parts such as toothed gears, chain gears, belts and pulleys. Many machine-tool makers have designed their machines so as to avoid the exposure of dangerous parts—for example, by the complete enclosure of gear wheels. The dies or tools of power presses have long been recognized as dangerous. Accidents are generally severe and usually result in permanent mutilation of the hand. Much thought and ingenuity have been devoted to the problem of protecting the operator. This has been made more difficult by the great variety of materials dealt with and the many different operations performed.

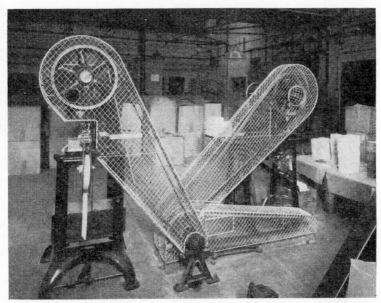

Fig. 428.—Metal Guards fitted over moving Belts
(*By courtesy of Frederick Braby & Co., Ltd.*)

A Temptation during Piece Work

Guards for power presses are of many kinds, including fixed, automatic and interlocked types. The guard most suitable for the job in hand must be carefully considered in each case and it is important that it should be impossible for the machine operator to displace or circumvent the guard and that it should cause the minimum possible interference with output. When machine operatives are paid on a piece-work basis, they may increase their earnings by reducing the time taken in removing completed work from their machine and in setting up new work. The time taken in moving the machine guard after each operation may tempt the operative to dispense with the guard in an effort to increase production.

Safety Devices regarded as Unprofessional

Unfortunately, certain workers are loath to use safety devices because they regard them as unworthy of an experienced worker and only fit for the young and inept. They feel that there is something unprofessional about them, in the same way that a barber will not demean himself by using a safety razor. Coercion is of little avail against such a feeling, for in trying to combat it we shall be up against that pride of achievement which is a man's chief incentive to action. If, however, we can show that true courage manifests itself more in putting up with the discomfort of a guard and so preserving a life that is useful to others than in running unnecessary risks, we are more likely to get the workers to use the guard provided than if coercion alone is attempted. In all industries, most production machines introduce risk in varying degree, and much effort has been devoted to guarding the dangerous parts to reduce to a minimum the chance of an accident occurring.

Care and Good Housekeeping in Factories

In the much wider field of accidents which are not caused by machinery, physical safeguards play an important part, but constant care and good housekeeping are essential. This applies particularly in the case where workers fall or where objects fall on to them (Duguid, 1949). In factories, special pathways indicated by two parallel white lines painted on the floor should be kept clear of any object whatsoever at all times.

Protective Clothing

In certain occupations protective clothing is of great value. Where its use is not obligatory it is often sold at reduced prices to the worker. Strong stiff hats (fig. 442), rubber aprons, coats, overalls, shin guards, rubber boots, gloves and goggles are standard articles used widely in handling chemical substances and in the mining industry. Where possible, equipment such as safety shoes should be handled in a special department. Reinforcement of the toecap by a steel arch is an excellent protective device for use in heavy industry (fig. 429). Drilling machines are the main cause of hair-entanglement accidents, of which 95 per cent happen to women and girls and 5 per cent to men and boys. Women workers should protect themselves against such scalping accidents by wearing turbans which completely enclose their hair (fig. 430). The slightest projection, even a small grub screw, on the drill renders such an accident more likely, but it is important to teach the worker that a revolving spindle which is perfectly smooth may be equally dangerous in its effects. In the manufacture (figs. 432 and 433) and handling of glass (fig. 434) special machinery and protective clothing are necessary.

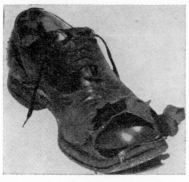

FIG. 429.—Undamaged Steel Toe-cap of Safety-shoe after 350-pound Crate fell on to a workman's Foot
(*By courtesy of Consolidated Edison Co., Inc.*)

The Safety Movement

By means of propaganda and education the Safety Movement has done good work to reduce accidents. It has spread to all civilized countries. It aims at protection through the education of the industrial worker by means of posters and lectures, advice to the employer as to safety methods and the formation of Works Safety Committees. By means of posters placed in prominent positions in factories, the attention of the workers is called to the grave results of accidents which may be due to their inattention, carelessness or failure to carry out instructions (figs. 435, 436 and 437). The posters are changed from time to time so that they may attract fresh attention and keep alive the workers' interest in accident prevention.

Suitable Topics for Accident Posters

A poster enjoining its target population to *Act Safely* or to *Mind your Hands* does not contain any clear directives as to the actual behaviour required. It assumes, quite arbitrarily, that the man already knows or recalls what is the safe way of handling any and every given situation. The instruc-

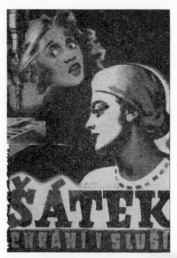

Fig. 430.—Correct Approach in Czech Poster aiming to reduce Scalping Accidents. *The Turban not only Protects you but also it is Becoming*
(*By courtesy of Dr. P. Pachner*)

tion *Mind your Head* in a bus is useful precisely because it refers to the immediate situation in which the passenger finds himself. The instruction *Mind your Hands* in a foundry or a steel works is useless because there are dozens of ways of minding one's hands and because a man absorbed in his job cannot divide his attention between the requirements of this job and the requirements of safety. Logically a poster should therefore be an extension, a reinforcement, a reminder, of training procedures, or a specific directive immediately applicable to the situation on the site where it is displayed. The instructions *Push this lever up before you start work*, or *This is how a sling must be fixed*, or *Throw the main switch BEFORE changing the fuse* tell the man exactly what is wanted of him. Any reference to caution, *Be Careful, Take Care*, should be avoided; there is good evidence to show that warnings of unknown and unspecified dangers tend to produce nervousness and reduce the level of skill and thereby may lead to accidents. Cautionary statements should therefore be supplanted by definite description. An instruction *Careful, Danger Within*, is ineffective and should be replaced by *Put out any bare lights and extinguish cigarettes, High Explosive Within*. Incidentally, the basic objections to so-called horror posters are that instead of the appropriate responses, emotional ones are evoked, which are known to affect skilful behaviour adversely (fig. 427.)

Safety Posters Specially Designed

Posters are widely used in the interests of accident prevention but little reliable information exists as to their efficacy. Not only are there few grounds for assuming that general posters with a vague message have an appreciable effect, but such effects as they may have are also difficult or impossible to measure. The same does not apply to accident poster specially designed to suit the needs of a particular industry. Their effect can be measured. A report by Laner and Sell (1960) from the Human Factors Section of the Operational Research Department, British Iron and Steel Research Association, suggests that appropriately chosen posters may appreciably reduce certain kinds of industrial hazard. They selected for study the hooking back of chain slings on to the crane hook when it is not in use (fig. 431). Omission of this action is potentially dangerous, especially

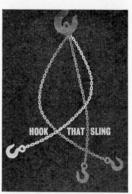

Fig. 431.—Poster specially designed for use in a controlled study of the behaviour of crane operatives

(*Laner, S., and Sell, R. G.,* Occupational Psychology, *1960,* 34, *153*)

in low-roofed shops, as the sling when left hanging from a moving crane can cause injury to anyone in the path of the crane; there are also instances on record when the dangling hook has caught on and dislocated machinery. For their experiment they used specially designed posters and they carried out their investigation in six steel works. They were able to show that the percentage of operations conforming with safety requirements averaged over a six-week period after display of the posters rose very appreciably, in some cases by more than 20 per cent. No comparable improvement was noted in a similar steel works in which no posters were displayed. Interestingly, the slingers often found it difficult to recall what the posters were and many doubted their efficacy. It is suggested that the effectiveness of the posters may have derived from their relevance to a specific working situation rather than to safety in general. This point should be borne in mind by all concerned with the design of safety propaganda.

Works' Safety Committees

One of the best methods of lessening accidents is the promotion of Works' Safety Committees on which the workers, the management and the works' medical officer are all represented. These committees inquire into the causes and circumstances attending accidents, and by their intimate knowledge of the working conditions in the factory they are able to make wise recommendations to prevent a repetition of such accidents. They are also well fitted to consider the advisability of adopting any suggestions sent in by the workers as to means of preventing accidents.

Voluntary Safety Organizations

The Royal Society for the Prevention of Accidents (RoSPA) and the Industrial Welfare Society have established many Area Committees to

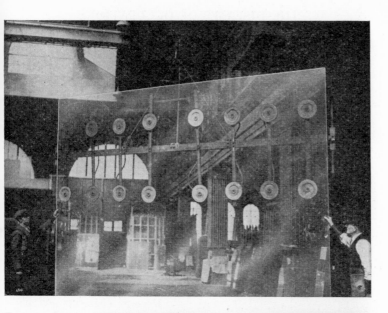

FIG. 432.—Large
Sheet of Plate-
glass lifted by
Sucker Crane

(*By courtesy of
Pilkington Bros.,
Ltd.*)

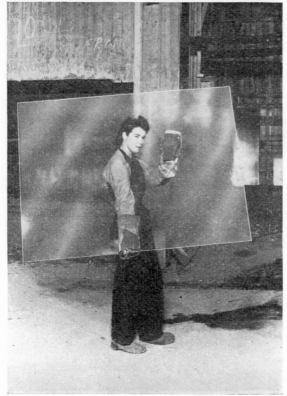

FIG. 433.—
Stout Leather
Gloves rein-
forced at Palm
and Wrist to
protect the
Hands against
Broken Glass

(*By courtesy of
Pilkington Bros.,
Ltd.*)

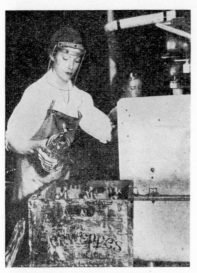

FIG. 434.—To protect against Cuts from Broken Glass the worker filling Soda-water Flasks wears a Face Mask
(By courtesy of Schweppes, Ltd.)

make inquiries and recommendations in such matters as prevention of sepsis; steps to promote the provision of a local Fracture Clinic; accidents to juveniles; effects of fumes from welding; breathing apparatus and gassing; eye injuries and use of goggles; traffic accidents; and electrical safeguards. These Committees and their parent Societies also carry on a campaign to reduce accidents by educational methods, exhibition of posters, conferences, lectures, competitions and award of prizes.

Research into Methods of Prevention

Doctors, engineers and physicists must constantly collaborate in efforts to improve schemes of safety and to devise new methods to protect the worker against injury. Certain automatic engineering devices which guarantee safety are now commonplace. Thus metal stamping machines are guarded in such a way that the electric circuit which operates the mechanism cannot be closed unless the worker is outside the guard and the guard locked (fig. 438). A safety unit has been developed which consists of a radioactive wristband worn by a machine operator and a detection instrument on the machine. If the operator's hand enters a dangerous area, the radiation emitted from the wristband operates a control which stops the machine (Dean, 1954).

ACCIDENTS AT DOCKS, WHARVES AND RAILWAY SIDINGS

A dock is an enclosed water area with facilities for the handling of ships, their passengers and their cargoes. There are two sorts, wet and dry. Wet docks are of two kinds, enclosed

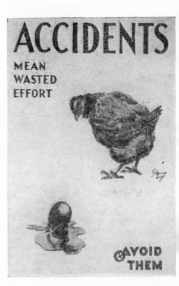

FIG. 435.—Witty Appeal to workmen about Accidents
(Royal Society for the Prevention of Accidents)

or open. In the enclosed kind, the water is impounded, and such a dock is commonly found where there is a considerable rise and fall of tide. The open kind is not fitted with dock gates and locks and is found where there is not much rise and fall. At Sunderland and Bristol, the main dock systems are enclosed; at Southampton and Glasgow they are open. Dry docks or graving docks are used by vessels undergoing survey or requiring underwater repairs.

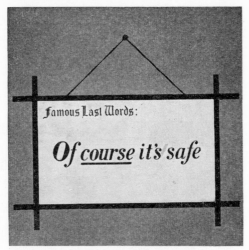

Fig. 436.—Poster warning against Breaches of Safety Regulations
(*Roya Society for the Prevention of Accidents*)

Types of Wharves and Sidings

Wharves are to be found along the containing walls of wet docks. They are frequently situated on the banks of rivers or canals; indeed, they existed in such places long before the first impounded water docks were constructed. Wharves are also variously known as quays, jetties, berths or staiths. In New York, berths are called piers because they are constructed on piers. Wharves may be open or they may be equipped with transit sheds, gear stores, offices and other ancillary buildings. They may have quay cranes or they may not. There will be bollards or mooring rings, probably railway lines, possibly one or more capstans, very often hydrants and sometimes pipe connections and valve pits for handling bulk oil. They may have any one of many different types of special equipment for special trades. Alongside the wharf there will be a sufficient

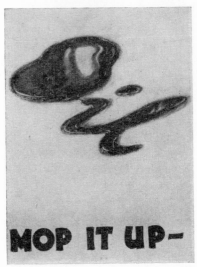

Fig. 437.—Poster using the Direct Appeal against Carelessness in Accident Causation
(*Royal Society for the Prevention of Accidents*)

minimum depth of water to accommodate the type and size of vessel for which the wharf is designed. There will normally be some form of lighting to enable work to proceed in hours of darkness. Railway sidings at docks include exchange sidings, sorting sidings, running lines, quayside tracks, standage sidings, loaded lines, light roads, gravitation sidings, sidings serving tenants' premises and hospital sidings for crippled wagons. The whole system may be owned and operated by the port, dock, quay or

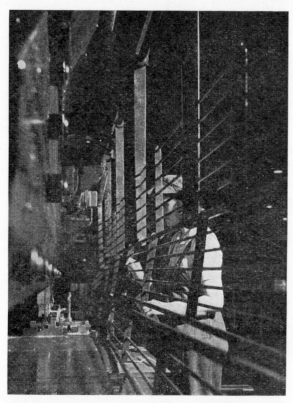

Fig. 438.—Metal-stamping Machine guarded in such a way that the Electric Circuit which operates the Mechanism cannot be closed unless the worker is outside the Guard and the Guard locked

(Crown Copyright: Central Office of Information)

wharf authority; or the complete service right up to the ship's side may be supplied by British Railways.

Jobs Involved and Workers Affected

The workers affected include ships' officers, crews and passengers; pilots and tugboat crews, harbour boatmen, sometimes called foy-boatmen, who perform the necessary work of handling ships' lines on or off bollards

or buoys; riggers, who in many ports are engaged to remove or replace
hatches and generally to prepare a cargo vessel for discharge, for loading
or for sailing; the general body of registered dock workers, especially
stevedores, controlled by the National Dock Labour Board and primarily
engaged in loading or discharging cargo or in working goods in or out of
sheds, warehouses, wagons and open storage wharfingers; checkers, winch-
men, hatchwaymen and capstanmen; crane drivers, locomotive drivers,
firemen, shunters, and tractor drivers; tillermen and lightermen; fresh-
water men working hydrants and water-boats; dock pilots, known on
the north-east coast as watermen; dock gatemen and hydraulic-machinery
men; watchmen at the landward entrances and at special points; coal
teemers, or tippers or hoistmen or boxmen; coal trimmers, whose work is
inboard; all the engineers' maintenance people, including tradesmen and
their labourers of many categories as well as a body of general labourers;
divers and their attendant labourers; all the crews who work the dredgers,
hoppers, launches and other harbour craft; dock office and traffic staff;
steamship agents and their clerks; policemen and fire-fighters belonging to
the borough or the port authority or a special force; tradespeople and other
persons authorised to visit ships; officers and servants of H.M. Customs,
the port health authority and the immigration department of the Home
Office; the principals, staff and workpeople of firms occupying tenancies
on the docks estate; visiting lorry drivers and their mates; staff and employees of contractors employed by the port authority; and members of
the general public to a greater or lesser extent.

Common Hazards arising at Work in Docks

People fall into docks and are drowned or injured. Cranes topple over
with great peril to the drivers and other persons. Railway wagons being
shunted or moved sometimes get out of control. Motorists, pedestrians and
cyclists are sometimes foolish or impatient and take risks when crossing
dock railway lines. Slinging of cargo is sometimes badly done, and heavy
objects fall from the slings or trays or nets when cranes are working.
Cargo-handling gear is sometimes faulty or ill-chosen and the load col-
lapses in transit between ship and shore. Dock workers handling cargo are
liable to injury moving in or out, or up and down, between the shore and
the bottom of ships' holds. Gantry girders have been known to collapse
with great peril to crane drivers and to persons working below them. A
winch-handle slipping out of control with a load on the fall puts the
operator and others in grave danger. A slipping foot on the brake pedal of a
lifting appliance similarly creates a dangerous situation for all concerned.
A crane driver can kill himself by suddenly braking to avoid dropping a
heavy load on persons working below him. The ballasting of the backstays
of derricks has been known to fail, involving the collapse of the whole
appliance. Divers can be trapped and drowned by the heavy weight of
their own protective equipment if the full safety drill is allowed to fail in
any particular. It is perhaps especially true of dock undertakings that

inevitably a large amount of general maintenance is always going on at the same time as the everyday work; ships must be turned round; cargo must be moved between ship and shore; any lack of liaison at all necessary levels, between the traffic manager on the one hand and the engineer on the other, is therefore extremely likely to produce dangerous conditions.

Conditions to be aimed at for Safety in Docks

To get as near to perfect safety as is humanly possible the following conditions should be present. First, all the requirements for safe working should be borne in mind from the beginning and incorporated in the design and layout of the facilities themselves. Secondly, similar requirements should mark the design, strength and fitness of all mechanical appliances, tools and gear. Thirdly, the facilities and the equipment must be continuously and properly maintained and regularly tested. Fourthly, entirely safe methods of working must be devised for all operations and must be efficiently taught to all operators concerned or likely to be concerned. And fifthly, the operators must use the safe methods and no others. Over the past 150 years scores of millions of pounds have been spent in building docks, wharves and railway sidings in the United Kingdom; in many cases, the broad lines of the original layout remain to this day. Unhappily with increased mechanization and modern changes in speed, method and purpose, the existing conditions are not always the best for safe working. Nevertheless, great opportunities to increase safety in layout do occur; extensions, improvements and modernization schemes are always going on; and, in particular, since 1945 the dock authorities in Great Britain have not been slow to grasp the special opportunity presented to them as the result of enemy action during the war, when damage in the docks, spread over 33 ports, amounted to £28,000,000.

Thoughtfulness, Alacrity and Watchfulness

Transcending protective restrictions, regulations and prohibitions is the mental attitude of the management, the supervisors and the workpeople to the whole problem of accidents. They must ever have in mind that men matter more than machines and more than money. The management must plan wisely, skilfully and safely; and they must appoint supervisors who will never, in their enthusiasm for the work, lose sight of the human beings upon whom the work depends. And finally, the workpeople themselves, knowing they are respected by those who direct the work, will respect themselves and one another, and, in consequence, there will grow among them a spirit of thoughtfulness instead of carelessness, cheerful alacrity instead of sluggish compliance, and keen-eyed watchfulness instead of the dangerous inattentiveness which produces more accidents than any other single cause (Bown, 1954).

Hazards of Work in Sewers

We have seen (p. 99) how Sir Edwin Chadwick advocated a main drainage scheme for London and how Sir Joseph Bazalgette in 1855 started work on a system which took 20 years to complete. The centenary of this work was celebrated in London in 1955. Since 1855 the population had increased from $2\frac{1}{4}$ to $4\frac{1}{2}$ millions of people. In 1955 during the working hours of any one day in London, drainage facilities were used by some 7 million people, and the daily consumption of water per head had gone up in 100 years from 20 to 50 gallons.

Vast Extent of Drainage Systems in Large Towns

The length of main sewers has increased from 163 to 403 miles. In the London main drainage area there are in addition some 3,000 miles of sewers maintained by local authorities. The sewage now treated is 103,336,000,000 gallons per annum, and 1,777,150 tons of sludge are sent to sea, to Black Deep 60 miles out from the mouth of the Thames (Rawlinson, 1955). A similar state of affairs applies in other large towns, for example Glasgow maintains 800 miles of public and common sewers which flow into the large intercepting sewers (Bell, 1952). Men working in sewers are liable to accidents causing physical injury, to drowning and to gassing accidents, including the explosion of mixtures of air with methane or petrol. The hazard of Weil's disease as it applies to sewer workers is discussed on p. 739.

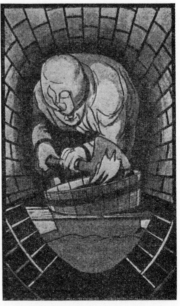

Fig. 439.—Removal of silt in a three-foot sewer
(*By courtesy of the Corporation of Glasgow*

Accidents Leading to Physical Injury

The sewers in which men work are usually 4 ft. 6 ins. or more in vertical diameter. In order to be self-flushing they are egg-shaped (fig. 439). The sewer flusher wades through water about ten inches deep and walks on a varying amount of solid silt. He wears leather-soled, hobnailed, rubber thigh-boots and gloves of cotton cloth. Accidents leading to physical injury occur from falls from ladders and foot-irons. Drowning is not unknown. Floods may result from storms, and the main drainage systems in towns usually include storm relief sewers. No man may enter a sewer alone and there must always be a man stationed on top of the manhole at the place where work is being carried out. Of course nobody works in a sewer while it is raining. The top man looks out for rain and when it begins to fall he signals to the men below by slamming down the manhole cover three times or by rattling a crowbar in the grating. Sounds of this sort travel a long way in the sewer. As soon as the men hear the signal they know they have but a few minutes to get out.

Safety Chains and Iron Guard Bars

Safety chains or iron bars are provided at the side entrance immediately below where the men are to work and these must be fixed across the sewer by the first man who enters it. In fast-flowing sewage or when the work is otherwise dangerous the men should be roped together by lifelines. Arrangements must be made for the top-men to be told of any storms, high tides or sudden large discharges from public baths, cooling tanks, ponds or water mains, so that the men in the sewers can be called up before the flood wave reaches them. Care should be taken that the men have a way out downstream of their working place. In the event of a man being caught by a flood, provided the guard-bars or chains are in position, he can let himself go with the flood without much risk.

Contamination of Sewage by Trade Effluents

To work in a sewer is to enter a lonely world of inky darkness and deathly silence. The atmosphere feels damp and has a faint sickly musty odour sometimes replaced by a more penetrating smell such as that of tar, paraffin, petrol, benzene or ammonia. Sewage is a mixture of liquids and solids of domestic and industrial origin which varies in composition from sewer to sewer and from hour to hour. Most of us think of sewage as being composed of kitchen water, bath water and human excreta, but to the sewermen working in industrial towns trade wastes are the important constituents. Engineering works contribute oils and grease as well as pickling acid, cyanides and suds, while garages are a common source of paraffin, petrol and diesel oil. From chemical works weak acid, weak alkali, spent carbide, resins and other materials enter the sewers. Ammoniacal liquors containing phenol and tar compounds gain access from steel works and gas generators. The paper industry and wool-scouring factories produce alkalis and soaps and many trades provide grease and other animal products. Although the discharge into sewers of most of these materials is prohibited by law, enforcement is difficult and so they appear from time to time (Bell, 1952).

The Hazard of Explosion

Inflammable and explosive gases and vapours occasionally found in sewers include coal-gas, methane (p. 651), acetylene, petrol and benzene. No man may take matches or a cigarette lighter into a sewer and no naked flame or fire is allowed within ten feet of any sewer entrance. To maintain ventilation during the course of work, the covers of the manholes upstream and downstream of the manhole from which work is in progress should be kept open. Under the general law special precautions must be taken to prevent the admission of petrol into sewers. Garages must have drains provided with petrol traps, but often they neglect to empty these. Such accidents as that resulting from a street collision during the transport of petrol in bulk may lead to an explosion. Arrangements should always be made to warn men in the sewers of such an accident. The sewer worker carries a flame safety lamp and he knows that the flame will cease to burn if he enters an area where there is insufficient oxygen to support life. He must be taught that even a small oxygen deficiency impairs co-ordination and leads to danger from failure to control the limbs accurately. He also uses the flame safety lamp to detect methane just as the coal miner does (p. 652).

Exposure to Toxic Gases and Vapours

In sewers with a low velocity flow the atmosphere may become contaminated with hydrogen sulphide from the decomposition of deposits of sewer solids. Dangerous concentrations of this gas may occur when acid wastes from manufacturing processes are discharged into sewage containing sulphides. For detecting H_2S the sewer worker is provided with lead acetate paper which he moistens and attaches to his flame safety lamp. Dangerous concentrations of hydrogen sulphide will blacken the paper. Hydrogen cyanide is a hazard in sewers because cyanides may be present in gas-works effluents and in trade wastes discharged from electroplating shops. Sewermen are instructed that should any unusual smell be met with in a sewer, especially a smell of almonds, all men shall leave the sewer at once and report to the superintendent. Unfortunately the almond odour of HCN can never be detected by numbers of people, including heavy smokers. In consequence its presence in sewers is a greater hazard than that of hydrogen sulphide. Other poisonous gases entering sewers from time to time are carbon dioxide, carbon monoxide, from leaking gas mains, ammonia from refrigerator plants, chlorine, phosgene, nitrous fumes, sulphur dioxide and carbon disulphide. Trouble can occur when removing sludge in which trichlorethylene or benzene has been entrapped.

The Morale of the Sewerman

Sewermen are generally of small build, cheery disposition and almost fearless. They display a remarkable team spirit and have in general the qualities found in miners. What attracts them to the job is the certainty of continued employment and the higher rate of pay for skilled work. Usually they are recruited from the general labour force engaged in road repairs. They are observed at work for several years and when a vacancy arises in the sewage squads a man who has proved his worth is then selected. Among Glasgow sewermen all are married and most have at least three children, about 50 per cent of them living in overcrowded houses without a bath. Periodic medical examination is essential, the local authority should launder the working clothing and provide at the depots wash-basins, showers, baths, hot water, soap and towels for all the men. Mechanical transport provided with proper facilities for washing in hot water should be a standard part of equipment. Rodent control should be improved in sewers and they should be better ventilated and better lighted. Electric handlamps should be issued in addition to flame safety lamps. The best electric lamp has two bulbs side by side, a white one for continuous use and a red one which lights up automatically in the presence of dangerous concentrations of toxic, asphyxiating or explosive gases. Sewermen should not be condemned to unemployment at 55 after 20 years of faithful service in this arduous task. Local authorities should find them alternative work and devise superannuation schemes to provide for their future (Bell, 1952).

TREATMENT OF INDUSTRIAL INJURIES

The objects of treatment in a case of industrial injury should be to secure the repair of the damaged part as quickly and completely as possible, and to do what may be necessary to replace the workman in remunerative employment, at his former job if possible, or in some other occupation, for which he may need training and assistance in placement. Such treatment may call for the application of one or more of the following procedures.

First-aid

The study of this important branch of surgery was greatly advanced during the Second World War, when much experience was gained of the efficacy of various methods of dealing on the spot with casualties from air raids and other forms of enemy action. In industry there may be special hazards when accidents occur from handling corrosive or toxic substances, or from electricity, radiant energy or extremes of temperature or pressure. The St. John Ambulance Association has recently published a text-book of industrial first-aid, in which special attention is given to these risks. *Section 45 of the Factories Act, 1937*, provides that in every factory—

> there shall be provided and maintained so as to be readily accessible a first-aid box or cupboard of the prescribed standard . . . under the charge of a responsible person who shall, in the case of a factory where more than fifty persons are employed, be trained in first-aid treatment.

There is no statutory definition of responsible person nor of what is meant by trained in first-aid treatment. In practice, the requirements of the Act are held to have been fulfilled if one or more of the workers in the factory holds a valid certificate in first-aid issued either by the British Red Cross Society or the St. John Ambulance Association.

Emergency Surgical Treatment

Emergency surgical treatment includes arrest of hæmorrhage, blood transfusion, cleansing and suture of wounds, radiography of suspected fractures and their reduction and fixation when present. Griffiths (1949) has shown, in the Albert Dock Hospital, London, how valuable time may be saved, and shock averted, by arranging for injured workers to be taken in a heated ambulance to a hospital at which the ambulance is driven directly into a heated resuscitation room equipped with all necessary apparatus for giving such emergency treatment at any hour of the day or night. The Slough Industrial Medical Service organizes similar facilities for a large trading estate, including over 300 firms, large and small; the equipment includes a travelling operating theatre. When, at the outbreak of the Second World War, Dr. George Riddoch was made Brigadier and Consultant Neurologist to the Home Army he at once took steps to provide a special hospital for the prompt and expert treatment of neuro-logical injuries, especially those of the spine, in sailors, soldiers and airmen. He succeeded in obtaining the services of Dr. (afterwards Sir Ludwig) Guttmann as Director and under his devoted and enthusiastic guidance the National Spinal Injuries Centre of the Stoke Mandeville Hospital became what it is today. A soldier shot in the neck by a terrorist in Aden in 1967 could be flown to England by the R.A.F., transferred to a helicopter, and arrive the same day in the helicopter bay at the hospital. As a result of such superb methods of transport he could be under treatment in bed already fitted with traction apparatus for the fracture of the cervical spine on the same day as the shooting took place. As part of rehabilitation patients with spinal injuries take part in the famous Stoke Mandeville games and these are transferred to Tokyo and other centres for the Olympic Games where paraplegic men and women of different nationalities compete at basket-ball in opposing teams in wheelchairs!

Treatment by Orthopædic Surgery and Physiotherapy

The measures include the further treatment of wounds or fractures, and operations for repair of damaged nerves, correction of deformities or elimination of infection. A particular industry may require the full time services of a surgeon with special skill and experience, for example, to suture the tendons at the wrist in the case of men who are injured while lifting and carrying sheets of plate glass. Physiotherapy includes heat, massage, electrical treatment and remedial exercises. In carrying out such treatment it is essential to secure the active co-operation of the patient. Physiotherapy commonly fails because it is carried out so infrequently. Böhler (1935) quotes a case in which a patient, in order to reach hospital, "'had to travel fifteen minutes by electric train, and then half an hour by the street tram. She was obliged to endure one and a half hour's cold in order to enjoy a quarter of an hour's hot air." At the Albert Dock Hospital patients attend the gymnasium all day and every day until they recover full working capacity.

Rehabilitation after Injury

The word rehabilitation is used in various senses. It is commonly meant to imply the refitting of the patient, after his injuries are healed, for remunerative employment and his placement in a suitable job. This may entail the provision of an appliance such as an artificial limb, or a course of training in a new occupation. Difficulties often arise over resumption of work owing to the lack of proper co-operation between those responsible for treatment and failure to consider the industrial environment to which the patient should return. Either he is discharged from hospital before he is fit to undertake the strain of work, or he continues attendance for long after he has reached a stage at which work would be the best form of treatment. If industrial injuries are to be treated effectively, it is necessary for the surgeon to make himself familiar with the physical requirements of the industries in which his patients work. He must maintain as close a liaison as possible with the management of the local industries and with the officers of the local Employment Exchange who are concerned with vocational training, placement and supervision. In these matters the surgeon will, of course, make full use of the services of the almoner and other social welfare workers, since the proper care of a case of industrial injury calls for team-work between those concerned with the medical, surgical, financial, social and even the legal consequences of the accident (Norris, 1951).

Research into Methods of Treatment

The best techniques for restoring the disabled are still being developed (Ling and O'Malley, 1958). Research work on methods of treatment applicable to industrial accidents has come from the Unit of the Medical Research Council at the Birmingham Accident Hospital. It has included the design of dressing-stations and the control of wound infection (Gissane, Miles and Williams, 1944), studies on added infection in industrial wounds (Clayton-Cooper and Williams, 1945), the incidence of sepsis in industry (Williams and Capel, 1945) and the bacterial flora of wounds and septic lesions of the hands (Williams and Miles, 1945). The treatment of burns has been especially studied by Colebrook, Duncan and Ross (1948) at the Burns Research Unit of the Medical Research Council at the same hospital. Here, work of much significance has been carried out; death-rates have been reduced by special procedures in plastic surgery, and by the use of an air-conditioned dressing-station which has greatly decreased the incidence of bacterial infection. In 1967 the Medical Research Council set up a Powered Limbs Research Unit at West Hendon Hospital, London, N.W.9, under the direction of Dr. A. B. Kinnier Wilson.

Dust Explosions in Factories

Besides coal dust (p. 1139), many other combustible dusts may produce explosions if thrown into suspension in air and ignited. Such explosions may take place in a wide variety of establishments, including grain elevators, wood-working plants, cereal mills, flour mills, sugar refineries, fertilizer plants, malt houses, cotton mills and plants producing starch products.

Dusts Concerned in Explosions

Explosions of combustible dusts may take place in plants where cork dust, pulverized coal, metal dust, sulphur dust, bark dust, coffee, cocoa and spice dusts, paper dust, gramophone-record dust, pitch and resin dust, rubber dust and soap powder are present. As a result of the increased use of metal powders in powder metallurgy and in military pyrotechnics, there has been an increase in metal-dust explosions. Such metal powders include magnesium, aluminium, cadmium, zinc, copper, iron, manganese, titanium, ferromanganese, antimony, zirconium and even tin and lead. Similarly, the number of explosions has increased in the rapidly expanding moulded plastics industry, in which many combustible synthetic resins, moulding compositions and fillers are used in powder form.

Conditions necessary for the Explosion

A dust explosion may be defined as the rapid combustion of a cloud or suspension of dust in air, during which heat is generated at a much higher rate than it is dissipated to the surroundings. This phenomenon, which is similar to that of a gas explosion, is characterized by the sudden development of pressure, which frequently causes the destruction of both the plant and the equipment containing the dust. The conditions necessary for the explosion are a sufficiently dense cloud and an ignition source intense enough to raise the temperature of part of the dust mixture to the ignition point. It should be pointed out that coarse dust of 710-micron size, as well as fine dust, may be involved in an explosion; it should be noted also that the dust concentrations necessary for explosions are much higher than those generally considered in toxicology (Pieters and Creyghton, 1951).

Causes of Industrial Dust Explosions

The following have been established as some of the definite causes of industrial dust explosions: electricity, such as sparks from motors, fuses, switches, short-circuits, static electrical discharges and the breaking of incandescent lights; frictional sparks from foreign materials going through grinding mills and into fans, from sledge hammers, from workmen's shoes and from grinding wheels and buffers; hot particles, such as glowing material fed to mills or dust collectors and sparks from boiler fires and locomotives; heated surfaces, such as overheated bearings and other moving parts of machines, dust which has settled on hot light-bulbs, dust on steam coils and on hot pipes in driers, friction in grain elevators; open flames and lights, such as lanterns, candles, gas-lights, torches, matches and smoking, and miscellaneous small-scale fires, including spontaneous ignition of waste and other materials, breaks in fuel lines and boiler backfires; small explosions of inflammable vapours and of dust blown into furnace and incinerator flues; and the disturbance of burning dust by the use of a water-hose (Hartmann, 1948).

ACCIDENTS IN MINES AND QUARRIES

In spite of efforts to reduce accidents in mines, mining remains amongst the most dangerous of our major industries. This is due to the natural conditions under which mining work is carried out, which have hitherto made it impossible to reduce the accident-rate to the average of that in other industries. In quarrying also, for similar reasons, the accident-rate remains high. The *Mines and Quarries Act, 1954,* which replaces the *Coal Mines Act, 1911,* tightens up the existing safety law bringing it into line with modern mining and quarrying practice.

Hazards of Work in Quarries

Great Britain is essentially a coal-mining country; the mining of tin and lead have been for years constantly diminishing. The only remaining branch of metalliferous mining is that for iron ore and, as we have seen (p. 156), much of this is done by opencast methods. Quarrying is carried out to obtain alabaster, chalk, chert, flint, granite, graphite, gravel, gypsum, kaolin, limestone, sand, sandstone and slate. The hazards met by the quarry worker include falls of ground detachment of rock, blasting accidents, falls from ladders or ledges, eye injuries from the dressing of stone, and accidents connected with tramways, the breaking of ropes or chains and the mismanagement of machinery.

Statistical Record of Accidents

One of the saddest documents published in Great Britain is the *Statistical Digest of the Ministry of Fuel and Power,* which sets forth annually the story of an immense amount of human suffering and loss of output due to accidents in mines. There is, however, a bright side to the story, since

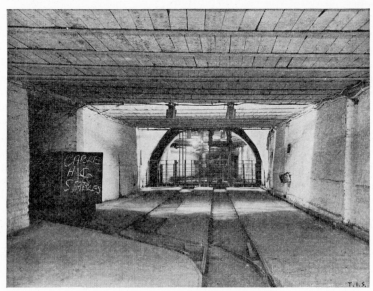

FIG. 440.—A well-lighted Pit Bottom
(By courtesy of Professor I. C. F. Statham)

during the last quarter of a century or so there has been a marked reduction in the number of men killed and seriously injured in our coal mines. This gratifying improvement has been specially noticeable during recent years. The total number of accidents in 1955 was the lowest recorded since 1949. The number of men killed during 1953 and 1954 was the lowest on record. The year 1955 unfortunately showed an increase, 421 against 392 and 371 respectively for all mines worked under the Coal Mines Act. From 1945 to 1947 there was a tendency for the number of comparatively minor accidents, causing disablement for more than three days, to decrease. This tendency was, however, reversed during the period 1948 to 1952 but it again decreased from 1953 to 1955, although the figure did not reach that recorded in 1945. Intensive campaigns are carried out amongst the miners with the object of persuading them to adopt precautions against sepsis following minor injuries. Continuous efforts are made to improve the lighting in the pits (figs. 440, 441) and, of course, miners wear protective clothing (fig. 442).

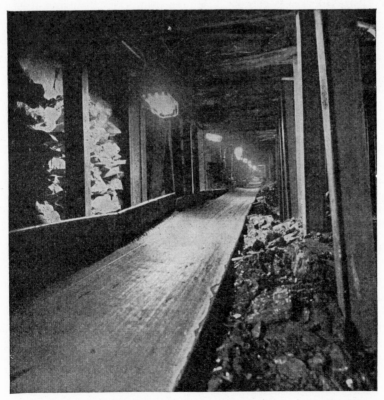

FIG. 441.—View along Conveyer Face lighted with Fluorescent Tube Fittings
(*By courtesy of Professor I. C. F. Statham*)

Causes of Accidents

It is incumbent upon all engaged in mining—workmen, management, trade-union leaders, inspectors and research workers alike—to do everything possible to attain that further improvement necessary to reduce the accident-rate, and to keep British mining in the proud place it has so long held, as the safest in the world. In this connexion it is often pointed out by H.M. Inspectors of Mines and others concerned with the safety of men working underground that many accidents would be avoided by the exercise of proper care on the part of the injured persons. This does not imply that all the avoidable accidents are due to gross errors or major and wilful contravention of the regulations. In many cases they arise from a commendable desire to obtain production even at the expense of safety, such as when a man continues to get or to load coal at the face instead of attending to support of the roof, with the result that he is injured by a comparatively small fall which might easily have been prevented. Not infrequently, however, accidents occur as the result of lack of forethought, of carelessness or even recklessness on the part of miners. If every worker underground took proper precautions at all times, the accident-rate in mines could be reduced to one-half of the present rate. This would mean not only a reduction in human suffering, but also an increase in output well worth the effort demanded.

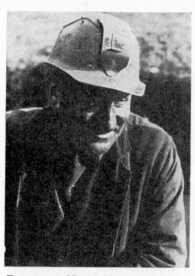

Fig. 442.—Hard, Plastic Protective Helmet worn by a Coal Miner
(*By courtesy of Philip Gee, Ltd.*)

Accidents from Falls of Ground

Falls of ground are responsible for about 50 per cent of the fatal accidents in coal mines, and over 40 per cent of the serious and non-fatal accidents. A large proportion of accidents from falls occurs under freshly exposed roof at or near the working face, where the excavation is newly made and the supports are usually of a temporary character. About 80 per cent of the accidents due to falls occur at or within 10 yards of the working face. Many of these accidents occur at the vicinity of the road-head. It is customary in this area to enlarge the roadways by ripping down the roof at what is called the ripping lip. As this lip is being constantly carried forward and exists in ground which is badly broken and still in the process of settling down, support of the roof calls for special care. This is shown by the fact that about 50 per cent of the accidents from falls in or near the face occur in this area. The precautions against accidents due to falls at or near the working-face include rigid compliance with the regulations and careful inspection and testing of the roof at frequent intervals. The early and systematic setting of all supports—sprags, props, chocks and packs—in accordance with the support rules is of the utmost importance; neglect and delay allow the roof to subside and become broken, making it difficult to support.

In his *Miners' Day* (1945), B. L. Coombes describes his personal experience of a fall of roof.

We were working at a place where the steel arches had been buckled up and were bending dangerously. It is first necessary to unbolt the fastening plates, a risky job, as they fly back when released and may travel through the air for fifteen or twenty yards; quite liable to harm harder things than heads in that buzzing flight of iron. The steel arches are sometimes forced a yard or more into the earth and are bent at all sorts of fantastic shapes. Not only is it difficult to get them free, but there is also the problem of getting them in trams and out to the surface. Space is limited and their bends are not. They are nasty things to handle, as they slip and crush any unwary fingers; besides, the surfaces get roughened and bits of rusty iron pierce our hands and bodies.

I feel they are better support than timber, for they rarely snap and do still hold some weight even when bent. We had dragged out a couple of arches and were preparing for the last. The timber laggings were hanging slightly downward and I was watching alertly in case they might slide and the loose stones above follow them down to where we were working. I put George on the upper and safer side because I wanted room to jump back, and George, despite all warnings, has not yet learned to give his mate a clear backward passage. Usually, when I jump back I crash into George, who has just then decided to come behind and have a look at what is going on.

It did happen suddenly, I know, but I was half prepared and was leaping back at the first crack. The road was rough and some empty trams were rather close. For a few seconds it seemed the world had closed in on me, and I instinctively rolled down alongside the trams for their shelter. Roof and laggings came down with a crash, forming a huge mound, under which was my lamp. As something, stone or timber, had caught me nicely in the solar plexus and knocked every pant out of me, I lay awhile in the dark, helpless and speechless.

Then I heard a horrible sound, not easy to describe. It seemed not human, a sort of animal moan mixed with a human scream. Some seconds passed before I realized it must be George, and that he must be hurt. More time passed before I could stand up and croak the message that I would be there in a minute. Then when I struggled forward and could see over the fall, I saw that George was not hurt but was running back and forth in his panic. He became more normal when he realized I was not badly hurt.

Poor old George! The crash, the silence from me and the disappearance of my light had convinced him I was buried. His first experience of that type of happening, he had no idea what to do. Later I gave him some tips from my experience. Not to attempt to help yourself in case of more falls, and because one man is usually impotent against large stones. Get the message to others quickly, and they will be there very quickly, never fear about that.

Withdrawal of Supports

Many of the supports at or near the coal face are of a temporary character and have to be withdrawn as the face advances. This applies especially to sprags, props and chocks, which are withdrawn, not only to conserve supplies of materials, but also to ensure effective roof control in the vicinity of the coal face and roadheads. The operation of withdrawing supports especially in packholes and wastes is skilled work, and calls for training, care and experience, as it is attended by a certain amount of danger. It should be undertaken only by qualified workers fully conversant with the correct methods of withdrawal practices. The Coal Mines (Support of Roof and Sides) Regulations, 1947, require that all workmen should be adequately trained in the work they have to perform.

Falls of Ground in Roadways

Something like 15 per cent of the accidents from falls occur in mine roadways. About half of these occur to men employed in repairing and enlarging the roadways, and the remainder to men employed on other duties or travelling on the roads. Accidents from falls on roadways are reduced by special care in the formation and support of the roadway at the time it is made and by efficient roof control at the face. The importance of the support and control of ripping lips and roadheads cannot be over emphasized. Approximately one third of the fatal accidents caused by falls of ground occur in this vicinity. Good roof control reduces the amount of fracturing of the roof strata and better and safer roads result. Although subsidence of the roof behind the face cannot be prevented, it can be controlled and the strata caused to subside without being unduly broken. In many cases the use of yielding supports, such as arches on stilts or sliding-girder arches, affords the safest means of supporting roads in the moving ground near the face. These yielding supports are removed and rigid supports inserted when the ground has finally settled (Statham, 1951).

Accidents due to Haulage

After falls of ground, the next most serious source of accidents in mines arises from injuries to men employed in haulage operations. Haulage is responsible for about 25 per cent of the total fatal and serious non-fatal accidents and for more than 20 per cent of all accidents. Although prior to 1938 the accident-rate due to haulage had remained almost stationary for over fifty years, since that date a substantial reduction in the serious-accident rate has been recorded.

Causes of Haulage Accidents

Haulage accidents arise from many causes; about 70 per cent occur to men during the actual performance of haulage operations, about 10 per cent to men travelling on haulage roads. The greatest number is due to men being crushed or run over by moving traffic, and runaways, and this is responsible for about 80 per cent of the deaths and upwards of 50 per cent of all accidents due to haulage. Restricted space and inadequate lighting have been the principal contributory factors. Comparatively few serious accidents are caused by breakages of ropes or draw gear. This is due to the careful choice and thorough examination of ropes or draw gear in practice, and to detailed investigations made into all cases when failure of these appliances occurs. Such investigations often suggest remedial measures.

Prevention of Haulage Accidents

The reduction in serious accidents due to haulage has been effected largely by detailed study of the problem by the various Mining Institutes in conjunction with the Safety in Mines Research Board, The National Coal Board, and by the circulation of illustrated pamphlets in which the causes of haulage accidents have been analysed, examples of safety devices and precautions described and recommendations made for increased safety in haulage operations. The prevention of such accidents calls for attention to many details. Special safety devices such as runaway switches or tub arresters should always be employed where there is danger of runaways. Such switches should be designed either to fall to safety or to be automatic. Backstays or drags should be attached to all sets ascending inclines, and should be of such a design that they cannot fall off or be over-ridden. Skotches and wheel lockers which do not fall out accidentally and which can be inserted without danger of the operator's fingers being trapped should be used. Coupling blocks should be hung between tubs or cars during coupling and uncoupling to avoid danger of injury to the operator's head if placed inadvertently between the tubs or cars, a practice which should always be avoided. Good track is essential to eliminate derailments, which are a common source of accidents. The provision of refuge holes, adequate means of lighting, efficient signalling equipment, the prohibition or limitation of travelling on haulage roads when vehicles are in motion, and the avoidance of interference with signals and other apparatus by unauthorized persons are other essential requirements for the safe and efficient running of haulages.

Locomotive Haulage and Trunk Conveyers

Owing to the more extensive use of trunk conveyers and locomotive haulage, there is reason to expect a considerable reduction in haulage accidents in newly opened and in reconstructed mines. The use of locomotives necessitates flat gradients, larger road clearances and improved tracks, more in line with surface railway practice, all of which tend to increase safety. The use of large mine-cars and the reduction of the number of men employed in haulage operations, together with the better lighting of haulage roadways, all will have a beneficial effect. These, in conjunction with adequate training of all haulage operatives in conformity with the regulations, should make underground haulage as safe and efficient as surface haulage. Not only should the accident-rate be reduced by these means, but conditions of work will be vastly improved and manual labour considerably reduced (Statham, 1951).

First-aid and Ambulance Services

The *First-aid Regulations, 1930*, call for adequate provision to be made at all mines for rendering first-aid in case of accident and for subsequent treatment of all injured persons. At every mine employing more than a hundred persons on a single shift, a suitable first-aid room, adequately equipped, must be provided at the surface, and must be in constant charge of a competent person. It is also required that a sufficient number of the persons employed below ground shall hold certificates of proficiency in first-aid. Thus, one person in every fifty in each district in charge of a deputy, and one in every thirty employed elsewhere, shall be so qualified. Dressings and antiseptics must either be carried by each workman, or in first-aid boxes, one of which must be carried by each first-aid man. In the latter case the first-aid boxes must be taken to the surface at the end of the shift and replenished as necessary. First-aid stations equipped with stretchers, splints, bandages, tourniquets and burn dressings must be provided at convenient places underground throughout the mine. Ambulance service must be available, and the manager must inspect the accommodation, equipment and materials at least once in every six months and see that defects, if any, are remedied.

Mine Rescue Services

The *Mines Rescue Regulations, 1928*, require that adequate provision for rescue shall be made at all mines employing more than ten men underground. For this purpose, properly equipped Central Rescue Stations must be provided. Each such station must be under the control of a fully trained and competent superintendent, must be within 15 miles of the mines served, and each mine must be in constant telephonic communication with the station. Central Rescue Stations are organized in two distinct ways: first, those which maintain a permanent rescue corps, similar to the staff of a fire station, ready for immediate action as required, and secondly, those which train rescue brigades from the collieries served by the station. In the latter case, when a disaster occurs the necessary rescue apparatus is brought from the Rescue Station and rescue teams are organised from the trained men at the colliery, generally under the supervision of the Rescue Station Superintendent who also makes arrangements for the testing and servicing of the rescue apparatus.

Use of Self-contained Breathing Apparatus

In both cases a specified number of trained men, depending upon the number employed below ground, must be employed at each colliery. Self-

:ontained breathing apparatus, which enables the wearer to enter and work in irrespirable atmospheres, is employed. It is of two types—the liquid-air type and the oxygen type. In both cases purifiers, which allow exhaled air to be rebreathed, are employed to conserve the liquid air or oxygen, and each type suffices for use for a period of two hours. The Mines Rescue Regulations specify in detail the methods to be adopted in the selection and training of rescue workers, the equipment to be provided and the general organization of rescue operations. Rescue Brigades deal with fires in mines (fig. 443) and perform valuable rescue work after explosions

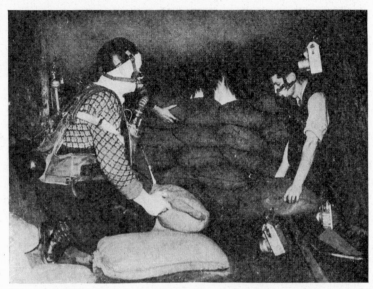

FIG. 443.—Miners wear Self-contained Breathing Apparatus while practising Sealing-off with Sandbags a Working which is on Fire
(*By courtesy of The Listener*)

and other accidents, often in circumstances of extreme danger. No praise can be too high for these men who volunteer for the work and are always ready to face peril in valiant attempts to save life and property.

Incidence of Injuries to the Limbs

An account of the National Coal Board Medical Service is given on p. 200. The medical inspectors and other doctors and nurses of this service take every care that the victim of an accident in a mine is given the best possible attention without delay. Among the total coal-mining population of Great Britain it is estimated that there are about 250,000 accidents per year, each causing absence of more than three days, a startling and appalling figure (McLintock, 1953). In 1951, among a population of 106,000 coal miners, injuries to the limbs accounted for 61 per cent of such accidents, the upper limb being involved in 36 per cent and the lower limb in 25 per cent of cases.

Rehabilitation of the Injured Miner

Under the *Miners' Welfare Commission* a rehabilitation scheme for trauma has been set up covering practically all coal miners. Problems of efficient treatment in the Rehabilitation Centres have been solved and the results, in terms of men restored to full work in the pits, are good. Six monthly conferences of orthopædic surgeons in the Commission's *Rehabilitation Service* have been arranged and are proving of value. But the social problems of resettlement of the injured miner have been solved only in part, and possibilities of successful rehabilitation of men disabled by pneumoconiosis, nystagmus and rheumatism are only now being explored. Meanwhile, the miners are proud and appreciative of their rehabilitation service, which is the best of its kind in the world (Nicoll, 1946).

The Problem of the Miner with Permanent Paraplegia

The problem of permanent paraplegia from spinal injury presents great difficulties. In time of peace 90 per cent of all such injuries occurring in Great Britain are due to accidents to miners while working underground. Indeed, the incidence of paraplegia in coal miners has been calculated at one case per 10,000 miners per annum (Nicoll, 1946). Since these men cannot be nursed at home, special institutions have been built for their treatment and rehabilitation. The Commission's *Miners' Rehabilitation Medical Committee* has recommended sixty beds as the optimum size for such centres, and work is in hand to ensure that Scotland, the North, the Midlands and the South will each possess its special Rehabilitation Centre.

Effects on Man-power and Recruitment

With an industrial medical service concentrating on the preventive side and a rehabilitation service concentrating on the curative side, the health hazards of coal mining are gradually being robbed of their disquieting effect on the mining community. This must ultimately have a good effect not only in reducing the toll on the skilled man-power of the industry but also in stimulating recruitment of new men for the pits.

FIREDAMP IN COAL MINES

The problem of eliminating the risk of explosions in the pits has been one of the main concerns of the coal-mining industry for three centuries. During the early part of the seventeenth century pits were sunk to coal seams lying at greater depths than had previously been worked, and in these deeper pits methane or firedamp began to be a greater hazard.

Firedamp ignited by the Fireman

At this time it was the custom for a specially selected miner to enter the pit early in the morning before his mates to fire the gas, a practice which led to the introduction of the term *fireman*. This man wrapped himself up in old clothing previously soaked in water and entered the mine carrying a long pole, to the end of which was fixed a lighted candle. Upon nearing an accumulation of gas, he dropped on all fours and, crawling forwards, pushed the candle towards the roof. This ignited the gas, the fireman meanwhile lying flat on his face until the flame had passed over him. He then rose and retreated from the mine, leaving it in a supposedly fit state for the men to enter.

The Use of Naked Lights

Knowledge of the dangers due to the presence of firedamp led naturally to attempts to make some form of safety-lamp. In the early days of mining, the lamps used by the miners were of the same type as those used in dwelling-houses. Many examples of these lamps in bronze and terra cotta have been left us by the Romans. In English mines where naked lights were allowed, a candle was carried in a lump of soft clay, which could be attached to any convenient part of the working or to the miner's hat (see fig. 386). Today an acetylene cap lamp is generally used.

The Flint and Steel Mill

The first safety-light was the flint and steel mill invented by Carlisle Spedding about 1760. The sharp edge of a flint was applied to a rapidly rotated toothed wheel of steel, and the sparks produced emitted considerable light (fig. 444). About 1795 attempts were made to use the light from phosphorescent materials such as decaying fish. In 1799 F. H. von Humbolt described a lamp which was supplied with air from a reservoir, a principle also employed by W. R. Clanny in 1813. While he was working at a Durham colliery in 1815 George Stephenson invented several safety-lamps, of which the third admitted air through tiny holes punched in a metal ring in its base. This lamp proved to be untrustworthy and was never widely used.

Invention of the Davy Lamp

The problem of the safety-lamp was solved when Sir Humphry Davy brought his powerful mind to bear on the subject (fig. 445). In all history there is to be found no finer contribution to industrial welfare than his work on the miner's safety-lamp. This was based upon scientific researches described by him to the Royal Society between 1815 and 1817. The investigations were undertaken at the request of a Society for Preventing Acci-

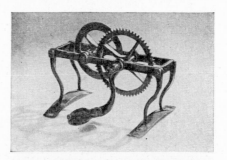

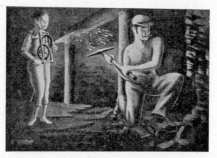

Fig. 444.—Flint and Steel Mill invented by Carlisle Spedding about 1760. The lower figure shows the Mill in use
(By courtesy of Professor I. C. F. Statham)

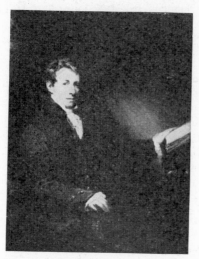

FIG. 445.—Sir Humphry Davy, Bart.,
1778–1829

dents in Mines formed in 1813 i
consequence of the increase of col
liery explosions as pits of greate
depth were worked. As the resul
of experiments Davy found that if
piece of metal gauze is interpose(
between a flame and an explosiv
gaseous mixture, the heat of th
flame is absorbed and conducte(
away by the metal gauze so that th
gaseous mixture does not explode

The Modern Flame Safety-lamp

His lamps were brought int(
use in the mines in 1816. For this
signal service to industry Davy received a baronetcy in 1818. No(
only was he the greatest chemist o(
many generations, but also he was
the finest of men, for he declined
the fortune he could have made by taking out a patent on his invention.
The original Davy lamp is obsolete (fig. 446). Owing to the obstruction
offered by the wire gauze, it gives a very poor illumination, and the flame
may be forced through the gauze when the current of air exceeds 5 feet
per second. In modern mines the air in some parts of the rapid ventilating roads may attain up to 30 feet
per second. Its modern equivalent, the flame safety-lamp, is in
daily use in coal mines where there
is the hazard of fire-damp or blackdamp (fig. 447) (see p. 652).

Prevalence of Explosions

During the period 1835 to
1850, no less than 643 explosions
took place in the coal mines in
Great Britain, an average of just
over forty a year. It was established that the explosions were
more frequent in the early part
of the week because of accumulation of firedamp during periods
of cessation of work when the
ventilation of the mine was
stagnant. It was also shown
that in the vast majority of cases

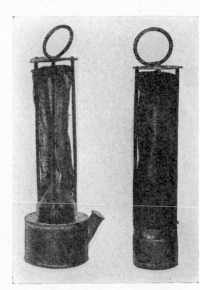

FIG. 446.—The original Davy Lamp

the ignition of the firedamp was brought about by the persistent use of naked lights in the fiery mines.

Effects of Serious Explosions

The noise of a serious explosion was often heard 3 or 4 miles away, and trembling of the earth felt for about half a mile round the workings. Immense quantities of dust and small coal accompanied the explosion, and rose high into the air in the form of an inverted cone. The heaviest part of the ejected matter, such as pieces of wood and small coal, fell near the pit,

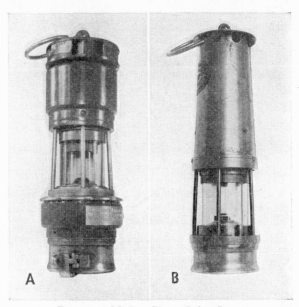

FIG. 447.—Modern Flame Safety Lamps
(A) The Hailwood Lamp   (B) The Davis Lamp
(By courtesy of Professor I. C. F. Statham)

but the dust borne away by the wind fell in a continual shower from the pit to distances even 2 miles away. Darkness like early twilight often enshrouded villages, and coal dust covered the roads so thickly that footsteps were strongly imprinted in it.

Violence and Gravity of Explosions

Often the heads of the shaft-frames were blown off, their sides set on fire and their pulleys shattered to pieces. The gravity of explosions was increased in many cases by the destruction of the brattice partitions (fig. 448) in the shafts, which blocked the pits and thus prevented the escape of possible survivors. It became established that explosions occurring in confined spaces were the most violent; that an explosion may be followed by others of a less violent character, and that by far the larger proportion of

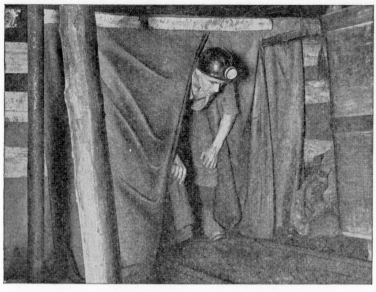

FIG. 448.—Brattice Sheet hung in Roadway of Coal Mine
(*By courtesy of Professor I. C. F. Statham*)

the victims were killed by breathing afterdamp, and not by the force of the explosion itself.

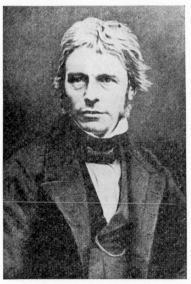

FIG. 449.—Michael Faraday,
1791–1867

Ventilation of Coal Mines

Ventilation was at first by fire, a system which consisted in erecting on the surface, within a few yards of the shaft, a large chimney. Near the bottom of this chimney was suspended an iron cradle containing burning coals which produced an upward current of air. It is known that the basket fire was employed to ventilate a colliery at Cheadle, Staffordshire, in the middle of the seventeenth century. Although the work of Stephen Hales had pointed the way in 1743, mechanical ventilation was not introduced into coalpits until 1807. Ventilation by means of centrifugal fans was introduced in 1860, and today fans circulate up to 400,000 cubic feet of air per minute (fig. 410). Such

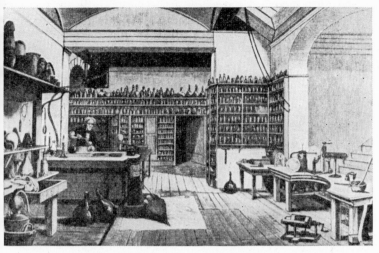

FIG. 450.—Michael Faraday in his Laboratory at the Royal Institution,
Albemarle Street, London
(*Water-colour by Harriet Moore, 1852*)

olumes of air are necessary for modern underground workings where two
ntake airways are required for each district, and the intake air must not
ontain less than 19 per cent of oxygen or more than 1·25 per cent of
arbon dioxide and 0·25 per cent of methane.

DUST EXPLOSIONS IN COAL MINES

The Haswell Colliery explosion which occurred in 1844 and caused
he deaths of ninety-five persons is of particular interest, since the Com-
nission appointed to inquire into the accident made new suggestions. The
Government appointed Professor Michael Faraday (figs. 449, 450) and others
o attend the inquest and report upon the cause of the catastrophe.

Report on the Haswell Colliery Explosion, 1844

In their report they stated that:

In considering the extent of the fire from the moment of explosion, it is not to be supposed that firedamp is its only fuel; the coal
dust swept by the rush of wind and flame from the floor, roof and
walls of the works would instantly take fire and burn, if there were
oxygen enough in the air present to support its combustion, and we
found the dust adhering to the face of the pillars, props and walls in
the direction of, and on the side towards the explosion, increasing
gradually to a certain distance, as we neared the place of ignition. This
deposit was in some parts half an inch, and in others almost an inch
thick; it adhered together in a friable coked state; when examined
with the glass it presented the fused, round form of burnt coal dust,

and when examined chemically, and compared with the coal itself reduced to powder, was found deprived of the greater portion of the bitumen, and in some instances entirely destitute of it. There is every reason to believe that much coal-gas was made from this dust in the very air itself of the mine by the flame of the firedamp, which raised and swept along; and much of the carbon of this dust remained unburnt only for want of air.

At first Faraday's discovery was almost universally doubted, and it took fifty years more to establish the fact that all great colliery explosions are due to ignition of mixtures of coal dust and air (Haldane, 1926).

Experimental Coal-dust Explosions, 1893

One of the principal actors in this drama was Dr. William Galloway of Cardiff who insisted that coal dust played an important part in causing the explosions. As a Junior Inspector of Mines he had opportunities of seeing the effects of several great explosions in Welsh collieries; and he drew the conclusion, expressed in several papers contributed by him to the Proceedings of the Royal Society, and giving also the results of experiments conducted by him with the co-operation of colliery owners, that it is coal dust which carries the flame with such disastrous effects along the roads of a colliery. This conclusion was so far from being in agreement with established existing theories, and was so unpopular, that Dr. Galloway found himself obliged to resign his appointment as Inspector. By degrees the new views made headway, and received the support of a Royal Commission, which reported in 1893 after various very convincing experiments had been made for it. These experiments showed that even where only small amounts of pure coal dust were present on the floor, roof timbers and sides of the gallery used, an explosion could easily be produced by a blasting shot in the complete absence of firedamp. Where experimental explosions were allowed to travel more than 100 yards along a boiler tube, the stout boiler plates near the open mouth of the tube were blown to pieces.

Violent Explosions stopped by Stone Dust

However, even such violent explosions were quickly stopped by stone dust. In proportion, moreover, as the percentage of stone dust mixed with the coal dust was made greater, the difficulty in starting an explosion became greater, until with 40 per cent of stone dust it was extremely difficult to initiate an explosion. Since varying percentages of stone dust are naturally present in the dust of coal mines, this discovery threw clear light on why certain coal mines and certain parts of them are much more liable to serious explosions than others.

Systematic Stone-dusting in Coal Mines

A systematic plan of stone-dusting was devised for mines. The stone dust used was from the soft shale cut away in the workings. Careful nquiry had shown that stone dust of this kind caused no injury to the lungs. About 1920, stone-dusting to such an extent as to prevent the proportion of the combustible matter in the dust along roadways from rising above 50 per cent was made legally obligatory, unless the dust is naturally wet or kept wet by watering. As a result of this far-reaching measure, there has been a great fall in the disastrous explosions which occurred at intervals over so long a period of British coal mining (Jones and Tideswell, 1947).

Safety in Mines Research Establishment

The organization known since 1950 as the Safety in Mines Research Establishment of the Ministry of Power has operated in one form or another since 1908. It has made noteworthy contributions to knowledge not only of the immediate problems of safety in mines connected with dusts, ventilation, inflammable gases, explosions, roof control, methods of working, lighting, health of the miner, electrical hazards, materials used in mining, and so forth, but also of fundamental scientific knowledge to a whole wide range of subjects which affect mining and mining conditions. These include physics of liquids and of fine particles, gas flow, ignition and combustion of gases and solids, flame propagation and explosions, metallurgy, coal constitution, palæobotany and medical science; this list is not exhaustive, but is a selection to show the breadth of interest of the Establishment as a whole. Smith (1960) has compiled a comprehensive bibliography of this work in which there are more than 1,500 entries. This shows the wide scope of the work of the Establishment touching as it does upon so many aspects of science and technology. The bibliography is of interest not only to practical doctors but also to workers in many fields of pure and applied science.

ELECTRICAL INJURIES

Electrical injuries may be received from lightning-stroke, from accidental contact with high-tension conductors on railways or in factories, mines, shipyards and farms, from faulty household electrical appliances or from judicial electrocution where this obtains. The first electrocution accident in industry occurred in England in 1879. In the 1960's accidental electric shock killed 1000 people a year in the U.S.A.

Effects of Electric Power applied to the Body

In Great Britain, electricity is usually supplied to householders at voltages of 250 or less. When the body is affected by electric power the severity of the injuries sustained in any given case depends upon the amount and path of the current flow through the victim. This is related both to the applied voltage and to the state of the body at the time. A potential of 500 volts under dry conditions would give rise to little current because of the high skin resistance and in the normal person the effect would be only the sensation of shock. A potential of 200 volts across the body through wet or sweating hands would cause a higher current which, acting in a vulnerable part of the body, might prove fatal. Generally, alternating voltages are more dangerous than direct voltages, partly because the usual frequency of 50 cycles per second is near to the optimum stimulation frequency of the heart. Voltages greater than 1,000 are spoken of as *high tension*. Any normal voltage source, provided it is capable of supplying a current of a few milliampères, can be dangerous under the right conditions. In judicial electrocution the victim is subjected to repeated discharges (4 to 8), each lasting some seconds (5 to 50), of alternately low and high potential (500 and 2,000 volts).

Effects of Lightning-stroke

A single lightning flash consists of from one to forty-two *main* strokes, each of which is preceded by a *leader* stroke. Current values of about 20,000 ampères operate over an average time of 30 microseconds. The potentials involved are of the order of thousands of millions of volts (Jex-Blake, 1945). Thus immense disruptive forces are liberated at each lightning flash, both electrical from the current flow itself and atmospheric from the disturbance of the air through which the current passes. When more than one object is struck by lightning, they are flung apart: a man is flung several yards from a tree under which he has been standing; or two men simultaneously struck are flung away from each other; a parcel held by an individual struck is hurled out of his grasp, and also his clothes are burst and torn off him in fragments, and he may be stripped naked. Within his body the same disruptive forces are at work and produce lesions in proportion to the rigidity and cohesion of the tissues. This accounts for the characteristic disruptive lesions found in the brain.

Acute Fatalities and Morbid Anatomy

In death from lightning-stroke the head is invariably struck. The body will be more or less stripped of clothes and streaks of *brushburn* may be found upon the skin. Leather garments, boots and belts may be burst. If a hat was worn, a hole will probably be found in it over the site of the scalp lesion. There is an effusion beneath the scalp without superficial abrasion. In the brain there are abnormal rents and fissures, the cerebrospinal spaces are distended, the perivascular spaces enlarged and the arteries at the base of the brain may show rupture of their muscular coats. In various situations the nerve cells show severe disruptive changes. Sometimes, if the victim was hurled or flung down, other signs of injury caused in this way may be found.

Lesions Compatible with Survival

Short of death, the effects of lightning stroke include burns, lacerations, fractures, conjunctivitis, paresis of accommodation, cataract, partial alopœcia, flaccid paralysis of the lower limbs and hysteria. Of all these lesions, the burn is the most common. It may occur in an unusual pattern as an arborescent marking known as a *brushburn*, or a series of long narrow lines on the skin. It is not a true burn, for it is painless and without inflammatory reaction. Metal objects in the pockets or in contact with the body, such as buckets and iron rods, may determine the site and severity of the lesions (Elwell, 1934).

A State of Suspended Animation

A person struck by lightning usually falls unconscious at once. He is pale and pulseless, and respiratory movements are suspended. This initial state of suspended animation or apparent death is common after lightning-stroke ,but not so frequent after accidental electrical injuries from contact with conductors. There may be powerful and generalized muscular spasm for a brief period, and the limbs may be in flexion. It is because of similar spasm in the heart and muscular arteries that the victim is pulseless and pale. Surface burns of varying severity are seen, and examination of the scalp will reveal a localized swelling at or near the vertex, with no cutaneous abrasion. As respiration becomes re-established, either spontaneously or after artificial respiration, the subject may become restless and resistive, crying with the pain of muscular spasm. Later, he becomes drowsy, has headache, and for one or more days may not be fully alert. Retrograde amnesia is common. Sometimes he speaks of having received a tremendous blow on the head, or of intense visual or auditory sensations, of pain in the trunk and limbs, or of giddiness.

Sequelæ of Lightning-stroke

Following lightning-stroke, the number of deaths is small in proportion to minor injuries; out of 300 persons in a church which was struck, 100 were made unconscious and injured, thirty had to take to bed, and only six were killed (Jex-Blake, 1945). Recovery from the average burn, laceration and fracture is prompt. Conjunctivitis and paresis of accommodation rapidly disappear. Flaccid paralysis of the lower trunk and limbs is temporary, power and sensation usually returning to normal after twelve hours. In cases of alopecia the hair grows again after six months. Hysterical deafness, blindness and aphonia should recover with adequate treatment. The only lesions which ever remain permanent are both rare—namely, cataract (p. 868) and a condition called spinal atrophic paralysis (Critchley, 1934). This consists of muscular atrophy with fibrillation without sensory disturbance in the distribution of the fourth to sixth cervical segments of the cord. It may progress and cripple the patient.

Contact with Live Conductors

If an individual merely touches a conducting element or a part of an electrical appliance which is not insulated, he receives a shock which causes a violent and unpleasant tingling sensation in the limb concerned or throughout his body, and this is quickly cut short by withdrawal of the part of his body from contact with the *live* object. The patient may feel faint but has no external injury. The serious cases are those in which the subject grasps a metal lamp-standard or other object which has become electrified as a result of a defect in the wiring. The flexor muscles of the grasping hand are at once thrown into strong spasm by the electrical stimulation, with the result that the patient cannot let go. The spasm quickly extends up the affected arm. Usually he brings up his other hand

and tries to release his first hand with it, and if he again catches the object by an electrified part, the muscles of both arms are quickly tetanized and the spasm spreads to his chest and other parts of his trunk.

Electrocution Accidents in the Bath

The patient becomes speechless and pale, then cyanosed and convulsed, he loses consciousness and may stop breathing. Unless the current can be switched off quickly death may result, but the severity of the effects varies according to the degree to which the patient is insulated. If the current is switched off within a few minutes, the patient usually recovers consciousness quickly but suffers from a variable degree of shock and muscular spasm. In another group of cases electrocution occurs in a bath. The subject, who is standing or sitting in the bath, may pick up an electric hair-dryer or touch an electric heater, probably with a dripping hand. Instantly electricity passes through and over the patient's wet body to the earth provided by the water and the bath. The symptoms which ensue are those already described, and unless the contact is broken, death may follow rapidly.

Electrical Necrosis

Severe electrical necrosis is an effect of heat which occurs with large currents, such as accidents with switchgear in generating stations or from accidentally touching overhead wires. The common accident is where a man approaches an electrode believing it to be *dead*, often with a spanner in his hands, and before he has touched it the current has made an arc from the electrode to the spanner or his flesh. This is followed by a violent explosion and mutual repulsion so that the man is blown away from the source. If he is working at a height he may be killed by the fall, but on the ground he will often be found running away from the scene of the accident. The heat generated is so great and the destruction so complete that it is often difficult to reconstruct the scene afterwards. Both spanner and electrode are vaporized and copper is deposited on the exposed parts of face and neck. The current may pass up the arm, find an exit from the shoulder, and become burnt out before it properly enters the body so that electrocution does not take place. If electrocution does occur, death as with lightning-stroke is instantaneous. The necrosis may be very severe. The heat calcines bone and carbonizes flesh, and beyond the area of complete necrosis muscles are roasted. In consequence the victim often loses a limb (Hughes, 1956).

Clinical Effects of Electric Shock

Electricians describe balls of light seen when a current is passing through their tissues, the so-called *electricians' moons*. After a shock a man may be apathetic or euphoric and experience a transitory hastening of the thought process. But more often the man is in an acute state of fear, violently trembling, pale and sweating. Cerebral œdema may lead to unconsciousness without more than momentary cessation of respiration or of the heart. Auditory hallucinations may occur and the patient may appear blinded or deafened for a period of minutes or hours. Loss of taste may be noticed. Paralysis of an affected limb for up to four hours is common, and subsequent pain and stiffness may continue for weeks or months. Flaccid paralysis may develop below the level of the shock, but generally resolves in two or three days. Permanent damage to the central nervous system is rare.

Sequelæ of Electric Shock

Arterial spasm in the form of Raynaud's syndrome or effort syndrome is not uncommon. The heart beat may be irregular, and a syndrome on *angina pectoris electrica* may occur, with retrosternal pain and tightness of effort persisting for weeks, but without specific electrocardiographic changes. Sudden blindness may occur from detachment of the retina, and arc-eye is usual with a major flash but clears up within a few days. A wide variety of late sequelæ is recorded. Cataract may appear days or months later (see p. 868). Pain at the insertion of muscles may persist for several months. There may be long-continued agitation, restlessness, confusion or dejection with low blood pressure. Confusional and psychotic states are usually temporary, and cerebral sclerosis with mental deficiency has been described. Less dramatic personality changes may occur and are said to last up to a year, but fear may have been the cause rather than electricity.

Protection against Lightning-stroke

Thunderstorms are less common in high latitudes than nearer the equator. On mountains and in open country, especially in the Tropics, it is important to know what to do when lightning comes near. It is safest to be inside a house, in a room with all the doors and windows closed, and away from the fireplace. In Great Britain telephones are fitted with lightning arresters and so may be used without danger. If there is no house, shed, cave or closed motor car available, the protection of a ditch or hollow should be sought. Crowds of people and the neighbourhood of domestic stock should be avoided, as should trees standing alone, wire fences, hedges, walls and the banks of rivers and ponds. The centre of a wood is fairly safe. If one has to be struck it is better to be wet through, for wet clothing may short-circuit most of the current (Jex-Blake, 1945).

The Standard of Design of Electrical Apparatus

Ignorance and negligence are responsible for a high proportion of electrical accidents. In factories, mines and shipyards, safety must be secured by the proper design of electrical apparatus, an active inspectorate and adequate safety-first propaganda. Since 1908 the use of electricity on factory premises for lighting, heating, motive power and other processes has been subject to Regulations under the Factories Acts. At that time the flimsiness of apparatus, the incomplete protection of fuse boards, the non-earthing of such metal work as motor frames, switch covers and lamp holders, and the faulty construction of portable hand lamps were the chief sources of danger.

Propaganda against Ignorance and Carelessness

Owing to ignorance, carelessness or a desire for economy, these faults continued to cause accidents. *The Electricity (Factories Act) Special Regulations, 1944,* have been effective in their intention, for since they came into force, although the units sold for power purposes in industry have increased by five times, the fatal-accident rate has remained nearly constant at about thirty per annum (Swann, 1949). Generators, transformers, motors and switchboards should be placed on a floor itself made of some insulating material and covered with insulating mats which must be kept dry and free from oil. No circuit should be worked upon until the power has been cut off and the switch padlocked. If it becomes absolutely necessary to handle a live circuit, care should be taken to work upon but one wire at a time and to wear rubber gloves. The standard of design, installation and maintenance of electrical plant is much higher than ever before. The chief cause of fatal accidents continues to be the breakdown of insulation during the use of portable electric hand-tools.

Accidents due to Mental Aberration

A less widely recognized factor in the causation of electrical injuries is a form of mental aberration. A number of fatalities has come about as a result of such lapses. Mistakes occur between live and dead sections of plant which, although of similar appearance, are considered sufficiently distinguished by position. An experienced switchboard attendant had occasion to open a number of cubicles to clean the auxiliary busbars of a large generating station. He knew the switchgear thoroughly but, in spite of safeguards, he obtained the key to an adjacent live cubicle, opened it and, disregarding the different layout of equipment from that in cubicles at which he had previously worked, he entered. He touched live 11-kilovolt conductors and received injuries from which he later died. The occurrence of accidents of this kind is one of the reasons why the regulations require that persons undertaking such work shall never be unaccompanied. A second man, either a mate or a supervising engineer, may remind a worker that he is about to make a mistake (Swann, 1946).

Adequate Guarding of Live Wires

Pylons carrying live wires must be provided with danger notices and fitted with metal spikes to discourage attempts to climb them. Where roads cross electric railways fitted with overhead conductor wires, screens must be erected in such a way as to prevent the electrocution through the stream of urine of small boys who engage in the ingenious but deadly pastime of aiming at the wires in this particular way from the bridges. In the home, bathrooms must never be fitted with electric-power points because of the danger involved in touching a defective electrical appliance with wet hands while standing in water in a metal bath.

Importance of Artificial Respiration

When the victim is unconscious, white and pulseless, artificial respiration must be undertaken at once and persevered with for at least eight hours before abandoning the patient. In factories, the majority of recoveries when artificial respiration is applied occur in the first ten minutes, but fewer after this period. There are few records of artificial respiration having been carried on in fatal cases for much longer than an hour, while many attempts are abandoned within half that time. Swallowing is the most reliable sign of the return of spontaneous breathing (Jellinek, 1932). Even when respiration is first resumed, it may fail again, and artificial respiration must be kept up and oxygen administered until the normal movements of breathing are fully established. To treat the shock, the patient must be kept warm and given fluids. He may complain of severe headache, which should be treated by anodynes, and of painful muscular cramp, for which massage is useful. Arc-eye and pain and stiffness in the limbs may be persistent and need hospital examination and treatment. Neurological symptoms and disabilities have to be dealt with according to their character and severity.

Treatment of Electrical Burns

The superficial linear burns of lightning-stroke are best covered by aseptic dressings, when they usually heal without scarring. The deeper burns from contact with live conductors should be covered with a clean sheet and the patient evacuated to hospital without delay. For the first two hours patients with burns travel well, and a journey no longer than this is justifiable to reach a hospital with a burns unit. Operations for excision of necrotic lesions and skin grafting may be necessary. By conservative treatment a surprising amount of function may be regained in individual cases, though at some risk to life from toxæmia and secondary hæmorrhage. Sequestra may form in bone and need removal.

The Management of Fear

In less severe cases where there may be coldness and pulselessness of a limb reassurance is necessary that this effect will last only a few hours. The most outstanding symptom in many cases is fear quite out of proportion to the severity of the accident, and this effect is found only when a current has passed through the body. Men with necrosis and flash burns, where the damage may have been severe, may cheerfully resume their work, but in many cases of electric shock much reassurance and modification of duties may be necessary in order to rehabilitate the man. Sometimes this dread is most difficult to treat and psychotherapy may be indicated (Hughes, 1956).

Accidents in Chemistry and Physics Laboratories

It is common knowledge that the handling of chemical substances and physics apparatus may involve certain hazards. From time to time over many years chemists and physicists and their technicians working in laboratories have met with injury and death by fire, explosion, radiation hazards and poisoning.

Death Roll of Chemists, Physicists and their Technicians

In 1811 the French chemist, Pierre Louis Dulong, discovered nitrogen trichloride, NCl_3, which is so dangerously explosive that during his experiments with it he lost an eye and three fingers. In 1847 in Turin the Italian chemist, Ascanio Sobrero, discovered nitroglycerine; when he heated a drop of it in a test-tube, it exploded with such violence that the glass splinters cut deep into his face and hands. In 1863 near Stockholm the young Swedish chemical engineer, Emil Oscar Nobel, was killed with four other people when the private laboratory belonging to his family was wrecked by the explosion of a quantity of nitroglycerine. We have seen (p. 152) how the English chemist, Charles Blachford Mansfield, was burnt to death when only thirty-five years of age. Accounts of sickness and death by poisoning of chemists and technicians are scattered through the various chapters of this book. The substances responsible are arseniuretted hydrogen (p. 344), dimethyl mercury (p. 314) and fluorine (p. 683). From time to time physicists and their technicians have died sometimes after great suffering from X-ray cancer (p. 902), mesothorium poisoning (p. 915), radium and polonium poisoning (p. 912) and chronic berylliosis (p. 431).

Good Housekeeping

Good housekeeping demands that aisles should not be blocked with boxes or other materials. Illumination should be sufficient and of even intensity in all sections of the laboratory to prevent dark spots and glare. For obvious reasons, horseplay in chemical laboratories must be absolutely forbidden. Spilt chemical substances should be removed from floors as soon as possible to prevent slipping. We have discussed at length (p. 677) the dangers which may be involved in dealing wrongly with spilt nitric acid. Some chemical substances should be neutralized or diluted before they are mopped up. Containers should be provided for the disposal of waste materials such as broken glassware, inflammable liquids, oily rags and dry chemical substances. It is inadvisable to store strong oxidizing and reducing agents or other pairs of reacting chemical substances near each other. This is of special importance in regions subject to earthquakes or tremors. Exits from workrooms and storage rooms of laboratories should be so arranged that technicians cannot be completely cut off should a fire, explosion or spill of corrosive material block the exit commonly used.

Mechanical Hazards

Goggles should be worn whenever glass is chipped, tools are ground or bottles whose stoppers are stuck are to be opened. Shields of safety glass should be used to protect operators during distillations and when working with equipment in which pressure or vacuum may develop. Laboratory tools such as cork borers, files and knives should be used in such a way that injury to the body will be avoided. For example, in boring a cork the hand holding it should not be placed opposite the borer. Instead, the cork should be held between the thumb and finger and allowed to rest against a block of wood. Similarly, knives used for cutting rubber tubing and other soft substances should be kept sharp and equipped with sturdy handles. In use, the cutting edge should be held away from the body. Glass tubing or thermometers should not be forced through stopper holes which are too small for them. Not only should the hole be of the proper size for a comfortable fit, but the glass should be lubricated with glycerine or water before it is pushed through the hole. In removing thermometers which are stuck in a stopper hole, it is often possible to accomplish the desired result without breaking equipment or injury to the operator by using a sharp cork borer just large enough to pass over the thermometer and by drilling into the stopper. Lubrication with glycerine in this operation facilitates the work and makes it safer (Pieters and Creyghton, 1957).

Hazards from Corrosive Substances

Strong acids, caustic alkalis, phenol, bromine and organic solvents are primary skin irritants. Where contact takes place, the skin may be dissolved, charred or cracked, resulting in painful injury. Contact of the skin with such substances must be avoided, but should it occur, the skin must be washed freely with running water immediately after the contact has been made. Carboys of strong acids and caustic alkalis should be mounted on a rocking device (fig. 451) and strict regulations enforced as to the use of personal protective equipment, including gloves to protect the hands, goggles to protect the eyes, or a splash shield to protect the entire face. Some chemical substances such as aniline, nitrobenzene, carbon disulphide, dimethyl sulphate, hydrocyanic acid and organic compounds of lead, mercury and arsenic may be absorbed through the skin to produce systemic damage to organs of the body other than the skin. Workers can be protected against these substances by preventing contact with them. If any such substance is spilled on the clothing, it should be removed immediately, since additional time of contact may be harmful and even cause death.

Hazards of Fire and Explosion

Inflammable liquids, if stored in glass containers, should be in bottles whose capacity does not exceed 1 litre. No more than one such bottle of each liquid should be kept in the laboratory proper, the remainder of the stock being stored in a fireproof vault. If more than 1 litre of an inflammable liquid is needed in the laboratory, metal safety containers should be used. Inflammable liquids should never be handled in the vicinity of open flames. Some highly inflammable liquids such as ether or carbon disulphide should not even be handled near hot bodies such as incandescent lights, hot plates or electric heaters. Distillation of inflammable liquids should never be carried out over a free flame. This operation is best performed over a water-bath with immersion electric heaters for the low-boiling liquids and over an enclosed electric hot-plate for the higher-boiling liquids. Inflammable liquids spilled on laboratory floors should be handled with caution. The atmosphere over such spilled liquid may contain an explosive concentration of the vapour. A spark created by an iron fitting of a mop hitting against a concrete floor, from a nail in a shoe against such a floor or any other source of ignition may be enough to produce a catastrophe. Spills of low-boiling liquids may be removed by first diluting with high-boiling petroleum

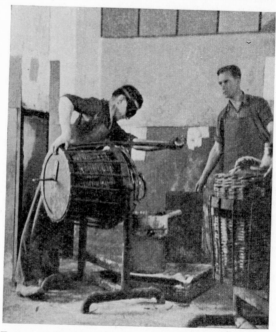

Fig. 451.—Inadequate protection of men handling strong acid. Although the carboy is mounted on a rocking device neither workman is wearing gloves and one of them has neither goggles nor splash shield to protect his face

naphtha or kerosene and then mopping up the liquid, or by evaporating the liquid completely into a portable, non-ferrous exhaust system equipped with a vapour-proof motor. The exhausted vapours should pass directly outdoors. Waste liquids which are inflammable should not be thrown into the sink, since evaporation with subsequent explosion might occur in sewers. Special covered metal containers should be provided for such wastes. These can then be moved to dumps for emptying. Fire extinguishers, preferably of the liquid CO_2 type, should be provided. A number of hand-size extinguishers should be distributed for convenience. In laboratories in which inflammable materials are commonly handled, a sprinkler system which operates automatically in case of fire should be installed. The doors of laboratories using cylinders of gases under pressure should bear pernanent notices warning the fire brigade and others of the hazard of xplosion.

Exposure to Toxic Substances

Chemists and other laboratory workers often handle highly toxic materials. Accidents or injury to health may be avoided by following a few rather simple rules. Beakers which have been used for chemical substances should never be used for drinking. Paper cups or a fountain should be provided for the purpose. Pipetting of solutions of poisonous or corrosive substances should be performed with a pipette filler which does not require the use of the mouth. Inhalation of noxious gases, vapours, mists, fumes or dusts can be avoided by performing all work in which such substances are used or formed in an efficient fume chamber. This should have air drawn into it, with all sliding doors open, at a rate not less than 100 linear feet per minute. The exhaust end of the duct should extend to a distance of at least 6 feet above the building and should be provided with a rain-cap. If large amounts of noxious gases are to be discharged from the laboratory, greater dilution with air, higher exhaust stacks or even air cleaning may be necessary to avoid creating a hazard or nuisance in the neighbourhood. Hydrogen sulphide is a common toxic gas, the extreme toxicity of which often goes unrecognized. Inexpensive equipment for testing the air of laboratories for this gas is readily obtainable. Chemical substances which interact to yield toxic gases should not be dumped into a sink without one being neutralized, if possible, and then flushed down completely before the other is added. Cyanides and acids are common offenders which must not be overlooked. In many instances, chemical substances of a low order of toxicity may be substituted for those which are more toxic. Three of the most toxic solvents used in chemical laboratories are carbon disulphide, benzene and carbon tetrachloride. While these are excellent solvents for many materials, they may often be replaced by petroleum naphtha, acetone or toluene. A solvent should not be used merely out of habit without inquiring whether there is a safe substitute. Where coal gas is used as fuel, burners, tubing and valves should be kept in excellent condition to prevent the risk of carbon-monoxide poisoning.

Hazard of Mercury Vapour

Mercury is a hazard which is often overlooked in the laboratory. Spilt mercury, and especially mercury in flooring cracks, may keep the atmosphere concentration of mercury vapour at a dangerously high level. Mercury should be handled over deep pans or over perforated table tops fitted with an inverted cone so that spilt mercury or mercury from broken apparatus can be collected readily. Should mercury get on a table or floor, it must be promptly removed by means of a suction hose fitted with a trap to prevent it from entering the pump. Mercury which cannot be removed completely by suction should be covered with powdered sulphur or calcium-hydrosulphide or polysulphide solution. Rooms which contain much spilt

mercury, especially in floor cracks, should be cleansed as thoroughly a
possible. This may necessitate lifting the floor boards. The flooring shoul
then be covered with sulphur or calcium-hydrosulphide solution, followe
by a well-sealed linoleum covering. After this, precautions to preven
further spillage will usually permit this room to be used in safety.

Hazards from Ionizing Radiation

We have seen how from time to time physicists and their technician
have died from the effects of X-rays (p. 902), mesothorium (p. 915)
radium and polonium (p. 912). X-ray technicians should be protected b
lead and leaded clothing and the laboratories should be monitored so tha
nobody will be over-exposed to the radiation. The use of the cyclotron an
the uranium pile for the production of radioactive isotopes has introduce
a serious potential hazard to some laboratories. For biochemical research
radioactive isotopes are used as tracers in metabolic experiments, especiall
those of carbon, phosphorus, iodine and calcium. Every laboratory engage
in such work should have a trained health physicist on its staff. Shieldin
with lead of required thickness, the use of remotely controlled equipmen
and adequate ventilation must be used to protect technicians from radia
tion and the absorption of radioactive material. Monitoring of laboratorie
is one of the requirements for safe operation. It is essential that all worker
wear film badges to indicate automatically the extent of radiation exposure
Ultra-violet and infra-red rays, although producing much less seriou
effects than the radiation of shorter wave-lengths, can also give rise to suc
disabilities as conjunctivitis and erythema. Workers exposed to such ray
must guard their eyes and skin to avoid disabilities.

Hazards from Laser Radiation

Laser radiation was produced by Maiman in 1960 and its uses i
medical research and surgery are still expanding. Light amplification b
the stimulated emission of radiation (hence the term laser) is achieve
by devices that emit a powerful and very pure kind of light called *coheren
light*; it is all of one wavelength and all waves are in phase and non-
divergent. These devices take several forms, some of which emit light ir
brief pulses and others as a continuous beam, but all produce light tha
can be focused to a fine point and to very high concentrations of energy
In fact, when the beam of certain lasers is focused with a lens system
momentary temperatures exceeding those on the sun's surface are said t
be produced at the point of focus. Nothing else is known to give powe
fluxes of such magnitude. Laser research may present hazards to th
workers involved. As instruments become more sophisticated and as th
shorter more biologically active wavelengths, such as the ultraviolet ones
are achieved, the eyes may be damaged. Corneal, iris, and lens injuries
flash blindness, and damage to enzyme systems in the rods and cones ar
possibilities. Moreover, ionizing radiation may be produced in the vicinity
of a laser-irradiated target. And there are indications that a microwave

eld of varying intensity exists around a laser while it operates: with
evices of higher power microwave effects may be induced in adjacent
iological systems. Such dangers plainly need to be watched.

Electrical Hazards

All electric wiring, extension wires, receptacles and sockets should be
waterproof and abrasion-resistant. Switches, motors and relays which must
perate in the presence of combustible materials should be dust and vapour-
roof. Incandescent lights also should be vapour-proof. High-tension
wiring and equipment should be surrounded by interlocking guards to
revent workers getting within contact distance of high-voltage conductors.
Such an interlock may consist of a switch which is automatically opened
hould anybody open the guard-fence door. High-tension equipment
which may act as a source of ozone should be mechanically ventilated to
revent this gas accumulating in a concentration of more than one part per
million by volume in the air. If the odour usually associated with ozone
an be detected, its concentration is excessive.

Education in Safe Procedure

Laboratory workers should make it an essential part of their education
o learn how to perform their work in the safest way possible. Knowledge
f the factors responsible for causing accidents makes it possible to avoid
uch accidents. All laboratory workers should be impressed with the fact
hat many dangerous materials are in common use and that hazardous
ituations may occur in laboratories. If these are treated with the respect
hey deserve, laboratory accidents can be prevented. It is the duty of the
lirectors of laboratories to inform their assistants what constitutes good,
afe procedure and to impress upon them the fact that he expects them to
onduct themselves accordingly at all times.

Design and Equipment of New Laboratories

It is the plain duty of teaching institutions, especially the universities
nd colleges of technology, to inculcate accident-awareness in their
tudents. The opportunity is being fully seized in the design and equipment of the numerous new university laboratories now being built in the
United Kingdom. Efficient fume extraction is provided in every laboratory,
carbon dioxide fire-extinguishers, frequently serviced by weighing the
emaining carbon dioxide, are available on every bench, and at convenient
key-points emergency showers release mains-pressure water at the turn
f a handle. The emergency shower is designed particularly as a precau-
ion against splashing with corrosive liquids; it is swift and efficient and
hould be followed up immediately by a warm bath. It is equally effective
or extinguishing fire on the clothing of a person splashed by burning
nflammable substances. The design of gas-masks, goggles, visors and
afety shields has enormously improved in recent years, and research
workers are well advised to wear safety glasses constantly at the bench;

they are no longer uncomfortable or unsightly. In the case of open labora
tories, workers should be encouraged to take the view that their precau
tions are as much against their neighbours' accidents as their own (Hunter
1961).

Safety Rules and First-aid

All employees, especially new ones, should be made to understand tha
they are expected to work safely for their own sake and for that of thei
colleagues. In large laboratories, printed instructions of safe practices ca
be issued. Such rules should not be expressed in general terms but mus
be quite specific for the type of work done in that laboratory. An adequat
first-aid room or cabinet should be provided. Materials kept in such a roon
or cabinet should never be allowed to become depleted. A chart showin
how to treat accidents and poisoning should hang in a position where it ca
be readily seen. Trained first-aid workers should be available, if possible
The name, address and telephone number of several nearby doctors an
hospitals with ambulance service should be prominently displayed. Ga
masks and respirators should be provided for use in emergency or fo
unusual operations. The various respiratory protective devices should b
of types approved for the purpose for which it is intended to use then
(Moskowitz, 1948).

HAZARDS FROM HANDLING PHARMACEUTICAL SUBSTANCES

Pharmaceutical chemists, pharmacologists, druggists, herb vendors
doctors, nurses, technicians and workmen are subject to special hazard
from contact with pharmaceutical substances. Contact with vegetable sub
stances, with the solvents used to extract the active principles and with th
finished products all have to be considered. Alkaloids present specia
hazards, notably in experimental pharmacology, where valuable lives hav
been lost in tests of new products. The saddest tragedies of all are thos
where the experimenter has developed addiction to a new alkaloid whos
properties at the time are largely unknown. In the manufacture of anti
venenes professional herpetologists, technicians and research worker
have been bitten by snakes (p. 1171). Dangers met with in the manu
facture of antisera will be described under bacteriological hazards (p. 1160)

Irritation of Nasal Mucosa and Conjunctiva

Noxious dusts are produced by the sorting, mixing and grinding of cer
tain vegetable substances used in pharmacy. The use of goggles and dus
masks is imperative both to get the work done and to protect the workers
The dusts of quillaia (*Quillaja saponaria*), sabadilla and *Veratrum albur*
cause sneezing, epistaxis, headache and irritation of the larynx and pharynx
Irritation of the conjunctiva and sometimes facial œdema occur from th
dusts of emetine, euphorbium, ipecacuanha, pulsatilla, pyrethrum, quillaia
rhubarb, senega and vanilla.

Keratitis and Opacity of the Cornea

Mustard oil causes conjunctival hyperæmia, lachrymation, photophobia and superficial vesicles on the cornea which may lead to corneal opacity. Workers who feed the root of podophyllin (*Podophyllum peltatum*) into grinders may suffer painful conjunctivitis and keratitis which is delayed in onset up to six hours after exposure and lasts several days. In its mild form it subsides spontaneously, but massive exposure may cause corneal ulceration.

Dermatitis Venenata

It was in 1713 in his *De Morbus Artificum Diatriba* that Ramazzini wrote his classic description of dermatitis venenata. An apothecary carried in his hand the root of an arum, "thereupon handling his privities was seized with so great an inflammation of the genitals, that it was followed by gangrene." Happily, contact dermatitis and the effects of sensitivity commonly produce much less drastic effects than this. Contact dermatitis occurs from handling emetine, ergot, ipecacuanha, phenothiazine and many alkaloids, including atropine, brucine, codeine, cocaine, hydrastine, opium, quinine and strychnine.

Sensitivity and Systemic Effects

Persons sensitized to some of these substances may suffer serious allergic reactions such as severe attacks of asthma provoked by inhalation of very small amounts of powdered ipecacuanha. Occasionally, systemic symptoms and signs appear—for example, insomnia from handling *d*-amphetamine sulphate, somnolence from inhalation of the dust of hops, giddiness from that of gall nuts and red urine and stools from handling the root of the madder plant (*Rubia tinctorum*). Anthrax pustule, an unlikely occurrence, affected two pharmacists engaged in cutting up leaves of *Datura stramonium* from Hungary.

Belladonna Poisoning

Belladonna poisoning, with dryness of the mouth and skin, widely dilated pupils and mental confusion, may occur from inhalation of dust when pure belladonna alkaloids are being handled without adequate protection, and similar cases have occurred during the grinding of belladonna leaves. The administration of neostigmine by subcutaneous injection results in rapid recovery, and ampoules containing 0·5 milligram per millilitre neostigmine methyl-sulphate should be available for use wherever there is a risk of belladonna poisoning (Watrous, 1947). A less serious effect of belladonna often attracts the attention of visitors to the pharmaceutical industry. This is the dilatation of one pupil due to direct contact with minute particles of one of the belladonna alkaloids which may result from slight exposure, such as walking through the manufacturing department. The affected eye should be irrigated thoroughly with normal saline and 0·25 per cent eserine ointment applied. The pupil then returns to normal size within a few hours.

Aconitine Poisoning

Unpleasant symptoms identical with those induced by the smoking of a strong cigar in a person unaccustomed to smoking have been observed following inhalation of pure aconitine hydrobromide in powder form. Pallor, weakness, nausea, vomiting and cold sweats lasting thirty minutes occurred in a man who weighed a small quantity of this alkaloid on an ordinary laboratory balance without using protective equipment.

Hazards of Organic Synthesis

Exposure to many potentially toxic substances may occur in the conditions in which organic chemical synthesis is used in the pharmaceutical industry. In contrast to the mass-production methods of the heavy chemical industry where it is economically possible to design equipment specially suited for one process and incorporating measures which ensure maximum safety and efficiency, the pharmaceutical industry is concerned with batch-process methods often of an experimental nature. Watrous (1947) points out that such methods result in many unexpected occurrences, strange chemical substances and unusual toxicological problems.

Hazard from Benzene Vapour

Large quantities of benzene are used in the extraction processes of the pharmaceutical industry especially for alkaloids. Careful supervision of these processes is necessary to prevent exposure to harmful concentrations of benzene. Workers should be examined at regular and frequent intervals. Laboratory research workers, in particular, need watching, for in spite of their scientific training they are apt to be careless in handling the reagents they use. In one works, leukopenia was found in five out of twenty research chemists, most of whom had Ph.D. degrees.

Chlorinating and Sulphonating Agents

Many of the substances used in organic synthesis of therapeutic agents are irritating to the skin, the mucous membranes or the lungs. Chlorinating agents include chlorine, phosphorus oxychloride, $POCl_3$, carbonyl chloride (phosgene), $COCl_2$, thionyl chloride, $SOCl_2$, and phosphorus pentachloride, PCl_5. All of these agents are irritant to mucous membranes and to the lungs, the effect upon the lungs being often delayed in onset and requiring prompt recognition and treatment. Sulphonating agents such as chlorsulphonic acid, essential in the synthesis of sulphonamides, and concentrated sulphuric acid are lung irritants.

Methylating Agents

It is important to make it clear that heat is evolved when concentrated sulphuric acid is mixed with water. Skin burns from splashes of concentrated sulphuric acid should be washed first with anhydrous ethyl alcohol. Dimethyl sulphate is a most potent cause of irritation to lungs, mucous membranes and skin, and other methylating agents such as nitrosomethylurethane and diazomethane cause irritation of the eyes with failure of accommodation. Dermatitis may develop after a latent interval of from five to ten days.

Acetylating Agents

There is risk in exposure also to alkyl halides such as methyl bromide, to sodium and potassium cyanide, and to organic cyanides such as benzyl cyanide and benzonitrile. The acetylating agents such as glacial acetic acid, acetic anhydride, monochloracetic and dichloracetic acids cause bullous dermatitis of delayed onset with extensive desquamation. There are no immediate symptoms, but skin splashes should be treated immediately by soaking for four hours in sodium-bicarbonate solution. Fortunately, the acetylating agents give good warning of their presence in the atmosphere and lung irritation seldom occurs.

Toxic Intermediate Products

Toxic intermediate products may also cause irritation of the lungs, mucous membranes and skin. Dichlorethyl acetate, an intermediate in the synthesis of sulphathiazole, may cause corneal ulceration and blistering of the skin, and is also a lung irritant. Aminothiazole causes urticaria, followed by painful swelling of joints resembling serum sickness, and there is some evidence that mild hypothyroidism may also develop from its absorption.

Hydrogen Sulphide and Carbon Monoxide

Hydrogen sulphide, mercaptans and other disagreeable-smelling compounds present in the purification of pentothal sodium are responsible for complaints of headache, nausea, vomiting, faintness and vertigo among workers. Carbon monoxide occurs in several processes and may be difficult to control where ampoules are sealed by gas flames in rooms which must be kept free of flying dust or low in moisture content of air. In such conditions it may be difficult to use conventional methods of exhaust ventilation.

Mepacrine and Emetine

Mepacrine causes conjunctivitis, rhinitis, stomatitis and dermatitis in a high proportion of cases. Mann (1947) found that workers making this substance complained of seeing blue haloes around lights. They had yellow pigmentation of the conjunctivæ, and she found that brown granules were present in the epithelial cells of the conjunctiva and cornea. When they were transferred to another department, all the symptoms and signs disappeared. Emetine hydrochloride may cause conjunctivitis from splashing in the eye of workers filling ampoules with a 6·5 per cent solution.

Arsphenamine and Neoarsphenamine

Arsphenamine dust blown into a worker's eye may cause a severe keratitis. No symptoms of arsenic poisoning were observed by Watrous

(1947) among workers exposed to concentrations of 0·001–0·015 milligrams per cubic foot in the manufacture of arsphenamine and its derivatives, but the arsenic content of urine and hair in these men was much above the accepted normal. A painful condition of the finger-nails is common among women who stick labels on ampoules of neoarsphenamine. Should an ampoule break, the solution is wiped up with a damp cloth. Oxidation occurs, and if the oxidized arsenic compound gets under the nails an exquisitely tender inflammatory process develops. This can be avoided by moistening the rags with sodium thiosulphate and changing them frequently.

Alkaloids and Mercury

There is evidence that absorption occurs in the preparation of tablets of morphine and codeine for hypodermic injection. These must be hand-moulded, because machine-pressed tablets would be too hard and would not dissolve readily. Drowsiness and lethargy have been observed, but there is no evidence that addiction results. Workers making amphetamine sulphate complain of insomnia. The risk of mercury poisoning exists in the manufacture of organic mercurial antiseptics, the moulding of mercury bichloride and mercury oxycyanide tablets, and in the use and maintenance of mercury manometers.

Gynæcomastia from Handling Stilbœstrol

In the final stages of purification of stilbœstrol by crystallization, spilling of the concentrated solution which dries and forms dust leads to absorption of amounts sufficient to cause gynæcomastia. This never results from handling the diluted forms for therapeutic use (Fitzsimons, 1944). Numerous hazards are mentioned by Watrous (1947), including the exposure to ultra-violet light of workers engaged in the manufacture of synthetic vitamin D from ergosterol, and to visible light of ampoule sealers. He also draws attention to the fact that enormous doses of toxic substances may be met with in the pharmaceutical industry when preparations for use in veterinary medicine are produced. A tonic powder for horses may contain as much as 2·5 per cent of white arsenic, and pure tetrachlorethane is used in vermifuge capsules.

Miscellaneous Sensitization Hazards

Sensitization to sulphaguanidine sometimes occurs resulting in asthma. It also occurs with chlorpromazine hydrochloride (largactil), a pink papular eruption appearing on the hands of workers handling cracked ampoules. Conjunctivitis and dermatitis are common from contact with acriflavine, and nicotinic acid causes a diffuse erythema resembling sunburn. Dry powdered penicillin may cause a follicular erythema, diffuse papular rashes on exposed parts or generalized urticaria. Local anæsthetics, particularly procaine, cause a mild papular contact dermatitis, and synthetic vitamin K, 2-methyl-1,4 naphthoquinone, leads to dark-brown staining of the skin nd an eczematous or papular rash. Disinfectants containing sulphon-chloramides cause dermatitis, rhinitis, conjunctivitis and bronchitis in ome individuals. Asthma may develop in susceptible persons.

Laboratory Infections

Certain laboratory workers are likely to be at risk of infection by virulent bacteria and viruses, and fatal accidents have occurred in the manufacture of vaccines where virulent cultures are handled in large quantities. Ielwig (1940) records several fatal infections with the virus of equine encephalomyelitis. A pharmacist who weighed 500 grams of pure desiccated scarlet-fever toxin, a light fluffy powder readily dispersed as dust, was affected next day by a sore throat, reddened strawberry tongue and an erythematous rash. There was no fever, and albuminuria did not develop. The symptoms subsided within forty-eight hours.

Early Experimenters become Cocaine Addicts

Soon after Karl Koller announced in Heidelberg in 1884 his discovery of the anæsthetic properties of cocaine when applied to the cornea, William S. Halsted and his two assistants Richard J. Hill and Frank Hartley at the Roosevelt Hospital, New York, began to experiment with this drug upon themselves. They demonstrated the superiority of endodermal as distinguished from the hypodermal injection method, the efficacy of dilute solutions of the analgesic drug when administered in large quantities, the prolongation of effect when the circulation of the part is reduced and most, important, the fact that sectional infiltration of a sensory or mixed nerve dulls sensation throughout the peripheral distribution of the nerve, the neuroregional method of anæsthesia. At the time the three experimenters little suspected the diabolic effects that cocaine can produce; all became addicts and the two assistants died.

William Stewart Halsted, 1852–1922

As a young man practising surgery in New York City, Halsted was a bold, spectacular surgeon, one of the most popular clinical teachers of his day, a prodigious worker and a keen athlete. When he worked on cocaine anæsthesia he was only thirty-two years of age, and the tragedy of addiction to the drug changed his whole life. Those who knew of it guarded the secret. It is difficult to learn anything very definite about it, but his close friends knew that he went through a terrible experience. About 1885 he was persuaded by Dr. Munroe to go to a hospital in Providence, Rhode Island, for a year. In the spring of 1886 he took a trip to the Windward Islands and then worked erratically in New York on the preparation of lectures which were never given.

A Personal Triumph over the Cocaine Habit

At the end of 1886 he was invited to Baltimore by Dr. Welch, where they lived together for a time, but even then Halsted had to go back to hospital in Providence. There he sent for the manager and asked him to make sure that he should have no money so that he could not buy any drug (Mac Callum, 1930). Through superhuman strength and determination he conquered the addiction and came back to a splendid life of achievement. As one of the famous four, which included W. H. Welch, William Osler and H. A. Kelly, he helped to build up the Medical School of the Johns Hopkins University from its foundations. He had become a recluse—modest, aloof shy and fastidious—but although he shunned publicity he always delighted in the company of his pupils. Not only was he the Lister of North America but also he was the greatest surgical philosopher that continent has ever produced, and he created a tradition in surgery which Harvey Cushing has compared to that of Billroth in Vienna.

ACCIDENTAL INFECTIONS IN BACTERIOLOGICAL LABORATORIES

The breakage of apparatus and spilling of cultures are sometimes responsible for infections in workers in bacteriological laboratories. Apart from such accidents, certain bacteria, rickettsiæ and viruses readily infect the laboratory worker, by passing through the respiratory tract, the skin or the conjunctiva. Laboratory infections have been recorded in men working with *Pasteurella pestis*, *Pfeifferella mallei*, meningoccocus *Brucella melitensis*, *Brucella abortus*, *Brucella suis*, *Francisella tularensis* and the viruses of louping-ill (p. 713), typhus, Q fever, psittacosis, lympho granuloma venereum, enzoötic abortion of ewes, foot-and-mouth disease the Newcastle disease of fowls, Rift-valley fever and yellow fever.

Plague, Glanders, Meningococcal Infections and Tularæmia

In 1903 a young Austrian doctor working in the Koch Institute for Infectious Diseases in Berlin died from plague following an accidental laboratory infection in which he splashed some fluid material from a guinea-pig infected with bubonic plague over an agar plate. In 1906 T. C. Parkinson, working with pneumonic plague at the Elstree branch of the Lister Institute, inhaled the organism and died. About 1905 in a laboratory at Czernowitz a man was centrifuging a glanders suspension when the centrifuge broke, scattering the culture. Four people were infected, and three of them died. It seems that the man responsible for the centrifuging was the one who recovered. In 1925 J. Šolc, of Prague died of acute glanders after inoculating guinea-pigs with material from a post-mortem on a horse (Šikl, 1947). In 1918 F. N. Thorborg died of meningococcal meningitis while employed in the manufacture of anti-meningococcal serum in the State Serum Institute of Copenhagen. At the same time F. Wülff was infected but fortunately recovered. Laboratory workers may become infected by any one of the three strains of undulant fever, but *Brucella melitensis* is the most likely one. Infection is often due to carelessness and poor technique, and it is dangerous to allow inexperienced and non-immune technicians to work with *Br. melitensis*. Tularæmia occurs in laboratory workers, who probably become infected by droplets rom the cough of experimental animals they handle (Ledingham and Fraser, 1924).

Psittacosis, Newcastle Disease and other Virus Infections

In world outbreaks of psittacosis, many bacteriologists and laboratory attendants have been infected while handling material from infected birds p. 716). Lymphogranuloma venereum has been acquired by labora-ory workers as an infection of the upper respiratory tract (Harrop and others, 1941). The virus of enzoötic abortion of ewes, previously un-recognized as a cause of human disease, gave rise to virus pneumonia in a lady doctor whose work involved inoculation of eggs with the virus and the preparation of suspensions from the infected yolk-sacs (Barwell, 1955). Louping-ill is a malady of sheep, endemic in some areas of Scotland. Since the virus was first isolated in 1928, no fewer than four laboratory workers have developed symptoms varying from a mild attack of what was called influenza to a definite encephalitis with headache, vomiting, delir-ium, tremor and lethargy (Rivers and Schwentker, 1934). The virus of the Newcastle disease of fowls has been transmitted to laboratory workers in three cases. The incubation period varied from a few hours to two days. The symptoms and signs were malaise, headache, unilateral superficial conjunctivitis, tenderness and enlargement of the corresponding pre-auricular lymph node, without fever. No involvement of the cornea occurred and all these patients recovered completely within two weeks (Burnet, 1943; Anderson, 1946).

Foot-and-mouth Disease in Laboratory Workers

Authentic cases of foot-and-mouth disease in man are very rare, and they have mostly occurred in laboratory workers. Pape, who with Wald-mann in 1921 discovered the method of infecting guinea-pigs with foot-and-mouth disease, cut his thumb with a broken glass vessel whilst col-lecting virus from a guinea-pig. Two days later he had slight headache and shivering. On the third day vesicles began to develop on the palms and soles and continued to appear at these sites, but not elsewhere, for two days. There were twenty-five vesicles in all, varying in size from 2 to 8 millimetres in diameter. They contained clear fluid and rapidly healed without suppuration. The only buccal lesion was a slight swelling and tenderness on the gum on one side at the time of the cutaneous eruption. This occurred before the discovery of the susceptibility of guinea-pigs, and no animals were inoculated, but Pape, when later inoculated with foot-and-mouth virus, proved to be immune. In 1922 several cases of vesicular stomatitis, sometimes with vesicles on the hands also, occurred in the prov-ince of Como, where there was an epizoötic of foot-and-mouth disease. Clear fluid from the vesicles of one of these patients with bullous stomatitis was taken to Milan and inoculated by Pancera into guinea-pigs and a calf, all of which developed typical lesions (Arkwright, 1928).

Danger from Neurotropic Viruses

The virus of Rift-valley fever has been responsible for numerou laboratory infections, although the mode of infection is unknown. The onset of the illness is abrupt, with malaise and headache. The temperature rises to 102° or 104° F., and pain occurs in the extremities and joints. There may be nausea, vomiting and epigastric discomfort associated with tender ness. Photophobia and conjunctival injection are common. The disease usually lasts only a few days and recovery is rapid. A fatal outcome is rare but unfortunately one of the laboratory workers died as a result of thrombo phlebitis in the seventh week of the illness (Schwentker and Rivers, 1934) The death of W. Brebner in 1932 led directly to the discovery of a new neurotropic virus. He was only twenty-nine years of age and was engaged in experimental work on poliomyelitis in New York. He was bitten slightly on the hand by an apparently healthy monkey, and a vesicular lesion ac companied by some lymphangitis appeared at the site of trauma. Thirteen days later he developed an ascending myelitis, to which he succumbed on the eighteenth day. His heroic death is recorded in the cold language of a scientific communication in which he is referred to as "the human case," thus, "in subsequent discussions the virus isolated from spleen, brain and cord of the human case will be called the B virus" (Sabin and Wright, 1934) The Brebner virus has since been responsible for another case of ascend ing myelitis in a laboratory attendant accustomed to handling monkeys

Direct Infection with Yellow Fever

Since the introduction of the rhesus monkey in the study of yellow fever various laboratory workers have acquired the disease, not through the agency of infected mosquitoes but by direct contamination with infective blood or tissues. Until 1928 investigations on yellow fever were invariably conducted in countries where it was endemic, and for this reason when members of the medical, laboratory and nursing staff developed the disease infection was attributed as a matter of course to the bite of the natural vector, *Aëdes argenteus* (*Stegomyia fasciata*). The tragic deaths of Guillet Adrian Stokes, William Young and Noguchi on the West Coast of Africa dramatically directed attention to the dangers of direct infection. As a result of the death of Adrian Stokes, who had not been working with in fected mosquitoes for several months, the passage of the virus through the skin of monkeys was investigated. It was shown that yellow fever resulted if infected blood was merely rubbed on the normal intact skin of the ab domen of *Macacus rhesus*. These experimental results did not determine whether the virus was capable of penetrating the unimpaired skin of the human hand, which is thicker and denser in texture than that of the monkey.

Yellow Fever in Clinical Laboratory Technicians

In the case of Adrian Stokes several abrasions were recorded as being present, but three cases have since been published which illustrate the important fact that in man the virus of yellow fever is capable of penetrating the intact skin of the hands. These three patients were laboratory workers in London who became directly infected with a Brazilian strain of yellow fever (Low and Fairley, 1931). The first patient was a youth aged seventeen who became infected by handling *Macacus rhesus* in the laboratory where experimental investigations on yellow fever were in progress. The second patient, a man of twenty-eight, estimated the bilirubin and urea on specimens of blood which had been collected from the first patient and sent from the ward to the laboratory. Both these men recovered. The third patient, a laboratory technician aged twenty-one, had performed a blood count of the second patient and for this purpose had collected the blood himself. After an incubation period of ten days he became severely ill with yellow fever, and in spite of the use of convalescent serum he died on the fifth day of the illness. These events emphasize the danger to those who make routine blood examinations in cases of yellow fever during the first four days of the illness, and probably also in the incubation period. In all cases where yellow fever is suspected, gloves should invariably be worn when blood is taken.

Death Roll of Scientific Workers

In addition to those mentioned above, the following lost their lives in investigating the diseases with which their names are associated: J. W. Lazear (yellow fever), D. A. Carrion (verrugas), T. Carbone and A. MacFadyen (Malta fever), J. E. Dutton (African relapsing fever), A. W. Bacot (typhus), T. B. McClintick (Rocky Mountain fever) and W. R. Price (kala-azar). A group of micro-organisms with characteristics intermediate between bacteria and viruses has been named rickettsiæ after Howard Taylor Ricketts, Professor of Pathology in the University of Chicago. In 1906 he demonstrated the transmission of Rocky Mountain fever by the bite of infected ticks and described the causative agent in their eggs. Four years later he went to Mexico to study tabardillo and found in this disease small organisms similar to those in Rocky Mountain spotted fever. He became infected with tabardillo, Mexican typhus, and died of it at the early age of 39. Stanislaus von Prowazek was an Austrian who studied in Prague and Vienna and became director of the zoological department at the Institute of Tropical Medicine in Hamburg. In 1914 he went to Belgrade and Constantinople to study typhus fever and in 1915 died of this disease when he was only 40. He found the typhus fever organisms identical with those which Ricketts had previously described. In honour of these two men the virus of louse-borne typhus has been named *Rickettsia prowazeki*.

Preventive Measures

The laboratory worker is often exposed to an atmosphere contaminated by infected droplets especially where techniques used in the study of viruses include the mechanical fragmentation of infected animal tissues.

Both the scientist and his technicians must be educated and regularly reminded to protect themselves and not merely their cultures against infection. Directors of laboratories should make it clear that they will not tolerate carelessness and poor technique, and they should never allow inexperienced technicians to handle hose animals, organisms or cultures which are known to be the most dangerous. Where possible, the worker

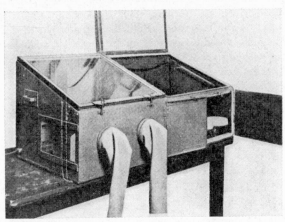

Fig. 452.—Ventilated Inoculation Box connected to a Chimney carrying a Gas Burner and an Exhaust Fan. Note Rubber Sleeves into which the Bacteriologist inserts his Hands

(*Van den Ende, M.* (1943), *J. Hyg.*, **43**, *189*)

must be immunized against the organism which he handles. Protective gowns, gloves and masks must be worn, and washed and sterilized at frequent intervals. Direct pipetting of cultures and other dangerous materials must be forbidden. Spilled material should be treated with a bactericidal agent, and glassware such as pipettes, tubes and rods placed in a bath containing an antiseptic solution immediately after use. Used petri dishes and flasks should also be placed in such baths or covered and autoclaved before being cleaned.

Safe Inoculation of Animals with Dangerous Pathogens

With dangerous pathogens such as the rickettsiæ of typhus fever, or the viruses of lymphogranuloma venereum and psittacosis, great care must be taken by the operator against the dissemination and inhalation of infective droplets. To minimize the risk to laboratory workers who employ the intranasal route of infection of mice with dangerous pathogens, van den Ende (1943) designed an inoculation box in which powerful through-draught ventilation was provided by a chimney carrying a gas burner and an exhaust fan. The operator wears a surgical gown and rubber gloves. His hands are introduced through rubber sleeves into the left-hand compartment of the box (fig. 452). Anæsthetized mice are handed in through a door on the left (fig. 453). When inoculated, the mice are placed in glass jars, which are then covered with lids and pushed across to the right-hand compartment. When he has finished the work the operator withdraws his arms and removes his gloves and gown for sterilization. As an additional

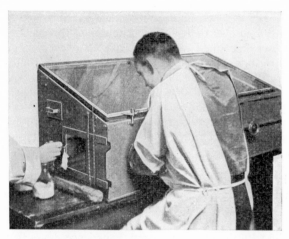

FIG. 453.—An Anæsthetized Mouse is about to be passed through the Door on the left. When he has inoculated it the Bacteriologist will place it in a Glass Jar, cover it with a lid and pass it across to the right-hand Compartment of the Box

(*Van den Ende, M.* (*1943*), *J. Hyg.*, **43**, *189*)

safeguard against the spread of infective droplets, each compartment is provided with a quartz-jacketed ultra-violet lamp which is turned on after the mice have been inoculated. They are exposed to the lamp for one hour before being removed from the box.

ACCIDENTS IN AGRICULTURAL WORK

Although the *Factory Act, 1833*, laid down that paid professional inspectors should be employed by the Government to make regular visits to factory premises, the agricultural labourer, forestry worker, herdsman, horticulturalist, nurseryman, gardener and farmer were neglected. Except for the *Threshing Machines Act, 1878*, and the *Chaff-Cutting Machines (Accidents) Act, 1897*, no further legislation was introduced to safeguard the health of such workers until the passing of the *Agriculture (Poisonous Substances) Act, 1952*, and the *Agriculture (Safety, Health and Welfare Provisions) Act, 1956*. In 1964 in the U.S.A. 8,300 farm workers died as a result of accidents on the land, while a further 760,000 suffered injuries, which were often severe, particularly those caused by machinery (Knapp, 1966).

Common Causes of Accidents

Because of the extremely wide variety of jobs done by a farmer o
farm-worker the risks to which he is exposed are infinitely varied. The
cover such things as the use of a wide range of field and barn machinery
the handling of animals, gunshot wounds, injuries to the back, falls o
every kind, cuts inflicted by hand tools, and electrocution. More super
vision is required over the defective condition of the floors of barns an
lofts, and over ropes and ladders which tend to rot for want of being kep
in dry places. Bridges which are unsafely constructed or unfenced resul
in injuries to farm workers. Physical safeguards such as hand-rail, mid
rail and toe-board should be standard fittings to all bridges and othe
elevated platforms. Serious eye injuries, often with loss of vision, occur i
hedging, ditching and working on stacks. All workers should be taught t
wear goggles while performing these tasks.

Danger from Bulls

The most dangerous animal on a farm is the bull. He is immensel
strong and quite unpredictable. There have been many instances wher
a bull has appeared to be quite docile for months and even years, the
suddenly for no apparent reason he has turned on the stockman an
mauled him with the utmost savagery. Experience shows that in genera
the small dairy breeds are more vicious than the larger and heavie
animals. Nevertheless, if proper precautions are taken the presence of
bull on a farm is not in itself a danger. He needs to be housed in condition
where he has light, shelter, facilities for exercise, and where he can se
other animals and men as they go about. The bull pen should be s
constructed that he can be fed and watered without anyone having to g
inside. Means should be available for securing him so that the pen ca
be cleaned out. Handling equipment, for example a bull pole, must b
strong enough for the purpose. Most accidents of this kind occur because
after a long period of good behaviour, the stockman is lulled into such
sense of security that he becomes careless in the precautions that h
knows he should take. In consequence, he is totally unprepared for tha
sudden savage attack that so often takes place without any warning. Goo
housing, sound equipment, and constant vigilance are essential to preven
accidents with bulls. Dehorning of cattle has been a feature of anima
husbandry practice for some years, and at one time it seemed that thi
would make the bull more or less harmless. The theory was that if yo
take away his capacity for goring people he would have no means left t
inflict serious harm on those who had to handle him and care for hi
necessities. To the surprise of some people, the bull changed his tactic
but not his nature. He still had his enormous strength, a head as hard a
iron, and his weight, and there continue to be incidents where the dehorne
bull butts his victim to the ground with blows like a battering ram an
then proceeds to kneel on him and at the same time deliver swinging blow
with his head. The consequences may be less spectacular but the resul

is that the victim is either killed or suffers severe crush injuries. Dehorning is no guarantee of safety, neither is it any substitute for good housing, careful handling, and constant vigilance. In recent years the bull population on farms has decreased as a result of artificial insemination. This has led to a reduction in bull accidents. In 1964 in Great Britain there were four fatal accidents and 102 non-fatal compared with six and 141 the previous year (Wilson, 1966).

Danger from other Farm Animals

The farm labourer frequently suffers injury when his foot is trodden on while he leads horses or cows. The provision of boots with a strong toecap would prevent this. It should be remembered that even cows and pigs can be vicious if molested when they have young. Pigs do not normally attack anyone, although the odd bad-tempered boar may occasionally do so. Caution is, however, needed when entering a pen containing a sow with a newly-born litter. She may well attack in the supposed defence of her young. A pig has two very long tusks in the lower jaw, and the attack consists of throwing the head upwards in such a way that one of the tusks can rip the leg of an intruder, causing a deep wound with the added risk that it may become infected. A light board carried by the stockman and held between the pig and his own leg gives adequate protection. The following unusual accidents are worth recording. A woman was attacked by a bantam cockerel which pecked viciously at her legs; a varicose vein was pierced and death followed. An elderly man was counting sheep as they followed each other through a gap in a hedge; four or five sheep made a rush for the gap knocking the man down. He broke his femur and died from shock.

Extension of Mechanization

Since about 1920 there has been a great increase in the use of tractors and other mechanical and electrical tools on farms and in dairies. Serious and fatal accidents are increasing with the extension of mechanization. Power-driven belts, shafting, chain and gear drives, saws, cutting blades and shears should be fitted with adequate guards. Electrocution accidents occur when elevators contact overhead electric wires during stack-building operations and when dairymen handle electrically operated pasteurizing plant which is not properly earthed. Exposure of machinery to the weather causes deterioration and sometimes snapping of parts, with the consequent risk of injury to the operator. Sack-lifters and jacks are constantly causing accidents because the ratchet or cogs have become worn.

Tractor Accidents

In 1955 there were 470,000 tractors in use on the farms of Great Britain leading to 25,000 accidents a year, 150 of them fatal. If allowed to stand in the open all night tractors frequently backfire, causing serious injury in some cases, whereas if they were adapted to the use of self-starters this risk would be avoided. A frequent cause of accidents when oiling up is the use of the grease gun with the engine running. Entanglement with the fan belt may then mean loss of fingers or a broken forearm. Tractor drivers, farmers and cowmen may be run over and killed by their own tractors. The most frequent cause of such accidents is the attempt to operate the clutch whilst dismounted in order to reverse the tractor slowly to couple it to a trailer. The existing clutch should be modified so that a hand lever working on the principle of the dead man's handle can be used for this purpose by a driver standing on the ground. The Ministry issues a free leaflet called *Why Tractors Overturn*, which lists the dangerous situations and how to avoid them. It gives this advice:

> Drive slowly over rough ground.
> Slow down before turning.
> Use a wide headland.
> Keep clear of ditches and banks.
> Avoid steep slopes.
> Extend the wheels in hilly country.
> Never hitch above drawbar level.
> See to regular maintenance.

In spite of the provisions of the *Act of 1956* the Ministry of Agriculture reported in 1961 that deaths from tractors overturning accounted for one-third of all deaths in agricultural work and that these figures were higher than those for 1960.

Urgent Need of Drastic Safety Measures

In an industry which is being increasingly mechanized and often manned by people new to the implements and plant employed, it is time that drastic safety measures were imposed by law. Since man failure is the prime cause of all accidents, methods for training farm workers in safety principles should be universally adopted. Nevertheless, at least 25 per cent of accidents are easily preventable by technical measures which are a safeguard even against ignorance, stupidity or wilful disregard of personal danger. We know that mechanical guarding and engineering revision are important factors in preventing the most serious injuries, and it is therefore an urgent matter that manufacturers should incorporate more safeguards in agricultural machinery. Systems should be inaugurated whereby farmers can get advice on hazards as well as skilled investigations of accidents that occur. Owing to the dispersal and mobility of both men and machines it is difficult to secure and maintain as high a standard of safety in agricultural work as it is in factories, but this is no excuse for apathy and inactivity (Botham and Winbolt, 1950).

An Act Safeguarding Agricultural Workers

Based on some of the recommendations made in 1949 by the Gowers Committee on health, welfare and safety in non-industrial employment, the *Agriculture (Safety, Health and Welfare Provisions) Act, 1956* enables the Agricultural Ministers to make protective regulations. These deal, among other things, with the safeguarding of workers from dangerous parts of machines, with the training or supervision of young persons when working with prescribed machines, and with the protection of workers from the risk of falls and strains. The maximum loads which workers may lift under different circumstances may be specified. The Act also provides for notices to be served requiring the provision of sanitary and washing facilities; and the Ministers may make regulations for the provision of movable sanitary facilities where workers are employed by a contractor or other person who is not the occupier of the land. In addition the Act provides that children under 13 years of age are prohibited from riding on or driving prescribed vehicles, machinery, or implements used in agriculture. All agricultural units are required to have a first-aid box whose contents are laid down by regulations. Regulations require the notification and keeping of records of accidents and certain diseases connected with agricultural work. The Act also makes certain rules concerning inquests on deaths which may have been caused by agricultural operations.

INJURIES FROM ANIMALS, REPTILES, INSECTS AND FISH

Various animals, reptiles, insects, fish and other marine creatures may attack or otherwise harm workmen, technicians and professional men and women carrying out their work.

Injuries from Animals

Men liable in the course of their work to be injured by animals include big-game hunters, biologists, brush salesmen, carters, cavalrymen, coachmen (p. 733), cowmen, explorers, farm labourers (p. 1165), forestry workers, fowlers, gamekeepers, grooms, horticultural workers (p. 1165), hunters, laboratory workers (p. 1160), missionaries, ostlers, postmen, poultry farmers (p. 716), shepherds (p. 713), stablemen, swineherds (p. 713), teamsters, trappers, veterinary surgeons, zoo keepers, breeders of dogs, cats, rabbits, birds, silver foxes, crocodiles and alligators, pet-shop salesmen (p. 711), wild-animal tamers, trainers and dealers, as well as sportsmen shooting deer and game. Not only are they exposed to the risk of being bitten by the animals concerned and to blows from hooves, horns and tails, but also they may be hurt by the instruments they use including firearms, knives, saws, shears, chaff-cutting and threshing machines, electrical equipment, tractors and traps (p. 1167). In 1843 in Bechuanaland the Rev. Dr. David Livingstone helping to rid a village in the Mabotsa Valley of marauding lions was mauled by the biggest lion in the neighbourhood (fig. 454). The animal sprang at him, seized him by the left shoulder, broke his humerus and shook him until he was dazed. He wrote in his diary—"Besides crunching the bone into splinters, he left eleven teeth wounds on the upper part of my arm. I have escaped

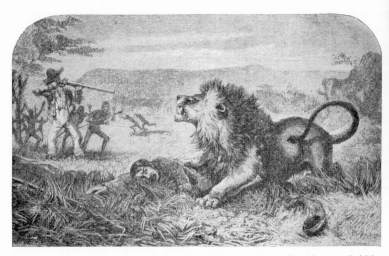

FIG. 454.—Escape of the Rev. Dr. David Livingstone from a lion that mauled him
(*After J. W. Whymper*)

with only the inconvenience of a false joint in my limb" (Livingstone, 1857). In 1850 a gentle lady Ellen Bright was fatally mauled by a lion she was taming in the famous circus of Lord John Sanger to whom she was distantly related.

Dog Bites infected with *Pasteurella septica*

In Great Britain dog bites are common, postmen, brush salesmen and veterinary surgeons being the favourite victims. Like all animal bites they tend to heal slowly. They are often infected, the usual organisms being *Pasteurella septica* and *Hæmophilus bronchisepticus* derived from the animal's mouth and they have caused tetanus. But since we have no rabies in Great Britain dog bites are not taken very seriously. Because of a large reservoir of wild canines, to say nothing of bats, it has been impossible so far to abolish rabies in North America, and for this reason every dog-bite has a significance which is absent in Great Britain (Parrish and others, 1959). *P. septica* has been reported as an upper-respiratory-tract commensal in dogs, cats, rabbits, pigs and other animals. Wounds infected by this organism are occasionally complicated by infection of underlying bone. Thus osteomyelitis of the jaw has sometimes been recorded following *P. septica* infection of a soft-tissue bite of the face. Infected dog-bites are characterized by prolonged treatment and unsightly scars. Since the bite commonly occurs on the face it is desirable to ensure healing with minimal scarring. All patients with dog-bites should be given tetanus toxoid or antiserum and if the wound is serious prophylactic penicillin therapy should be used. Surgical suture will often be necessary and sometimes the wound must be excised (Lee and Buhr, 1960).

Injuries from Venomous Reptiles

Breeders of snakes, herpetologists (p. 1154), serpent worshippers, snake charmers, fishermen, hunters and trappers may be bitten by various venomous reptiles including land snakes, water snakes, sea snakes, lizards, toads, salamanders and blood-sucking leeches and bats. Among the most deadly of the land snakes are the cobra (*Naja tripudians*), the daboia (*Vipera russelli*), the krait (*Bungarus fasciatus*) and the rattlesnake (*Crotalus terrificus*). Snakes bite man more often by accident than design and in snake country a little knowledge and common sense regarding the habits of snakes, the wearing of strong boots and leggings and the use of torches in walking along roads at night would greatly lessen the incidence of snakebite. Once a lethal dose of venom has been absorbed into the circulation a large dose of specific antivenene given to the patient intravenously and at once is the only measure that will save life. Fortunately poisonous snake-bite is not synonymous with snake-bite poisoning; many do not realize that poisonous snakes often bite without injecting significant venom. It can be assumed that when people accustomed to handling snakes are bitten it will be rare for much venom to be injected. For it often happens that professional herpetologists and snake-charmers are repeatedly bitten and yet survive; Ironmonger (1889) claimed to have been bitten forty-nine times. Poisonous sea snakes especially *Enhydrina schistosa* (Daudin) and *Hydrophis spiralis* (Shaw) abound round the shores of the Indian and western Pacific oceans. Fishermen handle them daily and are sometimes bitten. A survey of the fishing villages in north-west Malaya (Reid and Lim, 1957) showed that of 125 cases the effects were trivial in 55. In severe cases the symptoms and signs were paresis, trismus, dysphagia, ptosis oculi, muscle pains and tenderness and myoglobinuria. Among 44 severe cases, 24 victims returned to work within a week, 12 within one to two weeks, and 8 within one to three months. If paresis was mild, complete recovery occurred within a few days, but if it was moderate or severe it usually took several weeks. The case for the manufacture and use of a polyspecific antivenene is a clear one, but unhappily the work of those who wish to spread education and the means of treatment is often held up because the whole question is bedevilled by superstition and irrational fear. Indeed fear still causes many of the fishermen to hide the fact that they have been bitten at all. On the coast of Malaya sea snakes are readily distinguished from harmless water snakes which are often to be found at the mouths and along the shores of rivers. Of lizards all are harmless except the venomous *Heloderma horridum* which inhabits Mexico and Arizona.

Injuries from Insects

Biologists, apiarists, museum curators, explorers, missionaries, hunters and trappers may be bitten or stung by various insects including spiders, scorpions, centipedes, cockroaches, tarantulas, ants, biting flies, caterpillars, blistering beetles, midges, lice, fleas, bugs, mosquitoes, bees, wasps and hornets. Apart from being stung by insects other reactions are known to occur. Thus the blistering beetles *Cantharis vesicatoria, Mylabris sidæ, M. cichorii* and *M. pustulata* all produce cantharadin and can all cause vesication of the skin by contact. Inhalant allergic symptoms from contact with beetles, bees, flies, cockroaches, locusts and weevils are described on p. 1085. Of poisonous spiders *Latrodectus mactans*, known as the black widow, is dangerous to man. The female often weaves its web on the underside of privies and if disturbed is liable to bite man on the genitals, buttocks or thighs during the act of defæcation. Of poisonous centipedes the tropical species *Scolopendra morsitans* is the most feared. Usually the venoms of scorpions are not seriously toxic although in Manchuria *Buthus martensi* and at Durango in Mexico *Centruroides suffussus* are specially dreaded. Most tarantulas have a fairly innocent bite. Breeders of animals and birds, grooms, coachmen, veterinary surgeons and zoo keepers are liable to infection transmitted from animals and birds including anthrax (p. 721), glanders (p. 733), psittacosis (p. 716), tetanus, tuberculosis, tularæmia, and in some countries rabies. Gamekeepers, hunters and trappers are sometimes exposed to infestations by parasites including wood ticks (*Ixodes ricinus*), pigeon ticks (*Argas reflexus*) and bird lice (*Dermanyssus avium*). The ringworms transmissible to man from animals and birds are described on p. 710.

Athletes' Foot

Ringworm infestations of the glabrous skin may occur in people who frequent public swimming baths, Turkish baths, sports clubs and gymnasia. Unhappily they occur also in miners using pithead baths. *Trichophyton rubrum* is the commonest causative organism but occasionally other dermatophytes are encountered. *Tinea pedis* is spread especially where people mix in bare feet particularly if they share the same bath mats and towels. In the native laundries of India and China the Dhobi (Hindī, Dhōb, washing) often suffers from tinea pedis known as *Dhobi itch*, *Hongkong foot* or *laundrymen's itch*. This is perpetuated because he uses his feet in the process of washing clothes. Occasionally one of his clients develops ringworm of the skin of the chest because of contamination of his underclothing in the wash. *Tinea cruris* is fairly common principally on the inner side of the thighs and on the perineum. It is exacerbated by heat, perspiration and friction; it occurs also in cavalrymen. Athletes' foot is not confined to people living and working in hot climates. Outside the tropics it is kept going by the so-called subtropical micro-climate in rubber slippers or boots. Socks of synthetic fibres can aggravate the condition because the fibres do not imbibe sweat and are therefore responsible for its stagnation and the maceration of the skin. People who frequent swimming baths or Turkish baths should take their own slippers. Nobody should borrow slippers unless it is certain that disinfection has been carried out thoroughly. Persons affected with athletes' foot should be discouraged from frequenting swimming baths. In the home an infected member of the family should have towels, bath-mats, nail-brushes, sponges and soap kept apart for his own use. He should never share slippers with others or walk barefoot about the bedroom floor. In bed he should wear cotton socks to be washed at frequent intervals after boiling. The condition is difficult to cure especially if the toenails or fingernails have become affected. Whitfield's ointment or a cream containing salicylic and benzoic acids are often effective. A thin cotton sock makes a good dressing for the foot.

Attacks by Venomous Fish

Fishermen, sea anglers, shrimpers, bathers and naked divers may be injured by marine creatures. At least 150 varieties of fish, most of which inhabit tropical waters, secrete poisons which they can inject into the skin of man by their teeth, fins or barbs. In addition to painful lesions of the skin and other tissues, these poisons often cause constitutional symptoms. The venomous fish include the spiny dogfish (*Squalus acanthus*), cat-fish, bull trout, fortescue, red rock-cod, sting ray (*Trygon pastinaca*) and sea urchin (*Tripneustes esculentus*). The *Trachinidæ* or weevers inhabit the Atlantic coasts of Europe and Africa. The greater weever (*Trachinus draco*) is only 12 inches long. It hides in shingle at the bottom of the sea farther out than the lesser weever (*T. vipera*), which buries itself close inshore. Both have grooved spines connected with glands which secrete a poisonous fluid. The attack of these fish is followed by severe pain, local irritation, œdema, paralysis of the part, collapse, dyspnœa, delirium and even death within twenty-four hours. The wound may become infected, showing phlegmonous inflammation and even local gangrene. It should be washed with a 10 per cent aqueous solution of potassium permanganate. Infiltration of the tissues with 2 per cent procaine hydrochloride (novocaine) may be required for relief of pain, and morphine may prove necessary too. *Synanceia verrucosa*, found on the coral reefs of the Indian and Pacific Oceans. and also *Scorpæna scropha* may produce similar effects.

Attacks by Jelly-fish

The *Hydrozoa*, sometimes called *Hydromedusæ*, include the jelly-fish or sea-nettles. Jelly-fish life extends into many species. In general, the body, a mass of glossy jelly enclosed between the upper and lower sides of the bell or umbrella, bears a number of tentacles, some of which are provided with stinging-capsules or nematocysts. On contact, these are evaginated like the finger of a glove by a trigger mechanism, causing barbs to enter the skin of the victim, bearing with them a poison. The jelly-fish in the highest form of its development is seen in the *Siphonophora*, of which the genus *Physalia* in sky-blue, orange and other brilliant colours, is well known in the Atlantic, Pacific and Indian Oceans. When exposed to the wind *Physalia physalis* (Linn.) erects a crest resembling a sail so that it appears to swim with its companions in fleets. Since the latter part of the fifteenth century it has been known as the Portuguese man-of-war. It was the Portuguese in the time of Henry the Navigator who had fleets of the then curious, new, light ships called caravels, fitted with fore-and-aft lateen sails and well known to all seamen. The umbrella of *Physalia* is 6 inches in diameter and its stinging tentacles are from 3 to 30 feet long. Following stimulation they contract within a minute to 6 inches (Totton and Mackie, 1960).

Lesions caused by Stinging Tentacles

Its attack causes local inflammation of the skin, varying from a line of urticarial lesions to coagulation necrosis. There is erythema with œdema, itching and burning, sometimes followed by vesicular dermatitis. Systemic symptoms may follow rapidly, including lachrymation, coryza, muscular pains, a feeling of constriction in the chest and dyspnœa. Collapse and death are rare. The treatment for stings is the application of an anti-histamine cream or taking of anti-histamine tablets by mouth. Lane and Dodge (1958) report that nematocysts of *Physalia* on clothing or laboratory surfaces retain their reactivity for at least two weeks, and that surfaces, clothing and skin can be decontaminated by the application of 95 per cent ethyl alcohol. Unfortunately this treatment does not reduce the pain in the skin of stings already received. Small jelly-fish in great numbers frequently get into drift nets and cause painful intensely itching lesions of the skin through their toxin, *thalassine*. In mending such nets, men are at times affected with lachrymation and sneezing so severe as to force them to leave their work. These symptoms are evidently due to dust contaminated with the poison of the jelly-fish. Of the order *Hydroida*, the genus *Obelia* is a small free-swimming jelly-fish commonly found round the shores of Great Britain. Its sting is practically harmless.

Injuries to Naked Sponge-divers by a Sea-anemone

In the Mediterranean and Ægean, naked sponge-divers are often affected by what is known as *la maladie de Skevos Zervos* (1903), after the Greek physician who first established its cause. The men are stung by a sea-anemone, an actinia, *Sargarsia rosea*, which is parasitic on the roots of sponges. It is approximately 4 centimetres long, a polypoid hollow cylinder provided with two rows of graceful tentacles radially arranged which give it the shape of a flower. The sponge-fisherman severs the roots of the sponges with his knife and puts them into a net bag, which hangs around his neck and rests on his naked chest or abdomen. The disturbed actinia stabs its victim on his way to the surface, usually in the chest or abdominal wall, discharging from its mouth a white viscous venom. This produces immediate erythema, and vesicles develop within a few minutes. The initial lesion becomes red and swollen, and then changes to deep purple. Besides local pain, headache, nausea, vomiting, fever and rigors may occur. The wound is slow to heal and multiple abscesses and sloughing of the skin occur in some cases. In one instance exfoliation of the entire skin of the penis occurred. The initial lesion should be washed with a weak acid such as vinegar, and a bland oil applied.

Attacks on Man by the Shark and Other Fish

Of non-poisonous sea and river creatures, the shark, barracuda, caribi piranha, seal, conger-eel, skate and octopus occasionally attack men. Of the many hundreds of kinds of sharks only about ten or twelve are suspected of being man-killers. Probably the most dangerous is the great white shark (*Carcharodon rondeleti*). Shark attacks occur over large areas of the earth's surface. Most reports of attacks have come from South Africa, the Persian Gulf, Australia, the Caribbean, the United States and Central

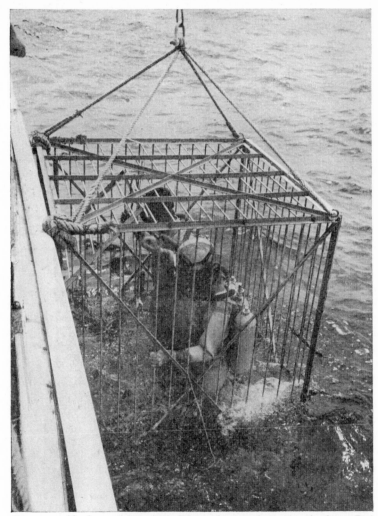

FIG. 455.—Shark-proof Cage. Two Divers about to descend to the Ocean Bed in an Oil Survey at Abu Dhabi
(*By courtesy of Anglo-Iranian Oil Co., Ltd.*)

America. Their victims include men, women, children, swimmers, skin divers, spearfishermen, pearl divers, shipwrecked sailors, ditched airmen and divers employed in off-shore drilling for oil companies (fig. 455). Sharks attack in all sorts of weather, calm or rough water, harbours, inlets, lakes and rivers in all depths of water and at distances varying from the open sea to a few feet from the shore. Wounds of shark victims are often baffling. Many of them are multiple and distributed over several parts of the body even after a single attack. Most are found on the legs, buttocks, arms and shoulders. Not all the injuries are due to bites. Sharks can also cause severe injuries and even amputation of portions of extremities by their fins or the impact of their rough speeding bodies against their victims. Rescuers frequently display great courage, although it is rare for them to be attacked or injured. The mortality rate of victims is high, chiefly on account of shock and loss of blood and the fact that most attacks occur in areas where little or no first aid facilities or skilled medical attention are available. Many victims die during rescue or on the way to hospital (Coppleson, 1965). Workers at the Oceanographic Research Institute at Durban, South Africa, deserve special mention for the remarkable success of their immediate first-aid methods. They treat the patient on the beach, allowing thirty minutes or even an hour to elapse before sending the victim to hospital. They rush the transfusions to the patient rather than the patient to the transfusions. As to the dress-diver he often carries a knife or spear as a defence against attack. Should a shark approach him he will not attempt to escape, for on the way up the shark might tear off his legs or kill him. So the diver will stand his ground because it is the safest thing to do, and usually he will scare the shark off by letting a great gush of air escape from the outlet valve of his helmet. Occasionally he has to fight a shark, and if he kills it he has its body hauled up to the salvage ship so that it will not attract other sharks. In tropical seas the octopus is large enough to hold a man in its tentacles, and this is what the diver really fears. If a large octopus seizes him, he must fight for his life. The tentacles, with their suckers, will wind all over him and so hamper his movements that his one hope is to reach the surface quickly. The men who have hauled him up must then hack the octopus to pieces to release him (Davis, 1951).

Conjunctivitis, Keratitis and Dermatitis in Fishermen

Fishermen and others who handle fish may suffer from conjunctivitis and erythema of the eyelids from toxic substances in the blood of eels. Keratitis sometimes occurs among fishmongers who deal in oysters, and is apparently due to minute fragments of shell which lodge in the eye during the process of opening oysters. *Dogger Bank itch* is an eczematous dermatitis observed in North Sea fishermen, particularly those fishing the Dogger Bank area. It is due to contact with the sea-chervil, a seaweed-like animal colony, *Alcyonidium hirsutum*. The sea-chervil is landed, sometimes in large quantities, in the nets with the fish and is thrown back into the sea. The dermatitis starts on the hands and clears when the fisherman goes ashore. On returning to fishing, increasingly severe attacks develop, with a blistered and œdematous eruption on the hands and arms, face and legs. Patch tests with material expressed from the chervil are positive in affected subjects and negative in controls. Both Weil's disease (p. 736) and erysipeloid of Rosenbach (p. 744) may occur in those who handle fish.

BIBLIOGRAPHY

ADAMSON, J. B. (1954), Personal communication.
ANDERSON, S. G. (1946), *Med. J. Aust.*, **1**, 371.
ARKWRIGHT, J. A. (1928), *Lancet*, **1**, 1191.
BARTLETT, SIR C. (1954), *Proc. Nat. Industr. Safety Conf.*, Ro.S.P.A., London, p. 5.
BARWELL, C. F. (1955), *Lancet*, **2**, 1369.
BELL, J. H. (1952), *The Sewerman at Work*, Highways Committee, Corporation of Glasgow.
BÖHLER, L. (1935), *The Treatment of Fractures*, 4th English Ed., Wright, Bristol.
BOTHAM, H., and WINBOLT, H. G. (1950), *The Farmer's Weekly*, **32**, 55.
BOWN, A. H. J. (1954), *Proc. Nat. Industr. Safety Conf.*, Ro.S.P.A., London, p. 52.
BURNET, F. M. (1943), *Med. J. Aust.*, **2**, 313.
CLAYTON-COOPER, B., and WILLIAMS, R. E. O. (1945), *Brit. J. industr. Med.*, **2**, 146.
COLEBROOK, L., DUNCAN, J. M., and ROSS, W. P. D. (1948), *Lancet*, **1**, 893.
COOMBES, B. L. (1945), *Miner's Day*, Penguin Books, London.
COPPLESON, SIR VICTOR M. (1965), *Roche Image*, London.
CRITCHLEY, M. (1934), *Lancet*, **1**, 68.
DAVIS, SIR R. H. (1951), *Deep Diving and Submarine Operations*, St. Catherine Press, London.
DEAN, G. (1954), *Report on the Atom*, Eyre and Spottiswoode, London.
DUGUID, L. N. (1949), Personal communication.
ELWELL, E. G. (1934), *Brit. med. J.*, **2**, 771.
VAN DEN ENDE, M. (1943), *J. Hyg.*, **43**, 189.
ENDEAN, R. (1967), Personal communication.
FARMER, E. (1932), *The Causes of Accidents*, London.
FARMER, E., and CHAMBERS, E. G. (1929), *Industr. Hlth. Res. Bd. Rep.*, No. 55.
FARMER, E., CHAMBERS, E. G., and KIRK, F. J. (1933), *Ibid.*, No. 68.
FITZSIMONS, M. P. (1944), *Brit. J. industr. Med.*, **1**, 235.
FREUD, S. (1922), *Introductory Lectures on Psychoanalysis*, Allen and Unwin, London.
GISSANE, W., MILES, A. A., and WILLIAMS, R. E. O. (1944), *Brit. J. industr. Med.*, **1**, 90.
GREENWOOD, M., and WOODS, H. M. (1919), *Industr. Fatig. Res. Bd., Rep.* No. 4.
GRIFFITHS, H. E. (1949), "The Burgeon in Industry," *Proc. Ninth Intern. Congr. Industr. Med., London*, Wright, Bristol.

HALDANE, J. S. (1926), *Historical Review of Coal Mining*, Fleetway Press, London, p. 266.

HARROP, G. A., RAKE, G. W., and SHAFFER, M. F. (1941), *Trans. Amer. Climat. (clin.) Ass.*, **56**, 154.

HARTMANN, I. (1948), in *Industrial Hygiene and Toxicology*, edited by Frank A. Patty, Interscience Publishers Inc., New York, Vol. 1, p. 439.

HELWIG, F. C. (1940), *J. Amer. med. Ass.*, **115**, 291.

HUGHES, J. P. W. (1956), *Brit. med. J.*, **1**, 852.

HUNTER, C. (1961), Personal communication.

HUNTER, L. (1961), Personal communication.

IRONMONGER, C. J. (1889), *Pacif. rur. Pr.*, **38**, 67.

JELLINEK, S. (1932), *Wien. klin. Wschr.*, **45**, 33.

JEX-BLAKE, A. J. (1945), *E. Afr. Med. J.*, **22**, 170.

JONES, S., and TIDESWELL, F. V. (1947), *The Prevention of Coal Dust Explosions*, Ministry of Fuel and Power, Safety in Mines Research Board, Paper No. 105, H.M.S.O., London.

JUNG, C. G. (1928), *Two Essays on Analytical Psychology*, London.

KNAPP, L. W. (1966), *Brit. med. J.*, **2**, 1132.

LANE, C. E., and DODGE, E. (1958), *Biol. Bull.*, **115**, 219.

LANER, S., and SELL, R. G. (1960), *Occupational Psychology*, **34**, 153.

LEDINGHAM, J. C. G., and FRASER, F. R. (1924), *Quart. J. Med.*, **17**, 365.

LEE, M. L. H., and BUHR, A. J. (1960), *Brit. med. J.*, **1**, 169.

LING, T. M., and O'MALLEY, C. J. S. (1958), *Rehabilitation after Illness and Accident*, Ballière, Tindall and Cox, London.

LIVINGSTONE, D. (1857), *Missionary Travels and Researches in South Africa*, John Murray, London, p. 11.

LOW, G. C., and FAIRLEY, N. M. (1931), *Brit. med. J.*, **1**, 125.

MacCALLUM, W. G. (1930), *William Stewart Halsted*, Johns Hopkins Press, Baltimore.

McCULLOUGH, T. W. (1961), *Ann. Rep. of the Chief Inspector of Factories for 1960*, Cmd. 1479, H.M.S.O., London.

McLINTOCK, J. S. (1953), *Brit. med. J.*, **1**, 1451.

MAIMAN, T. H. (1960), *Nature, Lond.*, **187**, 493.

MANN, I. (1947), *Brit. J. Ophthl.*, **31**, 40.

MOSCOWITZ, S. (1948), *New York State Department of Labor, Div. Industr. Hyg. Monthly Review*, **27**, 29.

NEWBOLD, E. M. (1926), *Industr. Fatig. Res. Bd. Rep.*, No. 34.

NICOLL, E. A. (1946), Personal communication.

NORRIS, D. C. (1951), "Industrial Injuries" in *Brit. Encyl. Med. Practice*, 2nd ed., **7**, 91.

PARRISH, H. M., CLACK, F. B., BROBST, D., and MOCK, J. F. (1959), *Publ. Hlth. Rep., Wash.*, **74**, 891.

PIETERS, H. A. J., and CREYGHTON, J. W. (1957), *Safety in the Chemical Laboratory*, 2nd ed., Butterworth, London.

RAWLINSON, J. (1955), *Centenary of London's Main Drainage*, London County Council, Staples Press, London.

REID, H. A., and LIM, K. J. (1957), *Brit. med. J.*, **2**, 1266.

RIVERS, T. M., and SCHWENTKER, F. F. (1934), *J. exp. Med.*, **59**, 669.

ROSS, T. A. (1937), *The Common Neuroses*, Arnold, London.

SABIN, A. B., and WRIGHT, A. M. (1934), *J. exp. Med.* **59**, 115.

SCHWENTKER, F. F., and RIVERS, T. M. (1934), *Ibid.*, **59**, 305.

ŠIKL, H. (1947), Personal communication.

SMITH, E. B. (1960), *Safety in Mines Research Establishment Bibliography*, 2nd ed., Ministry of Power, Sheffield.

STATHAM, I. C. F. (1951), *Coalmining*, English Universities Press, London.

SWANN, H. W. (1946), *Annual Report of the Chief Inspector of Factories for the Year 1945*, H.M.S.O., Cmd. 6992, p. 36; (1949), *Proc. Ninth Intern. Cong. Industr. Med., London*, Wright, Bristol, p. 1044.

TASKER, J. R. (1949), *Brit. med. J.*, **2**, 362.

TOTTON, A. K., and MACKIE, G. O. (1960), *Discovery Reports: Studies on Physalia physalis* (L.), **30**, 301, Cambridge University Press.

VERNON, H. M. (1918), *Accidents and Their Prevention*, Cambridge University Press, Cambridge.

WALSHE, Sir Francis (1958), *Medical Press*, **239**, 493.

WATROUS, R. M. (1947), *Brit. J. industr. Med.*, **4**, 111.

WHITFIELD, J. W. (1954), *Ibid.*, **11**, 126.

WILLIAMS, R. E. O., and CAPEL, E. H. (1945), *Ibid.*, **2**, 217.

WILLIAMS, R. E. O., and MILES, A. A. (1945), *J. Path. Bact.*, **57**, 27.

WILSON, G. S. (1966), *Brit. J. industr. Med.*, **23**, 1.

ZERVOS, S. (1903), *Comptes rendus du 2ᵉ Congrès médical panhéllénique à Athènes*, Athens, p. 365.

APPENDIX

At the time of going to press (10 Sept. 1968) sixteen medical men and one scientist working in occupational hygiene joined Professor Ronald E. Lane of Manchester in signing the following statement for publication in the medical press. Their combined experience of lead exposure and lead poisoning gathered in Great Britain, the U.S.A., France, Italy, Holland, Sweden and Yugoslavia is considerable.

The Diagnosis of Inorganic Lead Poisoning

Because of varying opinions on the diagnosis of inorganic lead poisoning which appear in the international literature, the signatories hope that the following statement may be of value. The statement is intended to provide guidance for hospital medical staff, industrial medical officers and other medical practitioners, in the examination of cases of suspected lead poisoning in adults.

A diagnosis of lead poisoning should be based on clinical findings and supported by biochemical evidence of excessive lead absorption, and if possible by evidence of unusual exposure.

There are varying degrees of lead absorption. The Table, which is based on personal experience and published data, lists biochemical tests for estimating the degree of lead absorption and the values likely to be found in four arbitrary categories of lead absorption. The values apply to estimations made *concurrently* with exposure and *concurrently* with the onset of symptoms. The values may be significantly lower a few weeks after cessation of exposure.

The four arbitrary categories are:

A. Absorption found in the 'normal' population when there has been no occupational or abnormal exposure.

B. Increased absorption resulting from occupational or abnormal exposure which is occupationally acceptable. At these levels of lead absorption the mild symptoms listed below, which are common to a number of minor complaints, are not attributable to lead.

C. Increased absorption from excessive occupational or other exposure which may be associated with mild symptoms or signs (see below) or, rarely, with severe symptoms or signs. Even in the absence of symptoms and signs these levels of absorption are unacceptable because of the possibility of toxic episodes and long term sequelae.

D. Dangerous absorption from occupational or other exposure in which mild, and severe, symptoms and also long term sequelae are increasingly probable.

Table VI

Categories of Lead Absorption

The values given below will not necessarily apply in cases where there is a lowered haemoglobin concentration, or where chelating agents, for example EDTA, have been used.

TEST	A Normal	B Acceptable	C Excessive	D Dangerous
Blood Lead	< 40 µg/100 ml	40–80 µg/100 ml	80–120 µg/100 ml	> 120 µg/100 ml
Urinary Lead	< 80 µg/l	80–150 µg/l	150–250 µg/l	> 250 µg/l
Urinary coproporphyrin	< 150 µg/l	150–500 µg/l	500–1500 µg/l	> 1500 µg/l
Urinary δ-aminolaevulinic acid	< 0·6 mg/100 ml	0·6–2 mg/100 ml	2–4 mg/100 ml	> 4 mg/100 ml

Blood and urinary lead determinations can only be relied upon when carried out in laboratories experienced in the techniques. Even so errors of ±10% may be expected.

Urinary samples of S. G. less than 1·010 are unreliable and should be rejected. 24 hr. samples or repeated spot samples are desirable.

A measurement of haemoglobin is important additional evidence; a lowered haemoglobin concentration is commonly found in lead poisoning and may be associated with categories C or D.

Punctate basophil counts, though still used, are less reliable than the tests shown in the Table, and are not advised.

Clinical Findings

Mild symptoms and signs of lead poisoning include: tiredness; lassitude; constipation; slight abdominal discomfort or pain; anorexia; altered sleep; irritability; anaemia; pallor; and, less frequently, diarrhoea and nausea. Many of these are symptoms of other, sometimes trivial, complaints and it is therefore essential for a correct diagnosis of lead poisoning that the symptoms and signs be associated with laboratory evidence of excessive absorption and that other causes be excluded.

The presence of a blue line in the gums and of a metallic taste are useful indicators of increased lead absorption.

Severe symptoms and signs include severe intermittent abdominal pain (colic); reduction of muscle power, e.g. wrist drop; muscle tenderness; paraethesiae; and other symptoms or signs of neuropathy, or encephalopathy. In a lead worker these is strong evidence of poisoning but supporting laboratory evidence of high lead absorption should be obtained.

Comments

The incidence of sequelae increases not only with an increase in absorption, when the latter is excessive, but also with the length of time that this absorption is allowed to continue. Therefore biochemical indications of excessive absorption, with or without clinical manifestations of poisoning, should be followed by appropriate industrial and/or medical action.

INDEX

Doyle, Sir A. Conan, 789
DPTF, 396
Drainage, 26, 33, 92, 93
Drapers' cramp, 879
Drebbel, Cornelius, 86
Drifter, 224, 982
Drikold, 654
Drinker respirator, the, 648
Drosophila melanogaster, 925
Druggets, 37
Drummers' cramp, 879
Drury Lane, 96
Dry batteries, 460, 461, 464
cleaning, 284, 579, 594, 603, 605, 607, 610, 613
ice, 654
murrain, 486
Drying of hats, 303
Drysalters' itch, 769
Dry shampoo, 607, 609
Dubini, Angelo, 750
Duck, 712
feathers, 767
fever, 767
Duckering process, 729
Duisberg, Carl, 153
Dukeron, 603
Dulong, Pierre Louis, 1148
Dunlop, J. B., 634
Dunraven, Lord, 139
Dupuytren's contracture, 757, 888
Duralumin, 164, 166, 1057
Durham oxen, 50
Dust,
altitude, effect on inhalation, 966
animal, 965, 1083–6
bone, 707, 1084
feathers, 707, 767
fur, 295, 707, 1084
hair, 707, 1084
horn, 707, 1084
ivory, 707, 1084
leather, 707
silk, 707, 1084
wool, 707, 1084
artificial corundum, 1058
bauxite, 1056
benign,
alabaster, 371–3
aluminium, 1008, 1055–8
oxide, 1055–8
anhydrite, 372
barium, 1053
calcium carbonate, 360
sulphate, 371
cement, 1051
chalk, 364–5
china clay, 1031–2
dolomite, 360
ferric oxide, 1051
fuller's earth, 1030
gypsum, 371–3
hæmatite, 9, 960, 981–2

iron, 1051–3
iron oxide, 1051–3
jewellers' rouge, 294, 1052
kaolin, 1031–2
limestone, 360, 1051
marble, 352
plaster of Paris, 362
silicon carbide, 1059
silver, 419
bird feather, 1085
duck, 1085
goose, 1085
coal, 1032–50
combustible, 1124–5
consumption, 954
corundum, 1058
electrostatic precipitation, 967
epoxy resins, 774
explosions,
factories, 1124–5
mines, 1139–41
explosive, 1124–5, 1139–41
antimony, 1124
bark, 1124
cadmium, 1124
coal, 1139–41
cocoa, 1124
coffee, 1124
copper, 1124
cork, 1124
ferromanganese, 1124
gramophone-record, 1124
iron, 1124
manganese, 1124
military pyrotechnics, 1124
moulding compositions, 1124
paper, 1124
pitch, 1124
plastics, 1124
powder metallurgy, 1124
resin, 1124
rubber, 1124
soap powders, 1124
spice, 1124
starch, 1124
sulphur, 1124
synthetic resins, 1124
tin, 1124
titanium, 1124
zinc, 1124
zirconium, 1124
foundry, 991
insect scales, 1172
bee, 1171
caddis fly, 1172
cockroach, 1171
dermestid, beetle, 1172
locust, 1172
May fly, 1172
water flea, 1172
masks, 1106, 1050, 1154
mechanization, 960
mineralogical composition, 969

Hippocrates, 11, 12, 29, 35, 80, 221,
  233, 235, 955
Hiroshima, 934
Histoplasmosis, 1047
Hodgkin, Thomas, 120
Hodmen's shoulder, 803
Hofmann, August W. von, 150, 152,
  504
Hogarth, William, 40
Hohenheim, A. T. B. von, 24, 28–31,
  33, 80, 767, 803
Holger, Nielson artificial respiration,
  646
Holkham sheepshearings, 50
Holman dryductor, 1001
Holmes, Oliver Wendell, 47
Holmes, Sherlock, 789
Holmgren, A. F., 78
Holothuroidea, 496
Home Office, 178, 183
  Lucifer Match Committee, 380
Homer, 15
Homogentisic acid, 529
Hongkong foot, 1172
Hood, Thomas, 136
Hookworm disease, 594, 749–55
Hoover dam, 854
Hop dermatitis, 777
  eye, 772
  gout, 809
  narcosis, 772, 1155
Hopcalite, 659
Hopper bale opener, cotton, 1061
Hoppers' eye, 772
  gout, 809
Hopton Wood stone, 225
Horn, 5, 9, 707, 721, 1084
Hornblende, 1010
Horner, Leonard, 125
Hornets, 1171
Horse,
  broken wind, 1078
  -bus driver, 733
  cavalry, 733
  coal mines, 738
  fly, 721
  glanders, 733
  herdsmen, 3
  inspectors, mines, 209
  ringworm, 710
  selenium poisoning, 486
  Steppes, 5
  -tram driver, 733
Horsehair,
  anthrax, 721
  sorter, 732
  sterilization, 726
Horticulture, 336, 1165, 1169
Hospital,
  Albert Dock, London, 1123
  Birmingham Accident, 1124
  Allgemeines Krankenhaus, Vienna,
  42

child-bed fever, 43
contracts with industry, 188
county, 41
fever, 43
filthy state of, 42
foundling, 39, 43, 44
Foundling, Florence, 43
Foundling, London, 44
gangrene, 43
gas gangrene, 42
Guy's, 42, 120
Hotel Dieu, Paris, 42
Llandough, 1039
London, The, (see London Hospital)
lying-in, 39, 41
maintained by industry, 180
Middlesex, The, 41
Moscow, 42
orphanages, 39
Priestman (Sir John), Finchale
  Abbey, 188
puerperal fever, 43
St. Bartholomew's, 41
St. George's, 41
St. Thomas's, 41
Stoke Mandeville, 1123
West Hendon, 1124
Westminster, The, 41
Hot gilding, 293
Hôtel Dieu, Paris, 42
House of Lords Committee, 1889,
  139–40
House painting, 123, 239
Household cleaning fluids, 612
Housemaids' knee, 222, 803
Houses of Parliament, 359
Housewife, 769, 773
Howell, Thomas, J., 125
Hudson tunnels, 658
Human relationships in industry, 192
Hume, Joseph, 99
Humpers' lump, 803
Hunt, Henry, 101
Hunter, John, 45
Hunters, 35, 1170
Huntsman, Benjamin, 56
Hutchinson, Sir Jonathan, 337
Hydro-blast, 1002
Hydrocarbon polymers, 161
Hydrochloric acid, 84, 148, 267, 391,
  458, 592, 679
  gas, 148
Hydrofluoric acid, 84, 436, 667, 683–6,
  687, 690
Hydrofluosilicic acid, 683, 685, 687
Hydrogen, 643, 649
  arsenide, 233, 345
  cyanide, 643, 655, 663–7
  fluoride, 643, 684, 686
    burns, 686
  halide, 593
  manufacture, 344
  peroxide, 685

selenide, 233, 489, 490
sulphide, 87, 256, 368, 373, 490,
  660–3, 1157
telluride, 233
Hydroida, 1174
Hydromedusa, 1173
Hydrophis spiralis, 1171
Hydroquinone, 203, 534, 773
  acetic acid, 534
Hydroxylamine, 539
Hydrozoa, 1173
Hygiene, 95, 97, 271, 278, 313
Hyperkeratosis, 793
Hypertension, 260
Hypertrichosis, 373
Hypothyroidism, 1157
Hysteria, 261, 1104

Iceland spar, 356
Idria, Yugoslavia, 291, 297, 306
Ignis fatuus, 651
Ilmarinen, 8
I.L.O., Geneva, 36
Immigrant workmen, 215
Immunotherapy, 46
Imperial,
  green, 334
  purple, 18
Incas, 3, 86, 293
Incendiary bomb, 376
Incentives in industry, 195
Independent Labour Party, 169
India,
  Bombay, 755
  Calcutta, 755
  Central India, 755
  cysticercosis, 755–64
  Deccan, 755
  endemic fluorosis, 701
  Madras, 701, 755
  manganese poisoning, 462
  Punjab, 701, 755
  United Provinces, 755
Indiarubber, See Rubber, 179, 788
Indian marking nut, 779
Indians, North American, 6
Indigo, 19, 579, 619
Indigofera anil, 19
Indium, 428
Indurite, 543
Industrial death benefits, 200
  fatigue, 1099
  Health Research Board, 193
  Health and Safety Centre, 1106
  incentives, 195, 197
  Injuries, 198
    and Burns Research Unit, MRC.,
      Birmingham Accident Hospital,
      1124
    Commissioner, 200
    Medical Appeal Tribunals, 199
      Boards, 198
    treatment, 1122–4

wild life, 398
morale, 195
nurse, 183, 184
Nursing Certificate, 184
Psychology Research Unit, MRC.,
  1106
Revolution, 22, 39, 52, 54, 60–88,
  147, 148, 157
training, 195
Welfare Society, 1112
Inecto, 572
Infections, 706, 764
Infective hæmorrhagic jaundice, 736
Infra-red radiation, 865
Ingot, 225
Inoculation, 45, 46
Insect,
  acarus, 784
  ant, 1171
  aphid, 397, 486, 561
    cotton, 524
    woolly, 560
  apple capsid bug, 560
    sucker, 560
  bean weevil, 1085
  bee, 1085, 1171
  beetle, 129, 397
    blistering, 1172
    dermestid, 1085
  bed bug, 599, 1171
  bird louse, 1171
  black widow spider, 1172
  blistering beetle, 1171
  bruke, 1085
  caddis fly, 1085
  caterpillar, 397, 784, 1171
  centipede, 1171
  cockroach, 524, 1085
  codling moth, 335
  cotton boll weevil, 342, 524
    aphid, 524
    flea hopper, 524
  dermestid beetle, 1172
  flea, 524, 1171
  fly, 397
    caddis, 1085
    horse, 721
    house, 524
    May-fly, 1085
    wheat bulb, 522
  froghopper, 397
  grain weevil, 599
  grub, 1073
  gypsy moth, 335
  head louse, 398
  hornet, 1171
  injuries from, 1171
  ladybird, 396
  leafhopper, 397
  locust, 1085
    larva, 1085
  louse, 397, 599, 784
    bird, 1171